Biotechnology

Dr. U. Satyanarayana
Dr. U. Chakrapani

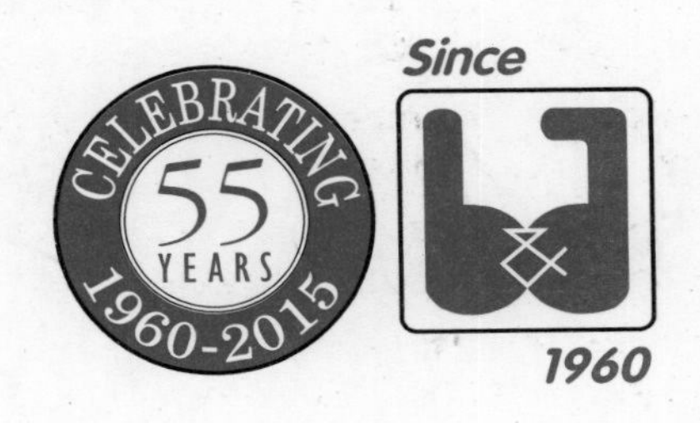

Biotechnology

Dr. U. Satyanarayana

M.Sc., Ph.D., F.I.C., F.A.C.B., F.A.C.B.I

Professor of Biochemistry & Director (Research)
Dr. Pinnamaneni Siddhartha Institute of Medical Sciences
(Dr. NTR University of Health Sciences)
Chinaoutpalli, Gannavaram (Mdl)
Krishna (Dist), A.P., India

Dr. U. Chakrapani

M.B.B.S., M.S., D.N.B.

BOOKS AND ALLIED (P) Ltd.

No.1-E(1) "Shubham Plaza" (1st Floor)
83/1, Beliaghata Main Road, Kolkata 700010 (India)
Tel : 8961053844 • 8274085530
e-mail : booksandallied1960@gmail.com, booksmktng@gmail.com

Biotechnology

First Published : 2005
Twelfth Printing : 2017
Revised Reprint : 2019

About Cover Design

Depicts the production of a recombinant DNA molecule, and its utility in modern Biotechnology with reference to microorganisms, plants and animals. (Note : This design is an oversimplification of the facts. For the sake of clarity, only a few helices of DNA structure are shown).

Publisher : Arunabha Sen
BOOKS AND ALLIED (P) LTD.
8/1 Chintamoni Das Lane, Kolkata 700009

Typesetter : BOOKS AND ALLIED (P) LTD.
8/1 Chintamoni Das Lane, Kolkata 700009

Printer : CALCUTTA ART STUDIO (P) LTD.
185/1 B. B. Ganguly Street, Kolkata 700012

Text Graphics : Shyamal Bhattacharya

Project Team : Shyamal Bhattacharya and Dinesh Bhunya

ISBN 81-87134-90-9

Price : ₹ **975.00**

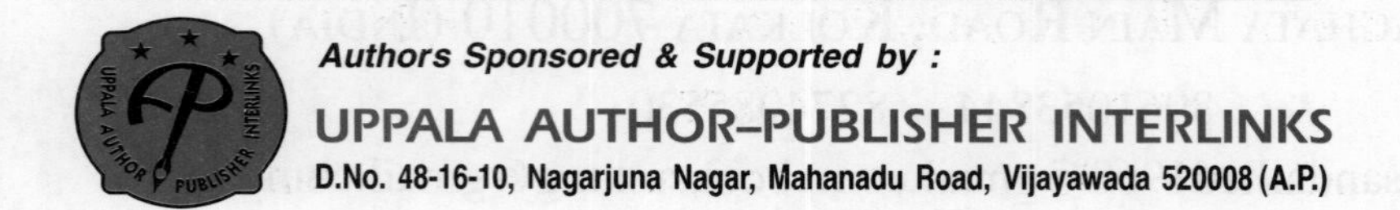

Preface

Biotechnology is an exciting, rapidly developing and revolutionary scientific discipline, with its roots in biological and technological sciences. During the past few years, the majority of scientific breakthroughs in biological sciences have come from biotechnology, particularly involving genetic engineering. Biotechnology impinges on everyone's life, and is truly regarded as the scientific technology of the twenty-first century.

THE NECESSITY FOR A COMPREHENSIVE BOOK ON BIOTECHNOLOGY

Biotechnology is a subject learnt by students with different backgrounds at the undergraduate and post-graduate levels. It is true that there are some books now available on biotechnology (by Indian and foreign authors). These books, however, deal with one or two specialized areas rather than covering the broad spectrum of biotechnology. Consequently, the students have to depend on many books for good and latest information on biotechnology. There is a long-felt need for a comprehensive book on biotechnology providing updated information on the subject.

THE BIRTH OF THE NEW BOOK

It will not be out of place to mention here how and when this book was born. The entire book was written in the early hours (between 2AM and 6AM, when the world around is fast asleep), during which period I carry out my intellectual activities. After a sound sleep, a fresh mind packed with creative ideas and innovative thoughts, has largely helped me to write this book in a novel and unique way. Truly, each page of this book was conceived in darkness and born at day break!

MAJOR HIGHLIGHTS OF THE BOOK 'BIOTECHNOLOGY'

The present book 'BIOTECHNOLOGY', in colour, with several novel features, is comprehensively written with latest advances in the subject to meet the needs of all categories of students learning biotechnology.

The section on 'Basics to learn Biotechnology' provides the most essential information needed to understand biotechnology. This is particularly useful to students from diverse backgrounds who are exposed to biotechnology all of a sudden. Molecular Biology is dealt with in good detail, as it lays the foundations for genetic engineering and modern biotechnology.

The other sections in this book include Recombinant DNA Technology, Medical/Pharmaceutical Biotechnology, Microbial/Industrial Biotechnology, Animal Cell/Animal Biotechnology, Plant/Agricultural Biotechnology and Environmental Biotechnology. Each section is carefully crafted to provide extensive, relevant and most recent information.

The book is written in a lucid style with colour illustrations, headings, sub-headings, tables and flow charts. Colours are useful for better understanding and easy reproducibility of the subject matter. An extensive glossary is added to the book to make the commonly used terms and words in biotechnology very clear.

Besides the student community, this book will immensely help the personnel working in biotechnology laboratories and industries. The language and contents of this book are made so simple and easy that even a lay man with a minimal knowledge of biological sciences will be able to understand the essence of biotechnology.

As the subject of biotechnology is multidisciplinary, books on the subject are written by authors with different backgrounds—botany, zoology, genetics, pharmacy, agriculture, engineering, etc. This results in an inevitable bias in the books. For instance, an author with a botany background tends to pay more attention to plant/agricultural biotechnolgy. The present book is free from such bias. Written by an author with biochemistry background, covering all aspects of life sciences, it is well balanced in the treatment of various branches of biotechnology. However, there is a perceptible bias in the book towards recent information on the applications of different branches of biotechnology to human healthcare, and for the ultimate benefit of mankind. This is justifiable from the fact that more than 70% of the budget earmarked for biotechnology research in developing countries goes towards healthcare research.

AN INVITATION TO READERS

This book is designed to cater to the needs of all categories of students learning biotechnology in various disciplines—life sciences, engineering and technology, medicine, agriculture, pharmacy, veterinary etc. Thus, this book may be regarded as a buffet table with something for everyone (in every discipline). It is ultimately for the reader to do appropriate self-service and enjoy the menu.

I invite the readers for the wonderful and exciting world of biotechnology, and learn the subject to maximum possible with ease and pleasure.

The subject of biotechnology is very vast, therefore it is not an easy job to prepare a concentrated capsule of biotechnology. As this book is intended to cater to the needs of students learning biotechnology from many different disciplines, there is a lot of scope to improve the book in future. This primarily depends on the feedback from the faculty and students with specific requests and ideas.

It is true that I represent a selected group of individuals authoring books, having some time at disposal, besides hard work, determination and dedication. I consider myself as an eternal learner and a regular student of biotechnology. However, it is beyond my capability to keep track of the evergrowing advances in biotechnology due to the exponential growth of the subject, and this makes me nervous. I honestly admit that I have to depend on mature readers for subsequent editions of this book.

I welcome constructive and helpful suggestions to improve the book.

DR. U. SATYANARAYANA

Acknowledgements

I owe a deep debt of gratitude to my parents, the late Sri U. Venkata Subbaiah, and Smt. Vajramma, for cultivating in me the habit of early rising. The writing of this book would never have been possible without this healthy habit. I am grateful to Dr. B. S. Narasinga Rao (former Director, National Institute of Nutrition, Hyderbad) for disciplining my professional life, and to my eldest brother, Dr. U. Gudaru (former Professor of Power systems, Walchand College of Engineering, Sangli), for disciplining my personal life.

My younger son, U. Amrutpani, has made a significant contribution at every stage in the preparation of this book—writing, verification, proof-reading, etc. My elder son, Dr. U. Chakrapani M.B.B.S, M.S., has helped me with his creative ideas and constructive suggestions to orient the book with adequate emphasis on human healthcare, besides involving himself in the verification and proof-reading of the book. I acknowledge the help of my friend, Dr. P. Ramanujam (Reader in English, Andhra Loyola College, Vijayawada), for his help at various stages of manuscript preparation.

I express my gratitude to Mr. Arunabha Sen (Executive Director, Books & Allied Pvt. Ltd., Kolkata) for his whole-hearted cooperation in bringing out this book to my satisfaction. I am grateful to Mr. Shyamal Bhattacharya for the excellent page-making and graphics-work in the book. I thank Mr. Dinesh Bhunya for proof-reading. I also thank Mr. Prasenjit Halder for the cover design of the book.

Last but not least, I thank my wife, Krishna Kumari, for her constant cooperation, support and encouragement.

I am grateful to Uppala Author-Publisher Interlinks, Vijayawada, for sponsoring and supporting me to write this book.

DR. U. SATYANARAYANA

Contents in Brief

SECTION VI

Animal Cell/Animal Biotechnology

SECTION VII

Plant/Agricultural Biotechnology

SECTION VIII

Environmental Biotechnology

SECTION IX

Biotechnology and Society

SECTION X

Basics to Learn Biotechnology

Appendices

Contents in Detail

SECTION III

Genetic Engineering/Recombinant DNA Technology

SECTION VII

Plant/Agricultural Biotechnology

SECTION IX

Biotechnology and Society

SECTION X

Basics to Learn Biotechnology

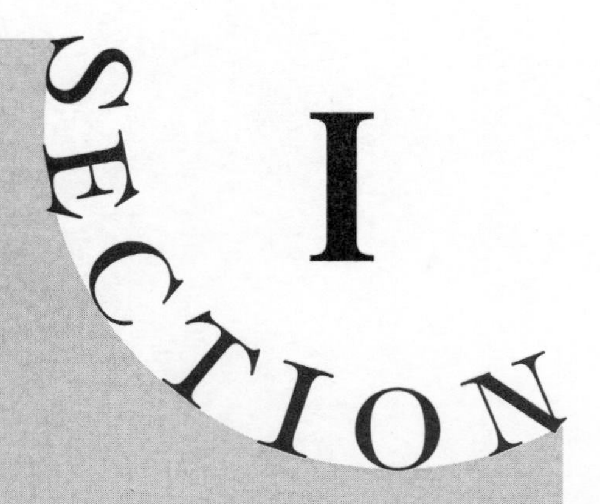

INTRODUCTION TO BIOTECHNOLOGY

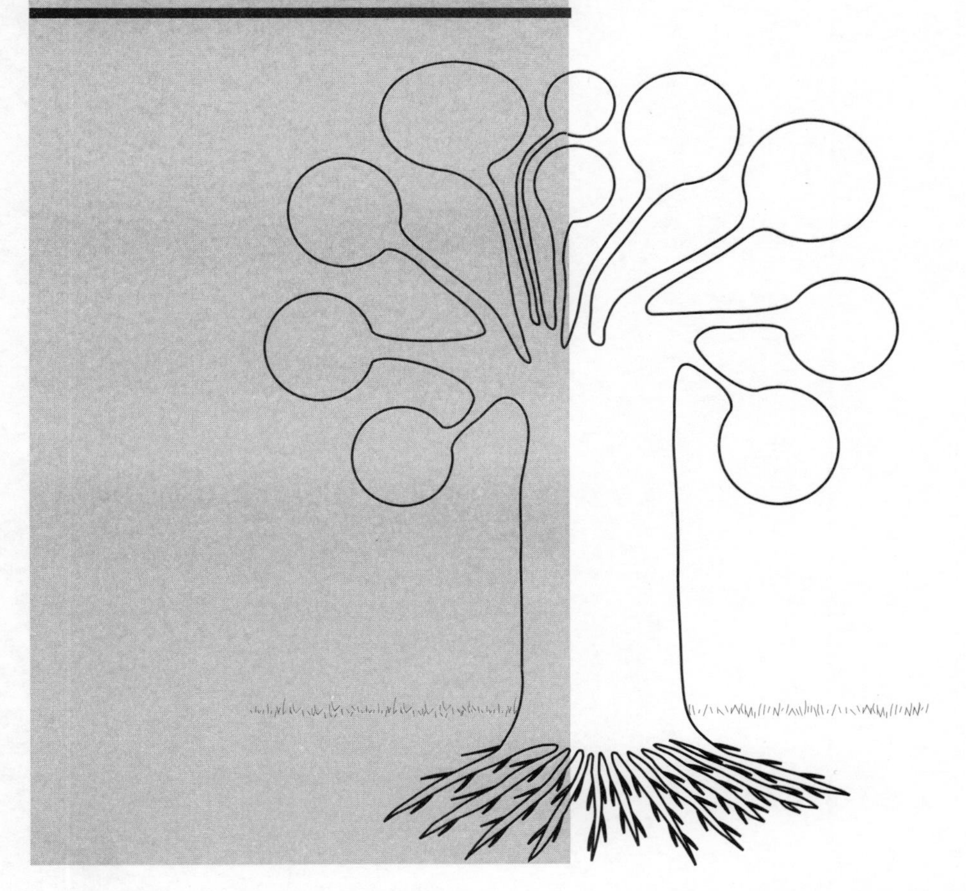

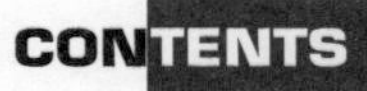

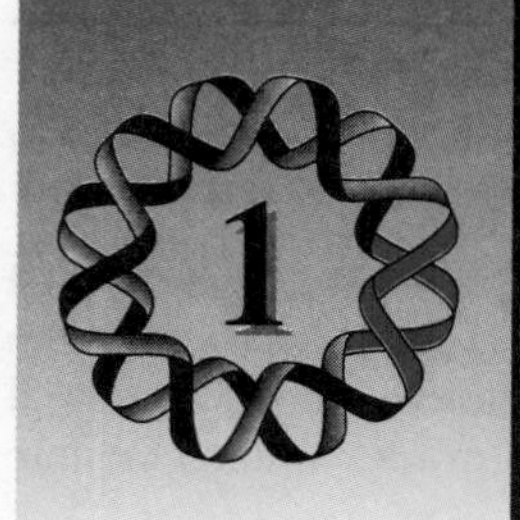

The Scope of Biotechnology

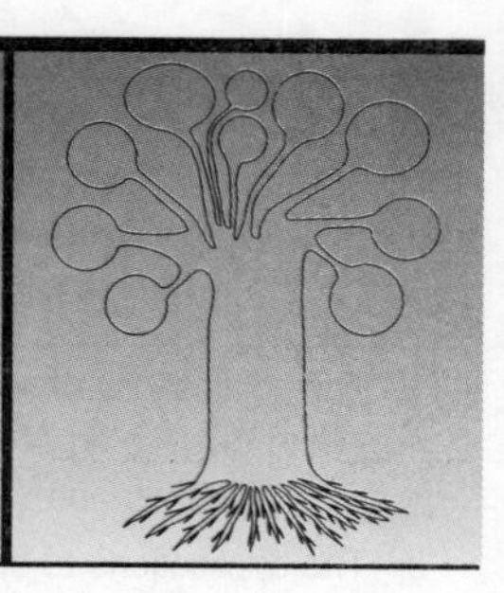

The term biotechnology represents a fusion or an alliance between ***biology*** and ***technology***. Frankly speaking, biotechnology is as old as human civilization, and is an integral part of human life. Thus, biotechnology is a ***newly discovered discipline for age-old practices***. There are records that wine and beer were prepared in as early as 6000 B.C., bread and curd in 4000 B.C. Today, we know that all these are the processes based on the natural capabilities of microorganisms.

OLD AND NEW BIOTECHNOLOGY

Many authors prefer to use the term ***old or traditional biotechnology*** to the ***natural processes*** that have been in use for many centuries to produce beer, wine, curd, cheese and many other foods.

The ***new or modern biotechnology*** embraces all the ***genetic manipulations***, cell fusion techniques and the improvements made in the old biotechnological processes.

We have to accept that the present day biotechnology is not something new, but it represents a series of technologies, some of them dating back to thousands of years e.g. production of foods, beverages, modification of plants and animals with desired tracts. It is only in recent years that these traditional practices are being subjected to scientific scrutiny, understood and improved, at least in some instances.

DEFINITION(S) OF BIOTECHNOLOGY

The term biotechnology was introduced in 1917 by a Hungarian engineer, Karl Ereky. He used the term for large-scale production of pigs by using sugar beets as the source of food. Ereky defined biotechnology as ***'all lines of work by which products are produced from raw materials with the aid of living things'***. This definition was almost ignored for many years. For most people, biotechnology represented two aspects of engineering—industrial fermentation and study of the efficiency at work place.

The fact that biotechnology is interdisciplinary in nature, with a wide range of applications has created some confusion with regard to its definition. This is mainly because scientists from each discipline have described the term from their own perspective. Around a dozen of the selected definitions of biotechnology are given in ***Table 1.1***.

The European Federation of Biotechnology (EFB) broadly considers biotechnology as "the integration of natural sciences and organisms, cells, parts thereof, and molecular analogues for products and services".

In whichever way the term biotechnology has been defined, it essentially represents ***the use of microbial, animal or plant cells or enzymes to synthesize, breakdown or transform materials***.

TABLE 1.1 Some selected definitions of biotechnology

1. The applications of scientific and engineering principles to the processing of materials by biological agents to provide goods and services.
2. The applications of biological organisms, systems and processes to manufacturing and service industries.
3. The controlled use of biological agents such as microorganisms or cellular components for beneficial purposes.
4. The integrated use of biochemistry, microbiology and engineering sciences in order to achieve technological application of the capabilities of microorganisms, cultured tissues/cells and parts thereof.
5. The use of living organisms and their components in agriculture, food, and other industries.
6. The use of biological organisms or their constituents for the transformation of inputs into commercial outputs.
7. A technology using biological phenomena for copying and manufacturing various kinds of useful substances.
8. Controlled and deliberate application of simple biological agents–living or dead or cell components–in technically useful operations, either of productive manufacture or as service operation.
9. The use of living organisms in systems or processes for manufacture of useful products. It may involve bacteria, algae, fungi, yeast, cells of higher plants or animals or subsystems of any of these or isolated components from living matter.
10. The use of living organisms to solve problems or make useful products.
11. The industrial production of goods and services by processes using biological organisms, systems and processes.
12. A set of techniques and processes involving biological materials.

HISTORY OF BIOTECHNOLOGY

From the historical perspective, the biotechnology dates back to the time (around 6000 BC) when the yeast was first used to produce beer and wine, and bacteria were first used to prepare yogurt.

Some researchers consider ***Louis Pasteur***, who identified the role of microorganisms in fermentation, (between 1857–1876) as the ***father of biotechnology***.

The development of biotechnology, in the first half of twentieth century is associated with the fields of applied microbiology and industrial fermentations (production of penicillin, organic solvents etc.)

The development of modern biotechnology is closely linked with the advances made in molecular biology. A selected list of historical foundations that contributed to the advancement of biotechnology is given in ***Table 1.2***.

The biotechnology revolution began in the 1970s and early 1980s when the scientists understood the genetic constitution of living organisms. A strong foundation of genetic engineering and modern biotechnology was laid down by Cohen and Boyer in 1973 when they could successfully introduce the desired genes of one organism into another, and clone the new genes (For more details, refer Chapter 6). It is an acknowledged fact that of all the scientific development, related ***recombinant DNA technology*** (***rDNA technology***) triggend the most significant and profound advancements in biotechnology. Thus, rDNA technology laid firm foundations for genetic engineering.

BIOTECHNOLOGY–A MULTIDISCIPLINARY GROWING TREE

Biotechnology is an interdisciplinary pursuit with multidisciplinary applications, and it may be represented as a growing biotechnology tree (***Fig. 1.1***). This figure gives an overview of biotechnology with special reference to the fundamental principles and scientific foundations, biotechnological tools and applications of biotechnology.

Scientific foundations of biotechnology

There is almost no discipline among the science subjects that has not contributed either directly or indirectly for the growth of biotechnology. About a dozen specialized branches of science that have predominantly provided the inputs for biotechnology are shown. These may be appropriately regarded as the ***roots of biotechnology***, and include biochemistry, genetics, molecular biology, chemical engineering and bioinformatics. A large number of scientists working in these specialities have contributed to the development of biotechnology.

Table 1.2 A selected list of historical foundations for the development of biotechnology

Year	Development
6000 BC	Wine preparation (using yeast)
4000 BC	Bread making (employing yeast)
1670–1680	Use of microorganisms for copper mining.
1865	Inheritance of genetic characters of Gregor Mendel.
1876	Louis Pasteur identified role microorganisms in fermentation.
1897	Extraction of enzymes from yeast by Edward Buchner.
1910	Sewage purification by employing microorganisms established.
1914	Production of industrial chemicals (acetone, butanol, glycerol) by using bacteria.
1917	The term biotechnology was coined by Karl Ereky.
1928	Discovery of penicillin by Alexander Flaming.
1943	Industrial production of penicillin.
1944	Identification of DNA as the genetic material (Avery, MacLeod and McCarty).
1953	Determination of DNA structure by Watson and Crick.
1958	Semiconservative replication of DNA by Messelson and Stahl.
1961	Lac operon model for gene regulation, proposed by Jacob and Monod.
1961	Launching of the Journal of Biotechnology and Bioengineering.
1962	Microbial mining of uranium.
1962–66	Entire genetic code deciphered.
1970	Isolation of the first restriction endonuclease enzyme.
1972	Synthesis of tRNA gene by Khorana *et al.*
1973	Establishment of recombinant DNA technology by Boyer and Cohen.
1975	Production of monoclonal antibodies by Kohler and Milstein.
1976	National Institute of Health, USA issued first guidelines for rDNA research.
1976	Sanger and Gilbert developed techniques to sequence DNA.
1977	First genome (of bacteriophage QX174) sequenced.
1978	Production of human insulin in *E. coli.*
1980	Site–directed mutagenesis by Gillam *et al.*
1980	U.S. Supreme Court rules that genetically engineered microorganisms can be patented (the case was fought by Anand Chakrabarty).
1981	First diagnostic kits based on monoclonal antibodies approved in U.S.
1981	First automated DNA synthesizers sold.
1982	U.S. approved humulin (human insulin), the first pharmaceutical product of rDNA technology, for human use.
1982	Approval given in Europe for the use of first animal vaccine produced by rDNA technology.
1983	Use of Ti plasmids to genetically transform plants.
1987	Gene transfer by biolistic transformation.
1988	Development of polymerase chain reaction.
1988	U.S. patent granted to genetically engineered mouse (susceptible to cancer).
1990	Approval granted in U.S. for trail of human somatic cell gene therapy.
1990	Official launching of human genome project.
1992	First chromosome (of yeast) sequenced.
1994–95	Genetic and physical maps of human chromosomes elucidated.
1996	First eukaryotic organism (*Saccharomyces cerevisiae*) sequenced.
1997	The first mammalian sheep, Dolly developed by nuclear cloning.
2000	First plant genome (of *Arabidopsis thaliana*) sequenced.
2001	Human genome, the first mammalian genome, sequenced.
2002	First crop plant (rice, *Oryza sativa*) genome sequenced.
2003	Mouse (*Mus musculis*) genome, the experimental animal closest model to man, sequenced.

Table 1.2 contd. next column

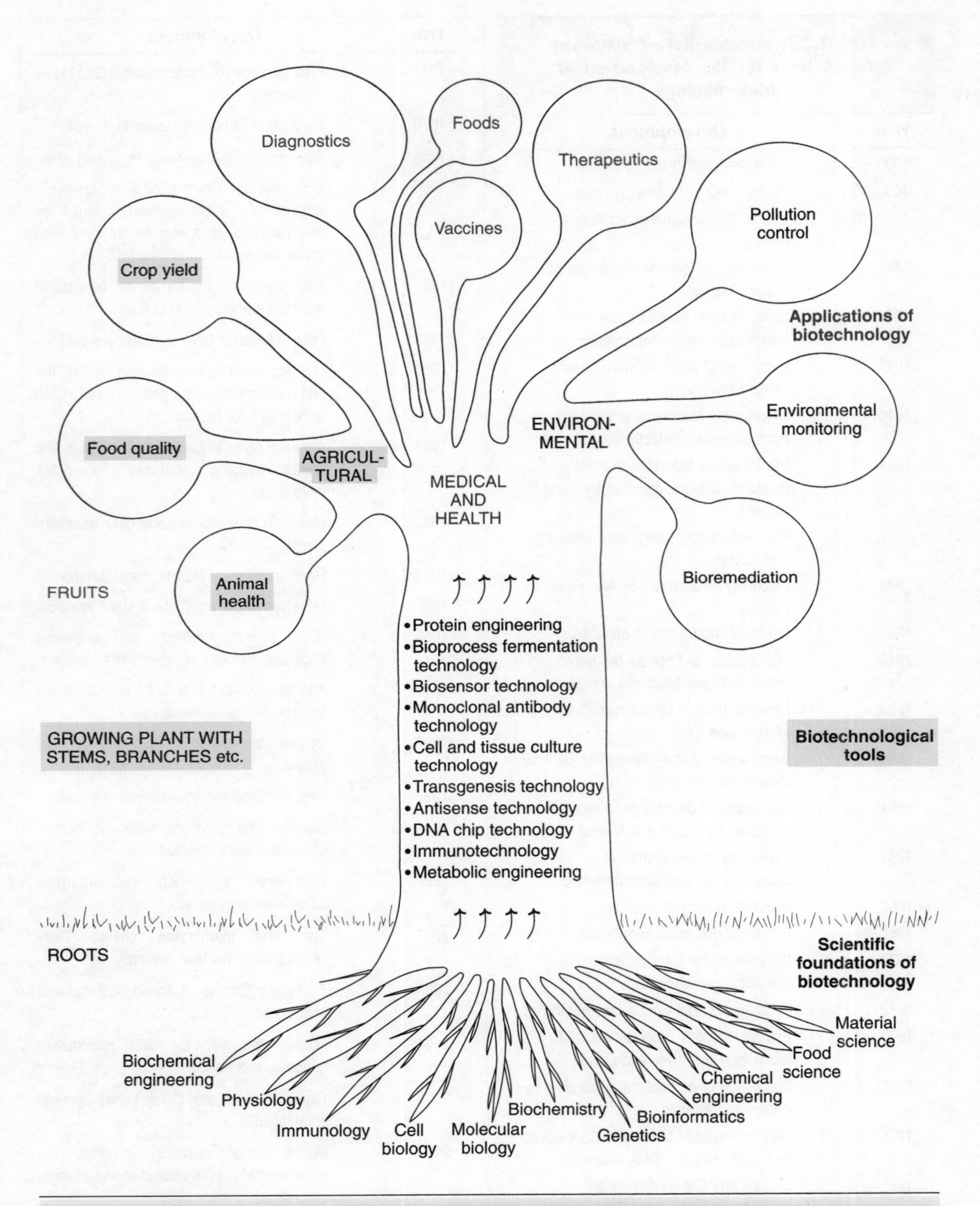

Fig. 1.1 : The biotechnology tree.

Biotechnological tools

Several methods, techniques or procedures which may be collectively called as biotechnological tools have been developed for transforming the scientific foundations into biotechnological applications. These tools include protein engineering, bioprocess/fermentation technology, cell and tissue culture technology, transgenesis and antisense technology.

Applications of biotechnology

The fruits of biotechnological research have wide range of applications. In fact, there is no other branch of science which has as many applications as biotechnology.

Biotechnology has benefited medical and health sciences (diagnostics, vaccines, therapeutics, foods), agricultural sciences (improved crop yield, food quality, improved animal health) and environmental sciences (pollution control, environmental monitoring, bioremediation).

It is desirable to describe at least one example of biotechnological achievement that has helped the mankind. Prior to 1982, insulin required for the treatment of diabetics was obtained from pig and cow pancreases. The procedure was tedious, and the use of animal insulin was frequently associated with complications. Then the human gene for insulin was isolated, cloned and expressed in microorganisms for the large scale production of insulin. ***Insulin was the first pharmaceutical product of recombinant DNA technology approved for human use.*** Millions of diabetics worldover are benefited by the biotechnology of insulin production.

COMMERCIALIZATION OF BIOTECHNOLOGY

The progress of biotechnology, to a great extent, is driven by economics. This is so since the ultimate objective of biotechnology is the development of commercial products. Due to high stakes in biotechnology, the business and research are closely associated. It is a fact that many biotechnology companies (besides the government-run institutions) have significantly contributed to the development of present day biotechnology. Most of the commercial developments of biotechnology have been centered in the United States and Europe. The biotechnology-based industries can be profitably run by brains than muscles. It is predicted that the twenty-first century will be dominated by ***biotechnology driven industries*** which may be considered as ***new money plants.***

PUBLIC PERCEPTION OF BIOTECHNOLOGY

Humans are the ultimate beneficieries of biotechnology. This may be through healthcare, transgenic plants and animals, pesticides, fertilizers, *in vitro* cultures etc. The public perceptions of biotechnology will significantly influence the rate and direction of future growth of biotechnology.

The use of recombinant DNA technology has raised safety concerns. The public attitudes to biotechnology are mostly related to matters of imaginary dangers of genetic manipulations. Some people argue against genetic engineering, and many times, the public and politicians are misled. There is a need for the biotechnology community to frequently interact with the media and public to clear the unwarranted fears about the genetic engineering and biotechnology.

THE FUTURE OF BIOTECHNOLOGY

Biotechnology, with much fanfare, has become a comprehensive scientific venture from the point of academic and commercial angles, within a short time with the sequencing of human genome and genomes of some other important organisms. The future developments in biotechnology will be exciting. It may be rather difficult to make any specific predictions, since new technical innovations are rapidly replacing the existing technologies.

It is expected that the development in biotechnology will lead to a new scientific revolution that could change the lives and future of the people. It has happend through industrial revolution and computer revolution. And now, it is the turn of biotechnology revolution that promises major changes in many aspects of modern life.

ORGANIZATION OF THE BOOK

As the subject of biotechnology is multidisciplinary in nature with several inputs, tools and outputs (see ***Fig. 1.1***), the organization of the book is as complicated as writing of the book. However, the complex subject of biotechnology has been made simpler and understandable by organizing the book into 10 Sections comprising 70 Chapters. Each section can be read independently as it is arranged in the heirarchical order of learning. It may however, be noted that each section or even a chapter cannot be treated in isolation as the subject of biotechnology is integrated, and interdependent on many other sections/chapters.

Section I (Chapter 1)

This section deals with the history, scope, ***relevance and importance*** of biotechnology.

Section II (Chapters 2-5)

The most important information on the ***molecular biology*** to equip the reader for a good understanding of modern biotechnology is given in this section. The chemistry and functions of nucleic acids (DNA and RNA) and gene regulation are described.

Section III (Chapters 6–12)

This section primarily deals with the basic and applied aspects of ***genetic engineering***. The methodology, polymerase chain reaction, gene libraries, site-directed mutagenesis, manipulation of gene expression, and human genome project are discussed in good detail.

Section IV (Chapters 13–18)

This section is directly concerned with biotechnology in human healthcare i.e. ***medical/ pharmaceutical biotechnology***. The advances in gene therapy, DNA in disease diagnosis and finger-printing, specialized products of DNA technology, and assisted reproductive technology are dealt with in this section.

Section V (Chapters 19–32)

The information on ***microbial/industrial biotechnology*** is given in this section. This includes the fermentation technology, downstream processing, enzyme technology, microbial production of organic solvents, organic acids, antibiotics, amino acids, vitamins, foods and beverages, and polysaccharides. Biomass and bioenergy, besides microbial mining are also described in this section.

Section VI (Chapters 33–41)

This section deals with ***animal cell/animal biotechnology***. The animal cell cultures—media, biology, characterization, cell-lines, scale-up, primary cultures, tissue engineering, and transgenic animals are described in this section.

Section VII (Chapters 42–53)

This section gives details on ***biotechnology*** directly concerned with ***plants and agriculture***. The plant tissue cultures, production of haploid plants, somaclonal variations, micropropagation, cryopreservation, methodology in the genetic engineering of plants, applications of transgenic plants etc., are described.

Section VIII (Chapters 54–60)

The information on ***biotechnology*** with reference to ***environment*** is furnished in this section. The various aspects of environmental pollution (air/water), and treatment modalities, besides the global environmental problems are given in good detail.

Section IX (Chapter 61)

The direct relevance of ***biotechnology*** to the ***society*** with particular reference to risks, ethics and patenting are described.

Section X (Chapters 62–70)

This section provides ***basic information on living systems***—cell, microorganisms, basic chemistry, biomolecules, enzymology, metabolisms, immunology, genetics, and bioinformatics. It makes the fundamentals clear and helps the reader to easily understand all aspects of biotechnology.

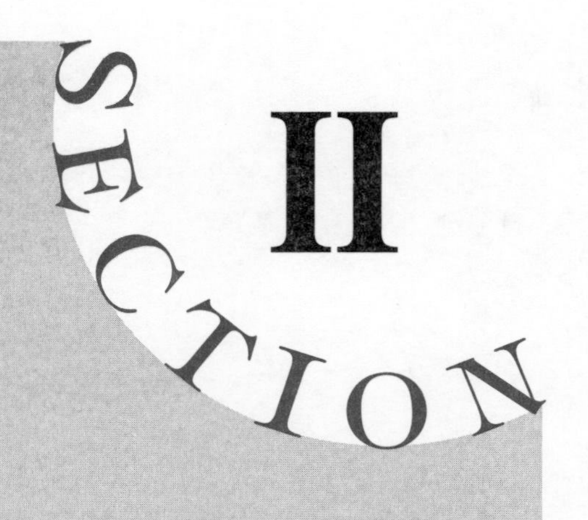

INTRODUCTION TO MOLECULAR BIOLOGY

CONTENTS

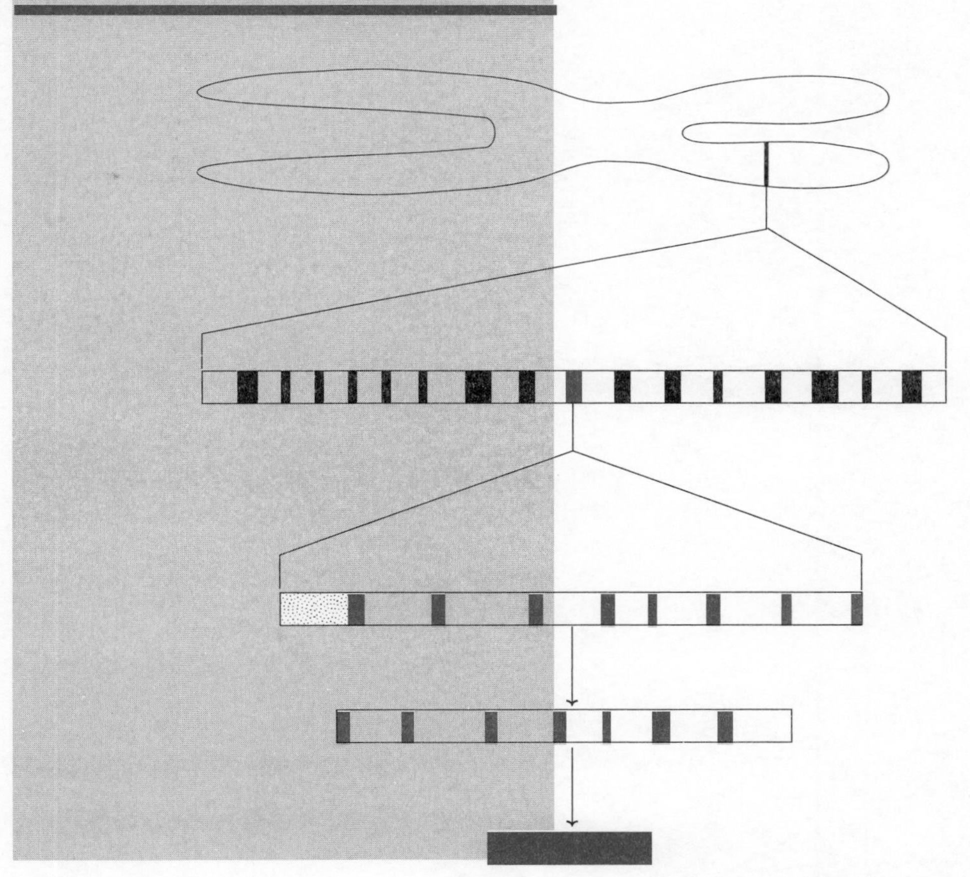

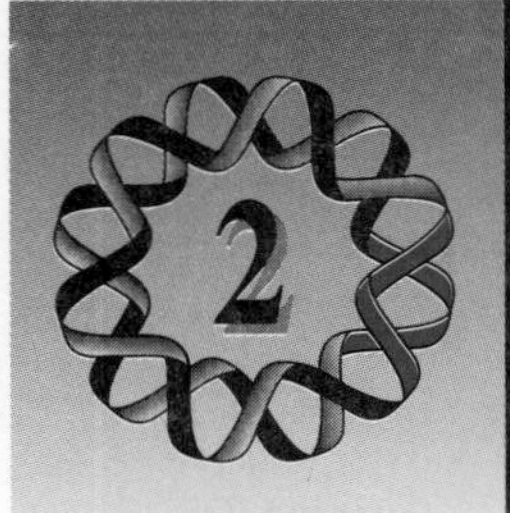

DNA and RNA — Composition and Structure

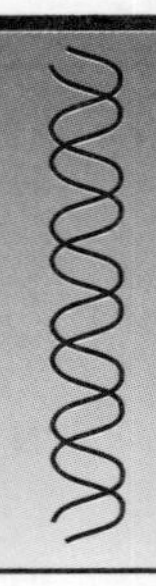

There are two types of nucleic acids, namely ***deoxyribonucleic acid*** (DNA) and ***ribonucleic acid*** (RNA). Primarily, nucleic acids serve as repositories and transmitters of genetic information.

Brief history

DNA was discovered in 1869 by Johann Friedrich Miescher, a Swiss researcher. The demonstration that DNA contained genetic information was first made in 1944, by Avery, Macleod and MacCary.

Functions of nucleic acids

DNA is the chemical basis of heredity and may be regarded as the reserve bank of genetic information. DNA is exclusively responsible for maintaining the identity of different species of organisms over millions of years. Further, every aspect of cellular function is under the control of DNA. The ***DNA*** is organized into ***genes***, the fundamental units of ***genetic information***. The genes control the protein synthesis through the mediation of RNA, as shown below

DNA ⟶ RNA ⟶ Protein

The interrelationship of these three classes of biomolecules (DNA, RNA and proteins) constitutes the ***central dogma of molecular biology*** or more commonly the ***central dogma of life***.

Components of nucleic acids

Nucleic acids are the polymers of nucleotides (polynucleotides) held by 3′ and 5′ phosphate bridges. In other words, nucleic acids are built up by the monomeric units—nucleotides (It may be recalled that protein is a polymer of amino acids).

NUCLEOTIDES

Nucleotides are composed of a ***nitrogenous base***, a ***pentose sugar*** and a ***phosphate***. Nucleotides perform a wide variety of functions in the living cells, besides being the building blocks or monomeric units in the nucleic acid (DNA and RNA) structure. These include their role as structural components of some coenzymes of B-complex vitamins (e.g. FAD, NAD^+), in the energy reactions of cells (ATP is the energy currency), and in the control of metabolic reactions.

STRUCTURE OF NUCLEOTIDES

As already stated, the nucleotide essentially consists of ***base***, ***sugar*** and ***phosphate***. The term nucleoside refers to base + sugar. Thus, nucleotide is nucleoside + phosphate.

Purines and pyrimidines

The nitrogenous bases found in nucleotides (and, therefore, nucleic acids) are ***aromatic heterocyclic compounds***. The bases are of two

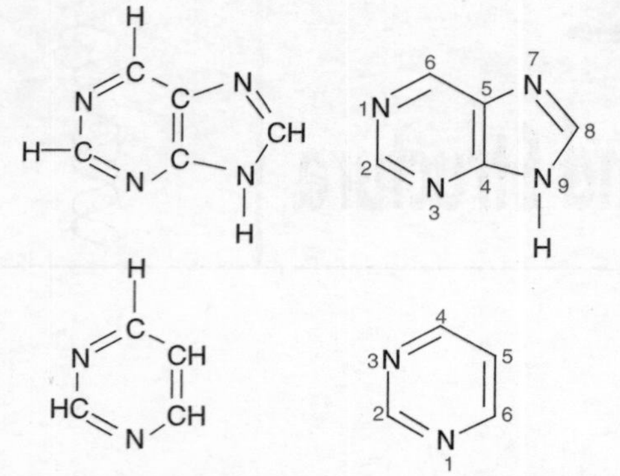

(A)

(B)

Fig. 2.1 : General structure of nitrogen bases (A) Purine (B) Pyrimidine (The positions are numbered according to the international system).

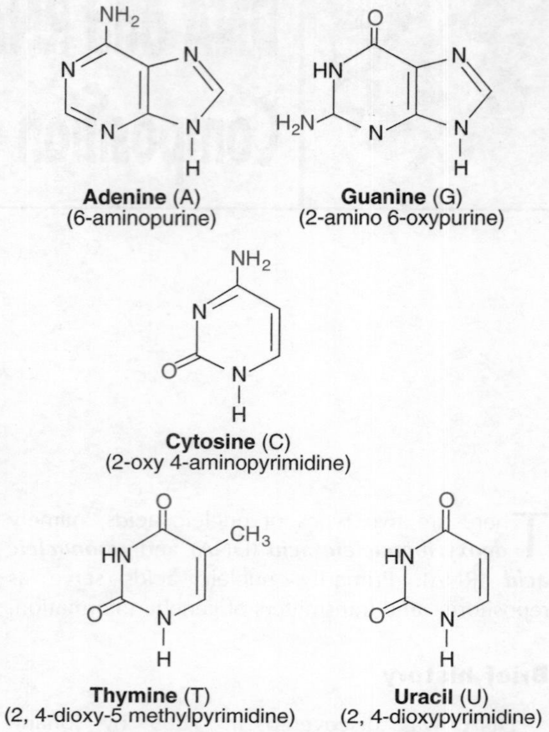

types—purines and pyrimidines. Their general structures are depicted in ***Fig. 2.1***. Purines are numbered in the anticlockwise direction while pyrimidines are numbered in the clockwise direction. And this is an internationally accepted system to represent the structure of bases.

Major bases in nucleic acids

The structures of major purines and pyrimidines found in nucleic acids are shown in ***Fig. 2.2***. DNA and RNA contain the same purines namely adenine (A) and guanine (G). Further, the pyrimidine cytosine (C) is found in both DNA and RNA. However, the nucleic acids differ with respect to the second pyrimidine base. ***DNA contains thymine (T) whereas RNA contains uracil (U)***. As is observed in the ***Fig. 2.2***, thymine and uracil differ in structure by the presence (in T) or absence (in U) of a methyl group.

Tautomeric forms of purines and pyrimidines

The existence of a molecule in a ***keto (lactam)*** and ***enol (lactim)*** form is known as tautomerism. The heterocyclic rings of purines and pyrimidines with ***oxo*** $\left(-\overset{O}{\overset{\|}{C}}-\right)$ functional groups exhibit tautomerism as simplified below.

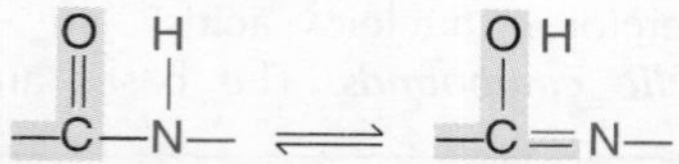

$$-\overset{O}{\overset{\|}{C}}-\overset{H}{\overset{|}{N}}- \rightleftharpoons -\overset{OH}{\overset{|}{C}}=N-$$

Lactam form **Lactim form**

Adenine (A) (6-aminopurine)

Guanine (G) (2-amino 6-oxypurine)

Cytosine (C) (2-oxy 4-aminopyrimidine)

Thymine (T) (2, 4-dioxy-5 methylpyrimidine)

Uracil (U) (2, 4-dioxypyrimidine)

Fig. 2.2 : Structures of major purines (A, G) and pyrimidines (C, T, U) found in nucleic acids.

The purine—guanine and pyrimidines-cytosine, thymine and uracil exhibit tautomerism. The lactam and lactim forms of cytosine are represented in *Fig. 2.3*.

At physiological pH, the lactam (keto) tautomeric forms are predominantly present.

Minor bases found in nucleic acids : Besides the bases described above, several minor and unusual bases are often found in DNA and RNA. These

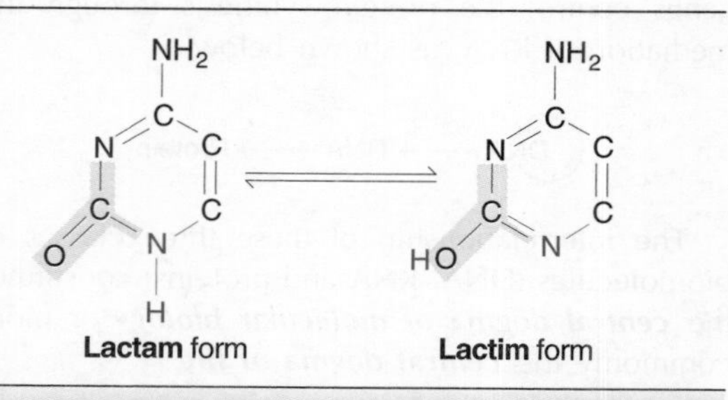

Fig. 2.3 : The tautomeric forms of cytosine.

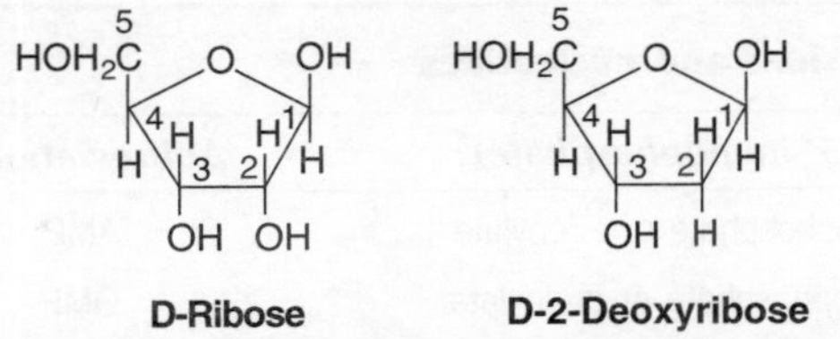

D-Ribose D-2-Deoxyribose

Fig. 2.4 : Structures of sugars present in nucleic acids (ribose is found in RNA and deoxyribose in DNA; Note the structural difference at C_2).

include 5-methylcytosine, N^4-acetylcytosine, N^6-methyladenine, N^6, N^6-dimethyladenine, pseudouracil etc. It is believed that the unusual bases in nucleic acids will help in the recognition of specific enzymes.

Sugars of nucleic acids

The five carbon monosaccharides (pentoses) are found in the nucleic acid structure. ***RNA*** contains ***D-ribose*** while ***DNA*** contains ***D-deoxyribose***. Ribose and deoxyribose differ in structure at C_2. Deoxyribose has one oxygen less at C_2 compared to ribose (***Fig. 2.4***).

Nomenclature of nucleotides

The addition of a pentose sugar to base produces a nucleoside. If the sugar is ribose, ribonucleosides are formed. Adenosine, guanosine, cytidine and uridine are the ribonucleosides of A, G, C and U respectively. If the sugar is a deoxyribose, deoxyribonucleosides are produced.

The term mononucleotide is used when a single phosphate moiety is added to a nucleoside. Thus adenosine monophosphate (AMP) contains adenine + ribose + phosphate.

The principal bases, their respective nucleosides and nucleotides found in the structure of nucleic acids are given in ***Table 2.1***. Note that the prefix 'd' is used to indicate if the sugar is deoxyribose (e.g. dAMP).

The binding of nucleotide components

The atoms in the purine ring are numbered as 1 to 9 and for pyrimidine as 1 to 6 (***Fig. 2.1***). The carbons of sugars are represented with an associated prime (′) for differentiation. Thus the pentose carbons are 1′ to 5′.

The pentoses are bound to nitrogenous bases by β-N-glycosidic bonds. The N^9 of a purine ring binds with $C_{1(1')}$ of a pentose sugar to form a covalent bond in the purine nucleoside. In case of pyrimidine nucleosides, the glycosidic linkage is between N^1 of a pyrimidine and C_1' of a pentose.

The hydroxyl groups of adenosine are esterified with phosphates to produce 5′- or 3′-monophosphates. 5′-Hydroxyl is the most commonly esterified, hence 5′ is usually omitted while writing nucleotide names. Thus AMP represents adenosine 5′-monophosphate. However, for adenosine 3′-monophosphate, the abbreviation 3′-AMP is used.

The structures of two selected nucleotides namely AMP and TMP are depicted in ***Fig. 2.5***.

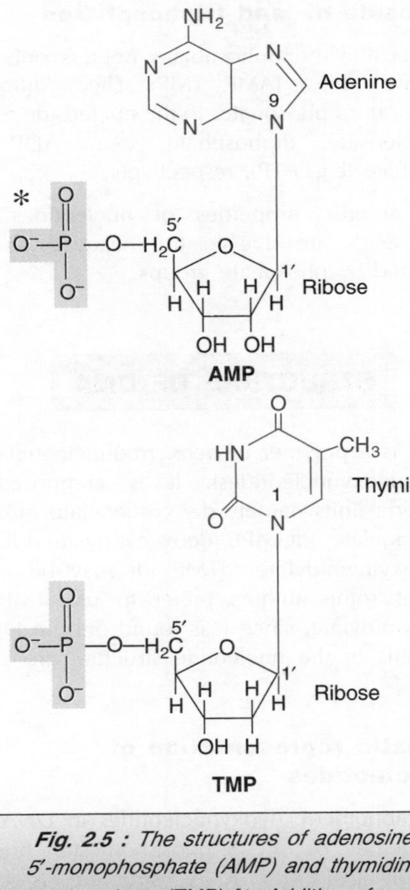

Adenine Ribose AMP Thymine Ribose TMP

Fig. 2.5 : The structures of adenosine 5′-monophosphate (AMP) and thymidine 5′-monophosphate (TMP) [-Addition of second or third phosphate gives adenosine diphosphate (ADP) and adenosine triphosphate (ATP) respectively].*

Table 2.1 Principal bases, nucleosides and nucleotides

Base	Ribonucleoside	Ribonucleotide (5′-monophosphate)	Abbreviation
Adenine (A)	Adenosine	Adenosine 5′-monophosphate or adenylate	AMP
Guanine (G)	Guanosine	Guanosine 5′-monophosphate or guanylate	GMP
Cytosine (C)	Cytidine	Cytidine 5′-monophosphate or cytidylate	CMP
Uracil (U)	Uridine	Uridine 5′-monophosphate or uridylate	UMP
Base	**Deoxyribonucleoside**	**Deoxyribonucleotide (5′-monophosphate)**	**Abbreviation**
Adenine (A)	Deoxyadenosine	Deoxyadenosine 5′-monophosphate or deoxyadenylate	dAMP
Guanine (G)	Deoxyguanosine	Deoxyguanosine 5′-monophosphate or deoxyguanylate	dGMP
Cytosine (C)	Deoxycytidine	Deoxycytidine 5′-monophosphate or deoxycytidylate	dCMP
Thymine (T)	Deoxythymidine	Deoxythymidine 5′-monophosphate or deoxythymidylate	dTMP

Nucleoside di- and triphosphates

Nucleoside monophosphates possess only one phosphate moiety (AMP, TMP). The addition of second or third phosphates to the nucleoside results in nucleoside diphosphate (e.g. ADP) or triphosphate (e.g. ATP), respectively.

The anionic properties of nucleotides and nucleic acids are due to the negative charges contributed by phosphate groups.

STRUCTURE OF DNA

DNA is a polymer of deoxyribonucleotides (or simply deoxynucleotides). It is composed of monomeric units namely deoxyadenylate (dAMP), deoxyguanylate (dGMP), deoxycytidylate (dCMP) and deoxythymidylate (dTMP) (It may be noted here that some authors prefer to use TMP for deoxythymidylate, since it is found only in DNA). The details of the nucleotide structure are given above.

Schematic representation of polynucleotides

The monomeric deoxynucleotides in DNA are held together by 3′, 5′-phosphodiester bridges (***Fig. 2.6***). DNA (or RNA) structure is often represented in a short-hand form. The horizontal line indicates the carbon chain of sugar with base attached to $C_{1'}$. Near the middle of the horizontal line is $C_{3'}$ phosphate linkage while at the other end of the line is $C_{5'}$ phosphate linkage (***Fig. 2.6***).

Chargaff's rule of DNA composition

Erwin Chargaff in late 1940s quantitatively analysed the DNA hydrolysates from different species. He observed that in all the species he studied DNA had equal numbers of adenine and thymine residues (A = T) and equal numbers of guanine and cytosine residues (G = C). This is known as Chargaff's rule of ***molar equivalence between the purines and pyrimidines in DNA*** structure. The significance of Chargaff's rule was not immediately realised. The double helical structure of DNA derives its strength from Chargaff's rule (discussed later).

Single-stranded DNA, and RNAs which are usually single-stranded, do not obey Chargaff's rule. However, double-stranded RNA which is the genetic material in certain viruses satisfies Chargaff's rule.

DNA DOUBLE HELIX

The double helical structure of DNA was proposed by ***James Watson*** and ***Francis Crick*** in 1953 (Nobel Prize, 1962). The elucidation of DNA structure is considered as a ***milestone in*** the era of ***modern biology***. The structure of DNA double helix is comparable to a twisted ladder. The salient features of Watson-Crick model of DNA (now known as B-DNA) are given below (***Fig. 2.7***).

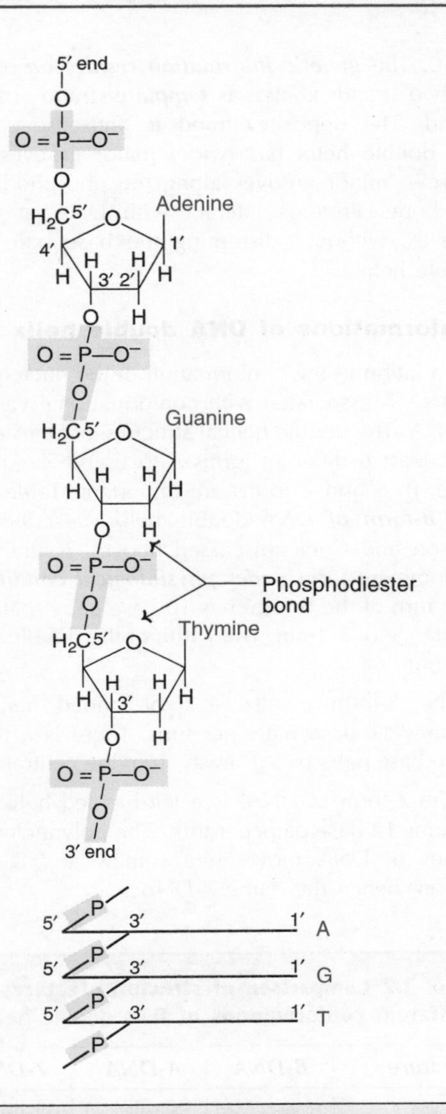

Fig. 2.6 : Structure of a polydeoxyribonucleotide segment held by phosphodiester bonds. On the lower part is the representation of short hand form of oligonucleotides.

1. The DNA is a right handed double helix. It consists of ***two polydeoxyribonucleotide chains*** (strands) twisted around each other on a common axis.

2. The two strands are ***antiparallel***, i.e., one strand runs in the 5′ to 3′ direction while the other in 3′ to 5′ direction. This is comparable to two parallel adjacent roads carrying traffic in opposite direction.

3. The width (or diameter) of a double helix is 20 A° (2 nm).

4. Each turn (pitch) of the helix is 34 A° (3.4 nm) with 10 pairs of nucleotides, each pair placed at a distance of about 3.4 A°.

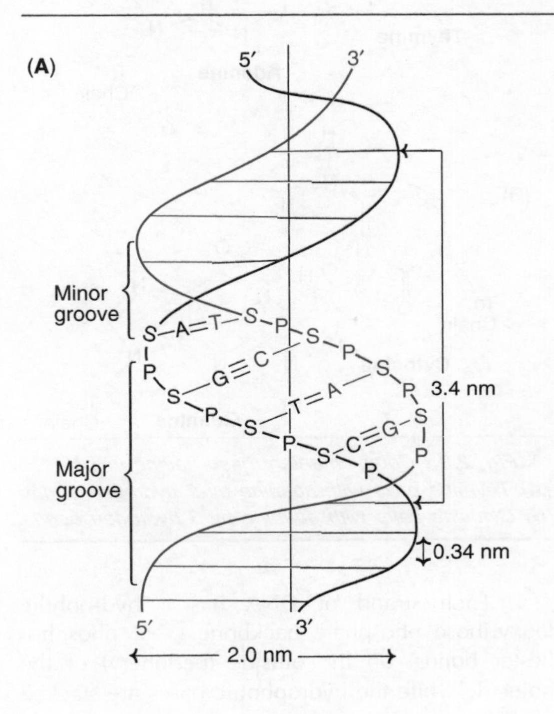

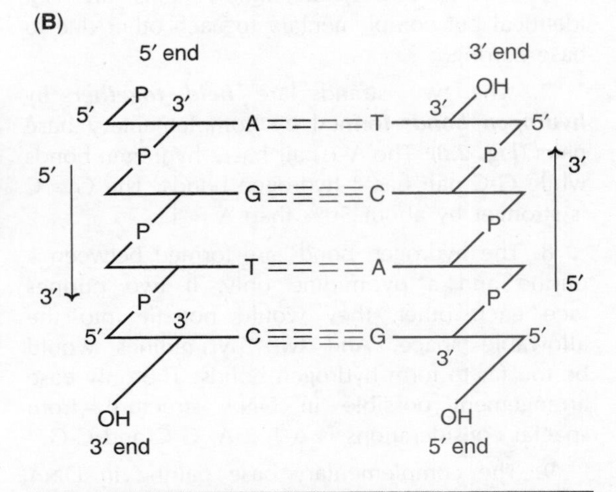

Fig. 2.7 : (A) Watson-Crick model of DNA helix (B) Complementary base pairing in DNA helix.

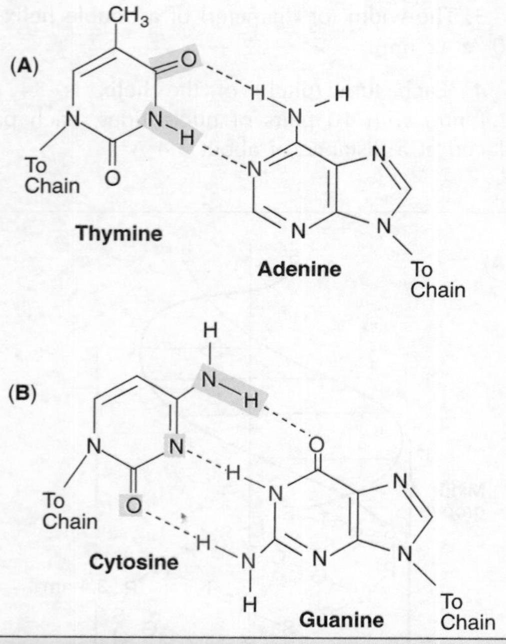

Fig. 2.8 : Complementary base pairing in DNA (A) Thymine pairs with adenine by 2 hydrogen bonds (B) Cytosine pairs with guanine by 3 hydrogen bonds.

5. Each strand of DNA has a hydrophilic deoxyribose phosphate backbone (3′-5′ phosphodiester bonds) on the outside (periphery) of the molecule while the hydrophobic bases are stacked inside (core).

6. The two polynucleotide chains are not identical but complementary to each other due to base pairing.

7. The two strands are ***held together by hydrogen bonds*** formed by complementary base pairs (***Fig. 2.8***). The A-T pair has 2 hydrogen bonds while G-C pair has 3 hydrogen bonds. The G ≡ C is stronger by about 50% than A = T.

8. The hydrogen bonds are formed between a purine and a pyrimidine only. If two purines face each other, they would not fit into the allowable space. And two pyrimidines would be too far to form hydrogen bonds. The only base arrangement possible in DNA structure, from spacial considerations is A-T, T-A, G-C and C-G.

9. The complementary base pairing in DNA helix proves ***Chargaff's rule***. The content of adenine equals to that of thymine (A = T) and guanine equals to that of cytosine (G = C).

10. The ***genetic information resides on*** one of the two strands known as ***template strand*** or sense strand. The opposite strand is antisense strand. The double helix has (wide) major grooves and (narrow) minor grooves along the phosphodiester backbone. Proteins interact with DNA at these grooves, without disrupting the base pairs and double helix.

Conformations of DNA double helix

Variation in the conformation of the nucleotides of DNA is associated with conformational variants of DNA. The double helical structure of DNA exists in at least 6 different forms-A to E and Z. Among these, B, A and Z forms are important (***Table 2.2***). The ***B-form of DNA*** double helix, described by Watson and Crick (discussed above), is the most predominant form ***under physiological conditions***. Each turn of the B-form has 10 base pairs spanning a distance of 3.4 nm. The width of the double helix is 2 nm.

The A-form is also a right-handed helix. It contains 11 base pairs per turn. There is a tilting of the base pairs by 20° away from the central axis.

The Z-form (Z-DNA) is a left-handed helix and contains 12 base pairs per turn. The polynucleotide strands of DNA move in a somewhat 'zig zag' fashion, hence the name Z-DNA.

TABLE 2.2 Comparison of structural features of different conformations of DNA double helix

Feature	*B-DNA*	*A-DNA*	*Z-DNA*
Helix type	Right-handed	Right-handed	Left-handed
Helical diameter (nm)	2.37	2.55	1.84
Distance per each complete turn (nm)	3.4	3.2	4.5
Rise per base pair (nm)	0.34	0.29	0.37
Number of base pairs per complete tern	10	11	12
Base pair tilt	+19°	–1.2° (variable)	–9°
Helix axis rotation	Major groove	Through base pairs (variable)	Minor groove

It is believed that transition between different helical forms of DNA plays a significant role in regulating gene expression.

OTHER TYPES OF DNA STRUCTURE

It is now recognized that besides double helical structure, DNA also exists in certain unusual structures. It is believed that such structures are important for molecular recognition of DNA by proteins and enzymes. This is in fact needed for the DNA to discharge its functions in an appropriate manner. Some selected ***unusual structures of DNA*** are briefly described.

Bent DNA

In general, adenine base containing DNA tracts are rigid and straight. Bent conformation of DNA occurs when A-tracts are replaced by other bases or a collapse of the helix into the minor groove of A-tract. Bending in DNA structure has also been reported due to photochemical damage or mispairing of bases.

Certain antitumor drugs (e.g. cisplatin) produce bent structure in DNA. Such changed structure can take up proteins that damage the DNA.

Triple-stranded DNA

Triple-stranded DNA formation may occur due to additional hydrogen bonds between the bases. Thus, a thymine can selectively form two ***Hoogsteen hydrogen bonds*** to the adenine of A-T pair to form ***T-A-T***. Likewise, a protonated cytosine can also form two hydrogen bonds with guanine of G–C pairs that results in C^+–G–C. An outline of Hoogsteen triple helix is depicted in ***Fig. 2.9***.

Triple-helical structure is less stable than double helix. This is due to the fact that the three negatively charged backbone strands in triple helix results in an increased electrostatic repulsion.

Four-stranded DNA

Polynucleotides with very high contents of guanine can form a novel tetrameric structure called ***G-quartets***. These structures are planar and are connected by Hoogsteen hydrogen bonds (***Fig. 2.10A***). Antiparaller four-stranded DNA structures, referred to as ***G-tetraplexs*** have also been reported (***Fig. 2.10B***).

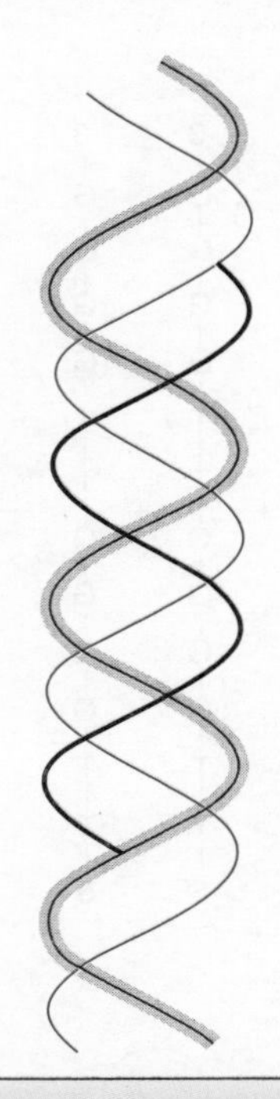

Fig. 2.9 : An outline of Hoogsteen triple helical structure of DNA.

The ends of eukaryotic chromosomes namely ***telomeres*** are rich in guanine, and therefore form G-tetraplexes. In recent years, telomeres have become the targets for anticancer chemotherapies.

G-tetraplexes have been implicated in the recombination of immunoglobulin genes, and in dimerization of double-stranded genomic RNA of the human immunodeficiency virus (HIV).

THE SIZE OF DNA MOLECULE-UNITS OF LENGTH

DNA molecules are huge in size. On an average, a pair of B-DNA with a thickness of 0.34 nm has a molecular weight of 660 daltons.

For the measurement of lengths, DNA double-stranded structure is considered, and expresssed in the form of ***base pairs*** (***bp***). A ***kilobase pair (kb)*** is 10^3 bp, and a ***megabase pair (Mb)*** is 10^6 bp and a gigabase pair (Gb) is 10^9 bp. The kb, Mb and Gb relations may be summarized as follows :

1 kb = 1000 bp

1 Mb = 1000 kb = 1,000,000 bp

1 Gb = 1000 Mb = 1,000,000,000 bp

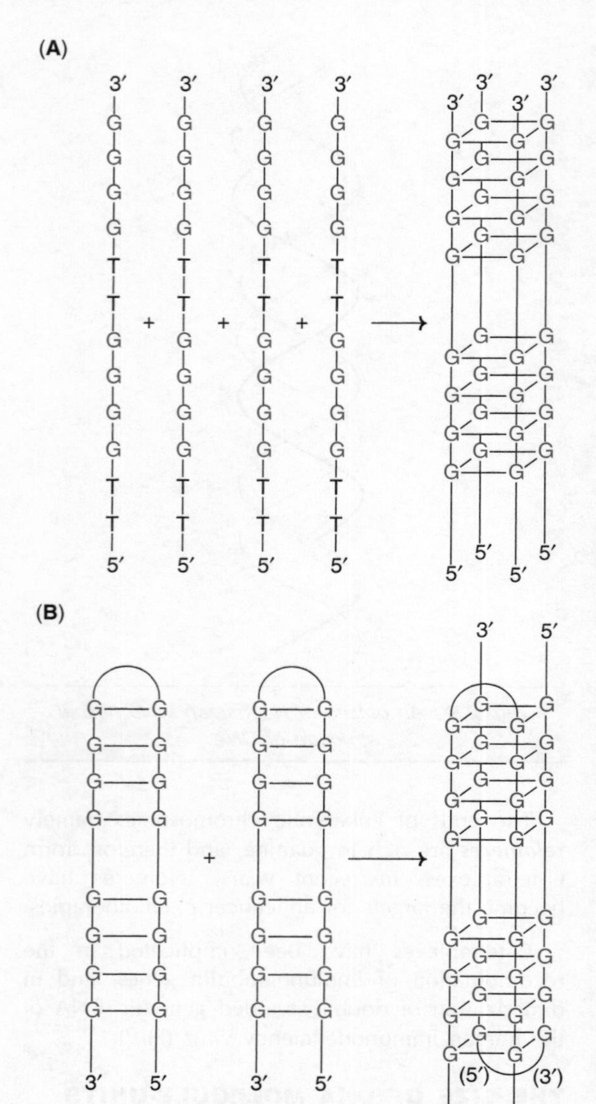

*Fig. 2.10 : Four–stranded DNA structure (**A**) Parallel G–quartets (**B**) Antiparallel G–tetraplex.*

It may be noted here that the lengths of RNA molecules (like DNA molecules) cannot be expressed in bp, since most of the RNAs are single-stranded.

The length of DNA varies from species to species, and is usually expressed in terms of base pair composition and ***contour length***. Contour length represents the total length of the genomic DNA in a cell. Some examples of organisms with bp and contour lengths are listed.

- λ phage virus — 4.8×10^4 bp — contour length 16.5 mm.
- *E. coli* — 4.6×10^6 bp — contour length 1.5 mm.
- Diploid human cell (46 chromosomes) — 6.0×10^9 bp — contour length 2 meters.

It may be noted that the genomic DNA size is usually much larger the size of the cell or nucleus containing it. For instance, in humans, a 2-meter long DNA is packed compactly in a nucleus of about 10μm diameter.

The genomic DNA may exist in linear or circular forms. Most DNAs in bacteria exist as closed circles. This includes the DNA of bacterial chromosomes and the extrachromosomal DNA of plasmids. Mitochondria and chloroplasts of eukaryotic cells also contain circular DNA.

Chromosomal DNAs in higher organisms are mostly linear. Individual human chromosomes contain a single DNA molecule with variable sizes compactly packed. Thus the smallest chromosome contains 34 Mb while the largest one has 263 Mb.

DENATURATION OF DNA STRANDS

The two strands of DNA helix are held together by hydrogen bonds. Disruption of hydrogen bonds (by change in pH or increase in temperature) results in the separation of polynucleotide strands. This phenomenon of ***loss of helical structure of DNA*** is known as ***denaturation*** (***Fig. 2.11***). The phosphodiester bonds are not broken by denaturation. Loss of helical structure can be measured by increase in absorbance at 260 nm (in a spectrophotometer).

Melting temperature (***Tm***) is defined as the temperature at which half of the helical structure of DNA is lost. Since G-C base pairs are more stable (due to 3 hydrogen bonds) than A-T base pairs (2 hydrogen bonds), the Tm is greater for DNAs with higher G-C content. Thus, the Tm is 65°C for 35% G-C content while it is 70°C for 50% G-C content. Formamide destabilizes hydrogen bonds of base pairs and, therefore, lowers Tm. This chemical compound is effectively used in recombinant DNA experiments.

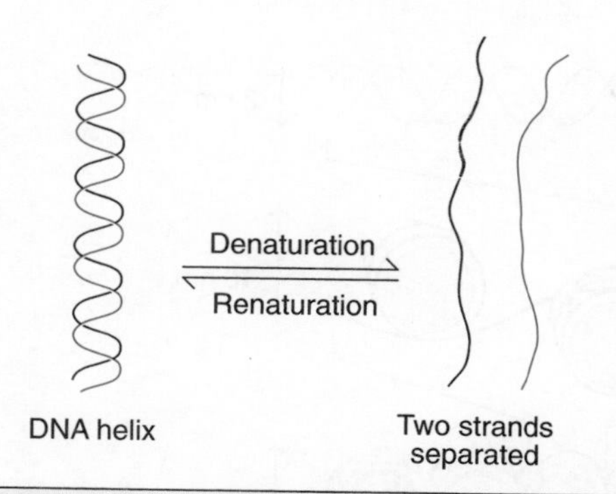

Fig. 2.11 : Diagrammatic representation of denaturation and renaturation of DNA.

Renaturation (or reannealing) is the process in which the separated complementary DNA strands can form a double helix.

ORGANIZATION OF DNA IN THE CELL

As already stated, the double-stranded DNA helix in each chromosome has a length that is thousands times the diameter of the nucleus. For instance, in humans, a 2-meter long DNA is packed in a nucleus of about 10 μm diameter! This is made possible by a compact and mavellous packaging, and organization of DNA inside in cell.

Organization of prokaryotic DNA

In prokaryotic cells, the DNA is organized as a single chromosome in the form of a double-stranded circle. These bacterial chromosomes are packed in the form of nucleoids, by interaction with proteins and certain cations (polyamines).

Organization of eukaryotic DNA

In the eukaryotic cells, the DNA is associated with various proteins to form ***chromatin*** which then gets ***organized into*** compact structures namely ***chromosomes*** (***Fig. 2.12***).

The DNA double helix is wrapped around the core proteins namely histones which are basic in nature. The core is composed of two molecules of histones (H2A, H2B, H3 and H4). Each core with two turns of DNA wrapped round it (approximately with 150 bp) is termed as a ***nucleosome***, the basic unit of chromatin. Nucleosomes are separated by spacer DNA to which histone H_1 is attached (***Fig. 2.13***). This continuous string of nucleosomes, representing beads-on-a string form of chromatin is termed as 10 nm fiber. The length of the DNA is considerably reduced by the formation of 10 nm fiber. This 10-nm fiber is further coiled to produce 30-nm fiber which has a solenoid structure with six nucleosomes to every turn. These 30-nm fibers are further organized into loops by anchoring the fiber at A/T-rich regions namely scafold-associated regions (SARS) to a protein scafold. During the course of mitosis, the loops are further coiled, the chromosomes condense and become visible.

STRUCTURE OF RNA

RNA is a polymer of ribonucleotides held together by 3′, 5′-phosphodiester bridges. Although RNA has certain similarities with DNA structure, they have several specific differences

1. **Pentose :** The sugar in RNA is ribose in contrast to deoxyribose in DNA.

2. **Pyrimidine :** RNA contains the pyrimidine uracil in place of thymine (in DNA).

3. **Single strand :** RNA is usually a single-stranded polynucleotide. However, this strand may fold at certain places to give a double-stranded structure, if complementary base pairs are in close proximity.

4. **Chargaff's rule—not obeyed :** Due to the single-stranded nature, there is no specific relation between purine and pyrimidine contents. Thus the guanine content is not equal to cytosine (as is the case in DNA).

5. **Susceptibility to alkali hydrolysis :** Alkali can hydrolyse RNA to 2′, 3′-cyclic diesters. This is possible due to the presence of a hydroxyl group at 2′ position. DNA cannot be subjected to alkali hydrolysis due to lack of this group.

6. **Orcinol colour reaction :** RNAs can be histologically identified by orcinol colour reaction due to the presence of ribose.

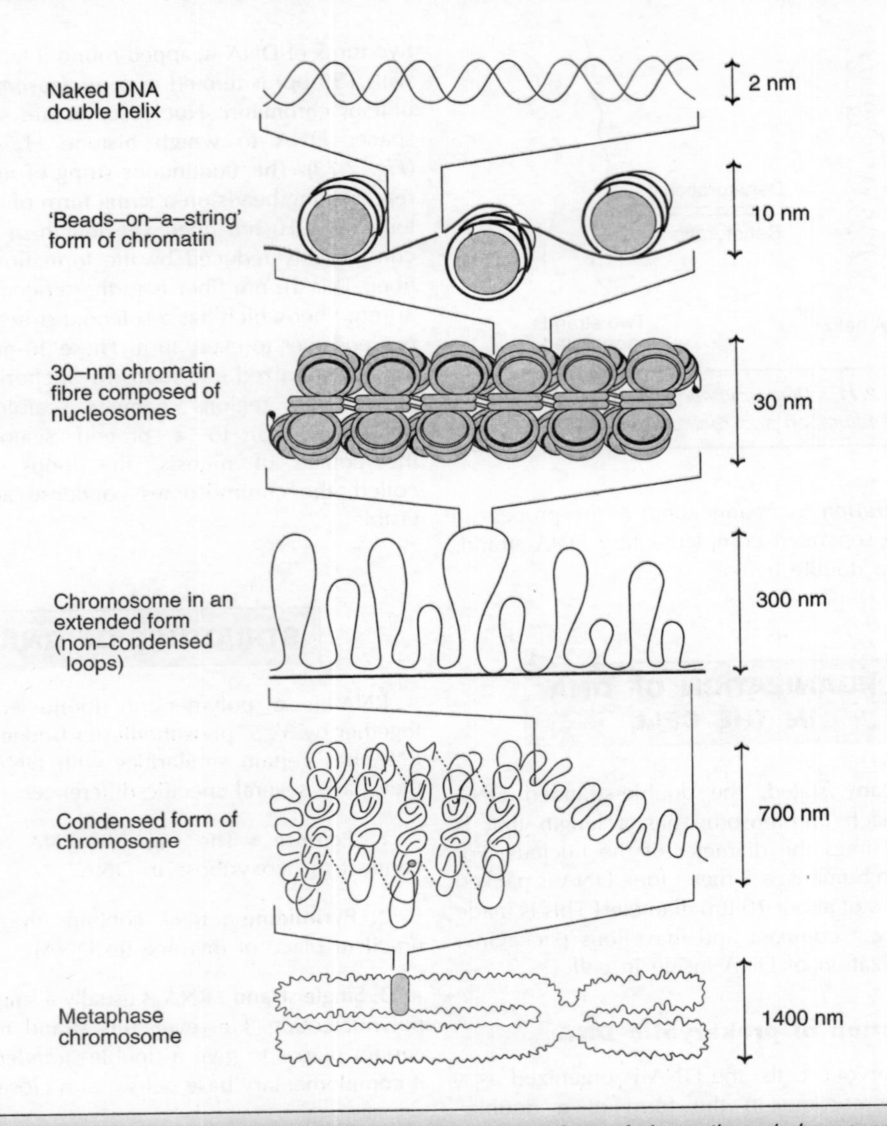

Fig. 2.12 : Organization of eukaryotic DNA structure in the form of chromatin and chromosomes.

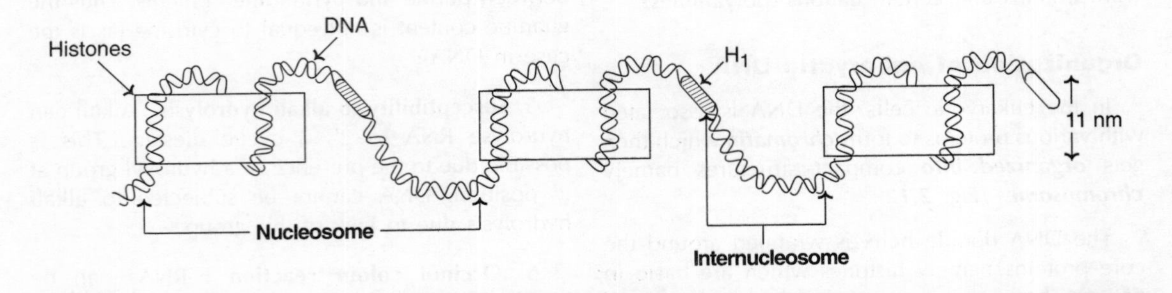

Fig. 2.13 : Structure of nucleosomes.

TABLE 2.3 Cellular RNAs and their function(s)

Type of RNA	*Abbreviation*	*Function(s)*
Messenger RNA	mRNA	Transfers genetic information from genes to ribosomes to synthesize proteins.
Heterogeneous nuclear RNA	hnRNA	Serves as precursor for mRNA and other RNAs.
Transfer RNA	tRNA	Transfers amino acid to mRNA for protein biosynthesis.
Ribosomal RNA	rRNA	Provides structural framework for ribosomes.
Small nuclear RNA	snRNA	Involved in mRNA processing.
Small nucleolar RNA	snoRNA	Plays a key role in the processing of rRNA molecules.
Small cytoplasmic RNA	scRNA	Involved in the selection of proteins for export.
Transfer–messenger RNA	tmRNA	Mostly present in bacteria. Adds short peptide tags to proteins to facilitate the degradation of incorrectly synthesized proteins.

TYPES OF RNA

The three major types of RNAs with their respective cellular composition are given below

1. **Messenger RNA** (mRNA) : 5–10%
2. **Transfer RNA** (tRNA) : 10–20%
3. **Ribosomal RNA** (rRNA) : 50–80%

Besides the three RNAs referred above, other RNAs are also present in the cells. These include heterogeneous nuclear RNA (hnRNA), small nuclear RNA (snRNA), small nucleolar RNA (snoRNA) and small cytoplasmic RNA (scRNA). The major functions of these RNAs are given in *Table 2.3*.

The RNAs are synthesized from DNA, and are primarily involved in the process of protein biosynthesis (Chapter 4). The RNAs vary in their structure and function. A brief description on the major RNAs is given.

Messenger RNA (mRNA)

The mRNA is synthesized in the nucleus (in eukaryotes) as ***heterogeneous nuclear RNA*** (hnRNA). hnRNA, on processing, liberates the functional mRNA which enters the cytoplasm to participate in ***protein synthesis***. mRNA has high molecular weight with a short half-life.

The eukaryotic mRNA is capped at the 5′-terminal end by 7-methylguanosine triphosphate. It is believed that this cap helps to prevent the hydrolysis of mRNA by 5′-exonucleases. Further, the cap may be also involved in the recognition of mRNA for protein synthesis.

The 3′-terminal end of mRNA contains a polymer of adenylate residues (20-250 nucleotides) which is known as ***poly (A) tail***. This tail may provide stability to mRNA, besides preventing it from the attack of 3′-exonucleases.

mRNA molecules often contain certain modified bases such as 6-methyladenylates in the internal structure.

Transfer RNA (tRNA)

Transfer RNA (***soluble RNA***) molecule contains 71-80 nucleotides (mostly 75) with a molecular weight of about 25,000. There are at least 20 species of tRNAs corresponding to 20 amino acids present in protein structure. The structure of tRNA (for alanine) was first elucidated by Holley.

The structure of tRNA depicted in ***Fig. 2.14*** resembles that of a clover leaf. tRNA contains mainly four arms, each arm with a base paired stem.

1. **The acceptor arm :** This arm is capped with a sequence CCA (5′ to 3′). The amino acid is attached to the acceptor arm.

2. **The anticodon arm :** This arm, with the three specific nucleotide bases (anticodon), is responsible for the recognition of triplet codon of mRNA. The

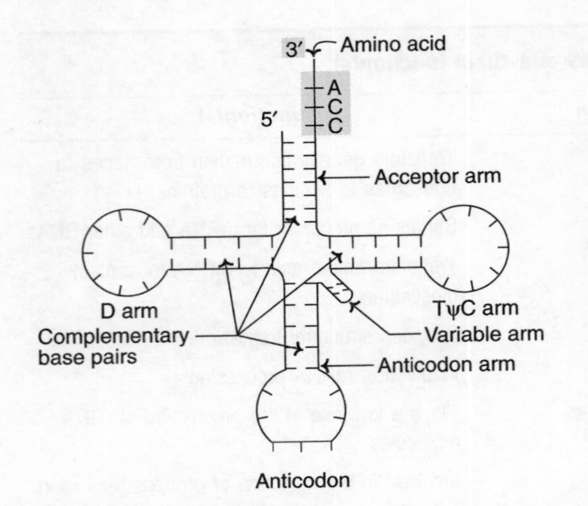

Fig. 2.14 : Structure of transfer RNA.

codon and anticodon are complementary to each other.

3. **The D arm :** It is so named due to the presence of dihydrouridine.

4. **The TΨC arm :** This arm contains a sequence of T, pseudouridine (represented by psi, Ψ) and C.

5. **The variable arm :** This arm is the most variable in tRNA. Based on this variability, tRNAs are classified into 2 categories :

(a) **Class I tRNAs :** The most predominant (about 75%) form with 3-5 base pairs length.

(b) **Class II tRNAs :** They contain 13-20 base pair long arm.

Base pairs in tRNA : The structure of tRNA is maintained due to the complementary base pairing in the arms. The four arms with their respective base pairs are given below

The acceptor arm	–	7 bp
The TΨC arm	–	5 bp
The anticodon arm	–	5 bp
The D arm	–	4 bp

Ribosomal RNA (rRNA)

The ribosomes are the factories of protein synthesis. The eukaryotic ribosomes are composed of two major nucleoprotein complexes–60S subunit and 40S subunit. The 60S subunit contains 28S rRNA, 5S rRNA and 5.8S rRNA while the 40S subunit contains 18S rRNA. The function of rRNAs in ribosomes is not clearly known. It is believed that they play a significant role in the binding of mRNA to ribosomes and protein synthesis.

Other RNAs

The various other RNAs and their functions are summarised in ***Table 2.3***.

CATALYTIC RNAs—RIBOZYMES

In certain instances, the RNA component of a ribonucleoprotein (RNA in association with protein) is catalytically active. Such RNAs are termed as ribozymes. At least five distinct species of RNA that act as catalysts have been identified. Three are involved in the self processings reactions of RNAs while the other two are regarded as true catalysts (RNase P and rRNA).

Ribonuclease P (RNase P) is a ribozyme containing protein and RNA component. It cleaves tRNA precursors to generate mature tRNA molecules.

RNA molecules are known to adapt tertiary structure just like proteins (i.e. enzymes). The specific conformation of RNA may be responsible for its function as biocatalyst. It is believed that ***ribozymes*** (RNAs) were functioning as ***catalysts before the occurrence of protein enzymes***, during the course of evolution.

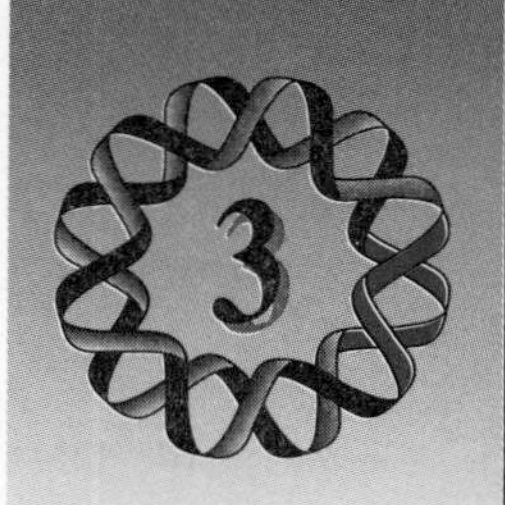

DNA — Replication, Recombination, and Repair

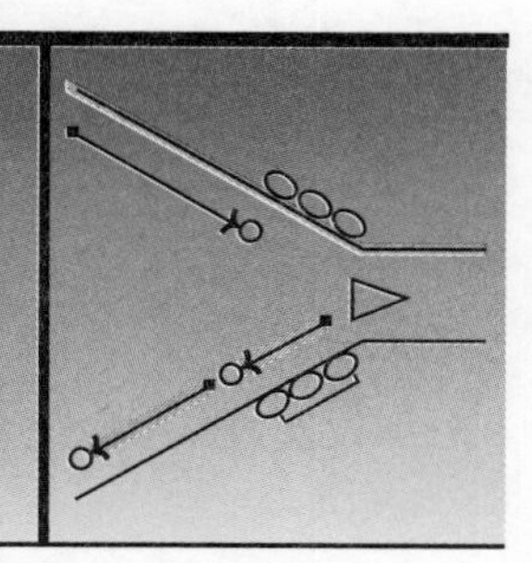

Deoxyribonucleic acid (DNA) is a macromolecule that carries genetic information from generation to generation. It is responsible to preserve the identity of the species over millions of years. ***DNA*** may be regarded as a ***reserve bank of genetic information*** or a memory bank.

A single mammalian fetal cell contains only a few picograms (10^{-12} g) of DNA. It is surprising that this little quantity of DNA stores information that will determine the differentiation and every function of an adult animal.

Why did DNA evolve as genetic material?

RNA molecules, in principle, can perform the cellular functions that are carried out by DNA. In fact, many viruses contain RNA as the genetic material. Chemically, DNA is more stable than RNA. Hence, during the course of evolution, DNA is preferred as a more suitable molecule for long-term repository of genetic information.

The central dogma of life

The ***biological information flows from DNA to RNA and from there to proteins***. This is the central dogma of life (***Fig. 3.1***). It is ultimately the DNA that controls every function of the cell through protein synthesis.

As the carrier of genetic information, DNA in a cell must be duplicated (replicated), maintained and passed down accurately to the daughter cells. Three distinct processes are designed for this purpose. The ***'three Rs' of DNA-r***eplication, ***r***ecombination, and ***r***epair, are dealt with in this chapter. There are certain common features between the three Rs.

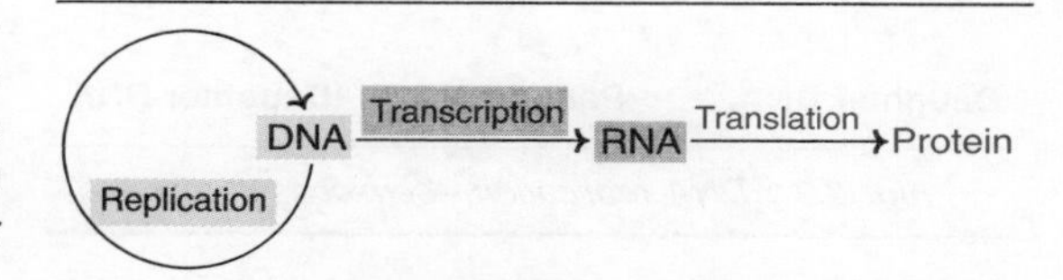

Fig. 3.1 : The central dogma of life.

- They act on the same substrate (DNA).
- They are primarily concerned with the making and breaking of phosphodiester bonds (the backbone of DNA structure).
- Enzymes used in the three processes are mostly similar/comparable.

REPLICATION OF DNA

DNA is the genetic material. When the cell divides, the daughter cells receive an identical copy of genetic information from the parent cell.

Replication is a ***process in which DNA copies itself to produce identical daughter molecules of DNA***. Replication is carried out with high fidelity

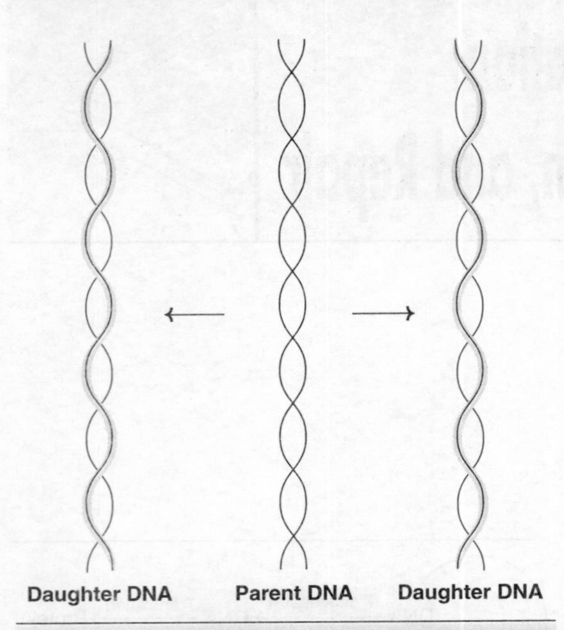

Fig. 3.2 : DNA replication—semiconservative.

which is essential for the survival of the species. Synthesis of a new DNA molecule is a complex process involving a series of steps.

The salient features of replication in prokaryotes are described first. This is followed by some recent information on the eukaryotic replication.

REPLICATION IN PROKARYOTES

Replication is semiconservative

The parent DNA has two strands complementary to each other. Both the strands undergo simultaneous replication to produce two daughter molecules. Each one of the newly synthesized DNA has one-half of the parental DNA (one strand from original) and one-half of new DNA (***Fig. 3.2***). This type of replication is known as semiconservative since ***half of the original DNA is conserved in the daughter DNA***. The first experimental evidence for the semiconservative DNA replication was provided by Meselson and Stahl (1958).

Initiation of replication

The initiation of DNA synthesis occurs at a site called origin of replication. In case of prokaryotes, there is a single site whereas in eukaryotes, there are multiple sites of origin. These sites mostly consist of a short sequence of A-T base pairs. A specific protein called ***dna A*** (20-50 monomers) binds with the site of origin for replication. This causes the double-stranded DNA to separate.

Replication bubbles

The two complementary strands of DNA separate at the site of replication to form a bubble. Multiple replication bubbles are formed in eukaryotic DNA molecules, which is essential for a rapid replication process (***Fig. 3.3***).

RNA primer

For the synthesis of new DNA, a short fragment of RNA (about 5-50 nucleotides, variable with species) is required as a primer. This primer is synthesized on the DNA template by a specific RNA polymerase called ***primase***. A constant synthesis and supply of RNA primers should occur on the lagging strand of DNA. This is in contrast to the leading strand which has almost a single RNA primer.

DNA synthesis is semidiscontinuous and bidirectional

The replication of DNA occurs in 5′ to 3′ directions, simultaneously, on both the strands of DNA. On one strand, the ***leading (continuous or forward) strand—the DNA synthesis is continuous***. On the other strand, the ***lagging (discontinuous or retrograde) strand—the synthesis of DNA is discontinuous***. Short pieces of DNA (15-250 nucleotides) are produced on the lagging strand.

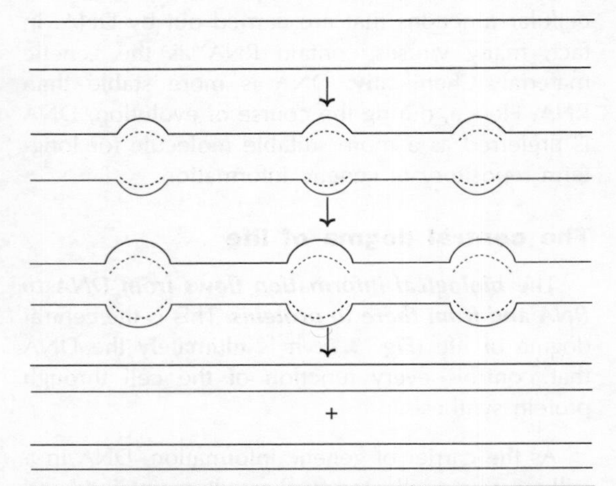

Fig. 3.3 : Schematic representation of multiple replication bubbles in DNA replication.

In the replication bubble, the DNA synthesis occurs in both the directions (bidirectional) from the point of origin.

Replication fork and DNA synthesis

The separation of the two strands of parent DNA results in the formation of a replication fork. The active synthesis of DNA occurs in this region. The replication fork moves along the parent DNA as the daughter DNA molecules are synthesized.

DNA helicases : These enzymes bind to both the DNA strands at the replication fork. Helicases move along the DNA helix and separate the strands. Their function is comparable with a ***zip opener***. Helicases are dependent on ATP for energy supply.

Single-stranded DNA binding (SSB) proteins : These are also known as DNA helix-destabilizing proteins. They possess no enzyme activity. SSB proteins bind only to single-stranded DNA (separated by helicases), keep the two strands separate and provide the template for new DNA synthesis. It is believed that SSB proteins also protect the single-stranded DNA degradation by nucleases.

DNA synthesis catalysed by DNA polymerase III

The synthesis of a new DNA strand, catalysed by DNA polymerase III, occurs in 5′→3′ direction. This is antiparallel to the parent template DNA strand. The presence of all the four deoxyribonucleoside triphosphates (dATP, dGTP, dCTP and dTTP) is an essential prerequisite for replication to take place.

The synthesis of two new DNA strands, simultaneously, takes place in the opposite direction—one is in a direction (5′→3′) towards the replication fork which is continuous, the other in a direction (5′→3′) away from the replication fork which is discontinuous (***Fig. 3.4***).

The incoming deoxyribonucleotides are added one after another, to 3′ end of the growing DNA chain (***Fig. 3.5***). A molecule of pyrophosphate (PPi) is removed with the addition of each nucleotide. The template DNA strand (the parent) determines the base sequence of the newly synthesized complementary DNA.

Polarity problem

The DNA strand (leading strand) with its 3′-end (3′-OH) oriented towards the fork can be elongated by sequential addition of new nucleotides. The other DNA strand (lagging strand) with 5′-end presents some problem, as there is no DNA polymerase enzyme (in any organism) that can catalyse the addition of nucleotides to the 5′ end (i.e. 3′→5′ direction) of the growing chain. This problem however is solved by synthesizing this strand as a series of small fragments. These pieces are made in the normal 5′→3′ direction, and later joined together.

Okazaki pieces : The small ***fragments of the discontinuously synthesized DNA*** are called Okazaki pieces. These are produced on the lagging strand of the parent DNA. Okazaki pieces are later joined to form a continuous strand of DNA. DNA polymerase I and DNA ligase are responsible for this process (details given later).

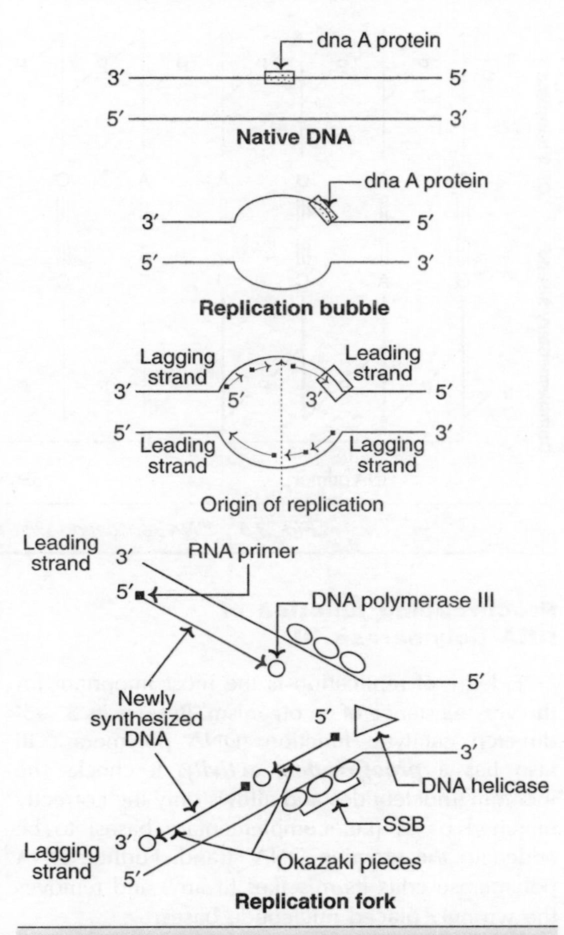

***Fig. 3.4 :** Overview of DNA replication process (SSB–Single-stranded binding protein).*

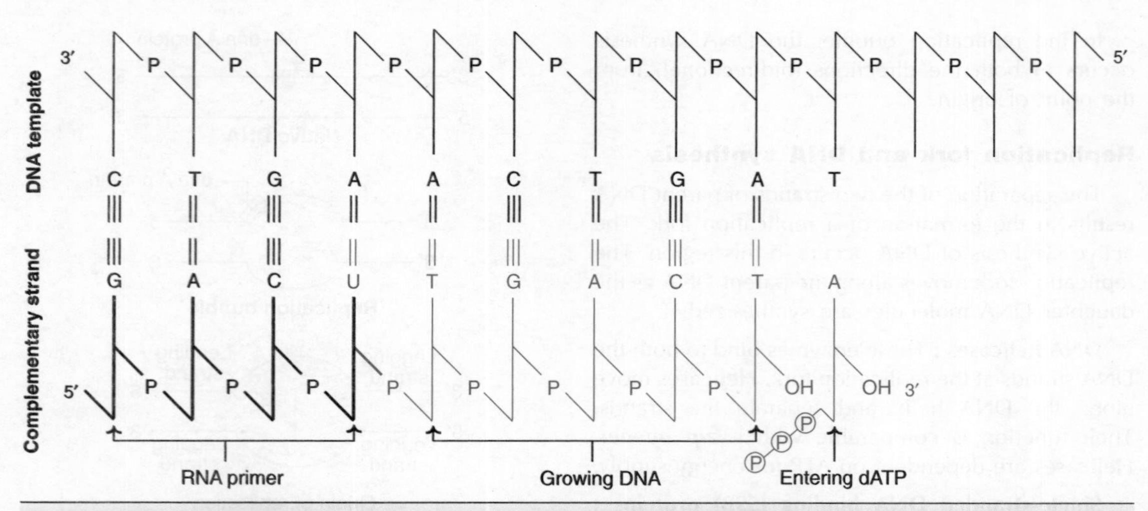

Fig. 3.5 : DNA replication with a growing complementary strand.

Proof-reading function of DNA polymerase III

Fidelity of replication is the most important for the very existence of an organism. Besides its 5′→3′ directed catalytic function, DNA polymerase III also has a ***proof-reading activity.*** It checks the incoming nucleotides and allows only the correctly matched bases (i.e. complementary bases) to be added to the growing DNA strand. Further, DNA polymerase edits its mistakes (if any) and removes the wrongly placed nucleotide bases.

Replacement of RNA primer by DNA

The synthesis of new DNA strand continues till it is in close proximity to RNA primer. Now the DNA polymerase I comes into picture. It removes the RNA primer and takes its position. DNA polymerase I catalyses the synthesis (5′→3′ direction) of a fragment of DNA that replaces RNA primer (***Fig. 3.6***).

The enzyme DNA ligase catalyses the formation of a phosphodiester linkage between the DNA synthesized by DNA polymerase III and the small fragments of DNA produced by DNA polymerase I. This process—nick sealing-requires energy, provided by the breakdown of ATP to AMP and PPi.

Another enzyme—DNA polymerase II—has been isolated. It participates in the DNA repair process.

Supercoils and DNA topoisomerases

As the double helix of DNA separates from one side and replication proceeds, supercoils are formed at the other side. The formation of supercoils can be better understood by comparing DNA helix with two twisted ropes tied at one end. Hold the ropes at the tied end in a fixed position. And let your friend pull the ropes apart from the other side. The formation of supercoils is clearly observed.

The problem of supercoils that comes in the way of DNA replication is solved by a group of enzymes called DNA topoisomerases. Type I DNA topoisomerase cuts the single DNA strand (nuclease

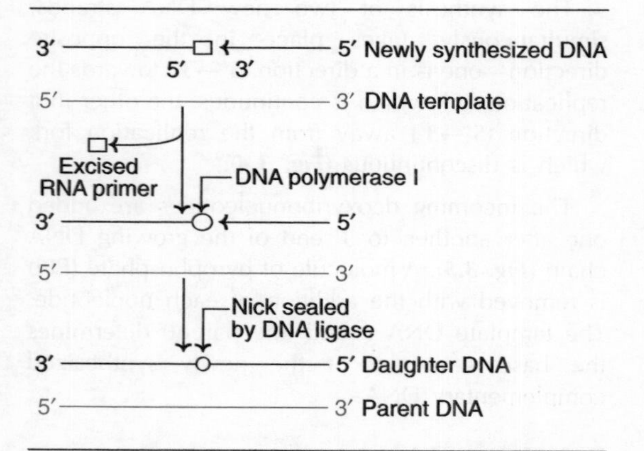

Fig. 3.6 : Overview of the action of DNA polymerase I and DNA ligase.

activity) to overcome the problem of supercoils and then reseals the strand (ligase activity). Type II DNA topoisomerase (also known as DNA gyrase) cuts both strands and reseals them to overcome the problem of supercoils.

REPLICATION IN EUKARYOTES

Replication of DNA in eukaryotes closely resembles that of prokaryotes. Certain differences, however, exist. Multiple origins of replication is a characteristic feature of eukaryotic cell. Further, at least ***five distinct DNA polymerases*** are known in eukaryotes. Greek letters are used to number these enzymes.

1. **DNA polymerase α** is responsible for the synthesis of RNA primer for both the leading and lagging strands of DNA.
2. **DNA polymerase β** is involved in the repair of DNA. Its function is comparable with DNA polymerase I found in prokaryotes.
3. **DNA polymerase γ**-this enzyme participates in the replication of mitochondrial DNA.
4. **DNA polymerase δ** is responsible for the replication on the leading strand of DNA. It also possesses proof-reading activity.
5. **DNA polymerase ε** is involved in DNA synthesis on the lagging strand and proof-reading function.

The differences in the DNA replication between bacteria and human cells, attributed to the enzymes, are successfully used in antibacterial therapy to target pathogen (bacterial) replication and spare the host (human) cells.

PROCESS OF REPLICATION IN EUKARYOTES

The replication on the leading (continuous) stand of DNA is rather simple, involving ***DNA polymerase* δ** and a sliding clamp called ***proliferating cell nuclear antigen (PCNA)***. PCNA is so named as it was first detected as an antigen in the nuclei of replicating cells. PCNA forms a ring around DNA to which DNA polymerase δ binds. Formation of this ring also requires another factor namely ***replication factor C (RFC)***.

The ***replication on the lagging*** (discontinuous) ***strand in eukaryotes is more complex*** when compared to prokaryotes or even the leading strand of eukaryotes. This is depicted in ***Fig. 3.7***, and briefly described hereunder.

The parental strands of DNA are separated by the enzyme helicase. A single-stranded DNA binding protein called ***replication protein A (RPA)*** binds to the exposed single-stranded template. This strand has been opened up by the replication fork (a previously formed Okazaki fragment with an RNA primer is also shown in ***Fig. 3.4***).

The enzyme primase forms a complex with DNA polymerase α which initiates the synthesis of Okazaki fragments. The primase activity of pol α-primase complex is capable of producing 10-bp RNA primer. The enzyme activity is then switched from primase to DNA polymerase α which elongates the primer by the addition of 20–30 deoxyribonucleotides. Thus, by the action of pol α-primase complex, short stretch of DNA attached to RNA is formed. And now the complex dissociates from the DNA.

The next step is the binding of replication factor C (RFC) to the elongated primer (short RNA-DNA). RFC serves as a clamp loader, and catalyses the assembly of proliferating cell nuclear antigen (PCNA) molecules. The DNA polymerase δ binds to the sliding clamp and elongates the Okazaki fragment to a final length of about 150–200 bp. By this elongation, the replication complex approaches the RNA primer of the previous Okazaki fragment.

The RNA primer removal is carried out by a pair of enzymes namely RNase H and flap endonuclease I (FENI). This gap created by RNA removal is filled by continued elongation of the new Okazaki fragment (carried out by polymerase δ, described above). The small nick that remains is finally sealed by DNA ligase.

Eukaryotic DNA is tightly bound to histones (basic proteins) to form nucleosomes which, in turn, organize into chromosomes. During the course of replication, the chromosomes are relaxed and the nucleosomes get loosened. The DNA strands separate for replication, and the parental histones associate with one of the parental strands. As the synthesis of new DNA strand proceeds, histones are also produced simultaneously, on the parent strand. At the end of replication, of the two daughter chromosomal DNAs formed, one contains the parental histones while the other has the newly synthesized histones.

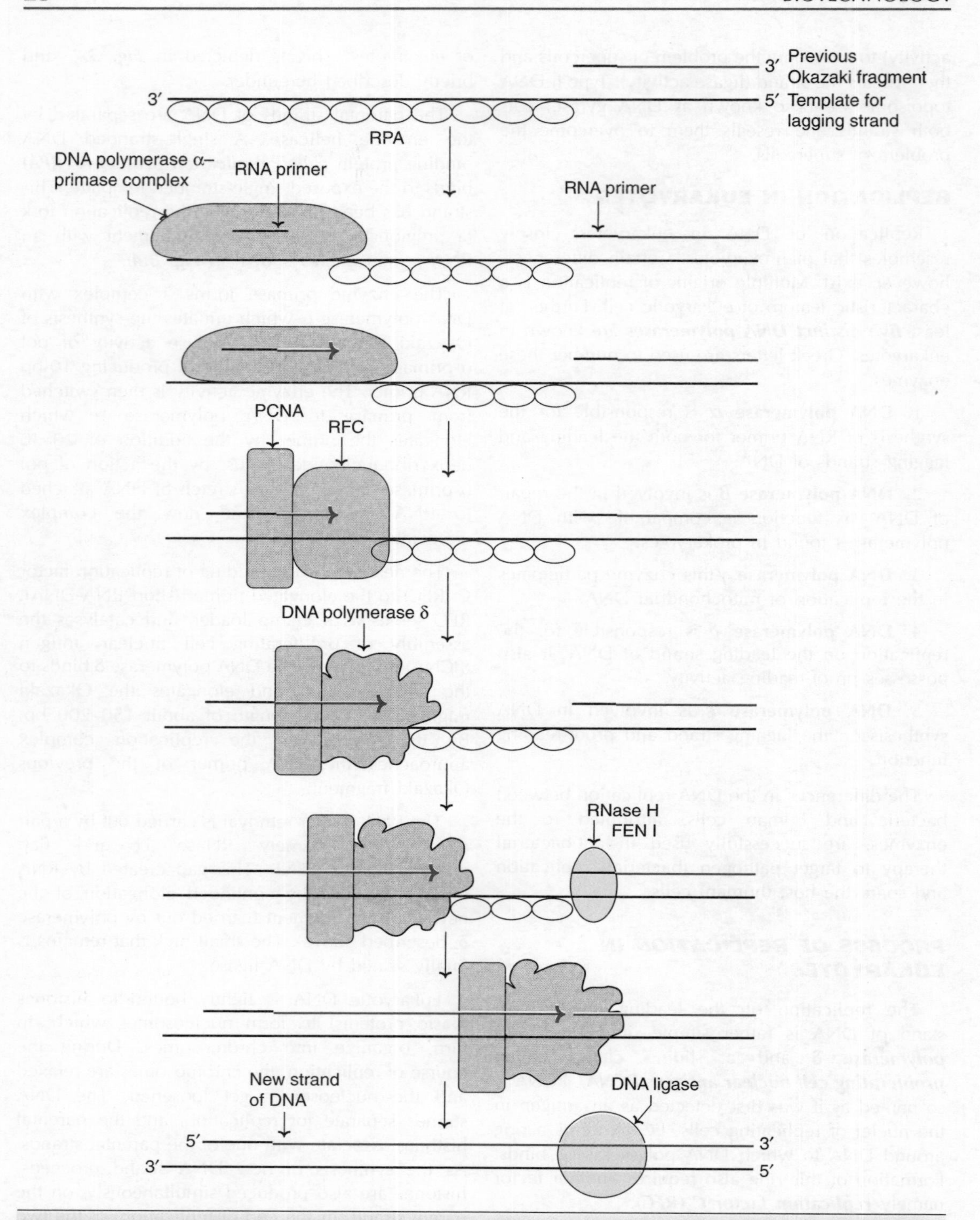

Fig. 3.7 : An outline of DNA replication on the lagging strand in eukaryotes (RPA–Replication protein A; PCNA–Proliferating cell nuclear antigen; RFC–Replication factor C; RNase H–Ribonuclease H; FENI–Flap endonuclease I; ***Note*** *: Leading strand not shown).*

INHIBITORS OF DNA REPLICATION

Bacteria contain a specific type II topoisomerase namely ***gyrase***. This enzyme cuts and reseals the circular DNA (of bacteria), and thus overcomes the problem of supercoils. Bacterial gyrase is inhibited by the antibiotics ciprofloxacin, novobiocin and nalidixic acid. These are widely used as antibacterial agents since they can effectively block the replication of DNA and multiplication of cells. These antibacterial agents have almost no effect on human enzymes.

Certain compounds that ***inhibit human topoisomerases*** are used as anticancer agents e.g. adriamycin, etoposide, doxorubicin. The nucleotide analogs that inhibit DNA replication are also used as anticancer drugs e.g. 6-mercaptopurine, 5-fluorouracil.

CELL CYCLE AND DNA REPLICATION

The cell cycle consists of four distinct phases in higher organisms—mitotic, G_1, S and G_2 phases (***Fig. 3.8***). When the cell is not growing, it exists in a dormant or undividing phase (G_0). G_1 phase is characterized by active protein synthesis.

Replication of DNA occurs only once in S-phase and the chromosomes get doubled i.e. diploid genome gets converted into tetraploid. The entire process of new DNA synthesis takes place in about 8–10 hours and a large number of DNA polymerases (500–1,000) are simultaneously involved in this process. It is believed that methylation of DNA serves as a marker to inhibit replication.

The G_2 phase is characterized by enlargement of cytoplasm and this is followed by the actual cell division that occurs in the mitotic phase.

Cyclins and cell cycle

Cyclins are a group of proteins that are closely ***associated with the transition of one phase of cell cycle to another***, hence they are so named. The most important cyclins are cyclin A, B, D and E. The concentrations of cyclins increase or decrease during the course of cell cycle. These cyclins act on cyclin-dependent kinases (CDKs) that phosphorylate certain substances essential for the transition of one cycle to another.

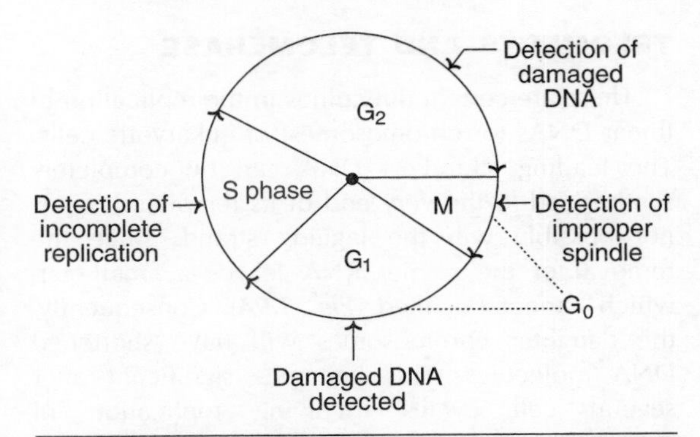

Fig. 3.8 : The cell cycle of a mammalian cell (M–Mitotic phase; G_1–Gap1 phase; G_0–Dormant phase; S phase — Period of replication; G_2–Gap 2 phase).

Cyclins and cyclin-dependent kinases (CDK1, CDK2, CDK4, CDK6) are intimately connected with the progression of cell cycle. For instance, cyclin D levels rise in late G1 phase which activate CDK4 and CDK6. This results in the assembly of nuclear proteins in a complex form in late G1 phase.

Cell cycle check points

As depicted in ***Fig. 3.8***, there occurs a continuous monitoring of the cell cycle with respect to DNA replication, chromosome segregation and integrity. If any damage to DNA is detected either in G1 or G2 phase of the cycle, or if there is a formation of defective spindle (i.e. incomplete chromosomal segregation), the cell cycle will not progress until appropriately corrected. If it is not possible to repair the damage done, the cells undergo ***apoptosis*** (programmed cell death).

Cancer and cell cycle

Cancer represents an excessive division of cells. In cancer, a large quantity of cells are in mitosis and most of them in S-phase.

Majority of the drugs used for cancer therapy are designed to block DNA replication or inhibit the enzymes that participate in replication (directly or indirectly). ***Methotrexate*** (inhibits dihydrofolate reductase) and ***5-fluorouracil*** (inhibits thymidylate synthase) block nucleotide synthesis.

In recent years, ***topoisomerase inhibitors*** are being used. They block the unwinding of parental DNA strands and prevent replication.

TELOMERES AND TELOMERASE

There are certain difficulties in the replication of linear DNAs (or chromosomes) of eukaryotic cells. The leading strand of DNA can be completely synthesized to the very end of its template. This is not possible wih the lagging strand, since the removal of the primer RNA leaves a small gap which cannot be filled (***Fig. 3.9A***). Consequently, the daughter chromosomes will have shortened DNA molecules. This becomes significant after several cell cycles involving replication of chromosomes. The result is that over a period of time, the chromosomes may lose certain essential genes and the cell dies. This is however, avoided to a large extent.

Telomeres are the special structures that prevent the continuous loss of DNA at the end of the chromosomes during the course of replication. Thus, they protect the ends of the chromosomes, and are also responsible to prevent the chromosomes from fusing with each other. Telomeres are many repeat sequences of six nucleotides present at the ends of eukaryotic chromosomes. Human telomeres contain thousands of ***repeat TTAGGG sequences***, which can be up to a length of 1500 bp.

Role of telomerase

Telomeres are maintained by the enzyme telomerase, also called as ***telomere terminal transferase***. Telomerase is an unusual enzyme as it is composed of both protein and RNA. In case of humans, the RNA component is 450 nucleotides in length, and at the 5′-terminal and it contains the sequence 5′-CUAACCCUAAC-3′. It may be noted that the central region of this sequence is complementary to the telomere repeat sequence 5′-TTAGGG-3′. The telomerase RNA sequence can be used as a template for extension of telomeres (***Fig. 3.9B***).

The telomerase RNA base pairs to the end of the DNA molecule with telomeres and extends to a small distance. Then translocation of telomerase occurs and a fresh extension of DNA takes place. This process of DNA synthesis and translocation is repeated several times until the chromosome gets sufficiently extended. The extension process gets completed through the participation of DNA polymerase and primase complex and sealing of the new DNA formed.

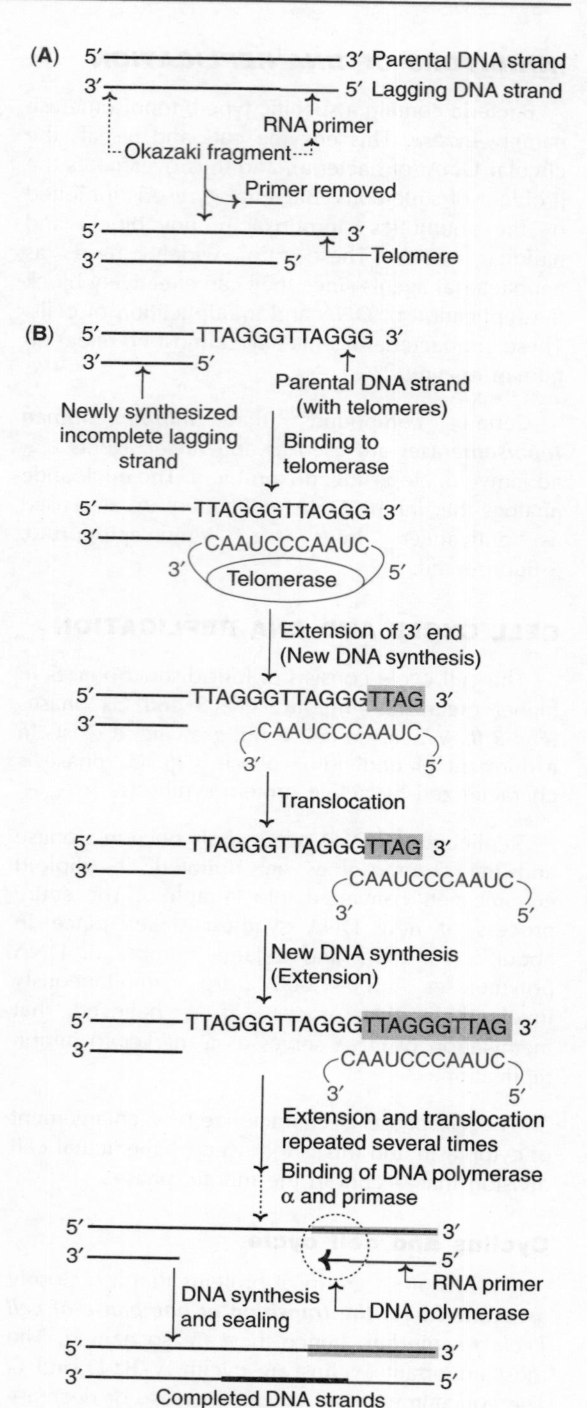

Fig. 3.9 : *Replication of DNA with telomeres (**A**) Formation of telomere (**B**) Role of telomerase in the replication of telomere (**Note :** Only 2/3 repeat sequences of telomere shown for clarity).*

It may be noted here that as such the telomeres do not encode proteins. Hence, when extended by telomerase, they need not have to remain the same length, and some shortening will not pose any problem. During the course of repeated cell cycles, there occurs ***progressive shortening of telomeres***, and this has to be ***prevented***, which is appropriately carried out ***by telomerase***.

TELOMERE IN SENESCENCE AND CANCER

Evidence is now forthcoming that telomerase is not active in all the mammalian cells. This is mainly because cells that have undergone differentiation no longer divide or divide only to a limited extent. Telomerase is highly active in the early embryo, and after birth it is active in the reproductive and stem cells. Stem cells divide continuously throughout the lifetime of an organism to produce new cells. These cells in turn are responsible to tissues and organs in the functional state e.g. hematopoietic stem cells of bone marrow.

Many biologists ***link the process of telomere shortening with cell senescence*** (i.e. cell death). This is mainly based on the observations made in the *in vitro* mammalian cell cultures. However, some researchers question this relation between telomere shortening and senescence.

Cancerous cells are able to divide continuously. There is a strong evidence to suggest that the absence of senescence in cancer cells is linked to the activation of the enzyme telomerase. Thus, telomere length is maintained throughout multiple cell divisions. It is however, not clear whether telomerase activation is a cause or an effect of cancer. There is however, evidence to suggest that telomerase activation is in fact the cause of certain cancers e.g. dyskeratosis congenita due to a mutation in the gene responsible for the RNA component of telomerase.

The enzyme ***telomerase is an attractive target for cancer chemotherapy***. The drugs have been designed to inactivate telomerase, and consequently induce senescence in the cancer cells. This in turn prevents the rapid cell proliferation.

RECOMBINATION

Recombination basically involves the exchange of genetic information. There are mainly two types of recombinations.

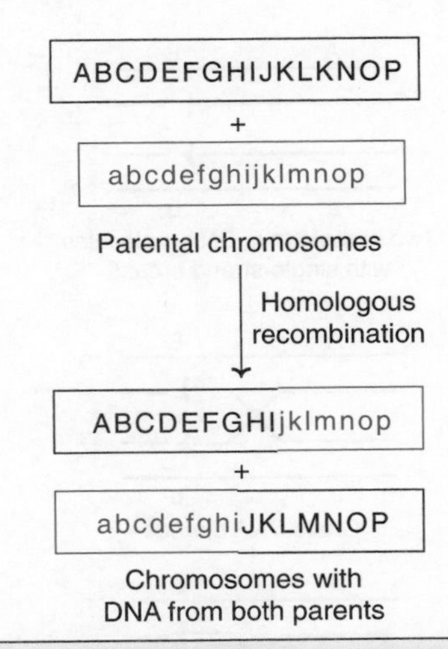

Fig. 3.10 : A diagrammatic representation of homologous recombination.

1. **Homologous recombination** : This is also called as ***general recombination***, and occurs between identical or nearly identical chromosomes (DNA sequences). The best example is the recombination between the paternal and maternal chromosomal pairs (***Fig. 3.10***).

2. **Non-homologous recombination** : This is regarded as ***illegitimate recombination*** and does not require any special homologous sequences. ***Transposition*** is a good example of non-homologous recombination. Random integration of outside genes into mammalian chromosomes is another example.

HOMOLOGOUS RECOMBINATION

It is a known fact that the chromosomes are not passed on intact from generation to generation. Instead, they are inherited from both the parents. This is possible due to homologous recombination. Three models have been put forth to explain homologous recombinations.

- Holliday model
- Meselson-Radding model
- Double-strand break model.

Holliday model

Holliday model (proposed by Holliday in 1964) is the simplest among the homologous recombination models. It is depicted in ***Fig. 3.11***, and briefly explained in the next page.

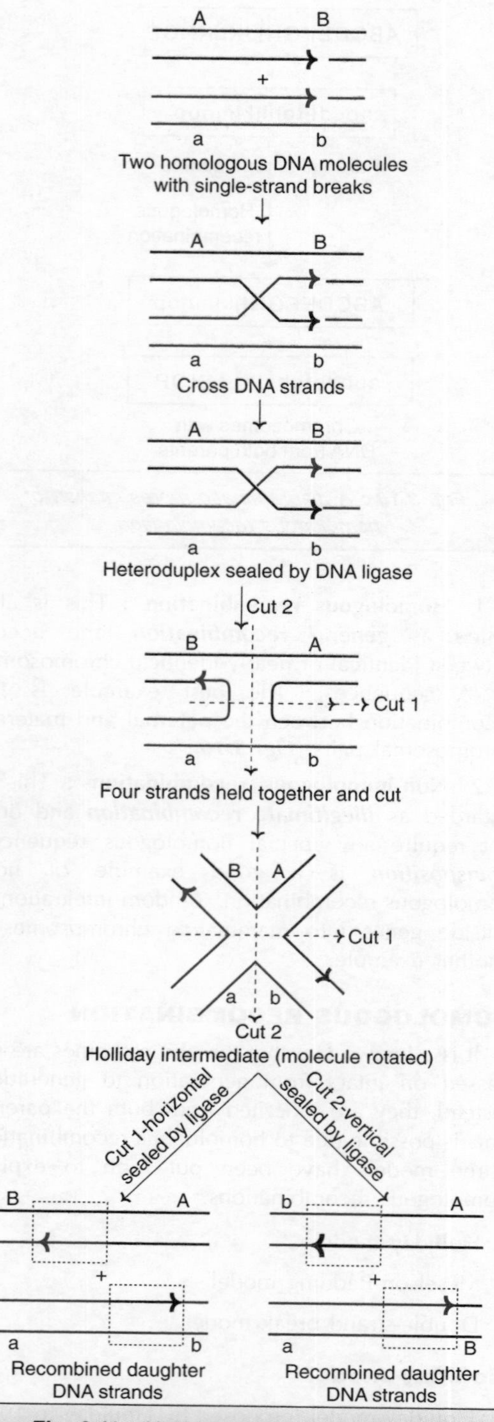

***Fig. 3.11 :** Holliday model for homologous recombination (**Note :** Heteroduplex regions are shown in dotted boxes).*

The two homologous chromosomes come closer, get properly aligned, and form single-strand breaks. This results in two aligned DNA duplexes. Now the strands of each duplex partly unwind and invade in the opposite direction to form a two strands cross between the DNA molecules.

There occurs simultaneous unwinding and rewinding of the duplexes in such a way that there is no net change in the amount of base pairing, but the position of crossover moves. This phenomenon referred to as ***branch migration***, results in the formation of ***heteroduplex DNA***. The enzyme DNA ligase seals the nick. The two DNA duplexes (4 strands of DNA), joined by a single crossover point can rotate to create a ***four-standed Holliday junction.*** Now the DNA molecules are subjected to symmetrical cuts in either of the two directions, and the cut ends are resealed by ligase.

The DNA exchange is determined by the direction of the cuts, which could be horizontal or vertical. If the corss strands are cut horizontally (cut 1), the flanking genes (or markers, i.e. AB/ab) remain intact, and no recombination occurs. On the other hand, if the parental strands are cut vertically (cut 2), the flanking genes get exchanged (i.e. Ab/aB) due to recombination.

NON-HOMOLOGOUS RECOMBINATION

The recombination process without any special homologous sequences of DNA is regarded as non-homologous recombination.

Transposition

Transposition primarily involves the ***movement of specific pieces of DNA in the genome***. The mobile segments of DNA are called ***transposons*** or ***transposable elements***. They were first discovered by Barbara McClintock (in 1950) in maize, and their significance was ignored for about two decades by other workers.

Transposons are mobile and can move almost to any place in the target chromosome. There are two modes of transposition. One that involves an RNA intermediate, and the other which does not involve RNA intermediate.

Retrotransposition : Transposition involving RNA intermediate represents retrotransposition (***Fig. 3.12***). By the normal process of transcription, a copy of RNA formed from a transposon (also

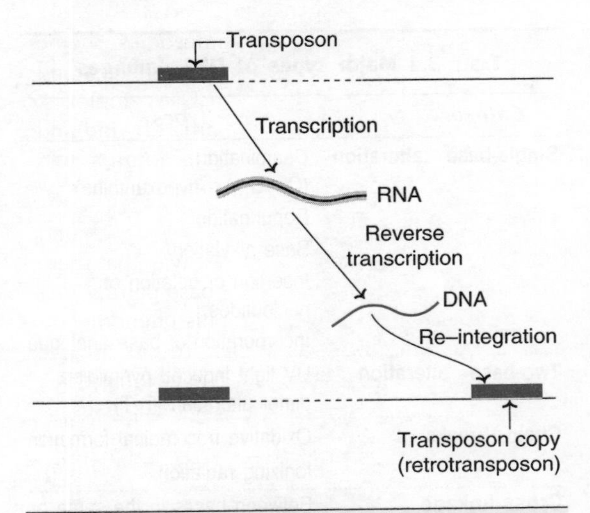

Fig. 3.12 : A diagrammatic representation of retrotransposition.

called as retrotransposon). Then by the enzyme reverse transcriptase, DNA is copied from the RNA. The newly formed DNA which is a copy of the transposon gets integrated into the genome. This integration may occur randomly on the same chromosome or, on a different chromosome. As a result of the retrotransposition, there are now two copies of the transposon, at different points on the genome.

DNA transposition : Some transposons are capable of direct transposition of DNA to DNA. This may occur either by replicative transposition or conservative transposition (***Fig. 3.13***). Both the mechanisms require enzymes that are mostly coded by the genes within the transposons.

In the ***replicative transposition,*** a direct interaction occurs between the donor transposon

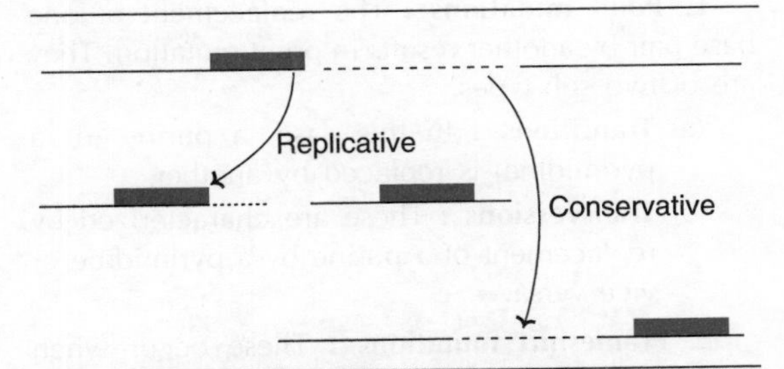

Fig. 3.13 : A diagrammatic representation of DNA transposition (coloured blocks represent transposons).

and the target site to result in ***copying of the donor element.***

In case of ***conservative transposition,*** the transposon is ***excised and reintegrated at a new site.***

DNA transposition is less common than retrotransposition in case of eukaryotes. However, in case of prokaryotes, DNA transposons are more important than RNA transposons.

Significance of transposition

It is now widely accepted that a large fraction of the human genome has resulted due to the accumulation of transposons. ***Short interspersed elements (SINEs)*** are repeats of DNA sequences which are present in about 500,000 copies per haploid human genome e.g. ***Alu sequences.***

Long interspersed elements (LINEs) are also repeated DNA sequences and are present in about 50,000 copies in the human genome e.g. L1 elements.

Some of the diseases caused by mutations are due to insertion of transpons into a genes.

DAMAGE AND REPAIR OF DNA

Being the carrier of genetic information, the cellular DNA must be replicated (duplicated), maintained, and passed down to the daughter cells accurately. In general, the accuracy of replication is extremely high. However, there do occur replication errors. It is estimated that approximately one error is introduced per billion base pairs during each cycle of replication. The cells do posses the capability to repair damages done to DNA to a large extent.

Consequences of DNA damage

Despite an efficient repair system for the damaged DNA, replication errors do accumulate that ultimately result in mutations. The human body possesses 10^{14} nucleated cells, each with 3×10^9 base pairs of DNA. It is estimated that about 10^{16} cell divisions occur in a lifetime. If 10^{-10} mutations per base pair per cell generation escape repair, this results in about one mutation per 10^6 base pairs in genome.

Besides the possible errors in replication, the DNA is constantly subjected to attack by both physical and chemical agents. These include radiation, free radicals, chemicals etc., which also result in mutations.

It is fortunate that a great majority of the mutations probably occur in the DNA that does not encode proteins, and consequently will not have any serious impact on the organism. This is not, however, all the time true, since mutations do occur in the coding regions of DNA also. There are situations in which the change in a single base pair in the human genome can cause a serious disease e.g. sickle-cell anemia.

TYPES OF DNA DAMAGES

The damage done to DNA by physical, chemical and environmental agents may be broadly classified into four categories with different types (***Table 3.1***).

The DNA damage may occur due to ***single-base alterations*** (e.g. depurination, deamination), ***two-base alterations*** (e.g. pyrimidine diamer) ***chain breaks*** (e.g. ionizing radiation) and ***cross-linkages*** (e.g. between bases). Some selected DNA damages are briefly described.

The occurrence of spontaneous deamination bases in aqueous solution at 37°C is well known. Cytosine gets deaminated to form uracil while adenine forms hypoxanthine.

Spontaneous depurination, due to cleavage of glycosyl bonds (that connect purines to the backbone) also occurs. It is estimated that 2000–10,000 purines may be lost per mammalian cell in 24 hours. The depurinated sites are called as ***abasic sites***. Originally, they were detected in purines, and called ***apurinic sites (AP sites)*** which represent lack of purine. Now, the term AP sites is generally used to represent ***any base lacking in DNA***.

The production of reactive oxygen species is often associated with alteration of bases e.g. formation of 8-hydroxy guanine. Free radical formation and oxidative damage to DNA increases with advancement of age.

Ultraviolet radiations result in the formation of covalent links between adjacent pyrimidines along the DNA strand to form ***pyrimidine dimers***. DNA chain breaks can be caused by ionizing radiations (e.g. X-rays).

TABLE 3.1 Major types of DNA damages

Category	*Types*
Single-base alteration	Deamination (C→U; A→hypoxanthine) Depurination Base alkylation Insertion or deletion of nucleotides Incorporation of base analogue
Two-base alteration	UV light induced pyrimidine dimer alteration (T–T)
Chain breaks	Oxidative free radical formation Ionizing radiation
Cross-linkage	Between bases in the same or opposite strands Between the DNA and protein molecules

MUTATIONS

The genetic macromolecule DNA is highly stable with regard to its base composition and sequence. However, DNA is not totally exempt from gradual change. A general picture of DNA damage and its repair is also described in this chapter.

Mutation refers to ***a change in the DNA structure of a gene***. The substances (chemicals) which can induce mutations are collectively known as ***mutagens***.

The changes that occur in DNA on mutation are reflected in replication, transcription and translation.

Types of mutations

Mutations are mainly of two major types—point mutations, frameshift mutations (***Fig. 3.14***).

1. **Point mutations :** The replacement of one base pair by another results in point mutation. They are of two sub-types.

(a) **Transitions :** In this case, a purine (or a pyrimidine) is replaced by another.

(b) **Transversions :** These are characterized by replacement of a purine by a pyrimidine or vice versa.

2. **Frameshift mutations :** These occur when one or more base pairs are inserted in or deleted from the DNA, respectively, causing ***insertion or deletion mutations.***

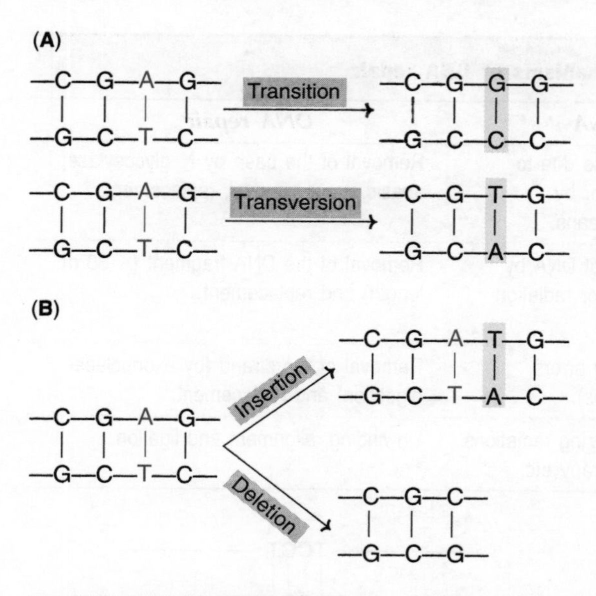

Fig. 3.14 : An illustration of mutations (A)-Point mutations; (B)-Frameshift mutations.

Consequences of point mutations

The change in a single base sequence in point mutation may cause one of the following (***Fig. 3.15***).

1. **Silent mutation :** The codon (of mRNA) containing the changed base may code for the same amino acid. For instance, *UCA* codes for serine and change in the third base *(UCU)* still codes for serine. This is due to degeneracy of the genetic code. Therefore, there are ***no detectable effects*** in silent mutation.

2. **Missense mutation :** In this case, the changed base may code for a different amino acid. For example, *UCA* codes for serine while *ACA* codes for threonine. The mistaken (or missense) amino acid may be ***acceptable***, ***partially acceptable*** or ***unacceptable*** with regard to the function of protein molecule. ***Sickle-cell anemia*** is a classical example of missense mutation.

3. **Nonsense mutation :** Sometimes, the codon with the altered base may become a ***termination*** (or nonsense) ***codon.*** For instance, change in the second base of serine codon *(UCA)* may result in *UAA*. The altered codon acts as a stop signal and causes termination of protein synthesis, at that point.

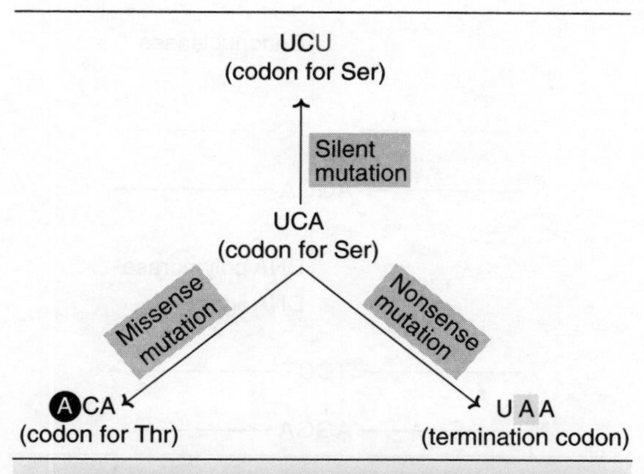

Fig. 3.15 : An illustration of point mutations (represented by a codon of mRNA).

Consequences of frameshift mutations

The insertion or deletion of a base in a gene results in an ***altered reading frame of the mRNA*** (hence the name frameshift). The machinery of mRNA (containing codons) does not recognize that a base was missing or a new base was added. Since there are no punctuations in the reading of codons, translation continues. The result is that the protein synthesized will have several altered amino acids and/or prematurely terminated protein.

Mutations and cancer

Mutations are permanent alterations in DNA structure, which have been implicated in the etiopathogenesis of cancer.

REPAIR OF DNA

As already stated, damage to DNA caused by replication errors or mutations may have serious consequences. The cell possesses an inbuilt system to repair the damaged DNA. This may be achieved by four distinct mechanisms (***Table 3.2***).

1. Base excision-repair
2. Nucleotide excision-repair
3. Mismatch repair
4. Double-strand break repair.

Base excision-repair

The bases cytosine, adenine and guanine can undergo spontaneous depurination to respectively form uracil, hypoxanthine and xanthine. These

TABLE 3.2 Major mechanisms of DNA repair

Mechanism	*Damage to DNA*	*DNA repair*
Base excision-repair	Damage to a single base due to spontaneous alteration or by chemical or radiation means.	Removal of the base by N–glycosylase; abasic sugar removal, replacement.
Nucleotide excision-repair	Damage to a segment of DNA by spontaneous, chemical or radiation means.	Removal of the DNA fragment (≈ 30 nt length) and replacement.
Mismatch repair	Damage due to copying errors (1-5 base unpaired loops).	Removal of the strand (by exonuclease digestion) and replacement.
Double-strand break repair	Damage caused by ionizing radiations, free radicals, chemotherapy etc.	Unwinding, alignment and ligation.

altered bases do not exist in the normal DNA, and therefore need to be removed. This is carried out by base excision repair (***Fig. 3.16***).

A defective DNA in which cytosine is deaminated to uracil is acted upon by the enzyme uracil DNA glycosylase. This results in the removal of the defective base uracil. An endonuclease cuts the backbone of DNA strand near the defect and removes a few bases. The gap so created is filled up by the action of repair DNA polymerase and DNA ligase.

Nucleotide excision-repair

The DNA damage due to ultraviolet light, ionizing radiation and other environmental factors often results in the modification of certain bases, strand breaks, cross-linkages etc. Nucleotide excision-repair is ideally suited for such large-scale defects in DNA. After the identification of the defective piece of the DNA, the DNA double helix is unwound to expose the damaged part. An ***excision nuclease*** (exinuclease) cuts the DNA on either side (upstream and downstream) of the damaged DNA. This defective piece is degraded. The gap created by the nucleotide excision is filled up by DNA polymerase which gets ligated by DNA ligase (***Fig. 3.17***).

Xeroderma pigmentosum (XP) is a rare autosomal recessive disease. The affected patients are photosensitive and susceptible to skin cancers. It is now recognized that XP is due to a defect in the nucleotide excision repair of the damaged DNA.

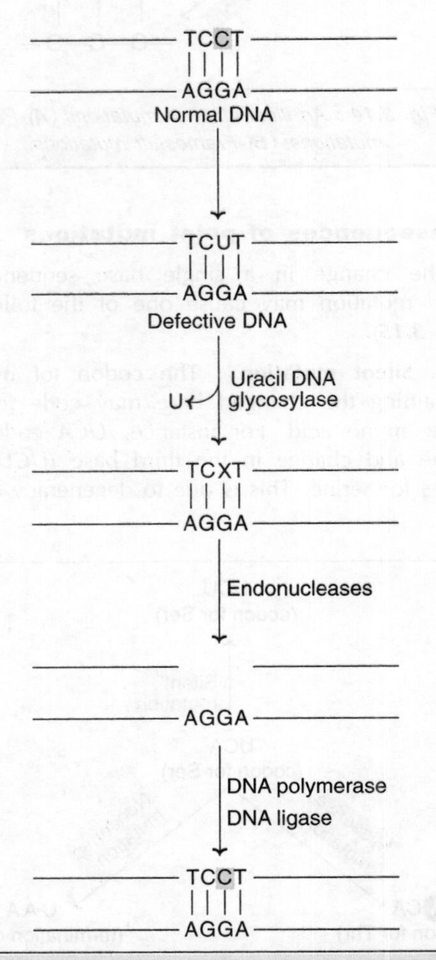

Fig. 3.16 : *A diagrammatic representation of base excision-repair of DNA.*

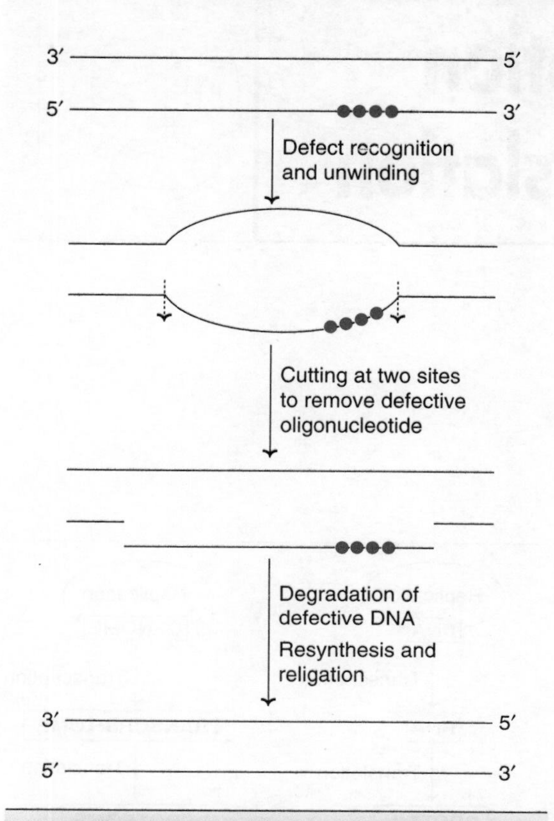

Fig. 3.17 : A diagrammatic representation of nucleotide excision-repair of DNA.

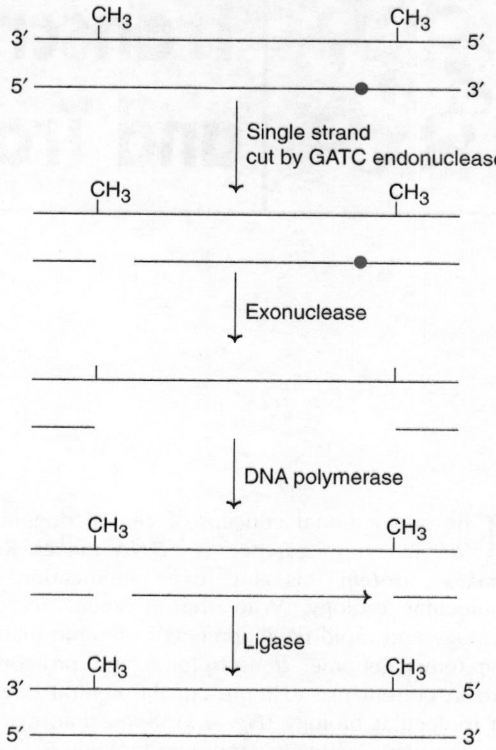

CH_3 CH_3
3′ 5′
5′ 3′
Single strand
cut by GATC endonuclease
CH_3 CH_3
Exonuclease
DNA polymerase
CH_3 CH_3
Ligase
CH_3 CH_3
3′ 5′
5′ 3′

Fig. 3.18 : A diagrammatic representation of mismatch repair of DNA.

Mismatch repair

Despite high accuracy in replication, defects do occur when the DNA is copied. For instance, cytosine (instead of thymine) could be incorporated opposite to adenine. Mismatch repair corrects a single mismatch base pair e.g. C to A, instead of T to A.

The template strand of the DNA exists in a methylated form, while the newly synthesized strand is not methylated. This difference allows the recognition of the new strands. The enzyme GATC endonuclease cuts the strand at an adjacent methylated GATC sequence (***Fig. 3.18***). This is followed by an exonuclease digestion of the defective strand, and thus its removal. A new DNA strand is now synthesized to replace the damaged one.

Hereditary nonpolyposis colon cancer (HNPCC) is one of the most common inherited cancers. This cancer is now linked with ***faulty mismatch repair*** of defective DNA.

Double-strand break repair

Double-strand breaks (DSBs) in DNA are dangerous. They result in genetic recombination which may lead to chromosomal translocation, broken chromosomes, and finally cell death. DSBs can be repaired by homologous recombination or non-homologous end joining. Homologous recombination occurs in yeasts while in mammals, non-homologous and joining dominates.

DEFECTS IN DNA REPAIR AND CANCER

Cancer develops when certain genes that regulate normal cell division fail or are altered. Defects in the genes encoding proteins involved in nucleotide-excision repair, mismatch repair and recombinational repair are linked to human cancers. For instance, as already referred above, HNPCC is due to a defect in mismatch repair.

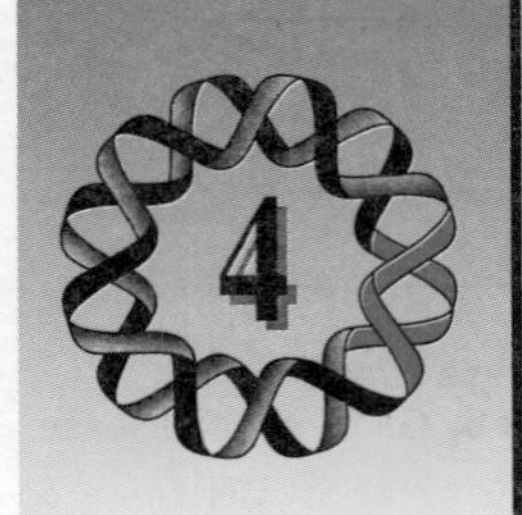

Transcription and Translation

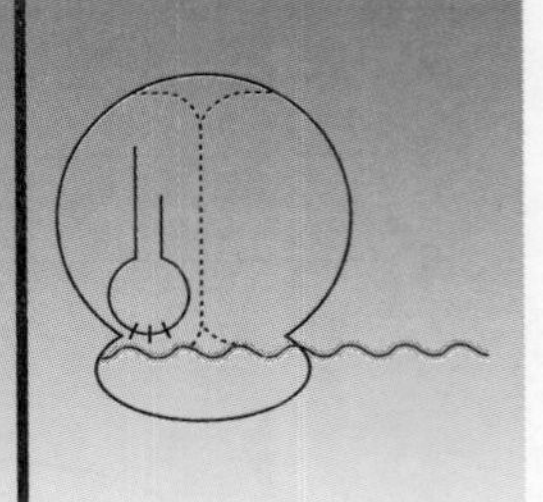

The conventional concept of central dogma of life which in essence is "***DNA makes RNA makes protein***" is an oversimplification of molecular biology. With the advances in cell biology and rapid developments in bioinformatics, the terms genome, transcriptome and proteomes are in current use to represent the central dogma of molecular biology (***Fig. 4.1***). Some information on the new concepts and terminology is given hereunder.

GENOME

The total DNA (genetic information) contained in an organism or a cell is regarded as the genome. Thus, the genome is the storehouse of biological information. It includes the chromosomes in the nucleus and the DNA in mitochondria, and chloroplasts.

Genomics : The study of the structure and function of genome is genomics. The term ***functional genomics*** is used to represent the gene expression and relationship of genes with gene products. ***Structural genomics*** refers to the structural motifs and complete protein structures. ***Comparative genomics*** involves the study of comparative gene function and phylogeny.

TRANSCRIPTOME

The RNA copies of the active protein coding genes represent transcriptome. Thus, transcriptome is the initial product of gene expression which directs the synthesis of proteins.

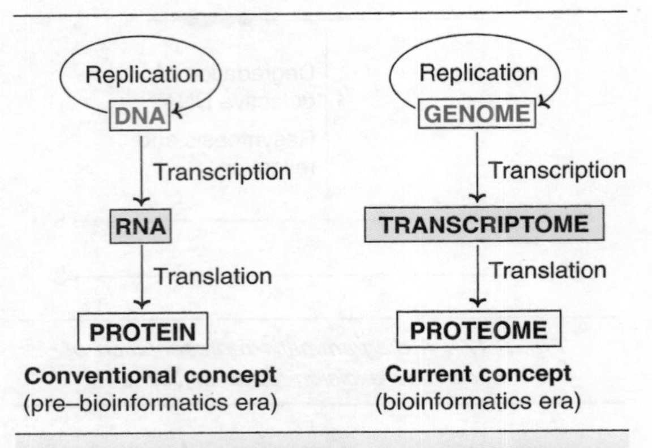

***Fig. 4.1 :** The central dogma of life (or molecular biology) represented in the form of conventional and current concepts.*

Transcriptomics : The study of transcriptome that involves all the RNA molecules made by a cell, tissue or an organism is transcriptomics.

PROTEOME

The cell's repertoire (repository/storehouse) of proteins with their nature and biological functions is regarded as proteome. Thus, proteome represents the entire range of proteins and their biological functions in a cell.

Proteomics : The study of the proteome.

Metabolomics : The use of genome sequence analysis for determining the capability of a cell, tissue or an organism to synthesize small molecules (metabolites) is metabolomics.

Whether the central dogma of life is represented in the conventional or more recent form, replication, transcription and translation are the key or core processes that ultimately control life. Replication of DNA has been described in Chapter 2, while transcription and translation are discussed in this chapter.

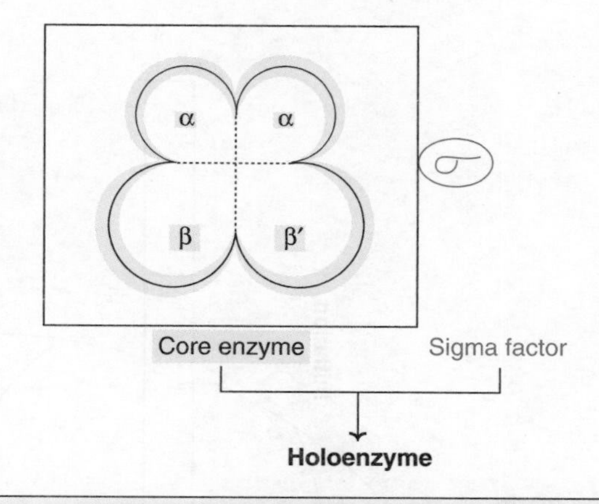

Fig. 4.2 : RNA polymerase of E. coli.

TRANSCRIPTION

Transcription is a process in which ribonucleic acid (RNA) is synthesized from DNA. The word ***gene*** refers to the ***functional unit of the DNA*** that can be transcribed. Thus, the genetic information stored in DNA is expressed through RNA. For this purpose, one of the two strands of DNA serves as a ***template*** (non-coding strand or sense strand) and produces ***working copies of RNA molecules***. The other DNA strand which does not participate in transcription is referred to as coding strand or antisense strand (frequently referred to as coding strand since with the exception of T for U, primary mRNA contains codons with the same base sequence).

Transcription is selective

The entire molecule of DNA is not expressed in transcription. RNAs are synthesized only for some selected regions of DNA. For certain other regions of DNA, there may not be any transcription at all. The exact reason for the selective transcription is not known. This may be due to some inbuilt signals in the DNA molecule.

The product formed in transcription is referred to as ***primary transcript.*** Most often, the primary RNA transcripts are inactive. They undergo certain alterations (splicing, terminal additions, base modifications etc.) commonly known as ***post-transcriptional modifications***, to produce functionally active RNA molecules.

There exist certain differences in the transcription between prokaryotes and eukaryotes. The RNA synthesis in prokaryotes is given in some detail. This is followed by a brief discussion on eukaryotic transcription.

TRANSCRIPTION IN PROKARYOTES

A single enzyme—DNA dependent RNA polymerase or simply ***RNA polymerase***—synthesizes all the RNAs in prokaryotes. RNA polymerase of *E. coli* is a complex holoenzyme (mol wt. 465 kDa) with five polypeptide subunits—2α, 1β and 1β′ and one sigma (σ) factor (***Fig. 4.2***). The enzyme without sigma factor is referred to as core enzyme ($\alpha_2\beta\beta'$).

An overview of RNA synthesis is depicted in ***Fig. 4.3***. Transcription involves three different stages—initiation, elongation and termination (***Fig. 4.4***).

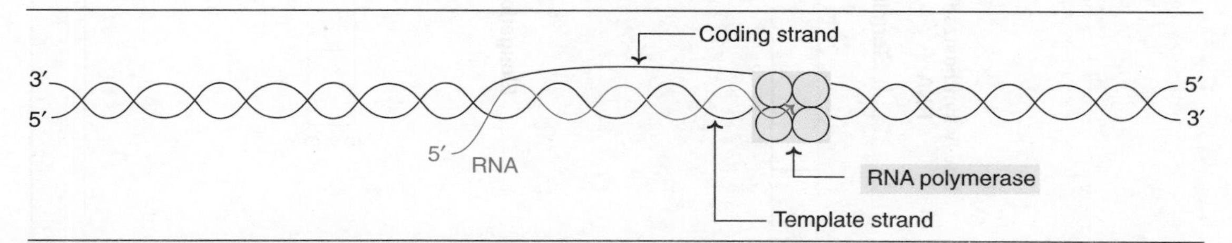

Fig. 4.3 : An overview of transcription.

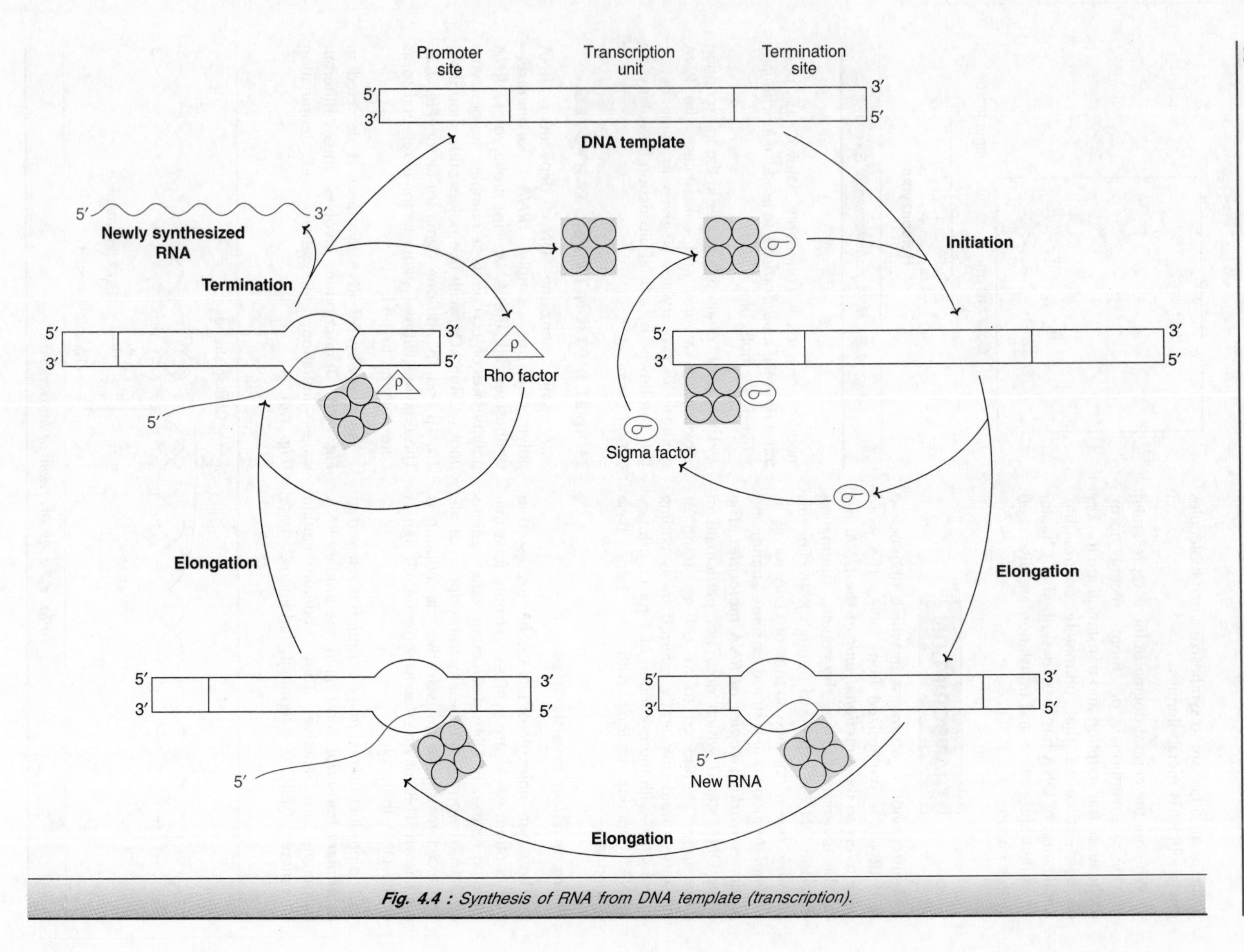

Fig. 4.4 : Synthesis of RNA from DNA template (transcription).

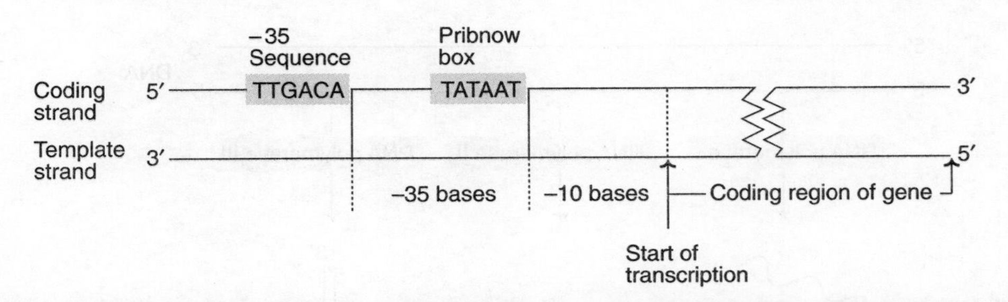

Fig. 4.5 : Promoter regions of DNA in prokaryotes.

Initiation

The binding of the enzyme RNA polymerase to DNA is the prerequisite for the transcription to start. The specific region on the DNA where the enzyme binds is known as ***promoter region.*** There are two base sequences on the ***coding DNA strand*** which the sigma factor of RNA polymerase can recognize for initiation of transcription (***Fig. 4.5***).

1. **Pribnow box (TATA box) :** This consists of 6 nucleotide bases (TATAAT), located on the left side about 10 bases away (upstream) from the starting point of transcription.

2. **The '-35' sequence :** This is the second recognition site in the promoter region of DNA. It contains a base sequence TTGACA, which is located about 35 bases (upstream, hence –35) away on the left side from the site of transcription start.

Elongation

As the holoenzyme, RNA polymerase recognizes the promoter region, the sigma factor is released and transcription proceeds. RNA is synthesized from 5′ end to 3′ end (5′→3′) antiparallel to the DNA template. RNA polymerase utilizes ribonucleotide triphosphates (ATP, GTP, CTP and UTP) for the formation of RNA. For the addition of each nucleotide to the growing chain, a pyrophosphate moiety is released.

The sequence of nucleotide bases in the mRNA is complementary to the template DNA strand. It is however, identical to that of coding strand except that RNA contains U in place of T in DNA (***Fig. 4.6***).

RNA polymerase differs from DNA polymerase in two aspects. No primer is required for RNA polymerase and, further, this enzyme does not possess endo- or exonuclease activity. Due to lack of the latter function (proof-reading activity), RNA polymerase has no ability to repair the mistakes in the RNA synthesized. This is in contrast to DNA replication which is carried out with high fidelity. It is, however, fortunate that mistakes in RNA synthesis are less dangerous, since they are not transmitted to the daughter cells.

The double helical structure of DNA unwinds as the transcription goes on, resulting in supercoils. The problem of supercoils is overcome by topoisomerases (more details given under replication).

Termination

The process of transcription stops by termination signals. Two types of termination are identified.

1. **Rho (ρ) dependent termination :** A specific protein, named ρ factor, binds to the growing RNA (and not to RNA polymerase) or weakly to DNA, and in the bound state it acts as ATPase and

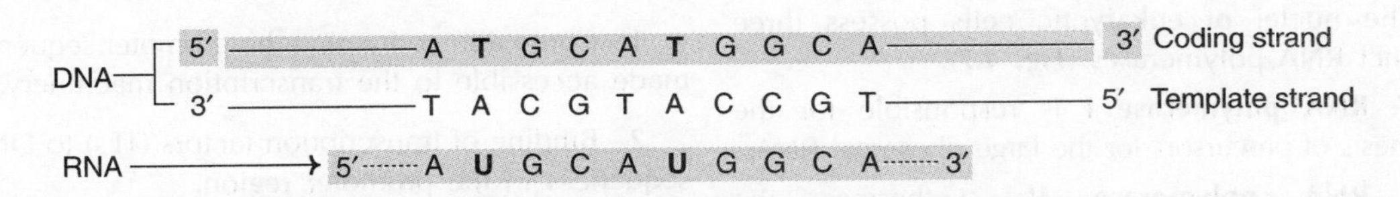

Fig. 4.6 : Promoter regions of DNA in prokaryotes.

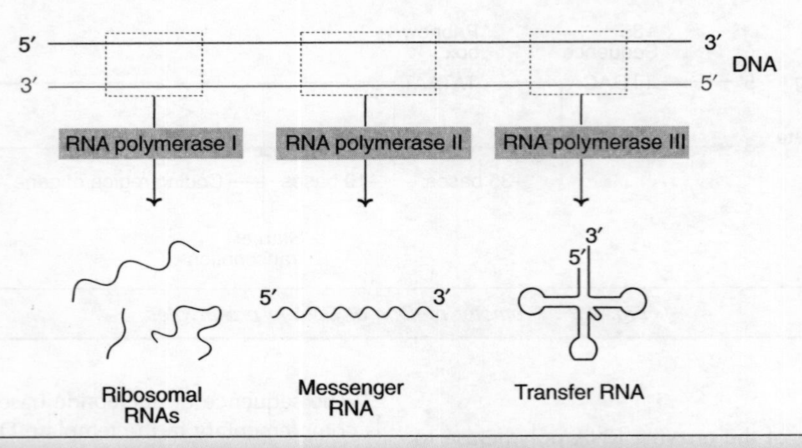

Fig. 4.7 : An overview of transcription in eukaryotes.

terminates transcription and releases RNA. The ρ factor is also responsible for the dissociation of RNA polymerase from DNA.

2. **Rho (ρ) independent termination :** The termination in this case is brought about by the formation of ***hairpins*** of newly synthesized RNA. This occurs due to the presence of ***palindromes***. A palindrome is a word that reads alike forward and backward e.g. madam, rotor. The presence of palindromes in the base sequence of DNA template (same when read in opposite direction) in the termination region is known. As a result of this, the newly synthesized RNA folds to form hairpins (due to complementary base pairing) that cause termination of transcription.

TRANSCRIPTION IN EUKARYOTES

RNA synthesis in eukaryotes is a much more complicated process than the transcription described above for prokaryotes. As such, all the details of eukaryotic transcription (particularly about termination) are not clearly known. The salient features of available information are given here.

RNA polymerases

The nuclei of eukaryotic cells possess three distinct RNA polymerases (***Fig. 4.7***).

1. **RNA polymerase I** is responsible for the synthesis of precursors for the large ribosomal RNAs.

2. **RNA polymerase II** synthesizes the precursors for mRNAs and small nuclear RNAs.

3. **RNA polymerase III** participates in the formation of tRNAs and small ribosomal RNAs.

Besides the three RNA polymerases found in the nucleus, there also exists a mitochondrial RNA polymerase in eukaryotes. The latter resembles prokaryotic RNA polymerase in structure and function.

Promoter sites

In eukaryotes, a sequence of DNA bases—which is almost identical to pribnow box of prokaryotes—is identified (***Fig. 4.8***). This sequence, known as ***Hogness box*** (or ***TATA box***), is located on the left about 25 nucleotides away (upstream) from the starting site of mRNA synthesis. There also exists another site of recognition between 70 and 80 nucleotides upstream from the start of transcription. This second site is referred to as ***CAAT box***. One of these two sites (or sometimes both) helps RNA polymerase II to recognize the requisite sequence on DNA for transcription.

Initiation of transcription

The molecular events required for the initiation of transcription in eukaryotes are complex, and broadly involve three stages.

1. Chromatin containing the promoter sequence made accessible to the transcription machinery.

2. Binding of transcription factors (TFs) to DNA sequences in the promoter region.

3. Stimulation of transcription by enhancers.

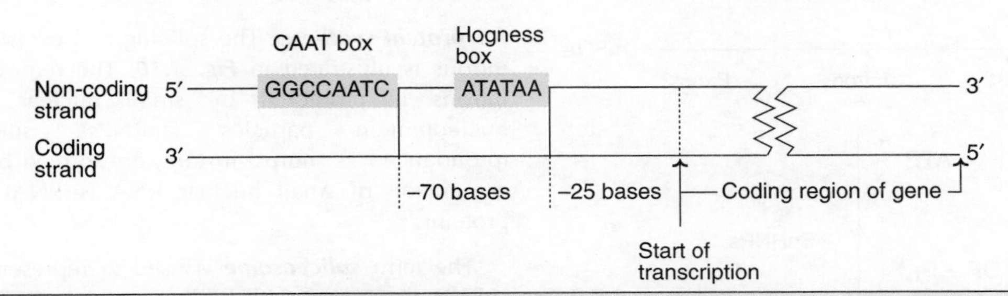

Fig. 4.8 : Promoter regions of DNA in eukaryotes.

A large number of ***transcription factors*** interact with eukaryotic promoter regions. In humans, about six transcription factors have been identified (TFIID, TFIIA, TFIIB, TFIIF, TFIIE, TFIIH). It is postulated that the TFs bind to each other, and in turn to the enzyme RNA polymerase.

Enhancer can increase gene expression by about 100 fold. This is made possible by binding to enhancers to transcription factors to form ***activators***. It is believed that the chromatin forms a loop that allows the promoter and enhancer to be close together in space to facilitate transcription.

Heterogeneous nuclear RNA (hnRNA)

The ***primary mRNA transcript*** produced by RNA polymerase II in eukaryotes is often referred to as heterogeneous nuclear RNA (hnRNA). This is then processed to produce mRNA needed for protein synthesis.

POST-TRANSCRIPTIONAL MODIFICATIONS

The RNAs produced during transcription are called primary transcripts. They undergo many alterations—***terminal base additions, base modifications, splicing*** etc., which are collectively referred to as post-transcriptional modifications. This process is required to convert the RNAs into the active forms. A group of enzymes, namely ribonucleases, are responsible for the processing of tRNAs and rRNAs of both prokaryotes and eukaryotes.

The prokaryotic mRNA synthesized in transcription is almost similar to the functional mRNA. In contrast, eukaryotic mRNA (i.e. hnRNA) undergoes extensive post-transcriptional changes.

An outline of the post-transcriptional modifications is given in ***Fig. 4.9***, and some highlights are described.

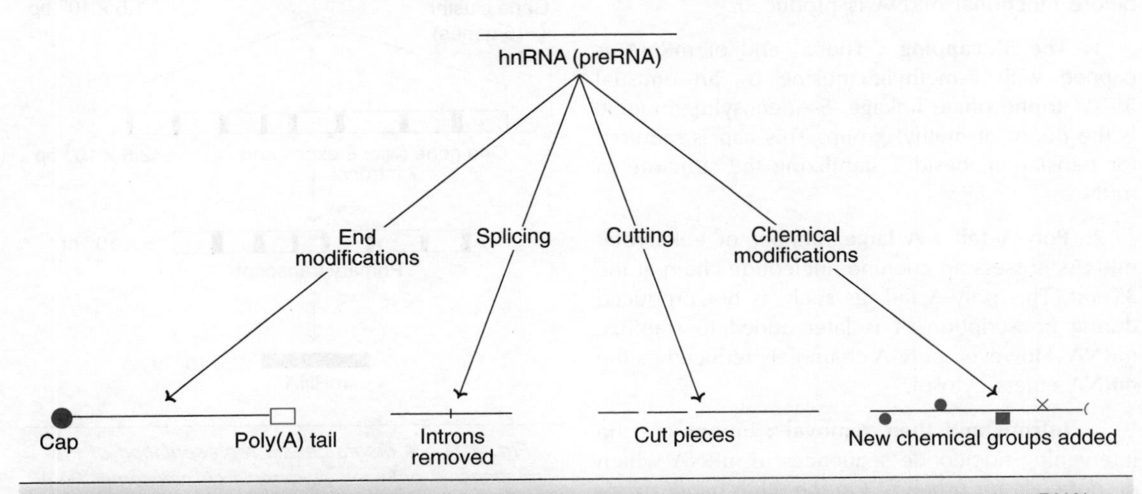

Fig. 4.9 : *An outline of post–transcriptional modifications of RNA (hnRNA-Heterogeneous nuclear RNA).*

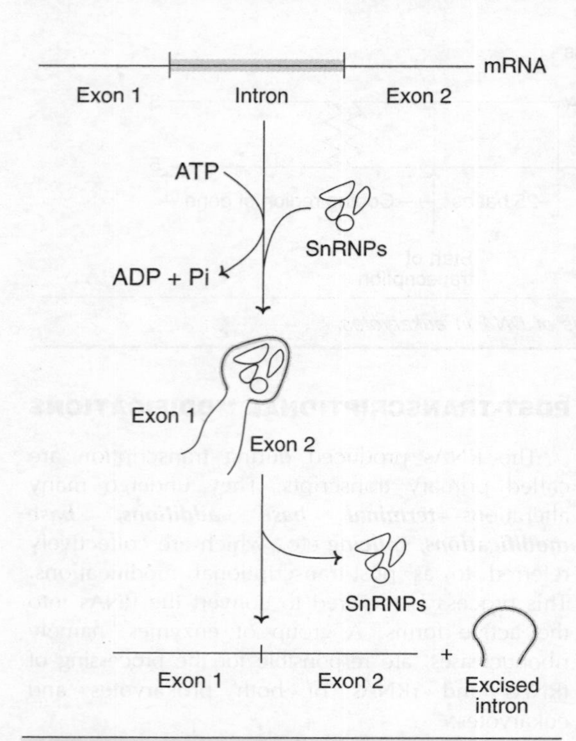

Fig. 4.10 : Formation of mature RNA from eukaryotic mRNA (SnRNPs–Small nuclear ribonucleoprotein particles).

Messenger RNA

The primary transcript of mRNA is the hnRNA in eukaryotes, which is subjected to many changes before functional mRNA is produced.

1. **The 5′ capping :** The 5′ end of mRNA is capped with 7-methylguanosine by an unusual 5′→5′ triphosphate linkage. S-Adenosylmethionine is the donor of methyl group. This cap is required for translation, besides stabilizing the structure of mRNA.

2. **Poly-A tail :** A large number of eukaryotic mRNAs possess an adenine nucleotide chain at the 3′-end. This poly-A tail, as such, is not produced during transcription. It is later added to stabilize mRNA. However, poly-A chain gets reduced as the mRNA enters cytosol.

3. **Introns and their removal :** Introns are the intervening nucleotide sequences in mRNA which do not code for proteins. On the other hand, ***exons of mRNA possess genetic code and are responsible for protein synthesis***. The splicing and excision of introns is illustrated in ***Fig. 4.10***. The removal of introns is promoted by small nuclear ribonucleoprotein particles (snRNPs). snRNPs, (pronounced as snurps) in turn, are formed by the association of small nuclear RNA (snRNA) with proteins.

The term ***spliceosome*** is used to represent the snRNP association with hnRNA at the exon-intron junction.

Post-transcriptional modifications of mRNA occurs in the nucleus. The mature RNA then enters the cytosol to perform its function (translation).

A diagrammatic representation of the relationship between eukaryotic chromosomal DNA and mRNA is depicted in ***Fig. 4.11***.

Different mRNAs produced by alternate splicing

Alternate patterns of hnRNA splicing result in different mRNA molecules which can produce

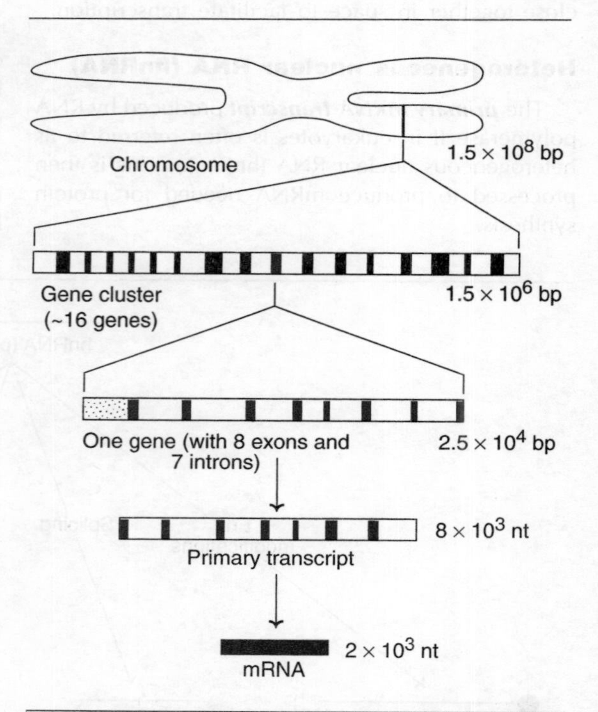

Fig. 4.11 : A diagrammatic representation of the relationship between eukaryotic chromosomal DNA and mRNA (bp–Base pair; nt–Nucleotides).

different proteins. Alternate splicing results in mRNA heterogeneity. In fact, the processing of hnRNA molecules becomes a site for the regulation of gene expression.

Faulty splicing can cause diseases : Splicing of hnRNA has to be performed with precision to produce functional mRNA. Faulty splicing may result in diseases. A good example is one type of ***β-thalassemia*** in humans. This is due to a mutation that results in a nucleotide change at an exon-intron junction. This leads to diminished or lack of synthesis of β-chain of hemoglobin, and consequently the disease β-thalassemia.

Transfer RNA

All the tRNAs of prokaryotes and eukaryotes undergo post-transcriptional modification. These include trimming, converting the existing bases into unusual ones, and addition of CCA nucleotides to 3′ terminal end of tRNAs.

Ribosomal RNA

The preribosomal RNAs originally synthesized are converted to ribosomal RNAs by a series of post-transcriptional changes.

Inhibitors of transcription

The synthesis of RNA is inhibited by certain antibiotics and toxins.

Actinomycin D : This is also known as dactinomycin. It is synthesized by *Streptomyces.* Actinomycin D binds with DNA template strand and blocks the movement of RNA polymerase. This was the very first antibiotic used for the treatment of tumors.

Rifampin : It is an antibiotic widely used for the treatment of tuberculosis and leprosy. Rifampin binds with the β-subunit of prokaryotic RNA polymerase and inhibits its activity.

α-Amanitin : It is a toxin produced by mushroom, *Amanita phalloides.* This mushroom is delicious in taste but poisonous due to the toxin α-amanitin which tightly binds with RNA polymerase II of eukaryotes and inhibits transcription.

CELLULAR RNA CONTENTS

A typical bacterium normally contains 0.05-0.10 pg of RNA which contributes to about 6% of the total weight. A mammalian cell, being larger in size, contains 20–30 pg RNA, and this represents only 1% of the cell weight. Transcriptome, representing the RNA derived from protein coding genes actually constitutes only 4%, while the remaining 96% is the non-coding RNA (***Fig. 4.12***). The different non-coding RNAs are ribosomal RNA, transfer RNA, small nuclear RNA, small nucleolar RNA and small cytoplasmic RNA. The functions of different RNAs are described in Chapter 2 (***Table 2.3***).

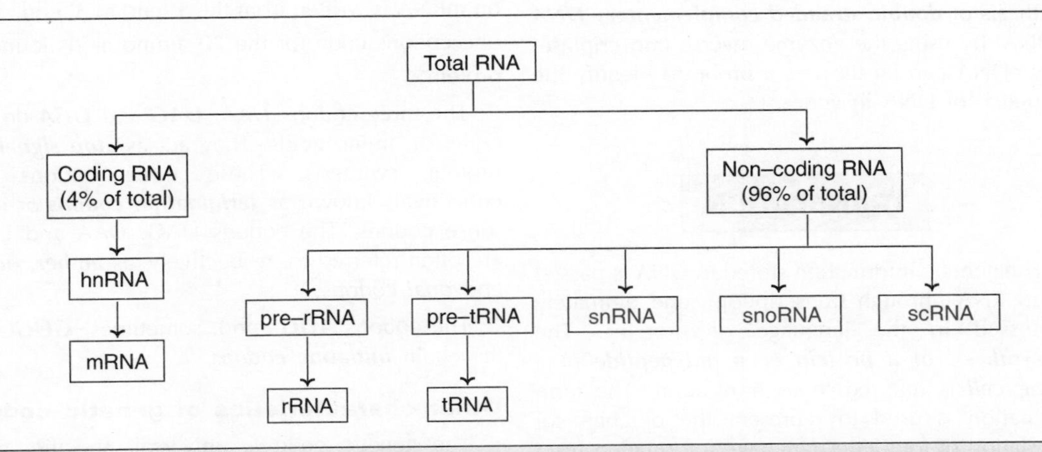

*Fig. 4.12 : A diagrammatic representation of RNA content of a cell (**Note :** RNAs represented in black are found in all organisms; RNAs in colour and exclusively present in eukaryotes only; hnRNA–Heterogeneous nuclear RNA; rRNA–Ribosomal RNA : tRNA–Transfer RNA; snRNA–Small nuclear RNA; snoRNA–Small nucleolar RNA; scRNA–Small cytoplasmic RNA).*

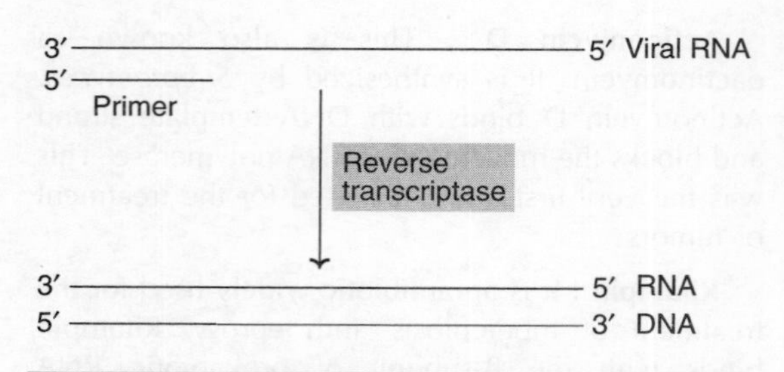

Fig. 4.13 : Reverse transcription of RNA virus.

REVERSE TRANSCRIPTION

Some of the viruses—known as ***retroviruses***—possess RNA as the genetic material. These viruses cause cancers in animals, hence known as ***oncogenic***. They are actually found in the transformed cells of the tumors.

The enzyme RNA dependent DNA polymerase —or simply ***reverse transcriptase***—is responsible for the formation of ***DNA from RNA*** (***Fig. 4.13***). This DNA is complementary (cDNA) to viral RNA and can be transmitted into host DNA.

Synthesis of cDNA from mRNA : As already described, the DNA expresses the genetic information in the form of RNA. And the mRNA determines the amino acid sequence in a protein. The mRNA can be utilized as a template for the synthesis of ***double-stranded complementary DNA*** (cDNA) by using the enzyme reverse transcriptase. This cDNA can be used as a probe to identify the sequence of DNA in genes.

TRANSLATION

The genetic information stored in DNA is passed on to RNA (through transcription), and ultimately expressed in the language of proteins. The ***biosynthesis of a protein or a polypeptide in a living cell*** is referred to as translation. The term translation is used to represent the biochemical translation of four-letter language information from nucleic acids (DNA and then RNA) to 20 letter language of proteins. The sequence of amino acids in the protein synthesized is determined by the nucleotide base sequence of mRNA.

Variability of cells in translation

There are wide variations in the cells with respect to the quality and quantity of proteins synthesized. This largely depends on the need and ability of the cells. ***Erythrocytes*** (red blood cells) lack the machinery for translation, and therefore ***cannot synthesize proteins***.

In general, the growing and dividing cells produce larger quantities of proteins. Some of the cells continuously synthesize proteins for export. For instance, liver cells produce albumin and blood clotting factors for export into the blood for circulation. The normal liver cells are very rich in the protein biosynthetic machinery, and thus the ***liver*** may be regarded as the ***protein factory in the human body***.

GENETIC CODE

The ***three nucleotide*** (triplet) ***base sequences in mRNA that act as code words for amino acids*** in protein constitute the genetic code or simply ***codons.*** The genetic code may be regarded as a dictionary of nucleotide bases (A, G, C and U) that determines the sequence of amino acids in proteins.

The codons are composed of the four nucleotide bases, namely the purines—adenine (A) and guanine (G), and the pyrimidines—cytosine (C) and uracil (U). These four bases produce 64 different combinations (4^3) of three base codons, as depicted in ***Table 4.1***. The nucleotide sequence of the codon on mRNA is written from the 5′-end to 3′ end. Sixty one codons code for the 20 amino acids found in protein.

The three codons ***UAA, UAG*** and ***UGA*** do not code for amino acids. They act as ***stop signals*** in protein synthesis. These three codons are collectively known as ***termination codons*** or non-sense codons. The codons UAG, UAA and UGA are often referred to, respectively, as ***amber***, ***ochre*** and ***opal*** codons.

The codons ***AUG***—and, sometimes, ***GUG***—are the chain ***initiating codons***.

Other characteristics of genetic code

The genetic code is universal, specific, non-overlapping and degenerate.

1. **Universality :** The same codons are used to code for the same amino acids in all the living organisms. Thus, the genetic code has been

conserved during the course of evolution. Hence genetic code is appropriately regarded as universal. There are, ***however, a few exceptions***. For instance, AUA is the codon for methionine in mitochondria. The same codon (AUA) codes for isoleucine in cytoplasm. With some exceptions noted, the genetic code is universal.

2. **Specificity :** A particular codon always codes for the same amino acid, hence the genetic code is highly specific or unambiguous e.g. UGG is the codon for tryptophan.

3. **Non-overlapping :** The genetic code is read from a fixed point as a continuous base sequence. It is non-overlapping, commaless and without any punctuations. For instance, UUUCUUAGAGGG is read as UUU/CUU/AGA/GGG. Addition or deletion of one or two bases will radically change the message sequence in mRNA. And the protein synthesized from such mRNA will be totally different. This is encountered in ***frameshift mutations*** which cause an alteration in the reading frame of mRNA.

4. **Degenerate :** Most of the amino acids have more than one codon. The codon is degenerate or redundant, since there are 61 codons available to code for only 20 amino acids. For instance, glycine has four codons. The codons that designate the same amino acid are called ***synonyms***. Most of the synonyms differ only in the third (3′ end) base of the codon.

The Wobble hypothesis explains codon degeneracy (described later).

TABLE 4.1 The genetic code along with respective amino acids

First base 5′end	*Second base (middle one)* U		C		A		G		*Third base 3′end*
	UUU	Phe	UCU		UAU	Try	UGU	Cys	U
	UUC		UCC	Ser	UAC		UGC		C
U	UUA	Leu	UCA		UAA	Stop	UGA	Stop	A
	UUG		UCG		UAG	Stop	UGG	Trp	G
	CUU		CCU		CAU	His	CGU		U
	CUC	Leu	CCC	Pro	CAC		CGC	Arg	C
C	CUA		CCA		CAA	Gln	CGA		A
	CUG		CCG		CAG		CGG		G
	AUU		ACU		AAU	Asn	AGU	Ser	U
	AUC	Ile	ACC	Thr	AAC		AGC		C
A	AUA		ACA		AAA	Lys	AGA	Arg	A
	AUG*	Met	ACG		AAG		AGG		G
	GUU		GCU		GAU	Asp	GGU		U
	GUC	Val	GCC	Ala	GAC		GGC	Gly	C
G	GUA		GCA		GAA	Glu	GGA		A
	GUG		GCG		GAG		GGG		G

*AUG serves as initiating codon, besides coding for methionine residue in protein synthesis; UAA, UAG and UGA called as nonsense codons, are responsible for termination of protein synthesis.

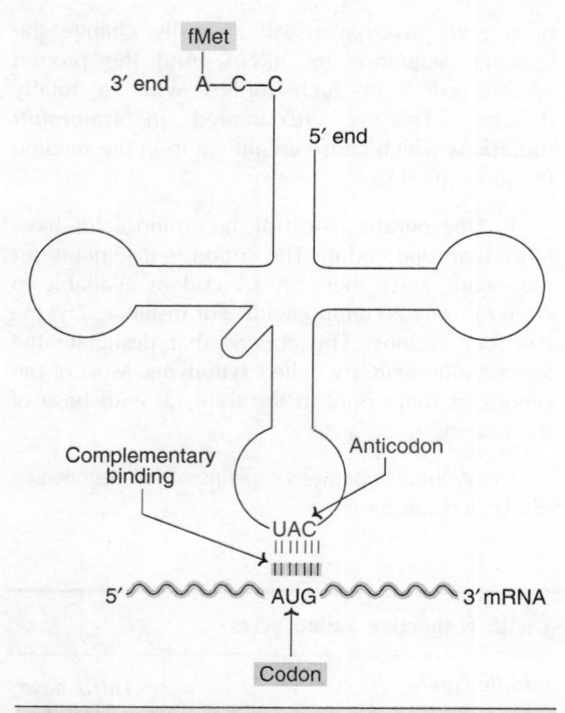

Fig. 4.14 : Complementary binding of codon (of mRNA) and anticodon (of tRNA).

Codon-anticodon recognition

The codon of the mRNA is recognized by the anticodon of tRNA (***Fig. 4.14***). They pair with each other in antiparallel direction (5′ →3′ of mRNA with 3′ →5′ of tRNA). The usual conventional complementary base pairing (A = U, C ≡ G) occurs between the first two bases of codon and the last two bases of anticodon. The third base of the codon is rather lenient or flexible with regard to the complementary base. The ***anticodon region*** of tRNA consists of seven nucleotides and it recognizes the three letter codon in mRNA.

Wobble hypothesis

Wobble hypothesis, put forth by Crick, is the phenomenon in which a ***single tRNA can recognize more than one codon***. This is due to the fact that the third base (3′-base) in the codon often fails to recognize the specific complementary base in the anticodon (5′-base). Wobbling is attributed to the difference in the spatial arrangement of the 5′-end of the anticodon. The possible pairing of 5′-end base of anticodon (of tRNA) with the 3′-end base of codon (mRNA) is given

Anticodon		Codon	
C	—	G	Conventional base pairing
A	—	U	
U	—	G or A	Non-conventional base (coloured) pairing
G	—	U or C	

Wobble hypothesis explains the degeneracy of the genetic code, i.e. existence of multiple codons for a single amino acid. Although there are 61 codons for amino acids, the number of tRNAs is far less (around 40) which is due to wobbling.

Mutations and genetic code

Mutations result in the change of nucleotide sequences in the DNA, and consequently in the RNA. The different types of mutations are described in Chapter 3. The ultimate effect of mutations is on the translation through the alterations in codons. Some of the mutations are harmful.

The occurrence of the disease ***sickle-cell anemia*** due to a single base alteration (CTC → CAC in DNA, and GAG → GUG in RNA) is a classical example of the seriousness of mutations. The result is that glutamate at the 6th position of β-chain of hemoglobin is replaced by valine. This happens since the altered codon GUG of mRNA codes for valine instead of glutamate (coded by GAG in normal people).

Frameshift mutations are caused by deletion or insertion of nucleotides in the DNA that generates altered mRNAs. As the reading frame of mRNA is continuous, the codons are read in continuation, and amino acids are added. This results in proteins that may contain several altered amino acids, or sometimes the protein synthesis may be terminated prematurely.

PROTEIN BIOSYNTHESIS

The ***protein synthesis*** which involves the translation of nucleotide base sequence of mRNA into the language of amino acid sequence may be divided into the ***following stages*** for the convenience of understanding.

I. Requirement of the components

II. Activation of amino acids

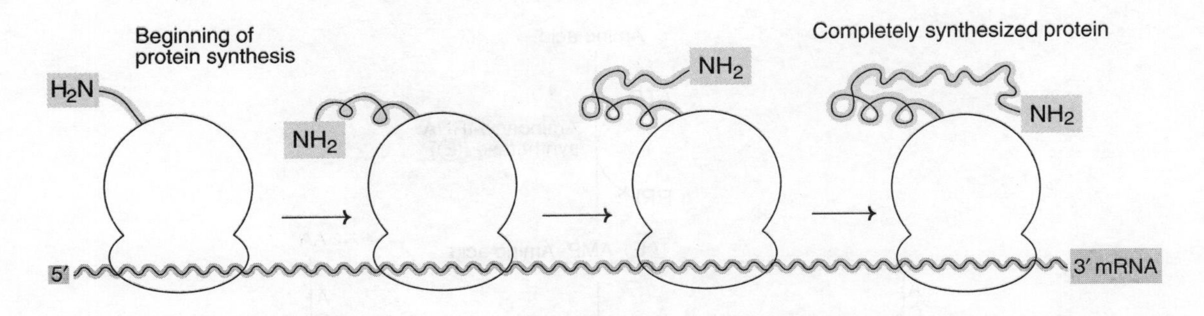

Fig. 4.15 : A polyribosome in protein synthesis.

III. Protein synthesis proper

IV. Chaperones and protein folding

V. Post-translational modifications.

I. REQUIREMENT OF THE COMPONENTS

The protein synthesis may be considered as a biochemical factory operating on the ribosomes. As a factory is dependent on the supply of raw materials to give a final product, the protein synthesis also requires many components.

1. **Amino acids :** Proteins are polymers of amino acids. Of the ***20 amino acids*** found ***in protein structure***, half of them (10) can be synthesized by man. About ***10 essential amino acids*** have to be provided through the diet. Protein synthesis can occur only when all the amino acids needed for a particular protein are available. If there is a deficiency in the dietary supply of any one of the essential amino acids, the translation stops. It is, therefore, necessary that a regular dietary supply of essential amino acids, in sufficient quantities, is maintained, as it is a prerequisite for protein synthesis.

As regards prokaryotes, there is no requirement of amino acids, since all the 20 are synthesized from the inorganic components.

2. **Ribosomes :** The functionally active ribosomes are the ***centres*** or ***factories for protein synthesis***. Ribosomes may also be considered as workbenches of translation. Ribosomes are huge complex structures (70S for prokaryotes and 80S for eukaryotes) of proteins and ribosomal RNAs. Each ribosome consists of two subunits—one big and one small. The functional ribosome has two sites—A site and P site. Each site covers both the subunits. ***A site*** is for binding of aminoacyl tRNA and ***P site*** is for binding peptidyl tRNA, during the course of translation. Some authors consider A site as acceptor site and P site as donor site. In case of eukaryotes, there is another site called ***exist site*** or ***E site***. Thus, eukaryotes contain three sites (A, P and E) on the ribosomes.

The ribosomes are located in the cytosomal fraction of the cell. They are found in association with rough endoplasmic reticulum (RER) to form clusters RER—ribosomes, where the protein synthesis occurs. The term ***polyribosome*** (polysome) is used when several ribosomes simultaneously translate on a single mRNA (***Fig. 4.15***).

3. **Messenger RNA (mRNA) :** The specific information required for the synthesis of a given protein is present on the mRNA. The DNA has passed on the genetic information in the form of ***codons*** to mRNA to translate into a protein sequence.

4. **Transfer RNAs (tRNAs) :** They carry the amino acids, and hand them over to the growing peptide chain. The amino acid is covalently bound to tRNA at the 3′-end. Each tRNA has a three nucleotide base sequence—the ***anticodon***, which is responsible to recognize the codon (complementary bases) of mRNA for protein synthesis.

In man, there are about 50 different tRNAs whereas in bacteria around 40 tRNAs are found. Some amino acids (particularly those with multiple codons) have more than one tRNA.

5. **Energy sources :** Both ***ATP*** and ***GTP*** are required for the supply of energy in protein synthesis. Some of the reactions involve the breakdown of ATP or GTP, respectively, to AMP and GMP with the liberation of pyrophosphate.

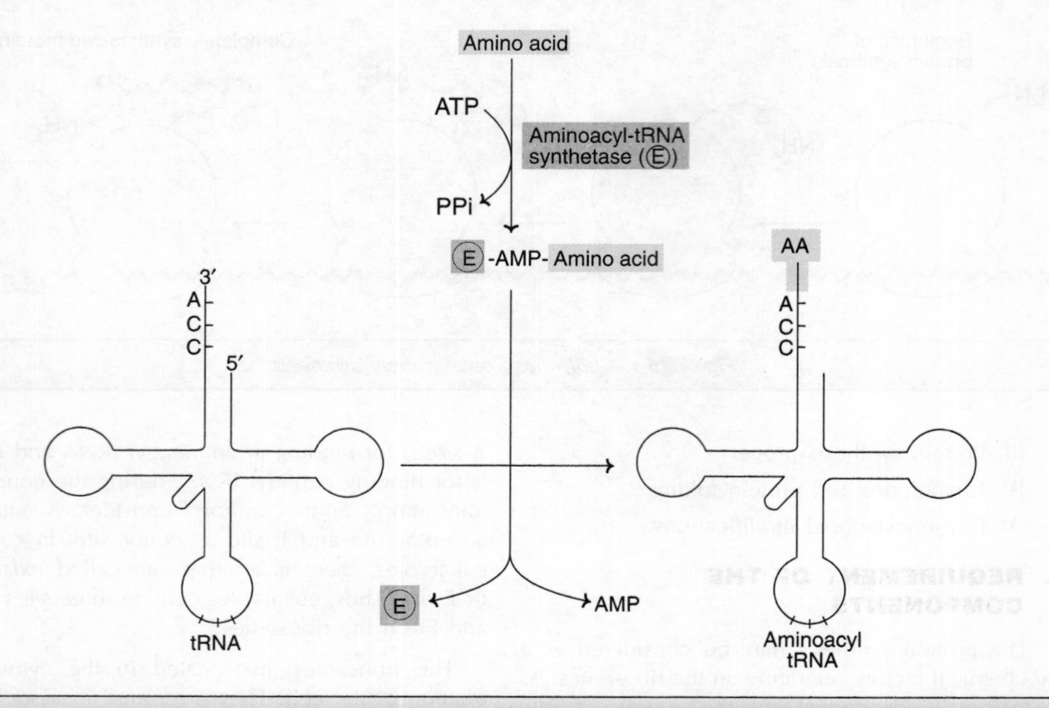

Fig. 4.16 : Formation of aminocacyl tRNA (AA–Amino acid; E–Enzyme).

Each one of these reactions consumes two high energy phosphates (equivalent to 2 ATP).

6. **Protein factors :** The process of translation involves a number of protein factors. These are needed for initiation, elongation and termination of protein synthesis. The protein factors are more complex in eukaryotes compared to prokaryotes.

II. ACTIVATION OF AMINO ACIDS

Amino acids are activated and attached to tRNAs in a two step reaction. A group of enzymes—namely aminoacyl tRNA synthetases—are required for this process. These enzymes are highly specific for the amino acid and the corresponding tRNA.

The amino acid is first attached to the enzyme utilizing ATP to form enzyme-AMP-amino acid complex. The amino acid is then transferred to the 3′ end of the tRNA to form aminoacyl tRNA (***Fig. 4.16***).

III. PROTEIN SYNTHESIS PROPER

The protein or polypeptide synthesis occurs on the ribosomes (rather polyribosomes). The ***mRNA is read in the 5′→3′ direction and the polypeptide synthesis proceeds from N-terminal end to C-terminal end***. Translation is directional and collinear with mRNA.

The prokaryotic mRNAs are ***polycistronic,*** since a single mRNA has many coding regions that code for different polypeptides. In contrast, eukaryotic mRNA is ***monocistronic,*** since it codes for a single polypeptide.

In case of prokaryotes, translation commences before the transcription of the gene is completed. Thus, simultaneous transcription and translation are possible. This is not so in case of eukaryotic organisms since transcription occurs in the nucleus whereas translation takes place in the cytosol. Further, the primary transcript (hnRNA) formed from DNA has to undergo several modifications to generate functional mRNA.

Protein synthesis is comparatively simple in case of prokaryotes compared to eukaryotes. Further, many steps in eukaryotic translation were not understood for quite sometime. For these reasons, majority of the textbooks earlier used to describe translation in prokaryotes in detail, and give most important and relevant information for eukaryotic translation. With the advances in molecular biology, the process of protein biosynthesis in eukaryotes is better understood now.

Translation in eukaryotes is briefly ***described here***, along with some relevant features of prokaryotic protein biosynthesis. Translation proper is divided into three stages—initiation, elongation and termination (as it is done for transcription).

INITIATION OF TRANSLATION

The initiation of translation in eukaryotes is complex, involving at least ***ten eukaryotic initiation factors (eIFs).*** Some of the eIFs contain multiple (3-8) subunits. The process of translation initiation can be divided into four steps (***Fig. 4.17***).

1. Ribosomal dissociation.
2. Formation of 43S preinitiation complex.
3. Formation of 48S initiation complex.
4. Formation of 80S initiation complex.

Ribosomal dissociation

The 80S ribosome dissociates to form 40S and 60S subunits. Two initiating factors namely eIF-3 and eIF-1A bind to the newly formed 40S subunit, and thereby block its reassociation with 60S subunit. For this reason, some workers name eIF-3 as ***anti-association factor***.

Formation of 43S preinitiation complex

A ternary complex containing met-tRNA^{i} and eIF-2 bound to GTP attaches to 40S ribosomal subunit to form 43S preinitiation complex. The presence of eIF-3 and eIF-1A stabilizes this complex (***Note :*** Met-tRNA is specifically involved in binding to the ***i***nitiation condon AUGs; hence the superscrip^{i} is used in met-tRNA^{i}).

Formation of 48S initiation complex

The binding of mRNA to 43S preinitiation complex results in the formation of 48S initiation complex through the intermediate 43S initiation complex. This, however, involves certain interactions between some of the eIFs and activation of mRNA.

eIF-4F complex is formed by the association of eIF-4G, eIF-4A with eIF-4E. The so formed eIF-4F (referred to as cap binding protein) binds to the cap of mRNA. Then eIF-4A and eIF-4B bind to mRNA and reduce its complex structure. This mRNA is then transferred to 43S complex. For the appropriate association of 43S preinitiation complex with mRNA, energy has to be supplied by ATP.

Recognition of initiation codon : The ribosomal initiation complex scans the mRNA for the identification of appropriate initiation codon. 5′-AUG is the initiation codon and its recognition is facilitated by a specific sequence of nucleotides surrounding it. This marker sequence for the identification of AUG is called as ***Kozak consensus sequences***. In case of prokaryotes the recognition sequence of initiation codon is referred to as ***Shine-Dalgarno sequence***.

Formation of 80S initiation complex

48S initiation complex binds to 60S ribosomal subunit to form 80S initiation complex. The binding involves the hydrolysis of GTP (bound to eIF-2). This step is facilitated by the involvement of eIF-5.

As the 80S complex is formed, the initiation factors bound to 48S initiation complex are released, and recycled. The activation of eIF-2 requires eIF-2B (also called as guanine nucleotide exchange factor) and GTP. The activated eIF-2 (i.e. bound to GTP) requires eIF-2C to form the ternary complex.

Regulation of initiation

The eIF-4F, a complex formed by the assembly of three initiation factors controls initiation, and thus the translation process. eIF-4E, a component of eIF-4F is primarily responsible for the recognition of mRNA cap. And this step is the rate-limiting in translation.

eIF-2 which is involved in the formation of 43S preinitiation complex also controls protein biosynthesis to some extent.

Initiation of translation in prokaryotes

The formation of translation initiation complex in prokaryotes is less complicated compared to eukaryotes. The 30S ribosomal subunit is bound to initiation factor 3 (IF-3) and attached to ternary complex of IF-2, formyl met-tRNA and GTP. Another initiation factor namely IF-I also participates in the formation of preinitiation complex. The recognition of initiation codon AUG is done through Shine-Dalgarno sequence. A 50S ribosome unit is now bound with the 30S unit to produce 70S initiation complex in prokaryotes.

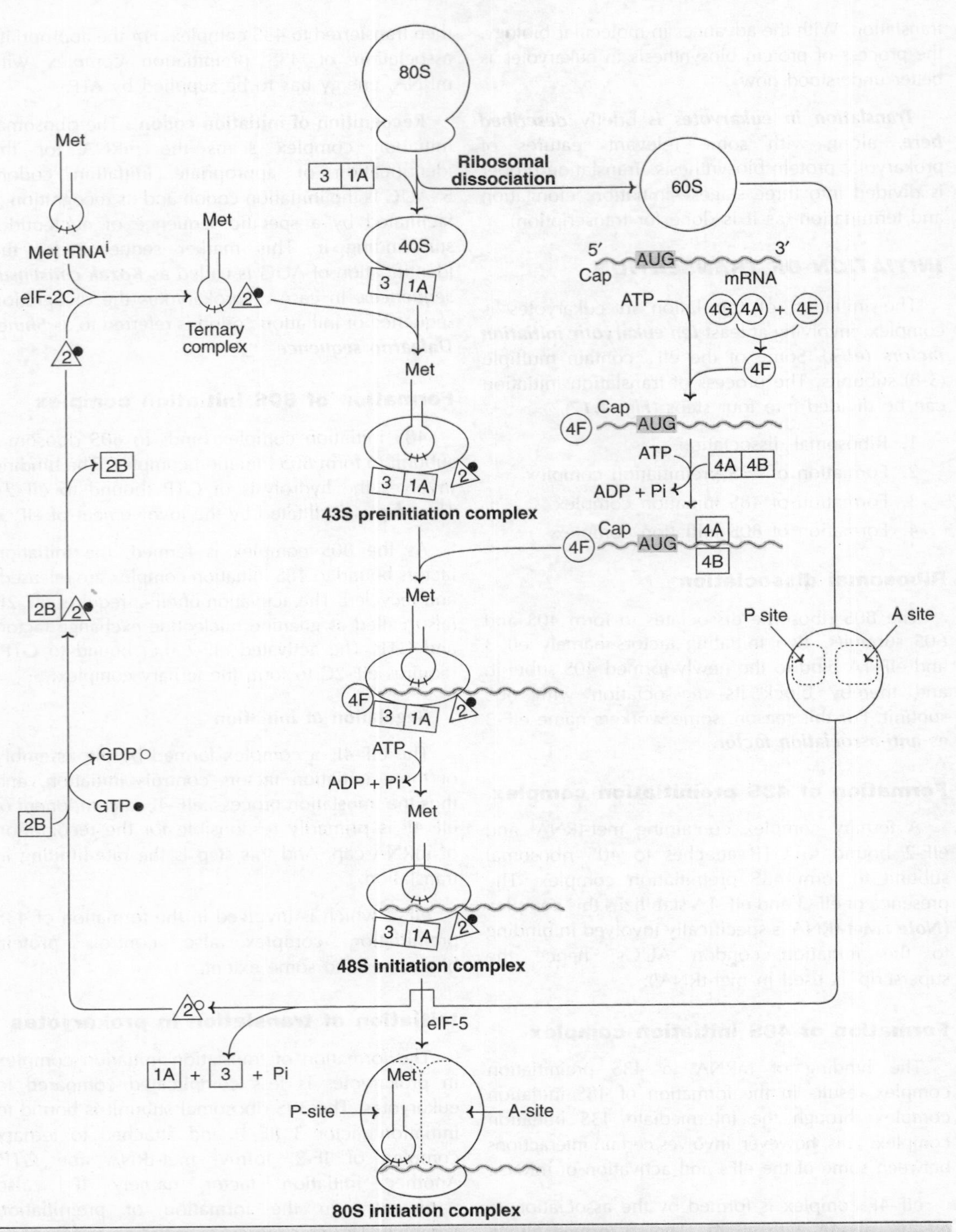

Fig. 4.17 : A diagrammatic representation of initiation of protein biosynthesis (translation) in eukaryotic cells (The eukaryotic initiation factors are represented by symbols ▢, △, and ◯. By prefixing with eIF, the full names of the factors are obtained e.g. ▢3 represents eIF–3).

ELONGATION OF TRANSLATION

Ribosomes elongate the polypeptide chain by a sequential addition of amino acids. The amino acid sequence is determined by the order of the codons in the specific mRNA. Elongation, a cyclic process involving certain elongation factors (EFs), may be divided into three steps (***Fig. 4.18***).

1. Binding of aminoacyl t-RNA to A-site.
2. Peptide bond formation.
3. Translocation.

Binding of aminoacyl—tRNA to A-site

The 80S initiation complex contains met-tRNA^{i} in the P-site, and the A-site is free. Another aminoacyl-tRNA is placed in the A-site. This requires proper codon recognition on the mRNA and the involvement of elongation factor 1α (EF-Iα) and supply of energy by GTP. As the aminoacyl-tRNA is placed in the A-site, EF-1α and GDP are recycled to bring another aminoacyl-tRNA.

Peptide bond formation

The enzyme ***peptidyltransferase*** catalyses the formation of peptide bond (***Fig. 4.19***). The activity of this enzyme lies on 28S RNA of 60S ribosomal subunit. It is therefore the ***rRNA*** (and not protein) referred to as ***ribozyme*** that catalyses the peptide bond formation. As the amino acid in the aminoacyl-tRNA is already activated, no additional energy is required for peptide bond formation.

The net result of peptide bond formation is the attachment of the growing peptide chain to the tRNA in the A-site.

Translocation

As the peptide bond formation occurs, the ribosome moves to the next codon of the mRNA (towards 3′-end). This process called translocation, basically involves the movement of growing peptide chain from A-site to P-site. Translocation requires EF-2 and GTP. GTP gets hydrolysed and supplies energy to move mRNA. EF-2 and GTP complex recycles for translocation.

In recent years, another site namely ***exist site*** (E-site) has been identified in eukaryotes. The deacylated tRNA moves into the E-site, from where it leaves the ribosome.

In case of prokaryotes, the elongation factors are different, and they are EF-Tu, EF-Ts (in place of of EF-1α) and EF-G (instead of EF-2).

Incorporation of amino acids

It is estimated that about ***six amino acids per second*** are incorporated during the course of elongation of translation ***in eukaryotes***. In case of prokaryotes, as many as 20 amino acids can be incorporated per second. Thus the process of protein/polypeptide synthesis in translation occurs with ***great speed*** and ***accurary***.

TERMINATION OF TRANSLATION

Termination is a simple process when compared to initiation and elongation. After several cycles of elongation, incorporating amino acids and the formation of the specific protein/polypeptide molecule, one of the ***stop or termination signals (UAA, UAG and UCA)*** terminates the growing polypeptide. The termination codons which act as stop signals do not have specific tRNAs to bind. As the termination codon occupies the ribosomal A-site, the release factor namely eRF recognizes the stop signal. eRF-GTP complex, in association with the enzyme peptidyltransferase, cleaves the peptide bond between the polypeptide and the tRNA occupying P-site. In this reaction, a water molecule, instead of an amino acid is added. This hydrolysis releases the protein and tRNA from the P-site. The 80S ribosome dissociates to form 40S and 60S subunits which are recycled. The mRNA is also released.

INHIBITORS OF PROTEIN SYNTHESIS

Translation is a complex process and it has become a favourite target for inhibition by antibiotics. Antibiotics are the substances produced by bacteria or fungi which inhibit the growth of other organisms. Majority of the antibiotics interfere with the bacterial protein synthesis and are harmless to higher organisms. This is due to the fact that the process of translation sufficiently differs between prokaryotes and eukaryotes. The action of a few important antibiotics on translation is described here.

Streptomycin : Initiation of protein synthesis is inhibited by streptomycin. It causes misreading of mRNA and interferes with the normal pairing between codons and anticodons.

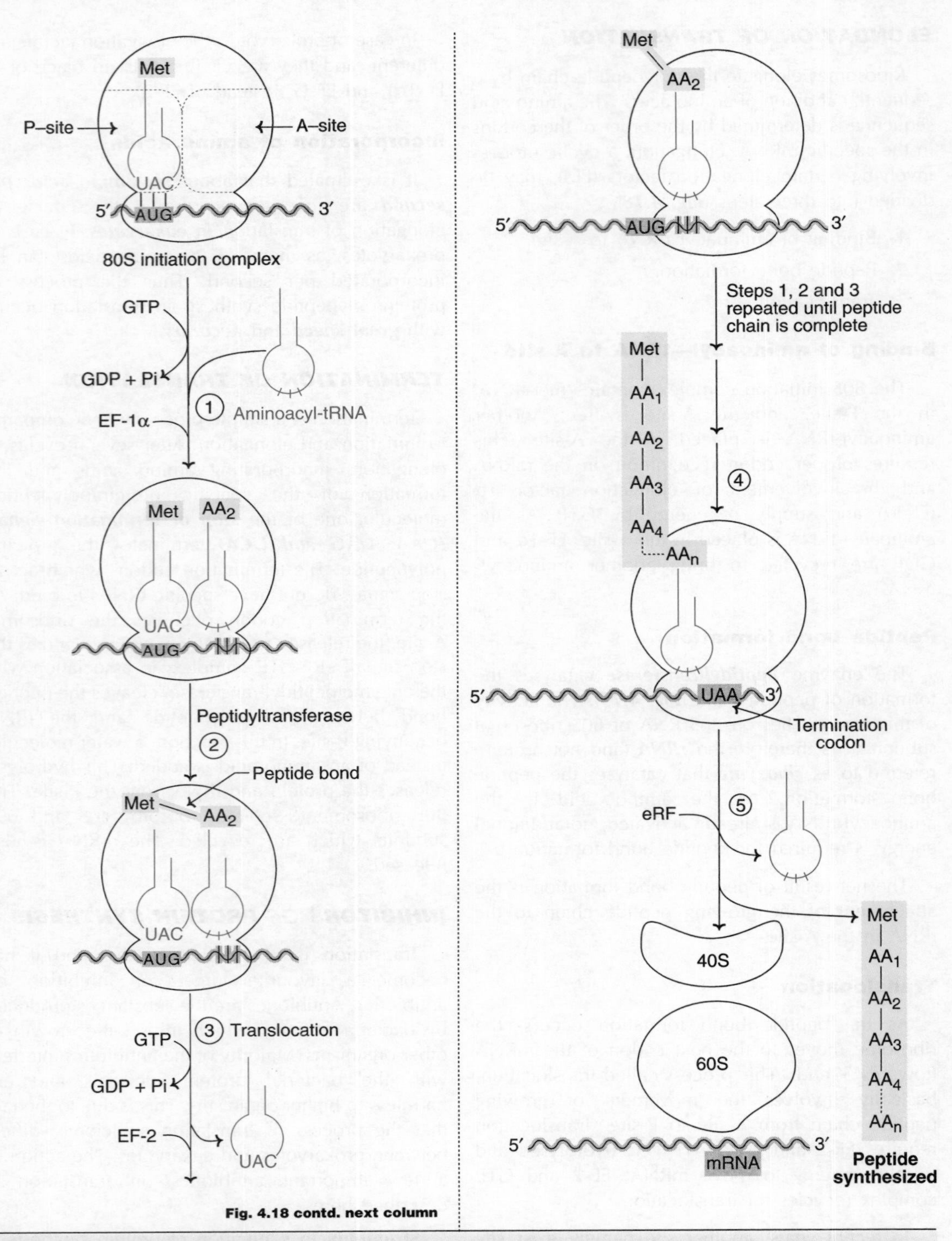

Fig. 4.18 : Protein biosynthesis — Elongation and termination (for initiation refer Fig. 4.17). Met-Methionine; P-site — Peptidyl tRNA binding site; A-site — Aminoacyl tRNA binding site. AA-Amino acid; EF-Elongation factor; RF-Releasing factor.

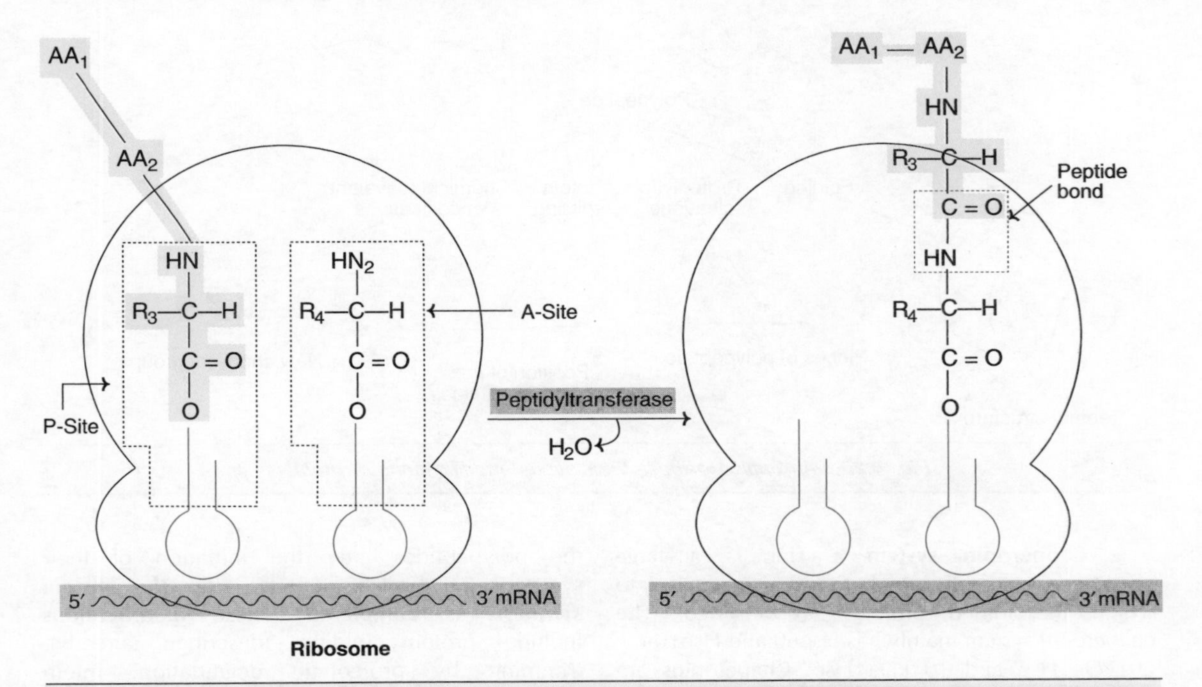

Fig. 4.19 : Formation of peptide bond in translation (P–site — Peptidyl tRNA site; A–site — Aminoacyl tRNA site).

Tetracycline : It inhibits the binding of aminoacyl tRNA to the ribosomal complex. In fact, tetracycline can also block eukaryotic protein synthesis. This, however, does not happen since eukaryotic cell membrane is not permeable to this drug.

Puromycin : This has a structural resemblance to aminoacyl tRNA. Puromycin enters the A site and gets incorporated into the growing peptide chain and causes its release. This antibiotic prevents protein synthesis in both prokaryotes and eukaryotes.

Chloramphenicol : It acts as a competitive inhibitor of the enzyme peptidyltransferase and thus interferes with elongation of peptide chain.

Erythromycin : It inhibits translocation by binding with 50S subunit of bacterial ribosome.

Diphtheria toxin : It prevents translocation in eukaryotic protein synthesis by inactivating elongation factor eEF_2.

IV CHAPERONES AND PROTEIN FOLDING

The three dimensional conformation of proteins is important for their biological functions. Some of the proteins can spontaneously generate the correct functionally active conformation e.g. danatured pancreatic ribonuclease. However, a vast majority of proteins can attain correct conformation, only through the assistance of certain proteins referred to as chaperones. Chaperones are ***heat shock proteins*** (originally discovered in response to heat shock). They facilitate and favour the interactions on the polypeptide surfaces to finally give the ***specific conformation of a protein***. Chaperones can reversibly bind to hydrophobic regions of unfolded proteins and folding intermediates. They can stabilize intermediates, prevent formation of incorrect intermediates, and also prevent undesirable interactions with other proteins. All these activities of chaperones help the protein to attain compact and biologically active conformation.

Types of chaperones

Chaperones are categorized into two major groups

1. **Hsp70 system :** This mainly consists of Hsp70 (70-kDa ***h***eat ***s***hock ***p***rotein) and Hsp40 (40-kDa Hsp). These proteins can bind individually to the substrate (protein) and help in the correct formation of protein folding.

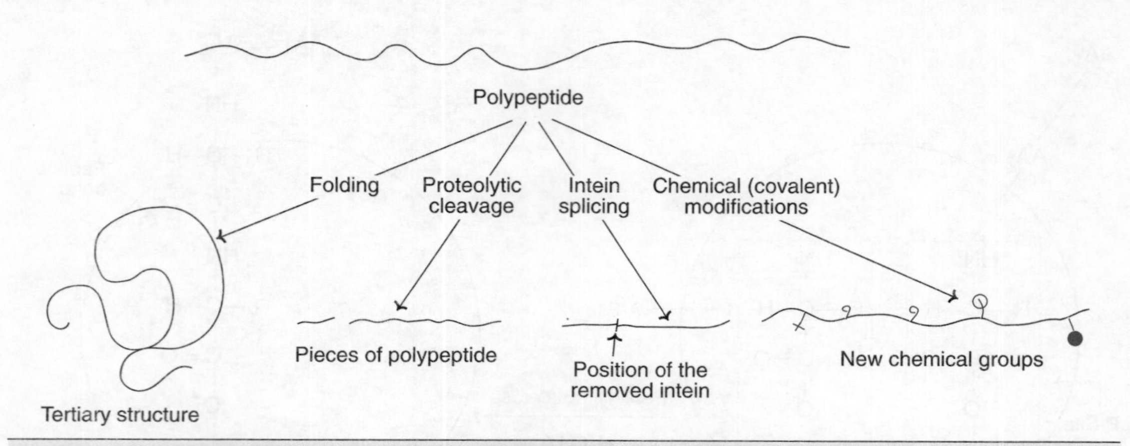

Fig. 4.20 : An outline of post–translational modifications of proteins.

2. **Chaperonin system :** This is a large oligomeric assembly which forms a structure into which the folded proteins are inserted. The chaperonin system mainly has Hsp60 and Hsp10 i.e. 60 kDa Hsp and 10 kDa Hsp. Chaperonins are required at a later part of the protein folding process, and often work in association with Hsp70 system.

Protein misfolding and diseases

The failure of a protein to fold properly generally leads to its rapid degradation. ***Cystic fibrosis*** (CF) is a common autosomal recessive disease. Some cases of CF with mutations that result in altered protein (cystic fibrosis transmembrane conductance regulator or in short CFTR) have been reported. Mutated CFTR cannot fold properly, besides not being able to get glycosylated or transported. Therefore, CFTR gets degraded.

Certain neurological diseases which are due to cellular accumulation of aggregates of misfolded proteins or their partially degraded products have been identified. The term ***prions*** (***pr***oteinous ***in***fectious agents) is used to collectively represent them.

Prions exhibit the characteristics of viral or microbial pathogens and have been implicated in many diseases. e.g. mad cow disease, Creutzfeldt-Jacob disease, Alzheimer's disease, Huntington's disease.

V. POST-TRANSLATIONAL MODIFICATIONS OF PROTEINS

The proteins synthesized in translation are, as such, not functional. Many changes take place in the polypeptides after the initiation of their synthesis or, most frequently, ***after the protein synthesis is completed***. These ***modifications*** include protein folding (described already), trimming by proteolytic degradation, intein splicing and covalent changes which are collectively known as post-translational modifications (***Fig. 4.20***).

Proteolytic degradation

Many proteins are synthesized as the precursors which are much bigger in size than the functional proteins. Some portions of precursor molecules are removed by proteolysis to liberate active proteins. This process—commonly referred to as trimming—may occur in Golgi apparatus, secretory vesicles and, sometimes, after the secretion of proteins. The formation of insulin from preproinsulin, conversion of ***zymogens*** (inactive digestive enzymes e.g. trypsinogen) to the active enzymes are some examples of trimming.

The synthesis of the proteins as inactive precursors and their later conversion into active form, may be, to protect the functional protein unit from the environmental insults.

Intein splicing

Inteins are ***intervening sequences in certain proteins***. These are comparable to introns in mRNAs. ***Inteins*** have to be ***removed***, ***and exteins ligated*** in the appropriate order for the protein to become active.

TABLE 4.2 Selected examples of post-translational modifications of proteins through their amino acids

Amino acid	*Post-translational modification(s)*
Amino-terminal amino acid	Glycosylation, acetylation, myristoylation, formylation.
Carboxy terminal amino acid	Methylation, ADP-ribosylation
Arginine	Methylation
Aspartic acid	Phosphorylation, hydroxylation
Cysteine (—SH)	Cystine (—S—S—) formation, selenocysteine formation, glycosylation.
Glutamic acid	Methylation, γ-carboxylation.
Histidine	Methylation, phosphorylation.
Lysine	Acetylation, methylation, hydroxylation, biotinylation.
Methionine	Sulfoxide formation.
Phenylalanine	Glycosylation, hydroxylation.
Proline	Hydroxylation, glycosylation.
Serine	Phosphorylation, glycosylation.
Threonine	Phosphorylation, methylation glycosylation.
Tryptophan	Hydroxylation.
Tyrosine	Hydroxylation, phosphorylation, sulfonylation, iodination.

Covalent modifications

The proteins synthesized in translation are subjected to many covalent changes. By these modifications in the amino acids, the proteins may be converted to active form or inactive form. Selected examples of covalent modifications are described below.

1. **Phosphorylation :** The hydroxyl group containing amino acids of proteins, namely serine, threonine and tyrosine are subjected to phosphorylation. The phosphorylation may either increase or decrease the activity of the proteins. A group of enzymes called ***protein kinases*** catalyse phosphorylation while protein phosphatases are responsible for dephosphorylation (removal of phosphate group). Many examples of enzymes that undergo phosphorylation or dephosphorylation are known in metabolisms.

2. **Hydroxylation :** During the formation of collagen, the amino acids proline and lysine are respectively converted to hydroxyproline and hydroxylysine. This hydroxylation occurs in the endoplasmic reticulum and requires vitamin C.

3. **Glycosylation :** The attachment of carbohydrate moiety is essential for some proteins to perform their functions. The complex carbohydrate moiety is attached to the amino acids, serine and threonine (O-linked) or to asparagine (N-linked), leading to the synthesis of glycoproteins.

Vitamin K dependent ***carboxylation*** of glutamic acid residues in certain clotting factors is also a post-translational modification.

In the ***Table 4.2***, selected examples of post-translational modification of proteins through their amino acids are given.

PROTEIN TRAGETING

The eukaryotic proteins (tens of thousands) are distributed between the cytosol, plasma membrane and a number of cellular organelles (nucleus, mitochondria, endoplasmic reticulum etc.). At the appropriate places, they perform their functions.

The proteins, synthesized in translation, have to ***reach*** their ***destination*** to exhibit their biological activity. This is carried out by a process called protein targeting or ***protein sorting*** or ***protein localization***. The proteins move from one compartment to another by multiple mechanisms.

The protein transport from the endoplasmic reticulum through the Golgi apparatus, and beyond uses carrier vesicles. It may be, however, noted that only the ***correctly folded proteins*** are recognized as the ***cargo for transport***. Protein targeting and post-translational modifications occur in a coordinated manner.

Certain glycoproteins are targeted to reach lysosomes, as the lysosomal proteins can recognize the glycosidic compounds e.g. N-acetyl-glucosamine phosphate.

For the transport of secretory proteins, a special mechanism is operative. A ***signal peptide*** containing 15–35 amino acids, located at the amino terminal end of the secretory proteins facilitates the transport.

Protein targeting to mitochondria

Most of the proteins of mitochondria are synthesized in the cytosol, and their transport to mitochondria is a complex process. Majority of the proteins are synthesized as larger preproteins with N-terminal presequences for the entry of these proteins into mitochondria. The transport of unfolded proteins is often facilitated by chaperones.

One protein namely ***mitochondrial matrix targeting signal***, involved in protein targeting has been identified. This protein can recognize mitochondrial receptor and transport certain proteins from cytosol to mitochondria. This is an energy-dependent process.

Protein targeting to other organelles

Specific signals for the transport of proteins to organelles such as nuclei and peroxisomes have been identified.

The smaller proteins can easily pass through nuclear pores. However, for larger proteins, ***nuclear localization*** *signals* are needed to facilitate their entry into nucleus.

MITOCHONDRIAL DNA, TRANSCRIPTION AND TRANSLATION

The mitochondrial DNA (mtDNA) has structural and functional resemblances with prokaryotic DNA. This fact supports the view that mitochondria are derivatives of prokaryotes. mtDNA is circular in nature and contains about 16,000 nucleotide bases.

A vast majority of structural and functional proteins of the mitochondria are synthesized in the cytosol, under the influence of nuclear DNA. However, certain proteins (around 13), most of them being the components of electron transport chain, are synthesized in the mitochondria. Transcription takes place in the mitochondria leading to the synthesis of mRNAs, tRNAs and rRNAs. Two types of rRNA and about 22 species of tRNA have been so far identified. This is followed by translation resulting in protein synthesis.

The mitochondria of the sperm cell do not enter the ovum during fertilization, therefore, ***mtDNA is inherited from the mother.*** Mitochondrial DNA is subjected to high rate of mutations (about 10 times more than nuclear DNA) that causes inherited defects in oxidative phosphorylation. The best known among them are certain mitochondrial myopathies and Leber's hereditary optic neuropathy. The latter is mostly found in males and is characterized by blindness due to loss of central vision as a result of neuroretinal degeneration. ***Leber's hereditary optic neuropathy*** is a consequence of single base mutation in mtDNA. Due to this, the amino acid histidine, in place of arginine, is incorporated into the enzyme NADH coenzyme Q reductase.

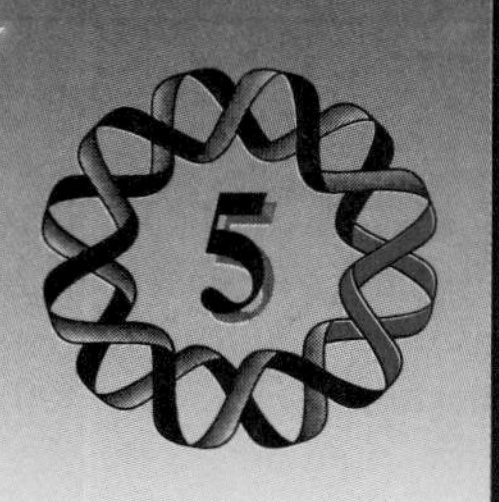

Regulation of Gene Expression

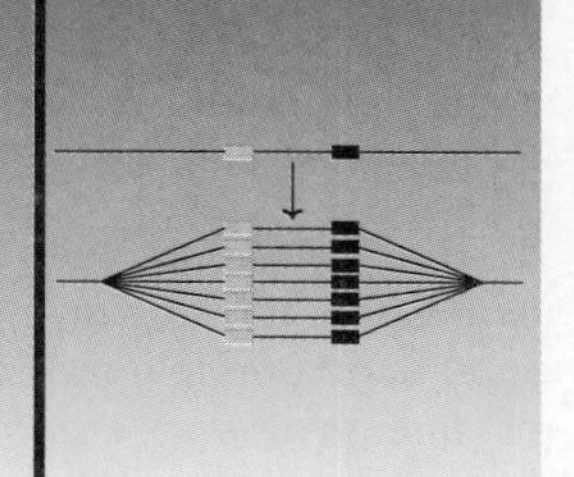

DNA, the chemical vehicle of heredity, is composed of ***functional units***, namely ***genes***. The term ***genome*** refers to the total genetic information contained in a cell. The bacterium *Escherichia coli* contains about 4,400 genes present on a single chromosome. The ***genome of humans*** is more complex, with 23 pairs of (diploid) chromosomes containing 6 billion (6×10^9) base pairs of DNA, with an estimated ***30,000–40,000 genes***. At any given time, only a fraction of the genome is expressed.

The living cells possess a remarkable property to adapt to changes in the environment by regulating the gene expression. For instance, insulin is synthesized by specialized cells of pancreas and not by cells of other organs (say kidney, liver), although the nuclei of all the cells of the body contain the insulin genes. Molecular regulatory mechanisms facilitate the expression of insulin gene in pancreas, while preventing its expression in other cells.

GENE REGULATION—GENERAL

The ***regulation of the expression of genes*** is absolutely ***essential for the growth, development, differentiation*** and the very existence of an organism. There are two types of gene regulation-positive and negative.

1. **Positive regulation :** The gene regulation is said to be positive when its expression is increased by a regulatory element (positive regulator).

2. **Negative regulation :** A decrease in the gene expression due to the presence of a regulatory element (negative regulator) is referred to as negative regulation.

It may be noted here that double negative effect on gene regulation results in a positive phenomenon.

Constitutive and inducible genes

The genes are generally considered under two categories.

1. **Constitutive genes :** The products (proteins) of these genes are required all the time in a cell. Therefore, the constitutive genes (or housekeeping genes) are expressed at more or less constant rate in almost all the cells and, further, they are not subjected to regulation e.g. the enzymes of citric acid cycle.

2. **Inducible genes :** The concentration of the proteins synthesized by inducible genes is regulated by various molecular signals. An inducer increases the expression of these genes while a repressor decreases, e.g. tryptophan pyrrolase of liver is induced by tryptophan.

One cistron-one subunit concept

The chemical product of a gene expression is a protein which may be an enzyme. It was originally believed that each gene codes for a specific enzyme, leading to the popular concept, one gene-one enzyme. This however, is not necessarily valid due to the fact that several enzymes (or proteins) are composed of two or more nonidentical subunits (polypeptide chains).

The cistron is the smallest unit of genetic expression. It is the fragment of DNA coding for the subunit of a protein molecule. The original concept of ***one gene-one enzyme is replaced by one cistron-one subunit.***

Models for the study of gene expression

Elucidation of the regulation of gene expression in prokaryotes has largely helped to understand the principles of the flow of information from genes to mRNA to synthesize specific proteins. Some important features of prokaryotic gene expression are described first. This is followed by a brief account of eukaryotic gene expression.

THE OPERON CONCEPT

The operon is the coordinated unit of genetic expression in bacteria. The concept of operon was introduced by Jacob and Monod in 1961 (Nobel Prize 1965), based on their observations on the regulation of lactose metabolism in *E. coli*. This is popularly known as ***lac operon***.

LACTOSE (LAC) OPERON

Structure of lac operon

The lac operon (***Fig. 5.1***) consists of a regulatory gene (I; I for inhibition), operator gene (O) and three structural genes (Z, Y, A). Besides these genes, there is a promoter site (P), next to the operator gene, where the enzyme RNA polymerase binds. The structural genes Z, Y and A respectively, code for the enzymes β-galactosidase, galactoside permease and galactoside acetylase. β-Galactosidase hydrolyses lactose (β-galactoside) to galactose and glucose while permease is responsible for the transport of lactose into the cell. The function of acetylase (coded by A gene) remains a mystery.

The structural genes Z, Y and A transcribe into a single large mRNA with 3 independent translation units for the synthesis of 3 distinct enzymes. An mRNA coding for more than one protein is known as ***polycistronic mRNA***. Prokaryotic organisms contain a large number of polycistronic mRNAs.

Repression of lac operon

The regulatory gene (I) is constitutive. It is expressed at a constant rate leading to the synthesis of lac repressor. Lac repressor is a tetrameric (4 subunits) regulatory protein (total mol. wt. 150,000) which specifically binds to the operator gene (O). This prevents the binding of the enzyme RNA polymerase to the promoter site (P), thereby blocking the transcription of structural genes (Z, Y and A). This is what happens in the absence of lactose in *E. coli*. The ***repressor molecule acts as a negative regulator of gene expression***.

Derepression of lac operon

In the presence of lactose (inducer) in the medium, a small amount of it can enter the *E. coli* cells. The repressor molecules have a high affinity for lactose. The lactose molecules bind and induce a conformational change in the repressor. The result is that the repressor gets inactivated and, therefore, cannot bind to the operator gene (O). The RNA polymerase attaches to the DNA at the promoter site and transcription proceeds, leading to the formation of polycistronic mRNA (for genes Z, Y and A) and, finally, the 3 enzymes. Thus, lactose induces the synthesis of the three enzymes β-galactosidase, galactoside permease and galactoside acetylase. ***Lactose acts by inactivating the repressor molecules***, hence this process is known as derepression of lac operon.

Gratuitous inducers : There are certain structural analogs of lactose which can induce the lac operon but are not the substrates for the enzyme β-galactosidase. Such substances are known as gratuitous inducers. Isopropylthiogalactoside (IPTG) is a gratuitous inducer, extensively used for the study of lac operon.

The catabolite gene activator protein : The cells of *E. coli* utilize glucose in preference to lactose; when both of them are present in the medium. After the depletion of glucose in the medium, utilization of lactose starts. This indicates that glucose somehow interferes with the induction of lac operon. This is explained as follows.

The attachment of RNA polymerase to the promoter site requires the presence of a ***catabolite gene activator protein (CAP)*** bound to cyclic AMP (***Fig. 5.2***). The presence of glucose lowers the intracellular concentration of cAMP by inactivating

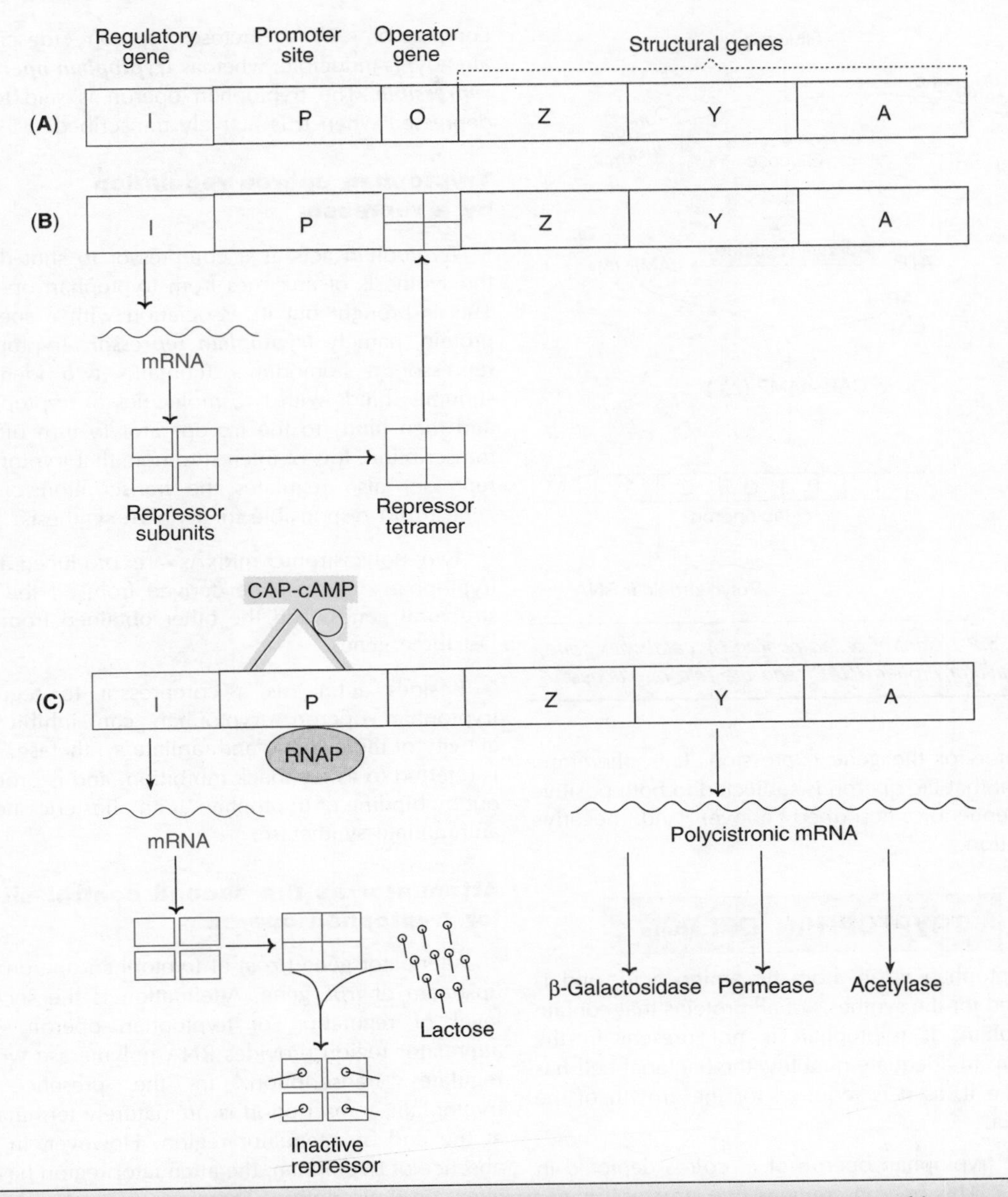

Fig. 5.1 : Model of lactose operon in E.coli *(A) Structure of lac operon (B) Repression of lac operon (C) Derepression of lac operon. (CAP—cAMP—catabolite gene activator protein bound to cAMP; RNAP—RNA polymerase).*

the enzyme adenylyl cyclase responsible for the synthesis of cAMP. Due to the diminished levels of cAMP, the formation of CAP-cAMP is low. Therefore, the binding of RNA polymerase to DNA (due to the absence of CAP-cAMP) and the transcription is almost negligible in the presence of glucose. Thus, glucose interferes with the expression of lac operon by depleting cAMP levels. Addition of exogenous cAMP is found to initiate the transcription of many inducible operons, including lac operon.

It is now clear that the presence of CAP-cAMP is essential for the transcription of structural genes of lac operon. Thus, CAP-cAMP acts as a positive

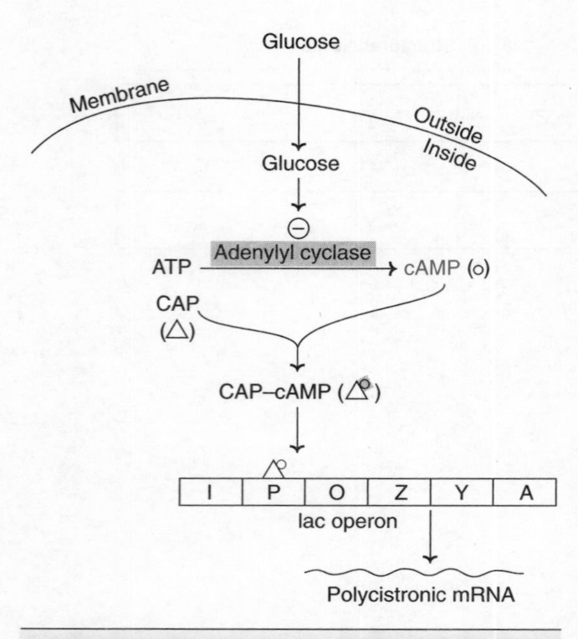

Fig. 5.2 : Control of lac operon by catabolite gene activator protein (CAP) and the role of glucose.

regulator for the gene expression. It is, therefore, evident that lac operon is subjected to both positive (by repressor, described above) and negative regulation.

TRYPTOPHAN OPERON

Tryptophan is an aromatic amino acid, and is required for the synthesis of all proteins that contain tryptophan. If tryptophan is not present in the medium in adequate quantity, the bacterial cell has to make it, as it is required for the growth of the bacteria.

The tryptophan operon of *E. coli* is depicted in ***Fig. 5.3***. This operon contains five structural genes (*trpE, trpD, trpC, trpB, trpA*), and the regulatory elements—primary promoter (*trpP*), operator (*trpO*), attenuator (*trpa*), secondary internal promoter ($TrpP_2$), and terminator (*trpt*).

The five structural genes of tryptophan operon code for three enzymes (two enzymes contain two different subunits) required for the synthesis of tryptophan from chlorismate.

The tryptophan repressor is always turned on, unless it is repressed by a specific molecule called corepressor. Thus lactose operon (described already) is inducible, whereas ***tryptophan operon is repressible***. The tryptophan operon is said to be depressed when it is actively transcribed.

Tryptophan operon regulation by a repressor

Tryptophan acts as a corepressor to shut down the synthesis of enzymes from tryptophan operon. This is brought out in association with a specific protein, namely ***tryptophan repressor***. Tryptophan repressor, a homodimer (contains two identical subunits) binds with two molecules of tryptophan, and then binds to the *trp* operator to turn off the transcription. It is of interest to note that tryptophan repressor also regulates the transcription of the gene (*trpR*) responsible for its own synthesis.

Two polycistronic mRNAs are produced from tryptophan operon—one derived from all the five structural genes, and the other obtained from the last three genes.

Besides acting as a corepressor to regulate tryptophan operon, tryptophan can inhibit the activity of the enzyme anthranilate synthetase. This is referred to as feedback inhibition, and is brought out by binding of tryptophan at an allosteric site on anthranilate synthetase.

Attenuator as the second control site for tryptophan operon

Attenuator gene (*trpa*) of tryptophan operon lies upstream of *trpE* gene. Attenuation is the second level of regulation of tryptophan operon. The attenuator region provides RNA polymerase which regulates transcription. In the presence of tryptophan, transcription is prematurely terminated at the end of attenuator region. However, in the absence of tryptophan, the attenuator region has no effect on transcription. Therefore, the polycistronic mRNA of the five structural genes can be synthesized.

GENE EXPRESSION IN EUKARYOTES

Each cell of the higher organism contains the entire genome. As in prokaryotes, gene expression in eukaryotes is regulated to provide the

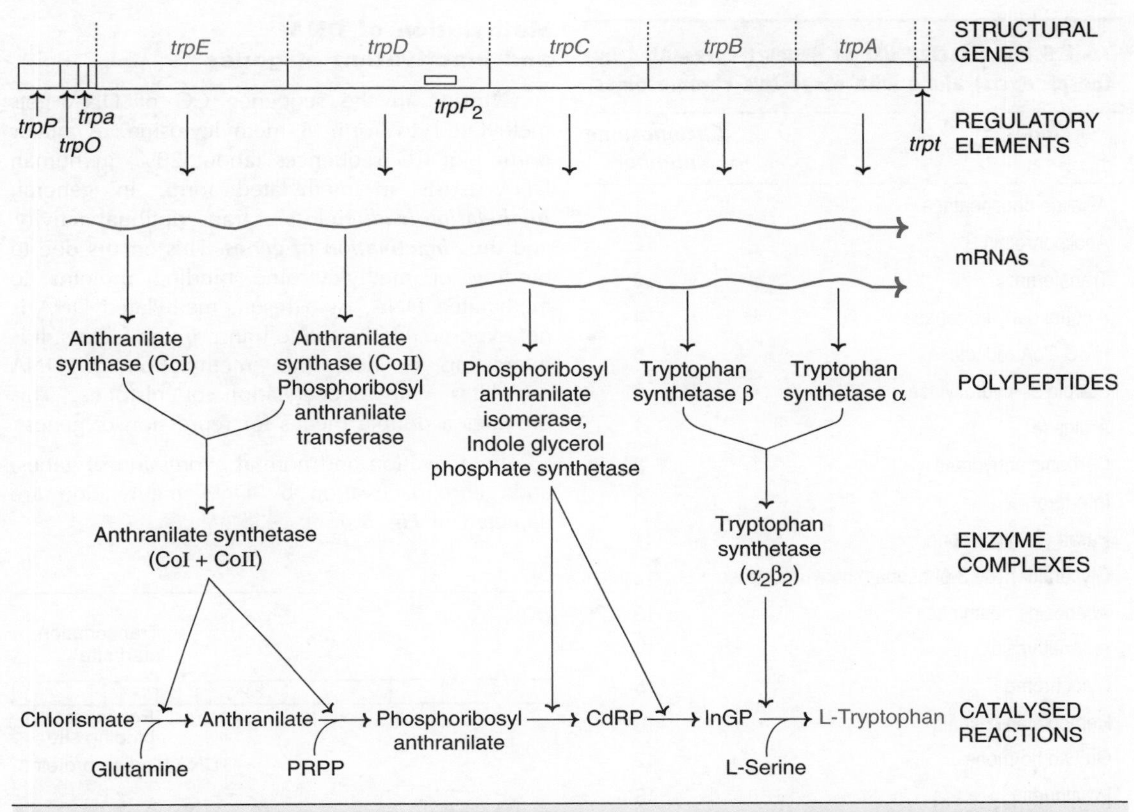

***Fig. 5.3 :** Tryptophan operon in* E.coli *[regulatory elements are promoter (trpP), operator (trpO), attenuator (trpa), secondary internal promoter (trpP$_2$) and terminator (trpt); CoI, CoII — Component I and component II; PRPP — 5-Phosphoribosyl 1-pyrophosphate; CdRP — Carboxyl-phenylamino 1 deoxyribulose 5-phosphate; InGP — Indole 3-glycerol phosphate].*

appropriate response to biological needs. This may occur in the following ways

- Expression of certain genes (housekeeping genes) in most of the cells.
- Activation of selected genes upon demand.
- Permanent inactivation of several genes in all but a few types.

In case of prokaryotic cells, most of the DNA is organized into genes which can be transcribed. In contrast, in mammals, ***very little of the total DNA is organized into genes*** and their associated regulatory sequences. The function of the bulk of the extra DNA is not known.

Eukaryotic gene expression and its regulation are highly complex. Some of the important aspects are briefly described.

CHROMATIN SRUCTURE AND GENE EXPRESSION

The DNA in higher organisms is extensively folded and packed to form ***protein-DNA complex*** called chromatin. The structural organization of DNA in the form of chromatin plays an important role in eukaryotic gene expression. In fact, chromatin structure provides an additional level of control of gene expression.

A selected list of genes (represented by the products) along with the respective chromosomes on which they are located is given in ***Table 5.1***.

In general, the genes that are transcribed within a particular cell are less condensed and more open in structure. This is in contrast to genes that are not transcribed which form highly condensed chromatin.

Table 5.1 A selected list of genes (represented by the products) along with respective chromosomes

Genes	*Chromosome number*
Alkaline phosphatase	1
Apolipoprotein B	2
Transferrin	3
Alcohol dehydrogenase	4
HMG CoA reductase	5
Steroid 21-hydroxylase	6
Arginase	7
Carbonic anhydrase	8
Interferon	9
Parathyroid hormone	11
Glyceraldehyde 3-phosphate dehydrogenase	12
Adenosine deaminase	13
α_1-Antitrypsin	14
Cytochrome P_{450}	15
Hemoglobin α-chain	16
Growth hormone	17
Prealbumin	18
Creatine phosphokinase (M chain)	19
Adenosine deaminase	20
Superoxide dismutase	21
Immunoglobulin (λ chain)	22
Glucose 6-phosphate dehydrogenase	X
Steroid sulfatase	Y

Histone acetylation and deacetylation

Eukaryotic DNA segments are wrapped around histone proteins to form nucleosome. Acetylation or deacetylation of histones is an ***important factor in determining the gene expression***. In general, acetylation of histones leads to activation of gene expression while deacetylation reverses the effect.

Acetylation predominantly occurs on the lysine residues in the amino terminal ends of histones. This modification in histones reduces the positive charges of terminal ends (tails), and decreases their binding affinity to negatively charged DNA. Consequently, nucleosome structure is disrupted to allow transcription.

Methylation of DNA and inactivation of genes

Cytosine in the sequence CG of DNA gets methylated to form 5′-methylcytosine. A major portion of CG sequences (about 20%) in human DNA exists in methylated form. In general, ***methylation leads to*** loss of transcriptional activity, and thus ***inactivation of genes***. This occurs due to binding of methylcytosine binding proteins to methylated DNA. As a result, methylated DNA is not exposed and bound to transcription factors. It is interesting to note that methylation of DNA correlates with deacetylation of histones. This provides a double means for repression of genes.

The activation and normal expression of genes, and gene inactivation by DNA methylation are depicted in ***Fig. 5.4***.

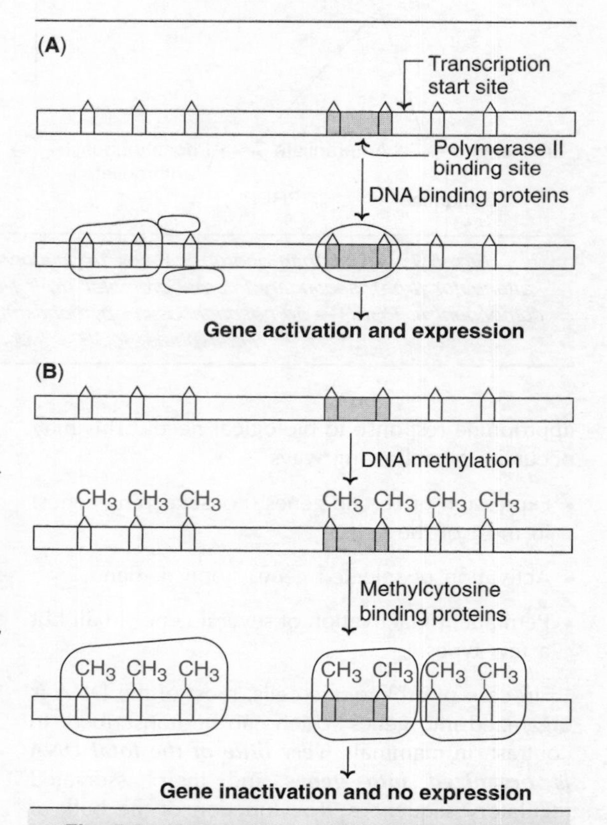

Fig. 5.4 : Methylation of DNA and inactivation of genes (A) Gene activation in the absence of DNA methylation (B) Gene inactivation due to methylation (⌂ represent CG sequences).

ENHANCERS AND TISSUE-SPECIFIC GENE EXPRESSION

Enhancers (or activators) are DNA elements that facilitate or ***enhance gene expression***. The enhancers provide binding sites for specific proteins that regulate transcription. They facilitate binding of the transcription complex to promoter regions. Enhancers differ from promoters in two distinct ways

1. Enhancers may be located thousands of base pairs away from the start of transcription site (promoters are close to the site of transcription).

2. They can work in either orientation i.e. enhancers can work upstream (5′) or downstream (3′) from the promoter.

Several eukaryotic genes containing enhancer elements at various locations relative to their coding regions have been identified.

Some of the enhancers possess the ability to promote transcription in a tissue-specific manner. For instance, gene expression in lymphoid cells for the production immunoglobulins (Ig) is promoted by the enhancer associated with Ig genes between J and C regions.

Transgenic animals are frequently used for the study of tissue-specific expression. The available evidence from various studies indicates that the ***tissue-specific gene expression is largely mediated through the involvement of enhancers***.

COMBINATION OF DNA ELEMENTS AND PROTEINS IN GENE EXPRESSION

Gene expression in mammals is a complicated process with several environmental stimuli on a single gene. The ultimate response of the gene which may be positive or negative is brought out by the association of DNA elements and proteins.

In the illustration given in the ***Fig. 5.5***, gene I is activated by a combination of activators 1, 2 and 3. Gene II is more effectively activated by the combined action of 1, 3 and 4. Activator 4 is not in direct contact with DNA, but it forms a bridge between activators 1 and 3, and activates gene II. As regards gene III, it gets inactivated by a combination of 1, 5 and 3. In this case, protein 5 interferes with the binding of protein 2 with the DNA and inactivates the gene.

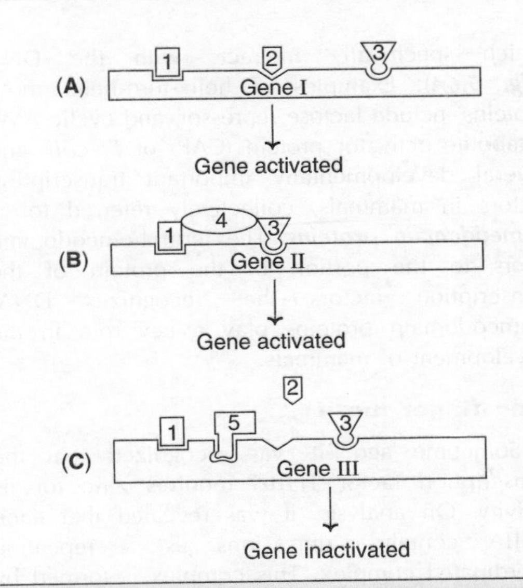

***Fig. 5.5 :** A diagrammatic representation of the association of DNA elements and proteins in gene regulation.* **A**, **B** *and* **C** *represent genes I, II and III (1...5 represent proteins).*

MOTIFS IN PROTEINS AND GENE EXPRESSION

A motif literally means a dominant element. Certain motifs in proteins mediate the binding of regulatory proteins (transcription factors) to DNA. The specific control of transcription occurs by the binding of regulatory proteins with high affinity to the correct regions of DNA.

A great majority of specific ***protein-DNA interactions*** are brought out by four unique motifs.

- Helix-turn-helix (HTH)
- Zinc finger
- Leucine zipper
- Helix-loop-helix (HLH).

The above listed ***amino acid motifs*** bind with high affinity to the specific site and low affinity to other parts of DNA. The motif-DNA interactions are maintained by hydrogen bonds and van der Waals forces.

Helix-turn-helix motif

The helix-turn-helix (***HTS***) motif is about 20 amino acids which represents a small part of a large protein. HTS is the domain part of the protein which specifically interacts with the DNA (***Fig. 5.6A***). Examples of helix-turn-helix motif proteins include lactose repressor, and cyclic AMP catabolite activator protein (CAP) of *E. coli*, and several developmentally important transcription factors in mammals, collectively referred to as ***homeodomain proteins***. The term homeodomain refers to the portion of the protein of the transcription factors that recognizes DNA. Homeodomain proteins play a key role in the development of mammals.

Zinc finger motif

Sometime ago, it was recognized that the transcription factor TFIIIA requires zinc for its activity. On analysis, it was revealed that each TFIIIA contains zinc ions as a repeating coordinated complex. This complex is formed by the closely spaced amino acids cysteine and cysteine, followed by a histidine—histidine pair. In some instances, His-His is replaced by a second Cys-Cys pair (***Fig. 5.6B***).

The zinc fingers bind to the major groove of DNA, and lie on the face of the DNA. This binding makes a contact with 5 bp of DNA. The ***steroid hormone receptor transcription factors*** use zinc finger motifs to bind to DNA.

The occurrence of a mutation resulting in a single amino acid change of zinc finger may lead to resistance to the action of certain hormones on gene expression. A mutated zinc finger resistant to the action of calcitriol (active form of vitamin D) has been identified. This may ultimately result in rickets (vitamin D deficiency).

Leucine zipper motif

The ***b***asic regions of leucine ***zip***per (bZIP) proteins are rich is the amino acid leucine. There occurs a periodic repeat of leucine residues at every seventh position. This type of repeat structure allows two identical monomers or heterodimers to ***zip together*** and form a dimeric complex. This protein-protein complex associates and interacts with DNA (***Fig. 5.6C***). Good examples of leucine zipper proteins are the enhancer binding proteins (EBP)—fos and jun.

Helix-loop-helix motif

Two amphipathic (literally means a feeling of closeness) α-helical segments of proteins can form helix-loop-helix motif and bind to DNA. The

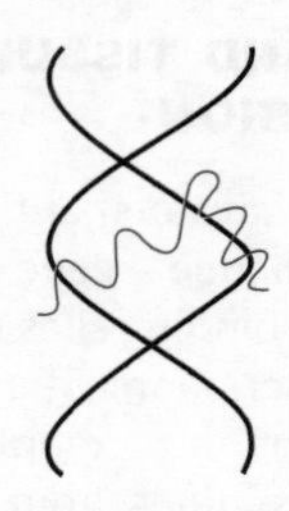

(A) Helix-turn-helix

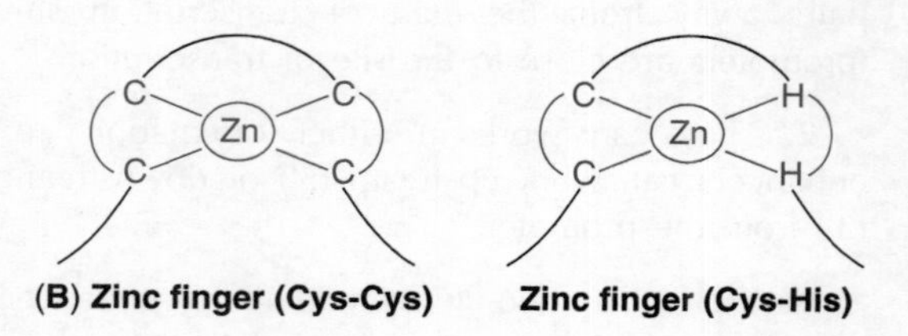

(B) Zinc finger (Cys-Cys) Zinc finger (Cys-His)

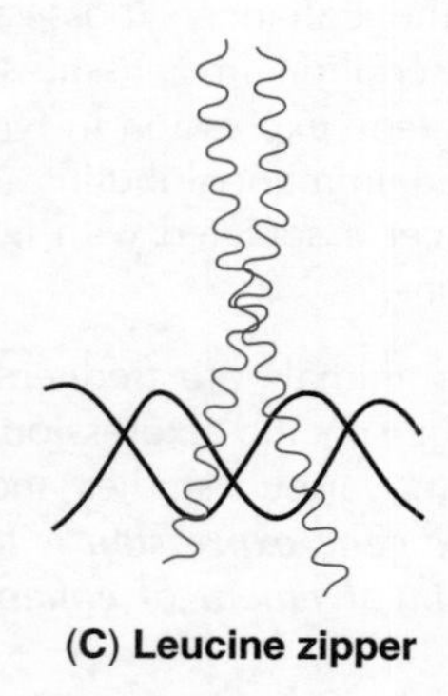

(C) Leucine zipper

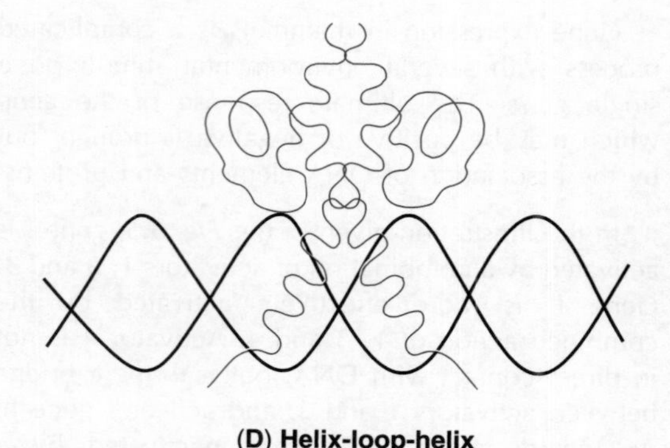

(D) Helix-loop-helix

Fig. 5.6 : Diagrammatic representation of common motifs in proteins interacting with DNA.

dimeric form of the protein actually binds to DNA (***Fig. 5.6D***).

GENE REGULATION IN EUKARYOTES

The important features of eukaryotic gene expression along with the regulatory aspects are described in the preceeding pages. Besides transcription, eukaryotic cells also employ variety of other mechanisms to regulate gene expression. The most important ones are listed below, and briefly described next.

1. Gene amplification
2. Gene rearrangement
3. Processing of RNA
4. Alternate mRNA splicing
5. Transport of mRNA from nucleus to cytoplasm
6. Degradation of mRNA.

Gene amplification

In this mechanism, the expression of a gene is increased several fold. This is commonly observed during the developmental stages of eukaryotic organisms. For instance, in fruit fly (*Drosophila*), the amplification of genes coding for egg shell proteins is observed during the course of oogenesis. The amplification of the gene (DNA) can be observed under electron microscope (***Fig. 5.7***).

The occurrence of gene amplification has also been reported in humans. Methotrexate is an anticancer drug which inhibits the enzyme dihydrofolate reductase. The malignant cells develop drug resistance to long term administration of methotrexate by amplifying the genes coding for dihydrofolate reductase.

Gene rearrangment

The body possesses an enormous capacity to synthesize a wide range of antibodies. It is estimated that the human body can produce about 10 billion (10^{10}) antibodies in response to antigen stimulations. The molecular mechanism of this antibody diversity was not understood for long. It is now explained on the basis of gene rearrangement or ***transposition of genes*** or ***somatic recombination of DNA***.

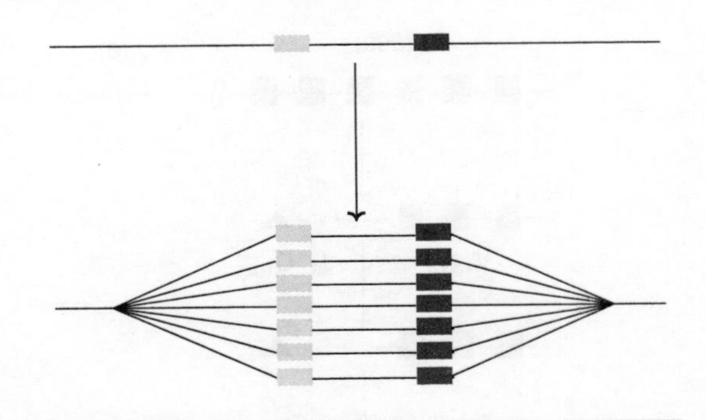

Fig. 5.7 : Diagrammatic representation of gene amplification (the genes are depicted in colour shade and colour).

The structure of a typical immunoglobulin molecule consists of two light (L) and two heavy (H) chains. Each one of these chains (L or H) contains an N-terminal variable (V) and C-terminal constant (C) regions. The V regions of immunoglobulins are responsible for the recognition of antigens. The phenomenon of gene rearrangement can be understood from the mechanism of the synthesis of light chains of immunoglobulins (***Fig. 5.8***).

Each light chain can be synthesized by three distinct DNA segments, namely the variable (V_L), the joining (J_L) and the constant (C_L). The mammalian genome contains about 500 V_L segments, 6 J_L segments and 20 C_L segments. During the course of differentiation of B-lymphocytes, one V_L segment (out of the 500) is brought closer to J_L and C_L segments. This occurs on the same chromosome. For the sake of illustration, 100th V_L, 3rd J_L and 10th C_L segments are rearranged in ***Fig. 5.8***. The rearranged DNA (with V_L, J_L and C_L fragments) is then transcribed to produce a single mRNA for the synthesis of a specific light chain of the antibody. By innumerable combinations of V_L, J_L and C_L segments, the body's immune system can generate millions of antigen specific immunoglobulin molecules.

The formation of heavy (H) chains of immunoglobulins also occurs by rearrangement of 4 distinct genes—variable (V_H), diversity (D), joining (J_H) and constant (C_H).

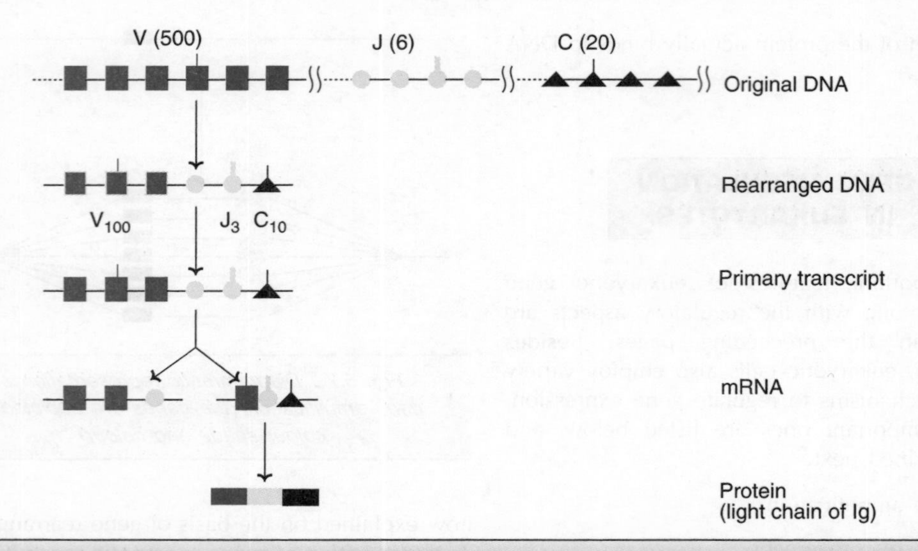

Fig. 5.8 : Diagrammatic representation of gene rearrangement for the synthesis of light chain of immunoglobulin.

Processing of RNA

The RNA synthesized in transcription undergoes modifications resulting in a functional RNA. The changes include intron-exon splicing, polyadenylation etc. (Chapter 4).

Alternate mRNA splicing

Eukaryotic cells are capable of carrying out alternate mRNA processing to control gene expression. Different mRNAs can be produced by alternate splicing which code for different proteins (for more details, Refer Chapter 4).

Degradation of mRNA

The expression of genes is indirectly influenced by the stability of mRNA. Certain hormones regulate the synthesis and degradation of some mRNAs. For instance, estradiol prolongs the half-life of vitellogenin mRNA from a few hours to about 200 hours.

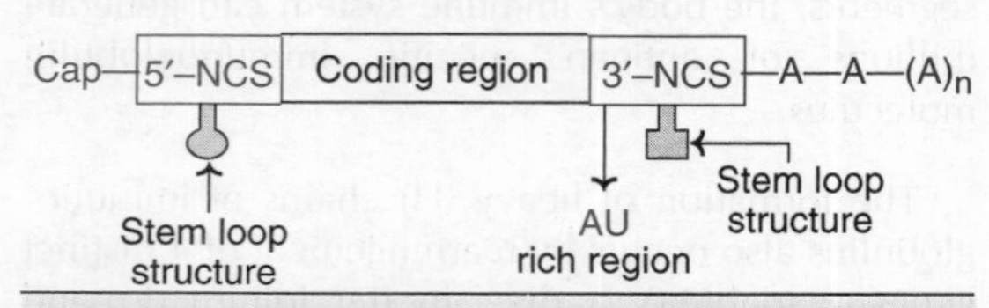

Fig. 5.9 : A diagrammatic representation of a typical eukaryotic mRNA. (NCS-Non-coding sequences)

It appears that the ends of mRNA molecules determine the stability of mRNA. A typical eukaryotic mRNA has 5′-non-coding sequences (5′-NCS), a coding region and a 3′-NCS. All the mRNAs are capped at the 5′ end, and most of them have a polyadenylate sequence at the 3′ end (***Fig. 5.9***). The 5′ cap and poly (A) tail protect the mRNA against the attack by exonuclease. Further, stem-loop structures in NCS regions, and AU rich regions in the 3′ NCS also provide stability to mRNA.

METHODS TO STUDY GENE EXPRESSION/REGULATION

Gene expression or gene regulation is usually studied at the transcriptional level, i.e. production of mRNA from the gene. The methods to elucidate gene expression are designed to provide information on one or more of the following

- Sequence of the gene
- Size of the transcript (mRNA)
- Starting and finishing points of genes to produce the transcript.
- Number and position of introns on the genes.
- The activity of the promoter.

Some of the important and general methods employed to study the gene regulation are briefly described.

Southern blot

Southern blot is a novel technique to detect a known fragment of DNA in the DNA preparation of an organism. This technique is particularly useful to detect the presence of a foreign DNA in the genetically modified organisms or to identify the presence and copy number of genes in an organism's genome. The details on this technique are given elsewhere (Chapter 7).

Northern blot

Northern blot specifically detects the size and sequence of the mRNA. The total mRNA is extracted from a cell or tissue suspension, and separated by agarose gel electrophoresis and then detected by hybridization (Refer Chapter 7).

Nuclease SI mapping

Nuclease SI is an enzyme that can specifically degrade single-stranded nucleic acids. Nuclease SI mapping is used *to* ***determine the number of introns*** present in a gene (***Fig. 5.10***).

The mature mRNA is hybridized with its corresponding gene (i.e. genomic DNA). The portion of the intron on the gene which is not transcribed is looped out. This looped-out intron can be specifically digested by nuclease SI, which degrades the single-stranded DNA. The number and presence of introns can be identified by analysing the fragmented DNAs.

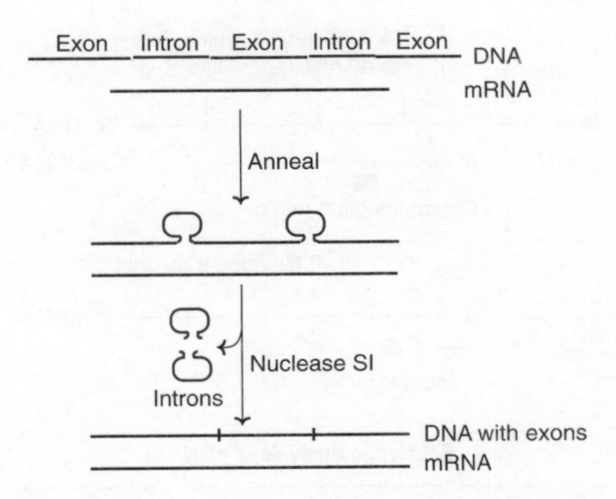

Fig. 5.10 : *A diagrammatic representation of mapping of introns by nuclease SI digestion.*

Nuclease protection assay

In nuclease protection assay, the test transcript (mRNA) is hybridized with excess quantities of *in vitro* synthesized and radioactively labeled DNA molecules (usually obtained from cloned genes). The annealed hybrids which are labeled, are subjected to digestion by nuclease SI which degrades single-stranded nucleic acids. The nuclease-treated and untreated hybridized molecules are separated by agar gel electrophoresis and identified (***Fig. 5.11***).

Nuclease protection assay is a variant of nuclease SI mapping and provides information as regards the presence of introns, transcriptional termini and the test transcript proper.

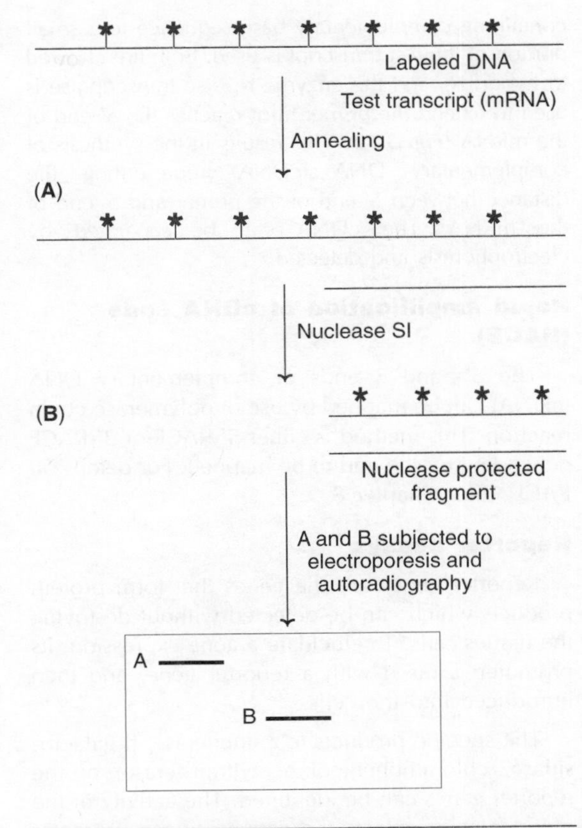

Fig. 5.11 : *A diagrammatic representation of nuclease protection assay **(A)** Hybridized DNA not treated with nuclease SI **(B)** Nuclease SI treated hybridized DNA.*

Primer extension

Primer extension method is a reliable technique to determine the 5′ end of the transcripts. For this purpose, a synthetic 5′-labeled oligonucleotide primer

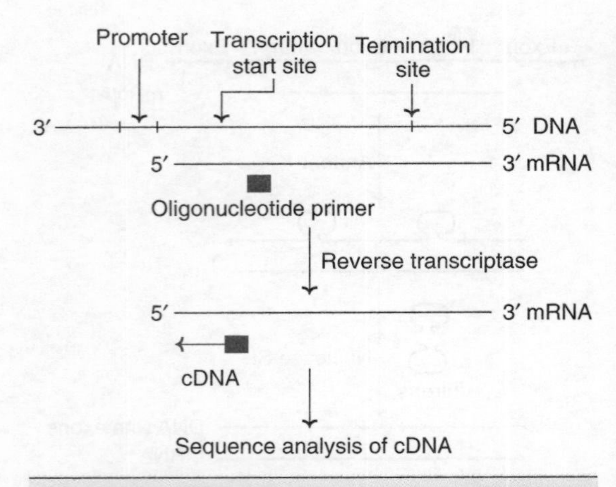

Fig. 5.12 : A diagrammatic representation of primer extension technique to detect the transcription start site.

containing complementary base sequence to a small portion of the test transcript is used. Both are allowed to hybridize, and the enzyme reverse transcriptase is used to extend the primer till it reaches the 5′ end of the mRNA (***Fig. 5.12***). This results in the synthesis of complementary DNA (cDNA) representing the distance between 5′-end of the primer and 5′-end of the mRNA. The cDNA can be separated by electrophoresis and detected.

Rapid amplification of cDNA ends (RACE)

The 5′- and 3′-ends of complementary DNA (cDNA) can be mapped by use of polymerase chain reaction. This method is either 5′-RACE or 3′-RACE depending on the end to be mapped. For details on RACE, refer Chapter 8.

Reporter assays

Reporter genes are the genes that form protein products which can be detected without destoying the tissues/cells. To elucidate a gene expression, its promoter is fused with a reporter gene, and then introduced into the cells.

The specific products (e.g. luciferase, β-galactosidase, chloramphenicol acetyltransferase) of the reporter genes can be identified. The activity of the reporter gene reflects the activity of the promoter gene, and consequently the gene expression.

Reporter assays are very useful for the study of gene expression *in vivo* in the tissues/cells.

GENE ANALYSIS BY T-DNA AND TRANSPOSON TAGGING

Gene tagging broadly involves the ***insertion of a recognizable DNA fragment within a gene*** so that the function of a gene is disrupted, and the gene is identified by virtue of the inserted DNA fragment.

T-DNA (transferred DNA) is the part of tumor-inducing plasmid (Ti plasmid) DNA found in the soil bacterium *Agrobacterium tumefaciens* (For details, Refer Chapter 49) Transposons or transposable elements are mobile genetic elements (DNA pieces) that can move from one place to another in a DNA molecule (Refer Chapter 3). Transposons or T-DNA can be used in gene tagging and gene analysis.

The transposon tagging of a gene is depicted in ***Fig. 5.13***. When a transposon in a plasmid is introduced into a cell, it gets incorporated into DNA, and the gene gets disrupted. Consequently, transposon insertion produces a mutant (A^-). This

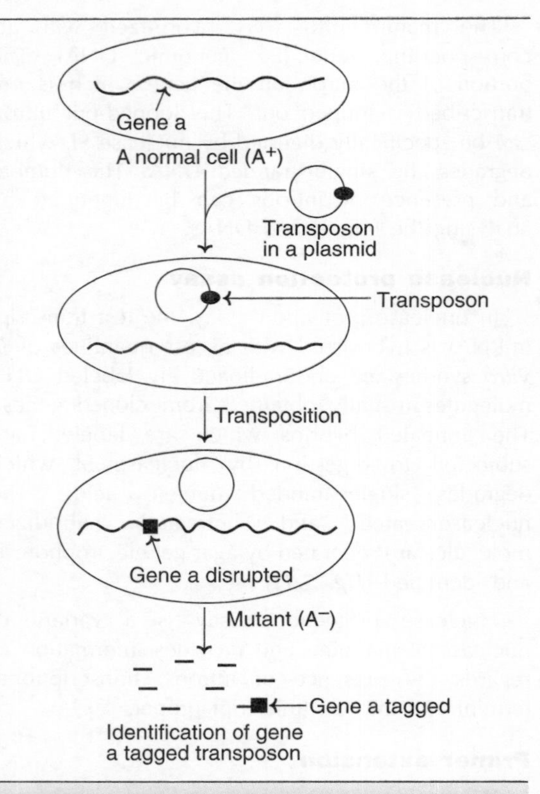

Fig. 5.13 : Transposon tagging of a gene in gene analysis.

mutant can be identified by its phenotype and a gene library. Further, the mutant can be screened for the presence of transposon. ***By identifying the location of insertion of transposon, the location of the specific gene can be identified.***

METHODS TO STUDY PROTEIN–PROTEIN INTERACTIONS

The operation of the genome can be evaluated by the study of proteome. Thus, by studying the functions of proteins, it is possible to understand how the genome operates and how a dysfunctional genome activity can result in disease states such as cancer.

Proteomics broadly involves the methodology for characterizing the protein content of the cell. This can be done by protein electrophoresis, mass spectrometry etc.

Identification of protein-protein interaction is a recent approach to study proteome. The ***protein interaction maps*** can be constructed to understand the relation between the proteome and cellular biochemistry. ***Phage display*** and ***yeast two-hybrid system are commonly used to study protein-protein interactions.***

PHAGE DISPLAY

Phage display is a novel technique to evaluate genome activity with particular reference to identify proteins that interact with one another. It basically involves insertion of a foreign DNA into phage genome, and its expression as fusion product with a phage coat protein (***Fig. 5.14A***). This is followed by screening of test protein by phage display library (***Fig. 5.14B***). The technique is briefly described below.

A special type of cloning vector such as a bacteriophage or filamentous bacteriophage (e.g. M13) are used for phage display. A fragment of DNA coding for the test protein is inserted into the vector DNA (adjacent to phage coat protein gene). After transformation of *E. coli,* this recombinant gene (fused frame of DNA) results in the synthesis of ***hybrid protein***. The new protein is made up of the test protein fused with the phage coat protein. The phage particles produced in the transformed *E. coli* display the test protein in their coats.

The test protein interaction can be identified by using a phage display library. For this purpose, the test protein is immobilized within a well of a

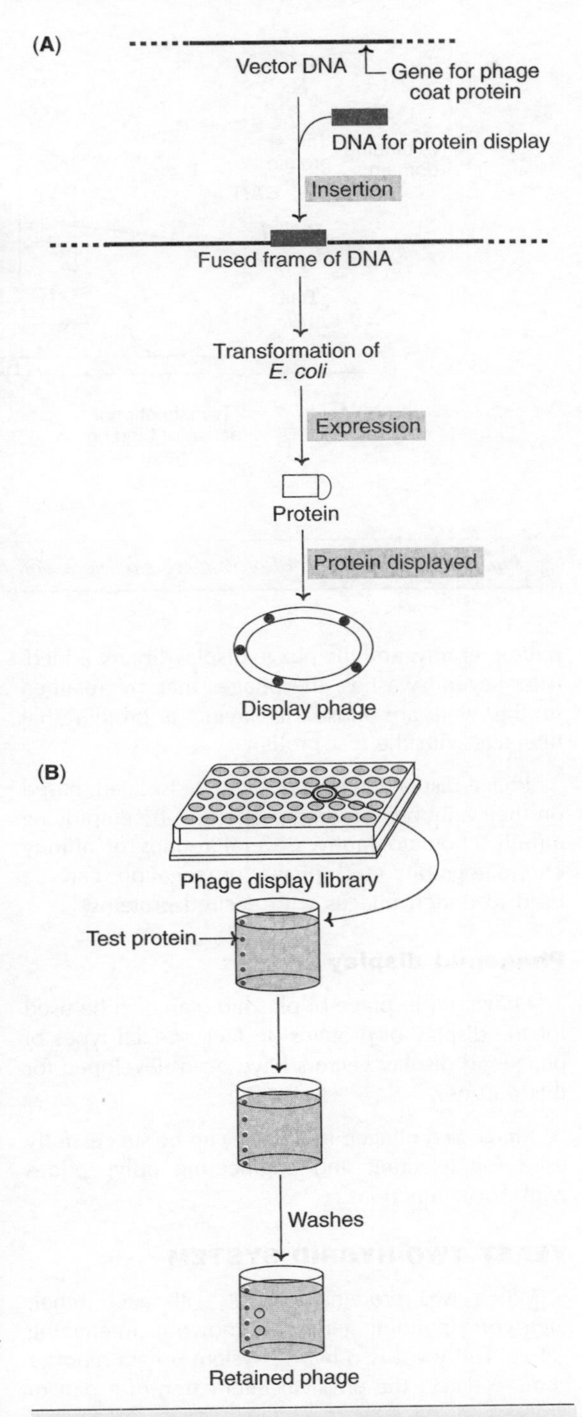

Fig. 5.14 : *Elucidation of protein–protein interaction by phage display **(A)** Production of fusion protein displayed on phage **(B)** Screening of test protein by phage display library.*

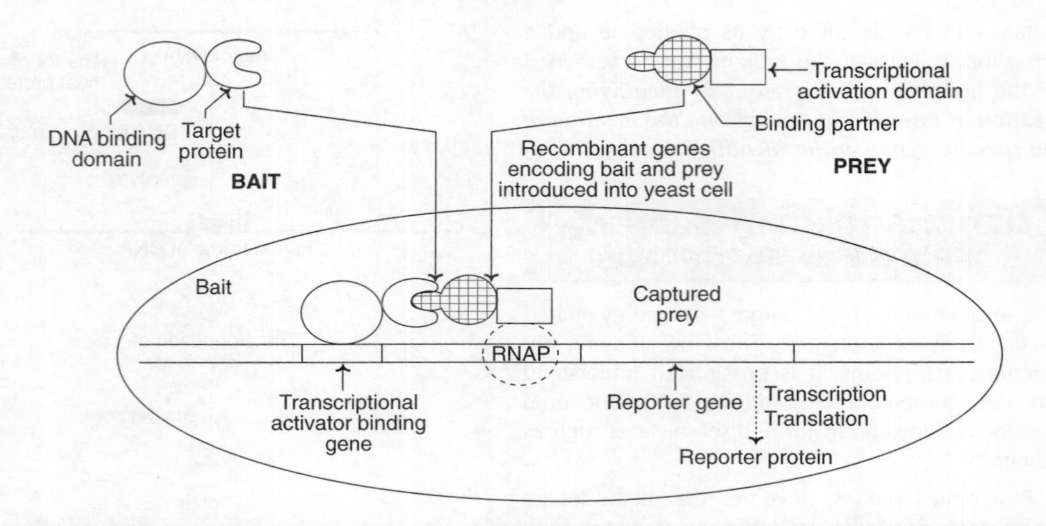

Fig. 5.15 : Elucidation of protein-protein interaction by yeast two-hybrid system (RNAP-RNA polymerase)

microtiter tray, and the phage display library added. After several washes, the phages that are retained in the well are those displaying a protein that interacts with the test protein.

Phage-displaying peptides can be isolated, based on their antibody-binding properties, by employing affinity chomatography. Several rounds of affinity chromatography and phage propagation can be used to enrich phages with desired proteins.

Phagemid display

Phagemid in place of plasmid, can also be used for the display of proteins. In fact, special types of phagemid display vectors have been developed for this purpose.

Phage and phagemid display can be successfully used for selecting and engineering polypeptides with novel functions.

YEAST TWO-HYBRID SYSTEM

When two proteins interact with each other, their corresponding genes are known as interacting genes. The yeast two-hybrid system uses a reporter gene to detect the physical interaction of a pair of proteins inside a yeast nucleus.

The two-hybrid method is based on the observation that most of the transcriptional proteins (i.e. the proteins involved in promoting transcription of a gene) contain two distinct domains — DNA binding domain and transcriptional activation domain. When these two domains are phyically separated, the protein loses its activity. However, the same protein can be reactivated when the domains are brought together. These proteins can bind to DNA and activate transcription.

The target protein is fused to a DNA-binding domain to form a ***bait***. When this target protein binds to another specifically designed protein namely the ***prey*** in the nucleus, they interact, which in turn switches on the expression of the reporter gene (***Fig. 5.15***). The reporter genes can be detected by growing the yeast on a selective medium.

It is possible to generate the bait and prey fusion proteins by standard recombinant DNA techniques. A single baid protein is frequently used to fish out interacting partners among the collection of prey proteins. A large number of prey proteins can be produced by ligating DNA encoding the activation domain of a transcriptional activator to a misture of DNA fragments from a cDNA library.

Yeast three-hybrid system

The interactions between protein and RNA molecules can be investigated by using a technique known as yeast three-hybrid system.

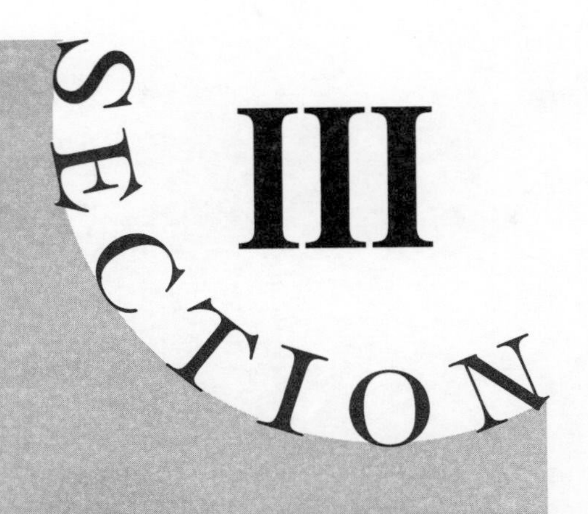

GENETIC ENGINEERING AND RECOMBINANT DNA TECHNOLOGY

CONTENTS

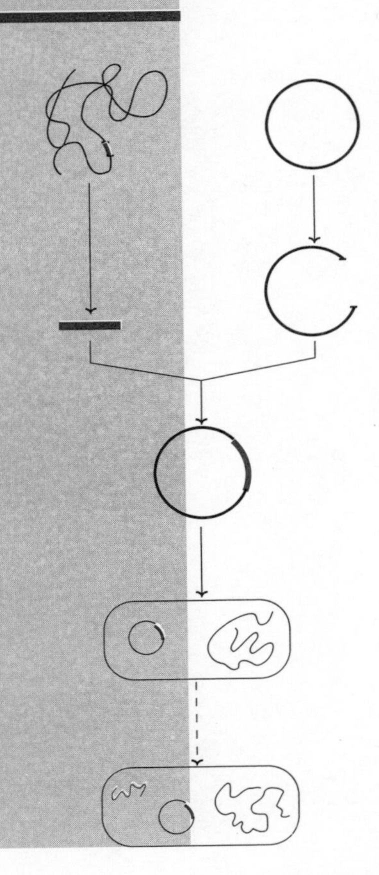

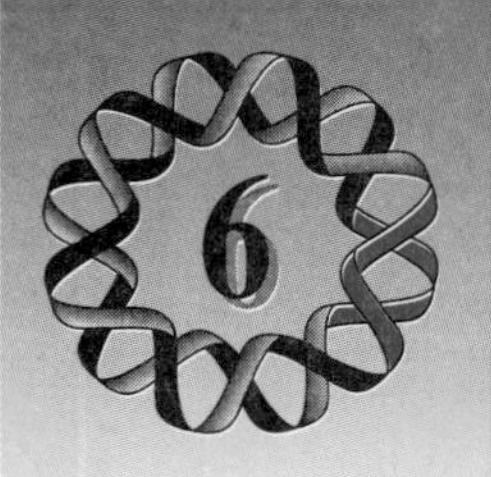

Introduction to Genetic Engineering

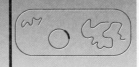

Genetic engineering primarily involves the ***manipulation of genetic material (DNA)*** to achieve the desired goal in a pre-determined way. Some ***other terms*** are also in common use to describe genetic engineering.

- ***Gene manipulation***
- ***Recombinant DNA (rDNA) technology***
- ***Gene cloning (molecular cloning)***
- ***Genetic modifications***
- ***New genetics.***

BRIEF HISTORY OF RECOMBINANT DNA TECHNOLOGY

The present day DNA technology has its roots in the experiments performed by ***Boyer and Cohen in 1973***. In their experiments, they successfully recombined two plasmids (pSC 101 and pSC 102) and cloned the new plasmid in *E.coli*. Plasmid pSC 101 possesses a gene resistant to antibiotic tetracycline while plasmid pSC 102 contains a gene resistant to another antibiotic kanamycin. The newly developed recombined plasmid when incorporated into the bacteria exhibited resistance to both the antibiotics-tetracycline and kanamycin.

The second set of experiments of Boyer and Cohen were more organized. A gene encoding a protein (required to form rRNA) was isolated from the cells of African clawed frog *Xenophs laevis*, by use of a restriction endonuclease enzyme (*ECoRI*). The same enzyme was used to cut open plasmid pSC 101 DNA. Frog DNA fragments and plasmid DNA fragments were mixed, and pairing occurred between the complementary base pairs. By the addition of the enzyme DNA ligase, a recombined plasmid DNA was developed. These new plasmids, when introduced into *E.coli*, and grown on a nutrient medium resulted in the production of an extra protein (i.e. the frog protein). Thus, the genes of a frog could be successfully transplanted, and expressed in *E.coli*. This made the real beginning of modern rDNA technology and laid foundations for the present day molecular biotechnology.

Some biotechnologists who admire Boyer-Cohen experiments divide the subject into two chronological categories.

1. ***BBC***-biotechnology ***B***efore ***B***oyer and ***C***ohen.
2. ***ABC***-biotechnology ***A***fter ***B***oyer and ***C***ohen.

More information on the historical developments of genetic engineering and biotechnology is given under the scope of biotechnology (Chapter 1).

An outline of recombinant DNA technology

There are many diverse and complex techniques involved in gene manipulation. However, the basic principles of recombinant DNA technology are reasonably simple, and broadly involve the following stages (***Fig. 6.1***).

1. Generation of DNA fragments and selection of the desired piece of DNA (e.g. a human gene).

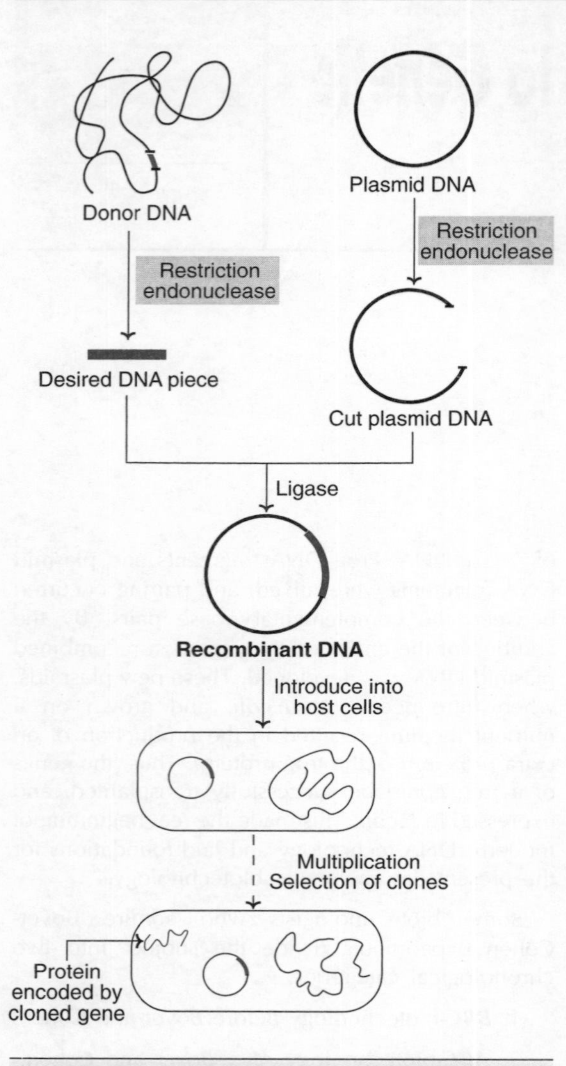

Fig. 6.1 : The basic principle of recombinant DNA technology.

2. Insertion of the selected DNA into a cloning vector (e.g. a plasmid) to create a ***recombinant DNA*** or ***chimeric DNA*** (Chimera is a monster in Greek mythology that has a lion's head, a goat's body and a serpent's tail. This may be comparable to Narasimha in Indian mythology).

3. Introduction of the recombinant vectors into host cells (e.g. bacteria).

4. Multiplication and selection of clones containing the recombinant molecules.

5. Expression of the gene to produce the desired product.

Recombinant DNA technology with special reference to the following aspects is described in this chapter.

1. Molecular tools of genetic engineering.
2. Host cells-the factories of cloning.
3. Vectors-the cloning vehicles.
4. Methods of gene transfer.
5. Gene cloning strategies.
6. Genetic engineering guidelines.
7. The future of genetic engineering.

MOLECULAR TOOLS OF GENETIC ENGINEERING

An engineer is a person who designs, constructs (e.g. bridges, canals, railways) and manipulates according to a set plan. The term genetic engineer may be appropriate for an individual who is involved in genetic manipulations. The ***genetic engineer's toolkit*** or molecular tools namely the enzymes most commonly used in recombinant DNA experiments are briefly described.

RESTRICTION ENDONUCLEASES— DNA CUTTING ENZYMES

Restriction endonucleases are one of the most important groups of enzymes for the manipulation of DNA. These are the bacterial enzymes that can cut/split DNA (from any source) at specific sites. They were first discovered in *E.coli* restricting the replication of bacteriophages, by cutting the viral DNA (The host *E.coli* DNA is protected from cleavage by addition of methyl groups). Thus, the enzymes that restrict the viral replication are known as ***restriction enzymes*** or restriction endonucleases.

Hundreds of restriction endonucleases have been isolated from bacteria, and some of them are commercially available. The progress and growth of biotechnology is unimaginable without the availability of restriction enzymes.

Nomenclature

Restriction endonucleases are named by a standard procedure, with particular reference to the bacteria from which they are isolated. The first letter (in italics) of the enzymes indicates the genus name, followed by the first two letters (also in italics) of the species, then comes the strain of the organism and finally a Roman numeral indicating the order of discovery. A couple of examples are given below.

EcoRI is from *Escherichia* (***E***) *coli* (***co***), strain Ry13 (***R***) and first endonuclease (***I***) to be discovered. ***HindIII*** is from ***Haemophilus*** (***H***) influenzae (***in***), strain Rd (***d***) and the third endonucleases (***III***) to be discovered.

Types of endonucleases

At least 4 different types of restriction endonucleases are known-type 1 (e.g *Ecok12*), type II (e.g. *EcoRI*), type III (e.g. *EcoPI*) and type IIs. Their characteristic features are given in ***Table 6.1***. Among these, type II restriction endonucleases are most commonly used in gene cloning.

TABLE 6.1 Characteristics of different types of restriction endonucleases

Type	*Salient features*
I	A single enzyme with 3 subunits for recognition, cleavage and methylation. It can cleave up to 1000 bp from recognition site.
II	Two different enzymes either to cleave or modify the recognition sequence. Cleavage site is the same or close to recognition site.
III	A single enzyme with 2 subunits for recognition and cleavage. Cleavage site is 24–26 bp from recognition site.
IIs	Two different enzymes, cleavage site is up to 20 bp from recognition site.

TABLE 6.2 Some restriction enzymes with sources, recognition sequences and the products formed

Enzyme (source)	*Recognition sequence*	*Products*
EcoRI (*Escherichia coli*)	5′......G✂A-A-T-T-C......3′ 3′......C-T-T-A-A✂G......5′	A-A-T-T-C...... G...... ......G C-T-T-A-A
BamHI (*Bacillus amylolique faciens*)	5′......G✂G-A-T-C-C......3′ 3′......C-C-T-A-G✂G......5′	G-A-T-C-C...... G...... ......G ......C-C-T-A-G
HaeIII (*Haemophilus aegyptius*)	5′......G-G✂C-C......3′ 3′......C-C✂G-G......5′	*C-C...... G-G...... ......*G-G ......C-C
HindIII (*Haemophilus influenzae*)	5′......A✂A-G-C-T-T......3′ 3′......T-T-C-G-A✂A......5′	A-G-C-T-T...... A...... ......A ......T-T-C-G-A
NotI (*Nocardia otitidis*)	5′......G-C✂G-G-C-C-G-C......3′ 3′......C-G-C-C-G-G✂C-G......5′	G-G-C-C-G-C...... C-G...... ......G-C ......C-G-C-C-G-G......

(**Note :** *Scissors indicate the sites of cleavage. * The products are with blunt ends while for the rest, the products are with sticky ends*).

Recognition sequences

Recognition sequence is the ***site where the DNA is cut*** by a restriction endonuclease. Restriction endonucleases can specifically recognize DNA with a particular sequence of 4-8 nucleotides and cleave. Each recognition sequence has two fold rotational symmetry i.e. the same nucleotide sequence occurs on both strands of DNA which run in opposite direction (***Table 6.2***). Such sequences are referred to as palindromes, since they read similar in both directions (forwards and backwards).

Cleavage patterns

Majority of restriction endonucleases (particularly type II) cut DNA at defined sites within recognition sequence. A selected list of enzymes, recognition sequences, and their products formed is given in ***Table 6.2.***

The cut DNA fragments by restriction endonucleases may have mostly ***sticky ends*** (cohesive ends) or ***blunt ends***, as given in Table 6.2. DNA fragments with sticky ends are particularly useful for recombinant DNA experiments. This is because the single-stranded sticky DNA ends can easily pair with any other DNA fragment having complementary sticky ends.

DNA LIGASES — DNA JOINING ENZYMES

The cut DNA fragments are covalently joined together by DNA ligases. These enzymes were originally isolated from viruses. They also occur in *E.coli* and eukaryotic cells. DNA ligases actively participated in cellular DNA repair process.

The action of DNA ligases is absolutely required to permanently hold DNA pieces. This is so since the hydrogen bonds formed between the complementary bases (of DNA strands) are not strong enough to hold the strands together. DNA ligase joins (seals) the DNA fragments by forming a phosphodiester bond between the phosphate group of 5′-carbon of one deoxyribose with the hydroxyl group 3′-carbon of another deoxyribose (***Fig. 6.2***).

Phage T4 DNA ligase requires ATP as a cofactor while *E.coli* DNA ligase is dependent on NAD^+. In each case, the cofactor (ATP or NAD^+) is split to form an enzyme—AMP complex that brings about the formation of phosphodiester bond. The action of DNA ligase is the ultimate step in the formation of a recombinant DNA molecule.

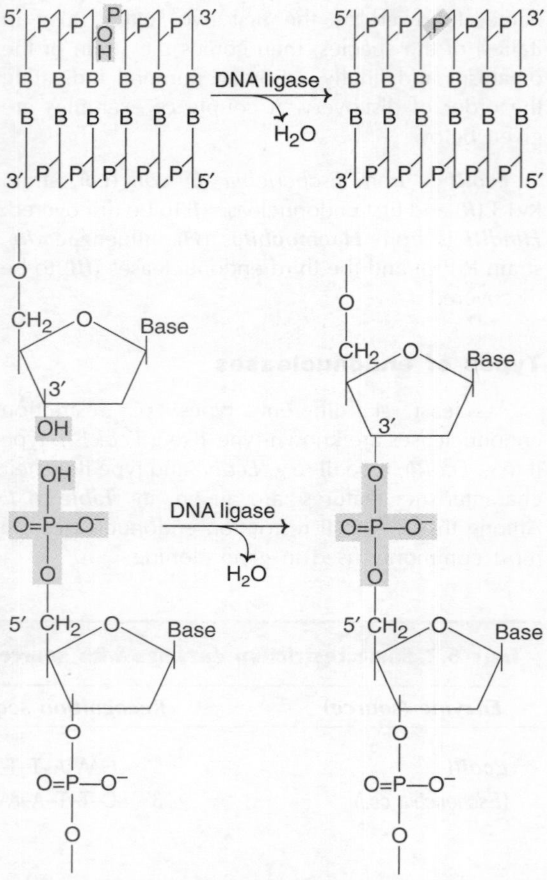

Fig. 6.2 : Action of DNA ligase in the formation of phosphodiester bond (B-base).

Homopolymer tailing

The complementary DNA strands can be joined together by ***annealing.*** This principle is utilized in homopolymer tailing. The technique involves the addition of oligo (dA) to 3′-ends of some DNA molecules and the addition of oligo (dT) to 3′-ends of other molecules. The homopolymer extensions (by adding 10-40 residues) can be synthesized by using terminal deoxynucleotidyltransferase (of calf thymus). Homopolymer tailing, achieved by annealing is illustrated in ***Fig. 6.3.***

Linkers and adaptors

Linkers and adaptors are ***chemically synthesized, short, double-stranded DNA molecules***. Linkers possess restriction enzyme cleavage sites. They can be ligated to blunt ends of any DNA molecule and cut with specific restriction enzymes to produce DNA fragments with sticky ends (***Fig. 6.4***).

Adaptors contain preformed sticky or cohesive ends. They are useful to be ligated to DNA fragments with blunt ends. The DNA fragments held to linkers or adaptors are finally ligated to vector DNA molecules (***Fig 6.4***).

ALKALINE PHOSPHATASE

Alkaline phosphatase is an enzyme involved in the removal of phosphate groups. This enzyme is useful to prevent the unwanted ligation of DNA molecules which is a frequent problem encountered in cloning experiments.

When the linear vector plasmid DNA is treated with alkaline phosphatase, the 5′-terminal phosphate is removed (***Fig 6.5***). This prevents both recircularization and plasmid DNA dimer formation. It is now possible to insert the foreign DNA through the participation of DNA ligase.

DNA MODIFYING ENZYMES

Some authors prefer to use the broad term DNA modifying enzymes to all the enzymes involved in recombinant DNA technology. These enzymes represent the ***cutting*** and ***joining*** functions in DNA manipulation. They are broadly categorized as nucleases, polymerases and enzymes modifying ends of DNA molecules, and briefly described below, and illustrated in ***Fig. 6.6***.

Nucleases

Nucleases are the enzymes that break the phosphodiester bonds (that hold nucleotides together) of DNA. ***Endonucleases*** act on the internal phosphodiester bonds while ***exonucleases*** degrade DNA from the terminal ends (***Fig 6.6A***). Restriction endonucleases, described already, are good examples of endonucleases. Some other examples of endo- and exonucleases are listed.

Endonucleases

- Nuclease S_1 specifically acts on single-stranded DNA or RNA molecules.
- Deoxyribonuclease I (DNase I) cuts either single or double-stranded DNA molecules at random sites.

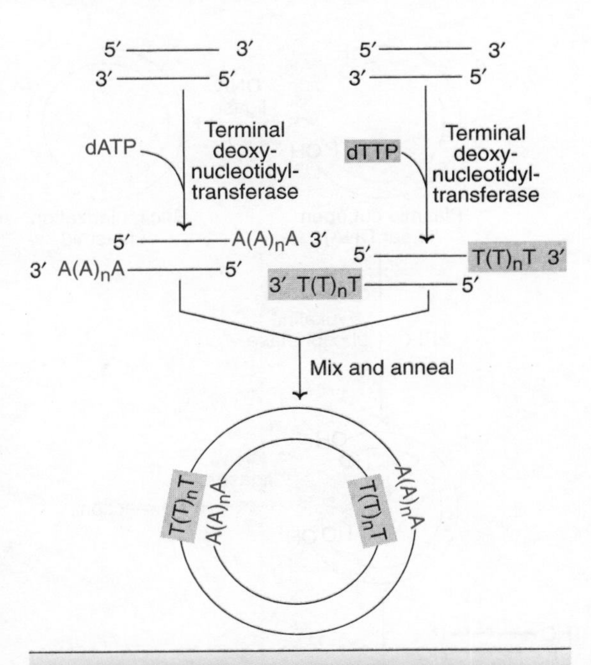

Fig. 6.3 : Homopolymer tailing.

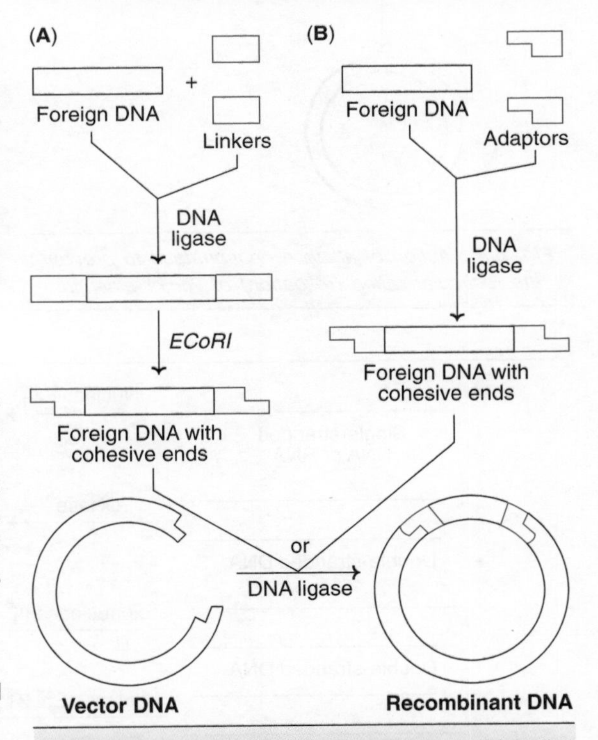

*Fig. 6.4 : Use of linkers (**A**) and adaptors (**B**) in the formation of recombinant DNA (Note that the linkers have blunt ends while adaptors have sticky ends).*

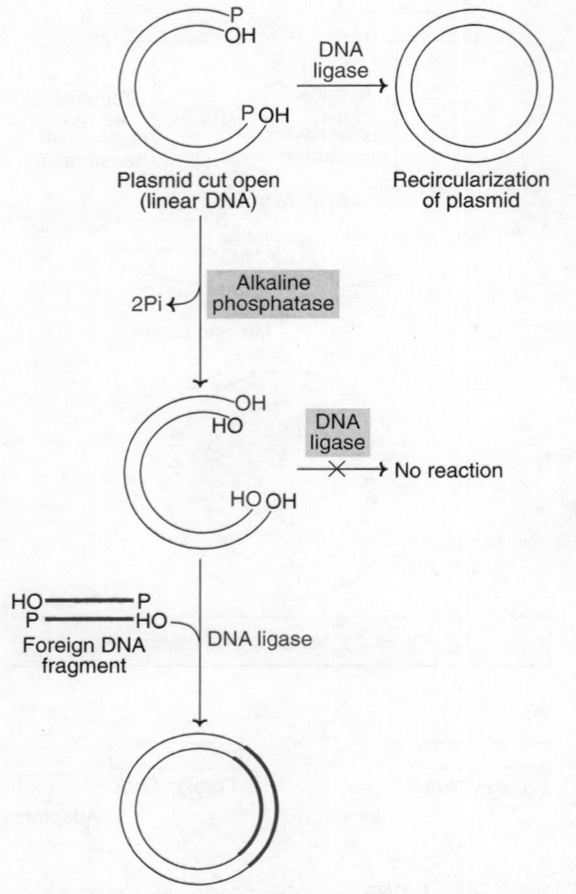

Fig. 6.5 : Action of alkaline phosphatase to prevent the recircularization (religation) of vector plasmid.

(A) Nucleases

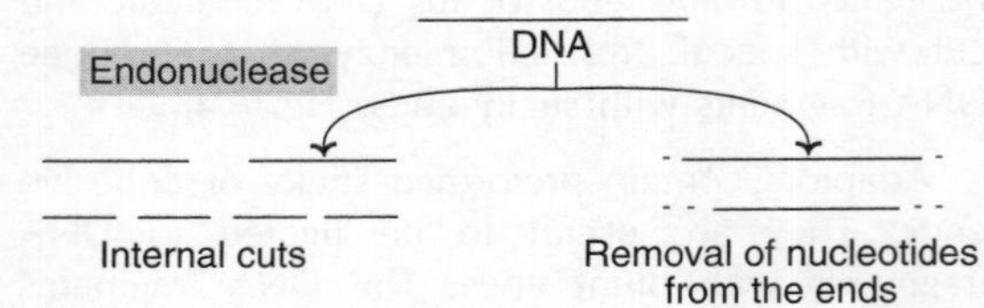

(B) DNA Polymerases

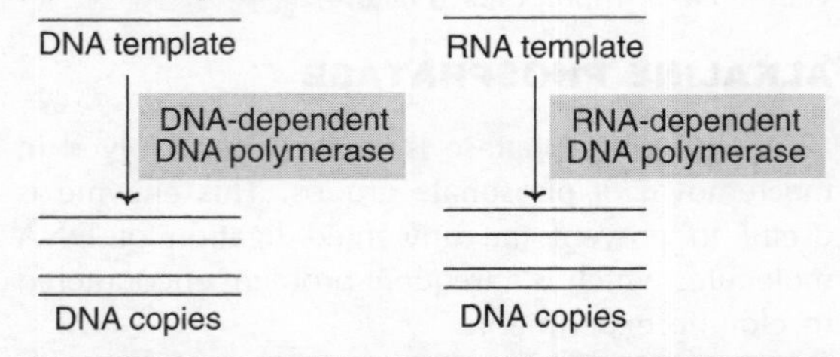

Fig. 6.6 : An outline of the activities of nucleases (A), and DNA polymerases (B).

Exonucleases

- Exonuclease III cuts DNA and generates molecules with protruding 5′-ends.
- Nuclease Bal 31 is a fast acting 3′-exonuclease. Its action is usually coupled with slow acting endonucleases.

A diagrammatic representation of the action of endo-and exonucleases is given in ***Fig. 6.7***.

Besides the DNA cutting enzymes, there are RNA specific nucleases, which are referred to as ***ribonucleases*** (***RNases***).

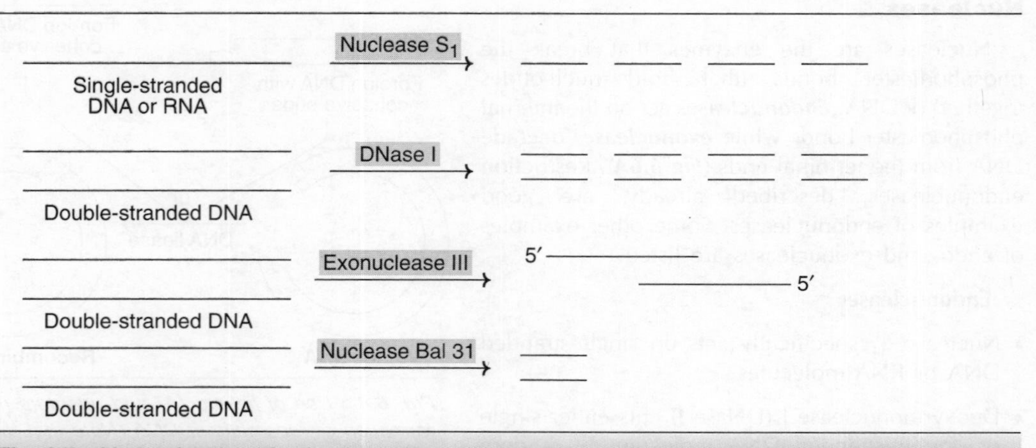

Fig. 6.7 : Mode of action of selected endo– and exonucleases (DNase I–Deoxyribonuclease I).

TABLE 6.3 The most commonly used enzymes in recombinant DNA technology/genetic engineering

Enzyme	*Use/reaction*
Alkaline phosphatase	Removes phosphate groups from 5′-ends of double/single-stranded DNA (or RNA).
Bal 31 nuclease	For the progressive shortening of DNA.
DNA ligase	Joins DNA molecules by forming phosphodiester linkages between DNA segments.
DNA polymerase I	Synthesizes DNA complementary to a DNA template.
DNase I	Produces single-stranded nicks in DNA.
Exonuclease III	Removes nucleotides from 3′-end of DNA.
λ exonuclease	Removes nucleotides from 5′-end of DNA.
Polynucleotide kinase	Transfers phosphate from ATP to 5′-OH ends of DNA or RNA.
Restriction enzymes	Cut double-stranded DNA with a specific recognition site.
Reverse transcriptase	Synthesizes DNA from RNA.
RNase A	Cleaves and digests RNA (and not DNA).
RNase H	Cleaves and digests the RNA strand of RNA-DNA heteroduplex.
Taq DNA polymerase	Used in polymerase chain reaction
SI nuclease	Degrades single-stranded DNA and RNA.
Terminal transferase	Adds nucleotides to the 3′-ends of DNA or RNA. Useful in homopolymer tailing.

Polymerases

The group of enzymes that catalyse the synthesis of nucleic acid molecules are collectively referred to as polymerases. It is customary to use the name of the nucleic acid template on which the polymerase acts (***Fig. 6.6B***). The three important polymerases are given below.

- ***DNA-dependent DNA polymerase*** that copies DNA from DNA.
- ***RNA-dependent DNA polymerase*** (reverse transcriptase) that synthesizes DNA from RNA.
- ***DNA-dependent RNA polymerase*** that produces RNA from DNA.

For more details on the functions of these enzymes, refer Chapter 4.

Enzymes modifying the ends of DNA

There are certain enzymes that act on the terminal ends of DNA and modify these molecules. The important ones are listed.

- ***Alkaline phosphatase*** that removes the terminal phosphate group (see ***Fig. 6.5***).
- ***Polynucleotide kinase*** involved in the addition of phosphate groups.
- ***Terminal transferase*** (also called terminal deoxynucleotidyl transferase) repeatedly adds nucleotides to any available 3′-terminal ends, the most suitable being the protruding 3′-ends. This enzyme is particularly useful to add homopolymer tails prior to the construction of recombinant DNA molecules.
- The most commonly used enzymes in recombinant DNA technology/genetic engineering are listed in ***Table 6.3***.

HOST CELLS — THE FACTORIES OF CLONING

The hosts are the ***living systems or cells*** in which the carrier of recombinant DNA molecule or ***vector can be propagated***. There are different types of host cells-prokaryotic (bacteria) and eukaryotic (fungi, animals and plants). Some examples of host cells used in genetic engineering are given in ***Table 6.4***.

Host cells, besides effectively incorporating the vector's genetic material, must be conveniently cultivated in the laboratory to collect the products. In general, ***microorganisms*** are ***preferred*** as host cells, since they ***multiply faster*** compared to cells of higher organism (plants or animals).

PROKARYOTIC HOSTS

Escherichia coli

The bacterium, *Escherichia coli* was the first organism used in the DNA technology experiments and continues to be ***the host of choice*** by many workers. Undoubtedly, *E.coli*, the simplest Gram negative bacterium (a common bacterium of human and animal intestine), has played a key role in the development of present day biotechnology. Under suitable environment, *E.coli* can double in number every 20 minutes. Thus, as the bacteria multiply, their plasmids (along with foreign DNA) also multiply to produce millions of copies, referred to as colony or in short ***clone.*** The term clone is broadly used to a mass of cells, organisms or genes that are produced by multiplication of a single cell, organism or gene.

Limitations of *E. coli* : There are certain limitations in using *E.coli* as a host. These include-causation of diarrhea by some strains, formation of endotoxins that are toxic, and a low export ability of proteins from the cell. Another ***major drawback*** is that *E.coli* (or even other prokaryotic organisms) ***cannot perform post-translational modifications***.

Bacillus subtilis

Bacillus subtilis is a rod shaped non-pathogenic bacterium. It has been used as a host in industry for the production of enzymes, antibiotics, insecticides etc. Some workers consider *B.subtilis* as an ***alternative to E.coli***.

EUKARYOTIC HOSTS

Eukaryotic organisms are preferred to produce human proteins since these hosts with complex structure (with distinct organelles) are more suitable to synthesize complex proteins. The ***most commonly used*** eukaryotic organism is the ***yeast, Saccharomyces cerevisiae***. It is a non-pathogenic organism routinely used in brewing and baking industry. Certain fungi have also been used in gene cloning experiments.

Mammalian cells

Despite the practical difficulties to work with and high cost factor, mammalian cells (such as mouse cells) are also employed as hosts. The advantage is that certain complex proteins which cannot be synthesized by bacteria can be produced by mammalian cells e.g. tissue plasminogen activator. This is mainly because the mammalian cells ***possess the machinery to modify the protein to its final form*** (post-translational modifications).

TABLE 6.4 Some examples of host cells used in genetic engineering

Group	Examples
Prokaryotic	
Bacteria	*Escherichia coli*
	Bacillus subtilis
	Streptomyces sp
Eurkaryotic	
Fungi	*Saccharomyces cerevisiae*
	Aspergillus nidulans
Animals	Insect cells
	Oocytes
	Mammalian cells
	Whole organisms
Plants	Protoplasts
	Intact cells
	Whole plants

It may be noted here that the gene manipulation experiments in higher animals and plants are usually carried out to alter the genetic make up of the organism to create transgenic animals (Chapter 41) and transgenic plants (Chapter 49), rather than to isolate genes for producing specific proteins.

VECTORS — THE CLONING VEHICLES

Vectors are the DNA molecules, which can ***carry a foreign DNA fragment to be cloned***. They are self-replicating in an appropriate host cell. The most important vectors are plasmids, bacteriophages, cosmids and phasmids.

Characteristics of an ideal vector

An ideal vector should be small in size, with a single restriction endonuclease site, an origin of replication and 1-2 genetic markers (to identify recipient cells carrying vectors). Naturally occurring plasmids rarely possess all these characteristics.

PLASMIDS

Plasmids are extrachromosomal, double-stranded, circular, self-replicating DNA molecules. Almost all the bacteria have plasmids containing a low copy number (1-4 per cell) or a high copy number (10-100 per cell). The size of the plasmids varies from 1 to 500 kb. Usually, plasmids contribute to about 0.5 to 5.0% of the total DNA of bacteria (**Note :** A few bacteria contain linear plasmids e.g. *Streptomyces* sp, *Borella burgdorferi*).

Types of plasmids

There are many ways of grouping plasmids. They are categorized as ***conjugative*** if they carry a set of transfer genes (*tra* genes) that facilitates bacterial conjugation, and ***non-conjugative***, if they do not possess such genes.

Another classification is based on the copy number. ***Stringent plasmids*** are present in a limited number (1-2 per cell) while ***relaxed plasmids*** occur in large number in each cell.

F-plasmids possess genes for their own transfer from one cell to another, while ***R-plasmids*** carry genes resistance to antibiotics.

In general, the conjugative plasmids are large, show stringent control of DNA replication, and are present in low numbers. On the other hand, non-conjugative plasmids are small, show relaxed control of DNA replication, and are present in high numbers.

Nomenclature of plasmids

It is a common practice to designate **p**lasmid by a lower case ***p***, followed by the first letter(s) of researcher(s) names and the numerical number given by the workers. Thus, ***pBR322*** is a **p**lasmid discovered by ***B***olivar and ***R***odriguez who designated it as ***322.*** Some plasmids are given names of the places where they are discovered e.g. ***pUC*** is **p**lasmid from ***U***niversity of ***C***alifornia.

pBR322 — the most common plasmid vector

pBR322 of *E.coli* is the most popular and widely used plasmid vector, and is appropriately regarded as the parent or grand parent of several other vectors.

pBR322 has a DNA sequence of 4,361 bp. It carries genes resistance for ampicillin (Amp^r) and

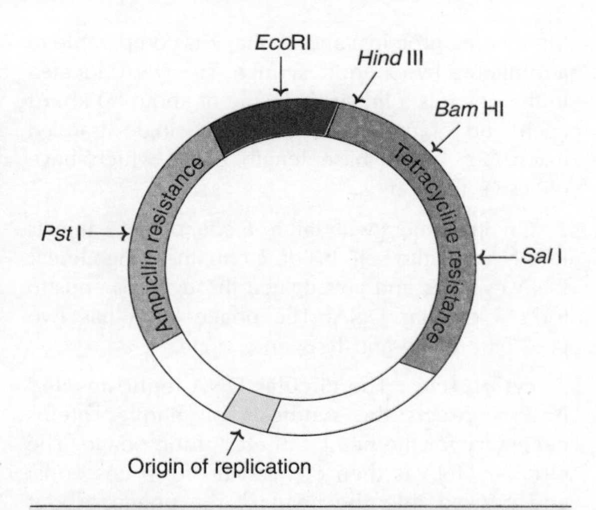

Fig. 6.8 : Genetic map of plasmid cloning vector pBR322.

tetracycline (Tel^r) that serve as markers for the identification of clones carrying plasmids. The plasmid has unique recognition sites for the action of restriction endonucleases such as *EcoRI, HindIII, BamHI, SalI* and *PstII* (***Fig. 6.8***).

Other plasmid cloning vectors

The other plasmids employed as cloning vectors include pUC19 (2,686 bp, with ampicillin resistance gene), and derivatives of pBR322–pBR325, pBR328 and pBR329.

BACTERIOPHAGES

Bacteriophages or simply ***phages*** are the ***viruses*** that ***replicate within the bacteria***. In case of certain phages, their DNA gets incorporated into the bacterial chromosome and remains there permanently. Phage vectors can accept short fragments of foreign DNA into their genomes. The advantage with phages is that they ***can take up larger DNA segments than plasmids***. Hence phage vectors are preferred for working with genomes of human cells.

Bacteriophage λ

Bacteriophage lambda (or simply ***phage λ***), a virus of *E.coli*, has been most thoroughly studied and developed as a vector. In order to understand how bacteriophage functions as a vector, it is desirable to know its structure and life cycle (***Fig. 6.9***). Phage λ consists of a head and a tail (both being proteins) and its shape is comparable to a miniature hypodermic syringe. The DNA, located in the head, is a linear molecule of about 50 kb. At each end of the DNA, there are single-stranded extensions of 12 base length each, which have cohesive (cos) ends.

On attachment with tail to *E.coli*, phage λ injects its DNA into the cell. Inside *E.coli*, the phage linear DNA cyclizes and gets ligated through cos ends to form a circular DNA. The phage DNA has two fates-lytic cycle and lysogenic cycle.

Lytic cycle : The circular DNA replicates and it also directs the synthesis of many proteins necessary for the head, tail etc, of the phage. The circular DNA is then cleaved (to form cos ends) and packed into the head of the phage. About 100 phage particles are produced within 20 minutes after the entry of phage into *E.coli*. The host cell is then subjected to lysis and the phages are released. Each progeny phage particle can infect a bacterial cell, and produce several hundreds of phages. It is estimated that by repeating the lytic cycle four times, a single phage can cause the death of more than one billion bacterial cells. ***If a foreign DNA is spliced into phage DNA, without causing harm to phage genes, the phage will reproduce (replicate the foreign DNA) when it infects bacterial cell.*** This has been exploited in phage vector employed cloning techniques.

Lysogenic cycle : In this case, the phage DNA (instead of independently replicating) becomes integrated into the *E.coli* chromosome and replicates along with the host genome. No phage particles are synthesized in this pathway.

Use of phage λ as a vector

Only about 50% of phage λ DNA is necessary for its multiplication and other functions. Thus, as much as 50% (i.e.up to 25kb) of the phage DNA can be replaced by a donor DNA for use in cloning experiments. However, several restriction sites are present on phage λ which is not by itself a suitable vector. The λ-based phage vectors are modifications of the natural phage with much reduced number of restriction sites. Some of them are discussed hereunder.

Insertion vectors : They have just one unique cleavage site, which can be cleaved, and a foreign DNA ligated in. It is essential that sufficient DNA (about 25%) has to be deleted from the vector to make space for the foreign DNA (about 18kb).

Replacement vectors : These vectors have a pair of restriction sites to remove the non-essential DNA (***stuffer DNA***) that will be replaced by a foreign DNA. Replacement vectors can accommodate up to 24kb, and propagate them.

Many phage vector derivations (insertion/ replacement) have been produced by researchers for use in recombinant DNA technology.

The main advantage of using phage vectors is that the foreign DNA can be packed into the phage (*in vitro* packaging), the latter in turn can be injected into the host cell very effectively (**Note :** No transformation is required).

Phage M_{13} vectors

Phage M_{13} (bacteriophage M_{13}) is a single-stranded DNA phage of *E.coli*. Inside the host cell, M_{13} synthesizes the complementary strand to form a double-stranded DNA (replicative form DNA; ***RF DNA***). For use as a vector, RF DNA is isolated and a foreign DNA can be inserted on it. This is then returned to the host cell as a plasmid. Single-stranded DNAs are recovered from the phage particles. Phage M_{13} is useful for sequencing DNA through Sanger's method (Refer Chapter 7).

COSMIDS

Cosmids are the vectors possessing the characteristics of both plasmid and bacteriophage λ. ***Cosmids*** can be constructed by adding a fragment of phage λ DNA including ***cos*** site, to plas***mids***. A foreign DNA (about 40 kb) can be inserted into cosmid DNA. The recombinant DNA so formed can be packed as phages and injected into *E.coli* (***Fig. 6.10***). Once inside the host cell, cosmids behave just like plasmids and replicate. The advantage with cosmids is that they can carry larger fragments of foreign DNA compared to plasmids.

Phasid vectors

Phasids are the combination of plasmid and phage and can function as either one (i.e as plasmid or phage). Phasids possess functional origins of replication of both plasmid and phage λ, and therefore can be propagated (as plasmid or phage) in appropriate *E.coli*. The vectors phasids may be used in many ways in cloning experiments.

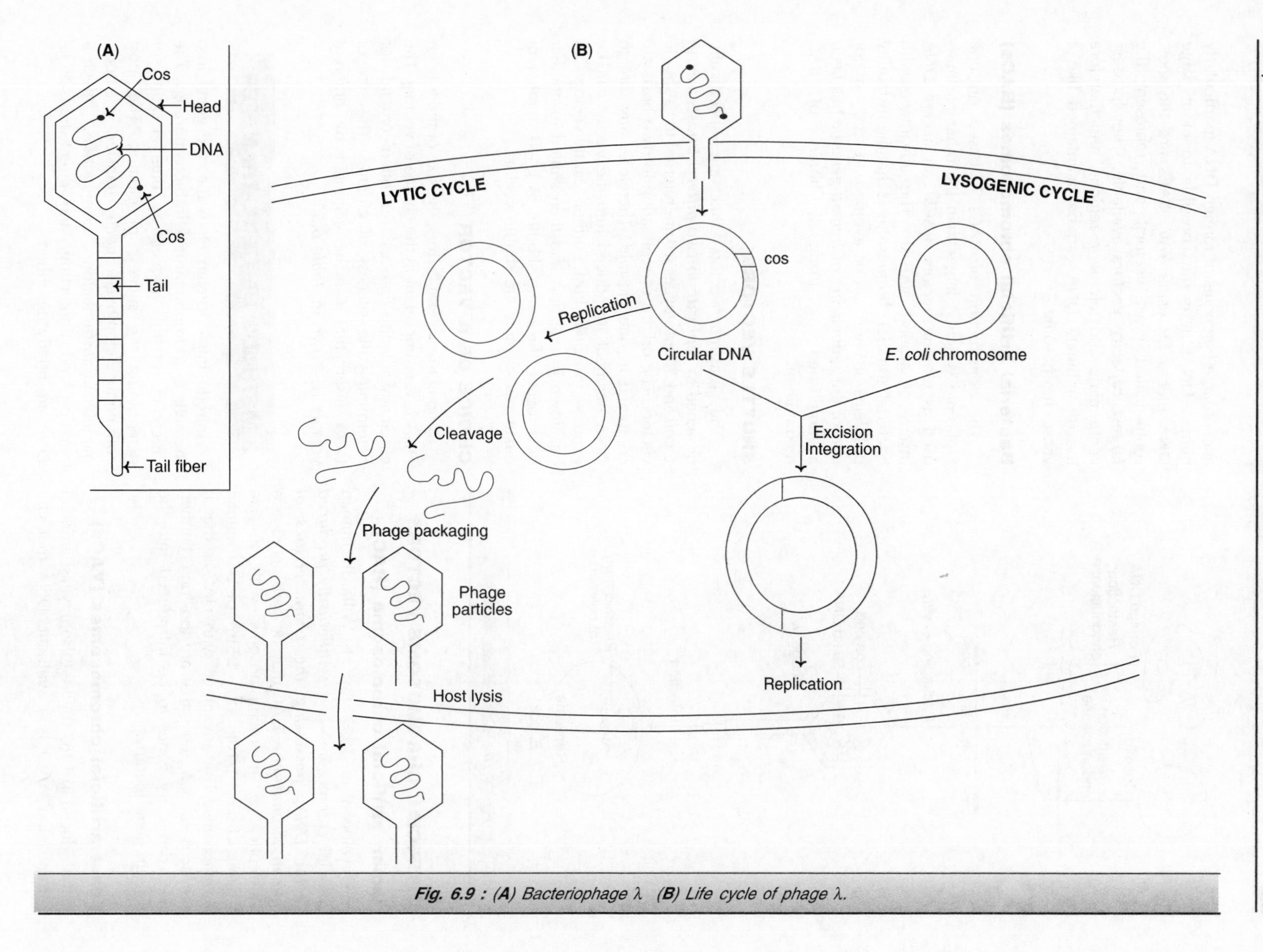

Fig. 6.9 : (A) Bacteriophage λ (B) Life cycle of phage λ.

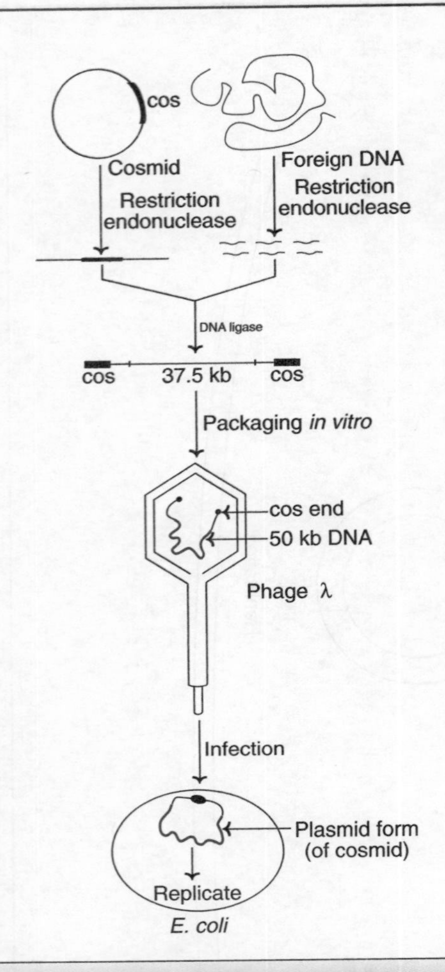

Fig. 6.10 : Cosmids as vectors.

ARTIFICIAL CHROMOSOME VECTORS

Human artificial chromosome (HAC)

Developed in 1997 (by H. Willard), human artificial chromosome is a ***synthetically produced vector DNA, possessing the characteristics of human chromosome***. HAC may be considered as a self-replicating microchromosome with a size ranging from 1/10th to 1/5th of a human chromosome. The advantage with HAC is that it can carry human genes that are too long. Further, HAC can carry genes to be introduced into the cells in gene therapy.

Yeast artificial chromosomes (YACs)

Introduced in 1987 (by M. Olson), yeast artificial chromosome (YAC) is a synthetic DNA that can accept large fragments of foreign DNA (particularly human DNA). It is thus possible to clone large DNA pieces by using YAC. YACs are the most sophisticated yeast vectors, and represent the ***largest capacity vectors*** available. They possess centromeric and telomeric regions, and therefore the recombinant DNA can be maintained like a yeast chromosome.

Bacterial artificial chromosomes (BACs)

The construction of BACs is based on one F-plasmid which is larger than the other plasmids used as cloning vectors. BACs can accept DNA inserts of around 300 kb. The advantage with bacterial artificial chromosome is that the instability problems of YACs can be avoided. In fact, a major part of the ***sequencing of human genome*** has been accomplished by using a library of BAC recombinant.

SHUTTLE VECTORS

The plasmid vectors that are specifically designed to ***replicate in two different hosts*** (say in *E.coli* and *Streptomyces* sp) are referred to as shuttle vectors. The origins of replication for two hosts are combined in one plasmid. Therefore, any foreign DNA fragment introduced into the vector can be expressed in either host. Further, shuttle vectors can be grown in one host and then shifted to another host (hence the name shuttle). A good number of eukaryotic vectors are shuttle vectors.

CHOICE OF A VECTOR

Among the several factors, the size of the foreign DNA is very important in the choice of vectors. The efficiency of this process in often crucial for determining the success of cloning. The size of DNA insert that can be accepted by different vectors is shown in ***Table 6.5***.

METHODS OF GENE TRANSFER

Introducing a foreign DNA (i.e. the gene) into the cells is an important task in biotechnology. The efficiency of this process is often crucial for determining the success of cloning. The most commonly employed gene transfer methods, namely transformation, conjugation, electroporation and lipofection, and direct transfer of DNA are briefly described.

TABLE 6.5 The different cloning vectors with the corresponding hosts and the sizes of foreign insert DNAs

Vector	*Host*	*Foreign insert DNA size*
Phage λ	*E. coli*	5–25 kb
Cosmid λ	*E. coli*	35–45 kb
Plasmid artifical chromosome (PAC)	*E. coli*	100–300 kb
Bacterial artificial chromosome (BAC)	*E. coli*	100–300 kb
Yeast chromosome	*S. cerevisiae*	200–2000 kb

TRANSFORMATION

Transformation is the method of introducing foreign DNA into bacterial cells (e.g. *E.coli*). The uptake of plasmid DNA by *E.coli* is carried out in ice-cold $CaCl_2$ (0-5°C), and a subsequent heat shock (37–45°C for about 90 sec). By this technique, the ***transformation frequency***, which refers to ***the fraction of cell population that can be transferred***, is reasonably good e.g. approximately one cell for 1000 (10^{-3}) cells.

Transformation efficiency : It refers to the number of transformants per microgram of added DNA. For *E.coli*, transformation by plasmid, the transformation efficiency is about 10^7 to 10^8 cells per microgram of intact plasmid DNA. The bacterial cells that can take up DNA are considered as competent. The competence can be enhanced by altering growth conditions.

The mechanism of the transformation process is not fully understood. It is believed that the $CaCl_2$ affects the cell wall, breaks at localized regions, and is also responsible for binding of DNA to cell surface. A brief heat shock (i.e. the sudden increase in temperature from 5°C to 40°C) stimulates DNA uptake. In general, large-sized DNAs are less efficient in transforming.

Other chemical methods for transformation

Calcium phosphate (in place of $CaCl_2$) is preferred for the transfer of DNA into cultured cells. Sometimes, calcium phosphate may result in precipitate and toxicity to the cells. Some workers use diethyl aminoethyl dextran (DEAE -dextran) for DNA transfer.

CONJUCTION

Conjugation is ***a natural microbial recombination process***. During conjugation, two live bacteria (a donor and a recipient) come together, join by cytoplasmic bridges and transfer single-stranded DNA (from donor to recipient). Inside the recipient cell, the new DNA may integrate with the chromosome (rather rare) or may remain free (as is the case with plasmids).

Conjugation can occur among the cells from different genera of bacteria (e.g *Salmonella* and *Shigella* cells). This is in contrast to transformation which takes place among the cells of a bacterial genus. Thus by conjugation, transfer of genes from two different and unrelated bacteria is possible.

The natural phenomenon of conjugation is exploited for gene transfer. This is achieved by transferring plasmid-insert DNA from one cell to another. In general, the plasmids lack conjugative functions and therefore, they are not as such capable of transferring DNA to the recipient cells. However, some plasmids with conjugative properties can be prepared and used.

ELECTROPORATION

Electroporation is based on the principle that high voltage electric pulses can induce cell plasma membranes to fuse. Thus, electroporation is a technique involving ***electric field-mediated membrane permeabilization.*** Electric shocks can also induce cellular uptake of exogenous DNA (believed to be via the pores formed by electric pulses) from the suspending solution. Electroporation is a simple and rapid technique for introducing genes into the cells from various organisms (microorganisms, plants and animals).

The basic technique of electroporation for transferring genes into mammalian cells is depicted in ***Fig. 6.11***. The cells are placed in a solution containing DNA and subjected to electrical shocks to cause holes in the membranes. The foreign DNA fragments enter through the holes into the cytoplasm and then to nucleus.

Electroporation is an effective way to transform *E.coli* cells containing plasmids with insert DNAs longer than 100 kb. The transformation efficiency is around 10^9 transformants per microgram of DNA

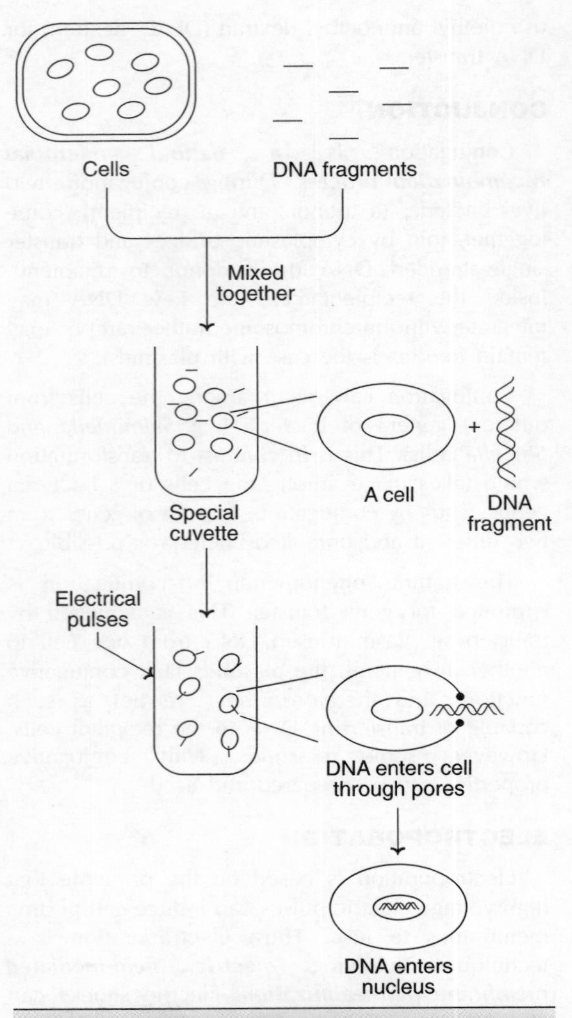

Fig. 6.11 : Gene transfer by electroporation. (Note : Magnification depicted on right side)

for small plasmids (about 3kb) and about 10^6 for large plasmids (about 130 kb).

LIPOSOME-MEDIATED GENE TRANSFER

Liposomes are circular lipid molecules, which have an aqueous interior that can carry nucleic acids. Several techniques have been developed to encapsulate DNA in liposomes. The liposome-mediated gene transfer, referred to as ***lipofection***, is depicted in ***Fig. 6.12***.

On treatment of DNA fragment with liposomes, the DNA pieces get encapsulated inside liposomes. These liposomes can adher to cell membranes and fuse with them to transfer DNA fragments. Thus, the DNA enters the cell and then to the nucleus. The positively charged liposomes very efficiently complex with DNA, bind to cells and transfer DNA rapidly.

Lipofection is a very efficient technique and is used for the transfer of genes to bacterial, animal and plant cells.

The different methods of gene transfer are briefly described above. More details are given in the respective chapters applying these techniques to achieve gene transfer.

TRANSDUCTION

Sometimes, the foreign DNA can be packed inside animal viruses. These viruses can naturally

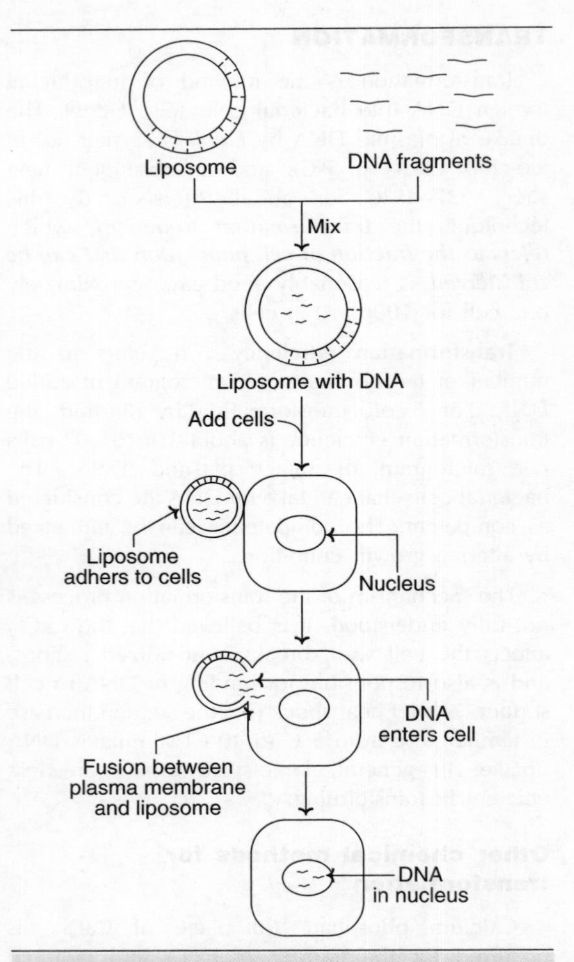

Fig. 6.12 : Liposome-mediated gene transfer (Note : For clarity, the native cell DNA is not shown).

infect the cells and introduce the DNA into host cells. The transfer of DNA by this approach is referred to as transduction.

DIRECT TRANSFER OF DNA

It is possible to directly transfer the DNA into the cell nucleus. Microinjection and particle bombardment are the two techniques commonly used for this purpose.

Microinjection

DNA transfer by microinjection is generally used for the cultured cells. This technique is also useful to introduce DNA into large cells such as oocytes, eggs and the cells of early embryos.

Some more details on gene transfer methods including particle bombardment are given in Chapter 49.

The term ***transfection is used for the transfer DNA into eukaryotic cells,*** by various physical or chemical means.

GENE CLONING STRATEGIES

A clone refers to ***a group of*** organisms, cells, ***molecules*** or other objects, ***arising from a single individual.*** Clone and colony are almost synonymous.

Gene cloning strategies in relation to recombinant DNA technology broadly involve the following aspects (***Fig. 6.13***).

- Generation of desired DNA fragments.
- Insertion of these fragments into a cloning vector.
- Introduction of the vectors into host cells.
- Selection or screening of the recipient cells for the recombinant DNA molecules.

It is obvious that for a good understanding (or account) of gene cloning strategies, this chapter has to be learnt in detail. In addition, the reader must invariably refer gene libraries (Chapter 9) for ***cloning of genes and screening strategies,*** and the ***polymerase chain reaction*** (Chapter 8) for *in vitro* generation of large quantities of DNA. Further, gene cloning also involves the expression of genes which is described under ***manipulation of gene expression in host cells*** (Chapter 11).

GENERATION OF DNA FRAGMENTS
(Restriction endonuclease digestion, cDNA synthesis, PCR, chemical synthesis)
↓
INSERTION INTO A CLONING VECTOR
(Ligation of blunt ends or cohesive ends, homopolymer tailing, linker molecules)
↓
INTRODUCTION INTO HOST CELLS
(Transformation, transfection, transduction)
↓
SELECTION OR SCREENING
(Hybridization, PCR, immonochemical methods, protein–protein interactions, functional complementation)

Fig. 6.13 : An overview of cloning strategies in recombinant DNA technology.

CLONING FROM GENOMIC DNA OR MRNA?

DNA represents the complete genetic material of an organism which is referred to as genome. Theoretically speaking, cloning from genomic DNA is supposed to be ideal. But the DNA contains non-coding sequences (introns), control regions and repetitive sequences. This complicates the cloning strategies, hence DNA as a source material is not preferred, by many workers. However, if the objective of cloning is to elucidate the control of gene expression, then genomic DNA has to be invariably used in cloning.

The use of mRNA in cloning is preferred for the following reasons.

- mRNA represents the actual genetic information being expressed.
- Selection and isolation mRNA is easy.
- As introns are removed during processing, mRNA reflects the coding sequence of the gene.
- The synthesis of recombinant protein is easy with mRNA cloning.

Besides the direct use of genomic DNA or mRNA, it is possible to synthesize DNA in the laboratory (Chapter 7), and use it in cloning experiments. This approach is useful if the gene sequence is short and the complete sequence of amino acids is known.

The different strategies for the cloning of genomic DNA and mRNA are described under gene libraries (Chapter 9).

GENETIC ENGINEERING OF PLANTS

For additional information on the genetic engineering of plants, the reader must refer Chapter 49. Some details on the following aspects are given in that chapter

- Gene transfer methods (vector-mediated gene transfer — T DNA, plant viruses; direct DNA transfer — physical and chemical methods).
- Marker genes for plant transformation.
- Promoters and terminators.
- Transgene stability, expression and gene silencing.
- Chloroplast transformation.

GENETIC ENGINEERING GUIDELINES

With the success of Boyer-Cohen experiments (in 1973), it was realised that recombinant DNA technology could be used to create organisms with novel genes. This created worldwide commotion (among scientists, public and government officials) about the safety, ethics and unforeseen consequences of genetic manipulations. Some of the phrases quoted in media in those days are given.

- Manipulation of life.
- Playing God.
- Man made evolution.
- The most threatening scientific research.

It was feared that some new organisms, created inadvertently or deliberately for warfare, would cause epidemics and environmental catastrophes. Due to the fears of the dangerous consequences, a cautious approach on recombinant DNA experiments was suggested.

In 1974, a group of ten scientists led by Paul Berg wrote a letter that simultaneously appeared in the prestigeous journals-Nature, Science and Proceedings of the National Academy of Sciences. The dangers of DNA technology were printed out in that letter (highlights given below) :

"Recent advances in techniques for isolation and rejoining of segments of DNA now permit construction of biologically active recombinant DNA molecules in vitro. Although such experiments are likely to facilitate the solution of important theoretical and practical biological problems, they would also result in creation of novel types of DNA elements whose biological properties cannot be completely predicted. There is a serious concern that some of these DNA molecules could prove biologically hazardous".

The letter also appealed to molecular biologists worldwide for a moratorium on many kinds of recombinant DNA research, particularly those involving pathogenic organisms.

ASILOMAR RECOMMENDATIONS

In February 1975, a group of 139 scientists from 17 countries held a conference at Asilomar, a conference center in California, USA. They assured the uneasy public that the microorganisms used in DNA experiments were specifically bred and could not survive outside the laboratory. These scientists ***formulated guidelines and recommendations for conducting experiments in genetic engineering.***

NIH GUIDELINES

National Institute of Health (NIH), USA constituted the ***Recombinant DNA Advisory Committee (RAC)*** which issued a set of stringent guidelines to conduct research on DNA. RAC was in fact overseeing the research projects involving gene splicing and recombinant DNA.

Some of the important original NIH recommendations on recombinant DNA research relate to the following aspects.

- Physical (laboratory) containment levels for conducting expermiments.
- Biological containment-the host into which foreign DNA is inserted should not proliferate outside the laboratory or transfer its DNA into other organisms.

- For research on pathogenic organisms, elaborate, controlled and self-contained rooms were recommended.
- For research on less dangerous organisms, units equipped with high quality filter systems should be used.
- No deliberate release of any organism containing recombinant DNA into the environment.

It may be noted here that although the NIH guidelines did not have the legal status, most institutions, companies and scientists voluntarily complied.

Relaxation of NIH guidelines

It was in 1980, the original NIH guidelines were considerably relaxed by NIH-RAC, based on the experience and experimental data obtained from the NIH-sponsored studies on recombinant DNA research. It was almost agreed that the original apprehensions on recombinant DNA research were unfounded.

It is a fact that the genetic engineering research flourished and progressed rapidly after relaxation of NIH guidelines. It may however be noted that NIH-RAC continues to be a watchdog over the DNA technology experiments.

Pharmaceutical products of recombinant DNA

As the recombinant DNA technology progressed, many pharmaceutical compounds of human health care are being produced through genetic manipulations. Most countries consider that the existing regulations for approval of pharmaceuticals of commercial use are adequate to ensure safety since the process by which the product manufactured is irrelevant. Thus, the recombinant DNA product (protein, vaccine, drug) is evaluated for its safety and efficacy like any other pharmaceutical product.

Genetically engineered organisms (GEOs)

Recombinant DNA research has resulted in the creation of many genetically engineered organisms. These include microorganisms, animals and plants. The latter two respectively result in transgenic animals and transgenic plants. The safety aspects and other related matters of GEOs are discussed at appropriate places in text, and some major highlights are given in Chapter 61.

THE FUTURE OF GENETIC ENGINEERING

DNA technology has largely helped scientists to understand the structure, function and regulation of genes. The development of new/modern biotechnology is primarily based on the success of DNA technology. Thus, the ***present biotechnology (more appropriately molecular biotechnology) has its main roots in molecular biology.***

Biotechnology is an interdisciplinary approach for applications to human health, agriculture, industry and environment. The major objective of biotechnology is to solve problems associated with human health, food production, energy production and environmental control.

The major contributions of genetic engineering through the new discipline biotechnology are given in this book.

It is an accepted fact that the recombinant DNA technology has entered the main stream of human life and has become one of the most significant applications of scientific research. ***Biotechnology is regarded as more an art than a science.***

After the successful sequencing of human genome, many breakthroughs in biotechnology are expected in future.

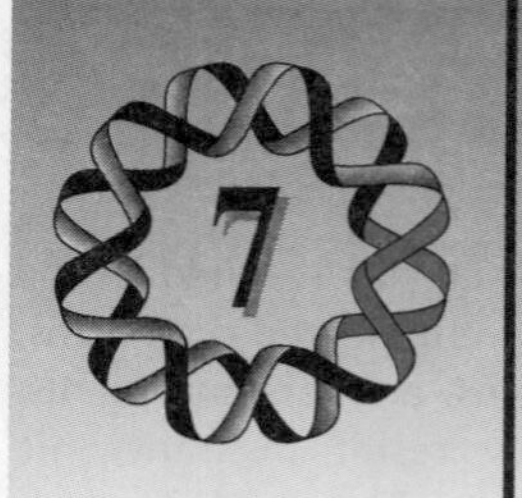

Basic Techniques in Genetic Engineering

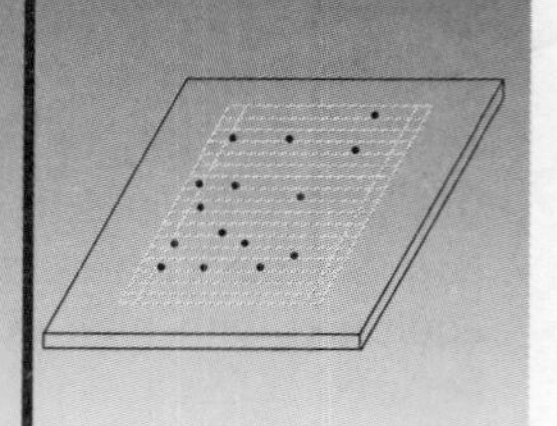

There are several techniques used in recombinant DNA technology or gene manipulation. The most frequently used methods are listed.

- Agarose gel electrophoresis.
- Isolation and purification of nucleic acids.
- Isolation of chromosomes.
- Nucleic acid blotting techniques.
- DNA sequencing.
- Alternate methods of DNA sequencing.
- Chemical synthesis of DNA.
- Methods of gene transfer (Chapters 6 and 49).
- Polymerase chain reaction (Chapter 8).
- Production of monoclonal antibodies (Chapter 17).
- Construction of gene library (Chapter 9).
- Radiolabeling of nucleic acids (Chapter 9).

Some details on the first seven techniques are described in this chapter while other technique are discussed elsewhere (as referred in the corresponding chapters). It may however, be noted that some specific applications of these techniques are frequently referred to as when needed in the corresponding chapters.

AGAROSE GEL ELECTROPHORESIS

Electrophoresis refers to the ***movement of charged molecules in an electric field.*** The negatively charged molecules move towards the positive electrode while the positively charged molecules migrate towards the negative electrode.

Gel electrophoresis is a routinely used analytical technique for the separation/purification of specific DNA fragments. The gel is composed of either polyacrylamide or agarose. Polyacrylamide gel electrophoresis (PAGE) is used for the separation of smaller DNA fragments while agarose electrophoresis is convenient for the separation of DNA fragments ranging in size from 100 base pairs to 20 kb pairs. Gel electrophoresis can also be used for the separation of RNA molecules.

Agarose is a ***polysaccharide*** derived from seaweeds. It forms a solid gel when dissolved in aqueous solution at concentrations between 0.5 and 2.0% (w/v). It may be noted here that the agarose used for electrophoresis is more purified form of agar when compared to that used for culture purposes.

A diagrammatic view of the agarose gel electrophoresis unit is shown in ***Fig. 7.1***.

The DNA samples are placed in the wells of the gel surface and the power supply is switched on. As the DNA is negatively charged, DNA fragments

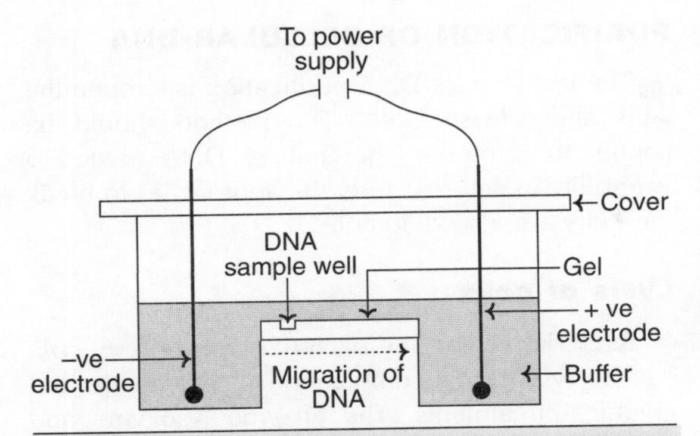

Fig. 7.1 : A diagrammatic representation of agarose gel electrophoresis system.

move through the gel towards the positive electrode. The rate of migration of DNA is dependent on the size and shape. In general, smaller linear fragments move faster than the larger ones. Hence, gel electrophoresis can be conveniently used for the separation of a mixture of DNA fragments, based on their size.

Agarose forms gels with pore sizes ranging from 100 to 300 nm in diameter. The actual pore size depends on the concentration of the agarose. The size of the pores determines the range of DNA fragments that can be separated on electrophoresis. For instance, a 0.3% agarose is used for the separation of DNA fragments between 5 and 50 kb, while a 5% agarose can separate 100–500 bp molecules.

The migration of DNA fragments during the course of electrophoresis can be monitored by using dyes with known migration rates. These dyes are added to the DNA samples before loading. The bands of the DNA can be detected by soaking the gel in ***ethidium bromide*** solution. When activated by ultraviolet radiation, DNA base pairs in association with ethidium bromide emit orange fluorescence. And in this way the DNA fragments separated in agarose electrophoresis can be identified (***Fig. 7.2***).

PULSED-FIELD GEL ELECTROPHORESIS (PFGE)

The large sized DNA molecules (~ 10 Mb) can be separated in agarose gels by using PFGE. This is made possible by periodically altering the direction of DNA migration by changing the orientation of electric field with respect to the gel. As the electric field orientation changes, the DNA molecules align themselves and migrate in new directions.

Limitation of PFGE : The major limitation of pulsed-field gel electrophoresis is that the samples do not migrate in straight lines. This makes the further analysis of DNA rather difficult.

CONTOUR-CLAMPED HOMOGENEOUS ELECTRICAL-FIELD ELECTROPHORESIS (CHEF)

CHEF is an improved method to apply alternating electrical fields to separate DNA molecules in electrophoresis. In this approach, the reorientation angle of electrical field is fixed at 120°C (or even at 90°) and electrophoresis carried out. By using CHEF, large DNA fragments (200–300 kb) can be routinely separated in a matter of hours.

POLYACRYLAMIDE GEL ELECTROPHORESIS (PAGE)

Polyacrylamide gel is composed of chains of acrylamide monomers cross-linked with methylenebisacrylamide units. The pore size of the gel is dependent on the total concentration of the monomers and the cross links.

Polyacrylamide gel electrophoresis (PAGE) is used ***for the separation of single-stranded DNA molecuels that differ in length by just one nucleotide***. Agarose gels cannot be used for this purpose. This is because polyacrylamide gels have

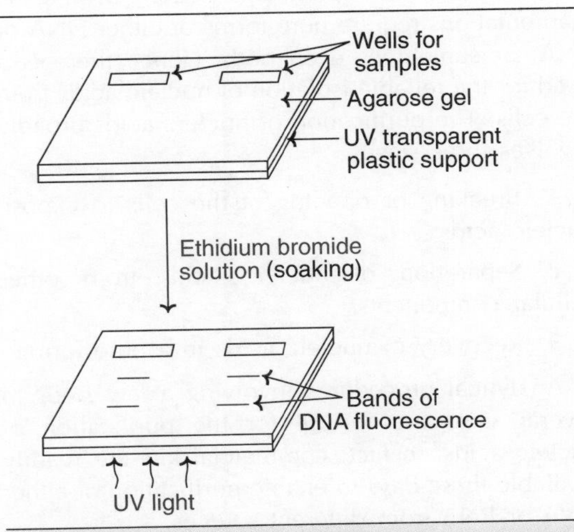

Fig. 7.2 : Identification of DNA bands separated by agarose gel electrophoresis.

smaller pore sizes than agarose gels and allow precise separation of DNA molecules from 10–1500 bp.

Polyacrylamide gel electrophoresis is a wonderful technique for the fine separation of DNA molecules that differ from each other even by 1-3 nucleotides. PAGE is used in DNA sequencing, and for the identification of amplified products of DNA by polymerase chain reaction (PCR).

OTHER USES OF GEL ELECTROPHORESIS

Besides the separation of DNA fragments, gel electrophoresis is also useful for understanding the molecular configuration of DNA molecules, and protein-nucleic acid interactions. The latter is based on the principle that binding of a protein to DNA usually results in the reduction of electrophoretic mobility.

The electrophoretic technique for protein-nucleic acid interaction involves the addition of a desired protein to double-stranded DNA fragments, separation of this complex and naked DNA by electrophoresis. The separated patterns can be visualized to understand the protein-nucleic acid interactions.

ISOLATION AND PURIFICATION OF NUCLEIC ACIDS

Almost all the experiments dealing with gene manipulations require pure forms of either DNA or RNA, or sometimes even both. Hence there is a need for the reliable isolation of nucleic acids from the cells. The purification of nucleic acids broadly involves three stages.

1. Breaking or opening of the cells to expose nucleic acids.

2. Separation of nucleic acids from other cellular components.

3. Recovery of nucleic acids in a pure form.

Analytical procedures involving a few steps to several steps are in use for the purification of nucleic acids. In fact, commercial kits are readily available these days to enable purification of either DNA or RNA from different sources.

The basic principles and procedures for nucleic acid purification are briefly described.

PURIFICATION OF CELLULAR DNA

The first step for DNA purification is to open the cells and release DNA. The method should be gentle to preserve the native DNA. Due to variability in cell structure, the approaches to break the cells are also different.

Lysis of cells

Bacterial cells : The bacterial cells (e.g. *E. coli*) can be lysed by a combination of enzymatic and chemical treatments. The enzyme lysozyme and the chemical ethylenediamine tetraacetate (EDTA) are used for this purpose. This is followed by the addition of a detergent such as sodium dodecyl sulfate (SDS).

Animal cells : Animal cells, particularly cultured animal cells, can be easily opened by direct treatment of cells with detergents (SDS).

Plant cells : Plant cells with strong cell walls require harsh treatment to break open. The cells are frozen and then ground in a morter and pestle. This is an effective way of breaking the cellulose walls.

Methods to purify DNA

There are two different approaches to purify DNA from the cellular extracts.

1. **Purification of DNA by removing cellular components :** This involves the degradation or complete removal of all the cellular components other than DNA. This approach is suitable if the cells do not contain large quantities of lipids and carbohydrates.

The cellular extract is centrifuged at a low speed to remove the debris (e.g. pieces of cell wall) that forms a pellet at the bottom of the tube. The supernatant is collected and treated with phenol to precipitate proteins at the interface between the organic and aqueous layers. The aqueous layer, containing the dissolved nucleic acids, is collected and treated with the enzyme ribonuclease (RNase). The RNA is degraded while the DNA remains intact. This DNA can be precipitated by adding ethanol and isolated after centrifugation, and suspended in an appropriate buffer.

2. **Direct purification of DNA :** In this approach, the DNA itself is selectively removed from the cellular extract and isolated. There are two ways for direct purification of DNA.

In one method, the addition of a detergent ***cetyltrimethyl ammonium*** (CTAB) results in the formation of an insoluble complex with nucleic acids. This complex, in the form of a precipitate is collected after centrifugation and suspended in a high-salt solution to release nucleic acids. By treatment with RNase, RNA is degraded. Pure DNA can be isolated by ethanol precipitation.

The second technique, is based on the principle of tight binding between DNA and silica particles in the presence of a denaturing agent such as guanidinium thiocyanate. The isolation of DNA can be achieved by the direct addition of silica particles and guanidinium thiocyanate to the cellular extract, followed by centrifugation. Alternately, a column chromatography containing silica can be used, and through this the extract and guanidinium thiocyanate are passed. The DNA binds to the silica particles in the column which can be recovered.

PURIFICATION OF PLASMID DNA

Pure forms of plasmid DNA are often required in genetic engineering experiments. The prerequisite for a successful isolation of plasmid DNA is the appropriate and gentle lysis of the host cells, so that the plasmid DNA is released without too much contamination of chromosomal DNA. The high molecular weight host cell chromosomal DNA can be removed along with the cell debris by high-speed centrifugation. This results in the formation of a ***cleared lysate*** from which pure plasmid DNA can be isolated. Of the several methods in use to isolate plasmid DNA, two are briefly described.

Isopycnic centrifugation method

The cleared lysate (referred above) is treated with a solution of cesium chloride (CsCl) containing ethidium bromide (EtBr). ***EtBr can bind with linear DNA molecules*** (chromosomal DNA fragments and open plasmid DNA) and not with circular plasmid DNA. The density of DNA-EtBr complex is much lower than the plasmid DNA. The circular plasmid DNA can be separated by isopycnic centrifugation in a CsCl-EtBr gradient (***Fig. 7.3***).

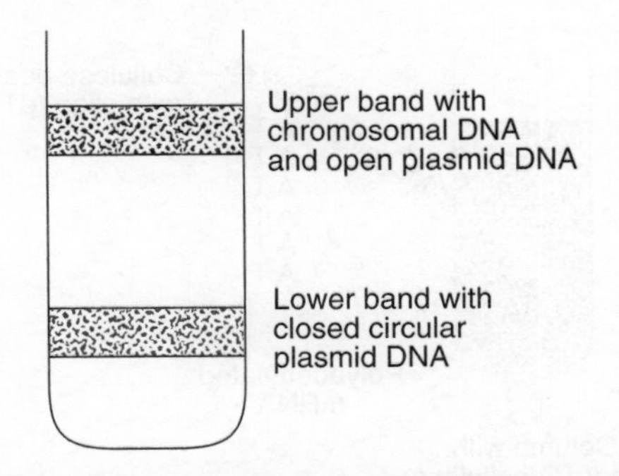

Fig. 7.3 : Purification of plasmid DNA by isopycnic centrifugation in CsCl-EtBr gradient.

Birnboim and Doly method

The technique developed by Birnboim and Doly (1979) is widely used for the purification of plasmid DNA. This method is based on the principle that there is a narrow range of ***pH (12.0–12.5) at which denaturation of linear DNA and not closed circular DNA occurs.***

When the cleared lysate is subjected to carefully monitored alkaline pH (12.0 to 12.5), the plasmid DNA molecules remain in solution while all other DNA molecules get denatured and precipitate. This precipitate can be removed by centrifugation. The plasmid DNA in the supernatant can be concentrated by ethanol precipitation. Sometimes, further purification of plasmid DNA may be necessary which can be achieved by gel filtration.

Factors affecting plasmid DNA purification

Several factors influence the purification of plasmid DNA. The most important ones are briefly described.

1. **Plasmid copy number :** The number of plasmids present in the host cells at the time of harvest is important. The copy number in turn is influenced by growth medium, genotype of host cell and the stage of growth. In general, the ***higher the copy number, the better is the yield of plasmid DNA on purification.***

2. **Preparation of cleared lysate :** The methodology adopted and the care taken for the lysis of the host cells to prepare cleared lysate is important.

3. **Host cells with *end A* gene :** The wild-type host cells posses *endA* gene that encodes the enzyme endonuclease I. The functions of this enzyme are not clearly known. It is however, observed that cell strains bearing *endA*

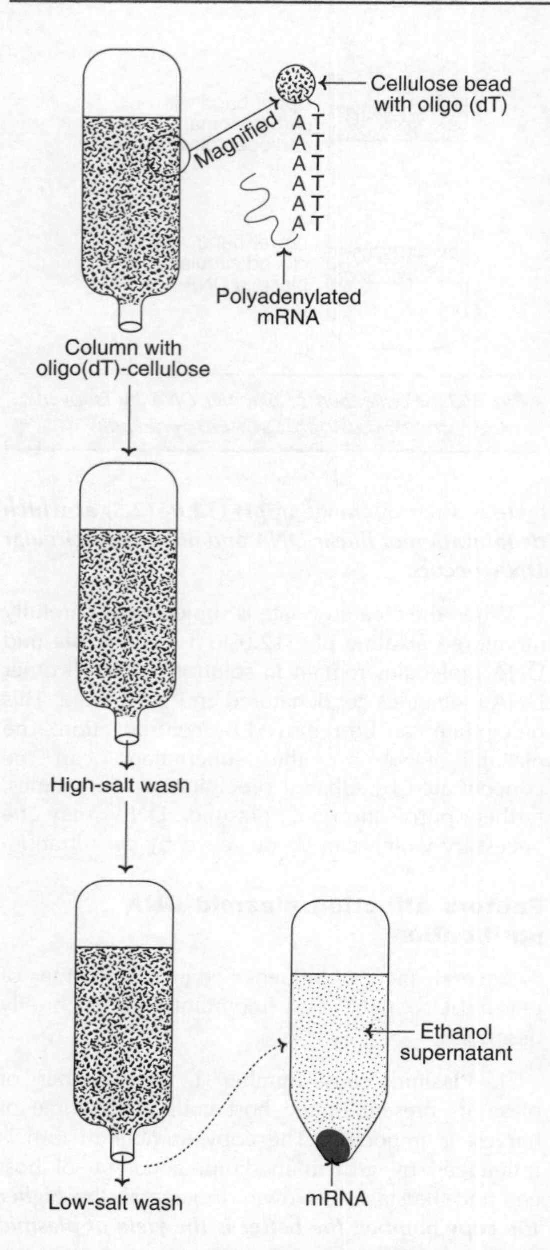

Fig. 7.4 : Purification of mRNA by affinity chromatography with oligo(dT)-cellulose.

mutations improve the stability and yield of plasmid DNA.

PURIFICATION OF mRNA

Among the RNAs, mRNA is frequently required in a pure form for genetic experiments.

After the cells are disrupted on lysis by different techniques (See p. 99), the cellular extract is deproteinised by treatment with phenol or phenol/ chloroform mixtures. On centrifugation, the nucleic acids get concentrated in the upper aqueous phase which may then be precipitated by using isopropanol or ethanol.

The purification of mRNA can be achieved by affinity chromatography using oligo (dT)-cellulose (***Fig. 7.4***). This is based on the principle that oligo (dT)-cellulose can specifically bind to the poly (A) tails of eukaryotic mRNA. Thus, by this approach, it is possible to isolate mRNA from DNA, rRNA and tRNA.

As the nucleic acid solution is passed through an affinity chromotographic column, the oligo(dT) binds to poly(A) tails of mRNA. By washing the column with high-salt buffer, DNA, rRNA and tRNA can be eluted, while the mRNA is tightly bound. This mRNA can be then eluted by washing with low-salt buffer. The mRNA is precipitated with ethanol and collected by centrifugation (***Fig. 7.4***).

ISOLATION OF CHROMOSOMES

Separation of large chromosomes of eukaryotes is not possible by conventional electrophoresis. The individual chromosomes of eukaryotes can be separated by ***fluorescence-activated cell sorting (FACS)***, also known as ***flow cytometry*** or ***flow karyotyping***.

FLUORESCENCE-ACTIVATED CELL SORTING

To carry out FACS, the dividing cells (with condensed chromosomes) are carefully broken open, and a mixture of intact chromosomes is prepared. These chromosomes are then stained with a fluorescent dye. The quantity of the dye that binds to a chromosome depends on its size. Thus, larger chromosomes (with more DNA) bind more dye and fluoresce more brightly than the smaller ones.

The dye-mixed chromosomes are diluted and passed through a fine aperture that results in the formation of a stream of droplets. Each droplet contains a single chromosome. The fluorescence of the chromosomes is detected by a laser. When the fluorescence indicates that the chromosome illuminated by the laser is the one desired,

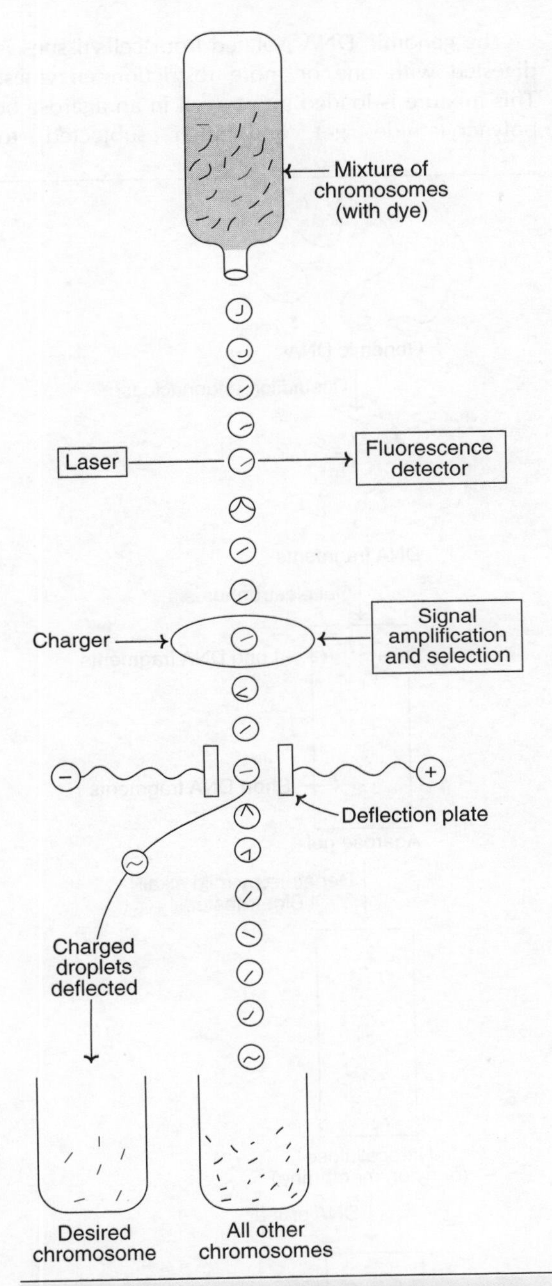

Fig. 7.5 : Separation of chromosomes by fluorescence-activated cell sorting (FACS).

electrical charge is specifically applied to these droplets (and no others) which get charged. This results in the deflection of the droplets with the desired chromosome which can be separated from the rest and collected (***Fig. 7.5***). Uncharged droplets that do not contain the desired chromosome pass through a waste collection vessel.

COLLECTION OF CHROMOSOMES WITH IDENTICAL SIZE

The direct application of FACS (described above) is not suitable for the separation of chromosomes with identical sizes. e.g. chromosomes 21 and 22 in humans. Collection of such chromosomes can be achieved by use of special dyes (e.g. Hoechst 33258 and chromomycin A_3) which bind to AT-rich DNA or GC-rich DNA. The rest of the procedure is the same that has been described.

It is convenient to separate two or more chromosomes with identical sizes by different dyes. This is possible since no two chromosomes are likely to contain identical GC/AT contents.

NUCLEIC ACID BLOTTING TECHNIQUES

Blotting techniques are very widely used analytical tools for the specific ***identification of desired DNA or RNA fragments*** from thousands of molecules. Blotting refers to the ***process of immobilization of sample nucleic acids or solid support*** (nitrocellulose or nylon membranes). The blotted nucleic acids are then used as targets in the hybridization experiments for their specific detection. An outline of the nucleic acid blotting technique is depicted in ***Fig. 7.6.***

Types of blotting techniques

The most comonly used blotting techniques are listed below

- Southern blotting (for DNA)
- Northern blotting (for RNA)
- Dot blotting (DNA/RNA)
- Colony and plaque hybridization (cells from colony).

The Southern blotting is named after the scientist Ed Southern (1975) who developed it. The other names Northern blotting and Western blotting are laboratory jargons which are now accepted. ***Western blotting involves the transfer of protein blots and their identification by using specific antibodies***.

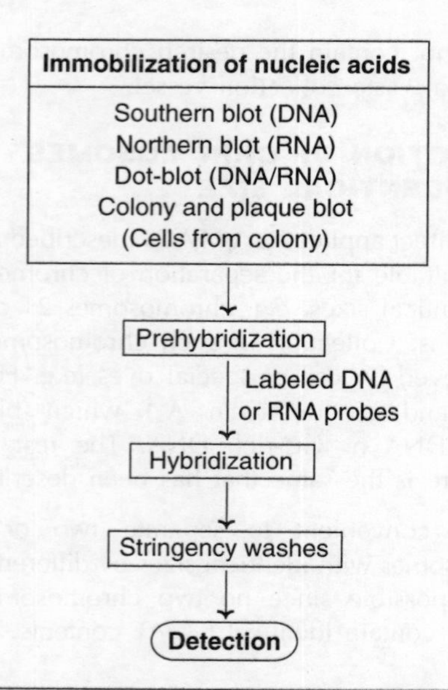

Fig. 7.6 : An outline of the nucleic acid blotting techniques.

A diagrammatic representation of a typical blotting apparatus is depicted in ***Fig. 7.7***.

SOUTHERN BLOTTING

Southern blotting technique is the first nucleic acid blotting procedure developed in 1975 by Southern. It is depicted in ***Fig. 7.8***, and briefly described.

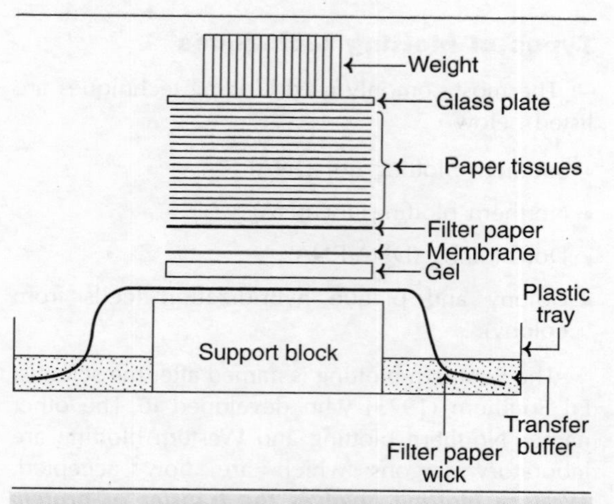

Fig. 7.7 : Diagrammatic representation of a typical blotting apparatus.

The genomic DNA isolated from cells/tissues is digested with one or more restriction enzymes. This mixture is loaded into a well in an agarose or polyacrylamide gel and then subjected to

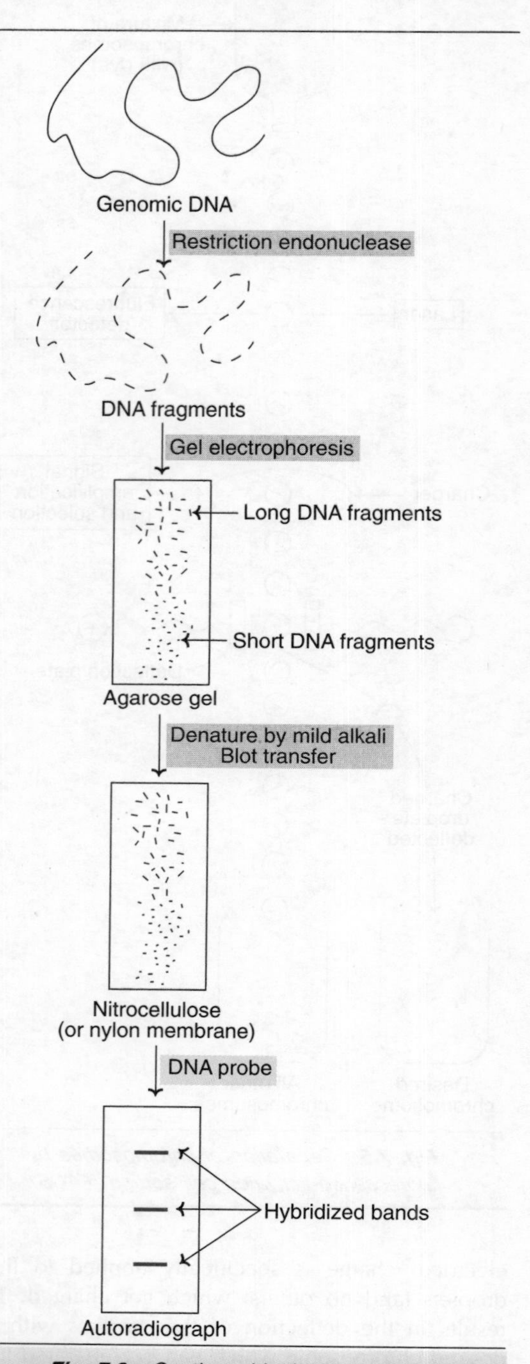

Fig. 7.8 : Southern blotting technique.

electrophoresis. DNA, being negatively charged migrates towards the anode (positively charged electrode); the smaller DNA fragments move faster.

The separated DNA molecules are denatured by exposure to a mild alkali and transferred to nitrocellulose or nylon paper. This results in an exact replica of the pattern of DNA fragments on the gel. The DNA can be annealed to the paper on exposure to heat (80°C). The nitrocellulose or nylon paper is then exposed to labeled cDNA probes. These probes hybridize with complementary DNA molecules on the paper.

The paper after thorough washing is exposed to X-ray film to develop autoradiograph. This reveals specific bands corresponding to the DNA fragments recognized by cDNA probe.

Factors affecting Southern blotting

1. **Stringent conditions (stringency control) :** Stringency refers to the specificity with which a particular DNA target sequence is detected by a probe. Thus, with high stringent conditions (elevated temperature and low salt concentration) only completely complementary DNA sequences will bind and hybridize. However, low stringent conditions will allow hybridization of partially matched sequences. Therefore, stringency control is very essential for specific detection of DNA molecules in Southern blotting. With good control of stringency, it is now possible to detect a DNA molecule just with a single base pair difference.

2. **Membranes for blot transfer :** In the early years, nitrocellulose was used for immobilization of DNA molecules during blot transfer. The drawback with nitrocellulose is that it is fragile and has to be carefully handled. In recent years, most laboratories use nylon membranes as they posses high tensile strength, and better binding capacity for nucleic acids.

Applications of Southern blotting

Southern blotting technique is extremely specific and sensitive, although it is a simple technique. Some of the applications are listed.

- It is an invaluable method in gene analysis.
- Important for the confirmation of DNA cloning results.
- Useful for mapping restriction sites around a single copy gene sequence.

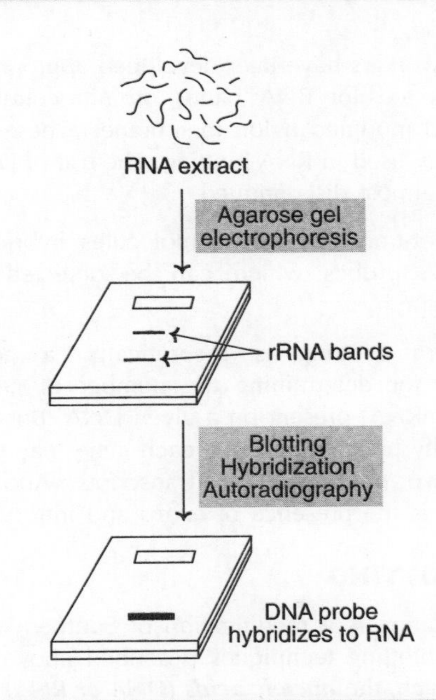

Fig. 7.9 : An outline of Northern blotting.

- Forensically applied to detect minute quantities of DNA (to identify parenthood, thieves, rapists etc.).
- Highly useful for the determination of restriction fragment length polymorphism (RFLP) associated with pathological conditions.
- DNA pieces from one species (e.g. human) can be used to detect DNA molecules from related species (e.g. chimpanze, cow). This technique is referred to as ***Zoo-blotting***.

NORTHERN BLOTTING

Northern blotting is the technique for the ***specific identification of RNA molecules***. The procedure adopted is almost similar to that described for Southern blotting and is depicted in ***Fig. 7.9***. RNA molecules are subjected to electrophoresis, followed by blot transfer, hybridization and autoradiography.

RNA molecules do not easily bind to nitrocellulose paper or nylon membranes. Blot-transfer of RNA molecules is carried out by using a chemically reactive paper prepared by diazotization of aminobenzyloxymethyl to create diazobenzyloxymethyl (DBM) paper. The RNA can covalently bind to DBM paper.

Some workers have later developed appropriate conditions to blot RNA bands on nitrocellulose paper, and modified nylon membranes. These are now widely used in RNA blotting. The use of DBM papers is almost discontinued.

The blot-transferred RNA molecules hybridize with DNA probes which can be detected by autoradiography.

Northern blotting is theoretically, a good technique for determining the number of genes (through mRNA) present on a given DNA. But this is not really practicable since each gene may give rise to two or more RNA transcripts. Another drawback is the presence of exons and introns.

DOT-BLOTTING

Dot-blotting is a modification of Southern and Northern blotting techniques described above. In this approach, the ***nucleic acids (DNA or RNA) are directly spotted onto the filters***, and not subjected to electrophoresis. The hybridization procedure is the same as in original blotting techniques.

Dot-blotting technique is particularly useful in obtaining quantitative data for the evaluation of gene expression.

WESTERN BLOTTING

Western blotting involves the ***identification of proteins***. It is to very useful to understand the nucleic acid functions, particularly during the course of gene manipulations.

The technique of Western blotting involves the transfer of electrophoresed protein bands from polyacrylamide gel to nylon or nitrocellulose membrane. These proteins can be detected by specific protein-ligand interactions. Antibodies or lectins are commonly used for this purpose.

AUTORADIOGRAPHY

Autoradiography is the process of ***localization and recording of a radiolabel*** within a solid specimen, with the production of an ***image in a photographic emulsion***. These emulsions are composed of silver halide crystals suspended in gelatin.

When a β-particle or a γ-ray from a radiolabel passes through the emulsions, silver ions are converted to metallic silver atoms. This results in the development of a visible image which can be easily detected.

Direct autoradiography

Direct autoradiography is ideally suited for the detection of weak to medium strength β-emitting radionuclides (^{3}H, ^{14}C, ^{35}S). In this technique, the sample is placed in direct contact with the film. The radioactive emissions result in the development of black areas.

Indirect autoradiography

For the detection of highly energetic β-particles (e.g. ^{32}P, ^{125}I), direct autoradiography is not suitable. This is because these emissions pass through and beyond the film, and a major part of the energy gets wasted.

Indirect autoradiography is useful for the detection of highly energetic β-particles. In this technique, the β-particle energy is first converted to light by a scintillator, which then emits photons on exposure to photographic emulsion.

Applications of autoradiography

As already described, autoradiography is closely associated with blotting techniques for the detection of DNA, RNA and proteins.

COLONY AND PLAQUE BLOTTING

Colony and plaque blotting is a process of hybridization for the specific ***identification and purification of colonies*** (e.g. bacterial clones). This technique is depicted in ***Fig. 7.10***, and briefly described hereunder.

The desired bacteria are grown as colonies on an agar plate. When a nitrocellulose filter paper is overlaid on the agar plate, the colonies get transferred. They are permanently fixed to the paper by heat. On treatment with alkali (NaOH), the cells lyse and the DNA gets denatured. When these DNA prints are exposed to specific probes (radiolabel), hybridization occurs. The hybrid complex can be localized and detected by autoradiography.

A similar strategy (described above for bacteria) can be used for the identification of phages and fragments of phage libraries.

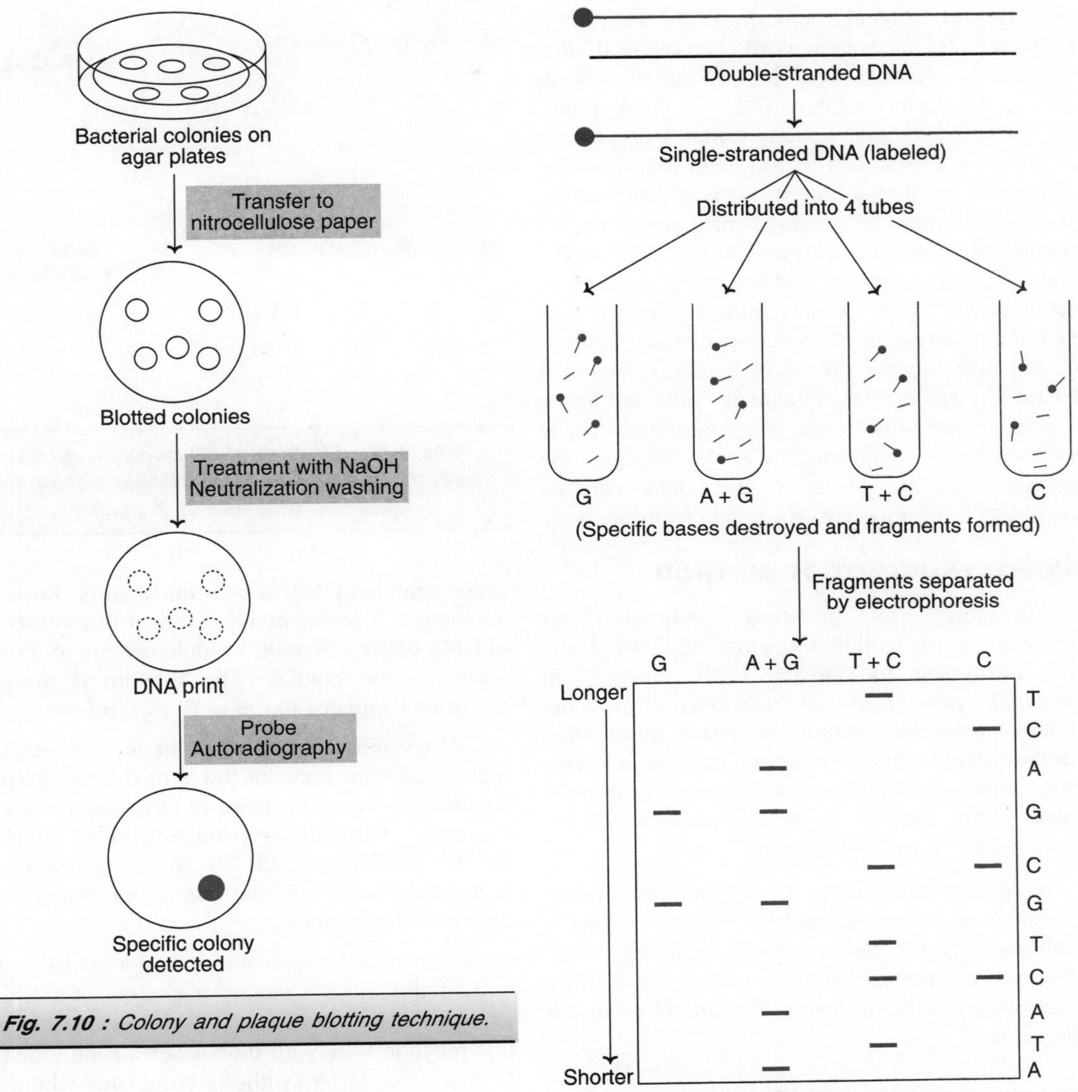

Fig. 7.10 : Colony and plaque blotting technique.

Fig. 7.11 : Maxam and Gilbert method for DNA sequencing.

DNA SEQUENCING

Determination of nucleotide sequence in a DNA molecule is the basic and fundamental requirement in biotechnology. DNA sequencing is important to understand the functions of genes, and basis of inherited disorders. Further, DNA cloning and gene manipulation invariably require knowledge of accurate nucleotide sequence.

MAXAM AND GILBERT TECHNIQUE

The first DNA sequencing technique, ***using chemical reagents***, was developed by Maxam and Gilbert (1977). This method is briefly described below (**Fig. 7.11**).

A strand of source DNA is labeled at one end with ^{32}P. The two strands of DNA are then separated. The labeled DNA is distributed into four samples (in separate tubes). Each sample is subjected to treatment with a chemical that specifically destroys one (G, C) or two bases (A + G, T + C) in the DNA. Thus, the DNA strands are partially digested in four samples at sites G, A + G, T + C and C. This results in the formation of a series of labeled fragments of varying lengths. The actual length of the fragment depends on the site at which the base is destroyed from the labeled end. Thus for instance, if there are C residues at positions 4, 7, and 10 away from the labeled end, then the treatment of DNA that specifically destroys C will give lebeled pieces of length 3, 6 and 9 bases. The labeled DNA fragments obtained in the four tubes are subjected to electrophoresis side by side and they are detected by autoradiograph. The sequence of the bases in the DNA can be constructed from the bands on the electrophoresis.

DIDEOXYNUCLEOTIDE METHOD

Currently, the preferred technique for determining nucleotide sequence in DNA is the one ***developed by Sanger*** (1980). This is an ***enzymatic procedure*** commonly referred to as the dideoxynucleotide method or ***chain termination method*** (**Note :** Fredrick Sanger won Nobel prize twice, once for determining the structure of protein, insulin; the second time for sequencing the nucleotides in an RNA virus).

A dideoxynucleotide is a laboratory-made chemical molecule that lacks a hydroxyl group at both the 2′ and 3′ carbons of the sugar (***Fig. 7.12***). This is in contrast to the natural deoxyribonucleotide that possesses at 3′ hydroxyl group on the sugar.

Termination role of dideoxynucleotide

In the normal process of DNA replication, an incoming nucleoside triphosphate is attached by its 5′-phosphate group to the 3′-hydroxyl group of the last nucleotide of the growing chain (Refer Chapter 3) when a dideoxynucleotide is incorporated to the growing chain, no further replication occurs. This is because dideoxynucleotide, lacking a 3′-hydroxyl group, cannot form a phosphodiester bond and thus the DNA synthesis terminates.

Sequencing method

The process of sequencing DNA by dideoxynucleotide method is briefly described. A single-stranded DNA to be sequenced is chosen as a template. It is attached to a primer (a short length of DNA oligonucleotide) complementary to a small section of the template. The 3′-hydroxyl group of the primer initiates the new DNA synthesis.

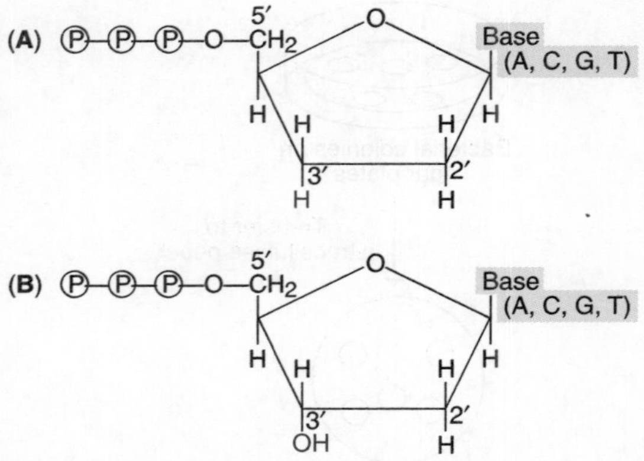

*Fig. 7.12 : Structure of **(A)** dideoxynucleotide triphosphate and **(B)** deoxynucleotide triphosphate (Note the difference at 3′-carbon).*

DNA synthesis is carried out in four reaction tubes. Each tube contains the primed DNA, ***Klenow subunit*** (the larger fragment of DNA polymerase of *E. coli*), four dideoxyribonucleotides (ddATP, ddCTP, ddGTP or ddTTP). It is necessary to radiolabel (with ^{32}P) the primer or one of the deoxyribonucleotides.

As the new DNA synthesis is completed, each one of the tubes contains fragments of DNA of varying length bound to primer. Let us consider the first reaction tube with dideoxyadenosine (ddATP). In this tube, DNA synthesis terminates whenever the growing chain incorporated ddA (complementary to dT on the template strand). Therefore, this tube will contain a series of different length DNA fragments, each ending with ddA. In a smilar fashion, for the other 3 reaction tubes, DNA synthesis stops as the respective dideoxynucleotides are incorporated.

The synthesis of new DNA fragments in the four tubes is depicted in ***Fig. 7.13***.

The DNA pieces are denatured to yield free strands with radiolabel. The samples from each tube are separated by polyacrylamide gel electrophoresis. This separation technique resolves DNA pieces, different in size even by a single

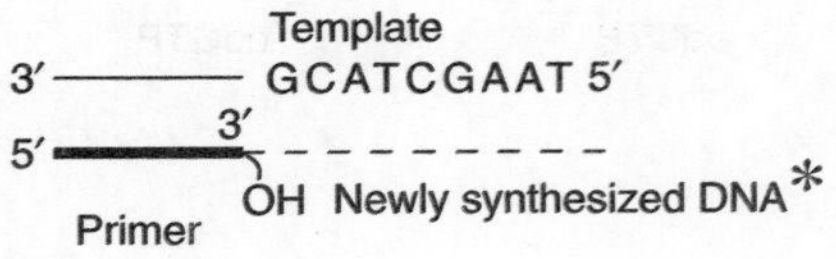

Template
3′ ——— GCATCGAAT 5′
3′
5′ ━━━ - - - - - - - - -
OH Newly synthesized DNA*
Primer

Reaction tube with dideoxynucleotide	Primer with nucleotide extended	Primer with sequence of nucleotides extended
ddATP	Primer + 4	Primer–CGTddA
	Primer + 9	Primer–CGTAGCTTddA
ddCTP	Primer + 1	Primer–ddC
	Primer + 6	Primer–CGTAGddC
ddGTP	Primer + 2	Primer–CddG
	Primer + 5	Primer–CGTAddG
ddTTP	Primer + 3	Primer–CGddT
	Primer + 7	Primer–CGTAGCddT
	Primer + 8	Primer–CGTAGCTddT

Fig. 7.13 : Synthesis of new DNA fragments in the presence of dideoxynucleotides (the size of the new DNA is variable, depending on the chain termination).*

nucleotide. The shortest DNA will be the fastest moving on the electrophoresis.

The sequence of bases in a DNA fragment is determined by identifying the electrophoretic (radiolabeled) bands by autoradiography. In the ***Fig. 7.14***, the sequence of the newly synthesized DNA fragment that is complementary to the original DNA piece is shown. It is conventional to read the bands from bottom to top in 5′ to 3′ direction. By noting the order of the bands first C, second G, third T and so on, the sequence of the DNA can be determined accurately. As many as 350 base sequences of a DNA fragment can be clearly identified by using autoradiographs.

Modifications of dideoxynucleotide method

Replacement of ^{32}P-radiolabel by ^{33}P or ^{35}S improves the sharpness of autoradiographic images. DNA polymerase of the thermophilic bacterium, *Thermus aquaticus* (in place of Klenow fragment of *E. coli* DNA polymerase I) or a modified form of phage T7 DNA polymerase (sequenase) improves the technique.

Limitations of dideoxynucleotide method

There are mainly two limitations in this techniques. The need for a single-stranded DNA template and the use of a primer to an unknown sequences. These problems can be overcome by using bacteriophage M_{13}.

BACTERIOPHAGE M_{13} AS A CLONING AND DNA SEQUENCING VECTOR

The life cycle of phage M_{13} is depicted in ***Fig. 7.15***. This virus contains a single-stranded circular DNA. When it infects *E. coli*, the double-stranded DNA is synthesized which is a replicative form (RF). RF DNA replicates until 50–100 copies are produced. Now the mode of replication is changed to synthesize single-stranded DNA (ssDNA) molecules. Each of the ssDNA of phage M_{13} is coated with a protein. The phage particles then freely pass through the membrane to be released out. Thus, the *E. coli* cells infected with M_{13} can continuously secrete infective particles, without undergoing lysis.

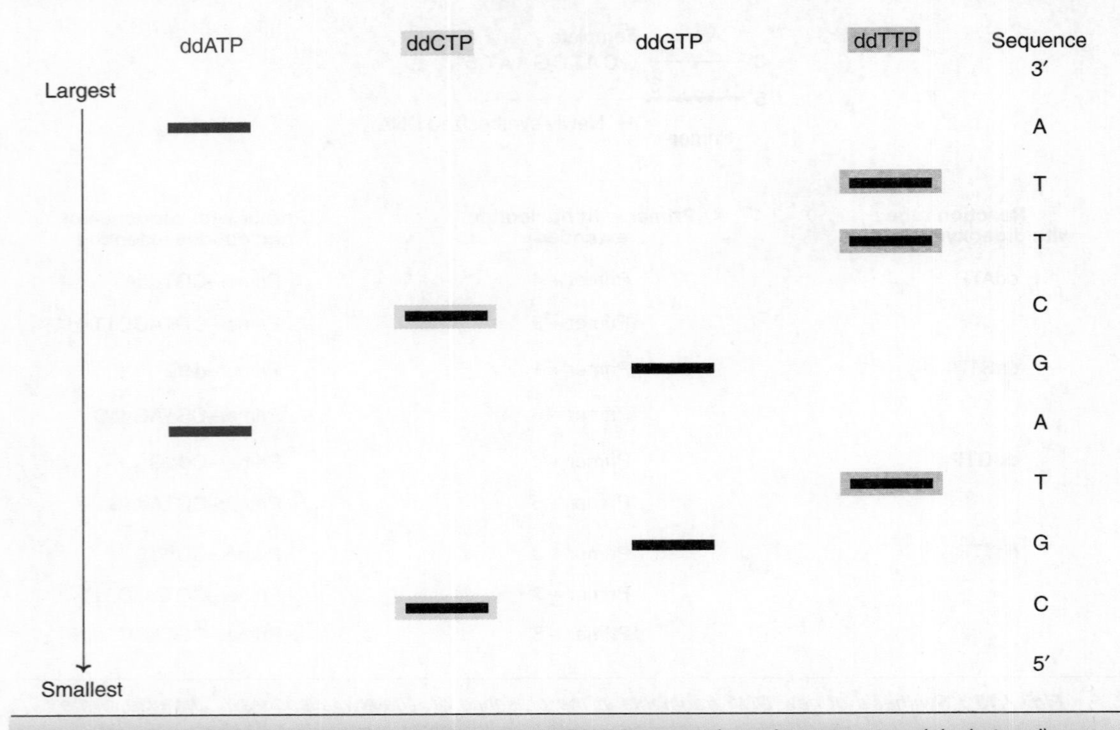

Fig. 7.14 : Sequence of the newly synthesized DNA fragment (complementary to original strand).

Bacteriophage M_{13} is employed as a cloning and DNA sequence determining vector. This is possible since the double-stranded replicative form can be isolated and used as a plasmid, while the single-stranded phage DNA can be employed as a template for DNA sequencing. Usually, a target DNA with less than 500 bp can be cloned and sequenced in phage M_{13}.

This double-stranded RF forms of phage M_{13} are isolated and the DNA to be cloned is inserted. This phage which is comparable to a plasmid is returned to *E. coli.* (The uptake of phages with inserts can be screened by using *lac Z* marker). As the phage undergoes its life cycle (***Fig. 7.15***), single-stranded DNA molecules of the inserted DNA are recovered. Sequence determination of the single-stranded DNA can be done by dideoxynucleotide method (See p. 102). The primer used is complementary to a part of phage M_{13} DNA which is close to the point of insertion. Therefore, a single primer can be used for different DNA molecules inserted.

For determining the sequence of a larger DNA (≤ 2,000 bp), it is necessary to clone different pieces of the DNA. From the sequences of these fragments (frequently overlapping), the final sequence can be built.

DNA SEQUENCING BY PRIMER WALKING

Primer walking or ***primer extension technique*** is employed for sequence determination of long pieces of DNA (≥ 5,000 bp). In this method, plasmid cloned DNA containing target DNA is annealed with a primer (synthetic oligonucleotide). The primer binds with the DNA close to the inserted DNA. Now the target DNA (250–350 nucleotides) is sequenced, most frequently by ***dideoxynucleotide method*** (described already).

From the base sequence of a fragment of the target DNA (determined in the first round), the second primer is chosen. It is an oligonucleotide to bind to a region approximately 300 nucleotides away from first primer binding. The next fragment of target DNA can be sequenced by another 250–300 bases (second round). This sequence will be useful to choose the third primer and determine the next 250–350 bases (third round). In this fashion, the primer walking is continued until the

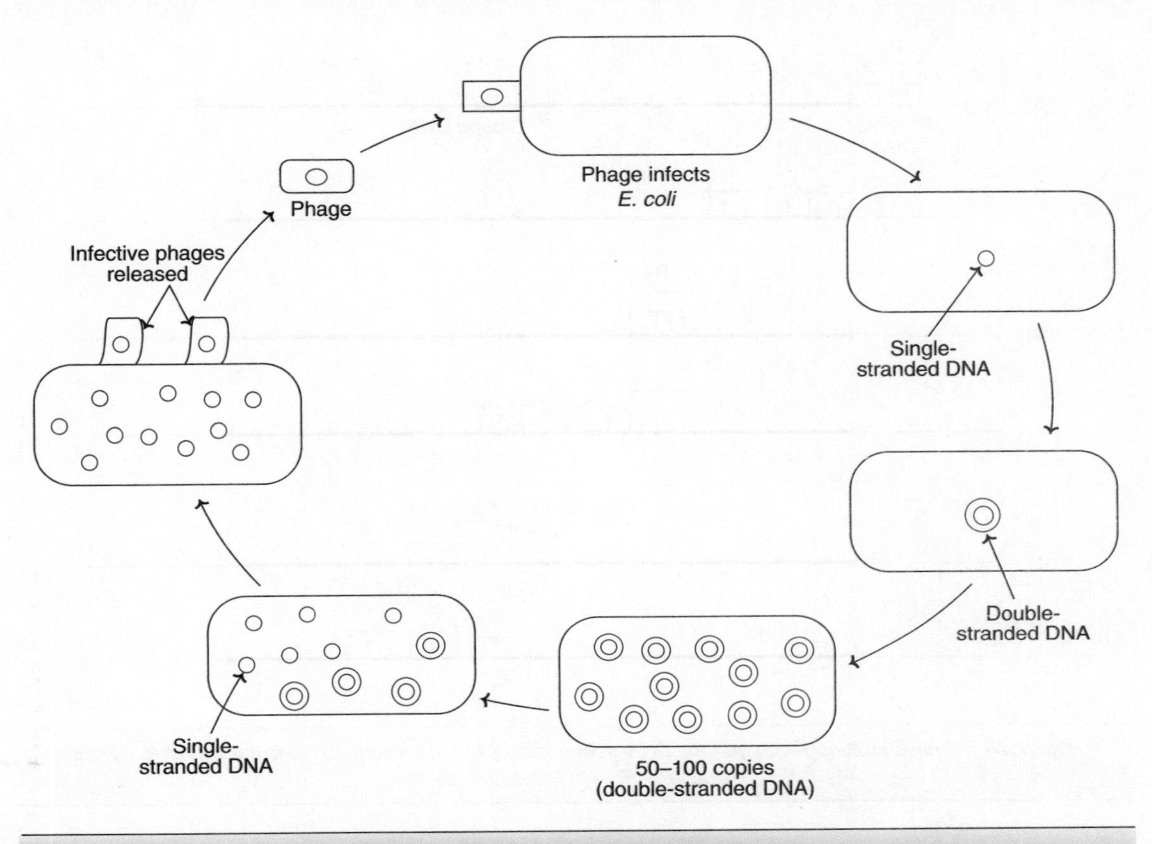

***Fig. 7.15** : The life cycle of bacteriophage M_{13}*

complete target DNA is sequenced. Three rounds of primer walking technique for DNA sequencing are depicted in ***Fig. 7.16***.

CHROMOSOME WALKING IN DNA SEQUENCING

Chromosome walking is a DNA base sequencing method in which the chromosome is analysed by extending one tip to reach the other. The technique basically involves systematically ***moving along the chromosome from a known location to an unknown location***, and thus ***determining the DNA sequence***. The method adopted in chromosome walking is depicted in ***Fig. 7.17***, and briefly described below.

A DNA fragment with approximately 40,000 base pairs can be sequenced. To start with a marker is used to identify the appropriate gene probe (from the DNA probe library). This gene probe must have a section of the base pair identical to the base pairs of the marker. This initial probe will hybridize only with the clones containing fragment A. This fragment A can be isolated, cloned and used as a probe to detect fragment B. This procedure of cloning and probing with fragments is repeated again and again until fragment D hybridizes with fragment E.

As is evident from the above description, chromosome walking uses probes derived from the ends of overlapping clones to facilitate a walk along with the DNA sequence. In the process of this walk, the sequence of the desired target gene can be identified.

Chromosome jumping

An improved strategy of chromosome walking is chromosome jumping. Many regions of DNA that are difficult to be cloned by walking can be jumped. The procedure involves the circularization of large genomic fragments generated by the

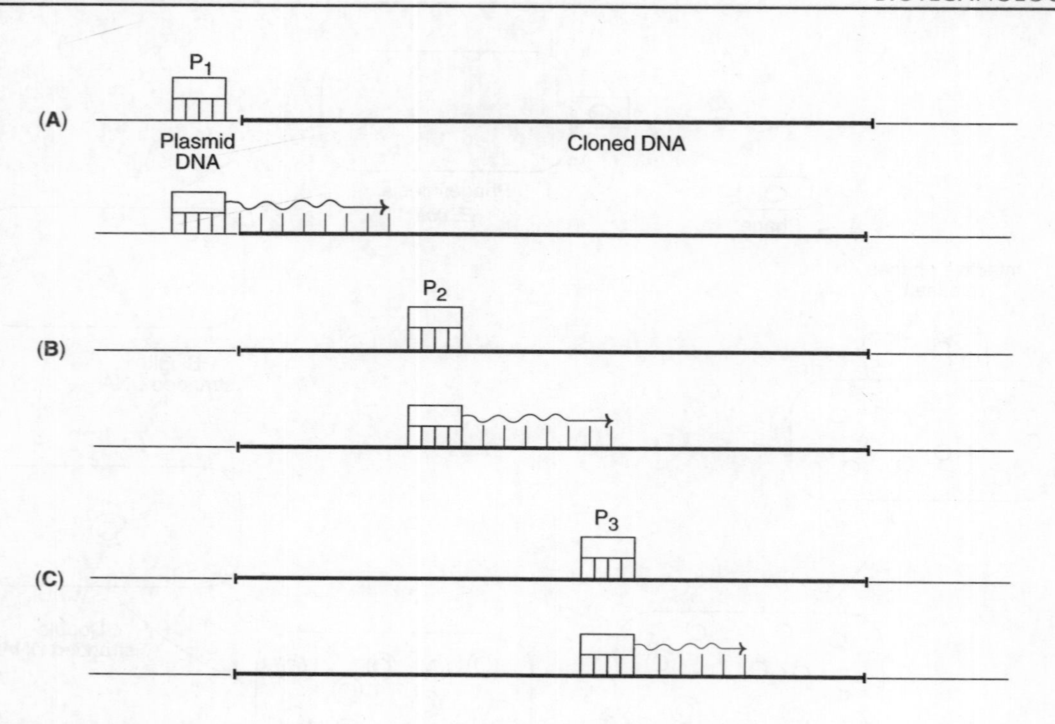

*Fig. 7.16 : Primer walking technique for DNA sequencing **(A)** First round **(B)** Second round **(C)** Third round (P_1, P_2, P_3–Primers 1, 2, 3).*

digestion of endonucleases. This is followed by cloning of the region lowering the closure of the fragment. By this approach, the ***DNA sequences located at far off places can be brought together and cloned***. A chromosome jumping can be constructed in this manner and used for long distance chromosome walks.

Applications of chromosome walking and jumping

The gene responsible for the disease ***cystic fibrosis (CF)*** has been ***identified*** by chromosome walking and jumping. The gene of protein responsible for CF is called cystic fibrosis transmembrane conductance regulator (CFTR) and is located on the long arm of chromosome 7.

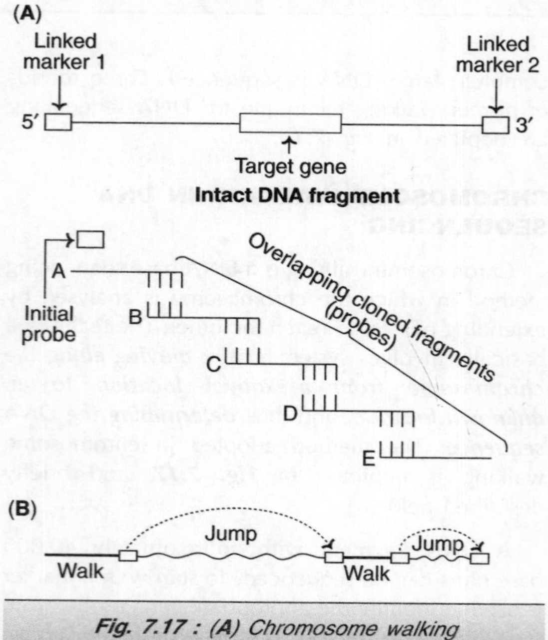

Fig. 7.17 : (A) Chromosome walking (B) Chromosome jumping.

AUTOMATED DNA SEQUENCING

DNA sequencing in the recent years is carried out by an ***automated DNA sequencer***. In this technique, flourescent tags are attached to chain-terminating nucleotides (dideoxynucleotides). This tag gets incorporated into the DNA molecules, while terminating new strand synthesis. Four different fluorescent dyes are used to identify chain-terminating reactions in a sequencing gel. The DNA bands are separated by electrophoresis and detected by their fluorescence. Recently, four dyes that exhibit strong absorption in laser are in use for automated sequencing.

Advantages of automated sequencing : It is a rapid and accurate technique. Automated DNA sequencer can accurately sequence up to 100,00 nucleotides per day. The cost works out to be not more than $0.2 per nucleotide. Automated DNA sequencing has been successfully ***used in the human genome project***.

ALTERNATIVE METHODS OF DNA SEQUENCING

Some groups of research workers have developed alternate methods to Sanger method for sequencing of DNA. Unfortunately, despite the initial excitement, most of these methods have disappeared from the scene. There are at least two methods with some promise for DNA sequencing- ***pyrosequencing***, and ***gene chips*** (microarrays).

PYROSEQUENCING

Pyrosequencing is a DNA sequencing method that is based on the principle of ***determining which one of the four bases (A, G, C, T) is incorporated at each step while a DNA template is copied***. In this technique, the template copies in a straight forward manner whithout added dideoxy-nucleotides (ddNTPs). As the new strand is synthesized, the order in which the deoxy-nucleotides (dNTPs) are incorporated is detected, and the sequence can be read as the reaction proceeds (***Fig. 7.18***). The identification of base addition becomes possible since the addition of a nucleotide is accompanied by the release of a molecule of pyrophosphate. This can be detected by chemiluminescence technique.

In the procedure of pyrosequencing, each dNTP is added individually (not all four together), along with a nucleotidase enzyme. This enzyme degrades the dNTP if it is not incorporated into the newly synthesized DNA strand. Once the appropriate nucleotide is incorporated into the new DNA strand, a molecule of pyrophosphate is released. This can be converted by the enzyme sulfurylase into a flash of light (chemiluminescence). By the addition of each dNTP separately, one after another, the order of the nucleotides added to the growing DNA strand can be followed, and the sequence can be identified.

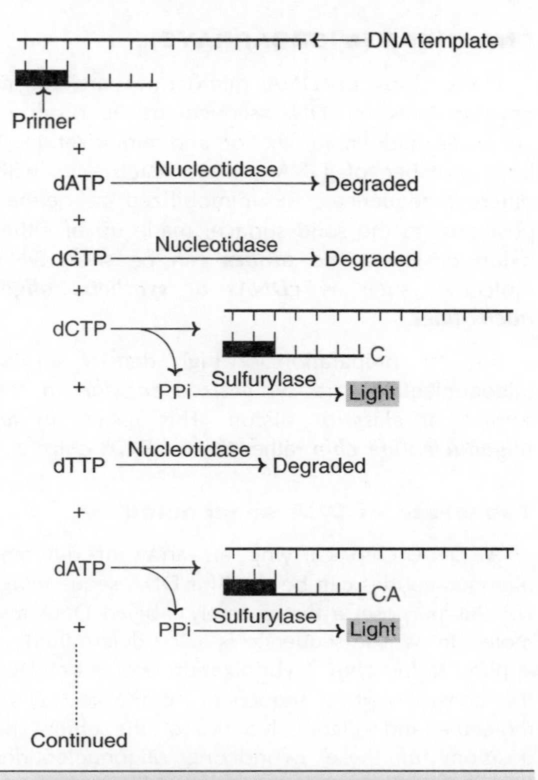

Fig. 7.18 : The technique of pyrosequencing.

Detection of the molecule ***pyro***phosphate is the basis of DNA ***sequencing***, hence the name ***pyrosequencing***. Since pyrosequencing does not require electrophoresis or any other DNA fragment separation technique, it is more rapid than chain termination sequencing.

The major ***limitation*** of pyrosequencing is that it is suitable to detect the ***sequence of about 200 nucleotides***. This is much less than the Sanger method. Many improvements are being made in pyrosequencing so that much longer DNA molecules can be sequenced. In fact, an automated system for pyrosequencing is also available now.

DNA CHIPS (MICROARRAYS)

DNA chips or DNA microarrays are recent developments for DNA sequencing as result of advances made in automation and miniarization. A large number of DNA probes, each one with different sequence, are immobilized at defined positions on the solid surface, made up of either nylon or glass. The ***probes*** can be short DNA molecules such as ***cDNAs or synthetic oligonucleotides***.

For the preparation of high density arrays, oligonucleotides are synthesized *in situ* on the surface of glass or silicon. This results in an ***oligonucleotide chip*** rather than a DNA chip.

Technique of DNA sequencing

A DNA chip carrying an array of different oligonucleotides can be used for DNA sequencing. For this purpose, a fluorescently labeled DNA test molecule, whose sequence is to be determined, is applied to the chip. Hybridization occurs between the complementary sequences of the test DNA molecule and oligonucleotides of the chip. The positions of these hybridizing oligonucleotides can be determined by confocal microscopy. Each hybridizing oligonucleotide represents an 8-nucleotide sequence that is present in the DNA probe. The sequence of the test DNA molecule can be deduced from the overlaps between the sequences of the hybridizing oligonucleotides (***Fig. 7.19***).

Applications of DNA chips

There have been many successes with this relatively new technology of DNA chips. Some of them are listed.

- Identification of genes responsible for the development of nervous systems.
- Detection of genes responsible for inflammatory diseases.
- Construction of microarrays for every gene in the genome of *E. coli*, and almost all the genes of the yeast *Saccharomyces cerevisiae*.
- Expression of several genes in prokaryotes has been identified.
- Detection and screening of single nucleotide polymorphisms (SNPs).

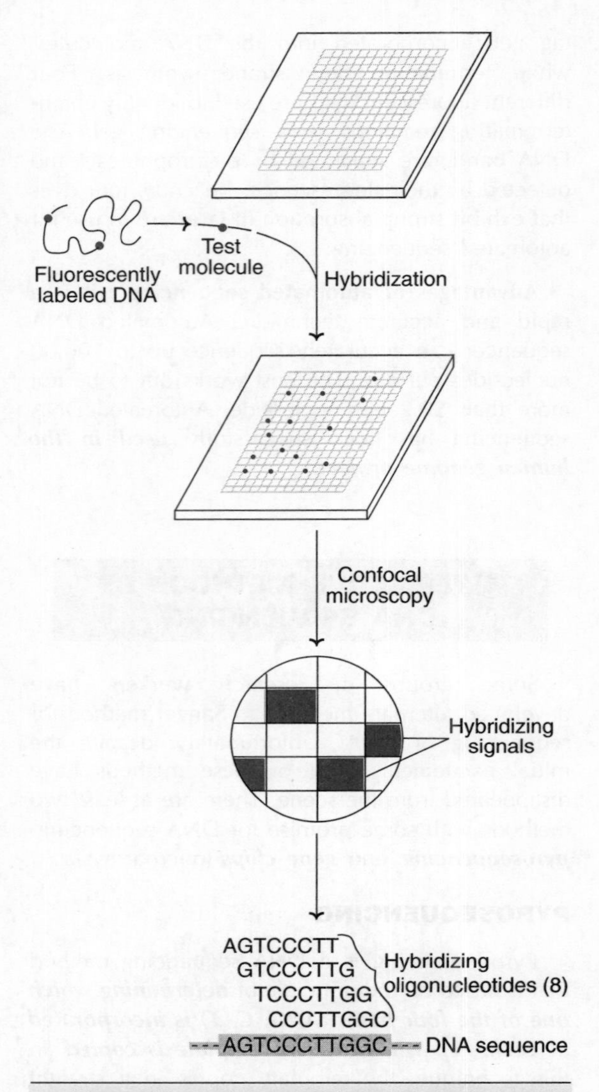

Fig. 7.19 : *Microarray (or chip) technology in DNA sequencing.*

- Rapid detection of microorganisms for environmental monitoring.

The future of DNA chips

The major limitation of DNA chips at present is the unavailability of complete genome arrays for higher eukaryotes, including humans. It is expected that within the next few years such DNA chips will be available. This will help the biotechnologists to capture the functional snapshots of the genome in action for higher organisms.

CHEMICAL SYNTHESIS OF DNA

Advances in the laboratory techniques have made it possible to chemically synthesize DNA in a short period. Thus, oligonucleotides of about 100 bases can be produced in about 10 hours. Laboratory synthesis of DNA (recently by use of ***DNA synthesizers or gene machines***) with specific sequence of nucleotides, rapidly and inexpensively, has significantly contributed to cloning. Chemical synthesis of DNA is based on the ability to protect the reactive – 5′ and – 3′ ends by blocking (protecting) them.

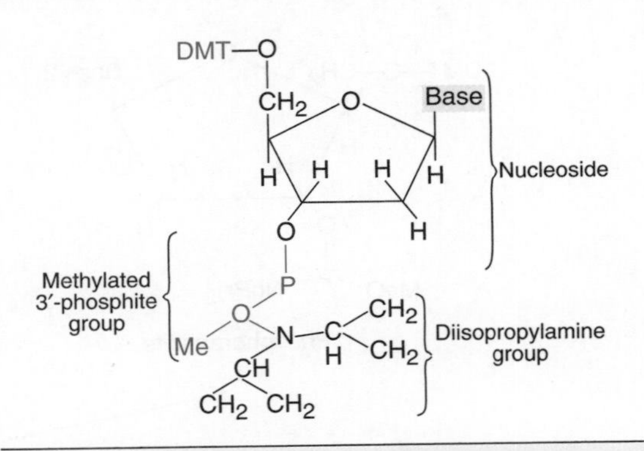

Fig. 7.20 : Structure of a phosphoramidite. (DMT-Dimethoxytrityl; Me-Methyl)

THE PHOSPHORAMIDITE METHOD

The phosphoramidite method is the technique of choice, currently in use, for the synthesis of DNA. The synthesis is carried out on a solid phase system i.e. by attaching the growing DNA strand to a solid support, in a reaction vessel. The procedure involves the following stages.

1. **Nucleoside attachment to solid support :** The initial nucleoside (base + sugar) is attached at 3′ end to an inert solid support, usually to glass beads with uniform pores, referred to as controlled pore glass (CPG) beads.

2. **Preparation of phosphoramidites :** For each one of the four bases (A, G, C and T), phosphoramidites can be synthesized. This is achieved by attaching dimethoxytrityl (DMT) group to the 5′-hydroxyl group of deoxyribose and a diisopropylamine group to the 3′-phosphite group of the nucleoside. A methyl residue protects the 3′-phosphite group. The general structure of phosphoramidite is depicted in ***Fig. 7.20***.

3. **Coupling :** A nucleotide precursor (i.e. a phosphoramidite) with its 3′-phosphorus couples with 5′-hydroxyl of the initial nucleoside bound to a CPG bead.

4. **Oxidation and deprotection :** The unstable trivalent phosphite is oxidized to pentavalent stable phosphate. This is followed by the removal of DMT that protects (deprotection) 5-hydroxyl group. For convenience, oxidation and deprotection are considered together in ***Fig. 7.21*** also, they are actually two independent reactions.

Another nucleotide precursor is now added and the reactions described in steps 3 and 4 are repeated.

Coupling, oxidation and deprotection are the three steps in the cyclic reaction for the DNA synthesis by phosphoramidite method. The cycles are repeated again and again to synthesise the desired DNA. At the end, the completed oligonucleotide is removed from the glass support and the groups protecting the bases and phosphates are cleaved.

Applications of synthesized oligonucleotides

Chemically synthesized oligonucleotides have a number of uses in biotechnology.

1. The linkers and adaptors are the oligonucleotides commonly employed in the preparation of recombinant DNA (Chapter 6).

2. Chemically synthesized DNAs with known sequences can be used for the synthesis of proteins/polypeptides.

3. DNA probes, particularly the single-stranded oligonucleotide probes, can be synthesized in the laboratory. This is based on the codon sequence of mRNA which in turn is dependent on the amino acid sequence.

4. Single-stranded oligonucleotides are used as primers in polymerase chain reaction (PCR).

5. For *in vitro* mutagenesis, single-stranded oligonucleotides are employed.

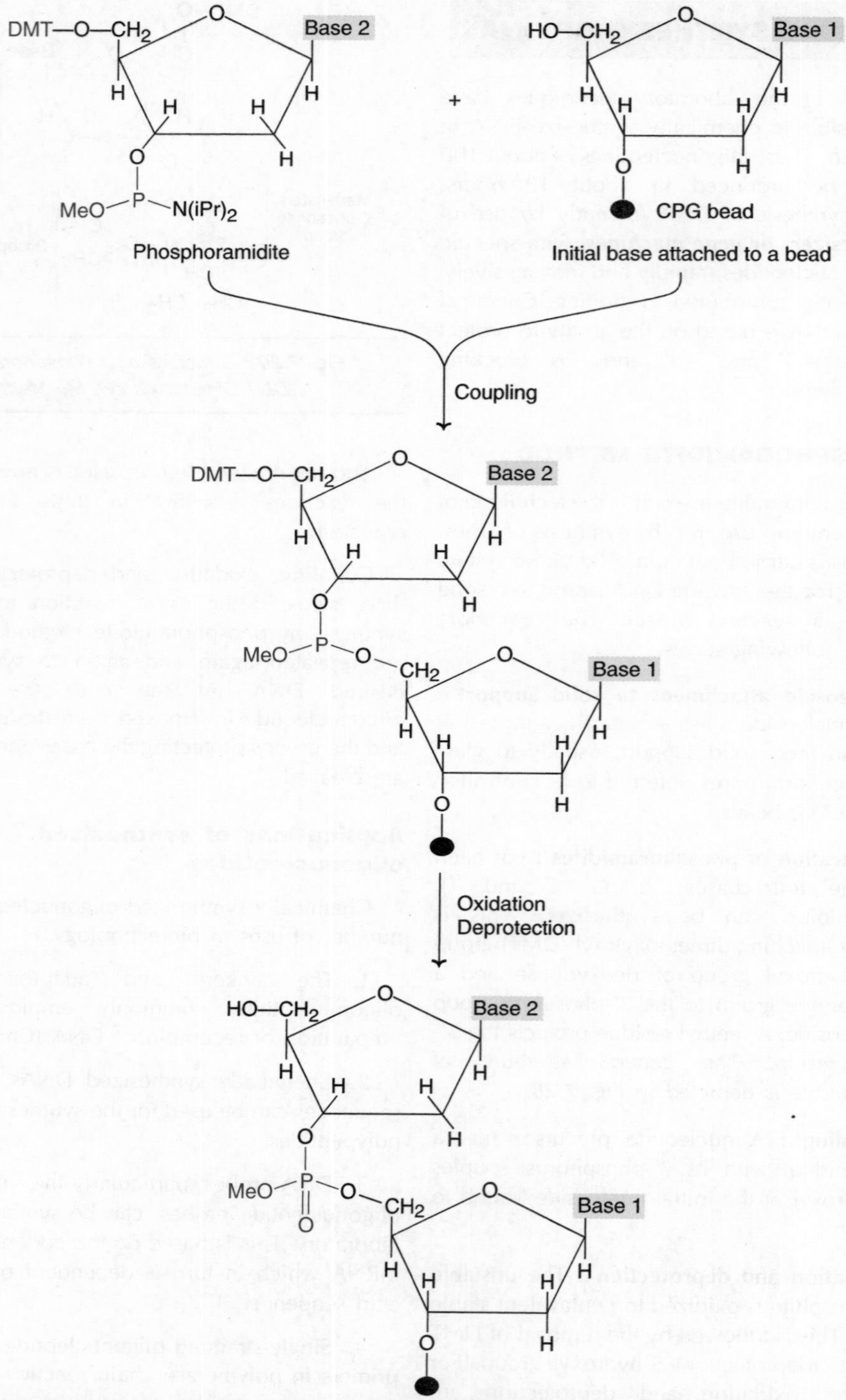

DMT—O—CH$_2$ Base 2

HO—CH$_2$ Base 1

MeO—P—N(iPr)$_2$

CPG bead

Phosphoramidite

Initial base attached to a bead

Coupling

Oxidation
Deprotection

Fig. 7.21 : Chemical synthesis of DNA by phosphoramidite method (CPG-Controlled pore glass; DMT-Dimethoxytrityl; Me-Methyl; N(iPr)$_2$-Diisopropylamine).

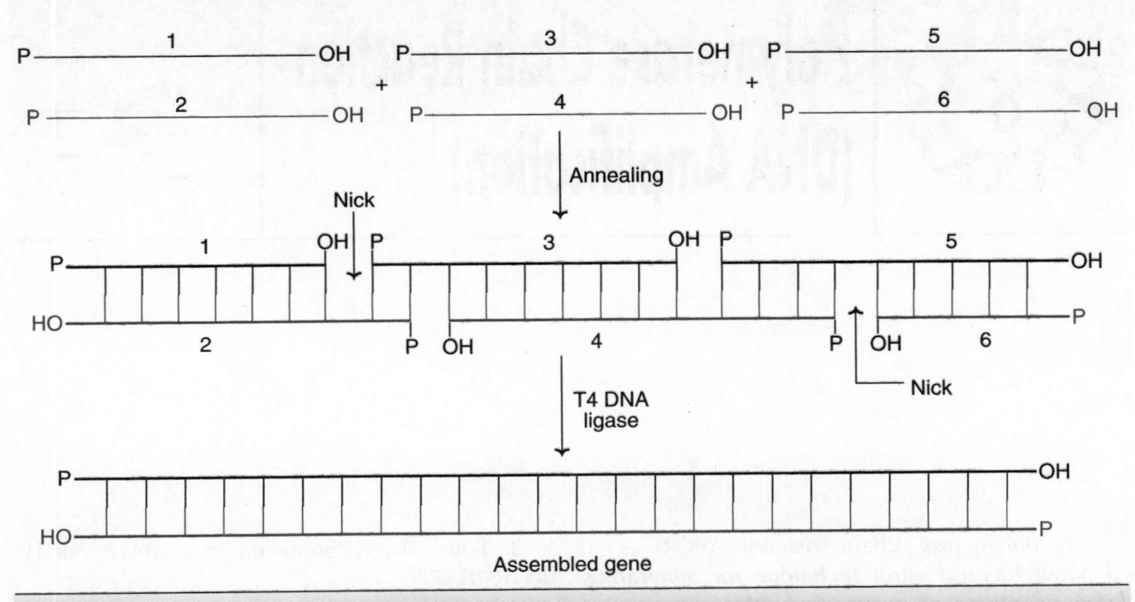

Fig. 7.22 : Chemical synthesis of a gene.

SYNTHESIS OF GENES

Gene is a double-stranded DNA; two single-stranded complementary oligonucleotides can be synthesized, separately, and on annealing they form double strands. This can be conveniently achieved for smaller genes (60–90 bp). However, the synthesis of longer genes (> 300 bp) is associated with some practical difficulties. This is mainly due to the fact that the coupling efficiency for the chemical synthesis of DNA is never 100%. To overcome this problem, small DNA fragments are synthesized and assembled (***Fig. 7.22***). Sealing of the nicks is achieved by use of T4 DNA ligase.

Another way of synthesizing genes is to produce overlapping oligonucleotides which on annealing contain large gaps. These gaps can be filled by enzymatic synthesis of DNA by DNA polymerase—while synthesizing genes in the laboratory, utmost care should be taken to see that the nucleotides are in the correct sequence (this can be checked by DNA sequence technique).

An Indian born and American settled scientist Har Gobind Khorana and his associates were the first to synthesize an entire tRNA gene for yeast alanyl tRNA in 1972.

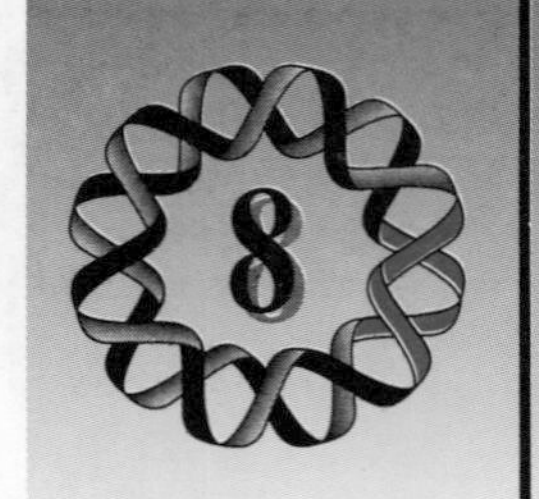

Polymerase Chain Reaction (DNA Amplification)

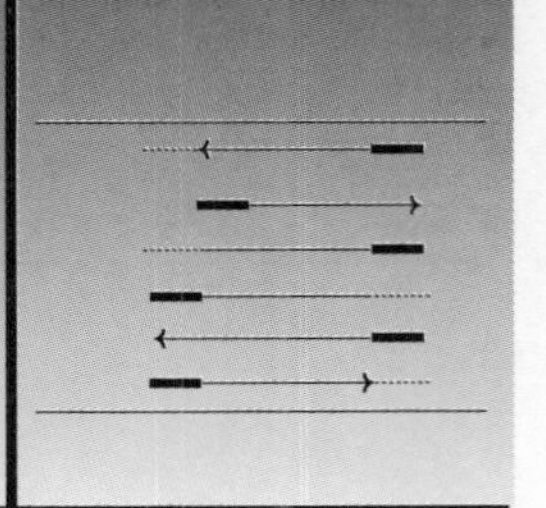

The polymerase chain reaction (PCR) is a laboratory (*in vitro*) ***technique for generating large quantities of a specified DNA***. Obviously, PCR is a ***cell-free amplification technique*** for synthesizing multiple identical copies (billions) of ***any DNA*** of interest. Developed in 1984 by Karry Mullis (Nobel laurate, 1993), PCR is now considered as a basic tool for the molecular biologist. As is a photocopier a basic requirement in an office, so is the PCR machine in a molecular biology laboratory!

Principle of PCR

The double-stranded DNA of interest is denatured to separate into two individual strands. Each strand is then allowed to hybridize with a primer (renaturation). The primer-template duplex is used for DNA synthesis (the enzyme-DNA polymerase). These three steps—***denaturation, renaturation*** and ***synthesis*** are repeated again and again to generate multiple forms of target DNA.

TECHNIQUE OF PCR

The essential requirements for PCR are listed below

1. A target DNA (100–35,000 bp in length).

2. Two primers (synthetic oligonucleotides of 17–30 nucleotides length) that are complementary to regions flanking the target DNA.

3. Four deoxyribonucleotides (dATP, dCTP, dGTP, dTTP).

4. A DNA polymerase that can withstand at a temperature upto 95° C (i.e., thermostable).

The reaction mixture contains the target DNA, two primers (in excess), a thermostable DNA polymerase (isolated from the bacterium *Thermus aquaticus* (i.e., *Taq* DNA polymerase) and four deoxyribonucleoties. The actual technique of PCR involves repeated cycles for amplification of target DNA. Each cycle has three stages.

1. **Denaturation :** On raising the temperature to about 95° C for about one minute, the DNA gets denatured and the two strands separate.

2. **Renaturation or annealing :** As the temperature of the mixutre is slowly cooled to about 55° C, the primers base pair with the complementary regions flanking target DNA strands. This process is called renaturation or annealing. High concentration of primer ensures annealing between each DNA strand and the primer rather than the two strands of DNA.

3. **Synthesis :** The initiation of DNA synthesis occurs at 3′-hydroxyl end of each primer. The primers are extended by joining the bases complementary to DNA strands. The synthetic process in PCR is quite comparable to the DNA replication of the leading strand (Refer Chapter 3). However, the temperature has to be kept optimal as required by the enzyme DNA polymerase. For *Taq*

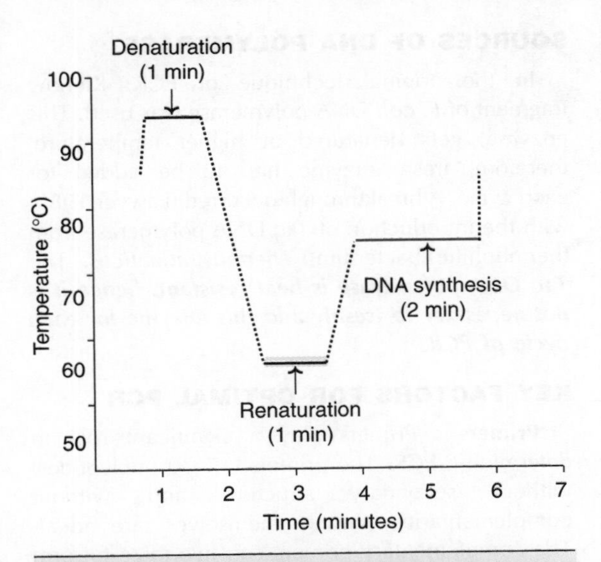

Fig. 8.1 : The three stages in each cycle of PCR in relation to temperature and time (Each cycle takes approximately 3-5 minutes).

DNA polymerase, the optimum temperature is around 75° C (for *E. coli* DNA polymerase, it is around 37° C). The reaction can be stopped by raising the temperature (to about 95° C).

The 3 stages of PCR in relation to temperature and time are depicted in ***Fig. 8.1***. Each cycle of PCR takes about 3-5 minutes. In the normal practice, the PCR is carried out in an automated machine.

As is evident from the ***Fig. 8.2*** (cycle I), the new DNA strand joined to each primer is beyond the sequence that is complementary to the second primer. These new strands are referred to as ***long templates*** and they will be used in the second cycle.

For the second cycle of PCR, the DNA strands (original + newly synthesized long template) are denatured, annealed with primers and subjected to DNA synthesis. At the end of second round, long templates, and short templates (DNA strands with primer sequence at one end, and sequence complementary to the other end primer) are formed.

In the third cycle of PCR, the original DNA strands along with long and short templates are the starting materials. The technique of denaturation, renaturation and synthesis are repeated. This procedure is repeated again and again for each cycle. It is estimated that at the end of 32nd cycle of PCR, about a million-fold target DNA is synthesized (***Table 8.1***). The short templates possessing precisely the target DNA as double-stranded molecules accumulate.

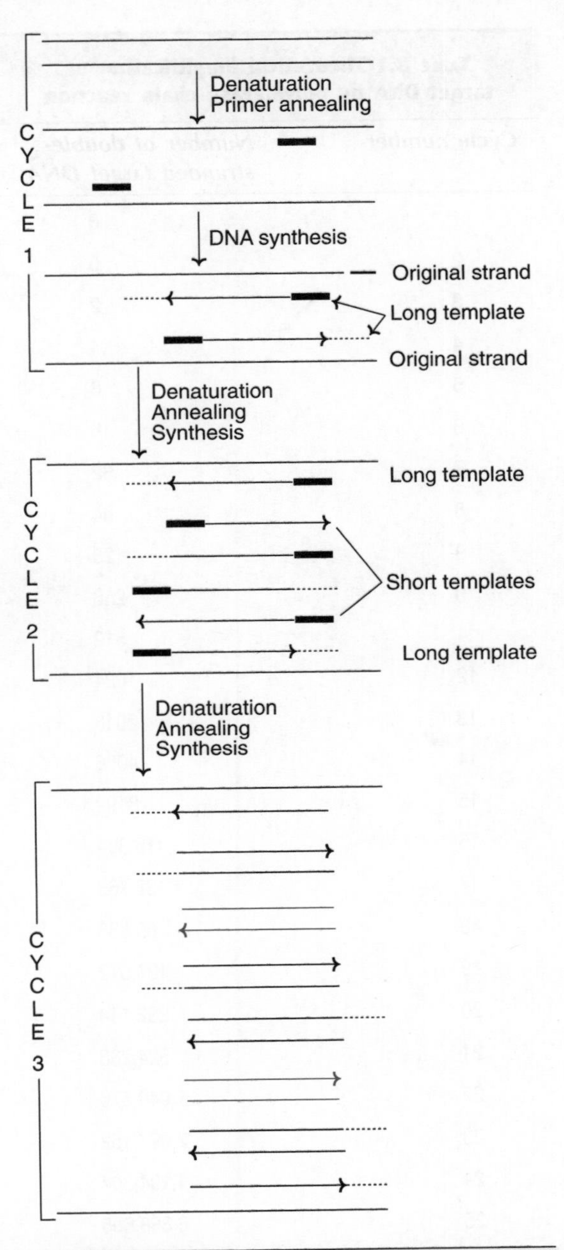

Fig. 8.2 : The polymerase chain reaction (PCR) representing the initial three cycles (▬ indicate primers).

Table 8.1 Theoretical amplification of target DNA by polymerase chain reaction

Cycle number	*Number of double-stranded target DNA*
1	0
2	0
3	2
4	4
5	8
6	16
7	32
8	64
9	128
10	256
11	512
12	1024
13	2048
14	4096
15	8192
16	16,384
17	32,768
18	65,536
19	131,072
20	262,144
21	524,288
22	1,048,576
23	2,097,152
24	4,194,304
25	8,388,608
26	16,777,216
27	33,544,432
28	67,108,864
29	134,217,728
30	268,435,456
31	536,870,912
32	1,073,741,824

SOURCES OF DNA POLYMERASE

In the original technique of PCR, Klenow fragment of *E. coli* DNA polymerase was used. This enzyme, gets denatured at higher temperature, therefore, fresh enzyme had to be added for each cycle. A breakthrough occurred (Lawyer 1989) with the introduction of *Taq* DNA polymerase from thermophilic bacterium, *Thermus aquaticus*. The ***Taq DNA polymerase is heat resistant, hence it is not necessary to freshly add this enzyme for each cycle of PCR***.

KEY FACTORS FOR OPTIMAL PCR

Primers : Primers play a significant role in determining PCR. The primers (17–30 nucleotides) without secondary structure and without complementarity among themselves are ideal. The complementary primers can hybridize to form ***primer dimer*** and get amplified in PCR. This prevents the multiplication of target DNA.

DNA polymerase : As already described, *Taq* DNA polymerase is preferred as it can withstand high temperature. In the ***hot-start protocol***, DNA polymerase is added after the heat denaturation step of the first cycle. This avoids the extension of the mismatched primers that usually occur at low temperature.

Taq polymerase lacks proof reading exonuclease (3′-5′) activity which might contribute to errors in the products of PCR. Some other thermostable DNA polymerases with proof-reading activity have been identified e.g., *Tma* DNA polymerase from *Thermotoga maritama; Pfu* DNA polymerase from *Pyrococcus furiosus*.

Target DNA : In general, the shorter the sequence of target DNA, the better is the efficiency of PCR. However, in recent years, amplification of DNA fragments upto 10 kb has been reported. The sequence of target DNA is also important in PCR. Thus, GC-rich regions of DNA strand hinder PCR.

Promoters and inhibitors : Addition of proteins such as bovine serum albumin (BSA) enhances PCR by protecting the enzyme DNA polymerase. Humic acids, frequently found in archeological samples of target DNA inhibit PCR.

VARIATIONS OF PCR

The basic technique of the PCR has been described. Being a versatile technique, PCR is

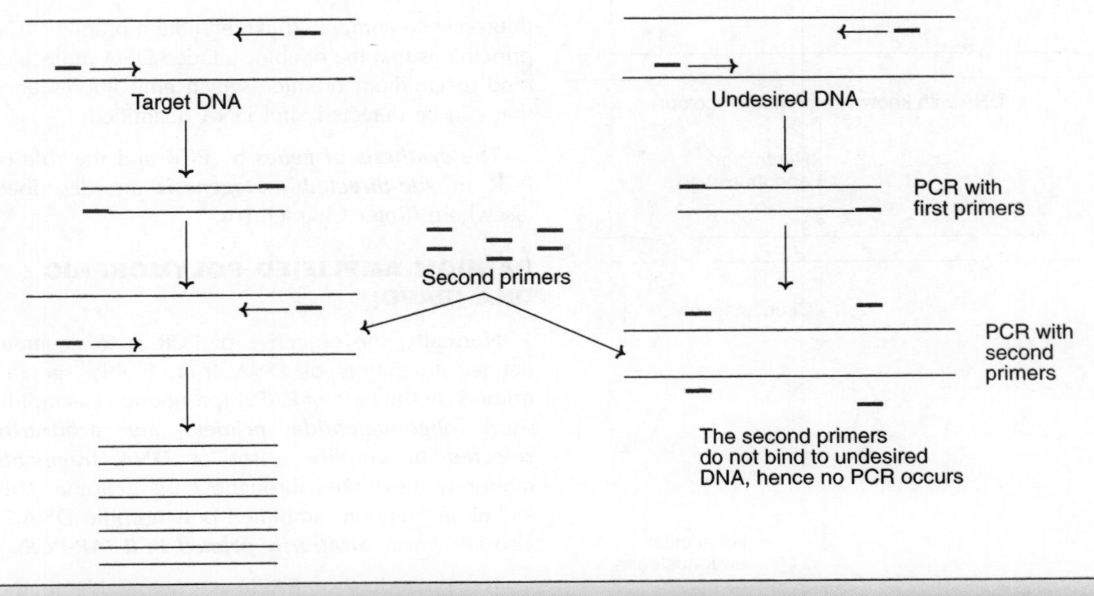

Fig. 8.3 : Nested polymerase chain reaction.

modified as per the specific demands of the situation. Thus, there are many variations in the original PCR, some of them are discussed, hereunder.

NESTED PCR

Sequence similarities between the target DNA and related DNA are very frequently seen. As a result of this, the primers may bind to both the DNAs and therefore even the undesired DNA also gets amplified in PCR. Use of ***nested primers*** increases the specificity of PCR, and selectively amplifies target DNA. Nested PCR is illustrated in ***Fig. 8.3***. In the first cycle of PCR, the products are both from target DNA and undesired DNA. A second set of internal primers is now used. They will selectively bind to target DNA and amplification proceeds.

INVERSE PCR

In the inverse PCR, amplification of DNA of the unknown sequences is carried out from the known sequence (***Fig. 8.4***). The target DNA is cleaved with a restriction endonuclease which does not cut the known sequence but cuts the unknown sequence on either side. The DNA fragments so formed are inverted and get circularized (DNA ligase is employed as a sealing agent). The circle containing the known sequences is now cut with another restriction enzyme. This cleaves only the known sequence. The target DNA so formed contains the known sequence at both the ends with target DNA at the middle. The PCR amplification can now be carried out. It may be noted that the primers are generated in the opposite direction to the normal, since the original sequence is inverted during circularization.

ANCHORED PCR

In the anchored PCR, a small sequence of nucleotides can be attached (tagged) to the target DNA i.e., the DNA is anchored. This is particularly useful when the sequence surrounding the target DNA is not known. The anchor is frequently a poly G tail to which a poly C primer is used. The anchoring can also be done by the use of adaptors. As the adaptors possess a known sequence, the primer can be chosen.

REVERSE TRANSCRIPTION PCR

The PCR technique can also be employed for the amplification of RNA molecules in which case it is referred to as reverse transcription — PCR (***RT-PCR***). For this purpose, the RNA molecule (mRNA) must be first converted to complementary DNA (cDNA) by the enzyme ***reverse transcriptase***. The cDNA then serves as the template for PCR. Different primers can be employed for the synthesis

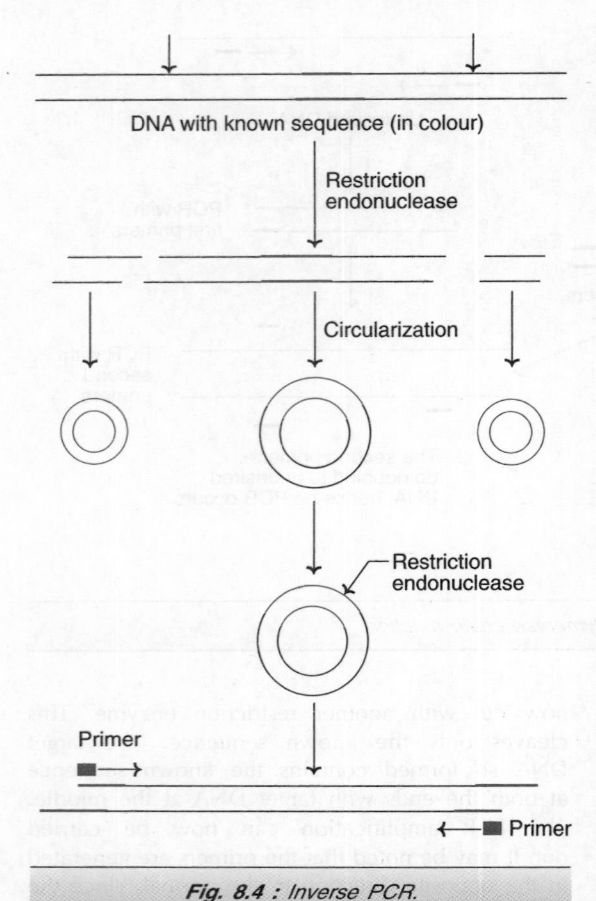

Fig. 8.4 : Inverse PCR.

of first strand of cDNA. These include the use of random primers, oligo dT primer and a sequence specific primer (*Fig. 8.5*).

ASYMMETRIC PCR

PCR technique can also be used for the synthesis of single-stranded DNA molecules, particularly useful for DNA sequencing (Chapter 7). In the asymmetric PCR, two primers in a ratio of 100 : 1 are used. After 20–25 cycles of PCR, one primer is exhausted. The result is that in the next 5–10 PCR cycles, only single-stranded DNAs are generated.

REAL-TIME QUANTITATIVE PCR

The quantification of PCR products in different cycles is not as simple as projected by thereotical considerations (*Table 8.1*). In practice, large variations occur. The most commonly used technique for measuring the quantity of PCR is by employing a fluorescence compound like eithidium bromide. The principle is that the double-stranded DNA molecules bind to ethidium bromide which emit fluorescence that can be detected, and DNA quantified.

The ***synthesis of genes*** by PCR and the role of PCR in ***site-directed mutagenesis*** are described elsewhere (Refer Chapter 10).

RANDOM AMPLIFIED POLYMORPHIC DNA (RAPD)

Normally, the objective of PCR is to generate defined fragments of DNA from highly specific primers. In the case of RAPD (pronounced as rapid), short ***oligonucleotide primers*** are ***arbitrarily selected to amplify*** a set of ***DNA fragments*** randomly distributed throughout the genome. This technique, random amplified polymorphic DNA is also known as ***arbitrarily primed PCR (AP-PCR)***.

The procedure of RAPD is comparable to the general technique of PCR. This method basically involves the use of a single primer at low stringency. A single short oligonucleotide (usually a 9–10 base primer) binds to many sites in the genome and the DNA fragments are amplified from them. The stringency of primer binding can be increased after a few PCR cycles. This allows the amplification of best mismatches. RAPD can be carefully designed so that it finally yields genome-specific band patterns that are useful for comparative analysis. This is possible since genomic DNA from two different individuals often produces different amplified patterns by RAPD. Thus, a particular DNA fragment may be generated for one individual and not for the other, and this represents DNA polymorphism which can be used as a genetic marker.

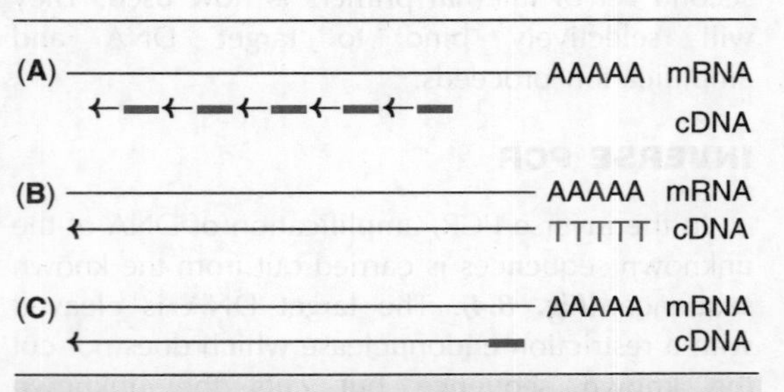

*Fig. 8.5 : Synthesis of first strand of cDNA in reverse transcription-PCR with different primers (**A**) Random primers (**B**) oligo dT primer (**C**) Sequence specific primer (**Note** : The primers are shown in colour).*

RAPD is widely used by plant molecular biologists for the ***genetic identification of plant species*** (Refer Chapter 53). For this purpose, different combinations of nucleotides, most of them random oligonucleotide primers have been designed and are commercially available. As each random primer anneals to a different region of DNA, many different regions of loci on the DNA can be identified. RAPD is thus useful for the construction of genetic maps and as a method for genomic fingerprinting.

Limitations of RAPD

The main problem of RAPD is associated with reproducibility. It is often difficult to obtain similar levels of primer binding in different experiments. It is therefore difficult to correlate results obtained by different research groups on RAPD.

AMPLIFIED FRAGMENT LENGTH POLYMORPHISM (AFLP)

AFLP is a very sensive method for detecting polymorphism in the genome. It is based on the principle of restriction fragment length polymorphism (RFLP, Refer Chapter 14) and RAPD. AFLP may be appropriately regarded as a diagnostic fingerprinting technique that detects genomic restriction fragments.

In the AFLP, PCR amplification rather than Southern blotting (mostly used in RFLP) is used for the detection of restriction fragments. It may be noted that AFLP is employed to detect the presence or absence of restriction fragments, and not the lengths of these fragments. This is the major difference between AFLP and RFLP. AFLP is very ***widely used in plant genetics***. It has not proved useful in the mapping of animal genomes, since this technique is mainly based on the presence of high rates of substitutional variations which are not found in animals. On the other hand, substitutional variations resulting in RFLPs are more common in plants.

The basic principle of AFLP involves the amplification of subsets of RFLPs using PCR (***Fig. 8.6***).

A genomic DNA is isolated and digested simultaneously with two different restriction endonucleases — *EcoRI* with a 6 base pair recognition site and *MseI* with a 4 base pair recognition site. These two enzymes can cleave the DNA and result in small fragments (< 1 kb) which can be amplified by PCR. For this purpose the DNA

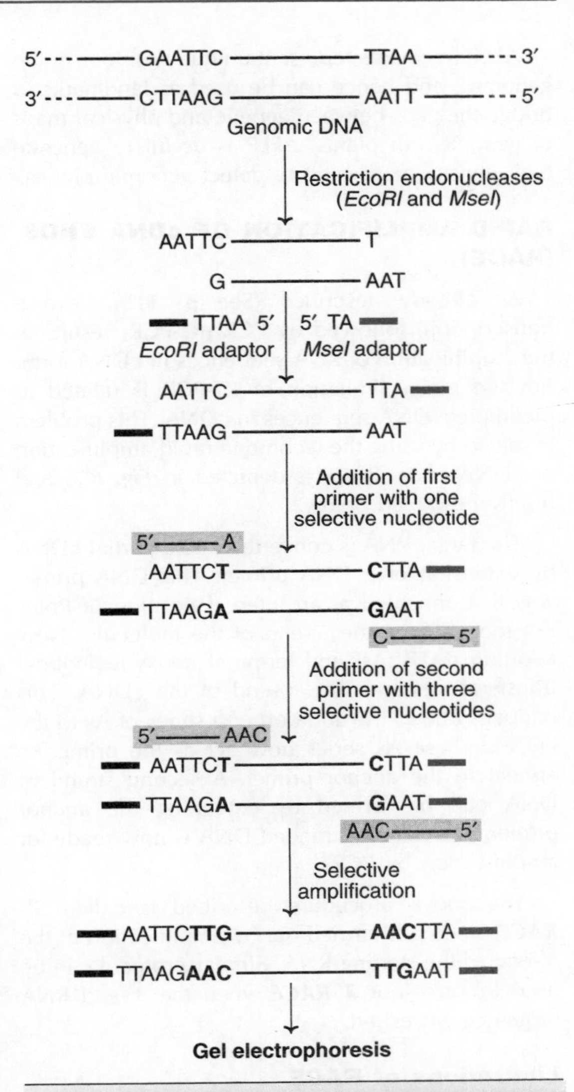

Fig. 8.6 : *The technique of amplified fragment length of polymorphism (AFLP).*

fragments are ligated with *EcoRI* and *MseI* adaptors. These common adaptor sequences (flanking genomic sequences) serve as primer binding sites on the restriction fragments. The DNA fragments can be amplified with AFLP primers each having only one selective nucleotide. These PCR products are diluted and used as templates for the selective amplification employing two new AFLP primers that have 2 or 3 selective nucleotides.

After the selective amplification by PCR, the DNA products are separated on a gel. The resultant DNA fingerprint is identified by autoradiography.

AFLP fragments represent unique positions in the genomes, and hence can be used as landmarks to bridge the gaps between genetic and physical maps of genomes. In plants, AFLP is useful to generate high density maps, and to detect genomic clones.

RAPID AMPLIFICATION OF cDNA ENDS (RACE)

As already described (See p. 115), reverse transcription, followed by PCR (RT-PCR) results in the amplification of RNA sequences in cDNA form. But the major limitation of RT-PCR is related to incomplete DNA sequences in cDNA. This problem is solved by using the technique rapid amplification of cDNA ends. RACE is depicted in ***Fig. 8.7***, and briefly described below.

The target RNA is converted into a partial cDNA by extension of a DNA primer. This DNA primer was first annealed at an interval position of RNA, not too far from the 5′-end of the molecule. Now addition dATP (As) and terminal deoxynucleotidyl transferase extends the 3′-end of the cDNA. This happens due to the addition of a series of As to the cDNA. These As series now act as the primer to anneal to the anchor primer. A second strand of DNA can be formed by extending the anchor primer. The double-stranded DNA is now ready for amplification by PCR.

The above procedure described is called ***5′-RACE***, since it is carried out by amplification of the 5′-end of the starting RNA. Similar protocol can be used to carry out ***3′-RACE*** when the 3′-end RNA sequence is desired.

Limitations of RACE

Since a specific primer is used, the specificity of amplification of RACE may not be very high. Another disadvantage is that the reverse transcriptase may not fully reach the 5′-ends of RNA, and this limits the utility of RACE. In recent years, some modifications have been done to improve RACE.

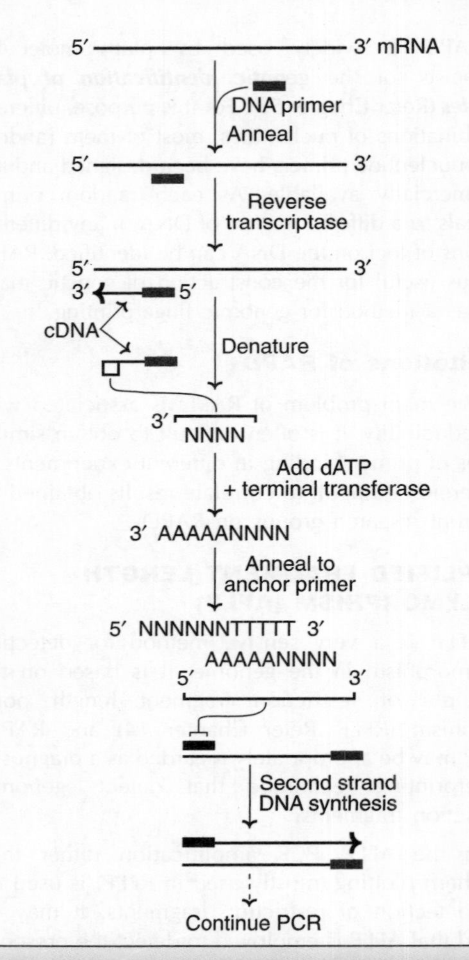

Fig. 8.7 : Rapid amplification of cDNA ends (RACE).

APPLICATIONS OF PCR

The advent of PCR had, and continues to have tremendous impact on molecular biology. The applications of PCR are too many to be listed here. Some of them are selectively and very briefly described. Other applications of PCR are discussed at appropriate places.

PCR IN CLINICAL DIAGNOSIS

The specificity and sensitivity of PCR is highly useful for the diagnosis of various diseases in humans. These include diagnosis of inherited disorders (genetic diseases), viral diseases, bacterial diseases etc.

The occurrence of genetic diseases frequently identified by restriction fragment length polymorphism (RFLP) can be employed only when there is a mutation resulting in a detectable change in the length of restriction fragment. Many genetic diseases occur without the involvement of RFLP.

For all such disorders, PCR technique is a real boon, as it provides direct information of DNA. This is done by amplification of DNA of the relevant region, followed by the direct analysis of PCR products.

Prenatal diagnosis of inherited diseases : PCR is employed in the prenatal diagnosis of inherited diseases by using chorionic villus samples or cells from amniocentesis. Thus, diseases like sickle-cell anemia, β-thalassemia and phenylketonuria can be detected by PCR in these samples.

Diagnosis of retroviral infections : PCR from cDNA is a valuable tool for diagnosis and monitoring of retroviral infections, e.g., HIV infection.

Diagnosis of bacterial infections : PCR is used for the detection of bacterial infection e.g., tuberculosis by *Mycobacterium tuberculosis.*

Diagnosis of cancers : Several virally-induced cancers (e.g., cervical cancer caused by human papilloma virus) can be detected by PCR. Further, some cancers which occur due to chromosomal translocation (chromosome 14 and 18 in follicular lymphoma) involving known genes are identified by PCR.

PCR in sex determination of embryos : Sex of human and live stock embryos fertilized *in vitro*, can be determined by PCR, by using primers and DNA probes specific for sex chromosomes. Further, this technique is also useful to detect sex — linked disorders in fertilized embryos.

PCR IN DNA SEQUENCING

As the PCR technique is much simpler and quicker to amplify the DNA, it is conveniently used for sequencing. For this purpose, single-strands of DNA are required. In asymmetric PCR (See p. 116), preferential amplification of a single-strand is carried out. In another method, ***strand removal*** can be achieved by digesting one strand (usually done by exonuclease by its action on 5′-phosphorylated strand).

PCR IN GENE MANIPULATION AND EXPRESSION STUDIES

The advantage with PCR is that the primers need not have complementary sequences for the target DNA. Therefore, the sequence of nucleotides in a piece of the gene (target DNA) can be manipulated and amplified by PCR. More details on this technique, referred to as ***site-directed mutagenesis***, are given elsewhere (Chapter 10). By using this method, coding sequence can be altered (thereby changing amino acids) to synthesize protein of interest. Further, gene manipulations are important in understanding the effects of promoters, initiators etc., in gene expression.

PCR is important in the study of mRNAs, the products of gene expression. This is carried out by reverse transcription — PCR.

PCR IN COMPARATIVE STUDIES OF GENOMES

The differences in the genomes of two organisms can be measured by PCR with random primers. The products are separated by electrophoresis for comparative identification. Two genomes from closely related organisms are expected to yield more similar bands. For more details, refer the technique random amplified polymorphic DNA (See p. 116).

PCR is very important in the study ***evolutionary biology***, more specifically referred to as ***phylogenetics***. As a technique which can amplify even minute quantities of DNA from any source (hair, mummified tissues, bone, or any fossilized material), PCR has revolutionized the studies in palaentology and archaelogy. The movie 'Jurassic Park', has created public awareness of the potential applications of PCR!

PCR IN FORENSIC MEDICINE

A single molecule of DNA from any source (blood strains, hair, semen etc.) of an individual is adequate for amplification by PCR. Thus, PCR is very important for identification of criminals.

The reader may refer DNA finger printing technique described elsewhere (Chapter 14).

PCR IN COMPARISON WITH GENE CLONING

PCR has several advantages over the traditional gene cloning techniques (Chapter 6). These include better efficiency, minute quantities of starting material (DNA), cost-effectiveness, minimal technical skill, time factor etc. In due course of time, PCR may take over most of the applications of gene cloning.

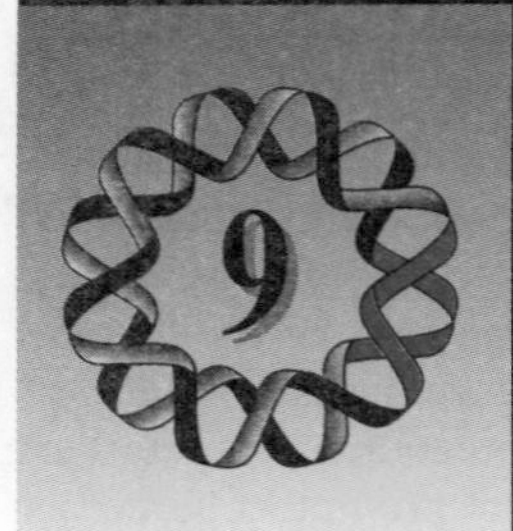

Gene Libraries

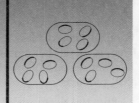

The ***collection of DNA fragments*** (specifically genes) from a particular species represents gene libraries. The creation or construction of gene libraries (broadly ***genomic libraries***) is accomplished by isolating the complete genome (entire DNA from a cell) which is cut into fragments, and cloned in suitable vectors. Then the specific clone carrying the desired (target) DNA can be identified, isolated and characterized. In this manner, a library of genes or clones (appropriately considered as ***gene bank***) for an the entire genome of a species can be constructed. The sizes of genomes in different species are variable (***Table 9.1***). A complete gene library for each organism contains all the genomic DNA.

Biotechnologists are particularly interested in the isolation of genes (and therefore creation of gene libraries) which encode for proteins. There is a distinct difference in the genes of prokaryotic and eukaryotic cells. In prokaryotic organisms, the structural genes coding for proteins are continuous. However, in case of eukaryotes, the coding regions (exons) of structural genes are separated by non-coding regions (introns). For this reason, the construction of gene libraries for eukaryotes is more complicated.

TABLE 9.1 Genome sizes of some organisms

Organism	*Genome size* (kb)*
Escherichia coli	4.0×10^3
Saccharomyces cerevisiae	1.35×10^4
Tobacco	1.6×10^6
Wheat	5.9×10^6
Drosophila melanogaster	1.8×10^5
Mouse	3.3×10^6
Human	3.2×10^6

*Haploid where appropriate

CREATING A GENE LIBRARY

The DNA from the source organism is digested by restriction endonuclease (e.g., *EcoRI*), to result in fragments. It is desirable to create conditions so that partial digestion and not complete digestion occurs. By this way, all possible DNA fragments of variable size can be produced. The partial digestion of a DNA with a restriction endonuclease is depicted in ***Fig. 9.1***. The cleavages occur at different sites to result in DNA fragments of varying lengths, some of them may be large while others are small. In practice, a combination of restriction enzymes are used to digest source DNA to release a large number of DNA fragments. The desired fragments can be isolated and cloned.

Some workers use the term shotgun experiment (or shotgun approach) for ceation of random clones; (without necessarily identifying all of them) from a genomic DNA. In ***shotgun approach, the DNA is subjected to random cleavage by restriction endonucleases.***

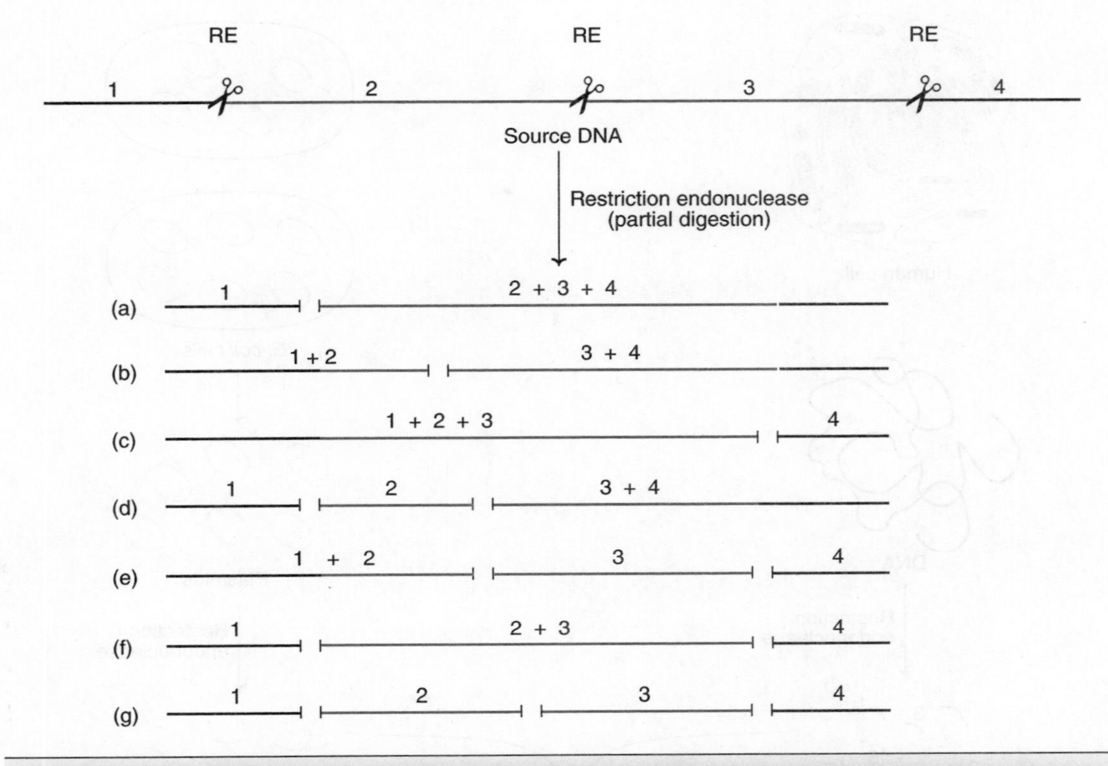

***Fig. 9.1** : Partial digestion of a DNA by the enzyme restriction endonuclease (RE) at three sites [**Note** : the coloured fragment represents the desired gene and it is one (shown in f) among several fragments formed].*

Maniatis technique for creating gene library

In the technique developed by Maniatis *et al* (1978), two restriction endonucleases are used to cut the target DNA. Partial digestion allows the formation of majority of DNA fragments with a length of 10–30 kb. The fragments are frequently overlapping and they can be fractionated by gel electrophoresis. The ***isolated fragments*** (approximately 20 kb in size) ***are inserted into λ phage vector and cloned***.

Establishing a gene library for humans

The human cellular DNA (the entire genome) may be subjected to digestion by restriction endonucleases (e.g., *EcoRI*). The fragments formed on an average are of about 4 kb size. (i.e., 4000 nitrogenes bases). Each human chromosome, containing approximately 100,000 kb can be cut into about 25,000 DNA fragments. As the humans have 23 different chromosomes (24 in man), there are a total of 575,000 fragments of 4 kb length formed. Among these 575,000 DNA fragments is the DNA or gene of interest (say insulin gene).

Now is the selection of a vector and cloning process. *E.coli*, a harmless bacterium to humans is most commonly used. The ***plasmids from E. coli*** are isolated. They are digested by the same restriction enzyme as was used for cutting human genome to form open plasmids. The human chromosomal DNA fragments and open plasmids are joined to produce recombined plasmids. These plasmids contain different DNA fragments of humans. The recombined plasmids are inserted into *E. coli* and the cells multiply (***Fig. 9.2***). The *E. coli* cells possess all the human DNA in fragments. It must, however be remembered that each ***E. coli cell contains different DNA fragments***. All the *E. coli* cells put together collectively represent ***genomic library*** (containing about 575,000 DNA fragments).

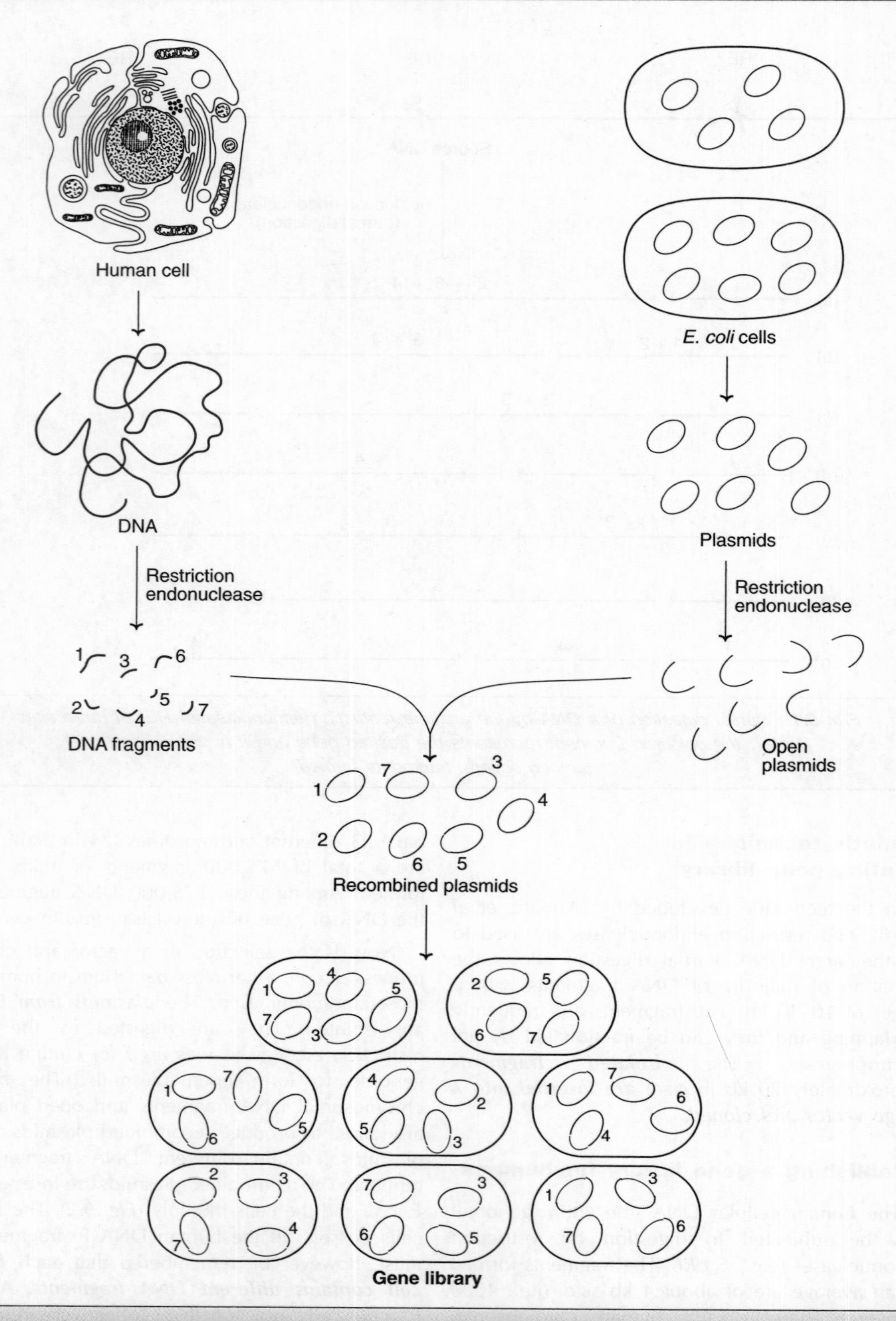

*Fig. 9.2 : Creation of a genomic library for humans. (**Note** : Double-stranded DNA is represented by single lines or circles for clarity; human DNA fragments are coloured).*

Other vectors for creating genomic libraries

In place of phages and plasmids, other vectors are in use for construction of large sized DNA libraries. These include ***cosmids, bacterial artificial chromosomes (BACs)*** and ***yeast artificial chromosomes (YACs)***. These are considered as high capacity vectors. Although they are ideal for construction of gene libraries, there are many practical difficulties associated with their use.

PCR AS AN ALTERNATIVE TO GENOMIC LIBRARY CONSTRUCTION

As already described in detail (Chapter 8), PCR is a technique for amplification of a specific DNA sequence. PCR with primers can be used to isolate target DNA directly from the genome. Thus, PCR serves as an alternative to DNA library (gene library) construction by cloning. This is not always possible since PCR technique can be employed for amplification of short length DNAs (usually 1-2 kb with a maximum of 5 kb). Further, the high temperature used in PCR, sometimes causes damage to bases and generates nicks in DNA strands.

Long PCR

With some modifications in the PCR, it is now possible to amplify DNA fragments up to a length of 22 kb from the human genomic DNA. This is achieved by using a combination of two DNA polymerase enzymes, besides lowering the reaction temperature. One of the DNA polymerases has proof-reading activity to remove the mismatched bases. Some commercial companies in fact provide enzyme cocktails ideally suited for long PCR e.g., TaqPlus Long PCR system marketed by ***Stratagene***. It contains *Taq* polymerase and the thermostable proof-reading enzyme *Pfee* polymerase.

Long PCR has been applied for the structured analysis of human genes and genomes of HIV.

Long PCR is unlikely to replace the construction of genomic libraries. This is because creation of DNA libraries is permanent while long PCR is temporary. Further, PCR can be employed for amplifying selected DNA fragments (of interest) from genomic libraries.

Fragment libraries

Biotechnologists often come across minute quantities of starting materials e.g., single cells, fixed tissues, fossils etc. It is quite difficult to apply traditional technique for construction of genomic libraries from such samples. PCR is ideally suited for isolation and amplification of genes from very small samples. Thus, PCR can be used for the creation of random genomic fragment libraries.

COMPLEMENTARY DNA LIBRARIES

Cloning of eukaryotic genes is rather complicated and requires special techniques. This is mainly due to the non-coding sequences (introns) in the DNA. In the eukaryotic cell as the gene is transcribed, the RNA undergoes several changes in the nucleus (referred to as splicing) to release a mature and functional mRNA into the cytoplasm. In this manner, the introns are removed. In some genes, introns form a major bulk of the gene. For instance, in the human dystrophin gene, as much as 99% of the DNA sequence is composed of introns. There are as many as 79 introns!

The prokaryotes, particularly the bacteria, do not possess the ability to remove the introns. Hence the functional mRNA is not correctly formed in a prokaryotic cell for an eukaryotic gene. Thus, cloning of eukaryotic genes becomes a difficult task.

Synthesis of complementary DNA

Complementary DNA (cDNA) is a double-stranded complement of an mRNA. cDNA can be synthesized from mRNA by ***reverse transcription***. An eukaryotic functional mRNA which does not have introns possesses a G cap at 5′ and a poly (A) tail at the 3′ end (approximately 200 adenine residues).

The requisite mRNA is isolated and purified (particularly from cells which are rich in the specific mRNA e.g., pancreatic cells for insulin mRNA). An oligo-dT primer is added to bind to the short segment of poly A tail region (by annealing). This primer provides 3′-hydroxyl group for the synthesis of a DNA strand. With the addition of the enzyme reverse transcriptase and four deoxynucleotides (dATP, dTTP, dGTP and dCTP), DNA synthesis proceeds. For the bases ***A, G, C*** and

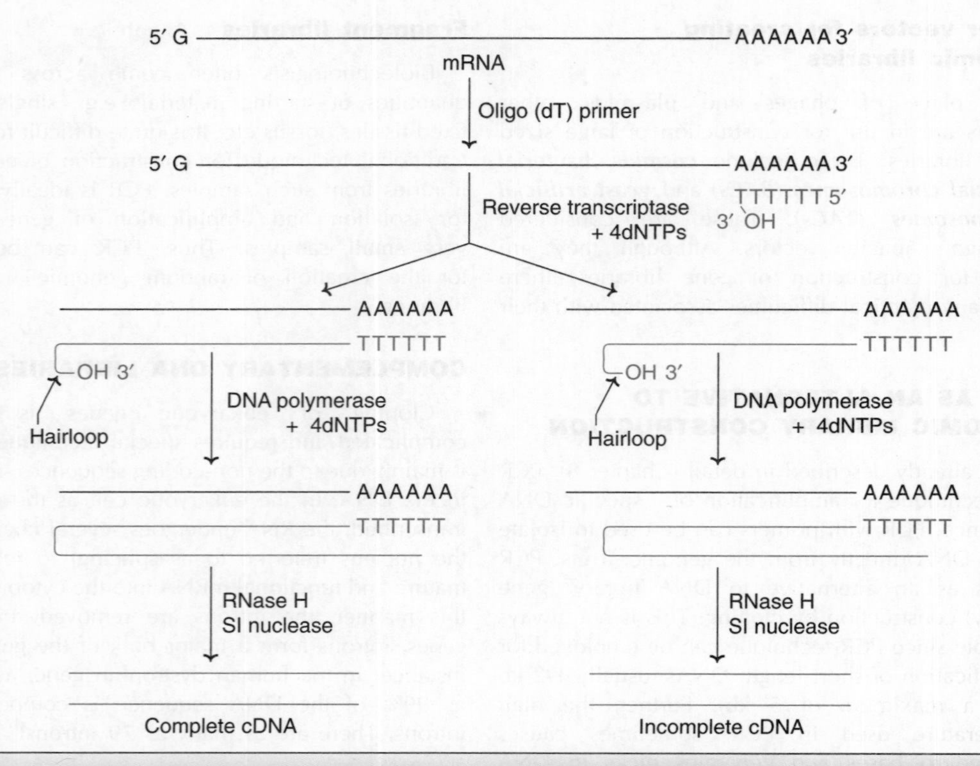

Fig. 9.3 : Synthesis of complementary DNA (cDNA).

U in the template (mRNA), the ***corresponding complementary bases*** in DNA respectively are ***T***, ***C***, ***G*** and ***A***. The newly synthesized first DNA strand has a tendency to fold back on to itself for a few nucleotides to form a hairpin loop (***Fig. 9.3***).

The loop of the first DNA strand serves as the template for the synthesis of second DNA strand. By the addition of *E. coli* DNA polymerase (Klenow fragment), the second DNA strand synthesis occurs starting from the end of the hairpin loop. On treatment with the enzyme RNase H, mRNA molecules are degraded. The enzyme SI nuclease cleaves the hairpin loops and degrades single-stranded DNA extensions. The final products are complementary DNA copies of original mRNA, some of them are complete while others are incomplete.

Limitation of the technique : The main disadvantage with the hairpin method is the loss of a small sequence at the 5′ end of cDNA due to cleavage by SI nuclease.

Improved method for cDNA synthesis

To overcome the limitation described above, some improvements have been made in cDNA synthesis. One such improved technique is shown in ***Fig. 9.4***.

As the first strand of cDNA is synthesized, it is ***tailed with cytidine residues*** with the help of the enzyme terminal transferase. The mRNA strand is hydrolysed with alkali, and the full length cDNA is recovered. A synthetic oligo-dG primer is then annealed to oligo-dC. This in turn enables the synthesis of the second strand of cDNA. By this improved technique, a full length of cDNA corresponding to mRNA (in turn the gene) is obtained. But the efficiency of this method is comparatively lower.

Construction of cDNA libraries

The complementary DNA molecules can be cloned in cloning vector (e.g., plasmid), for creating cDNA libraries. The cDNA insertion into the vector should have correct orientation. This is achieved by

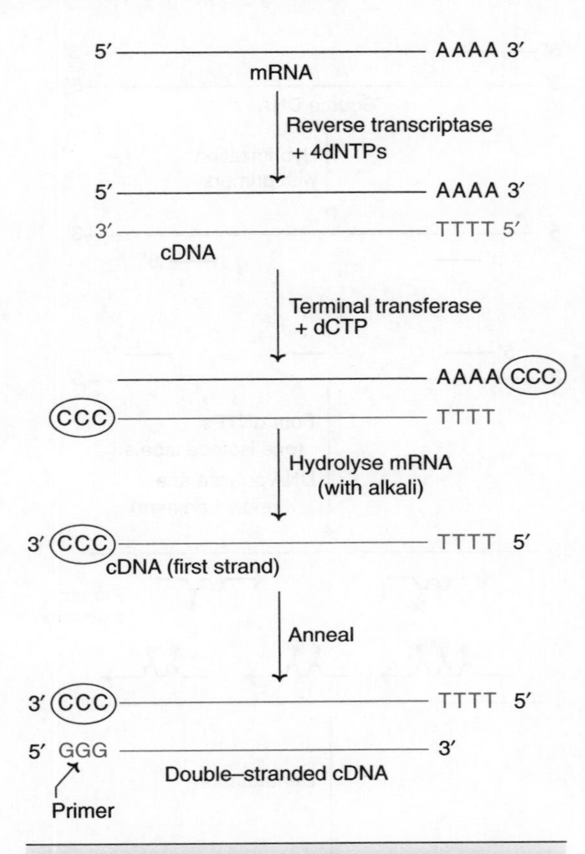

Fig. 9.4 : Improved method for complementary DNA synthesis.

the addition of a synthetic linker to the double-stranded cDNA.

In a technique developed by Okayama and Berg (1982), the mRNA is first linked to the plasmid cloning vector and then cDNA synthesis is carried out.

RT-PCR as an alternative to cDNA cloning

Reverse transcription followed by PCR (RT-PCR) can amplify the mRNA to give cDNA (For details Refer Chapter 8).

RT-PCR is very rapid hence cDNA molecules can be obtained in a short period. Further, even the long length mRNAs can be conveniently used in RT-PCR.

There are some disadvantages also in RT-PCR. The DNA polymerase used in RT-PCR is error-prone, and even a very minute contamination of mRNA (with other mRNAs) will give false results.

SCREENING STRATEGIES

Once a DNA library or a cDNA library is created, the clones (i.e., the cell lines) must be screened for identification of specific clones. The screening techniques are mostly based on the sequence of the clone or the structure/function of its product.

SCREENING BY DNA HYBRIDIZATION

The target sequence in a DNA can be determined with a ***DNA probe*** (***Fig. 9.5***). To start with, the double-stranded DNA of interest is converted into single strands by heat or alkali (denaturation). The two DNA strands are kept apart by binding to solid matrix such as nitrocellulose or nylon membrane. Now, the single strands of DNA probe (100–1,000 bp) labeled with radioisotope are added. Hybridization (i.e., base pairing) occurs between the complementary nucleotide sequences

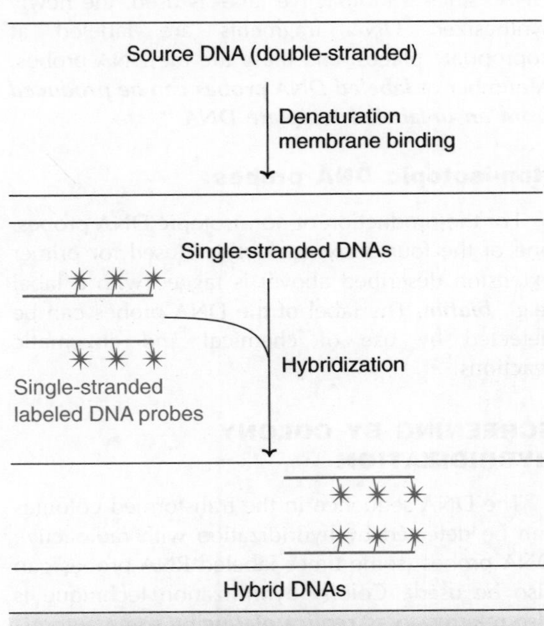

Fig. 9.5 : Screening by DNA hybridization (✳ indicates radioisotope label in the DNA probe)

of the target DNA and the probe. For a stable base pairing, at least 80% of the bases in the two strands (target DNA and the probe) should be matching. The hybridized DNA can be detected by ***autoradiography***.

DNA PROBES

The DNA probes used for screening purpose can be synthesized in many ways.

Random primer method

Radioisotope labeled DNA primers can be produced by this technique (***Fig. 9.6***). The double-stranded DNA containing the sequence needed to serve as a probe is denatured. ***A mixture of synthetic oligonucleotides, with all possible combinations of bases*** (*A, G, C* and *T*), with a length of 6 nucleotides each ***serve as primers***. Some of these primers with complementary sequences will hybridize with the template DNA. This occurrence is entirely by chance and the probability is reasonably good.

By the addition of four deoxyribonucleotides (one of them is radiolabeled) and in the presence of the enzyme DNA polymerase of *E. coli* (Klenow fragment), the primers are extended on the template DNA. Since a radioactive label is used, the newly synthesized DNA fragments are labeled at appropriate places, and these are the DNA probes. A number of ***labeled DNA probes can be produced from an unlabeled template DNA***.

Non-isotopic DNA probes

For the production of non-isotopic DNA probes, one of the four deoxynucleotides (used for primer extension described above) is tagged with a label (e.g., ***biotin***). The label of the DNA probes can be detected by use of chemical and enzymatic reactions.

SCREENING BY COLONY HYBRIDIZATION

The DNA sequence in the transformed colonies can be detected by hydridization with radioactive DNA probes (some times labeled RNA probes can also be used). Colony hybridization technique is also referred to as ***replica plating*** by some authors. The technique depicted in ***Fig. 9.7*** is briefly described.

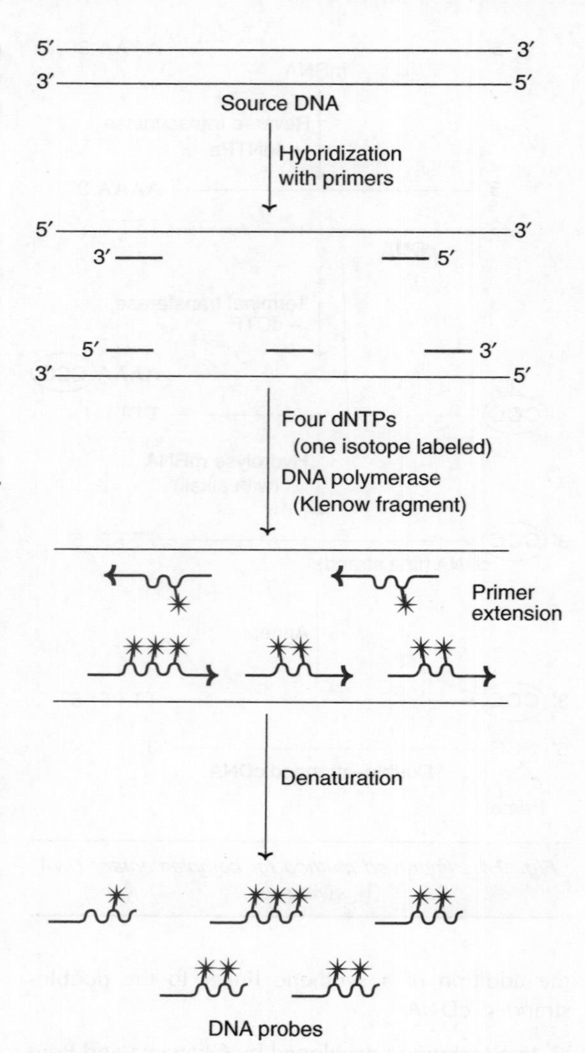

Fig. 9.6 : *Synthesis of radioisotope labeled DNA probes (**Note :** Non-isotopic DNA probes can be prepared by tagging with chemical labels e.g. biotin)*

The transformed cells are grown as colonies on a master plate. Samples of each colony are transferred to a solid matrix such as nitrocellulose or nylon membrane. The transfer is carefully carried out to retain the pattern of the colonies on the master plate. Thus, the nitrocellulose paper contains a photocopy pattern of the master plate colonies. The colony cells are lysed and deproteinized. The DNA is denatured and irreversibly bound to matrix. Now a radiolabeled DNA probe is added which hybridizes with the

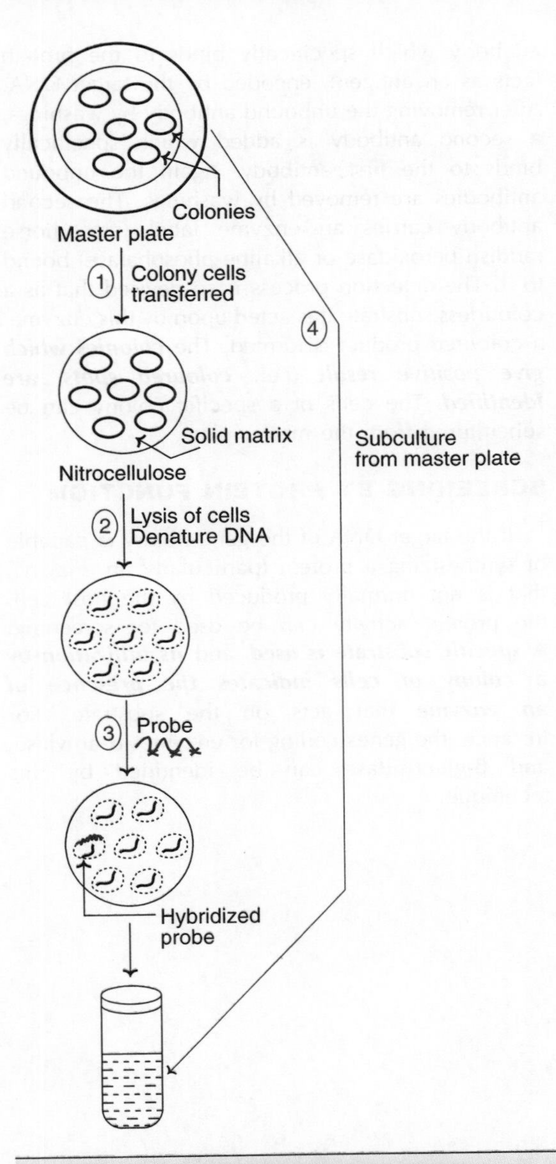

*Fig. 9.7 : Screening by colony hybridization (**Note** : Step 4 is carried out for the colony identified in step 3).*

complementary target DNA. The non-hybridized probe molecules are washed away. The colony with hybridized probe can be identified on autoradiograph. The cells of this colony (from the master plate) can be isolated and cultured.

Many a times multiple colonies are detected on hybridization by a DNA probe. This is due to overlapping sequences. To identify which colony has the complete sequence of the target gene, data observed from the restriction endonuclease analysis will be helpful.

Modifications of colony hybridization technique

Several improvements in the colony hybridization technique, described above, have been made in recent years. In the ***plaque lift technique***, nitrocellulose paper is directly applied on the upper surface of master agar plate making a direct contact. By this way, plaques can be lifted and several identical DNA prints can be made from a single plate. This technique increases reliability. More recently, screening of DNA libraries is carried out by automated techniques.

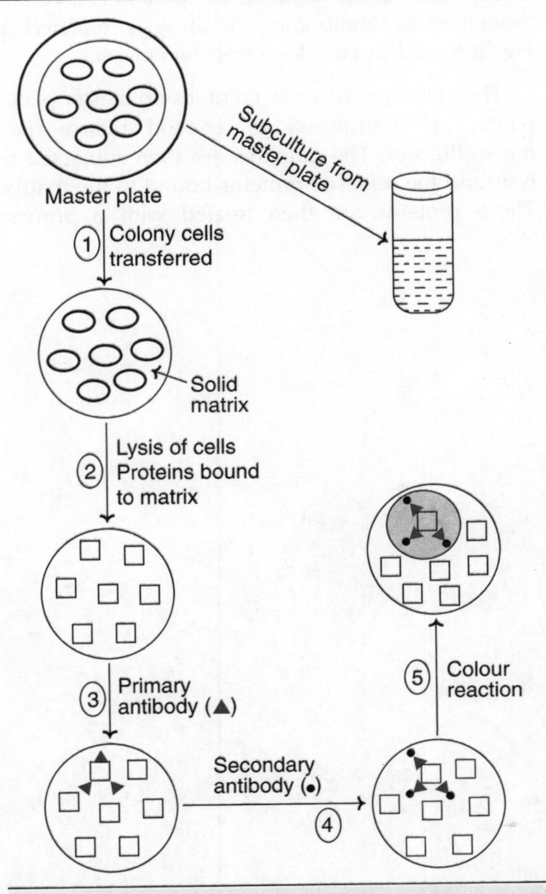

Fig. 9.8 : Immunological assay for screening a gene library.

SCREENING BY PCR

Polymerase chain reaction (PCR) is as good as hybridization technique for screening DNA libraries. But adequate information (on the franking sequences of target DNA) must be available to prepare primers for this method. The colonies are maintained in multiwell plates, each well is screened by PCR and the positive wells are identified.

SCREENING BY IMMUNOLOGICAL ASSAY

Immunological techniques can be used for the detection of a protein or a polypeptide, synthesized by a gene (through transcription followed by translation). The procedure adopted for immunological assay and hybridization technique (described already) are quite comparable. Screening procedure by immunological assay is depicted in ***Fig. 9.8***, and briefly described hereunder.

The cells are grown as colonies on master plates which are transferred to a solid matrix (i.e., nitrocellulose). The colonies are then subjected to lysis and the released proteins bound to the matrix. These proteins are then treated with a primary antibody which specifically binds to the protein (acts as an antigen), encoded by the target DNA. After removing the unbound antibody by washings, a second antibody is added which specifically binds to the first antibody. Again the unbound antibodies are removed by washings. The second antibody carries an enzyme label (e.g., horse raddish peroxidase or alkaline phosphatase) bound to it. The detection process is so devised that as a colourless substrate it is acted upon by this enzyme, a coloured product is formed. The ***colonies which give positive result*** (i.e., ***coloured spots***) ***are identified***. The cells of a specific colony can be subcultured from the master plate.

SCREENING BY PROTEIN FUNCTION

If the target DNA of the gene library is capable of synthesizing a protein (particularly an enzyme) that is not normally produced by the host cell, the protein activity can be used for screening. A ***specific substrate is used***, and ***its utilization by a colony of cells indicates the presence of an enzyme*** that acts on the substrate. For instance, the genes coding for enzymes α-amylase, and β-glucosidase can be identified by this technique.

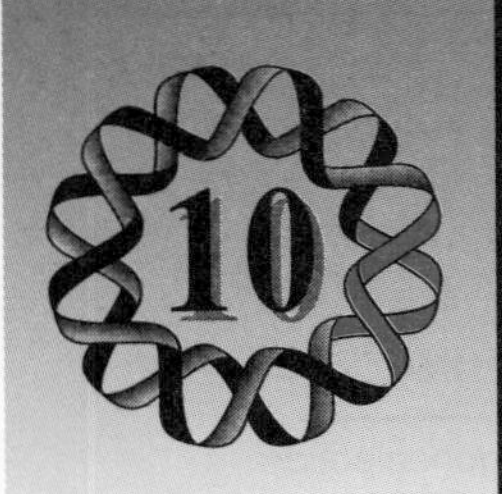

Site-directed Mutagenesis and Protein Engineering

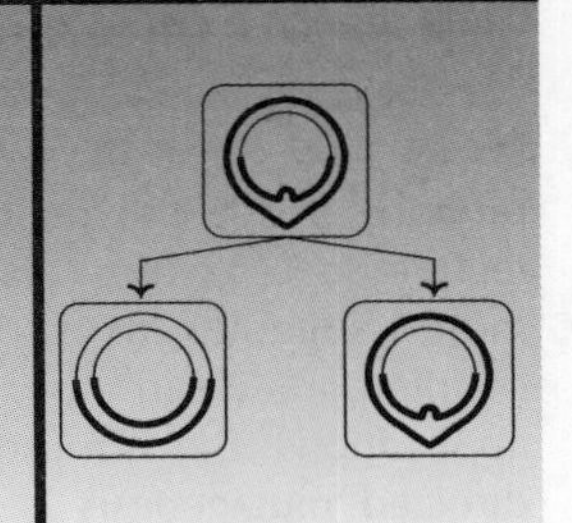

With the advances in genetic engineering, genes can be isolated (from any organism) and used for the synthesis of naturally occurring proteins. Some of these proteins serve as enzymes (i.e., biocatalysts), and a selected few of them have industrial applications. Thus, ***of the 2000 natural enzymes, around 20 are used in food, and pharmaceutical industries*** e.g., α-amylase, cellulase, papain. The industrial enzymes enjoy a special status in biotechnology.

The natural enzymes are not well suited for industrial applications due to unnatural and unphysiological environments such as high temperature, unsuitable pH, the presence of certain chemicals (organic solvents) etc. Many attempts are made to improve the efficiency of natural enzymes for industrial use e.g., immobilization (Refer Chapter 21), chemical modifications. But these have very limited impact.

STRATEGIES TO IMPROVE *IN VITRO* ACTIVITIES OF ENZYMES

Several possibilities can be thought of to improve the *in vitro* activities of the enzymes. Some of them are listed below.

- Increasing substrate affinity to enzyme.
- Making the enzyme thermal tolerant (active at high temperature) and/or pH stable.
- Enhancing the substrate specificity by modifying the substrate binding site of the enzyme.
- Designing the enzyme to make it resistant to proteolytic degradation.
- Synthesizing enzyme that is stable and active in non-aqueous solvents.
- Changing the enzyme in order to make it independent of cofactor(s) for its function.
- Eliminating allosteric sites in the enzyme so that it is not controlled by feedback inhibition.
- Improving the stability of the enzyme to heavy metals.
- Fusing the enzymes (making a multienzyme complex) needed in the reactions to give a final product.

Although the above possibilities appear to be more theoretical than practical, some achievements have been made for more efficient use of industrial enzymes. By subjecting the proteins to chemical modifications, suitable changes can be made in enzyme activity. Chemical manipulation of enzymes are non-specific, harsh and should be done repeatedly, hence not preferred.

Modifications in the DNA sequence of a gene are ideal to create a protein with desired properties. ***Site-directed mutagenesis is the technique for generating amino acid coding changes in the DNA (gene)***. By this approach ***specific (site-directed) change (mutagenesis)*** can be made in the base (or bases) of the gene ***to produce a desired enzyme***. The net result in site-directed mutagenesis is incorporation of a desired amino acid (of one's choice) in place of a specific amino acid in a protein or a polypeptide. By employing this technique, enzymes that are more efficient and more suitable than the naturally occurring counterparts can be created for industrial applications. But it must be remembered that site-directed mutagenesis is a trial and error method that may or may not result in a better protein. Further, the detailed information on the structure and functions of a protein are desirable to undertake site-directed mutagenesis. It is customary to give emphasis for the creation of enzymes by this technique because of their commercial value through industrial use. The fact is that any naturally occurring protein with improved functions can be synthesized by site-directed mutagenesis.

There are many methods employing site-directed mutagenesis. A selected few of them are briefly described.

OLIGONUCLEOTIDE-DIRECTED MUTAGENESIS

In the technique of oligonucleotide-directed mutagenesis, ***the primer is a chemically synthesized oligonucleotide*** (7–20 nucleotides long). It is complementary to a position of a gene around the site to be mutated. But it contains mismatch for the base to be mutated.

The basic technique is depicted in ***Fig. 10.1***. The starting material is a single-stranded DNA (to be mutated) carried in an M_{13} phage vector. On mixing this DNA with primer, the oligonucleotide hybridizes with the complementary sequences, except at the point of mismatched nucleotide. Hybridization (despite a single base mismatch) is possible by mixing at low temperature with excess of primer, and in the presence of high salt concentration.

By the addition of 4-deoxyribonucleoside triphosphates and DNA polymerase (usually Klenow fragment of *E.coli* DNA polymerase) replication occurs. Thus the oligonucleotide primer is extended to form a complementary strand of the DNA. The ends of the newly synthesized DNA are sealed by the enzyme DNA ligase. The double- stranded DNA (i.e., M_{13} phage molecule) containing the mismatched nucleotides is introduced into *E. coli* by transformation. The infected *E. coli* cells produce M_{13} virus particles containing either the original wild type sequence or the mutant sequence. The virus particles lyse the cells and form plaques.

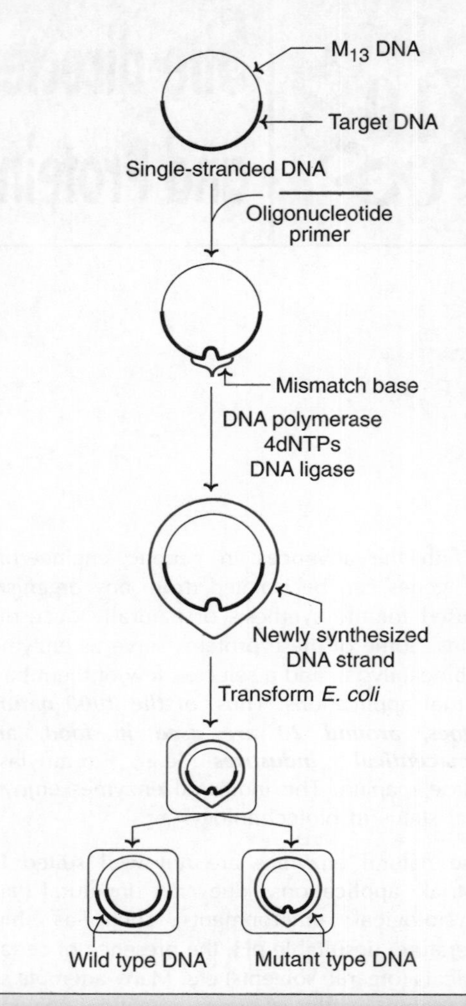

Fig. 10.1 : Oligonucleotide-directed mutagenesis (dNTPs–Deoxyribonucleoside triphosphates)

Theoretically, it is expected that half of the phage M_{13} particles should carry wild type sequence while the other half mutant sequence (since the DNA replicates semiconservatively). But in actual practice, due to technical reasons, only ***1-5% of the viruses with mutated sequences are recovered***.

The double-stranded DNAs of M_{13} are isolated. The mutated genes are cut with restriction enzymes,

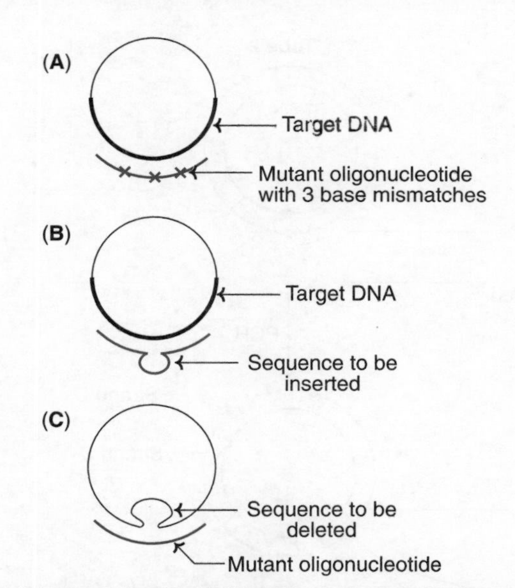

*Fig. 10.2 : Variations in oligonucleotide-directed mutagenesis **(A)** Multiple point mutagenesis **(B)** Insertion mutagenesis **(C)** Deletion mutagenesis.*

ligated to a plasmid vector of *E. coli.* The altered protein is produced in the *E. coli* which can be isolated and purified.

Oligonucleotide-directed mutagenesis by using plasmid DNA (instead of M_{13}) is also in use. This technique reduces the number of steps since mutagenesis and cloning the target DNA are in the same vector.

Variations in oligonucleotide-directed mutagenesis

There are some variations in use in the oligonucleotide-directed mutagenesis, as the situation demands.

1. **Multiple point mutagenesis :** Oligonucleotide-directed mutagenesis can be used to create DNAs with multiple point mutations with the requisite number of base mismatches (***Fig. 10.2A***).

2. **Insertion mutagenesis :** In this case, the mutant oligonucleotide carries a sequence to be inserted (sandwiched between two sites with complementary sequences). This can bind with the target DNA on either side (***Fig. 10.2B***).

3. **Deletion mutagenesis :** The mutant oligonucleotide binds to two separate sites on either side of the target DNA. This enables a small position of target DNA to be deleted (***Fig. 10.2C***).

CASETTEE MUTAGENESIS

In casettee mutagenesis, a synthetic double-stranded oligonucleotide (a small DNA fragment i.e., casettee) containing the requisite/desired mutant sequence is used. It replaces the corresponding sequence in the wild type DNA. ***Casettee mutagenesis is possible if the fragment of the gene to be mutated lies between two restriction enzyme cleavage sites.*** This intervening sequence can be cut and replaced by the synthetic oligonucleotide (with mutation).

The outline of the casettee mutagenesis technique is depicted in ***Fig. 10.3***. The plasmid DNA is cut with restriction enzymes (such as *EcoR1* and *Hind111*). The synthetic oligonucleotide containing mutant sequence is also cleaved and ligated to plasmid DNA. The recombinant plasmids that multiply in *E. coli* are all mutants.

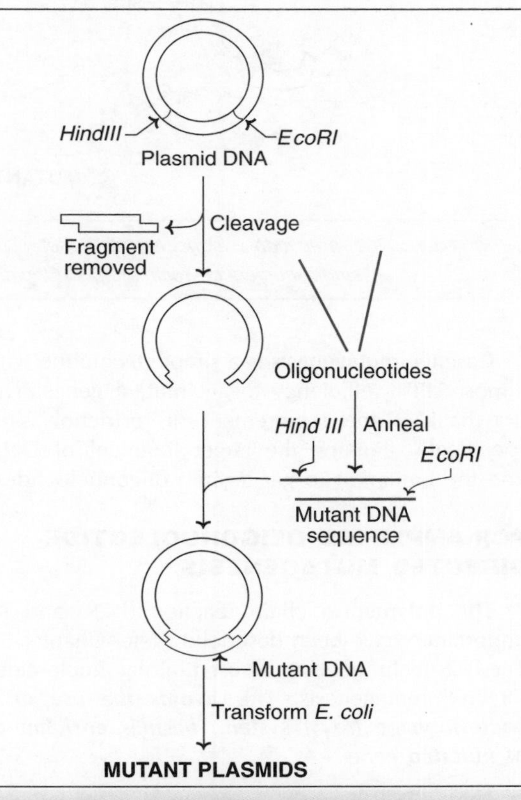

Fig. 10.3 : Casettee mutagenesis.

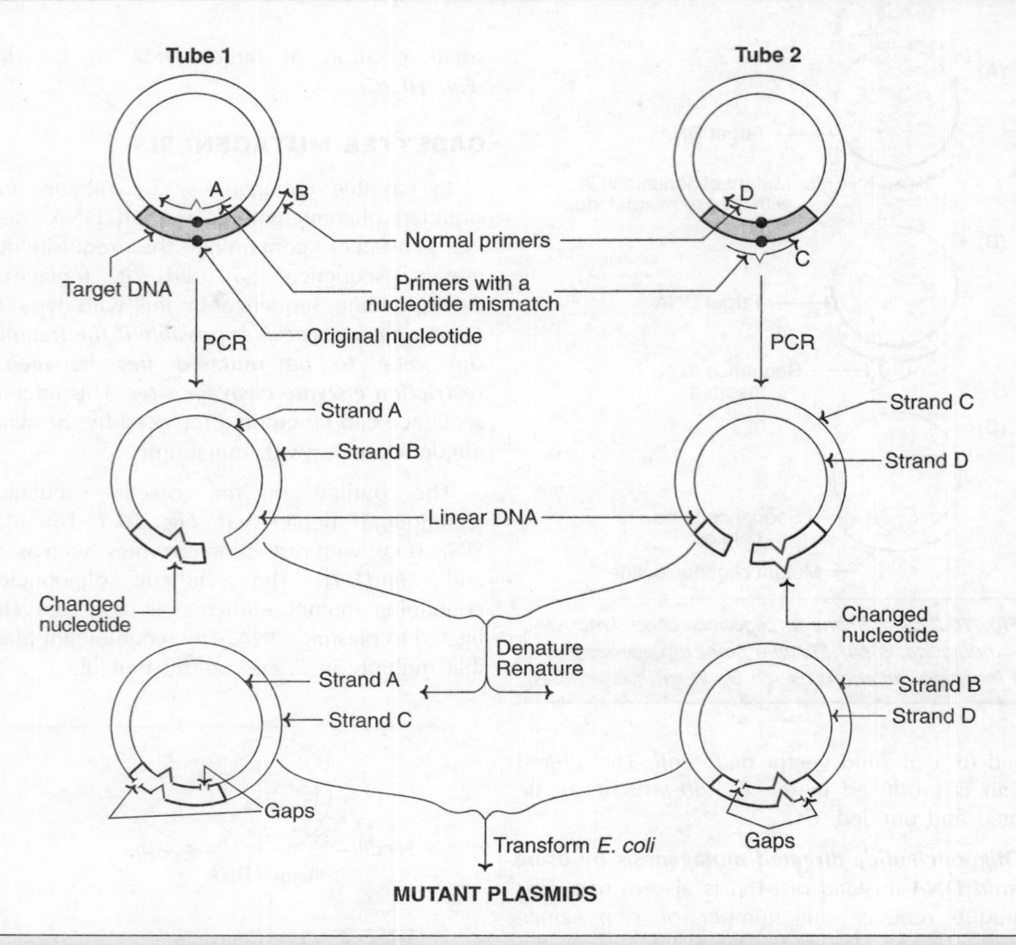

Fig. 10.4 : PCR-amplified oligonucleotide-directed mutagenesis (⟶ -Normal primers; ⟶ -Primers with a single nucleotide mismatch; ● -Original nucleotides; ═⌃═ -Changed nucleotides).

Casettee mutagenesis is a simple technique with almost 100% efficiency to get mutant genes. The drawback is the requirement of restriction sites specifically flanking the target fragment of DNA and the limitation to get desired oligonucleotides.

PCR-AMPLIFIED OLIGONUCLEOTIDE-DIRECTED MUTAGENESIS

The polymerase chain reaction (PCR) and its importance have been described (Refer Chapter 8). The PCR technique can be used in oligonucleotide-directed mutagenesis. This ***avoids the use of a bacteriophage (M_{13}) system, besides enrichment of mutated gene***.

The PCR-based mutagenesis technique commonly employed is depicted in ***Fig. 10.4***. First the target DNA (gene) is cloned on to a plasmid vector and distributed into two reaction tubes. To each tube are added two primers (oligonucleotides synthesized by using PCR). One primer (A in tube 1 and C in tube 2) is complementary to a region in one strand of the cloned gene except for one nucleotide mismatch (i.e., the one targeted for a change). The other primer (B in tube 1 and D in tube 2) is fully complementary to a sequence in the other strand, within or adjacent to the cloned gene. The placement of primers for hybridization (with the DNA strands) in each tube is done in opposite direction. Now, the PCR technique is carried out for amplification of the DNA molecules. These DNAs are actually linear. In ***Fig. 10.4***, they are shown as discontinuous circles for understanding subsequent steps.

The products of PCR in the two reaction tubes are mixed. The DNA molecules undergo denaturation and renaturation. A strand from one reaction tube (strand A) hybridizes with its complementary strand from other reaction tube (strand C). They form circles with nicks (gaps). The circular plasmids (containing mutant DNA) with nicks are introduced into *E. coli* by transformation. The nicks are sealed *in vivo* by host cell enzymes and the plasmids are propagated indefinitely.

PROTEIN ENGINEERING

One of the most exciting aspects of genetic engineering is to design, develop and produce ***proteins with improved operating characteristics*** (increased stability, improved kinetics etc.), besides sometimes ***creating even novel proteins***. The techniques such as site-directed mutagenesis and gene cloning are utilized for this pupose.

INCREASING THE STABILITY AND BIOLOGICAL ACTIVITY OF PROTEINS

By increasing the half-lives or thermostability of enzymes/proteins, their industrial applications or therapeutic uses can be more appropriately met. Some of the approaches for producing proteins with enhanced stability are described below.

ADDITION OF DISULFIDE BONDS

Significant ***increase in the thermostability of enzymes*** is observed ***by adding disulfide bonds***. However, the additional disulfide bonds should not interfere with the normal enzyme function.

In general, the new protein with added disulfide bonds does not readily unfold at high temperatures, and further it is resistant to denaturation at non-physiological conditions (high pH, presence of organic solvents). These characteristics are particularly important for industrial applications of certain enzymes.

T4 Lysozyme

This an enzyme of bacteriophage T4. Good success has been achieved in introducing disulfide bonds in T4 lysozyme. This was done by changing two, four or six amino acids (in close proximity) to cysteine residues to respectively form one, two or three disulfide bonds.

In the wild type (native) T4 lysozyme, there are two cysteine residues at positions 54 and 97 which however are not held together by a disulfide bond. By oligonucleotide-directed mutagenesis, cysteine residues created disulfide bonds between positions (numbered form N-terminal end) 3 and 97, 9 and 164, and 21 and 142 of the enzyme. Introduction of disulfide bonds increases the folded structure and thermostability of the enzyme. Thus, ***T4 lysozyme with three disulfide bonds is very stable with good biological activity***. (**Note :** T4 lysozyme has no industrial or therapeutic applications. It is discussed here due to the success achieved in protein engineering).

Xylanase

This is an enzyme used in the industry for manufacture of paper from wood pulp. Xylanase has to be catalytically active at high temperature. Introduction of ***disulfide bonds*** (one, two or three) makes it thermostable, and substantially ***improves its functional efficiency***.

CHANGING ASPARAGINE TO OTHER AMINO ACIDS

At high temperature, the amino acids ***asparagine*** and also ***glutamine*** are likely to ***undergo deamidation*** (releasing ammonia) to respectively form aspartic acid and glutamic acid. These alterations are often associated with changes in the protein folding and ***loss of biological activity***.

Triosephosphate isomerase

This is a dimeric enzyme with identical subunits, each one having two asparagine residues which are thermosensitive (undergo deamidation). Oligonucleotide-directed mutagenesis was used to ***introduce threonine or isoleucine in place of asparagine*** at positions 14 and 78. The new enzyme was found to be ***thermostable***. On the other hand, when the asparagine residues were replaced by aspartic acid, the enzyme was unstable even at low temperature, with reduced activity.

REDUCING THE FREE SULFHYDRYL GROUPS

Sometimes, the presence of free sulfhydryl groups (contributed by cysteine residues) in more

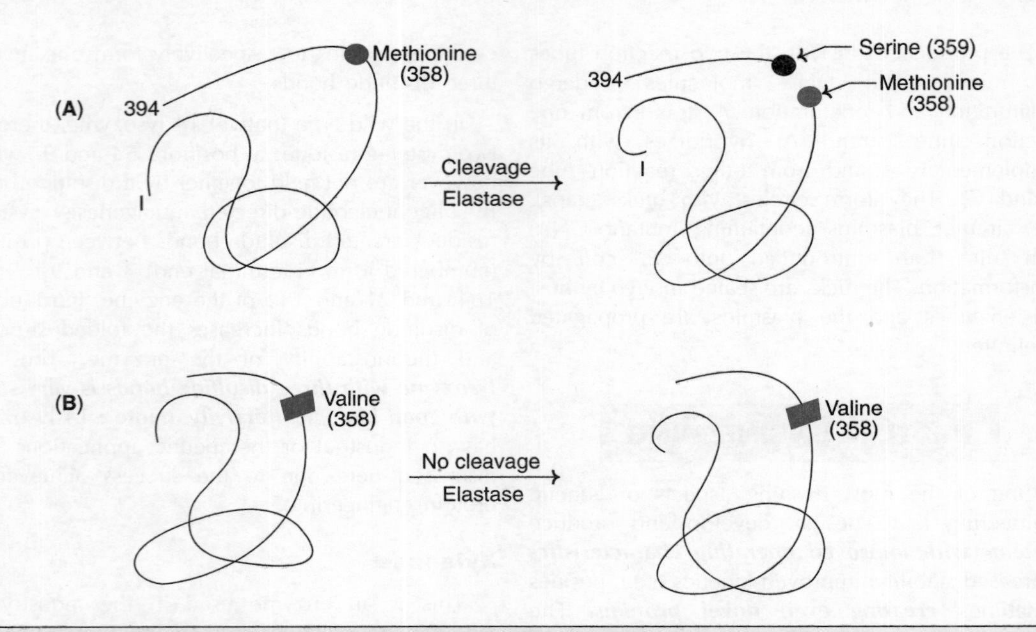

Fig. 10.5 : (A) The cleavage of α_1–antitrypsin by binding to elastase (B) No cleavage occurs when methionine (358) is replaced by valine.

numbers may be responsible for the low activity of the protein. In such a case, the protein or ***enzyme stability and its activity can be increased by reducing the number of sulfhydryl groups***.

Human β-interferon

The antiviral activity of human β-interferon (IFN β) produced in *E. coli* by genetic engineering was found to be only 10% of the original glycosylated form. Further, IFN β was found to exist as dimers and oligomers which are almost inactive. In fact, the cysteine residues were involved in intermolecular disulfide bonding resulting in the formation of dimers and oligomers. This happens in *E. coli* cells and not in human cells. This problem was successfully overcome by replacing cysteine residues by serine. It may be noted that the structures of these two amino acids are similar except that serine has oxygen in place of sulfur in cysteine. Consequently, ***introduction of serine in place of cysteine reduces free sulfhydryl groups***.

By the above process, IFN β with increased stability and good biological activity can be produced. Increased stability is in fact required for storage and therapeutic use of proteins such as interferons.

SINGLE AMINO ACID CHANGES

Some of the recombinant proteins can be improved in their stability and biology activity by a second generation variants. These have been frequently achieved by a single amino acid change.

α_1-Antitrypsin

α_1-Antitrypsin inhibits the action of neutrophil elastase (elastase is an enzyme that damages the lung tissues, often resulting in emphysema i.e. abnormal distension of lungs by air). α_1-Antitrypsin binds to elastase and prevents its action. In this process, α_1-antitrypsin gets cleaved between serine (359 residue) and methionine (358 residue). The free methionine is oxidized to methionine sulfoxide, making α_1-antitrypsin a poor inhibitor of elastase.

By ***replacing methionine at 358 position by valine, an oxidative-resistant variant of α_1-antitrypsin has been created (Fig. 10.5)***. This new enzyme is particularly important in treating patients with genetic deficiency of α_1-antitrypsin.

Insulin

In the neutral solution, therapeutic insulin is present mostly as zinc—containing hexamer. By introducing single amino acid substitutions, insulins were found to be in monomeric state with good stability and biological activity.

Tissue plasminogen activator (tPA)

Tissue plasminogen activator is therapeutically used to lyse the blood clots that cause myocardial infarction. Due to its shorter half-life (around 5 minutes), tPA has to be repeatedly administered. By ***replacing asparagine residue*** (at position 120) ***with glutamine, the half-life of tPA can be substantially increased***. This is due to the fact that glutamine is less glycosylated than asparagine and this makes a difference in the half-life of tPA.

Hirudin

Hirudin is a protein secreted by leech salivary gland, and is a strong thrombin inhibitor (i.e., acts as an anticoagulant). By ***replacing asparagine*** (at 47 position) ***with lysine, the potency of hirudin can be increased*** several-fold.

Dihydrofolate reductase

The enzyme dihydrofolate reductase (DHFR) catalyses the conversion of 7, 8-dihydrofolate to 5, 6, 7, 8-tetrahydrofolate. The latter coenzyme is closely involved in one carbon metabolism, which ultimately results in the synthesis of nucleic acids and amino acids. The inhibition of DHFR (conventionally by folate analogues such as methotrexate) will restrict the growth of tumor cells. Therefore the enzyme DHFR has some therapeutic applications.

By employing site-directed mutagenesis, ***replacement of glycine*** (at position 95) ***by alanine*** **was found to produce *DHFR* which is *completely inactive***.

T4 lysozyme

Replacement of glycine by any other amino acid in the protein structure, in general, decreases the stability. On the other hand, proline residues increase protein stability. In T4 lysozyme, substitution of glycine (at position 77) by alanine, and alanine (at position 82) by proline are found to increase the enzyme stability.

IMPROVING KINETIC PROPERTIES OF ENZYMES

It is possible to improve the functional activities of enzymes, by improving their kinetic properties (K_m, specificity etc.) through oligonucleotide-directed mutagenesis. This is particularly required for enzymes with industrial and therapeutic applications.

Subtilisin

Subtilisin is a major industrial enzyme secreted by Gram-positive bacteria (*Bacillus* species). It is a serine protease very widely ***used as an enzyme detergent*** (cleaning agent in laundries). However, the large scale industrial use of native subtilisin is restricted due to the oxidative inactivation of this enzyme. This occurs in a manner analogous to that already discussed for α_1-antitrypsin. The reason being that ***methionine*** (at position 222) lying close to the active site ***gets oxidized, making the enzyme inactive***. Logically, ***replacement of methionine*** (at position 222) ***by other amino acids will solve the problem***. This has been done, and in fact, all the 19 other amino acids have been tried as substitutes for methionine, with varying success.

Subtilisin is an enzyme that has been extensively exploited for genetic manipulations over the past 15 years. The result is that ***about 50% of the native amino acids of this enzyme have been changed by in vitro mutagenesis***. And almost every property of subtilisin has been altered. These include its stability, substrate specificity, thermal and alkaline inactivation.

Modifying metal requirement of subtilisin : The enzyme subtilisin binds to calcium and gets stabilized. But in many industries where subtilisin is used, metal-chelating agents are also employed. They bind to calcium and the enzyme becomes inactive. This problem can be solved by oligonucleotide-directed mutagenesis. The nucleotide sequence in the DNA encoding for the amino acids (residues 75 to 83) that bind to calcium is removed. Then, several other amino acids are modified in subtilisin by trial and error method. In fact, success has been achieved in creating calcium-free subtilisin with good stability and activity.

Asparaginase

This is an enzyme used ***in the control of leukemia*** (uncontrolled growth of white blood cells). Intravenous administration of asparaginase cleaves asparagine to aspartate (the reduced availability of asparagine restricts cell prolifiration).

Surprisingly, the asparaginases from different sources exhibited differences in their effectiveness to control leukemia. This is due to the variations in the kinetic properties. Thus, the ***asparaginase with a low K_m value*** (i.e., with high affinity for asparagine hence more breakdown) has to be selected ***for therapeutic use in the control of leukemia***.

Tyrosyl t-RNA synthetase

The enzyme tyrosyl t-RNA synthetase from *Bacillus stearothermophilus* has been modified with regard to substrate binding i.e., K_m value. This enzyme catalyses the two reactions given below to finally give tyrosine t-RNA.

Tyrosine + ATP ⟶ Tyrosyladenylate + PPi

Tyrosyladenylate + t-RNA ⟶ Tyrosine t-RNA + AMP

Replacement of threonine (at position 51), ***by*** either ***alanine or proline***, variants of tyrosyl t-RNA synthetase have been produced. Alanine variant has a two fold binding affinity (low K_m) for ATP. And for proline variant ATP binds about 100-fold more tightly (very low K_m). (**Note :** The proline in general distorts the helical structure and reduces the enzyme affinity to the substrate. The one mentioned here is surprisingly, an exception).

Restriction endonucleases

The protein engineering studies can be successfully employed for modifying enzyme specificities. This is what has been achieved in oligonucleotide-directed mutagenesis with respect to restriction endonucleases.

So far, about 2500 restriction endonucleases are known. However, since most of these enzymes recognize the same sequence on the DNA for their action, there are only about 200 different recognition sites. Thus there is an overlap in the recognition sites of several restriction enzymes. As such, there are two types of restriction endonucleases—the ***frequent cutters*** which recognize a sequence of 4-6 bp and ***rare cutters*** recognizing a sequence above 8 bp. The rare cutters are more useful for producing large DNA fragments.

By ***using protein engineering technique***, the existing ***restriction endonucleases have been suitably modified to produce rare cutters***.

PROTEIN ENGINEERING BY USE OF GENE FAMILIES

The recent development in protein engineering is ***DNA shuffling***, also known as ***molecular breeding*** (developed by Nesse in 2000). This method can be applied to a protein if it belongs to a known protein family. The technique primarily involves isolation of genes from each species, and then creation of hybrids in different combinations. While applying this approach to subtilisin, genes from 26 species were mixed to create a library. Among these, 4 enzymes were found to have improved properties.

PROTEIN ENGINEERING THROUGH CHEMICAL MODIFICATIONS

Although with limited success, chemical modifications of proteins have been attempted to increase the stability of proteins to high temperature and organic solvents. The amino acid lysine residues can be cross-linked by use of chemical linkers.

The most extensively used ***protein cross linker*** is ***glutaraldehyde***. It stabilizes the proteins in solutions. By using glutaraldehyde, certain proteins (hemoglobin, insulin, phosphofructokinase, lactate dehydrogenase) have been stabilized.

PROTEIN ENGINEERING—AN EVER EXPANDING FIELD

Selected examples of protein engineering are described above only to highlight the scope of protein engineering. The techniques of enzyme engineering are rapidly expanding and several newer developments are in the offing to develop proteins / enzymes for industrial and therapeutic purposes.

The question before biotechnologists specialized in protein engineering is not 'what modifications are possible', but 'how do I achieve the modifications I wish to make'.

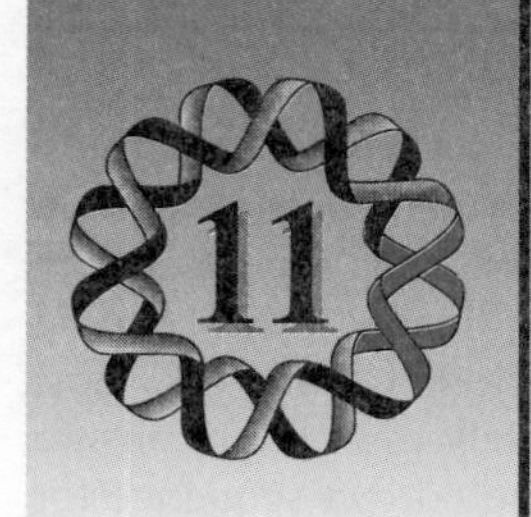

Manipulation of Gene Expression in Host Cells

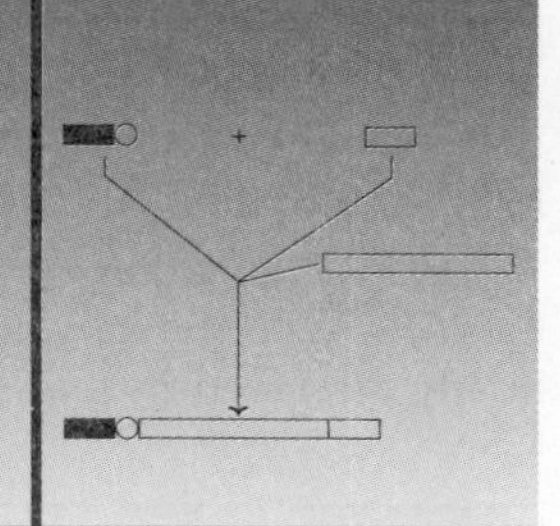

The preparation of recombinant DNAs, their insertion into vectors, and the cloning methods have been described (Chapter 6). The expression of cloned genes in the host organisms is dealt with in this chapter.

SELECTION OF HOST CELLS FOR GENE EXPRESSION

The nature of a host cell or an organism is as important as the nature of a vector. The most important requirements of a good host include its suitable cultivation in the laboratory, besides incorporating the vector's genetic material. Several prokaryotes and eukaryotes are employed as hosts to express foreign genes (Refer Chapter 6).

Prokaryotic hosts

The bacterium ***Escherichia coli*** was the first organism to be used in recombinant DNA technology experiments, and continues to be ***a host of choice for commercial production of proteins***. The extensive use of *E. coli* is mainly due to its high rate of reproduction (the cells double in number, every twenty minutes), besides good knowledge on its biochemistry, physiology and molecular biology. There are a few disadvantages also in using *E. coli* as a host. These include a relatively poor export system for proteins and the production of endotoxins which are often difficult to remove (from other useful products).

The other host bacterium in use is *Bacillus subtilis.* This organism is widely employed for commercial production of antibiotics, industrial enzymes, insecticides etc.

Eukaryotic hosts

It is often desirable to use eukaryotic organisms, with a well defined nucleus and celluar organelles, as hosts. The ***main advantage*** with eukaryotes is that they bring about several ***post-translational modifications*** to make viable and functional proteins. Further, use of eukaryotic hosts is not associated with the generation and interference of toxins which is the case with some prokaryotes. Thus, eukaryotic gene expression systems are preferred for the production of proteins and therapeutic agents that are useful for humans and animals.

The yeast ***Saccharomyces cerevisiae is widely used*** as a host for the expression of cloned eukaryotic genes. The other yeasts in use include *Kluveromyces lactis, Schizosaccharomyces pombe* and *Picha pastoris.*

The ***insect cells*** which are ***infected by baculovirus*** are in use as hosts in recent years. The baculovirus system can carry and express hundreds of genes in insect cells. Another advantage is that the safety factor since baculoviruses do not infect humans, other vertebrates or plants.

Mammalian cells such as ***mouse cells*** can be used as hosts to produce complex proteins with optimal biological functions. But the limitations with mammalian cells are that the techniques are tedious, often difficult, and also expensive.

The manipulation of gene expression, as it is carried out, in prokaryotic and eukaryotic cells is briefly discussed in the following pages.

MANIPULATION OF GENE EXPRESSION IN PROKARYOTES

The ***prime objective of gene cloning*** is to finally result in the ***large scale production of proteins*** for a variety of purposes (industrial, commercial, human health and welfare). This is achieved by the maximal expression of cloned genes through manipulations. The following are the important features of gene expression that can be considered for manipulation.

- The presence of regulatable promoters.
- The number of copies of cloned genes.
- The location of the cloned genes whether inserted into a plasmid or integrated into host genome.
- The translation efficiency of the host.
- The cellular location of the foreign protein and its stability in the host cell.

Some of the strategies that are employed for the manipulation of gene expression in *E. coli* are discussed hereunder.

Regulatable promoters

The presence of a strong regulatable promoter sequence is essential for an effective expression of a cloned gene. This is achieved by employing the promoters of *E. coli lac* (lactose) operon or *trp* (tryptophan) operon. These promoters have strong affinity for RNA polymerase, and consequently the dounstream region (of cloned gene) is transcribed. The promoters thus provide a switch for turning on or turning off the transcription of a cloned gene.

Fusion proteins

The ***combination of a foreign protein*** (encoded by a cloned gene) ***with the host protein*** is referred to as a fusion protein.

In general, the foreign proteins synthesized are rapidly degraded. This can be reduced by covalently linking a stable host protein to the foreign proteins (i.e., fusion proteins). The fusion proteins in fact protect the proteolytic degradation of cloned gene product. The synthesis of fusion proteins is achieved by ligating the coding sequences of two genes (cloned gene and host gene). However, it is absolutely essential to ensure that cloned gene contains the correct sequence for the synthesis of the target protein.

Cleavage of fusion proteins : The fusion proteins, as such, interfere with the biological activity of the target protein. Therefore, these proteins should be cleaved to release the specific desired functional proteins.

Uses of fusion proteins : The purification of recombinant proteins is much easier in the form of fusion proteins. Fusion proteins are also useful for generating antibodies against target proteins.

Tandem gene arrays

In general, increase in the number of plasmids (containing cloned gene) proportionately increases the production of recombinant protein. This has a drawback. As the plasmid number increases, the genes coding for antibiotic resistance also increase. The overall effect is that the regular metabolic activites of the host cell are disturbed for the synthesis of plasmid proteins. Consequently, the yield of cloned gene product is not optimum.

An alternative approach is to clone ***multiple copies of the target gene on a single plasmid*** (instead of a single gene on a plasmid). In this manner, tandem arrays of a gene can be created. However, each sequence of the genes should be in correct orientation for transcription and translation.

Efficiency of translation

The quantity of the cloned gene product produced depends on the efficiency of translation. In general, the binding ability of mRNA with the ribosomal RNA, at translational initiation signal called ***ribosome binding site determines translation***. Thus, the efficiency of translation is better if the binding of mRNA to rRNA is stronger. The actual binding between mRNA and rRNA occurs by complementary base pairing of a sequence of 6-8 nucleotides.

To achieve maximum translation, the *E. coli* expression vectors are designed to possess a strong ribsome binding site.

Stability of proteins

The half-lives of recombinant proteins are highly variable, ranging from minutes to hours. The stability of proteins can be increased by adding amino acids at the N-terminal end of the proteins. Thus, by attaching methionine, serine and alanine to the N-terminal end, the half-life of β-galactosidase can be increased from 2 minutes to 20 hours! Frequently, a single ***amino acid addition at N-terminal end stabilizes the protein***. The yield of recombinant DNA proteins can be enhanced by increasing half-lives.

Secretion of proteins

The stability of a protein and its secretion are interrelated. An amino acid sequence (signal peptide) may be attached to a protein to facilitate its secretion through cell membrane. Recombinant proteins secreted into the growth medium can be easily purified.

Integration of cloned DNA into the host chromosome

The use of plasmids for transcription and translation of cloned DNA imposes a metabolic load (discussed later) on the host. In addition, there is often a chance of losing plasmids during cell multiplication. These problems can be overcome by integrating the cloned DNA directly into host chromosomal DNA. Once the ***cloned DNA becomes a part of genome, it can be maintained for several generations***.

Cloned DNA integration into the host DNA is possible only when there is a complementary sequence of about 50 nucleotides between them. The exchange of DNAs occurs by a recombination process (***Fig. 11.1***). The cloned DNA lies in the middle of plasmid DNA. On physical contact with chromosomal DNA, base pairing occurs between plasmid DNA (x and y) and chromosomal DNA (x′ and y′). And the cloned DNA is transferred to host chromosomal DNA by a physical exchange i.e., recombination.

Metabolic load

The presence of ***cloned DNA alters the metabolism*** and cellular functions ***of the host organism***. Such metabolic changes are collectively referred to as metabolic load, ***metabolic drain or metabolic burden***. There are several causes for the

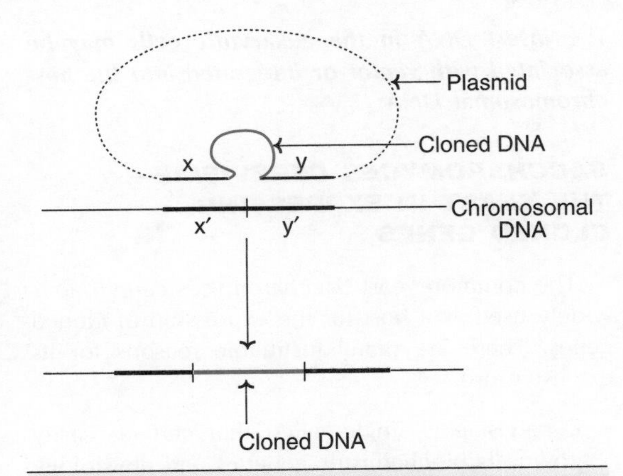

Fig. 11.1 *: Integration of a cloned DNA into chromosomal DNA.*

metabolic load. These include increased utilization of energy for replication and maintenance of plasmids, overproduction of proteins (also drains amino acids, tRNAs), and interference of foreign proteins on the host cell function.

MANIPULATION OF GENE EXPRESSION IN EUKARYOTES

Expression of cloned genes in eukaryotes has certain ***advantages***. The most important being the ***ability of eukaryotic organisms to bring about post-translational modifications***—glycosylation, phosphorylation, correct disulfide bond formation, proteolytic cleavage etc. Eukaryotic expression systems produce stable and biologically active proteins. This is in contrast to the prokaryotic expression of cloned genes.

In general, the eukaryotic expression of cloned genes is quite comparable to that occurs in the prokaryotes. However, from the technical perspective, it is more difficult to conduct experiments with eukaryotic cells. Many a times, vectors with two distinct origins of replication are used. They serve as shuttle vectors and function in prokaryotic as well as eukaryotic hosts.

The insertion of a foreign DNA into bacterial and yeast cells is referred to as ***transformation*** (Refer Chapter 6). The term ***transfection*** is used for the introduction of a foreign DNA into animal cells.

The ***insert DNA in the eukaryotic cells may be associated with vector or integrated into the host chromosomal DNA.***

SACCHAROMYCES CEREVISIAE— THE YEAST IN EXPRESSING CLONED GENES

The common yeast *Saccharomyces cerevisiae* is widely used as a host for the expression of cloned genes. There are many justifiable reasons for its extensive use.

- *S. cervisiae* is single-celled that can be easily grown. Its biochemistry, genetics and physiology are quite known.
- It has a naturally occurring plasmid and strong promoters for efficient expression.
- *S. cerevisiae* can bring about many post-translational changes in proteins.
- The secreted recombinant proteins can be easily isolated, since very few host proteins are secreted.
- The U.S. Food and Drug Administration has certified *S. cerevisiae* as a ***generally recognized as a safe*** (***GRAS***) organism.

As such, *S. cerevisiae* has been in use for several decades in baking and brewing industries. Biotechnologists work quite comfortably with this yeast to ***produce a large number of recombinant proteins***. These include ***insulin, α_1-antitrypsin, hepatitis B virus surface antigen***, platelet derived growth factor, fibroblast growth factor and HIV-I antigens. These products are in use as diagnostic agents, vaccines, and therapeutic agents.

Vectors for *S. cerevisiae*

There are three types of vectors for *S. cerevisiae* :

1. Episomal or plasmid vectors.
2. Integrating vectors.
3. Yeast artificial chromosomes (YACs).

1. **Plasmid vectors :** Among the vectors, plasmids with single cloned genes are widely used. Manipulation with growth conditions increase the vector stability and expression efficiency. Use of tandem gene arrays has not met with success, since they are unstable.

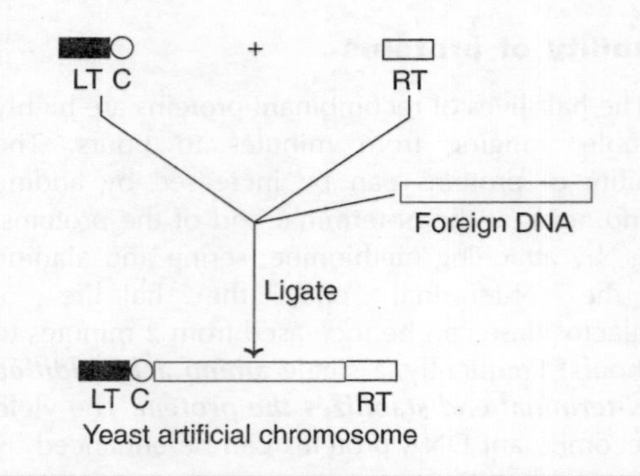

Fig. 11.2 : Construction of yeast artificial chromosome (LT-Left telomere; C-Centromere; RT-Right telomere).

2. **Integrating vectors :** They are basically the integration of cloned genes with chromosomal DNA. These are not frequently used, since the protein production is low.

3. **Yeast artificial chromosome (YAC) :** Introduced in 1987, YAC is a fragment of yeast DNA that will accept a foreign DNA of about 250–500 kb in length. In fact, the yeast DNA is only about 1% of the total DNA which however, is very important, since it contains three essential genes required for replication. These are the genes for ***telomere*** (that protects DNA from nuclease degradation and thus maintains stability), ***centromere*** (forms spindles during cell division) and the ***origin of replication*** (where DNA polymerase initiates replication). YAC behaves just like a chromosome and replicates.

The construction of the yeast artificial chromosome is depicted in ***Fig. 11.2***. Two opposite ends of a yeast chromosome namely the left telomere and right telomere are chosen. The left telomere is then attached to a centromere. A large segment of the foreign DNA is added and all the three are ligated. Unlike the plasmid vectors, the stability of YAC increases as the size of insert DNA increases.

YACs have not been used for commercial production of recombinant proteins. However, they have been employed successfully for physical mapping of genomic DNAs, particularly in human genome project, (For details, Refer Chapter 12).

Post-translational modifications by *S. cerevisiae*

The heterologous proteins synthesized by *S. cerevisiae* undergo post-translational changes while they are being exported into the extracellular environment. To facilitate protein secretion, a single (leader) peptide is attached to the protein. This peptide is removed by the yeast endoprotease.

OTHER YEAST EXPRESSION SYSTEMS

Despite the very successful use of *S. cerevisiae* for generating recombinant proteins, there are certain limitations. These include a very low or a limited yield, difficulty in secretion of some proteins and hyperglycosylation. Attempts are being made to explore the utility of other yeasts for the production of hepatitis B virus surface antigen (HBsAg) and bovine lysozyme. The yeast, ***Hansenula polymorpha***, is employed for the ***synthesis of α- and β-globin chains of human hemoglobin***.

INSECT CELL EXPRESSION SYSTEMS

Cultured insect cells are in use for expressing cloned DNAs. *Baculoviruses* exclusively infect insect cells. The DNA of these viruses encode for several products and their productivity in cells is very high to the extent of more than 10,000 times compared to mammalian cells. Besides carrying a large number of foreign genes, the baculoviruses can effectively express and process the products formed. Another advantage with these viruses is that they ***cannot infect humans***, other vertebrates or plants. Thus, ***baculoviruses are safe vectors***.

Polyhedrin gene of baculovirus

The polyhedrin gene is responsible for the synthesis of a matrix protein-polyhedrin. This protein is synthesized in large quantities by baculovirus during the infection cycle. Polyhedrin protects the virus from being inactivated by environmental agents. The promoter for polyhedrin gene is very strong. However, the life-cycle of baculovirus does not depend on the presence of this gene. Polyhedrin gene can be replaced by a cloned gene, and the genetically engineered baculovirus can infect the cultured insect cells. The cloned gene expresses, and large quantities of recombinant proteins are produced. Because of a close similarity in the post-translational modifications between insects and mammals, biologically active proteins can be produced by this approach. And in fact, by using baculovirus as an expression vector system, a good number of mammalian and viral proteins have been synthesized (***Table 11.1***).

Table 11.1 Selected examples of recombinant proteins produced by baculovirus expression vector system

Adenosine deaminase
Alkaline phosphatase
Amyloid precursor protein
Anthrax antigen
DNA polymerase α
Erythropoietin
HIV-I envelope protein
Interferons (α, β)
Interleukin-2
Malaria proteins
Pancreatic lipase
Polio virus proteins
Rabies virus proteins
Rhodopsin
Simian rotavirus capsid antigen
Tissue plasminogen activator

Baculovirus expression vector system

The most commonly used baculovirus is ***Autographa californica multiple nuclear polyhedrosis virus (AcMNPV)***. It can grow on the insect cell lines (e.g., derived from fall army worm) and produce high levels of polyhedrin or a recombinant protein.

The organization of a baculovirus (AcMNPV) transfer vector is shown in ***Fig. 11.3A***. It consists of an *E. coli*-based plasmid vector along with the DNA of baculovirus. This in turn has AcMNPV DNA, a polyhedrin promoter region, cloning site for insert DNA and polyhedrin termination region.

When the insect culture cells, transfected with AcMNPV are mixed with transfer vector carrying a cloned gene, a double crossover occurs. The result is that the cloned gene with polyhedrin promoter and termination sequences gets integrated into

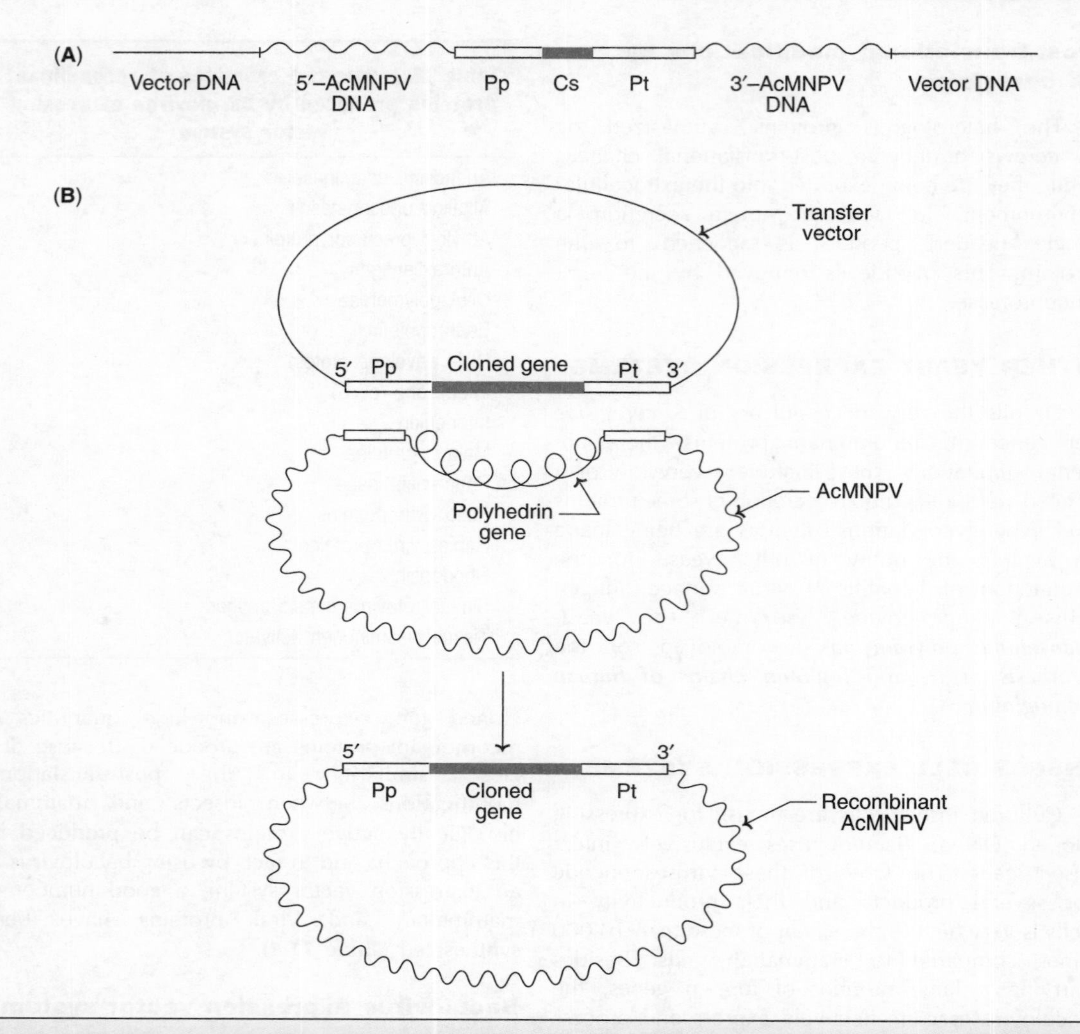

*Fig. 11.3 : Baculovirus expression vector system **(A)** Organization of baculovirus transfer vector **(B)** Replacement of the polyhedrin gene of baculovirus with a cloned gene from a transfer vector (AcMNPV–*Autographa californica *multiple nuclear polyhedrosis virus; Pp–Polyhydrin gene promoter; Cs–Cloning site; Pt–Polyhedrin gene termination; **Note :** The coding region of polyhedrin gene not shown in A).*

AcMNPV DNA (***Fig. 11.3B***). In this process, polyhedrin gene is lost. The recombinant baculovirus containing cloned gene is isolated.

The host insect culture cells, on infection with recombinant baculovirus, produce heterologous proteins. A large number and a wide variety of recombinant proteins (around 500) have been synthesized in the laboratory. A majority of them (>95%) have the requisite post-translational modifications. A selected list of recombinant proteins is given in ***Table 11.1***.

Modifications in the production of recombinant baculovirus

The original method of creating recombinant baculovirus has undergone several changes. Incorporation of a unique Bsu 361 restriction endonuclease site on the polyhedrin gene increases the yield of recombinant baculovirus production to about 30% from the normal 1%.

Bacmid : This is shuttle vector for *E. coli* and insect cell baculovirus. Construction of a recombinant bacmid is a novel approach to carry

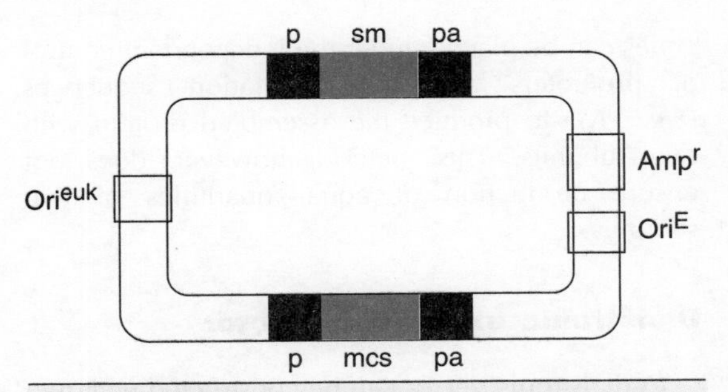

Fig. 11.4 : A diagrammatic representation of mammalian expression vector (p–Promoter sequence; Pa–polyadenylation sequence; mcs–Multiple cloning site; sm-Selectable marker gene; Ori^{euk}–Origin of eukaryotic replication; Ori^{E}–Origin of E. coli *replication; Amp^{r}–Ampicilin resistant marker gene).*

out all the genetic manipulations including the expression of baculovirus vector in *E. coli.*

Use of yeast cells : The genetic manipulations of AcMNPV genome can be done in yeast cells with yeast-insect shuttle vector. Then the recombinant baculovirus is introduced into insect cells.

MAMMALIAN CELL EXPRESSION VECTORS

Mammalian expression vectors are ***useful for the production*** of specific and authentic ***recombinant proteins*** (for use as therapeutic agents). In addition, they are also helpful for studying the function and regulation of mammalian genes. In general, the mammalian expression vectors are quite comparable to other eukaryotic expression vectors. However, large-scale production of recombinant proteins with engineered mammalian cells is costly.

A diagrammatic representation of mammalian vector is shown in ***Fig. 11.4***. It contains a eukaryotic origin of replication from an animal virus such as Simian virus 40 (SV40) and a prokaryotic origin of replication (from *E. coli*). The mammalian vector has a multiple cloning site and a selectable marker gene. Both of them are under the control of eukaryotic promoter and polyadenylation sequences. These sequences are obtained from either animal viruses (SV40, herpes simplex virus) or mammalian genes (growth hormone, metallothionein). The promoter sequences facilitate the transcription of cloned genes (at the multiple cloning site) and the selectable marker genes. On the other hand, the polyadenylation sequences terminate the transcription. Ampicillin resistant marker gene can be used for selecting the transformed *E. coli* cells.

Markers for mammalian expression vectors

There are several markers in use for the selection of transformed mammalian cells. The bacterial gene (Neo^{r}) that encodes for neomycin phosphotransferase is frequently used. The other markers are the genes that encode for the enzyme dihydrofolate reductase (DHFR), and glutamine synthetase (GS).

GENE EXPRESSION TO PRODUCE PROTEINS

Several proteins have been produced by mammalian expression vectors. The yield of protein synthesis in some cases, is increased by inserting an intron between the promoter and the cloned gene. However, the reason for this is not clear.

Coordinated expression

By coordinating the expression of a cloned gene and a selected marker, the production of recombinant protein can be increased.

The coordinated expression of DHFR (marker) and a cloned gene is illustrated in ***Fig. 11.5***. The DHFR gene is inserted close to a cloned gene and both of them are under the control of a single promoter and termination (polyadenylation) sequences. The DHFR gene is flanked by intron-removing sequence. As the genes are expressed, DHFR is synthesized by primary transcript while the recombinant protein is formed from spliced mRNA.

Expression of two cloned genes

Some proteins are composed of two or more subunits. For example, hemoglobin is a tetramer with two copies of each subunit i.e., $\alpha_2\beta_2$. Each subunit can be separately synthesized by the corresponding cloned gene, and they are then mixed to form the multimeric protein *in vitro*. This method is not very satisfactory since the *in vitro* assembly of multimeric proteins is not efficient. Techniques have been developed in recent years to produce two different proteins (i.e., subunits of a multimeric protein) in the same cell simultaneously.

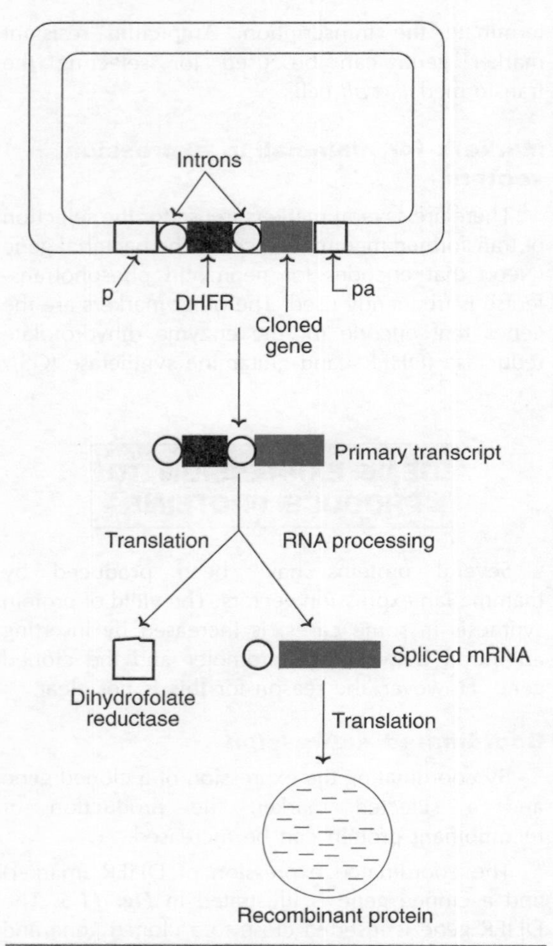

Fig. 11.5 : Coordinated expression of DHFR and a cloned gene (DHFR–Dihydrofolate reductase; p–Promoter sequence; pa–Polyadenylation sequence).

Two-vector expression system

Two expression vectors, each carrying a cloned gene for each subunit, are co-transfected into host cells (***Fig. 11.6***). These genes encode for the corresponding protein subunits. They then assemble to form a functional protein. The two-vector expression system has certain limitations — loss of one vector, overexpression of cloned gene in one of the vectors. This causes an imbalance in the formation and assembly of subunits.

Two-gene expression vector

A single vector carrying two cloned genes is used to overcome the above problem. The two genes can be placed under the independent control of promoters and polyadenylation sequences (***Fig. 11.7***) to produce the assembled protein with two subunits. This method, however, does not ensure production of equal quantities of two subunits.

Dicistronic expression vector

A dicistronic vector can be constructed with two cloned genes joined together to a small sequence of DNA that contains an ***internal ribosomal entry site*** (***IRES***). IRESs, found in mammalian viruses, allow a simultaneous transcription and translation to produce the assembled protein (***Fig. 11.8***). The transcription of gene-IRES-gene is under the control of a singe promoter and termination signals. By using dicistronic expression vector, ***the synthesis of equal amounts of the protein subunits can be achieved.***

COLLECTION AND PURIFICATION OF RECOMBINANT PROTEINS

As the recombinant proteins are produced by the cloned genes, they start accumulating. The next task is to collect and purify the specific gene product i.e., the requisite protein. This is not an easy job since many a times the recombinant protein is foreign to the host cell which possesses an enzyme machinery to degrade the outside proteins. Thus, human insulin produced in the bacterial host cells can be degraded by the proteases. This problem can be solved by using bacterial strains (e.g., *E. coli*) deficient in proteases. But there is a disadvantage since the proteases are defensive enzymes and hence the new strains lacking these enzymes are susceptible for easy destruction.

In an alternative approach, the ***recombinant proteins are fused with the native host proteins*** (Refer fusion proteins p. 138). The fusion proteins are ***resistant to protease activity***. Some times, foreign proteins accumulate as aggregates in the host organism, minimizing the protease degradation. The problem with protein aggregates is that the biological activity may be lost while extracting the protein from the aggregates.

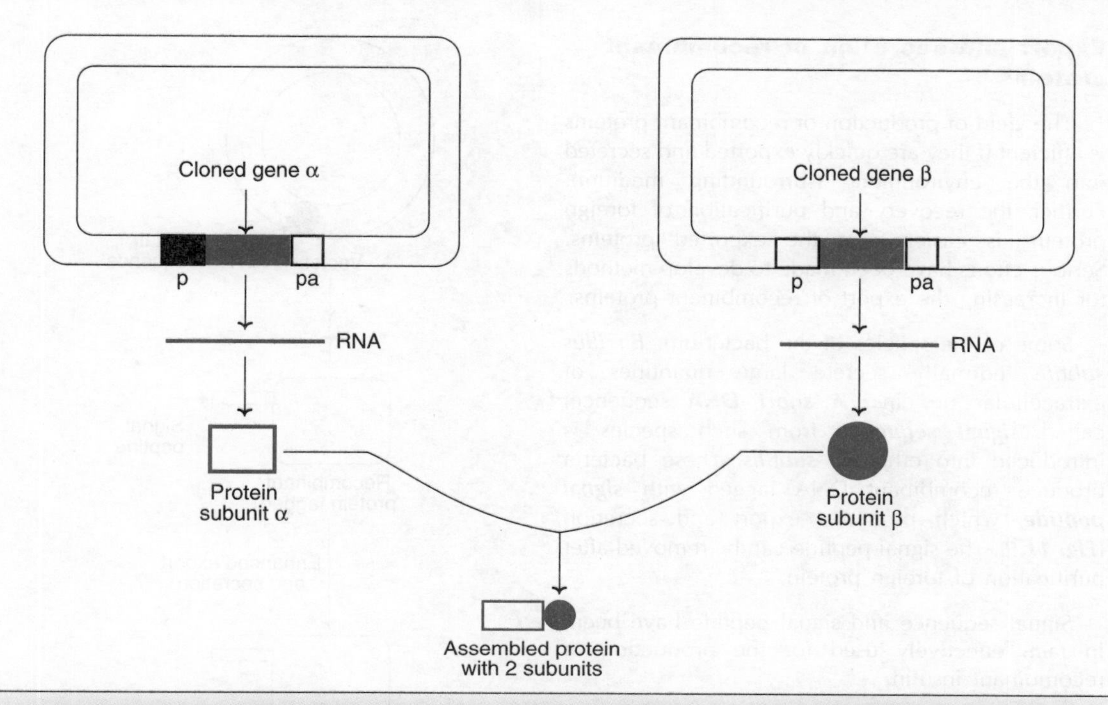

Fig. 11.6 : Two–vector expression system for producing a dimeric protein (p–Promoter sequence; pa–Polyadenylation sequence)

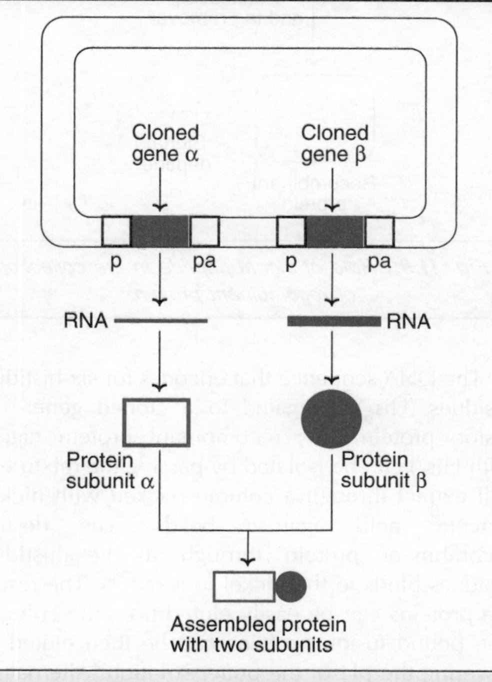

Fig. 11.7 : Two–gene expression vector for producing a dimeric protein (p–Promoter sequence; pa–Polyadenylation sequence).

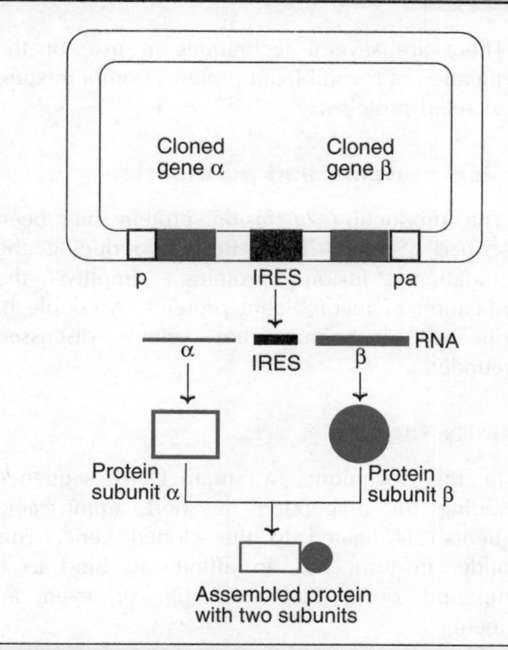

Fig. 11.8 : Dicistronic expression vector for producing a dimeric protein (p–Promoter sequence; pa–Polyadenylation sequence; IRES–Internal ribosomal entry site).

Export and secretion of recombinant proteins

The yield of production of recombinant proteins is efficient if they are quickly exported and secreted into the environment (surrounding medium). Further, the recovery and purification of foreign proteins is easier from the exported proteins. Serious efforts have been made to develop methods for increasing the export of recombinant proteins.

Some of the species of the bacterium, *Bacillus subtilis* normally secrete large quantities of extracellular proteins. ***A short DNA*** sequence, called ***signal sequence*** from such species is introduced into other *B. subtilis.* These bacteria produce recombinant DNA tagged with ***signal peptide***, which promotes export and secretion (***Fig. 11.9***). The signal peptide can be removed after purification of foreign protein.

Signal sequence and signal peptide have been, in fact, effectively used for the production of recombinant insulin.

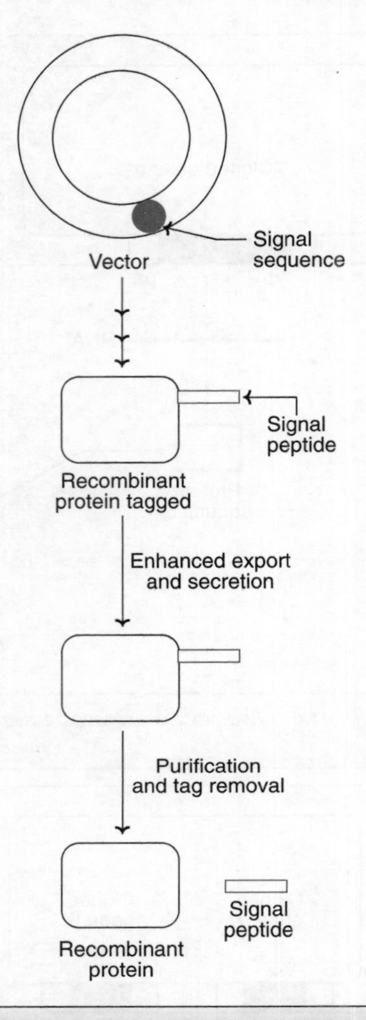

Fig. 11.9 : *Role of signal peptide in the collection of recombinant protein.*

PURIFICATION OF RECOMBINANT PROTEINS

There are several techniques in use for the purification of recombinant proteins from a mixture of secreted proteins.

Fusion proteins and purification

The production of fusion protein has been described (See p. 138). Besides reducing the degradation, fusion proteins simplify the purification of recombinant proteins. A couple of purification techniques are briefly discussed hereunder.

Affinity tagging

In this technique, a small DNA sequence encoding for a peptide (a short amino acid sequence) is ligated to the cloned gene. This peptide, in turn, has an affinity to bind to a compound or a macromolecule or even an element.

The tagged amino acid sequence, which forms a part of the recombinant protein acts as an ***affinity tag*** or ***identification tag***. The use of ***hexahistidine tag*** is briefly described in the next column.

The DNA sequence that encodes for six histidine residues (His_6) is ligated to a cloned gene. The fusion protein (i.e., recombinant protein tagged with His_6) can be isolated by passing the mixture of cell extract through a column packed with nickel-triacetic acid agarose beads. The desired recombinant protein through its hexahistidine residues binds to the nickel ions (Ni^{2+}). The rest of the proteins can be easily eluted from the column. The bound fusion proteins can be then eluted by lowering the pH of the buffer solution. Alternately, the fusion proteins can be selectively removed by binding of heaxahistidine tag to a competitor compound such as imidazole.

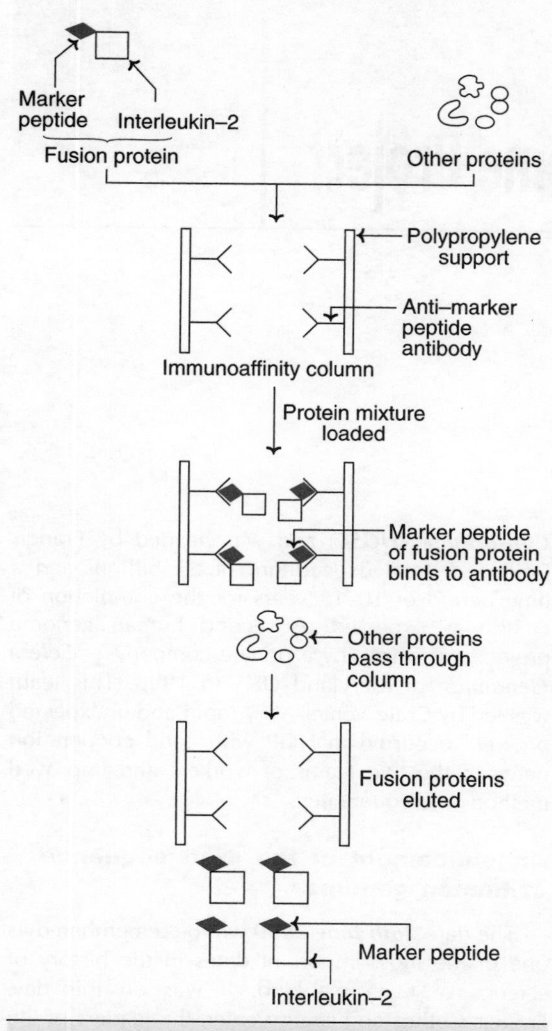

***Fig. 11.10 :** Immunoaffinity chromatographic purification of a fusion protein (Interleukin-tagged with marker peptide).*

The next step is to remove the hexahistidine tag. This can be done by digestion with proteases which specifically act at the site of the tag. There is a need ***to remove hexahistidine residues only if the recombinant protein is being used as a therapeutic agent***. For all other purposes, hexahistidine tag is acceptable, since it does not interfere in the normal structure and function of the proteins.

Immunoaffinity purification

The immunoaffinity chromatographic purification technique of fusion proteins with special reference to human interleukin-2 is described.

Interleukin-2 gene joined to a small DNA sequence encoding a marker peptide (that synthesizes 8 amino acids, Asp-Tyr-Lys-Asp-Asp-Asp-Asp-Lys) produces a fusion protein in yeast (*S. cerevisiae*). The marker peptide has a dual function-reduces the degradation of interleukin-2, besides helping in its purification (**Note :** The eight-amino acid marker peptide is commercially available under the brand name ***Flag peptide***).

The fusion protein, interleukin-2 joined to a marker peptide can be purified by immunoaffinity chromatography (***Fig. 11.10***). The specific monoclonal antibodies (MAb) against the marker peptide, are immobilized on a polypropylene support. These ***MAb serve as the ligand*** (anti-marker peptide antibodies) and ***selectively bind to fusion proteins*** tagged with marker peptide. However, the remaining proteins pass through the immunoaffinity column. The immunopurified fusion proteins can be eluted later from the column.

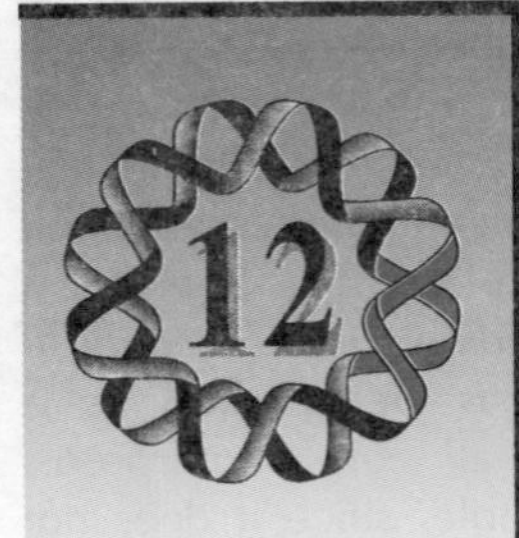

Human Genome Project

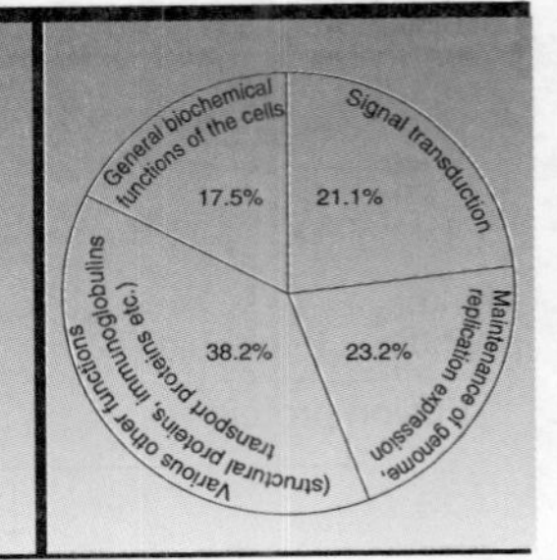

The most important features of a DNA molecule are the nucleotide sequences, and the identification of genes and their activities. Since 1920, scientists have been working to determine the sequences of pieces of DNA. This was further extended for the complete sequence determination of genome of certain lower organisms e.g. plasmid pBR 322 in 1979. The mitochondrial genome was sequenced in 1981.

THE BIRTH AND ACTIVITY OF HUMAN GENOME PROJECT

The human genome project (***HGP***) was conceived in 1984, and officially begun in earnest in October 1990. The primary objective of HGP was to determine the nucleotide sequence of the entire human nuclear genome. In addition, HGP was also entrusted to elucidate the genomes of several other model organisms e.g. *Escherichia coli*, *Saccharomyces cerevisiae* (yeast), *Caenorhabditis elegans* (roundworm), *Mus musculus* (mouse). James Watson (who elucidated DNA structure) was the first Director of HGP.

In 1997, United States established the ***National Human Genome Research Institute*** (***NHGRI***). The HGP was an international venture involving research groups from six countries — USA, UK, France, Germany, Japan and China, and several individual laboratories and a large number of scientists and technicians from various disciplines. This collaborative venture was named as ***International Human Genome Sequencing Consortium*** (***IHGSC***) and was headed by Francis Collins. A total expenditure of $3 billion, and a time period of 10–15 years for the completion of HGP was expected. A second human genome project was set up by a private company — ***Celera Genomics***, of Maryland USA in 1998. This team was led by Craig Venter. Very rapid and unexpected progress occurred in HGP with good cooperation between the two teams of workers and improved methods in sequencing.

Announcement of the draft sequence of human genome

The date ***26th June 2000*** will be remembered as one of the most important dates in the history of science or even mankind. It was on this day, Francis Collins and Craig Venter, the leaders of the two human genome projects, in the presence of the President of U.S., jointly announced the working drafts of human genome sequence. The detailed results of the teams were later published in February 2001 in scientific journals Nature (IHGSC) and Science (Celera Genomics).

The human genome project results attracted worldwide attention. This achievement was hailed with many descriptions in the media.

- The mystery of life unravelled.
- The library of life.
- The periodic table of life.
- The Holy grail of human genetics.

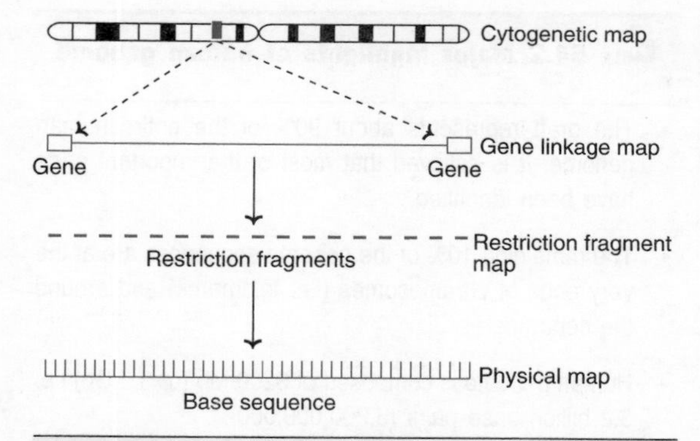

Fig. 12.1 : Different types of genome maps.

It may however, be noted that the draft human genome sequences were not complete, and may represent around 90%. The remaining 10% is made up of sequence where few genes are located.

MAPPING OF THE HUMAN GENOME

The most important objective of human genome project was to construct a series of maps for each chromosome. In ***Fig. 12.1***, an outline of the different types of maps is given.

1. **Cytogenetic map :** This is a map of the chromosome in which the active genes respond to a chemical dye and display themselves as bands on the chromosome.

2. **Gene linkage map :** A chromosome map in which the active genes are identified by locating closely associated marker genes. The most commonly used DNA markers are ***restriction fragment length polymorphism (RFLP), variable number tandems repeats (VNTRs) and short tandem repeats (STRs)***. VNTRs are also called as ***minisatellites*** while STRs are ***microsatellites***.

3. **Restriction fragment map :** This consists of the random DNA fragments that have been sequenced.

4. **Physical map :** This is the ultimate map of the chromosome with highest resolution base sequence. The methods for DNA sequencing are given in Chapter 7. Physical map depicts the location of the active genes and the number of bases between the active genes.

APPROACHES FOR GENOME SEQUENCING

A list of different methods used for mapping of human genomes is given in ***Table 12.1***. These techniques are also useful for the detection of normal and disease genes in humans.

For elucidating human genome, different approaches were used by the two HGP groups. ***IHGSC*** predominantly employed map first and sequence later approach. The principal method was ***heirarchical shotgun sequencing***. This technique involves fragmentation of the genome into small fragments (100–200 kb), inserting them into vectors (mostly bacterial artificial chromosomes, BACs) and cloning. The cloned fragments could be sequenced.

Celera Genomics used ***whole genome shotgun approach***. This bypasses the mapping step and saves time. Further, Celera group was lucky to have ***high-throughput sequenators*** and ***powerful computer programmes*** that helped for the early completion of human genome sequence.

Whose genome was sequenced?

One of the intriguing questions of human genome project is whose genome is being sequenced and how will it relate to the 6 billion or so population with variations in world? There is no simple answer to this question. However, looking from the positive side, it does not matter whose genome is sequenced, since the phenotypic differences between individuals are due to variations in just 0.1% of the total genome sequences. Therefore many individual genomes can be used as source material for sequencing.

Much of the human genome work was performed on the material supplied by the Centre for Human Polymorphism in Paris, France. This institute had collected cell lines from sixty different French families, each spanning three generations. The material supplied from Paris was used for human genome sequencing.

HUMAN GENOME SEQUENCE-RESULTS SUMMARISED

The information on the human genome projects is too vast, and only some highlights can be given (***Table 12.2***). Some of them are briefly described.

TABLE 12.1 A list of principal methods used for mapping of genomes (and also normal and disease genes in humans)

Method	*Comments*
DNA sequencing	Physical map of DNA can be identified with highest resolution.
Use of probes	To identify RFLPs, STS and SNPs.
Radiation hybrid mapping	Fragment genome into large pieces and locate markers and genes. Requires somatic cell hybrids.
Fluorescence *in situ* hybridization (FISH)	To localize a gene on chromosome.
Sequence tagged site (STS) mapping	Applicable to any part of DNA sequence if some sequence information is available.
Expressed sequence tag (EST) mapping	A variant of STS mapping; expressed genes are actually mapped and located.
Pulsed-field gel electrophoresis (PFGE)	For the separation and isolation of large DNA fragments.
Cloning in vectors (plasmids, phages, cosmids, YACs, BACs)	To isolate DNA fragments of variable lengths.
Polymerase chain reaction (PCR)	To amplify gene fragments
Chromosome walking	Useful for cloning of overlapping DNA fragments (restricted to about 200 kb).
Chromosome jumping	DNA can be cut into large fragments and circularized for use in chromosome walking.
Detection of cytogenetic abnormalities	Certain genetic diseases can be identified by cloning the affected genes e.g. Duchenne muscular dystrophy.
Databases	Existing databases facilitate gene identification by comparison of DNA and protein sequences.

(RFLP–Restriction fragment length polymorphism; STS–Sequence tagged site; SNP–Single nucleotide polymorphism; YAC–Yeast artificial chromosome; BAC–Bacterial artificial chromosome)

TABLE 54.2 Major highlights of human genome

- The draft represents about 90% of the entire human genome. It is believed that most of the important parts have been identified.
- The remaining 10% of the genome sequences are at the very ends of chromosomes (i.e. telomeres) and around the centromeres.
- Human genome is composed of 3200 Mb (or 3.2 Gb) i.e. 3.2 billion base pairs (3,200,000,000).
- Approximately 1.1 to 1.5% of the genome codes for proteins.
- Approximately 24% of the total genome is composed of introns that split the coding regions (exons), and appear as repeating sequences with no specific functions.
- The number of protein coding genes is in the range of 30,000–40,000.
- An average gene consists of 3000 bases, the sizes however vary greatly. Dystrophin gene is the larget known human gene with 2.4 million bases.
- Chromosome 1 (the larget human chromosome) contains the highest number of genes (2968), while the Y chromosome has the lowest. Chromosomes also differ in their GC content and number of transposable elements.
- Genes and DNA sequences associated with many diseases such as breast cancer, muscle diseases, deafness and blindness have been identified.
- About 100 coding regions appear to have been copied and moved by RNA–based transposition (retro-transposons).
- Repeated sequences constitute about 50% of the human genome.
- A vast majority of the genome (~ 97%) has no known functions.
- Between the humans, the DNA differs only by 0.2% or one in 500 bases.
- More than 3 million single nucleotide polymorphisms (SNPs) have been identified.
- Human DNA is about 98% identical to that of chimpanzees.
- About 200 genes are close to that found in bacteria.

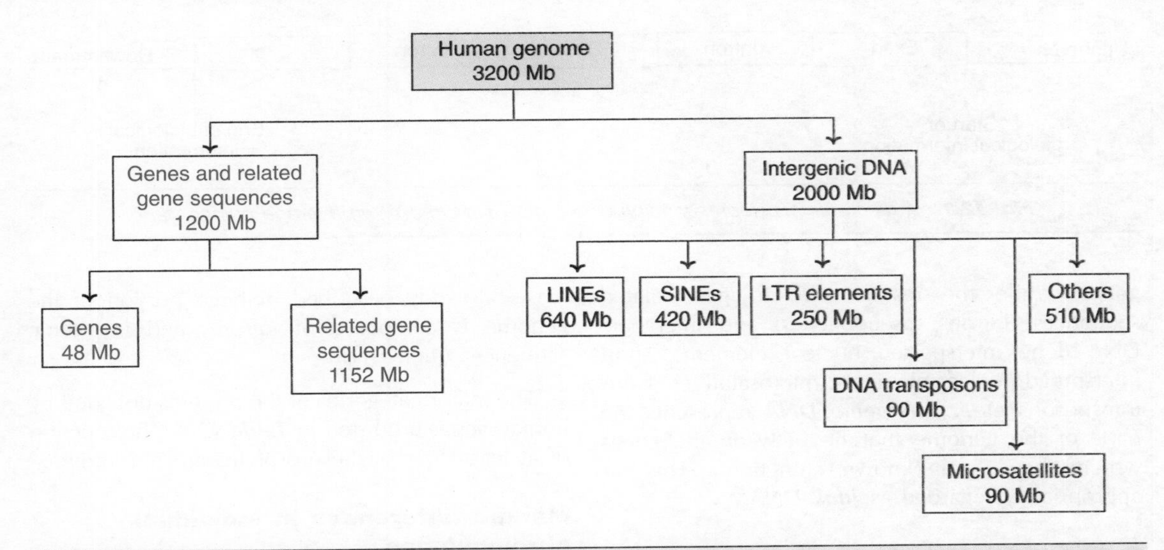

Fig. 12.2 : An overview of the organization of human genome (LINEs-Long interspersed nuclear elements; SINEs–Short interspersed nuclear elements; LTR-Long terminal repeats).

TABLE 12.3 Some interesting analogs/sidelights about human genome

- The base sequence in human genome would fill about 200 telephone books of 1000 pages each.
- If the genome is recited at the rate of one base per second for 24 hours a day, it would take a century to recite the book of life.
- If a typist types at the rate of 60 words per minute (i.e. 360 letters) for 8 hours a day, he/she would take around 50 years to type human genome.
- If the DNA sequence is typed in lines 10 cm containing 60 nucleotide bases and printed the human genome sequence (from a single cell) would stretch a distance of 5000 km.
- If the DNA in the entire human body is put end to end, it would reach to the sun and back over 600 times (**Note :** The human body contains 100 trillion cells; the length of DNA in a cell is 6 feet; the distance between the sun and earth is 93 million miles).
- The total expenditure for human genome project was $3 billion. The magnitude of this huge amount has to be appreciated. If one starts counting at a non–stop rate of a dollar per second, it would take about 90 years to complete.

Most of the genome sequence is identified

About 90% of the human genome has been sequenced. It is composed of 3.2 billion base pairs (3200 Mb or 3.2 Gb). If written in the format of a telephone book, the base sequence of human genome would fill about 200 telephone books of 1000 pages each. Some other interesting analogs/ sidelights of genome are given in ***Table 12.3***.

Individual differences in genomes : It has to be remembered that every individual, except identical twins, have their own versions of genome sequences. The differences between individuals are largely due to ***single nucleotide polymorphisms (SNPs)***. SNPs represent positions in the genome where some individuals have one nucleotide (i.e. an A), and others have a different nucleotide (i.e. a G). The frequency of occurrence of SNPs is estimated to be one per 1000 base pairs. About 3 million SNPs are believed to be present and at least half of them have been identified.

Organization of human genome

An outline of the organization of the human genome is given in ***Fig. 12.2***. Of the 3200 Mb, only a small fraction (48 Mb) represents the actual

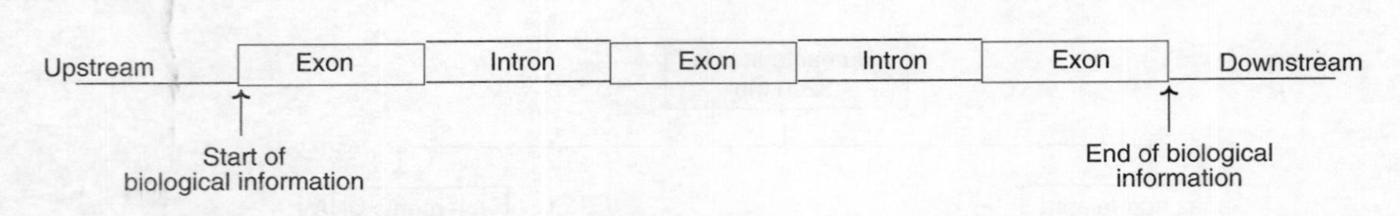

Fig. 12.3 : A diagrammatic representation of a typical structure of an average human gene.

genes, while the rest is due to gene-related sequences (introns, pseudogenes) and intergenic DNA (long interspersed nuclear elements, short interspread nuclear elements, microsatellites, DNA transposons etc.). ***Intergenic DNA*** represents the parts of the genome that lie between the genes which have no known function. This is appropriately regarded as ***junk DNA***.

Genes present in human genome

The two genome projects differ in their estimates of the total number of genes in humans. Their figures are in the range of 30,000–40,000 genes. The main reason for this variation is that it is rather difficult to specifically recognize the DNA sequences which are genes and which are not.

Before the results of the HGP were announced, the best guess of human genes was in the range of 80,000–100,000. This estimate was based on the fact that the number of proteins in human cells are 80,000–100,000, and thus so many genes expected. The fact that the number of genes is much lower than the proteins suggests that the ***RNA editing*** (RNA processing) is widespread, so that a single mRNA may code for more than one protein.

A diagrammatic representation of a typical structure of an average human gene is given in ***Fig. 12.3***. It has exons and introns.

A broad categorization of human gene catalog in the form of a pie chart is depicted in ***Fig. 12.4***. About 17.5% of the genes participate in the general biochemical functions of the cells, 23% in the maintenance of genome, 21% in signal transduction while the remaining 38% are involved in the production of structural proteins, transport proteins, immunoglobins etc.

Human genes encoding proteins

It is now clear that only 1.1-1.5% of the human genome codes for proteins. Thus, this figure 1.1-1.5% represents exons of genome.

As alreaddy described, a huge portion of the genome is composed of introns, and intergenic sequences (junk DNA).

The major categories of the proteins encoded by human genes are listed in ***Table 12.4***. The function of at least 40% of these proteins are not known.

Marked differences in individual chromosomes

The landscape of human chromosomes varies widely. This includes many features such as gene number per megabase, GC content, density of SNPs and number of transposable elements. For instance, chromosome 19 has the richest gene content (23 genes per megabase) while chromosome 13 and Y chromosome have the least gene content (5 genes per megabase).

Other interesting / important features of human genome

For more interesting features of human genome, refer ***Table 12.3***.

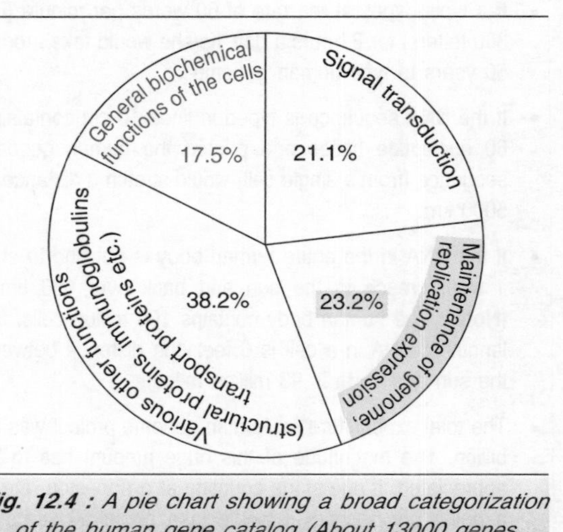

Fig. 12.4 : A pie chart showing a broad categorization of the human gene catalog (About 13000 genes whose functions are not known are not included).

TABLE 12.4 Different categories of proteins encoded by human genes (*based on the Human Genome Project report, 2001*)

Category of proteins	*Percentage*	*Actual number of genes*
Unknown functions	41.0%	12,809
Nucleic acid enzymes	7.5%	2,308
Transcription factors	6.0%	1,850
Receptors	5.0%	1,543
Hydrolases	4.0%	1,227
Regulatory proteins (G-proteins, cell cycle regulators etc.)	3.2%	988
Protooncogenes	2.9%	902
Structural proteins of cytoskeleton	2.8%	876
Kinases	2.8%	868

(Note : This table is based on the rough draft of human genome reported by Celera Genomics. The percentages are derived from a total of 26,383 genes)

- It is surprising to note that the number of genes found in humans is only twice that present in the roundworm (19,099) and thrice that of fruit fly (13,001).
- Around 200 genes appear to have been derived from bacteria by lateral transfer. Surprisingly, none of these genes are present in non-vertebrate eukaryotes.
- The proteins encoded by human genes are more complex than that of invertebrates.
- The flood of the data of human genome projects will be highly useful for bioinformatics and biotechnology.

GENOMES OF SOME OTHER ORGANISMS SEQUENCED

Sequencing of genomes is not confined to humans. For obvious reasons and significance, human genome sequencing attracted worldwide attention.

In fact, the first genome sequence of the bacteriophage QX174 was determined in 1977. Yeast was the first eukaryotic organism to be sequenced (1986). Recently, the mouse, an animal model closest to human has been sequenced. A selected list of genomes that have been sequenced is given in *Table 12.5*.

BENEFITS/APPLICATIONS OF HUMAN GENOME SEQUENCING

It is expected that the sequencing of human genome, and the genomes of other organisms will dramatically change our understanding and perceptions of biology and medicine. Some of the benefits of human genome project are given.

Identification of human genes and their functions

Analysis of genomes has helped to identify the genes, and functions of some of the genes. The functions of other genes and the interaction between the gene products needs to be further elucidated.

TABLE 12.5 A selected list of genomes that have been sequenced

Name of the species	*Genome size (Mb/kb)*	*Comments (year)*
Bacteriophage QX174	5.38 kb	First genome sequenced (1977).
Plasmid pBR 322	4.3 kb	First plasmid sequenced (1979).
Yeast chromosome III	315 kb	First chromosome sequenced (1992).
Haemophilus influenzae	1.8 Mb	First genome of cellular organism to be sequenced (1995).
Saccharomyces cerevisiae	12 MB	First eukaryotic organism to be sequenced (1996).
Arabidopsis thaliana	125 MB	First plant genome to be sequenced (2000).
Homo sapiens (human)	3200 MB	First mammalian genome to be sequenced (2001).
Oryza sativa (rice)	430 MB	First crop plant genome to be sequenced (2002).
Mus musculis (mouse)	3300 MB	Animal model closest to human (2003).

Understanding of polygenic disorders

The biochemistry and genetics of many single-gene disorders have been elucidated e.g. sickle-cell anemia, cystic fibrosis, retinoblastoma. A majority of the common diseases in humans, however, are polygenic in nature e.g. cancer, hypertension, diabetes. At present, we have very little knowledge about the causes of these diseases. The information on the genome sequence will certainly help to unravel the mysteries surrounding polygenic diseases.

Improvements in gene therapy

At present, human gene therapy is in its infancy for various reasons. Genome sequence knowledge will certainly help for more effective treatment of genetic diseases by gene therapy.

Improved diagnosis of diseases

In the near future, probes for many genetic diseases will be available for specific identification and appropriate treatment.

Development of pharmacogenomics

The drugs may be tailored to treat the individual patients. This will become possible considering the variations in enzymes and other proteins involved in drug action, and the metabolism of the individuals.

Genetic basis of psychiatric disorders

By studying the genes involved in behavioural patterns, the causation of psychiatric diseases can be understood. This will help for the better treatment of these disorders.

Understanding of complex social trait

With the genome sequence now in hand, the complex social traits can be better understood. For instance, recently genes controlling speech have been identified.

Knowledge on mutations

Many events leading to the mutations can be uncovered with the knowledge of genome.

Better understanding of developmental biology

By determining the biology of human genome and its regulatory control, it will be possible to understand how humans develop from a fertilized eggs to adults.

Comparative genomics

Genomes from many organisms have been sequenced, and the number will increase in the coming years. The information on the genomes of different species will throw light on the major stages in evolution.

Development of biotechnology

The data on the human genome sequence will spur the development of biotechnology in various spheres.

ETHICS AND HUMAN GENOME

The research on human genomes will make very sensitive data available that will affect the personal and private lives of individuals. For instance, once it is known that a person carries genes for an incurable disease, what would be the strategy of an insurance company? How will the society treat him/her? There is a possibility that ***individuals with substandard genome sequences may be discriminated***. Human genome results may also promote racial discrimination categorizing the people with ***good*** and ***bad genome sequences***. Considering the gravity of ethics related to a human genome, about 3% of the HGP budget was earmarked for ethical research.

In the 1990s, there was a move by some scientists to patent the genes they discovered. This created an uproar in the public and scientific community. Fortunately, the idea of patenting genes (of human genome sequencing) was dropped. The fear still exists that genetic information will be used for commercial purposes.

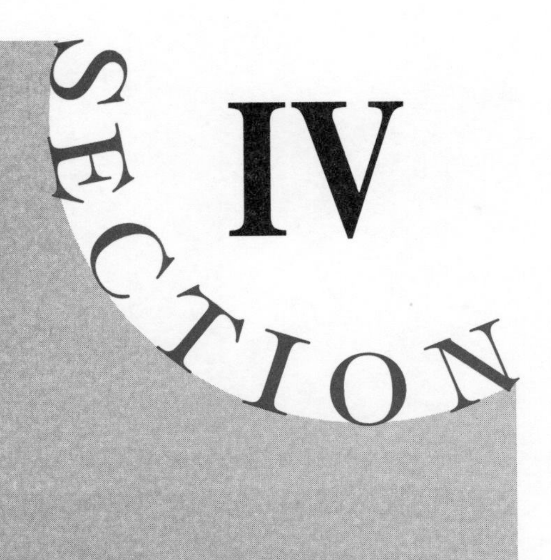

MEDICAL/ PHARMACEUTICAL BIOTECHNOLOGY (BIOTECHNOLOGY IN HEALTHCARE)

CONTENTS

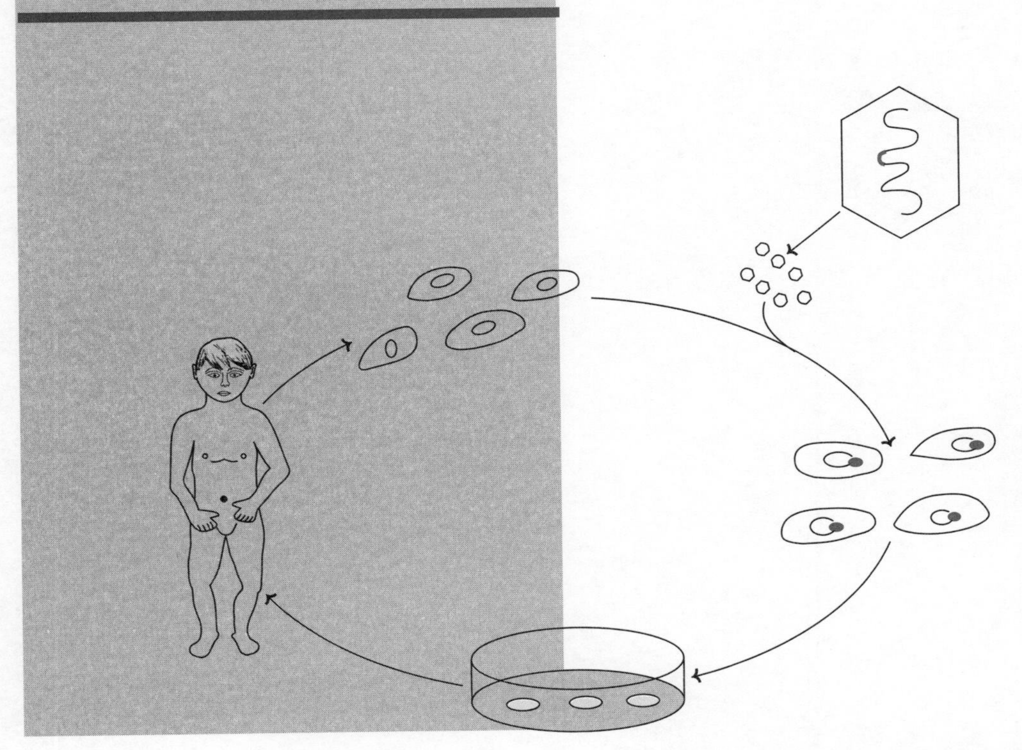

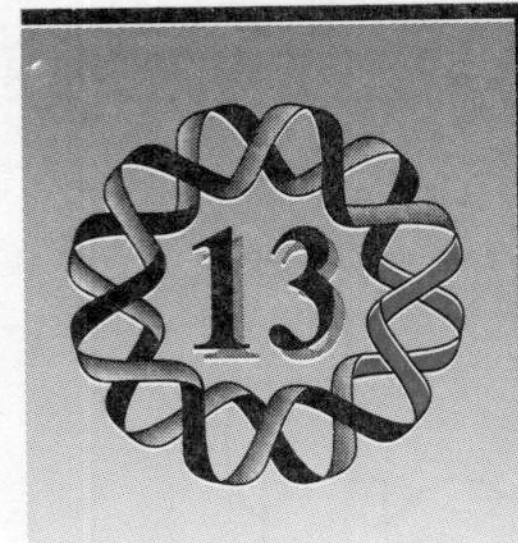

Gene Therapy

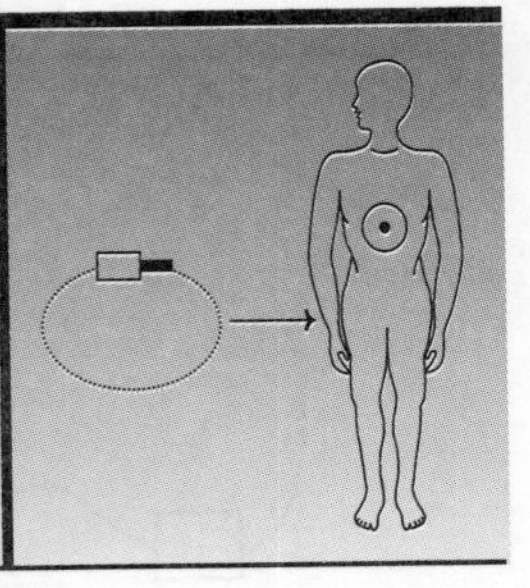

Advances in biochemistry and molecular biology have helped to understand the genetic basis of inherited diseases. It was a dream of the researchers to replace the defective genes with good ones, and cure the genetic disorders.

Gene therapy is the process of inserting genes into cells to treat diseases. The newly introduced genes will encode proteins and correct the deficiencies that occur in genetic diseases. Thus, gene therapy primarily involves ***genetic manipulations*** in animals or humans ***to correct a disease***, and keep the organism in good health. The initial experiments on gene therapy are carried out in animals, and then in humans. Obviously, the goal of the researchers is to benefit the mankind and improve their health.

An overview of gene therapy strategies is depicted in ***Fig. 13.1***. In ***gene augmentation therapy***, a DNA is inserted into the genome to replace the missing gene product. In case of ***gene inhibition therapy***, the antisense gene inhibits the expression of the dominant gene.

APPROACHES FOR GENE THERAPY

There are two approaches to achieve gene therapy.

1. **Somatic cell gene therapy :** The ***non-reproductive (non-sex) cells*** of an organism are referred to as somatic cells. These are the cells of an organism other than sperm or eggs cells, e.g., bone marrow cells, blood cells, skin cells, intestinal cells. At present, all the research on gene therapy is directed to correct the genetic defects in somatic cells. In essence, somatic cell gene therapy involves the ***insertion of a fully*** functional and ***expressible gene into a target somatic cell*** to correct a genetic disease permanently.

2. **Germ cell gene therapy :** The ***reproductive (sex) cells*** of an organism constitute germ cell line. Gene therapy involving the introduction of DNA into germ cells is passed on to the successive generations. For safety, ethical and technical reasons, germ cell gene therapy is not being attempted at present.

The genetic alterations in somatic cells are not carried to the next generations. Therefore, ***somatic cell gene therapy is preferred*** and extensively studied with an ultimate objective of correcting human diseases.

Development of gene therapy in humans for any specific disease involves the following steps. In fact, this is a general format for introducing any therapeutic agent for human use.

1. *In vitro* experiments and research on laboratory animals (pre-clinical trials).

2. Phase I trials with a small number (5–10) of human subjects to test safety of the product.

3. Phase II trials with more human subjects to assess whether the product is helpful.

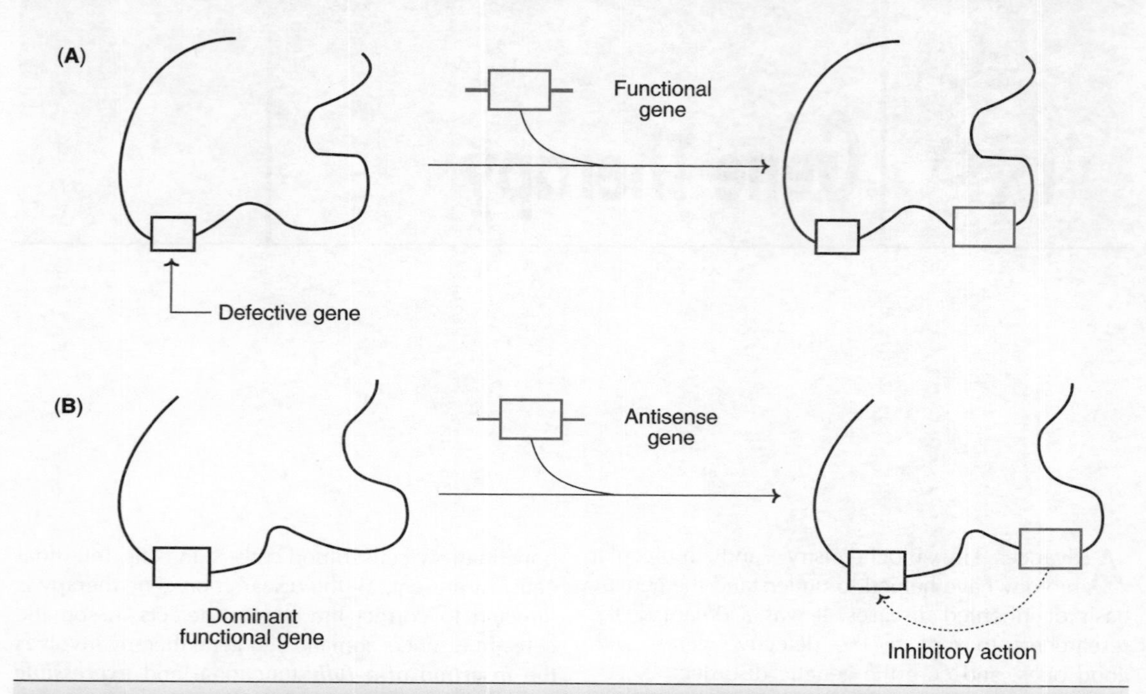

Fig. 13.1 : Overview of two major gene therapy strategies (A) Gene augmentation therapy (B) Gene inhibition therapy.

4. Phase III trials in large human samples for a final and comprehensive analysis of the safety and efficacy of the product.

As such, gene therapy involves a great risk. There are several regulatory agencies whose permission must be sought before undertaking any work related to gene therapy. ***Recombinant DNA Advisory Committee (RAC)*** is the supervisory body of the National Institute of Health, U.S.A., that clears proposals on experiments involving gene therapy. A large number of genetic disorders and other diseases are currently at various stages of gene therapy trials. A selected list of some important ones is given in ***Table 13.1***.

There are two types of gene therapies.

I. ***Ex vivo* gene therapy :** This involves the ***transfer of genes in cultured cells*** (e.g., bone marrow cells) which are then reintroduced into the patient.

II. ***In vivo* gene therapy :** The ***direct delivery of genes into the cells*** of a particular tissue is referred to as *in vivo* gene therapy.

EX VIVO GENE THERAPY

The *ex vivo* gene therapy can be applied to only selected tissues (e.g., bone marrow) whose cells can be cultured in the laboratory.

The technique of *ex vivo* gene therapy involves the following steps (***Fig. 13.2***).

1. Isolate cells with genetic defect from a patient.

2. Grow the cells in culture.

3. Introduce the therapeutic gene to correct gene defect.

4. Select the genetically corrected cells (stable transformants) and grow.

5. Transplant the modified cells to the patient.

The procedure basically involves the ***use of the patient's own cells for culture and genetic correction, and then their return back to the patient***. This technique is therefore, not associated with adverse immunological responses after transplanting the cells. *Ex vivo* gene therapy is

Table 13.1 Human gene therapy trials

Disease	*Gene therapy*
Severe combined immunodeficiency (SCID)	Adenosine deaminase (ADA).
Cystic fibrosis	Cystic fibrosis transmembrane regulator (CFTR).
Familial hypercholesterolemia	Low density lipoprotein (LDL) receptor.
Emphysema	α_1-Antitrypsin
Hemophilia B	Factor IX
Thalassemia	α- or β-Globin
Sickle-cell anemia	β-Globin
Lesch-Nyhan syndrome	Hypoxanthine-guanine phosphoribosyltransferase (HGPRT).
Gaucher's disease	Glucocerebrosidase
Peripheral artery disease	Vascular endothelial growth factor (VEGF)
Fanconi anemia	Fanconi anemia C
Melanoma	Tumor necrosis factor (TNF)
Melanoma, renal cancer	Interleukin-2 (IL-2)
Glioblastoma (brain tumor), AIDS, ovarian cancer	Thymidine kinase (herpes simplex virus)
Head and neck cancer	p^{53}
Breast cancer	Multidrug resistance I
AIDS	*rev* and *env*
Colorectal cancer, melanoma, renal cancer	Histocompatability locus antigen-B_7 (HLA-B_7)
Duchenne muscular dystrophy	Dystrophin
Short stature*	Growth hormone
Diabetes*	Glucose transporter-2, (GLUT-2), glucokinase
Phenylketonuria*	Phenylalanine hydroxylase
Citrullinemia*	Arginosuccinate synthetase

* *Mostly confined to animal experiments*

efficient only, if the therapeutic gene (remedial gene) is stably incorporated and continuously expressed. This can be achieved by use of vectors.

VECTORS IN GENE THERAPY

The ***carrier particles or molecules used to deliver genes to somatic cells*** are referred to as vectors. The important vectors employed in *ex vivo* gene therapy are listed below and briefly described next.

- Viruses
- Human artificial chromosome
- Bone marrow cells.

VIRUSES

The vectors frequently used in gene therapy are viruses, particularly ***retroviruses***. RNA is the genetic material in retroviruses. As the retrovirus enters the host cell, it synthesizes DNA from RNA (by reverse transcription). The so formed viral DNA (referred to as provirus) gets incorporated into the DNA of the host cell. The proviruses are normally harmless. However, there is a tremendous risk, since some of the retroviruses can convert normal cells into cancerous ones. Therefore, it is absolutely essential to ensure that such a thing does not happen.

Making retroviruses harmless

Researchers employ certain biochemical methods to convert harmful retroviruses to harmless ones, before using them as vectors. For instance, by artificially ***removing a gene that encodes for the viral envelope, the retrovirus*** can be crippled and ***made harmless***. This is because, without the

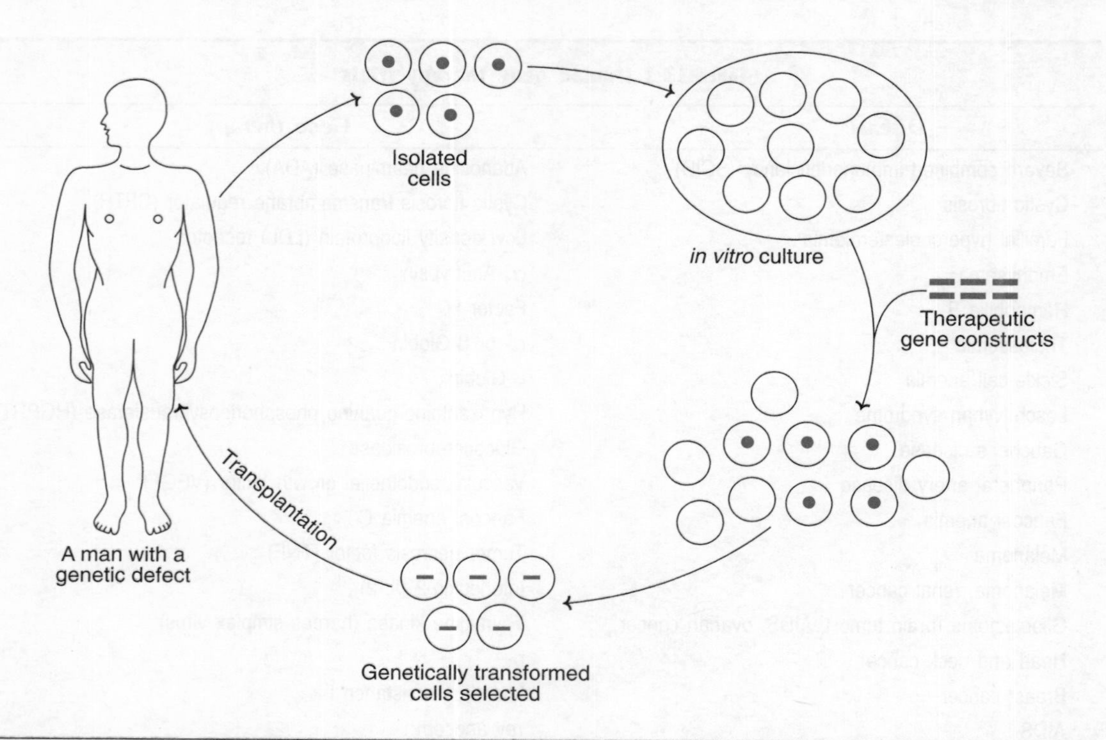

Fig. 13.2 : The procedure for ex vivo *gene therapy.*

envelope, retrovirus cannot enter the host cell. The production of a large number (billions) of viral particles can be achieved, starting from a single envelope defective retrovirus (***Fig. 13.3***). This is made possible by using helper viruses which contain normal gene for envelope formation. Along with the helper virus, the vector (with defective envelope gene) can enter the host cell and both of them multiply. By repeated multiplication in host cells, billions of vector and helper viruses are produced. The vector viruses can be separated from the helper viruses and purified. Isolation of vector viruses, totally free from helper viruses, is absolutely essential. Contamination of helper viruses is a big threat to the health of the patients undergoing gene therapy.

Retroviruses in gene therapy

The genetic map of a typical retrovirus is depicted in ***Fig. 13.4A***. In general, the retrovirus particle has RNA as a genome organized into six regions. It has a 5′-long terminal repeat (5′-LTR), a non-coding sequence required for packaging RNA designated as psi (Ψ), a gene ***gag*** coding for structural protein, a gene ***pol*** that codes for reverse transcriptase, a gene ***env*** coding for envelope protein and a 3-LTR sequence.

For use of a retrovirus as a vector, the structural genes ***gag*** and ***pol*** are deleted (besides ***env*** gene, as described above). These genes are actually adjacent to Ψ region. In addition, a promoter gene is also included (***Fig. 13.4B***). This vector design allows the synthesis of cloned genes. A ***retroviral vector can carry a therapeutic DNA of maximum size of 8 kb.***

A retroviral vector DNA can be used to transform the cells. However, the efficiency of delivery and integration of therapeutic DNA are very low. In recent years, techniques have been developed to deliver the vector RNA to host cells at a high frequency. For this purposes, packaged retroviral RNA particles are used. This technique allows a high efficiency of integration of pharmaceutical DNA into host genome.

Several ***modified viral vectors*** have been developed in recent years for gene therapy. These include ***oncoretrovirus***, ***adenovirus***, ***adeno-***

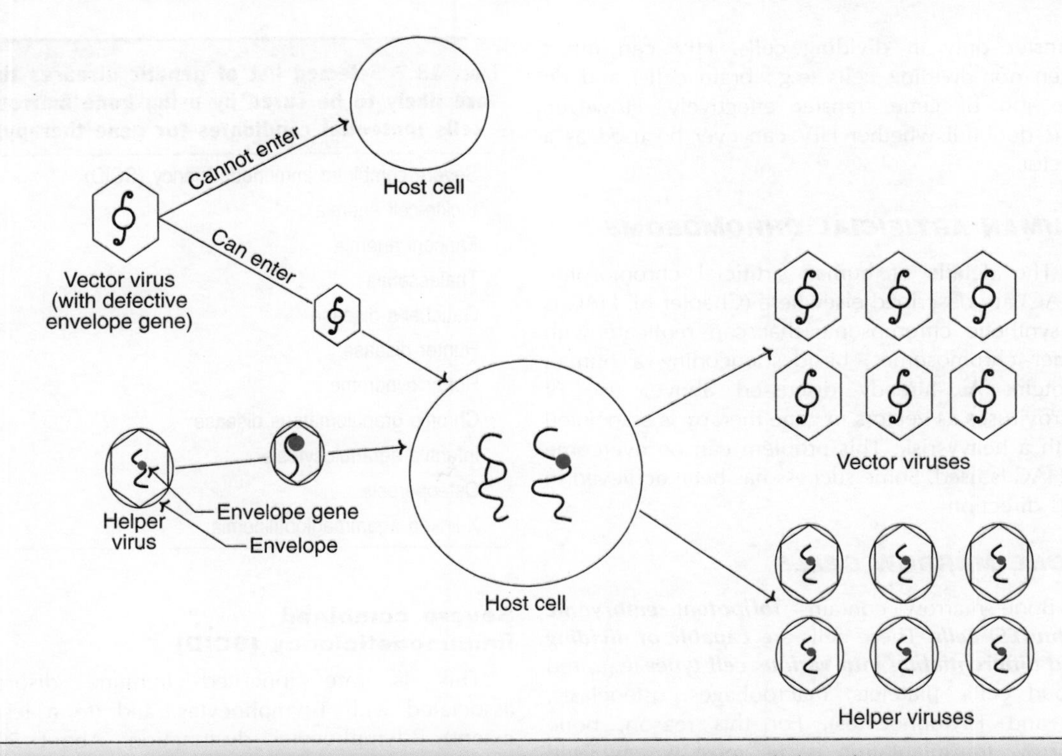

Fig. 13.3 : *Large scale production of vector viruses by using helper viruses.*

associated virus, herpes virus and a number of hybrid vectors combining the good characters of the parental vectors.

Murine leukemia viruses in gene therapy

This is a retrovirus that causes a type of leukemia in mice. It can react with human cells as well as the mouse cells, due to a similarity in the surface receptor protein. Murine leukemia virus (MLV) is frequently used in gene transfer.

AIDS virus in gene therapy?

It is suggested that the human immunodeficiency virus (HIV) can be used as a vector in gene transfer. But this is ***bound to create public uproar***. Some workers have been successful in creating a harmless HIV (crippled HIV) by removing all the genes related to reproduction. At the same time, the essential genes required for gene transfer are retained. There is a distinct advantage with HIV when compared with MLV. MLV is capable of bringing out gene

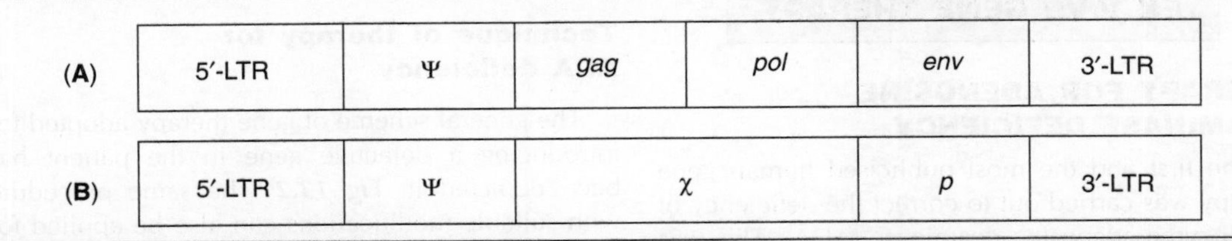

Fig. 13.4 : *A retrovirus used in gene therapy.* ***(A)*** *General map of a typical retrovirus* ***(B)*** *Gene map of a modified retrovirus for use in gene therapy (LTR-Long terminal repeat; Ψ-Packaging signal sequence;* gag-*Coding sequence for structural protein;* pol-*Coding sequence for reverse transcriptase;* env-*Envelope protein coding sequence; χ-Therapeutic gene; p–Promoter gene).*

transfer only in dividing cells. HIV can infect even non-dividing cells (e.g., brain cells) and do the job of gene transfer effectively. However, it is doubtful whether HIV can ever be used as a vector.

HUMAN ARTIFICIAL CHROMOSOME

The details of human artificial chromosome (HAC) are described elsewhere (Chapter 6). HAC is a synthetic chromosome that can replicate with other chromosomes, besides encoding a human protein. As already discussed above, use of retroviruses as vectors in gene therapy is associated with a heavy risk. This problem can be overcome if HAC is used. Some success has been achieved in this direction.

BONE MARROW CELLS

Bone marrow contains ***totipotent embryonic stem (ES) cells***. These cells are ***capable of dividing and differentiating into various cell types*** (e.g., red blood cells, platelets, macrophages, osteoclasts, B- and T-lymphocytes). For this reason, bone marrow transplantation is the most widely used technique for several genetic diseases. And there is every reason to believe that the genetic disorders that respond to bone marrow transplantation are likely to respond to ***ex vivo*** gene therapy also (***Table 13.2***). For instance, if there is a gene mutation that interferes with the function of erythrocytes (e.g., sickle-cell anemia), bone marrow transplantation is done. Bone marrow cells are the potential candidates for gene therapy of sickle-cell anemia. However, this is not as simple as theoretically stated.

TABLE 13.2 Selected list of genetic diseases that are likely to be cured by using bone marrow cells (potential candidates for gene therapy)

Severe combined immunodeficiency (SCID)
Sickle-cell anemia
Fanconi anemia
Thalassemia
Gaucher's disease
Hunter disease
Hurler syndrome
Chronic granulomatous disease
Infantile agranulocytosis
Osteoporosis
X-linked agammaglobulinemia

SELECTED EXAMPLES OF *EX VIVO* GENE THERAPY

THERAPY FOR ADENOSINE DEAMINASE DEFICIENCY

The first and the most publicised human gene therapy was carried out to correct the deficiency of the enzyme adenosine deaminase (ADA). This was done on September 14, 1990 by a team of workers led by Blaese and Anderson at the National Institute of Health, USA (The girl's name is Ashanti, 4 years old then).

Severe combined immunodeficiency (SCID)

This is rare inherited immune disorder associated with T-lymphocytes, and (to a lesser extent) B-lymphocytes dysfunction. About 50% of SCID patients have a defect in the gene (located on chromosome 20, and has 32,000 base pairs and 12 exons) that encodes for adenosine deaminase. In the deficiency of ADA, deoxyadenosine and its metabolites (primarily deoxyadenosine 5′-triphosphate) accumulate and destroy T-lymphocytes. T-Lymphocytes are essential for body's immunity. Besides participating directly in body's defense, they promote the function of B-lymphocytes to produce antibodies. Thus, the ***patients of SCID*** (lacking ADA) ***suffer from infectious diseases and die at an young age***. Previously, the children suffering from SCID were treated with conjugated bovine ADA, or by bone marrow transplantation.

Technique of therapy for ADA deficiency

The general scheme of gene therapy adopted for introducing a defective gene in the patient has been depicted in ***Fig 13.2***. The same procedure with suitable modifications can also be applied for other gene therapies.

A plasmid vector bearing a proviral DNA is selected. A part of the proviral DNA is replaced by the ADA gene and a gene (G 418) coding for

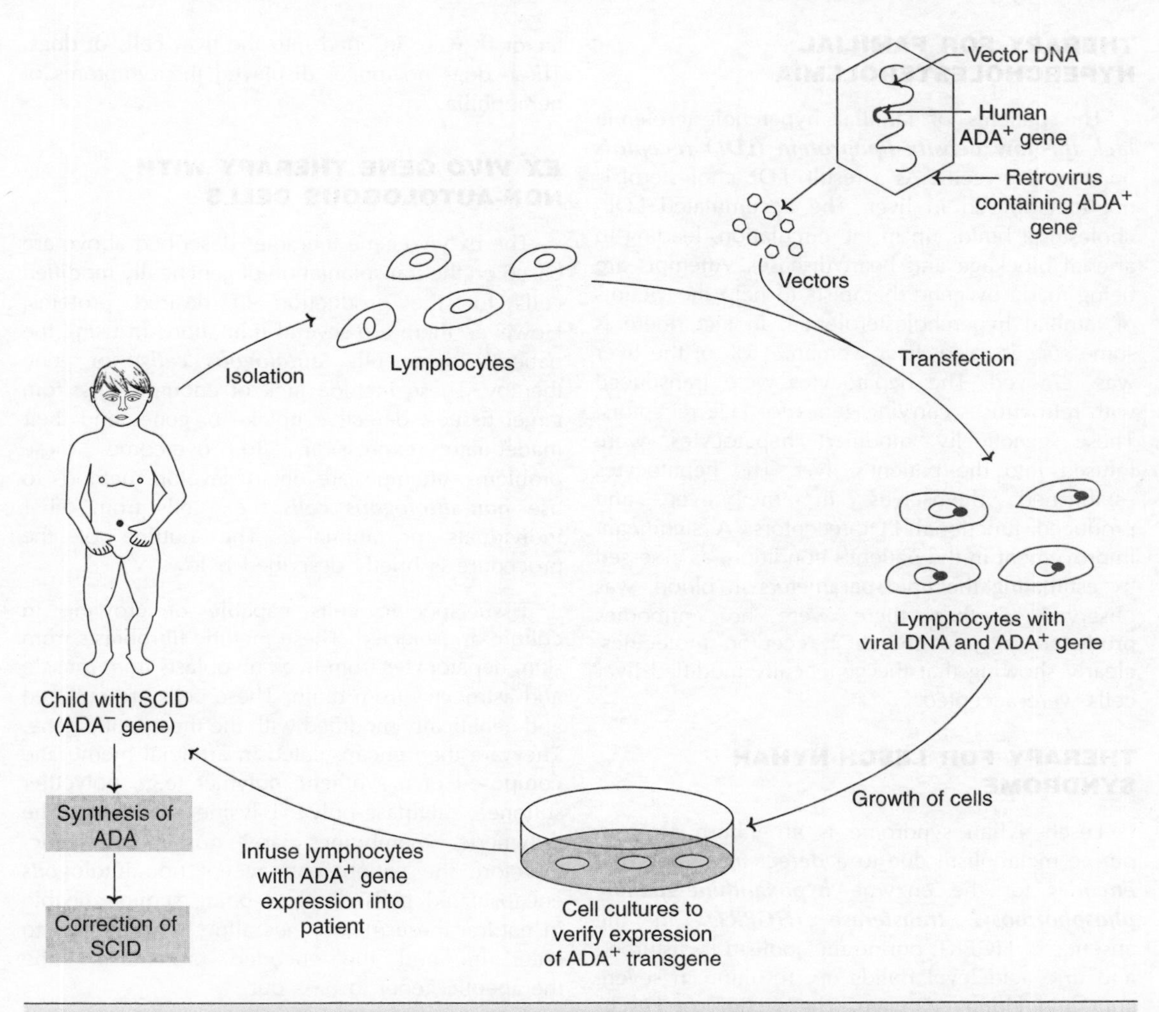

***Fig. 13.5 :** Treatment of adenosine deaminase (ADA) deficient patient by somatic* ex vivo *gene therapy (SCID-Severe combined immunodeficiency disease).*

antibiotic resistance, and then cloned. The antibiotic resistance gene will help to select the desired clones with ADA gene.

A diagrammatic representation of the treatment of ADP deficient patient is depicted in ***Fig. 13.5***.

Circulating lymphocytes are removed from a patient suffering from ADA deficiency. These cells are transfected with ADA gene by exposing to billions of retroviruses carrying the said gene. The genetically-modified lymphocytes are grown in cultures to confirm the expression of ADA gene and returned to the patient. These lymphocytes persist in the circulation and synthesize ADA. Consequently, the ability of the patient to produce antibodies is increased. However, there is a limitation. The lymphocytes have a short life span (just live for a few months), hence the transfusions have to be carried out frequently.

Transfer of ADA gene into stem cells

In 1995, ADA gene was transfered into the stem cells, obtained from the umbilical cord blood, at the time of baby's delivery. Four days after birth, the infant received the modified cells back. By this way, a permanent population of ADA gene producing cells was established.

THERAPY FOR FAMILIAL HYPERCHOLESTEROLEMIA

The patients of familial hypercholesterolemia ***lack the low density lipoprotein (LDL) receptors*** on their liver cells. As a result, LDL cholesterol is not metabolised in liver. The accumulated LDL-cholesterol builds up in the circulation, leading to arterial blockage and heart diseases. Attempts are being made by gene therapists to help the victims of familial hypercholesterolemia. In fact, there is some success also. In a woman, 15% of the liver was removed. The hepatocytes were transduced with retroviruses carrying genes for LDL receptors. These genetically modified hepatocytes were infused into the patient's liver. The hepatocytes established themselves in the liver and produced functional LDL-receptors. A significant improvement in the patient's condition, as assessed by estimating the lipid parameters in blood, was observed. Further, there were no antibodies produced against the LDL-receptor molecules, clearly showing that the genetically modified liver cells were accepted.

THERAPY FOR LESCH-NYHAN SYNDROME

Lesch-Nyhan syndrome is an inborn error in purine metabolism due to a ***defect in a gene that encodes*** for the enzyme ***hypoxanthine-guanine phosphoribosyl transferase (HGPRT)***. In the absence of HGPRT, purine metabolism is disturbed and uric acid level builds up, resulting in severe gout and kidney damage. The victims of Lesch-Nyhan syndrome exhibit symptoms of mental retardation, besides an urge to bite lips and fingers, causing self-mutilation.

By using retroviral vector system, HGPRT producing genes were successfully inserted into cultured human bone marrow cells. The major problem in humans is the involvement of brain. Experiments conducted in animals are encouraging. However, it is doubtful whether good success can be achieved by gene therapy for Lesch-Nyhan syndrome in humans, in the near future.

THERAPY FOR HEMOPHILIA

Hemophilia is a genetic disease due ***lack of a gene that encodes for clotting factor IX***. It is characterized by excessive bleeding. By using a retroviral vector system, genes for the synthesis of factor IX were inserted into the liver cells of dogs. These dogs no longer displayed the symptoms of hemophilia.

EX VIVO GENE THERAPY WITH NON-AUTOLOGOUS CELLS

The *ex vivo* gene therapies described above are based on the transplantation of genetically modified cells for the production of desired proteins. However, there are several limitations in using the patient's own cells (***autologous cells***) for gene therapy. These include lack of enough cells from target tissues, defective uptake of genes and their inadequate expression. To overcome these problems, attempts are on to develop methods to use ***non-autologous cells*** (i.e., cells from other individuals or animals). The outline of the procedure is briefly described below.

Tissue-specific cells capable of growing in culture are selected. These include fibroblasts from skin, hepatocytes from liver, myoblasts from muscle and astrocytes from brain. These cells are cultured and genetically modified with the therapeutic gene. They are then encapsulated in artificial membrane composed of a synthetic polymer (e.g., polyether sulfone, alginase-poly L-lysine-alginate). The polymeric membranes are non-immunogenic, therefore the patient can accept non-autologous encapsulated cells. Further, being semipermeable in nature, these membranes allow the nutrients to enter in, and the encoded protein (by the therapeutic gene) to pass out.

Experiments conducted in animals have shown some encouraging results for using non-autologous cells in gene therapy. The encapsulated cells were found to proliferate and produce the required protein. However, the success has been very limited in human trials.

IN VIVO GENE THERAPY

The ***direct delivery of the therapeutic gene*** (DNA) ***into the target cells*** of a particular tissue of a patient constitutes *in vivo* gene therapy (***Fig. 13.6***). Many tissues are the potential candidates for this approach. These include liver, muscle, skin, spleen, lung, brain and blood cells. Gene delivery can be carried out by ***viral*** or ***non-***

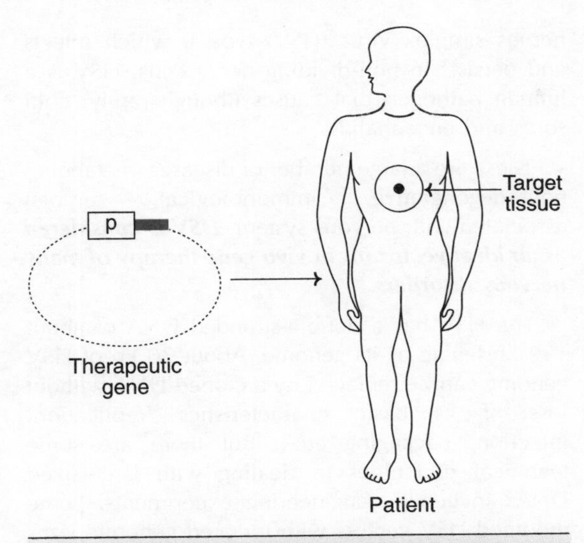

Fig. 13.6 : Diagrammatic representation of in vivo *gene therapy. (p-Promoter gene specific for therapeutic gene)*

viral vector systems. The success of ***in vivo*** gene therapy mostly depends on the following parameters

- The efficiency of the uptake of the remedial (therapeutic) gene by the target cells.
- Intracellular degradation of the gene and its uptake by nucleus.
- The expression capability of the gene.

In vivo gene therapy with special reference to gene delivery systems (viral, non-viral) with suitable examples is described.

GENE DELIVERY BY VIRUSES

Many viral vector systems have been developed for gene delivery. These include retroviruses, adenoviruses, adeno-associated viruses and herpes simplex virus.

Retrovirus vector system

Replication defective retrovirus vectors that are harmless are being used (See p. 159). A ***plasmid in association with a retrovirus, a therapeutic gene and a promoter is referred to as plasmovirus***. The plasmovirus is capable of carrying a DNA (therapeutic gene) of size less than 3.4 kb. Replication defective virus particles can be produced from the plasmovirus.

As such, for the delivery of genes by retroviral vectors, the target cells must be in a dividing stage. But majority of the body cells are quiescent. In recent years, viral vectors have been engineered to infect non-dividing cells. Further, attempts are on to include a DNA in the retroviral vectors (by engineering *env* gene) that encodes for cell receptor protein. If this is successfully achieved, the retroviral vector will specifically infect the target tissues.

Adenoviral vector system

Adenoviruses (with a ***DNA genome***) are considered to be good vectors for gene delivery because they ***can infect most of the non-dividing human cells***. A common cold adenovirus is a frequently used vector. As the target cells are infected with a recombinant adenovirus, the therapeutic gene (DNA) enters the nucleus and expresses itself. However, this DNA does not integrate into the host genome. Consequently, adenoviral based gene therapy required periodic administration of recombinant viruses.

The efficiency of gene delivery by adenoviruses can be enhanced by developing a virus that can specifically infect target cells. This is possible by incorporating a DNA encoding a cell receptor protein.

Adeno-associated virus vector system

Adeno-associated virus is a human virus that can integrate into chromosome 19. It is a single-stranded, non-pathogenic small DNA virus (4.7 kb). As the adeno-associated virus enters the host cell, the DNA becomes double-stranded, gets integrated into chromosome and expresses.

Adeno-associated viruses can serve as good vectors for the delivery of therapeutic genes. Recombinant viruses are created by using two plasmids and an adenovirus (i.e., helper virus) by a special technique. Some attempts were made to use therapeutic genes for the treatment of the human diseases-hemophilia (for production of blood clotting factor IX) and cystic fibrosis (for synthesis of cystic fibrosis transmembrane regulator protein) by employing adeno-associated viruses.

Therapy for cystic fibrosis

Cystic fibrosis (CF) is one of the most common (frequence 1 : 2,500) and fatal genetic diseases. It is characterized by the accumulation of sticky, dehydrated mucus in the respiratory tract and lungs. Patients of CF are highly susceptible to bacterial infections in their lungs and most of them die before reaching the age of thirty.

Cystic fibrosis can be traced in European folklore, the following statement used to be said "Woe to that child which when kissed on the forehead tastes salty. He is be witched and soon must die".

Biochemical basis : In the normal persons the chloride ions of the cells are pushed out through the participation of a protein called ***cystic fibrosis transmembrane regulator (CFTR)***. In the patients of cystic fibrosis, the CFTR protein is not produced due to a gene defect. Consequently, the chloride ions concentrate within the cells which draw water from the surroundings. As a result, the respiratory tract and the lungs become dehydrated with sicky mucus, an ideal environment for bacterial infections.

Gene therapy : As the defective gene for cystic fibrosis was identified in 1989, researchers immediately started working on gene therapy for this disease. Adenoviral vector systems have been used, although the success has been limited. The major drawback is that the benefits are short-lived, since the adenoviruses do not integrate themselves into host cells. Multiple administration of recombinant adenovirus caused immunological responses that destroyed the cells.

By using adeno-associated virus vector system, ***some encouraging results were reported in the gene therapy of CF***. In the phase I clinical trials with CF patients, the vector persisted for about 70 days and some improvement was observed in the patients.

Some researchers are trying to insert CF gene into the developing fetal cells (in experimental animals such as mice) to produce CFTR protein. But ***a major breakthrough is yet to come***.

Herpes simplex virus vector system

The retroviruses and adenoviruses (discussed above) employed in *in vivo* gene therapy are engineered to infect specific target cells. There are some viruses which have a natural tendency to infect a particular type of cells. The best example is herpes simplex virus (HSV) type I, which infects and persists in non-dividing nerve cells. HSV is a human pathogen that causes (though rarely) cold sores and encephalitis.

These are a large number of diseases (metabolic, neurodegenerative, immunological, tumors) associated with nervous system. ***HSV is considered as an ideal vector for in vivo gene therapy of many nervous disorders.***

The HSV has a double-stranded DNA of about 152 kb length as its genome. About 30 kb of HSV genome can be replaced by a cloned DNA without loss of its basic characteristics (replication, infection, packaging etc.). But there are some technical difficulties in dealing with large-sized DNAs in genetic engineering experiments. Some modified HSV vectors with reduced genomic sizes have been developed.

Most of the work on the gene therapy, related to the use of HSV as a vector, is being conducted in experimental animals. And the results are quite encouraging. HSV vectors could deliver therapeutic genes to the brain and other parts of nervous system. These genes are well expressed and maintained for long periods. More research, however, is needed before going for human trials.

If successful, HSV may help to treat many neurodegenerative syndromes such as Parkinson's disease and Alzheimer's disease by gene therapy.

GENE DELIVERY BY NON-VIRAL SYSTEMS

There are certain limitations in using viral vectors in gene therapy. In addition to the prohibitive cost of maintaining the viruses, the viral proteins often induce inflammatory responses in the host. Therefore, there is a continuous search by researchers to find alternatives to viral vector systems.

Pure DNA constructs

The ***direct introduction of pure DNA constructs into the target tissue*** is quite simple. However, the efficiency of DNA uptake by the cells and its expression are rather low. Consequently, large quantities of DNA have to be injected periodically. The therapeutic genes produce the proteins in the target cells which enter the circulation and often get degraded.

Lipoplexes

The ***lipid-DNA complexes*** are referred to as lipoplexes or more commonly ***liposomes***. They have a DNA construct surrounded by artificial lipid layers. A large number of lipoplexes have been prepared and used. They are non-toxic and non-immunogenic. The major limitation with the use of lipoplexes is that as the DNA is taken up by the cells, most of it gets degraded by the lysosomes. Thus, the efficiency of gene delivery by lipoplex is very low.

Some clinical trials using liposome-CFTR gene complex showed that the gene expression was very short-lived.

DNA-molecular conjugates

The use of DNA-molecular conjugates avoids the lysosomal breakdown of DNA. Another advantage of using conjugates is that large-sized therapeutic DNAs (> 10 kb) can be delivered to the target tissues. The most commonly used synthetic conjugate is ***poly-L-lysine***, bound to a specific target cell receptor. The therapeutic DNA is then made to combine with the conjugate to form a complex (***Fig. 13.7***). This DNA molecular conjugate binds to specific cell receptor on the target cells. It is engulfed by the cell membrane to form an endosome which protects the DNA from being degraded. The DNA released from the endosome enters the nucleus where the therapeutic gene is expressed.

Human artificial chromosome

Human artificial chromosome (***HAC***) which can carry a large DNA (one or more therapeutic genes with regulatory elements) is ***a good and ideal vector***. Studies conducted in cell cultures using HAC are encouraging. But the major ***problem is the delivery*** of the large-sized chromosome ***into the target cells***. Researchers are working to produce cells containing genetically engineered HAC. There exists a possibility of encapsulating and implanting these cells in the target tissue. But a long way to go!

Efficiency of gene delivery by non-viral vectors

Although the efforts are continuously on to find suitable non-viral vectors for gene delivery, the success has been very limited. This is mainly due to the following two reasons.

1. The efficiency of transfection is very low.

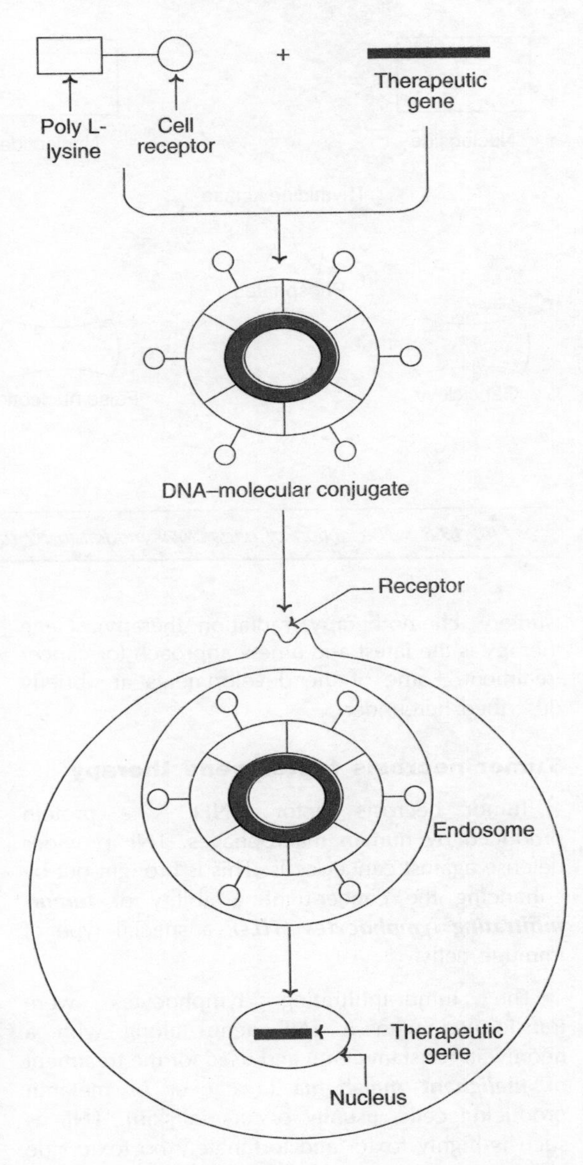

Fig. 13.7 : DNA-molecular conjugate in the delivery of therapeutic gene.

2. The expression of the therapeutic gene is for a very short period, consequently there is no effective treatment of the disease.

GENE THERAPY STRATEGIES FOR CANCER

Cancer is the leading cause of death throughout the world, despite the intensive treatment strategies

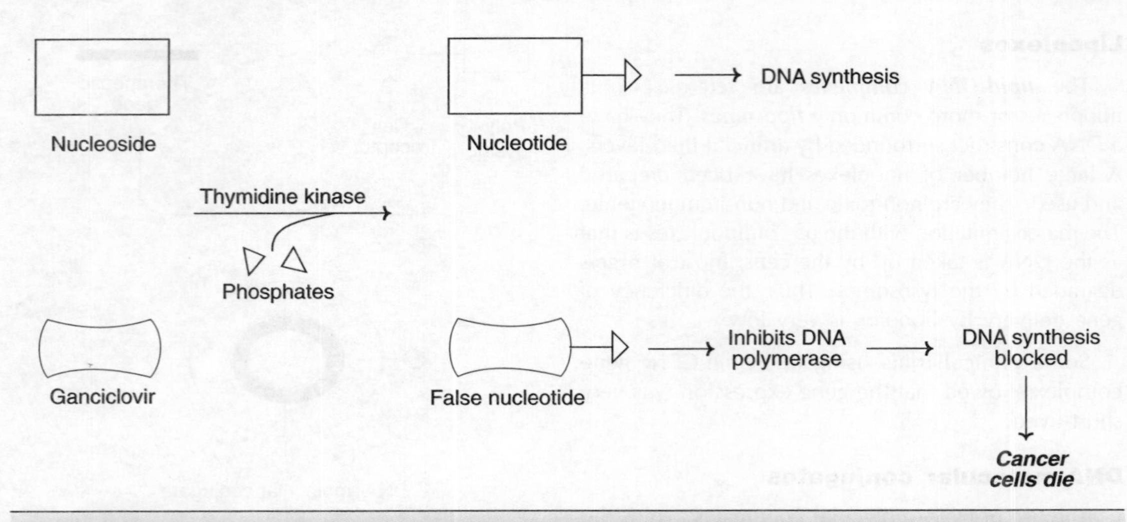

Fig. 13.8 : The action of ganciclovir mediated by thymidine kinase to inhibit the growth of cancer cells.

(surgery, chemotherapy, radiation therapy). Gene therapy is the latest and a new approach for cancer treatment. Some of the developments are briefly described hereunder.

Tumor necrosis factor gene therapy

Tumor necrosis factor (TNF) is a protein produced by human macrophages. TNF provides defense against cancer cells. This is brought out by enhancing the cancer-fighting ability of ***tumor-infiltrating lymphocytes (TILs)***, a special type of immune cells.

The tumor-infiltrating lymphocytes were transformed with a TNF gene (along with a neomycin resistant gene) and used for the treatment of ***malignant melanoma*** (a cancer of melanin producing cells, usually occurs in skin). TNF as such is highly toxic, and fortunately no toxic side effects were detected in the melanoma patients injected with genetically altered TILs with TNF gene. Some improvement in the cancer patients was observed.

Suicide gene therapy

The gene encoding the enzyme ***thymidine kinase*** is often referred to as suicide gene, and is used for the treatment of certain cancers.

Thymidine kinase (TK) phosphorylates nucleosides to form nucleotides which are used for the synthesis of DNA during cell division. The drug ***ganciclovir*** (***GCV***) bears a close structural resemblance to certain nucleosides (thymidine). By mistake, TK phosphorylates ganciclovir to form triphosphate-GCV, a false and unsuitable nucleotide for DNA synthesis. ***Triphosphate-GCV inhibits DNA polymerase (Fig. 13.8)***. The result is that the elongation of the DNA molecule abruptly stops at a point containing the false nucleotide (of ganciclovir). Further, the triphospate-GCV can enter and kill the neighbouring cancer cells, a phenomenon referred to as ***bystander effect***. The ultimate result is that the cancer cells cannot multiply, and therefore die. Thus, the drug ganciclovir can be used to kill the cancer cells.

Ganciclovir is frequently referred to as a ***prodrug*** and this type of approach is called ***prodrug activation gene therapy***. Ganciclovir has been used for treatment of brain tumors (e.g., glioblastoma, a cancer of glial cells in brain), although with a limited success.

In the suicide gene therapy, the ***vector used*** is ***herpes simplex virus (HSV)*** with a gene for thymidine kinase (TK) inserted in its genome. Normal brain cells do not divide while the brain tumor cells go on dividing unchecked. Thus, there is a continuous DNA replication in tumor cells. By using GCV-HSVTK suicide gene therapy, some reduction in proliferating tumor cells was reported. Several new strategies are being developed to increase the delivery of HSVTK gene to all the cells throughout a tumor.

Two-gene cancer therapy

For treatment of certain cancers, two gene systems are put together and used. For instance, ***TK suicide gene*** (i.e., GCV-HSVTK) is clubed with ***interleukin-2 gene*** (i.e. a gene promoting immunotherapy). Interleukin-2 produced mobilizes immune response. It is believed that certain proteins are released from the tumor cells on their death. These proteins, in association with immune cells, reach the tumor and initiate immunological reactions directed against the cancer cells.

Two-gene therapies have been carried out in experimental animals with colon cancer and liver cancer, and the results are encouraging.

Gene replacement therapy

A gene named ***p^{53}*** codes for a ***p***rotein with a molecular weight of ***53*** kilodaltons (hence p^{53}). p^{53} is considered to be a ***tumor-suppressor gene***, since the protein it encodes binds with DNA and inhibits replication. The tumor cells of several tissues (breast, brain, lung, skin, bladder, colon, bone) were found to have altered genes of p^{53} (mutated p^{53}), synthesizing different proteins from the original. These altered proteins cannot inhibit DNA replication. It is believed that the damaged p^{53} gene may be a causative factor in tumor development.

Some workers have tried to replace the damaged p^{53} gene by a normal gene by employing adenovirus vector systems (See p. 165). There are some encouraging results in the patients with liver cancer.

The antisense therapy for cancer is discussed elsewhere (See p. 170).

GENE THERAPY FOR AIDS

AIDS is a global disease with an alarming increase in the incidence every year. It is invariably fatal, since there is no cure. Attempts are being made to relieve the effects of AIDS by gene therapy. Some of the approaches are discussed hereunder.

rev and *env* genes

A mutant strain of human immunodeficiency virus (HIV), lacking ***rev*** and ***env*** genes has been developed. The regulatory and envelope proteins of HIV are respectively produced by ***rev*** and ***env*** genes. Due to lack of these genes, the virus cannot replicate.

Researchers have used HIV lacking ***rev*** and ***env*** genes for therapeutic purposes. T-Lymphocytes from HIV-infected patients are removed, and mutant viruses are inserted into them. The modified T-lymphocytes are cultivated and injected into the patients. Due to lack of essential genes, the viruses (HIV) cannot multiply, but they can stimulate the production of CD_8 (cluster determinant antigen 8) cells of T-lymphocytes. CD_8 cells are the killer lymphocytes. It is proved in the laboratory studies that these lymphocytes destroy the HIV-infected cells.

Genes of HIV proteins

Some genes synthesizing HIV proteins are attached to DNA of mouse viruses. These genetically-modified viruses are injected to AIDS patients with clinical manifestations of the disease. It is believed that the HIV genes stimulate normal body cells to produce HIV proteins. The latter in turn stimulate the production of anti-HIV antibodies which prevent the HIV replication in AIDS patients.

Gene to inactivate *gp120*

gp120 is a ***g***lyco***p***rotein (molecular weight ***120*** kilodaltons) present in the envelope of HIV. It is absolutely essential for binding of virus to the host cell and to bring replication. Researchers have synthesized a gene (called F105) to produce an antibody that can inactivate gp120. In the ***anti-AIDS therapy, HIV-infected cells are engineered to produce anti-HIV antibodies*** when injected into the organism.

Studies conducted in experimental animals showed a drastic reduction in the synthesis of gp120 due to anti-AIDS therapy. The production of HIV particles was also very reduced. There are some attempts to prevent AIDS by antisense therapy (See p. 171).

ANTIGENE AND ANTISENSE THERAPY

In general, gene therapy is carried out by introducing a therapeutic gene to produce the defective or the lacking protein. But there are certain disorders (cancer, viral and parasitic infections, inflammatory diseases) which result in an overproduction of certain normal proteins. It is possible to treat these diseases by ***blocking transcription*** using a single-stranded nucleotide sequence (antigene oligonucleotide) that hybridizes with the specific gene, and this is called ***antigene therapy***. ***Antisense therapy*** refers to the ***inhibition of translation*** by using a single-stranded nucleotide (antisense oligonucleotide). Further, it is also possible to inhibit both transcription and translation by blocking (with oligonucleotides) the transcription factor responsbile for the specific gene expression.

Nucleic acid therapy refers to the ***use of DNA or RNA molecules for therapeutic purposes***, as stated above. The naturally occurring sequences of DNA and RNA (with suitable modifications) or the synthetic ones can be employed in nucleic acid therapy. Theoretically, there is a vast potential for use of nucleic acids as therapeutic agents. But most of the work that is being carried out relates to the use of RNA in antisense therapy. Some of these are described below (**Note :** Some authors use antisense therapy in a broad sense to reflect antigene therapy as well as antisense therapy, discussed in the previous paragraph).

ANTISENSE THERAPY FOR CANCER

Oncogenes are the genes responsible for the causation of cancer. The dominantly acting oncogenes can be targeted in antisense technology by using antisense transgenes or oligonucleotides. Antisense oligonucleotides are used for the treatment of myeloid leukemia in as early as 1991.

Antisense RNA molecules are more frequently used in cancer therapy. This approach is effective only if the antisense oligonucleotide (antisense mRNA) specifically binds to the target mRNA and blocks protein biosynthesis (translation). This can be achieved in two ways, as illustrated in ***Fig. 13.9***.

The antisense cDNA can be cloned and transfected into cells. Antisense mRNA is synthesized by transcription. This can readily bind with the specific mRNA and block translation (***Fig. 13.9A***). The mRNA is actually formed by a gene containing exons and introns through transcription, followed by processing.

The other way to block translation is to directly introduce antisense RNA into the cells. This hybridizes with target mRNA and blocks translation (***Fig. 13.9B***).

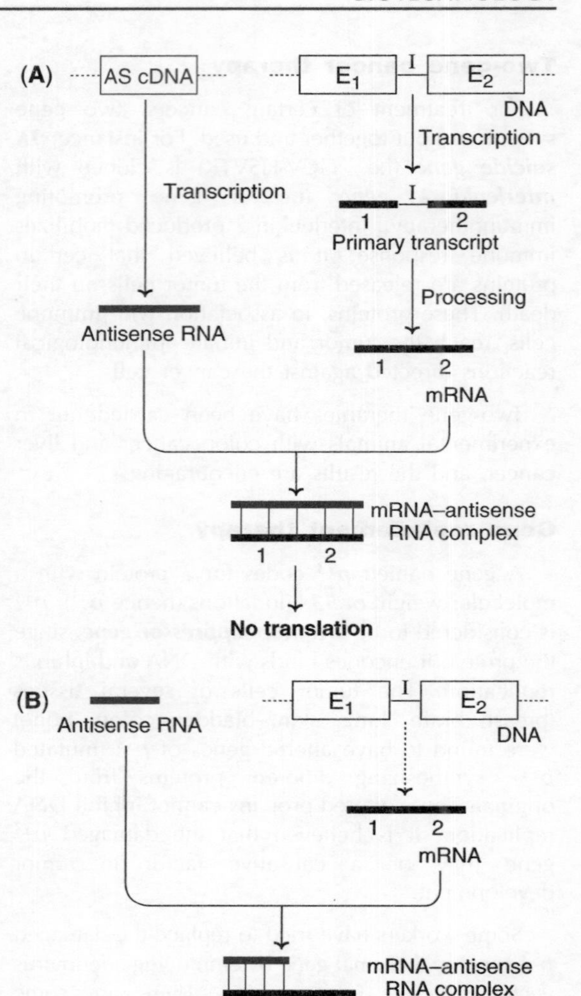

***Fig. 13.9 :** Inhibition of translation by antisense RNA (**A**) The cloned AS cDNA introduced into cells to produce antisense RNA (**B**) Antisense RNA directly introduced into cells. (AS cDNA = Antisense complementary DNA; E_1, E_2-Exons in a gene; I-Intron)*

The antisense mRNA therapy was tried for the treatment of a brain tumor namely malignant glioma and the cancer of prostate gland. In case malignant glioma, the protein insulin-like growth factor I (IGF-I) is overproduced, while in prostate cancer, insulin-like growth factor I receptor (IGF-IR) protein is more synthesized. For both these cancers, the respective antisense cDNAs can be used to synthesize, antisense mRNA molecules. These in turn, are used to block translation, as briefly described above and illustrated in ***Fig. 13.9***.

ANTISENSE THERAPY FOR AIDS

Attempts are also being made to prevent HIV infection through antisense therapy. The basic principle is briefly described (***Fig. 13.10***).

The target cells for HIV infection are genetically engineered to contain a gene that can express a complementary copy of HIV genome. This gene produces antisense RNA. When the cells containing antisense RNA are infected by HIV, it binds to viral RNA forming a double-stranded RNA-RNA hybrid molecules. This double-stranded molecule cannot be used by the enzyme reverse transcriptase. Consequently, a DNA copy of the HIV genome cannot be made and incorporated into the genome.

ANTISENSE OLIGONUCLEOTIDES AS THERAPEUTIC AGENTS

It is found that oligodeoxynucleotides (with about 15-20 units) can hybridize with specific mRNA and block translation with an ultimate effect of reducing the specific protein. Oligonucleotides can hybridize with different types of RNA transcripts-mRNAs, intron-exons, double-stranded RNAs. The major limitation of using naturally occurring oligonucleotides is that they are degraded by intracellular nucleases.

Certain modifications in the nucleotides (bases or sugars, phosphate) without affecting their hybridization ability have been prepared. However, these modified oligonucleotides are resistant to degradation by nucleases. The most widely used antisense oligonucleotide has a sulfur group in place of the free oxygen in phosphodiester bond. The modified bond is referred to as ***phosphorothioate linkage***. These phosphorothioate antisense oligonucleotides are resistant to degradation by nucleases, besides being water soluble. Some other modifications of oligonucleotides are with phosphoramidite linkage and 2-0-methylribose (***Fig. 13.11***). The modified antisense oligonucleotides are in fact used as therapeutic agents in the clinical trials for the treatment of certain cancers, bowel disease, AIDS, malaria and viral infections.

The free oligonucleotides do not readily enter the cells. Therefore, they are encapsulated in liposomes for efficient delivery to inhibit the mRNA translation.

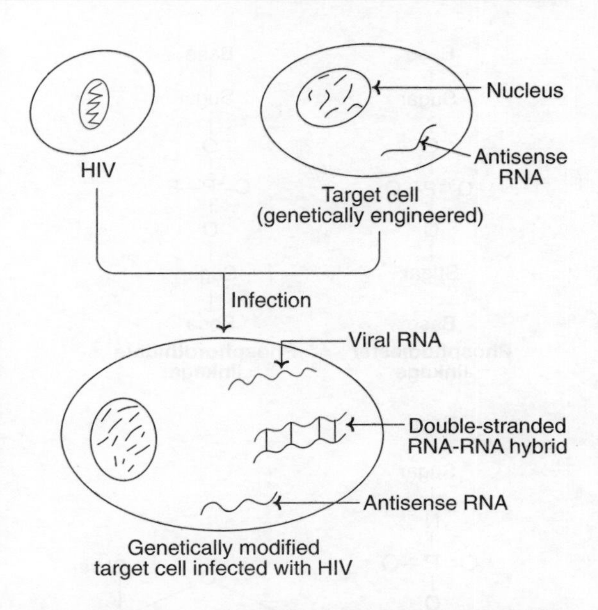

Fig. 13.10 : Antisense therapy to prevent AIDS (HIV-Human immunodeficiency virus)

Possible inhibition of smooth muscle cell proliferation : Proliferation of smooth muscle cells (along with secretion of extracellular matrix) has been implicated in hypertension, failure of coronary bypass grafts, hypertension and atherosclerosis. There exists a possibility of controlling smooth muscle cell proliferation by using antisense therapy.

CHIMERIC OLIGONUCLEOTIDES IN GENE CORRECTION

Many genetic diseases are due to single base pair mutations. A strategy has been devised to correct such defects by using a ***chimeric oligonucleotides*** composed of RNA-DNA oligonucleotide with 68 units. This chimeric oligonucleotide has hairpin caps and methylated ribose sugars (at 2nd carbon). The hairpin caps protect the molecule from the degradation by exonucleases while methylated ribose prevents digestion by RNase.

The correction of a single base pair mutation by using a chimeric oligonucleotide is depicted in ***Fig. 13.12***. The RNA-DNA molecules (chimeric oligonucleotides) bind more readily with duplex DNA and bring about the correction in the mutated base pair.

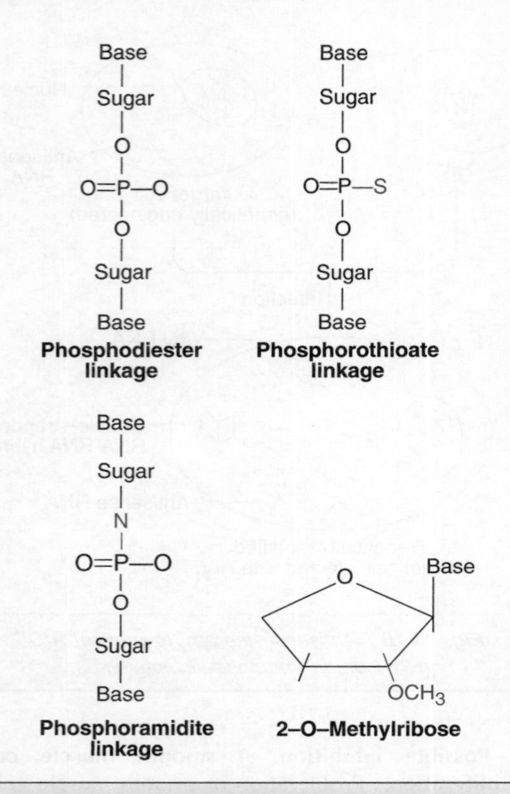

Fig. 13.11 : Certain modifications in antisense oligonucleotides.

APTAMERS AS THERAPEUTIC AGENTS

A special type of ***oligonucleotides*** that can specifically ***bind to target proteins*** and not to nucleic acids are referred to as aptamers. Aptamers are useful as therapeutic agents. For instance, an aptamer that can bind to thrombin inhibits blood clotting. Such oligonucleotides can be used in surgical procedures.

RIBOZYMES AS THERAPEUTIC AGENTS

RNA molecules that can serve as ***enzymes*** (biocatalysts) are referred to as ribozymes. The naturally occurring ribozymes are to be modified so that they can specifically hybridize with mRNA sequences and block protein biosynthesis (translation). There is a limitation however, in directly inserting ribozymes into target cells, as they are easily degraded. This can be overcome by binding ribozyme with an oligodeoxynucleotide. There is a possibility of treating certain cancers and viral diseases by genetically engineered ribozymes.

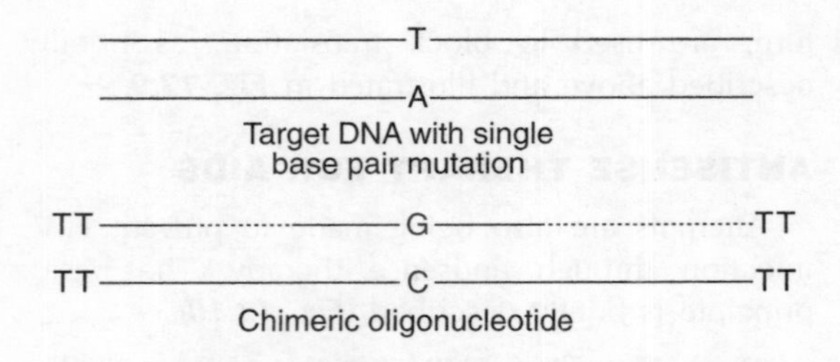

Fig. 13.12 : Chimeric oligonucleotide in gene correction (The dotted lines represent ribonucleotides while the continuous lines correspond to deoxyribonucleotides; the coloured base pair is the correct one to replace the mutated base pair)

THE FUTURE OF GENE THERAPY

Theoretically, gene therapy is ***the permanent solution for genetic diseases***. But it is not as simple as it appears since gene therapy has several inbuilt complexicities. Gene therapy broadly involves isolation of a specific gene, making its copies, inserting them into target tissue cells to make the desired protein. The story does not end here. It is absolutely essential to ensure that the gene is harmless to the patient and it is appropriately expressed (too much or too little will be no good). Another concern in gene therapy is the body's immune system which reacts to the foreign proteins produced by the new genes.

The public, in general, have an ***exaggerated expectations*** on gene therapy. The researchers, at least for the present, are ***unable to satisfy them***. As per the records, by 1999 about 1000 Americans had undergone clinical trails involving various gene therapies. Unfortunately, the gene therapists are unable to categorically claim that gene therapy has permanently cured any one of these patients! Some people in the media (leading news papers and magazines) have openly questioned whether it is worth to continue research on gene therapy!!

It may be true that as of now, gene therapy due to several limitations, has not progressed the way it should, despite intensive research. But ***a break-through may come anytime***, and of course, this is only possible with persistent research. And a day may come (it might take some years) when almost every disease will have a gene therapy, as one of the treatment modalities. And gene therapy will revolutionize the practice of medicine!

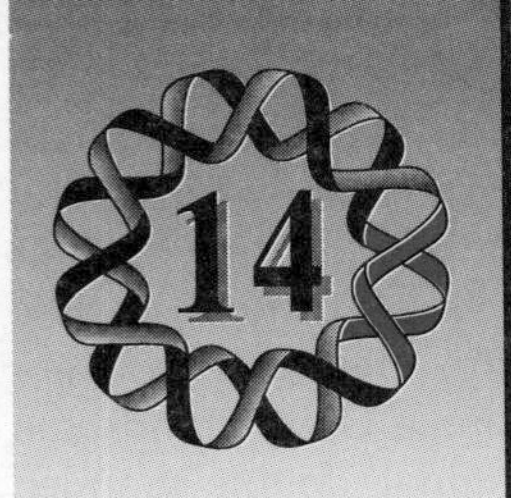

DNA in Disease Diagnosis and Medical Forensics

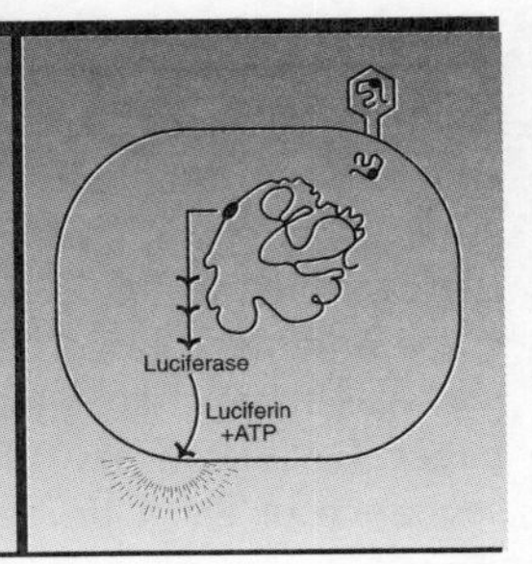

Diagnosis of diseases due to pathogens (bacteria, viruses, fungi etc.) or due to inherent genetic defects is necessary for appropriate treatment. Traditional diagnostic methods for parasite infections include microscopic examination, *in vitro* culture, and detection of antibodies in serum. And for the genetic diseases, the procedures such as estimation of metabolites (blood/urine) and enzyme assays are employed. These laboratory techniques are indirect and not always specific. Scientists are in continuous search for specific, sensitive and simple diagnostic techniques for identification of diseases.

DNA, being the genetic material of the living organisms, contains the information that contributes to various characteristic features of the specific organism. Thus, ***the presence of a disease-causing pathogen can be detected by identifing a gene or a set of genes of the organism***. Likewise an ***inherited genetic defect can be diagnosed by identifying the alterations in the gene***. In the modern laboratory diagnostics, DNA analysis is a very useful and sensitive tool.

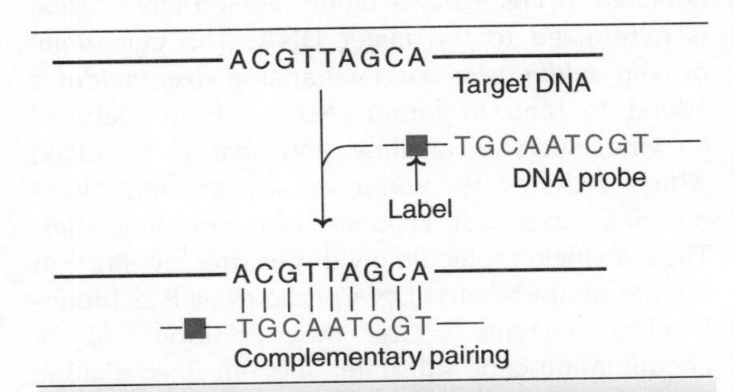

Fig. 14.1 : Hybridization of target DNA with DNA probe (with radioactive isotope label).

The basic principles underlying the DNA diagnostic systems, and their use in the diagnosis of certain pathogenic and genetic diseases are described. Besides these, the various approaches for DNA fingerprinting (or DNA profiling) are also discussed.

METHODS OF DNA ASSAY

The specific ***identification of the DNA sequence*** is absolutely ***essential in the laboratory diagnostics***. This can be achieved by employing the following principles/tools.

NUCLEIC ACID HYBRIDIZATION

Hybridization of nucleic acids (particularly DNA) is the basis for reliable DNA analysis. Hybridization is based on the principle that a single-stranded DNA molecule recognizes and specifically binds to a complementary DNA strand amid a mixture of other DNA strands. This is comparable to a specific key and lock relationship. The general procedure adopted for nucleic acid hybridization is as follows (***Fig. 14.1***).

The single-stranded target DNA is bound to a membrane support. Now the DNA probe (single-stranded and labeled with a detector substance) is added. Under appropriate conditions (temperature, ionic strength), the DNA probe pairs with the complementary target DNA. The unbound DNA probe is removed. Sequence of nucleotides in the target DNA can be identified from the known sequence of DNA probe.

There are two types of DNA hybridization-radioactive and non-radioactive respectively using DNA probes labeled with isotopes and non-isotopes (discussed below) as detectors.

DNA PROBES

A DNA probe or a ***gene probe*** is a synthetic, ***single-stranded DNA molecule that can recognize and specifically bind to a target DNA*** (by complementary base pairing) in a mixture of biomolecules. DNA probes are either long (> 100 nucleotides) or short (< 50 nucleotides), and may bind to the total or a small portion of the target DNA. There is a wide variation in the size of DNA probes used (may range from 10 bases to 10,000 bases). The most important requirement is their specific and stable binding with target DNAs.

Methods employed to obtain DNA probes

A great majority of DNA probes are chemically synthesized in the laboratory. There are, however, many other ways of obtaining them-isolation of selected regions of genes, cloning of intact genes, producing from mRNAs.

Isolation of selected regions of genes : The DNA from an organism (say a pathogen) can be cut by using restriction endonucleases. These DNA fragments are cloned in vectors and the DNA probes can be selected by screening.

Synthesis of DNA probes from mRNA : The mRNA molecules specific to a particular DNA sequence (encoding a protein) are isolated. By using the enzyme reverse transcriptase, complementary DNA (cDNA) molecules are synthesized. This ***cDNA*** can be used ***as a probe*** to detect the target DNA.

Mechanism of action of DNA probes

The basic principle of DNA probes is based on the ***denaturation and renaturation (hybridization) of DNA***. When a double-stranded DNA molecule is subjected to physical (temperature > 95°C or pH < 10.5) or chemical (addition of urea or formaldehyde) changes, the hydrogen bonds break and the complementary strands get separated. This process is called denaturation. Under suitable conditions (i.e., temperature, pH, salt concentration), the two separated single DNA strands can reassemble to form the original double-stranded DNA, and this phenomenon is referred to as renaturation or hybridization.

Radioactive detection system

The ***DNA probe*** is usually ***tagged with a radioactive isotope*** (commonly phosphorus-32). The target DNA is purified and denatured, and mixed with DNA probe. The isotope labeled DNA molecules specifically hybridizes with the target DNA (***Fig. 14.1***). The non-hybridized probe DNA is washed away. The presence of radioactivity in the hybridized DNA can be detected by autoradiography. This reveals the presence of any bound (hybridized) probe molecules and thus the complementary DNA sequences in the target DNA.

Non-radioactive detection system

The disadvantage with the use of radioactive label is that the isotopes have short half-lives and involve risks in handling, besides requiring special laboratory equipment. So, non-radioactive detection systems (e.g., biotinylation) have also been developed. ***Biotin-labeled (biotinylated) nucleotides are incorporated into the DNA probe***. The detection system is based on the enzymatic conversion of a chromogenic (colour producing) or chemiluminescent (light emitting) substrates.

The procedure commonly adopted for chemiluminescent detection of target DNA is depicted in ***Fig. 14.2***. A biotin labeled DNA probe is hybridized to the target DNA. The egg white protein ***avidin*** or its bacterial analog ***streptavidin*** is added to bind to biotin. Now a biotin labeled enzyme, such as alkaline phosphatase is added which attaches to avidin or streptavidin. These proteins have four separate biotin-binding sites. Thus, a single molecule (avidin or streptavidin) can bind to biotin-labeled DNA probe as well as biotin-labeled enzyme. On the addition of a chemiluminescent substrate, the enzyme alkaline phosphatase acts and converts it to a light emitting product which can be measured. (**Note :** When the enzyme peroxidase is employed in place of alkaline phosphatase, chromogenic substrates will be used, and the colour of the product formed is measured).

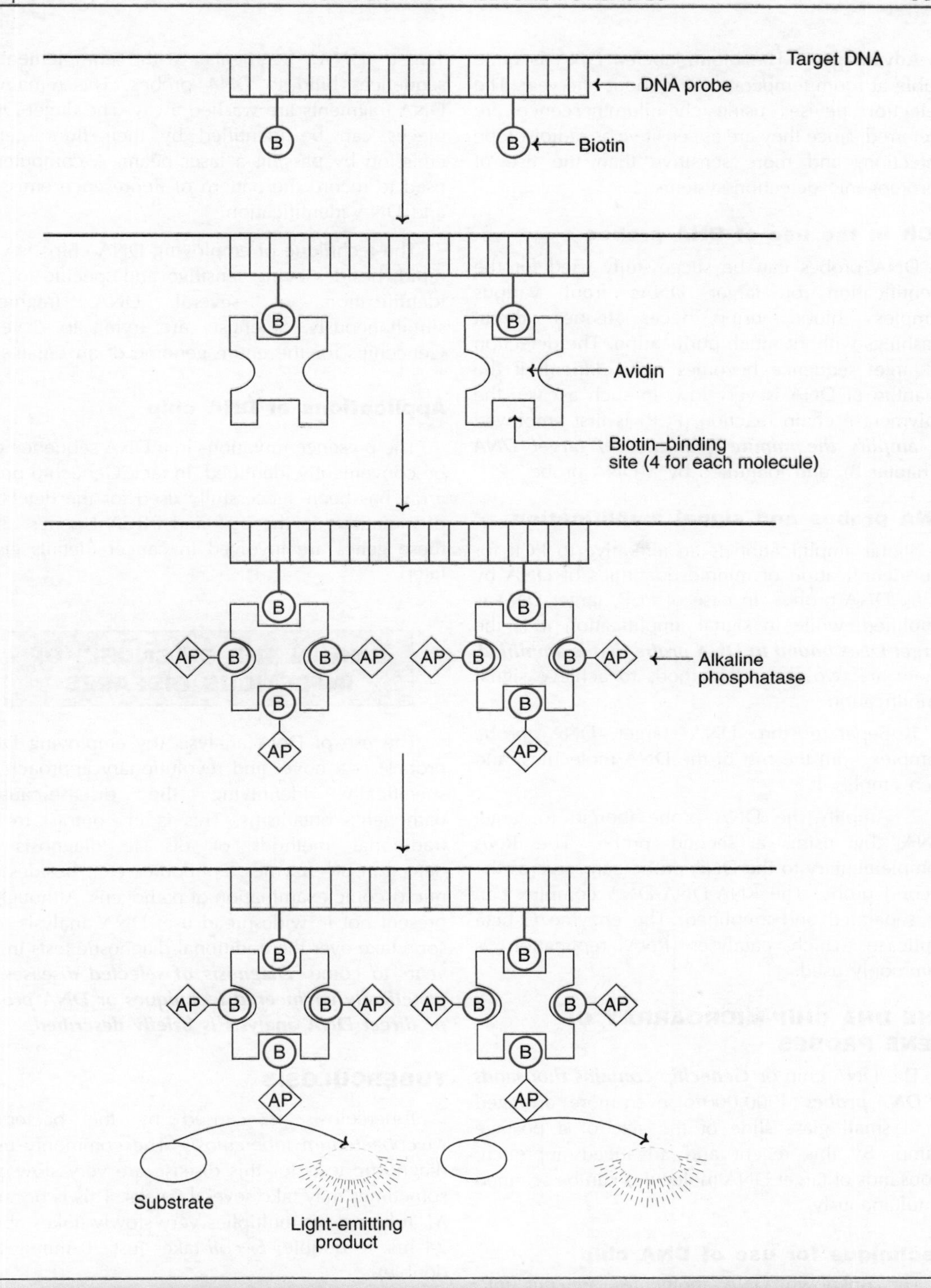

***Fig. 14.2 :** Non-radioactive detection system of target DNA by using biotin-labeled DNA probe (**Note :** Chemiluminescent detection is illustrated; for chromogenic detection, the enzyme peroxidase and a chromogenic substrate are used)*

Advantages : The biotin-labeled DNA is quite stable at room temperature for about one year. The detection devises using chemiluminescence are preferred, since they are as sensitive as radioisotope detection, and more sensitive than the use of chromogenic detection systems.

PCR in the use of DNA probes

DNA probes can be successfully used for the identification of target DNAs from various samples — blood, urine, feces, tissues, throat washings without much purification. The detection of target sequence becomes quite difficult if the quantity of DNA is very low. In such a case, the polymerase chain reaction (PCR) is first employed to ***amplify the minute quantities of target DNA*** (Chapter 8), and identified by a DNA probe.

DNA probes and signal amplification

Signal amplification is an alterative to PCR for the identification of minute quantities of DNA by using DNA probes. In case of PCR, target DNA is amplified, while in signal amplification it is the ***target DNA bound to DNA probe that is amplified.*** There are two general methods to achieve signal amplification.

1. Separate the DNA target—DNA probe complex from the rest of the DNA molecules, and then amplify it.

2. Amplify the DNA probe (bound to target DNA) by using a second probe. The RNA complementary to the DNA probe can serve as the second probe. The RNA-DNA-DNA complex can be separated and amplified. The enzyme O-beta replicase which catalyses RNA replication is commonly used.

THE DNA CHIP-MICROARRAY OF GENE PROBES

The DNA chip or ***Genechip contains thousands of DNA probes*** (4000,000 or even more) arranged on a small glass slide of the size of a postage stamp. By this recent and advanced approach, thousands of target DNA molecules can be scanned simultaneously.

Technique for use of DNA chip

The unknown DNA molecules are cut into fragments by restriction endonucleases. Fluorescent markers are attached to these DNA fragments. They are allowed to react to the probes of the DNA chip. Target DNA fragments with complementary sequences bind to DNA probes. The remaining DNA fragments are washed away. The target DNA pieces can be identified by their fluorescence emission by passing a laser beam. A computer is used to record the pattern of fluoresence emission and DNA identification.

The technique of employing DNA chips is very rapid, besides being sensitive and specific for the identification of several DNA fragments simultaneously. Scientists are trying to develop Genechips for the entire genome of an organism.

Applications of DNA chip

The presence mutations in a DNA sequence can be conveniently identified. In fact, Genechip probe array has been successfully used for the detection of mutations in the p53 and BRCA I genes. Both these genes are involved in cancer (details given later).

DNA IN THE DIAGNOSIS OF INFECTIOUS DISEASES

The use of DNA analysis (by employing DNA probes) is a novel and revolutionary approach for specifically identifying the disease-causing pathogenic organisms. This is in contrast to the traditional methods of disease diagnosis by detection of enzymes, antibodies etc., besides the microscopic examination of pathogens. Although at present not in widespread use, DNA analysis may soon take over the traditional diagnostic tests in the years to come. ***Diagnosis of selected diseases by genetically engineered techniques or DNA probes or direct DNA analysis is briefly described.***

TUBERCULOSIS

Tuberculosis is caused by the bacterium *Mycobacterium tuberculosis*. The commonly used diagnostic tests for this disease are very slow and sometimes may take several weeks. This is because *M. tuberculosis* multiplies very slowly (takes about 24 hrs. to double; *E. coli* takes just 20 minutes to double).

A novel diagnostic test for tuberculosis was developed by genetic engineering, and is illustrated in ***Fig. 14.3***. A gene from ***firefly***, encoding the

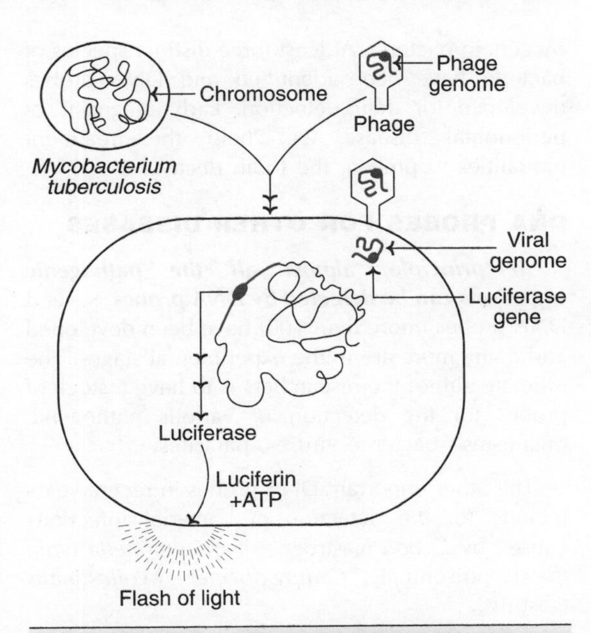

Fig. 14.3 : Diagnosis of tuberculosis by using a genetically engineered bacteriophage (phage).

enzyme ***luciferase*** is introduced into the bacteriophage specific for *M. tuberculosis*. The bacteriophage is a bacterial virus, frequently referred to as ***luciferase reporter phage or mycophage***. The genetically engineered phage is added to the culture of *M. tuberculosis*. The phage attaches to the bacterial cell wall, penetrates inside, and inserts its gene (along with luciferase gene) into the *M. tuberculosis* chromosome. The enzyme luciferase is produced by the bacterium. When luciferin and ATP are added to the culture medium, luciferase cleaves luciferin. This reaction is accompanied by a flash of light which can be detected by a luminometer. This diagnostic test is quite sensitive for the confirmation of tuberculosis.

The ***flash of light is specific for the identification of M. tuberculosis*** in the culture. For other bacteria, the genetically engineered phage cannot attach and enter in, hence no flash of light would be detected.

MALARIA

Malaria, mainly caused by *Plasmodium falciparum* and *P. vivax*, affects about one-third of the world's population. The commonly used laboratory tests for the diagnosis of malaria include microscopic examination of blood smears, and detection of antibodies in the circulation. While the former is time consuming and frequently gives false-negative tests, the latter cannot distinguish between the past and present infections.

A ***specific DNA diagnostic test*** for identification of the current infection of *P. falciparum* has been developed. This is carried out by ***using a DNA probe that can bind and hybridize with a DNA fragment of P. falciparum genome*** and not with other species of *Plasmodium*. It is reported that this DNA probe can detect as little as 1 ng of *P. falciparum* in blood or 10 pg of its purified DNA.

CHAGAS' DISEASE

The protozoan parasite *Trypanosoma cruzi* causes Chagas' disease. This disease is characterized by destruction of several tissues (liver, spleen, brain, lymph nodes) by the invading parasite. Chagas' disease is diagnosed by the microscopic examination of the fresh blood samples. Immunological tests, although available, are not commonly used, since they frequently give false-positive results.

Scientists have identified a DNA fragment with 188-base pair length present in *T. cruzi* genome. This is however, not found in any other related parasite. A PCR technique is employed to amplify the 188 bp DNA fragment. This can be detected by using polyacrylamide gel electrophoresis. Thus, PCR-based amplification can be effectively used for the diagnosis of Chagas' disease.

ACQUIRED IMMUNODEFICIENCY SYNDROME (AIDS)

AIDS is caused by the virus, ***human immunodeficiency virus*** (***HIV***). The commonly used laboratory test for detection of AIDS is the detection of HIV antibodies. However, it might take several weeks for the body to respond and produce sufficient HIV antibodies. Consequently, the antibodies test may be negative (i.e., false-negative), although HIV is present in the body. During this period, being a carrier, he/she can transmit HIV to others.

DNA probes, with radioisotope label, for HIV DNA are now available. By ***using PCR and DNA probes, AIDS can be specifically diagnosed in the laboratory***. During the course of infection cycle,

HIV exists as a segment of DNA integrated into the T-lymphocytes of the host. The T-lymphocytes of a suspected AIDS patient are isolated and disrupted to release DNA. The so obtained DNA is amplified by PCR, and to this DNA probes are added. If the HIV DNA is present, it hybridizes with the complementary sequence of the labeled DNA probe which can be detected by its radioactivity. The advantage of DNA probe is that it can detect the virus when there are no detectable antibodies in the circulation.

HIV diagnosis in the newborn

Detection of antibodies is of no use in the newborn to ascertain whether AIDS has been transmitted from the mother. This is because the antibodies might have come from the mother but not from the virus. This problem can be solved by using DNA probes to detect HIV DNA in the newborn.

HUMAN PAPILLOMA VIRUS

Human papilloma virus (HPV) causes ***genital warts***. HPV is also associated with the cervical cancer in women. The ***DNA probe*** (trade name ***Virapap*** detection kit) that specifically detects HPV has been developed. The tissue samples obtained from woman's cervix are used. HPV DNA, when present hybridizes with DNA probe by complementary base pairing, and this is the positive test.

LYME DISEASE

Lyme disease is caused by the bacterium, *Borrelia burgdorferi*. This disease is characterized by fever, skin rash, arthritis and neurological manifestations.

The diagnosis of Lyme disease is rather difficult, since it is not possible to see *B. burgdorferi* under microscope and the antibody detection tests are not very reliable.

Some workers have used PCR to amplify the DNA of *B. burgdorferi*. By using appropriate DNA probes, the bacterium causing Lyme disease can be specifically detected.

PERIODONTAL DISEASE

Periodontal disease is characterized by the degenerative infection of gums that may ultimately lead to tooth decay and loss. This disease is caused by certain bacteria. At least three distinct species of bacteria have been identified and DNA probes developed for their detection. Early diagnosis of periodontal disease will help the treatment modalities to prevent the tooth decay.

DNA PROBES FOR OTHER DISEASES

In principle, almost all the pathogenic organisms can be detected by DNA probes. Several DNA probes (more than 100) have been developed and many more are in the experimental stages. The ultimate aim of the researchers is to have a stock of probes for the detection of various pathogenic organisms—bacteria, viruses, parasites.

The other important DNA probes in recent years include for the detection of bacterial infections caused by *E. coli* (gastroenteritis) *Salmonella typhi* (food poisoning), *Campylobacter hyoitestinalis* (gastritis).

Diagnosis of tropical diseases

Malaria, filariasis, tuberculosis, leprosy, schistosomiasis, leishmaniasis and trypanosomiasis are the tropical diseases affecting millions of people throughout the world. As already described (See p. 177), for the diagnosis of malaria caused by *P. falciparum*, a DNA probe has been developed. A novel diagnostic test, by genetic manipulations, has been devised for the diagnosis of tuberculosis (See p. 176). Scientists are continuously working to develop better diagnostic techniques for other tropical diseases.

DNA IN THE DIAGNOSIS OF GENETIC DISEASES

Traditional laboratory tests for the diagnosis of genetic diseases are mostly based on the estimation of metabolites and/or enzymes. This is usually done after the onset of symptoms.

The laboratory tests based on DNA analysis can specifically diagnose the inherited diseases at the genetic level. DNA-based tests are useful to discover, well in advance, whether the individuals or their offsprings are at risk for any genetic disease. Further, such tests can also be employed for the prenatal diagnosis of hereditary disorders, besides identifying the carriers of genetic diseases.

By knowing the genetic basis of the diseases, the individuals can be advised on how to limit the transmission of the disease to their offsprings. It may also be possible, in due course of time, to treat genetic diseases by appropriate gene therapies.

Theoretically, it is possible to develop screening tests for all single-gene diseases. Some of the important genetic diseases for which DNA analysis is used for diagnosis are briefly described.

CYSTIC FIBROSIS

Cystic fibrosis (CF) is a common and fatal hereditary disease. The patients produce thick and sticky mucus that clogs lungs and respiratory tract (For some more details on CF, refer Chapter 13). Cystic fibrosis is due to a defect in *cftr* gene that encodes ***cystic fibrosis transmembrane regulator protein***. *cftr* gene is located on chromosome 7 in humans, and a DNA probe has been developed to identify this gene.

The genetic disease cystic fibrosis is inherited by a recessive pattern, i.e., the disease develops when two recessive genes are present. It is now possible to detect CF genes in duplicate in the fetal cells obtained from samples of amniotic fluid. As the test can be done months before birth, it is possible to know whether the offspring will be a victim of CF. One group of researchers have reported that CF gene can be detected in the eight-celled embryo obtained through *in vitro* fertilization.

SICKLE-CELL ANEMIA

Sickle-cell anemia is a genetic disease characterized by the irregular sickle (crescent like) shape of the erythrocytes. Biochemically, this disease results in severe anemia and progressive damage to major organs in the body (heart, brain, lungs, joints).

Sickle-cell anemia occurs due to a single amino acid change in the β-chain of hemoglobin. Specifically, the amino acid ***glutamate at the 6th position of β-chain is replaced by valine***. At the molecular level, sickle-cell anemia is due to a single-nucleotide change (***A → T***) in the β-globin gene of coding (or antisense) strand. In the normal β-globin gene the DNA sequence is CCTGAGGAG, while in sickle-cell anemia, the sequence is CCTGTGGAG. This single-base mutation can be detected by using restriction enzyme *MstII* to cut

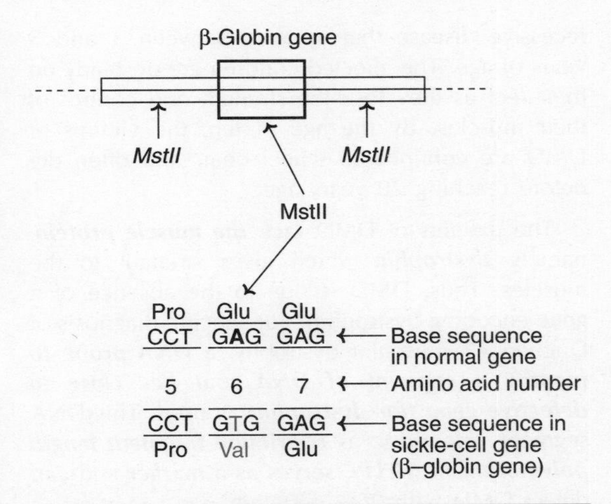

Fig. 14.4 : *Single-base change resulting in sickle-cell anemia.* ***(Note :*** *A small and relevant DNA fragment of β-globin gene magnified and shown with encoded amino acids).*

DNA fragments in and around β-globin gene, followed by the electrophoretic pattern of the DNA fragments formed. The change in the base from A to T in the β-globin gene destroys the recognition site (CCTGAGG) for *MstII* (***Fig. 14.4***). Consequently, the DNA fragments formed from a sickle-cell anemia patient for β-globin gene differ from that of a normal person. Thus, sickle-cell anemia can be detected by digesting mutant and normal β-globin gene by restriction enzyme and performing a ***hybridization with a cloned β-globin DNA probe***.

Single-nucleotide polymorphisms

The ***single base changes*** that occur in some of the genetic diseases (e.g., sickle-cell anemia) are collectively referred to as single-nucleotide polymorphisms (***SNPs***, pronounced ***snips***). It is estimated that the frequency of SNPs is about one in every 1000 bases. Sometimes SNPs are associated with amino acid change in the protein that is encoded. A point mutation in α_1-antitrypsin gene is also a good example of SNPs, besides sickle-cell anemia.

DUCHENNE'S MUSCULAR DYSTROPHY

Duchenne's muscular dystrophy (***DMD***) is a genetic abnormality characterized by progressive wasting of leg and pelvic muscles. It is a sex-linked recessive disease that appears between 3 and 5 years of age. The affected children are unsteady on their feet as they lose the strength and control of their muscles. By the age of ten, the victims of DMD are confined to wheel chair and often die before reaching 20 years age.

The patients of DMD ***lack the muscle protein***, namely ***dystrophin*** which gives strength to the muscles. Thus, DMD is due to the absence of a gene encoding dystrophin. For specific diagnosis of Duchenne's muscular dystrophy, a ***DNA probe to identify a segment of DNA that lies close to defective gene (for dystrophin)*** is used. This DNA segment, referred to as ***restriction fragment length polymorphism (RFLP), serves as a marker*** and can detect DMD with 95% certainity.

In the DNA diagnostic test using RFLP for DMD, DNA samples must be obtained from as many blood relatives (parents, grand-parents, uncles, aunts etc.) as possible. The RFLP patterns, constructed for the entire family are thoroughly checked for the affected and unaffected relatives. This is required since there is a wide variation in RFLPs from family to family. Thus, there is no single identifying test for the diagnosis of genetic diseases based on RFLPs analysis.

HUNTINGTON'S DISEASE

Huntington's disease is a genetic disease (caused by a dominant gene) characterized by progressive deterioration of the nervous system, particularly the destruction of brain cells. The victims of this disease (usually above 50 years of age) exhibit thrashing (jerky) movements and then insanity [older name was Huntington's chorea; *chorea (Greek) means to dance]*. Huntington's disease is invariably fatal.

The molecular basis of Huntington's disease has been identified. The gene responsible for this disease lies on chromosome number 4, and is characterized by ***excessive repetition of the base triplet CAG***. The victims of Huntington's disease have CAG triplet repeated 42–66 times, against the normal 11–34 times. The ***triplet CAG encodes*** for the amino acid ***glutamine***. It is believed that the ***abnormal protein*** (with very high content of glutamine) ***causes the death of cells*** in the basal ganglia (the part of the brain responsible for motor function).

Huntington's disease can be detected by the analysis of RFLPs in blood related individuals. The clinical manifestations of this disease are observed after middle age, and by then the person might have already passed on the defective gene to his/her offsprings.

FRAGILE X SYNDROME

Fragile X syndrome, as the name indicates, is due to a genetic defect in X chromosome (a sex chromosome) and affects both males and females. The victims of this disease are characterized by mental retardation.

Researchers have found that sufferers of fragile X syndrome have the three nucleotide bases (***CGG***) repeated again and again. It is believed that these ***trinucleotide repeats block the transcription process resulting in a protein deficiency***. This protein is involved in the normal function of the nerve cells, and its deficiency results in mental retardation.

A ***DNA probe*** has been developed for the detection of fragile X syndrome in the laboratory.

OTHER TRIPLE REPEAT DISEASES

Excessive ***repetition*** of ***triplet bases*** in DNA are now known to result in several diseases which are collectively referred to as triple repeat diseases. Besides Huntington's disease and fragile X syndrome (discussed above), some more triple repeats are given below.

Friedreich's ataxia

The trinucleotide GAA repeats 200 to 900 times on chromosome 9 in Friedreich's ataxia. This disease is associated with degradation of spinal cord. ***Spinocerebellar ataxia*** is another triplet disease, characterized by neuromuscular disorder, and is due to trinucleotide repeats of CAG by 40 to 80 times on chromosome 6.

There are a few triple repeat diseases in which the repeats tend to increase with each generation and the diseases become more severe. This also results in the onset of clinical manifestations at early ages. ***Kennedy's disease***, also called ***spinobulbar muscular atropy*** (***CAG repeat***) and ***myotonic dystrophy*** (***CTG***) are good examples.

Are triple repeat diseases confined to humans?

Triple repeat diseases have so far not been detected in any other organisms (bacteria, fruit flies, other mammals) except in humans. More studies however, may be needed to confirm this. The occurrence of triple repeat diseases indicates that the structure of DNA may be rather unstable and dynamic. This is in contrast to what molecular biologists have been thinking all along.

ALZHEIMER'S DISEASE

Alzheimer's disease is characterized by loss of memory and impaired intellectual function (dementia). The victims of this disease cannot properly attend to their basic needs, besides being unable to speak and walk.

The patients of Alzheimer's disease were found to have a specific protein, namely ***amyloid*** in the plaques (or clumps) of dead nerve fibers in their brains. A group of researchers have identified a specific ***gene on chromosome 21*** that is believed to be ***responsible for familial Alzheimer's disease***.

A ***DNA probe*** has been developed to locate the genetic marker for Alzheimer's disease. The present belief is that many environmental factors, and a virus may also be responsible for the development of this disease. It may be possible that in the individuals with genetic predisposition, the outside factors may be stimulatory for the onset of the disease.

AMYOTROPHIC LATERAL SCLEROSIS

Amyotrophic lateral sclerosis (***ALS***) is characterized by degenerative changes in the motor neurons of brain and spinal cord. A gene to explain the inherited pattern of ALS was discovered.

The gene, known as ***sodI***, encoding for the enzyme ***superoxide dismutase*** is located on chromosome 21. This gene was found to be defective in families suffering from amyotrophic lateral sclerosis. In fact, certain point mutations in the *sodI* resulting in single amino acid changes in superoxide dismutase have been identified.

Superoxide dismutase is a key enzyme in eliminating the highly toxic free radicals that damage the cells (free radicals have been implicated in aging and several disease e.g. cancer, cataract, Parkinson's disease, Alzheimer's disease). On the basis of the function of superoxide dismutase, it is presumed that ALS occurs as a result of free radical accumulation due to a defective enzyme (as a consequence of mutated gene *sodI*). The deleterious effects of free radicals can be reduced by administering certain compounds such as vitamins C and E.

Another group of workers have reported that the defective superoxide dismutase cannot control a transporter protein responsible for the removal of the amino acid glutamate from the nerve cells. As a result, large quantities of glutamate accumulate in the nervous tissue leading to degenerative changes.

CANCERS

It is now agreed that there is some degree of genetic predisposition for the occurrence of cancers, although the influence of environmental factors cannot be underestimated. In fact, cancer susceptible genes have been identified in some families e.g., genes for melanoma susceptibility in humans are located on chromosomes 1 and 9.

p^{53} gene

The gene p^{53} encodes for a ***p***rotein with a molecular weight ***53*** kilodaltons (hence the name). It is believed that the protein produced by this gene helps DNA repair and suppresses cancer development. Certain damages that occur in DNA may lead to unlimited replication and uncontrolled multiplication of cells. In such a situation, the protein encoded by p^{53} gene binds to DNA and blocks replication. Further, it facilitates the faulty DNA to get repaired. The result is that the cancerous cells are not allowed to establish and multiply. Thus, ***p^{53} is a cancer-suppressor gene*** and acts as a guardian of cellular DNA.

Any ***mutation in the gene p^{53}*** is likely to alter its tumor suppressor function that ***lead to cancer development***. And in fact, the altered forms of p^{53} recovered from the various tumor cells (breast, bone, brain, colon, bladder, skin, lung) confirm the protective function of p^{53} gene against cancers.

It is believed that the environmental factors may cause mutations in p^{53} gene which may ultimately lead to cancer. Some of the mutations of p^{53} gene may be inherited, which probably explains the occurrence of certain cancers in some families.

Genes of breast cancer

Two ***genes***, namely ***BRCAI*** and ***BRCAII***, implicated in certain ***hereditary forms of breast cancer*** in women, have been identified. It is estimated that about 80% of inherited breast cancers are due to mutations in either one of these two genes — BRCAI or BRCAII. In addition, there is a high risk for ovarian cancer due to mutations in BRCAI.

It is suggested that the normal genes BRCAI and BRCAII encode proteins (with 1863 and 3418 amino acids respectively) that function in a manner comparable to gene p^{53} protein (as described above). As such, BRCAI and BRCAII are DNA-repair and tumor-suppressor genes. Some researchers believe that these two proteins act as gene regulators.

Diagnostic tests for the analysis of the genes BRCAI and BRCAII were developed. Unfortunately, their utility is very limited, since there could be hundreds of variations in the base sequence of these genes.

Genes of colon cancer

The occurrence of colon cancer appears to be genetically linked since it runs in some families. Some researchers have identified a gene linked with ***hereditary nonpolyposis colon cancer*** or ***HNPCC*** (some times called ***Lynch syndrome***). This gene encoded a protein that acts as a guardian and brings about DNA repair whenever there is a damage to it. However, as and when there is a mutation to this protective gene, an altered protein is produced which cannot undo the damage done to DNA. This leads to HNPCC. It is estimated that the occurrence of this altered gene is one in every 200 people in general population.

Microsatellite marker genes

Microsatellites refer to the short repetitive sequences of DNA that can be employed as markers for the identification of certain genes. For colon cancer, microsatellite marker genes have been identified on chromosome 2 in humans. There is a lot of variability in the sequence of microsatellites (as is the case with RFLPs described on p. 185).

Early detection of the risk for colon cancer by DNA analysis is a boon for the would be victims of this disease. The suspected individuals can be periodically monitored for the signs and treated appropriately. Unlike many other cancers, the chances of cure for colon cancer are reasonably good.

Gene of retinoblastoma

Retinoblastoma is a rare cancer of the eye. If detected early, it can be cured by radiation therapy and laser surgery or else the eyeball has to be removed.

Scientists have identified a missing or a defective (mutated) gene on chromosome number 13, being responsible for retinoblastoma. The normal gene when present on chromosome 13 is anticancer and does not allow retinoblastoma to develop.

DIABETES

Diabetes mellitus is a clinical condition characterized by ***increased blood glucose level (hyperglycemia)*** due to insufficient or inefficient (incompetent) insulin. In other words, individuals with diabetes cannot utilize glucose properly in their body.

A rare form of ***type II diabetes*** (i.e., non-insulin dependent diabetes mellitus, NIDDM) is ***maturity onset diabetes of the young (MODY)***. MODY, occurring in adolescents and teenagers, is found to have a genetic basis. A ***gene, synthesizing the enzyme glucokinase***, located on chromosome 7, is found to be ***defective in MODY patients***.

Glucokinase is a key enzyme in glucose metabolism. Besides its involvement in the metabolism, glucokinase in the pancreatic cells serves as a detector for glucose concentration in the blood. This detection stimulates β-cells of the pancreas to secrete insulin. A gene modification that results in a defective or an altered glucokinase hampers pancreatic insulin secretion. Later work has shown that glucokinase gene is defective in the common form of type II diabetes.

DNA probes for type II diabetes

The glucokinase genes from normal and type II diabetes patients were cloned and scanned with DNA probes. It was found that ***a single base mutation of the gene led to a defective glucokinase production that is largely responsible for MODY***, and also a majority of individuals with type II diabetes. Later, some workers reported a possibility of at least a dozen mutations (though less important than the one discussed) in glucokinase gene for type II diabetes.

Genes responsible for type I diabetes

Type I diabetes or insulin-dependent diabetes mellitus (IDDM) mainly occurs in childhood, particularly between 12–15 years of age. IDDM is characterized by almost total deficiency of insulin. Researchers have identified at least 18 different chromosome regions linked with type I diabetes. These DNA sequences are located on chromosomes 6, 11 and 18.

OBESITY

Obesity is an abnormal increase in the body weight due to fat deposition. Men and women are considered obese if their weight due to fat, respectively exceeds more than 20% and 25% of the body weight. Obesity increases the risk of high blood pressure, diabetes, atherosclerosis and other life-threatening conditions.

Although many believed that obesity could be genetically inherited, the molecular basis was not known for long. It was in 1994, a group of workers identified a mutated gene that caused obesity in mice. Later, a similar gene was found in humans also.

The gene designated ***ob*** (for ***ob***ese) is located on chromosome 6 in mouse. The DNA of ob gene contains 650 kb and encodes a protein with 167 amino acids in adipose tissue. This protein is responsible to keep the weight of the animals under control. The genetically ***obese mice have mutated ob gene*** and therefore the weight-control protein is not produced. It is believed that this protein functions like a hormone, acts on the hypothalamus, and controls the site of hunger and energy metabolism (these two factors are intimately linked with obesity).

With the discovery of ***ob*** gene, the treatment for inherited obesity may soon become a reality. In fact, one multinational biotechnology company has started producing ***ob protein*** that can be used for weight reduction in experimental mice.

Besides the ***ob*** gene, a few other genes (***fat*** gene, ***tub*** gene) that might be associated with obesity have also been discovered.

DNA ANALYSIS FOR OTHER HUMAN DISEASES

There is a continuous search for the identification of more and more genes that are responsible for human diseases. Such an approach will ultimately help in the specific diagnosis of these diseases before their actual occurrence. In addition to human diseases described above, some more are given below.

Deafness

The deafness, inherited in some families, has genetic basis. A team of workers have identified a gene on chromosome 5, encoding a protein that facilitates the assembly of actin (protein) molecules in the cochlea of inner ear. The association of actin is very essential for the detection of sound waves by the ear. A mutation of the gene on chromosome 5 results in a defective protein synthesis and non-assembly of actin molecules which cause deafness. Some other genes, besides the one described here, have also been found to be associated with deafness.

Glaucoma

Glaucoma is a disease of the eye that may often lead to blindness. It occurs as a result of damage to the optic nerve due to pressure that builds up in the eye. A gene responsible for the hereditary glaucoma in teenagers has been detected on chromosome 1. Another group of researchers have found a gene on chromosome 3 which is linked with the adult-onset glaucoma.

Baldness

There is an inherited form of baldness, called ***alopecia universalis***. This is found to be associated with a gene located on chromosome 12.

Parkinson's disease

Parkinson's disease is a common disorder in many elderly people, with about 1% of the population above 60 years being affected. It is characterized by muscular regidity, tremors, expressionless face, lethargy, involuntary movements etc. In the victims of Parkinson's disease, there is ***degeneration of brain cells, besides a low concentration of dopamine*** (a neuro-transmitter). Researchers have identified that a gene-encoded protein namely ***α-synuclein*** plays a significant role in the development of Parkinson's disease. An altered form of α-synuclein (due to a mutation in the gene) accumulates in the brain as ***Lewy bodies***. This is responsible for nerve cells degeneration and their death in the Parkinson's disease.

Hemochromatosis

Hemochromatosis is an iron-overload disease in which iron is directly deposited in the tissues (liver, spleen, heart, pancreas and skin). An abnormal gene on chromosome 6 is linked with hemochromatosis. The amino acid ***tyrosine***, in the normal protein encoded by this gene is ***replaced by cysteine***. This abnormal protein is responsible for ***excessive iron absorption*** from the intestine which accumulates in the various tissues leading to their damage and malfunction.

Menke's disease

Menke's disease, a copper deficiency disorder, is characterized by decreased copper in plasma, depigmentation of hair, degeneration of nerve cells and mental retardation. A gene located on X-chromosome, encoding a transport protein, is linked with Menke's disease. A defect in the gene, consequently in the protein, impairs copper absorption from the intestine.

GENE BANKS — A NOVEL CONCEPT

As the search continues by scientists for the identification of more and more genes responsible for various diseases, the enlightened public (particularly in the developed countries), is very keen to enjoy the fruits of this research outcome. As of now, DNA probes are available for the detection a limited number of diseases. Researchers continue to develop DNA probes for a large number of genetically predisposed disorders.

Gene banks are the centres for the storage of individual's DNAs for future use to diagnose diseases. For this purpose, the DNA isolated from a person's cells (usually white blood cells) is stored. As and when a DNA probe for the detection of a specific disease is available, the stored DNA can be used for the diagnosis or risk assessment of the said genetic disease.

In fact, some institutions have established gene banks. They store the DNA samples of the interested customers at a fee (one firm was charging $ 200) for a specified period (say around 20–25 years). For the risk assessment of any disease, it is advisable to have the DNAs from close relatives of at least 2-3 generations.

DNA ANALYSIS FOR ENVIRONMENTAL MONITORING

Environmental pollution (particularly water and foods) by pathogenic microorganisms and viruses is a common occurrence. In the traditional approach, the pathogens are identified by cultivating them in the laboratory. In recent years, techniques have been developed for their detection by DNA analysis.

WATER QUALITY TESTING

The quality of potable water can be tested by detecting the ***indicator bacteria*** such as ***Escherichia coli***. For the DNA analysis, water is filtered and the bacteria trapped on the filter are broken to release DNA. By use of DNA probes to detect specific genes, the presence of *E. coli* can be specifically detected. The DNA analysis technique is very sensitive and is capable of identifying a single *E. coli* cell in 100 ml of water. It is also possible to detect other pathogenic organisms such as *Salmonella, Vibrio* and *Shigella* in due course of time.

DNA analysis can also be employed for the specific detection of ***viruses and protozoal pathogens***.

DNA FINGERPRINTING OR DNA PROFILING

DNA fingerprinting is the present day ***genetic detective*** in the practice ***of modern medical forensics***. The underlying principles of DNA fingerprinting are briefly described.

The structure of each person's genome is unique. The only exception being monozygotic identical twins (twins developed from a single fertilized ovum). The unique nature of genome structure provides a good opportunity for the specific identification of an individual.

It may be remembered here that in the traditional fingerprint technique, the individual is identified by preparing an ink impression of the skin folds at the tip of the person's finger. This is based on the fact that the nature of these skin folds is genetically determined, and thus the fingerprint is unique for an individual. In contrast, the ***DNA fingerprint is an analysis of the nitrogenous base sequence in the DNA of an individual***.

History and terminology

The original DNA fingerprinting technique was developed by Alec Jaffreys in 1985. Although the DNA fingerprinting is commonly used, a more general term ***DNA profiling*** is preferred. This is due to the fact that a wide range of tests can be carried out by DNA sequencing with improved technology.

Applications of DNA fingerprinting

The amount of DNA required for DNA fingerprint is remarkably small. The ***minute quantities of DNA*** from blood strains, body fluids, hair fiber or skin fragments ***are enough***. ***Polymerase chain reaction is used to amplify*** this DNA for use in fingerprinting. DNA profiling has wide range of applications—most of them related to medical forensics. Some important ones are listed below.

- Identification of criminals, rapists, thieves etc.
- Settlement of paternity disputes.
- Use in immigration test cases and disputes.

In general, the fingerprinting technique is carried out by collecting the DNA from a suspect (or a person in a paternity or immigration dispute) and matching it with that of a reference sample (from the victim of a crime, or a close relative in a civil case).

DNA MARKERS IN DISEASE DIAGNOSIS AND FINGERPRINTING

The ***DNA markers are highly useful for genetic mapping of genomes***. There are four types of DNA sequences which can be used as markers.

1. Restriction fragment length polymorphisms (***RFLFs***, pronounced as rif-lips).

2. Minisatellites or variable number tandem repeats (***VNTRs***, pronounced as vinters).

3. Microsatellites or simple tandem repeats (***STRs***).

4. Single nucleotide polymorphisms (***SNPs***, pronounced as snips).

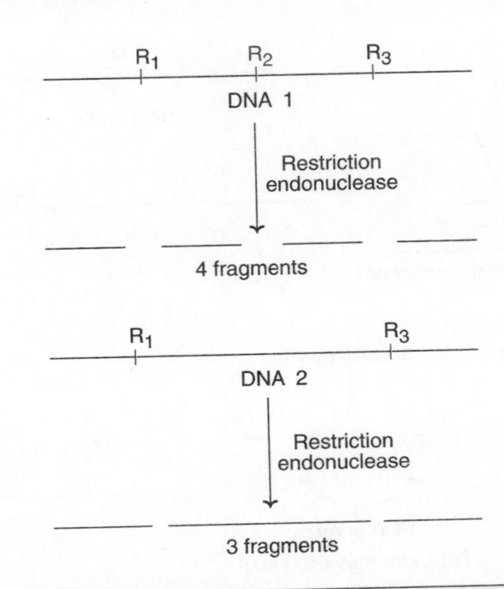

***Fig. 14.5** : An outline of the restriction fragment length polymorphism (RFLP) (R_1, R_2, R_3 represent the sites for the action of restriction endonucleases).*

The general aspects of the above DNA markers are described along with their utility in disease diagnosis and DNA fingerprinting.

RESTRICTION FRAGMENT LENGTH POLYMORPHISMS (RFLPs)

A RFLP represents a stretch of DNA that serves as a marker for mapping a specified gene. RFLPs are located randomly throughout a person's chromosomes and have no apparent function.

A DNA molecule can be cut into different fragments by a group of enzymes called restriction endonucleases (For details, Refer Chapter 6). These fragments are called ***polymorphisms*** (literally means ***many forms***).

An outline of RFLP is depicted in ***Fig. 14.5***. The DNA molecule 1 has three restriction sites (R_1, R_2, R_3), and when cleaved by restriction endonucleases forms 4 fragments. Let us now consider DNA 2 with an inherited mutation (or a genetic change) that has altered some base pairs. As a result, the site (R_2) for the recognition by restriction endonuclease is lost. This DNA molecule 2 when cut by restriction endonuclease forms only 3 fragments (instead of 4 in DNA 1).

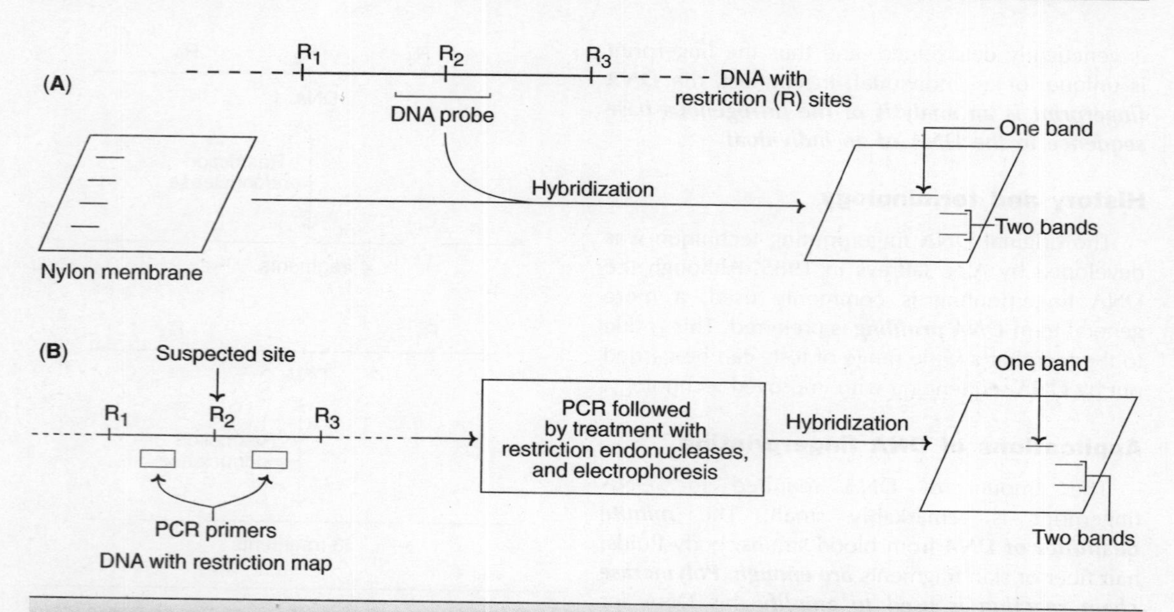

Fig. 14.6 : Two common methods used for scoring restriction fragment length polymorphism (RFLP) (A) RFLP by Southern hybridization (B) RFLP by polymerase chain reaction (PCR).

As is evident from the above description, a stretch of DNA exists in ***fragments*** of various ***lengths*** (***polymorphisms***), derived by the action of ***restriction*** enzymes, hence the name restriction fragment length polymorphisms.

RFLPs in the diagnosis of diseases

If the RFLP lies within or even close to the locus of a gene that causes a particular disease, it is possible to trace the defective gene by the analysis of RFLP in DNA. The person's cellular DNA is isolated and treated with restriction enzymes. The DNA fragments so obtained are separated by electrophoresis. The RFLP patterns of the disease suspected individuals can be compared with that of normal people (preferably with the relatives in the same family). By this approach, it is possible to determine whether the individual has the marker RFLP and the disease gene. With 95% certainity, RFLPs can ***detect single gene-based diseases***.

Methods of RFLP scoring : Two methods are in common use for the detection of RFLPs (***Fig. 14.5***).

1. **Southern hybridization :** The DNA is digested with appropriate restriction enzyme, and separated by agarose gel electrophoresis. The so obtained DNA fragments are transferred to a nylon membrane. A DNA probe that spans the suspected restriction site is now added, and the hybridized bands are detected by autoradiograph. If the restriction site is absent, then only a single restriction fragment is detected. If the site is present, then two fragments are detected (***Fig. 14.6A***).

2. **Polymerase chain reaction :** RFLPs can also be scored by PCR. For this purpose, PCR primers that can anneal on either side of the suspected restriction site are used. After amplification by PCR, the DNA molecules are treated with restriction enzyme and then analysed by agarose gel electrophoresis. If the restriction site is absent only one band is seen while two bands are found if the site is found (***Fig. 14.6B***).

Applications of RFLPs : The approach by RFLP is very powerful and has helped many genes to be mapped on the chromosomes. e.g. sickle-cell anemia (chromosome 11), cystic fibrosis (chromosome 7), Huntington's desease (chromosome 4), retinoblastoma (chromosome 13), Alzheimer's disease (chromosome 21).

VARIABLE NUMBER TANDEM REPEATS (VNTRs)

VNTRs, also known as minisatellites, like RFLPs, are DNA fragments of different length. The main

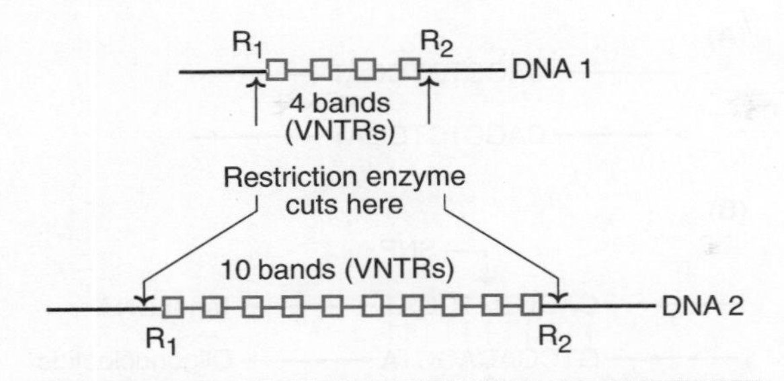

Fig. 14.7 : A diagrammatic representation of variable number tandem repeats (VNTRs). Each band (or copy) represents a repeating sequence in the DNA (e.g. 100 base pairs each). R_1 and R_2 indicate the sites cut by a restriction enzyme.

difference is that RFLPs develop from random mutations at the site of restriction enzyme activity while VNTRs are formed due to different number of base sequences between two points of a DNA molecule. In general, VNTRs are made up of tandem repeats of short base sequences (10–100 base pairs). The number of elements in a given region may vary, hence they are known as variable number tandem repeats.

An individual's genome has many different VNTRs and RFLPs which are unique to the individual. The ***pattern of VNTRs and RFLPs forms the basis of DNA fingerprinting*** or DNA profiling.

In the ***Fig. 14.7***, two different DNA molecules with different number of copies (bands) of VNTRs are shown. When these molecules are subjected to restriction endonuclease action (at two sites R_1 and R_2), the VNTR sequences are released, and they can be detected due to variability in repeat sequence copies. These can be used in mapping of genomes, besides their utility in DNA fingerprinting.

VNTRs are useful for the detection of certain genetic diseases associated with alterations in the degree of repetition of microsatellites e.g. Huntington's chorea is a disorder which is found when the VNTRs exceed 40 repeat units.

Limitations of VNTRs : The major drawback of VNTRs is that they are not evenly distributed throughout the genome. VNTRs tend to be localized in the telomeric regions at the ends of the chromosomes.

Use of RFLPs and VNTRs in genetic fingerprinting

RFLPs caused by variations in the number of VNTRs between two restriction sites can be detected (***Fig. 14.8***). The DNAs from three individuals with different VNTRs are cut by the specific restriction endonuclease. The DNA fragments are separated by electrophoresis, and identified after hybridization with a probe complementary to a specific sequence on the fragments.

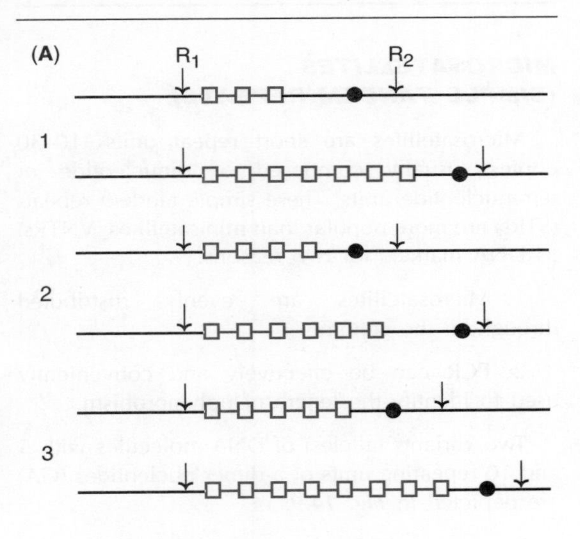

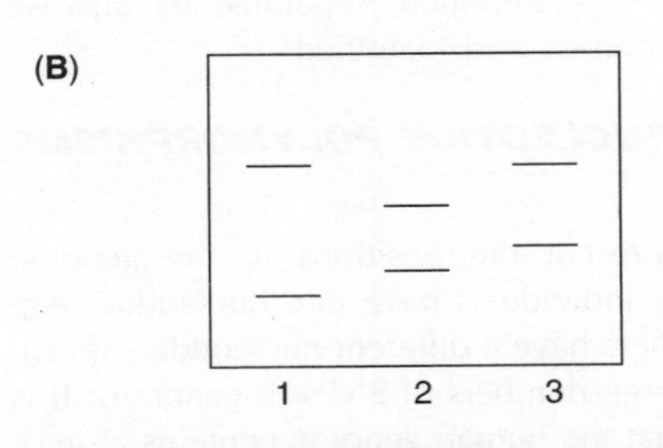

*Fig. 14.8 : Use of restriction fragment length polymorphisms (RFLPs) caused by variable number tandem repeats (VNTRs) in genetic fingerprinting **(A)** An illustration of DNA structure from three individuals **(B)** Hybridized pattern of DNA fragment with a probe complementary to the sequence shown in black circles (1, 2 and 3 represent the individuals; R_1 and R_2 indicate restriction sites; coloured squares are the number of VNTRs)*

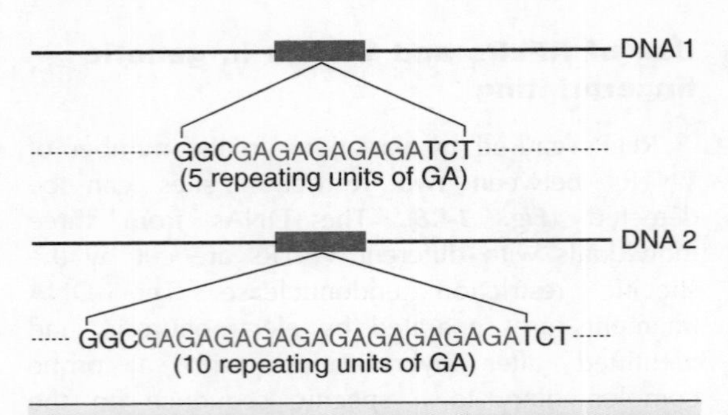

Fig. 14.9 : Two alleles of DNA molecules representing 5 and 10 dimer repeating units.

MICROSATELLITES (SIMPLE TANDEM REPEATS)

Microsatellites are short repeat units (10–30 copies) usually composed of dinucleotide or tetranucleotide units. These simple tandem repeats (STRs) are more popular than minisatellites (VNTRs) as DNA markers for two reasons.

1. Microsatellites are evenly distributed throughout the genome.

2. PCR can be effectively and conveniently used to identify the length of polymorphism.

Two variants (alleles) of DNA molecules with 5 and 10 repeating units of a dimer nucleotides (GA) are depicted in ***Fig. 14.9***.

By use of PCR, the region surrounding the microsatellites is amplified, separated by agarose gel electrophoresis and identified.

SINGLE NUCLEOTIDE POLYMORPHISMS (SNPs)

SNPs represent the positions in the genome where some individuals have one nucleotide (e.g. G) while others have a different nucleotide (e.g. C). There are large numbers of SNPs in genomes. It is estimated that the human genome contains at least 3 million SNPs. Some of these SNPs may give rise to RFLPs.

SNPs are highly useful as DNA markers since there is no need for gel electrophoresis and this saves a lot of time and labour. The detection of SNPs is based on the oligonucleotide hybridization analysis (***Fig. 14.10***).

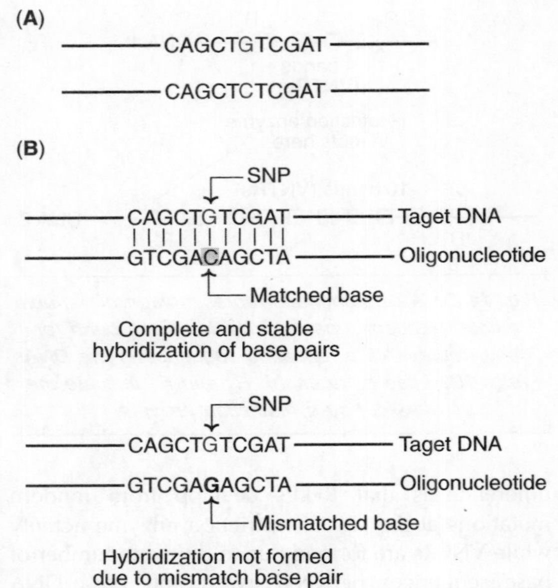

Fig. 14.10 : (A) An illustration of single nucleotide polymorphism (SNP) (B) Oligonucleotide hybridization to detect SNP.

An oligonucleotide is a short single-stranded DNA molecule synthesized in the laboratory with a length not usually exceeding 50 nucleotides. Under appropriate conditions, this nucleotide sequence will hybridize with a target DNA strand if both have completely base paired structure. Even a single mismatch in base pair will not allow the hybridization to occur.

DNA chip technology is most commonly used to screen SNPs hybridization with oligonucleotide (Refer Chapter 7).

CURRENT TECHNOLOGY OF DNA FINGERPRINTING

In the forensic analysis of DNA, the original techniques based on RFLPs and VNTRs are now largely replaced by microsatellites (short tandem repeats). The basic principle involves the amplification of microsatellites by polymerase chain reaction followed by their detection.

It is now possible to generate a DNA profile by automated DNA detection system (comparable to the DNA sequencing equipment).

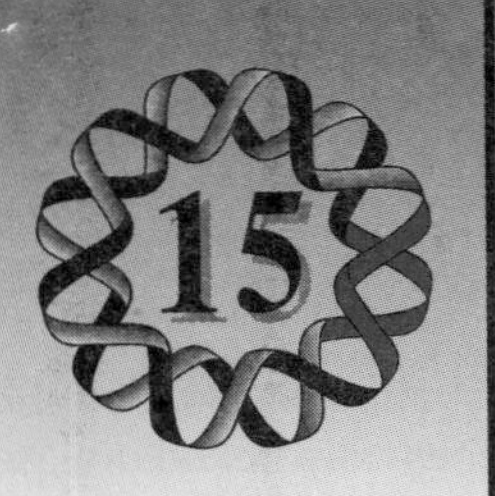

Pharmaceutical Products of DNA Technology

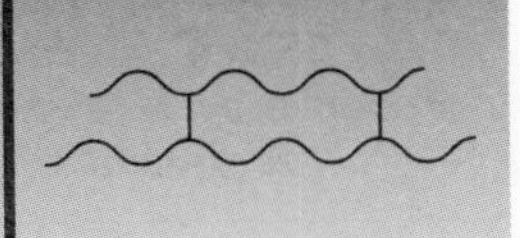

A few decades ago, it was realised that certain proteins could be used as pharmaceutical agents for the treatment of human diseases. e.g. insulin for diabetes mellitus, interferon for viral diseases. However, the availability of such therapeutic/pharmaceutical products was very limited due to costly and cumbersome procedures involved in their isolation/production. Further, their use in humans was associated with several complications. For instance, administration of pig insulin to diabetic patients results in the development of antibodies.

The advent of recombinant DNA technology heralded a new chapter for the production of a wide range of therapeutic agents in sufficient quantities for human use. The commercial exploitation of ***recombinant DNA (rDNA) technology*** began in late 1970s by a few biotechnological companies to produce proteins. There are at least 400 different proteins being produced (by DNA technology) which may serve as therapeutic agents for humans. A selected list of some important human proteins produced by recombinant DNA technology potential for the treatment of human disorders is given in ***Table 15.1***. As of now, only a selected few of them (around 30) have been approved for human use, and the most important among these are given in ***Table 15.2***.

The pharmaceutical products of recombinant DNA technology are broadly divided into the following three categories and briefly discussed with important examples.

1. Human protein replacements.
2. Therapeutic agents for human diseases.
3. Vaccines.

Some authors do not make such categorization and consider all of them together as pharmaceutically important products of biotechnology.

HUMAN PROTEIN REPLACEMENTS

The synthesis of the cellular proteins is ultimately under the control of genes. Any defect in a gene produces an incorrect protein or no protein at all. Sometimes, the occurrence of a defective (i.e. functionally ineffective) or deficient protein may cause a disease. Thus, gene defects will result in inherited or genetically linked diseases.

Identification of defective or deficient proteins in the causation of inherited diseases is very important. The ***recombinant DNA technology can be fruitfully employed to produce human proteins that can be used for the treatment of genetically linked diseases***. This is referred to as human protein replacement strategy in biotechnology.

INSULIN

The hormone insulin is produced by the β-cells of islets of Langerhans of pancreas. Human insulin contains 51 amino acids, arranged in two polypeptide chains. The chain A has 21 amino

Table 15.1 A selected list of human proteins produced by recombinant DNA technology for treatment of human disorders

Disorder	*Recombinant protein(s)*
Anemia	Hemoglobin, erythropoietin
Asthma	Interleukin-I receptor
Atherosclerosis	Platelet-derived growth factor
Delivery	Relaxin
Blood clots	Tissue plasminogen activator, urokinase
Burns	Epidermal growth factor
Cancer	Interferons, tumor necrosis factor, colony stimulating factors, interleukins, lymphotoxin, macrophage-activating factor
Diabetes	Insulin, insulin-like growth factor
Emphysema	α_1-Antitrypsin
Female infertility	Chorionic gonadotropin
Free radical damage (minimizing)	Superoxide dismutase
Growth defects	Growth hormone, growth hormone-releasing factor, somatomedin-C
Heart attacks	Prourokinase
Hemophilia A	Factor VIII
Hemophilia B	Factor IX
Hepatitis B	Hepatitis B vaccine
Hypoalbuminemia	Serum albumin
Immune disorders	Interleukins, β-cell growth factors
Kidney disorders	Erythropoietin
Low Gehrig's disease (amytrophic lateral sclerosis)	Brain-derived neurotropic factor
Multiple sclerosis	Interferons (α, β, γ)
Nerve damage	Nerve growth factor
Osteomalacia	Calcitonin
Pain	Endorphins and enkephalins
Rheumatic disease	Adrenocorticotropic hormone
Ulcers	Urogastrone
Viral infections	Interferons (α, β, γ)

acids while B has 30 amino acids. Both are held together by disulfide bonds.

Diabetes mellitus

Diabetes mellitus affects about 2–3% of the general population. It is a genetically linked disease characterized by ***increased blood glucose concentration (hyperglycemia)***. The occurrence of diabetes is due to insufficient or inefficient (incompetent) insulin. Insulin facilitates the cellular uptake and utilization of glucose for the release of energy. In the absence of insulin, glucose accumulates in the blood stream at higher concentration, usually when the blood glucose concentration exceeds about 180 mg/dl, glucose is excreted into urine. The patients of diabetes are weak and tired since the production of energy (i.e. ATP) is very much depressed.

Table 15.2 A selected list of recombinant proteins that have been approved for human use by U.S. Food and Drug Administration

Recombinant protein	*Disorder(s) treated*
Coagulation factor VIII	Hemophilia A
Coagulation factor IX	Christmas disease
DNase I	Cystic fibrosis
Erythropoietin	Anemia, kidney disease
Glucocerebrosidase	Gaucher's disease
Growth hormone	Growth defects in children
Granulocyte colony stimulating factor	Cancer
Hepatitis B surface antigen (vaccine)	Hepatitis B
Insulin	Diabetes mellitus
Interferon α	Leukemia, kaposi sarcoma genital warts, hepatitis B
Interferon β	Multiple sclerosis
Interferon γ	Chronic granulomatous disease
Interleukin-2	Renal cell carcinoma
Interleukin-10	Thrombocytopenia
Somatotropin	Growth defects
Tissue plasminogen activator	Acute myocardial infarction, pulmonary embolism

The more serious complications of uncontrolled diabetes include kidney damage (nephropathy), eye damage (retinopathy), nerve diseases (neuropathy) and circulatory diseases (atherosclerosis, stroke). In fact, diabetes is the third leading cause of death (after heart disease and cancer) in many developed countries.

In the early years, insulin isolated and purified from the pancreases of pigs and cows was used for the treatment of diabetics. There is a slight difference (by one to three amino acids) in the structure of animal insulin compared to human insulin. This resulted in allergy in some of the diabetics when animal insulin was administered. Another problem with animal insulin is that large number of animals have to be sacrificed for extracting insulin from their pancreases. For instance, about 70 pigs (giving about 5 kg pancreatic tissue) have to be killed to get insulin for treating a single diabetic patient just for one year!

Production of recombinant insulin

Attemps to produce insulin by recombinant DNA technology started in late 1970s. The ***basic technique consisted of inserting human insulin gene and the promoter gene of lac operon on to the plasmids of E. coli.*** By this method human insulin was produced. It was in July 1980, seventeen human volunteers were, for the first time, administered recombinant insulin for treatment of diabetes at Guy's Hospital, London. And in fact, insulin was the first ever pharmaceutical product of recombinant DNA technology administered to humans. Recombinant insulin worked well, and this gave hope to scientists that DNA technology could be successfully employed to produce substances of medical and commercial importance. An ***approval***, by the concerned authorities, for using recombinant insulin for the treatment of diabetes mellitus was ***given in 1982***. And in 1986, Eli Lilly company received approval ***to market hum***an ins***ulin*** under the trade name ***Humulin***.

Technique for recombinant insulin production : The orginal technique (described briefly above) of insulin synthesis in *E. coli* has undergone several changes, for improving the yield. e.g. addition of signal peptide, synthesis of A and B chains separately etc.

The procedure employed for the synthesis of two insulin chains A and B is illustrated in

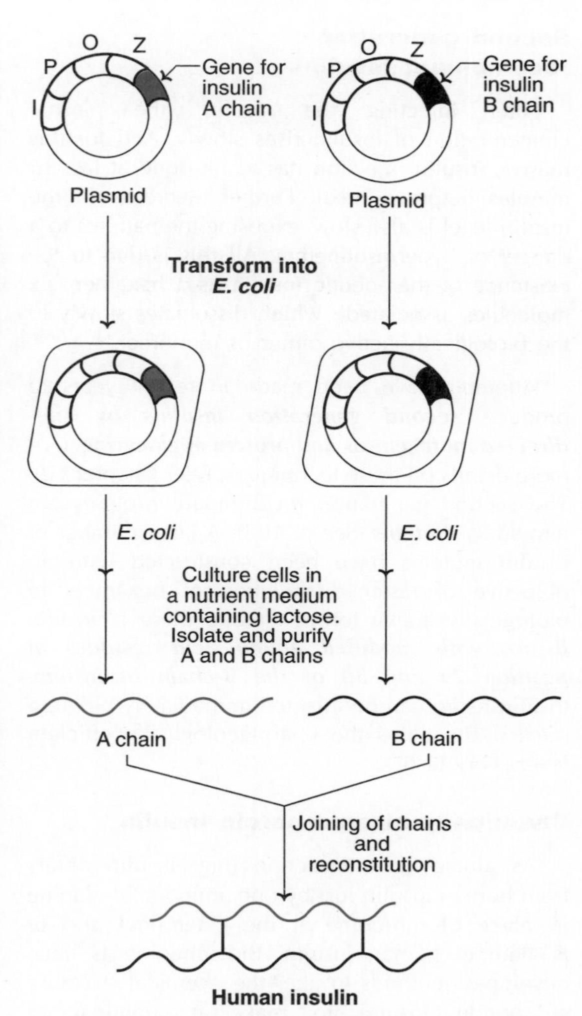

***Fig. 15.1 :** The production of recombinant insulin in* E. coli *(I-Inducer gene, P-Promoter gene, O-Operator gene, Z-β-Galactosidase gene; all these genes are of lac operon system).*

Fig. 15.1. The genes for insulin A chain and B chain are separately inserted to the plasmids of two different *E. coli* cultures. The *lac* operon system (consisting of inducer gene, promoter gene, operator gene and structural gene Z for β-galactosidase) is used for expression of both the genes. The presence of lactose in the culture medium induces the synthesis of insulin A and B chains in separate cultures. The so formed insulin chains can be isolated, purified and joined together to give a full-pledged human insulin.

Second generation recombinant insulins

After injecting the insulin, the plasma concentration of insulin rises slowly. And for this reason, insulin injection has to be done at last 15 minutes before a meal. Further, decrease in the insulin level is also slow, exposing the patients to a danger of hyperinsulinemia. All this is due to the existence of therapeutic insulin as a hexamer (six molecules associated), which dissociates slowly to the biologically active dimer or monomer.

Attempts have been made in recent years to produce ***second generation insulins by site-directed mutagenesis and protein engineering***. (For more details on these techniques, refer Chapter 10). The second generation recombinant proteins are termed as ***muteins*** (See p. 198). A large number of insulin muteins have been constructed with an objective of faster dissociation of hexamers to biologically active forms. Among these is ***insulin lispro, with modified amino acid residues at position 29 and 30 of the B-chain of insulin***. Insulin lispro can be injected immediately before a meal as it attains the pharmacologically efficient levels very fast.

Chemically altered porcin insulin

As already stated, porcin (pig) insulin differs from human insulin just by one amino acid-alanine in place of threonine at the C-terminal and of B-chain of human insulin. Biotechnologists have developed methods to alter the chemical structure of porcin insulin to make it identical to human insulin. And this chemically modified porcin insulin can also be employed for the treatment diabetes mellitus.

HUMAN GROWTH HORMONE

Growth hormone is produced by the pituitary gland. It regulates the growth and development. Growth hormone stimulates overall body growth by increasing the cellular uptake of amino acids, and protein synthesis, and promoting the use of fat as body fuel.

Insufficient human growth hormone (hGH) in young children results in retarded growth, clinically referred to as ***pituitary dwarfism***. The child usually is less than four feet in height, and has chubby face and abundant fat around the waist.

Traditional treatment for dwarfism : The children of pituitary dwarfism were treated with regular ***injections of growth hormone extracted from the brains of deceased humans***. It may be noted that only human growth hormone is effective for treatment of dwarfism. (This is in contrast to diabetes where animal insulins are employed). At least eight pituitary glands from cadavers must be extracted to get hGH adequate for treating a dwarf child just for one year! And such treatment has to be continued for 8–10 years!! Further, administration hGH isolated from human brains exposes the children to a great risk of transmitting the cadaver brain diseases (through virus or viral-like agents) e.g. Creuzfeldt-Jacob (CJ) syndrome characterized by convulsions, wasting of muscle etc.

Production of recombinant hGH

Biotechnologists can now produce hGH by genetic engineering. The technique adopted is quite comparable with that of insulin production. The procedure essentially consists of inserting hGH gene into *E. coli* plasmid, culturing the cells and isolation of the hGH from the extracellular medium.

Limitation in hGH production : The hGH is a protein comprised of 191 amino acids. During the course of its natural synthesis in the body, hGH is tagged with a single peptide (with 26 amino acids). The signal peptide is removed during secretion to release the active hGH for biological functions. The entire process of hGH synthesis goes on in an orderly fashion in the body. However, ***signal peptide interrupts hGH production by recombinant technology***. The complementary DNA (cDNA) synthesized from the mRNA encoding hGH is inserted into the plasmid. The plasmid containing *E. coli* when cultured, produces full length hGH along with signal peptide. But *E. coli* cannot remove the signal peptide. Further, it is also quite difficult to get rid of signal peptide by various other means. Theoretically, cDNA encoding signal peptide can be cut to solve these problems. Unfortunately, there is no restriction endonuclease to do this job, hence this is not possible.

A novel approach for hGH production : Biotechnologists have resolved the problem of signal peptide interruption by a novel approach (***Fig. 15.2***). The base sequence in cDNA encoding signal peptide (26 amino acids) plus the neighbouring 24 amino acids (i.e. a total 50 amino

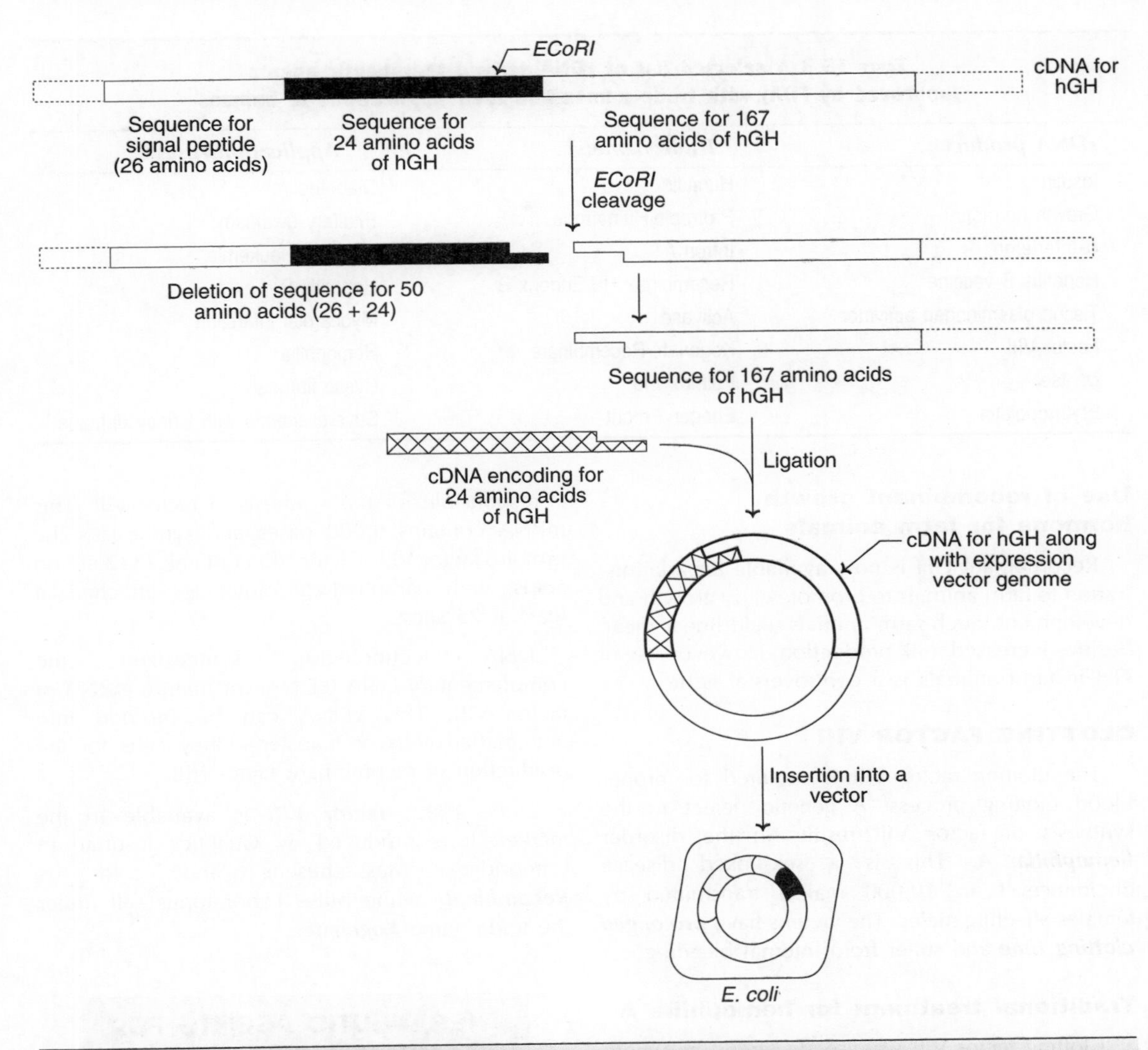

Fig. 15.2 : The production of recombinant human growth hormone (cDNA–Complementary DNA, hGH–Human growth hormone)

acids) is cut by restriction endonuclease *ECoRI*. Now a gene (cDNA) for 24 amino acid sequence of hGH (that has been deleted) is freshly synthesized and ligated to the remaining hGH cDNA. The so constitued cDNA, attached to a vector, is inserted into a bacterium such as *E. coli* for culture and production of hGH. In this manner, the biologically functional hGH can be produced by DNA technology.

Recombinant hGH was approved for human use in 1985. It is marketed as ***Protropin*** by Genetech company and ***Humatrope*** by Eri Lilly company.

Controversy over the use of hGH

Recombinant hGH can be administered to children of very short stature. It has to be given daily for many years with an annual cost of about $ 20,000. Some workers have reported substantial increase in the height of growth retarded children. One group of workers observed that the normal growth pattern in children was not restored on hGH administration, although there was an initial spurt. Another big question raised by the opponents of hGH therapy is whether it is necessary to consider short stature as a disorder at all for treatment!

Table 15.3 A selected list of rDNA-derived therapeutic agents (approved by FDA) with trade names and their applications in humans

rDNA product	*Trade name(s)*	*Applications/uses*
Insulin	Humulin	Diabetes
Growth hormone	Protropin/Humatrope	Pituitary dwarfism
α-Interferon	Intron A	Hairy cell leukemia
Hepatitis B vaccine	Recombinax HB/Engerix B	Hepatitis B
Tissue plasminogen activator	Activase	Myocardial infarction
Factor VIII	Kogenate/Recombinate	Hemophilia
DNase	Pulmozyme	Cystic fibrosis
Erythropoietin	Epogen/Procrit	Severe anemia with kidney damage

Use of recombinant growth hormone for farm animals

Recombinant GH is now available for administration to farm animals to promote early growth and development. Such farm animals yield linear meat, besides increased milk production. However, use of GH in farm animals is a controversial issue.

CLOTTING FACTOR VIII

The clotting factor VIII is required for proper blood clotting process. A genetic defect in the synthesis of factor VIII results in the disorder ***hemophilia A***. This is a sex-linked disease (incidence 1 in 10,000 males) transmitted by females affecting males. The victims have ***prolonged clotting time*** and suffer from internal bleeding.

Traditional treatment for hemophilia A

Clotting factor VIII was isolated from the whole blood and administered to the patients of hemophilia A. This approach requires large quantities of blood. Another problem is the risk of transmission of certain diseases like AIDS to the hemophiliacs.

Production of recombinant factor VIII

The gene for the formation of factor VIII is located on X chromosome. It is a complex gene of 186 kb (i.e., 186,000 base pairs) in size, organized into 26 exons of varying length. In between the exons, many introns are present. The introns vary in their size, starting from 200 base pairs to as high as 32,000 base pairs.

Biotechnologists were able to isolate mature mRNA (containing only exons and no introns) that is responsible for the synthesis of factor VIII. This mRNA contains 9,000 bases and synthesizes the protein, factor VIII. Factor VIII contains 2332 amino acids, with carbohydrate molecules attached at least at 25 sites.

DNA technologists synthesized the complementary DNA (cDNA) for mature mRNA of factor VIII. This cDNA can be inserted into mammalian cells or hamster kidney cells for the production of recombinant factor VIII.

Since 1992, ***factor VIII*** is available in the market. It is produced by Genetics Institute in Cambridge, Massachusetts and sold as ***Recombinate*** while Miles Laboratories sell under the trade name ***Kogenate***.

THERAPEUTIC AGENTS FOR HUMAN DISEASES

Biotechnology is very useful for the production of several therapeutic products for treating human diseases. A selected list of rDNA-derived therapeutic agents along with trade names and their uses in humans are given in ***Table 15.3***. Some of these are described above (under human protein replacements) while the remaining are discussed below.

TISSUE PLASMINOGEN ACTIVATOR

Tissue plasminogen activator (tPA) is a naturally occurring protease enzyme that helps ***to dissolve blood clots***. tPA is a boon for ***patients suffering from thrombosis***.

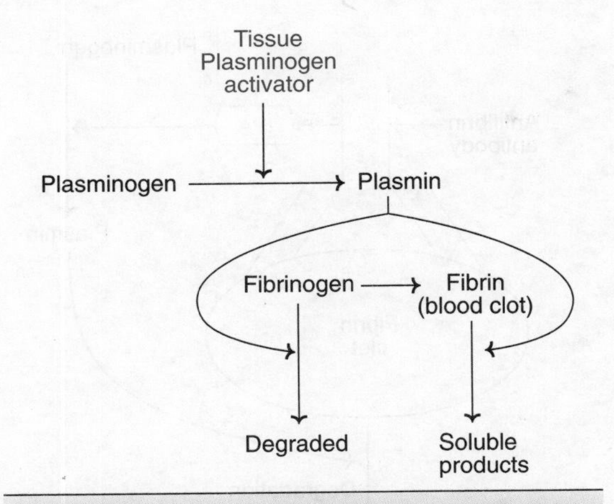

Fig. 15.3 : Role of tissue plasminogen activator in dissolving blood clots.

The majority of natural deaths worldwide are due to a blockade of cerebral or coronary artery by a blood clot, technically called as thrombus. The phenomenon of thrombus blockage of blood vessels is referred to as thrombosis.

Chemically, thrombus consists of a network of fibrin, formed from the fibrinogen. In the normal circumstances, plasmin degrades fibrin and dissolves blood clots. This plasmin is actually produced by activation of plasminogen by tissue plasminogen activator (***Fig. 15.3***). The natural biological systems is however, not that efficient to remove the blood clots through this machinery. Tissue plasminogen activator is very useful as a therapeutic agent in dissolving blood clots (thrombi) by activating plasminogen. By removing the arterial, thrombi, the possible damage caused by them on heart and brain could be reduced.

Production of recombinant tPA

DNA technologists synthesized the complementary DNA (cDNA) molecule for tissue plasminogen activator. This cDNA was then attached to a synthetic plasmid and introduced into mammalian cells (***Fig. 15.4***). They were cultured and tPA-producing cells were selected by using methotrexate to the medium. tPA-producing cells were transferred to an industrial tank (fermenter). tPA, secreted into the culture medium, is isolated for therapeutic purpose. It may be noted here that ***tPA was the first pharmaceutical product to be produced by mammalian cell culture***.

Recombinant tPA has been in use since 1987 for ***treatment of patients with acute myocardial infarction or stroke.*** Genetech was the first to market tPA with a trade name ***Activase***.

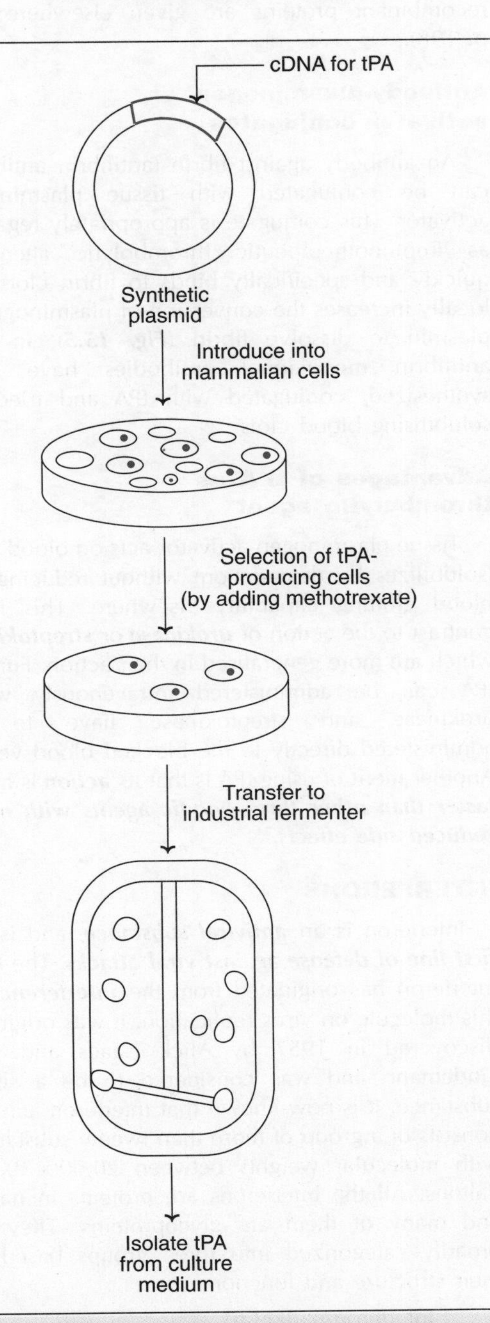

Fig. 15.4 : The production of recombinant tissue plasminogen activator (tPA).

Alteplase and Reteplase : These are the second generation recombinant tPAs. They have ***increased in vivo half-lives*** and are functionally more efficient. The general aspects of second generation recombinant proteins are given elsewhere (See p. 198).

Antibody-plasminogen activator conjugates

An antibody against fibrin (antifibrin antibody) can be conjugated with tissue plasminogen activator. This conjugate is appropriately regarded as immunotherapeutic thrombolytic agent. It quickly and specifically binds to fibrin clots and locally increases the conversion of plasminogen to plasmin to dissolve fibrin (***Fig. 15.5***). In fact, antifibrin monoclonal antibodies have been synthesized, conjugated with tPA and tried for solubilising blood clots.

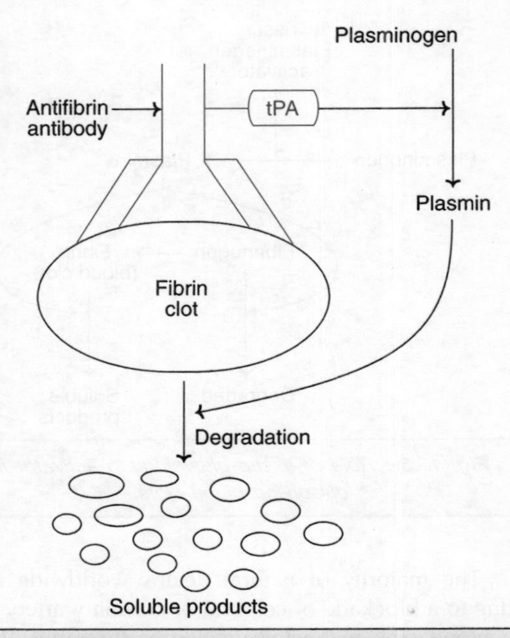

Fig. 15.5 : Action of antifibrin antibody—tPA conjugate in dissolving blood clot (tPA–tissue plasminogen activator).

Advantages of tPA as thrombolytic agent

Tissue plasminogen activator acts on blood clots (solubilizes by degradation) without reducing the blood clotting capability elsewhere. This is in contrast to the action of ***urokinase*** or ***streptokinase*** which are more generalised in their action. Further, tPA can be administered intravenously while urokinase and streptokinase have to be administered directly to the blocked blood vessel. Another merit of using tPA is that its ***action*** is much ***faster than other thrombolytic agents with much reduced side effects***.

INTERFERONS

Interferon is an ***antiviral substance***, and is the ***first line of defense against viral attacks***. The term interferon has originated from the ***interference*** of this molecule on virus replication. It was originally discovered in 1957 by Alick Isaacs and Jean Lindemann and was considered to be a single substance. It is now known that interferon actually consists of a group of more than twenty substances with molecular weights between 20,000–30,000 daltons. All the interferons are proteins in nature and many of them are glycoproteins. They are broadly categorized into three groups based on their structure and function

Interferon-α (IFN-α)
Interferon-β (IFN-β)
Interferon-γ (IFN-γ)

Mechanism of action of interferons

Interferons are produced by mammalian cells when infected by viruses. As the virus releases its nucleic acid into cellular cytoplasm, it stimulates the host DNA to produce interferons. These interferons, secreted by the cells, bind to the adjacent cells. Here, they stimulate the cellular DNA to produce a series of antiviral enzymes. The so formed proteins inhibit viral replication and protect the cells (***Fig. 15.6***). It is believed that the protective (enzymes) proteins bind to mRNA of viruses and block their protein synthesis. The action of interferons appears to be species specific. Thus, human interferons operate in humans. Other animal (dog, mouse) interferons are ineffective in man.

Isolation of interferons in the early years

Blood was the only source of interferons earlier. The procedure was very tedious and the quantity of interferons isolated was very little. Thus, as much as 50,000 litres of human blood was required to get just 100 mg of interferons! Therefore, it was very difficult to conduct research or use interferons for therapeutic purposes.

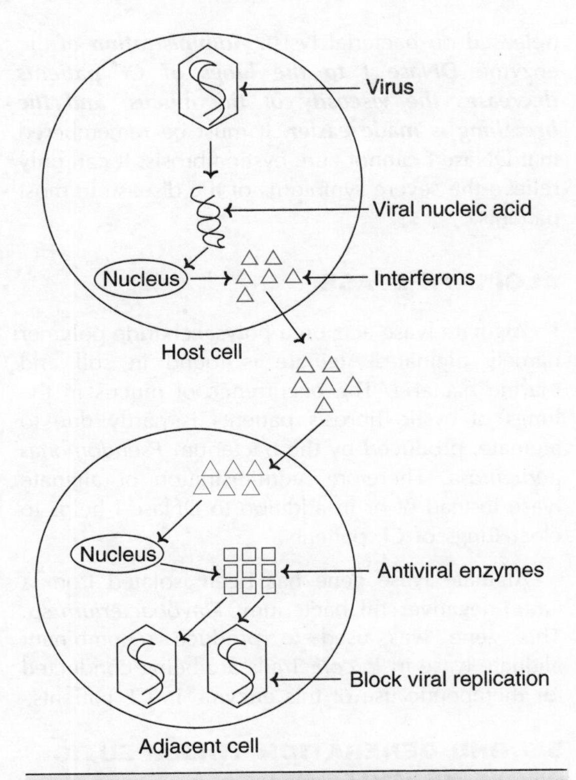

Fig. 15.6 : The mechanism of action of interferons.

Production of recombinant interferons

The complementary DNA (cDNA) was synthesized from the mRNA of a specific interferon. This is inserted to a vector (say plasmid) which is introduced into *E. coli* or other cells. The interferon can be isolated from the culture medium. This is the basic mechanism of producing recombinant interferons.

The production of interferons is relatively less in bacterial hosts, although *E. coli* was the first to be used. This is mainly because most interferons are glycoproteins in nature and bacteria do not possess the machinery for glycosylation of proteins.

Production interferons by yeasts : The yeast *Saccharomyces cerevisiae* is more suitable for the production of recombinant interferons. This is mainly because the yeast possess the mechanism to carry out glycosylation of proteins, similar to that occurs in mammalian cells. The DNA sequence coding for specific human interferon can be attached to the yeast alcohol dehydrogenase gene in a plasmid and introduced into 4 yeast cells. The yield of interferons is several fold higher compared to *E. coli.*

Production of hybrid interferons : Several attempts have been made to produce hybrid interferons. This is advantageous since ***different interferons with different antiviral activities can be combined to produce a more efficient interferon.*** Further, the glycosylation step can be bypassed, and bacteria can be used to produce hybrid interferons. The hybrid interferons are more reactive in performing their function.

The creation of hybrid genes from the genes of IFN-α_2 and IFN-α_3 is illustrated in ***Fig. 15.7***. These genes are digested by restriction endonucleases. The resulting fragments are ligated to generate hybrid genes. The appropriate hybrid genes can be selected and used for producing hybrid interferons. As already stated, *E. coli* can be employed for this purpose.

Therapeutic applications of interferons

Interferons-α, -β and -γ were respectively approved for therapeutic use in humans in the years 1986, 1993 and 1990. A Swiss biotechnology firm was the first to market ***interferon-α*** with a ***trade name Intron***. Interferons are used for the treatment of a large number of viral diseases and cancers. The cancers include leukemia, kaposis sarcoma, bladder cancer, head and neck cancer, renal cell carcinoma, skin cancer and multiple myeloma. The other diseases employing interferon therapy are AIDS, multiple sclerosis, genital warts, hepatitis C, herpes zoster etc.

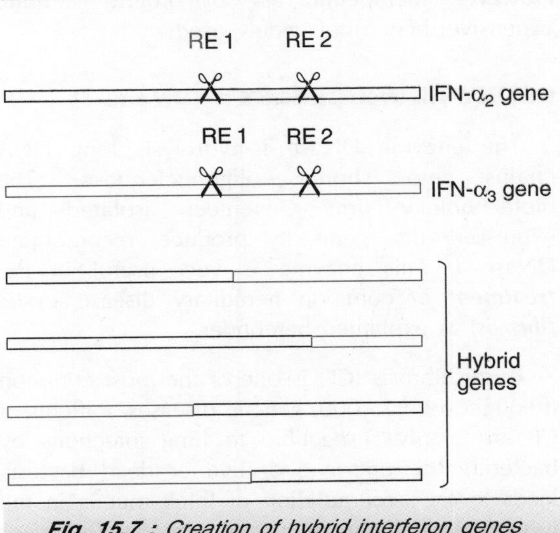

Fig. 15.7 : Creation of hybrid interferon genes (RE-Restriction endonuclease, IFN-Interferon).

Interferons are also employed in the treatment of common colds and influenza. For this purpose, interferons can be used as nasal sprays.

The basic mechanism of action of interferons against viruses has already been described. Interferons are found to cause the death of cancerous cells. This is brought out by stimulating the action of ***natural killer (NK) cells***, a specialised form of lymphocytes that can destroy cancerous cells.

Despite the widespread therapeutic applications of interferons, they are not within the reach of a large number of common people due to the cost factor (the cost of production being very high).

ERYTHROPOIETIN

Erythropoietin is a hormone synthesized by the kidneys. It stimulates the stem cells of bone marrow to produce mature erythrocytes. Biotechnologists were successful in producing recombinant erythropoietin. An approval for its therapeutic use in humans was obtained in the year 1989. Amgen Inc. first ***marked erythropoietin*** with a trade name ***Epogen***. It is useful in treating the patients with severe anemia that accompanies kidney disease. Another firm Ortho-Biotech company produced ***Procrit***, a genetically engineered erythropoietin in 1997. Procrit acts like the natural hormone and stimulates the production of erythrocytes. It is used in anemic patients undergoing non-cardiac, non-vascular surgery. Procrit administration before surgery serves as an alternative to blood transfusion. However, therapeutic use of procrit is quite expensive, hence not widely used.

DEOXYRIBONUCLEASE I (DNase I)

The enzyme DNase I hydrolysis long DNA chains into shorter oligonucleotides. The biotechnology firm Genentech isolated and expressed the gene to produce recombinant DNase I. This enzyme is very useful in the ***treatment of*** common hereditary disease ***cystic fibrosis***, as explained hereunder.

Cystic fibrosis (CF) is one of the most common (frequency 1 : 25,000) genetic diseases. Patients of CF are highly susceptible to lung infections by bacteria. The presence of live or dead bacteria leads to the accumulation of thick mucus in the lungs making the breathing very difficult. The major constituent of this mucus is the bacterial DNA (released on bacterial lysis). ***Administration of*** the enzyme ***DNase I to the lungs of CF patients decreases the viscosity of the mucus, and the breathing is made easier***. It must be remembered that DNase I cannot cure cystic fibrosis. It can only relieve the severe symptoms of the disease in most patients.

ALGINATE LYASE

Alginate lyase acts on a polysaccharide polymer namely alginate. Alginate is found in soil and marine bacteria. The occurrence of mucus in the lungs of cystic fibrosis patients is partly due to alginate, produced by the bacterium *Pseudomonas aeruginosa*. Therefore, administration of alginate lyase instead of or in addition to DNase I helps to clear lungs of CF patients.

Alginate lyase gene has been isolated from a Gram-negative soil bacterium, *Flavobacterium* sp. This gene was used to produce recombinant alginate lyase in *E. coli*. Trails are being conducted for therapeutic use of this enzyme in CF patients.

SECOND GENERATION THERAPEUTIC PROTEINS (MUTEINS)

By employing ***site-directed mutagenesis***, the amino acid sequence of a recombinant protein can be suitably modified as desired, by a technique referred to as ***protein engineering*** (For details Refer Chapter 10). The mutated proteins are collectively referred to as ***muteins***. Protein engineering is a rational approach to modify a protein with regard to its stability, solubility, specificity, substrate affinity, pharmacokinetics etc.

The muteins obtained by protein engineering technique are considered as ***Second generation of therapeutic proteins***. Selected examples of such proteins (e.g. ***insulin lispro***, ***Alteplase***) are already described (See p. 192 and p. 196).

VACCINES

Vaccines are another important group of pharmaceutical products of recombinant DNA technology. They are separately dealt with in Chapter 16. However, the reader must treat and learn vaccines also as a part of this chapter.

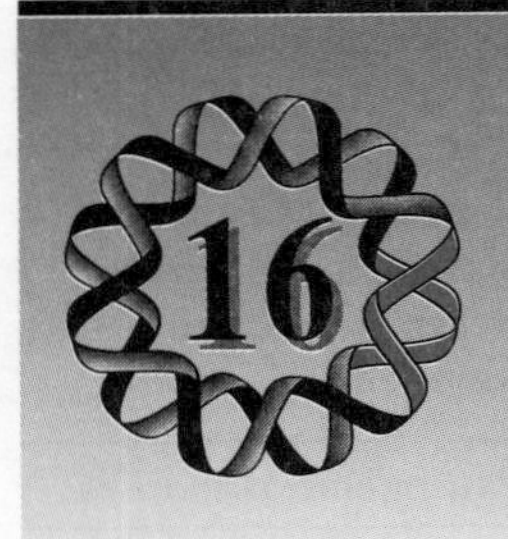

Recombinant Vaccines

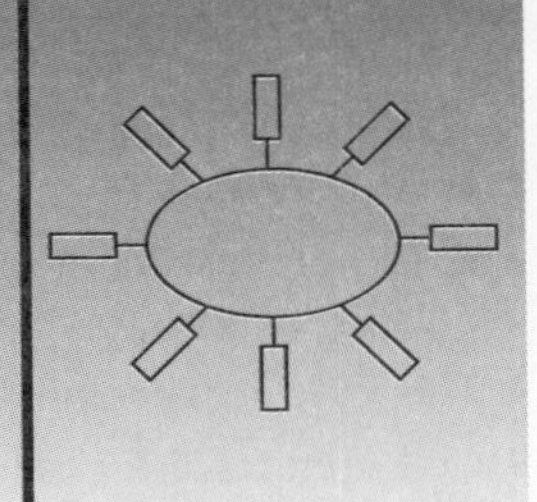

Vaccination is the phenomenon of preventive immunization. In the modern concept, vaccination involves the ***administration*** (injection or oral) ***of an antigen to elicit an antibody response that will protect the organism against future infections.***

Vaccines, although in a very crude form, were used in a peculiar manner by Chinese in as early as eleventh century. They used to remove the dried scabs of smallpox patients and ground them. The so prepared powder was sprayed in the noses of healthy people. It was observed that these people were less susceptible to smallpox when there was an outbreak of epidemic.

Smallpox is a virulent disease with a high death rate. Even the survivors become victims of permanent disfigurement, blindness and mental retardation. Edward Jenner, an English Physician, observed that the farmers and milkmaids working with cows developed a mild form of smallpox called cowpox or vaccinia. And the cowpox infection could protect these people from the infection of smallpox. It was in 1796, Jenner experimentally tested this observation. He inoculated an 8–year old boy with exudate from a cowpox lesion, and he repeated it twice with a gap of some weeks. He then inoculated more human volunteers. Jenner noted that smallpox did not develop in these volunteers. This was the first discovery of the principle of vaccination.

It took nearly hundred years for the scientists to clearly understand the basis of smallpox immunity. We now know that cowpox viruses (vaccinia) inoculated by Jenner, stimulate the body's immune system to produce antibodies which neutralise the cowpox as well as smallpox viruses. The present day vaccines which are more refined work in a similar fashion.

Vaccines are mainly of three types.

1. ***Dead bacteria or inactivated viruses.***
2. ***Live non-virulent or weakened (attenuated) bacteria/or viruses.***
3. ***Viral fragments or bacterial molecules (subunit vaccines).***

A vaccine triggers the body's immune system to produce antibodies against a specific disease—causing organism (virus, bacterium or other parasite). This provides surveillance against future exposure to such an organism and thus protects the body. Many communicable diseases (smallpox, cholera, typhoid, tuberculosis, poliomyelitis) have been brought under control through vaccination. However, as on today, for several diseases, there are no vaccines e.g., AIDS, leprosy, filariasis.

TRADITIONAL VACCINES

The disease producing organisms (infectious agents) are grown in culture. They are then purified and either killed (inactivated) or made non-virulent (attenuated). This has to be carefully done without the loss of the organism's ability to evoke immune response against a virulent form of disease-causing organism.

The traditional production of vaccines has several drawbacks.

- It is not possible to develop vaccines for the organisms not grown in culture.
- The yield of vaccines is very low.
- Cell cultures are costly to maintain.
- There is a danger of non-virulent organisms getting converted to virulent ones. Vaccinations by such organisms may cause the disease itself.
- It is not possible to prevent all the diseases by use of traditional vaccines e.g., AIDS.

Purified antigen vaccines

Some improvements in traditional vaccines have been made by isolating the antigens from the pathogenic organisms. The antigens of bacterial cell walls (e.g., *Streptococcus pneumoniae* causing pneumonia), and the endotoxins are good examples of purified vaccines. The endotoxins that do not possess toxicity but retain immunogenecity are referred to as ***toxoids*** e.g. toxods of tetanus, diphtheria etc.

RECOMBINANT VACCINES—GENERAL

Recombinant DNA technology in recent years, has become a boon to produce ***new generation vaccines***. By this approach, some of the limitations (listed above) of traditional vaccine production could be overcome. In addition, several new strategies, involving gene manipulation are being tried to create novel recombinant vaccines.

The list of diseases for which recombinant vaccines are developed or being developed is given in ***Table 16.1***. It may be stated here that due to very stringent regulatory requirements to use in humans, the new generation vaccines are first tried in animals, and it may ***take some more years before most of them are approved for use in humans***.

Types of recombinant vaccines

The recombinant vaccines may be broadly categorized into three groups :

1. **Subunit recombinant vaccines :** These are the components of the pathogenic organisms. Subunit vaccines include proteins, peptides and DNA.

2. **Attenuated recombinant vaccines :** These are the genetically modified pathogenic organisms (bacteria or viruses) that are made non-pathogenic and used as vaccines.

TABLE 16.1 A selected list of diseases along with the pathogenic organisms for which recombinant vaccines are developed or being developed

Disease	*Pathogenic organism*
Viral diseases	
Accute infantile gastroenteritis	Rotavirus
Acute respiratory diseases	Influenza A and B viruses
AIDS	Human immunodeficiency virus
Chicken pox	Viricella–zoster virus
Encephalitis	Japanese encephalitis virus
Genital ulcers	Herpes simplex virus type–2
Hemorrhagic fever	Dengue virus
Liver damage	Hepatitis A virus
Liver damage	Hepatitis B virus
Upper and lower respiratory tract lesions	Yellow fever virus
Bacterial diseases	
Cholera	*Vibrio cholerae*
Diarrhea	*E. coli*
Dysentery	*Shigella* strain
Gonorrhea	*Neissria gonorroheae*
Leprosy	*Mycobacterium leprae*
Meningitis	*Neisseria meningitidis*
Pneumonia	*Streptococcus pneumoniae*
Rheumatic fever	*Streptococcus* group A
Tetanus	*Clostridium tetani*
Tuberculosis	*Mycobacterium tuberculosis*
Typhoid	*Salmonella typhi*
Urogenital tract infection	*Streptococcus* group B
Parasitic diseases	
Filariasis	*Wuchereria bancrofti*
Malaria	*Plasmodium* sp
River blindness	*Onchocerca volvulus*
Schistosomiasis	*Schistosoma mansoni*
Sleeping sickness	*Trypanosoma* sp

3. **Vector recombinant vaccines :** These are the genetically modified viral vectors that can be used as vaccines against certain pathogens.

Some of the developments made in the production of recombinant vaccines against certain diseases are briefly described.

SUBUNIT VACCINES

As already stated, subunit recombinant vaccines are the ***components (proteins, peptides, DNAs) of the pathogenic organisms***. The advantages of these vaccines include their purity in preparation, stability and safe use. The disadvantages are— high cost factor and possible alteration in native conformation. Scientists carefully evaluate the pros and cons of subunit vaccines for each disease, and proceed on the considered merits.

HEPATITIS B

Hepatitis B is a widespread disease in man. It primarily affects liver causing ***chronic hepatitis, cirrhosis and liver cancer***. Hepatitis B virus is a 42 nm particle, called ***Dane particle***. It consists of a core containing a viral genome (DNA) surrounded by a phospholipid envelope carrying surface antigens (***Fig. 16.1A***). Infection with hepatitis B virus produced Dane particles and 22 nm sized particles. The latter contain surface antigens which are more immunogenic. It is however, very difficult to grow hepatitis B virus in mammalian cell culture and produce surface antigens.

The gene encoding for ***hepatitis B surface antigen (HBsAg)*** has been identified. ***Recombinant hepatitis B vaccine as a subunit vaccine, is produced by cloning HbsAg gene in yeast cells.*** *Saccharomyces cerevisiae*, a harmless baking and brewing yeast, is used for this purpose (***Fig. 16.1B***). The gene for HBsAg is inserted (pMA 56) which is linked to the alcohol dehydrogenase promoter. These plasmids are then transferred and cultured. The cells grown in tryptophan, free medium are selected and cloned. The yeast cells are cultured. The HBsAg gene is expressed to produce 2nm sized particles similar to those found in patients infected with hepatitis B. (These particles are immunoreactive with anti-HBsAg antibodies). The subunit HBsAg as 22 nm particles can be isolated and used to immunize individuals against hepatitis B.

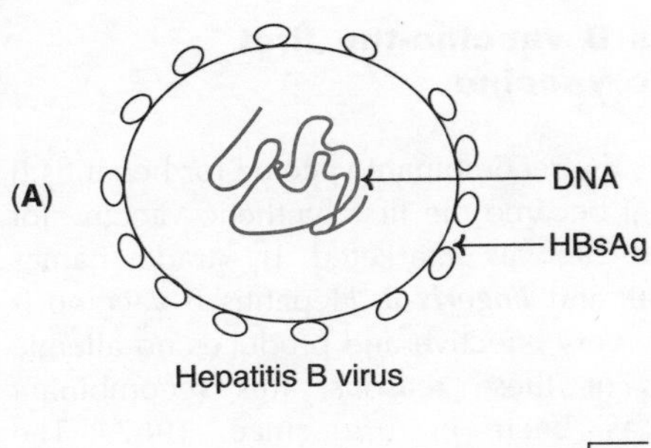

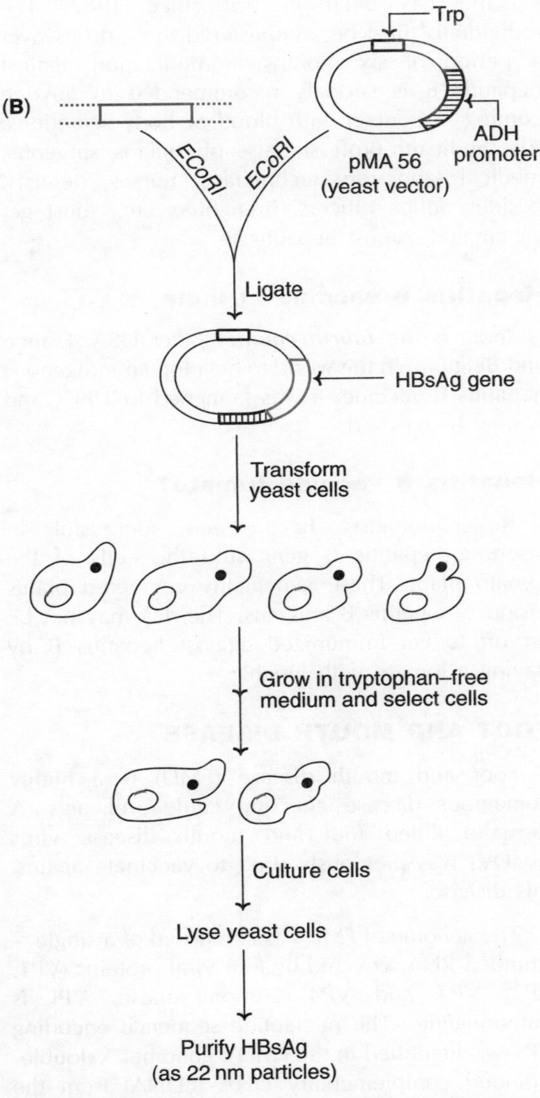

*Fig. 16.1 : **(A)** Hepatitis B virus–Dane particle (42 nm particle); **(B)** Production of hepatitis B surface antigen (HBsAg) in yeast cells (Trp–Tryptophan, ADH–Alcohol dehydrogenase).*

Hepatitis B vaccine-the first synthetic vaccine

In 1987, the recombinant vaccine for hepatitis B (i.e. HBsAg) became the first synthetic vaccine for public use. It was marketed by trade names ***Recombivax*** and ***Engerix-B***. Hepatitis B vaccine is safe to use, very effective and produces no allergic reactions. For these reasons, this recombinant vaccine has been in use since 1987. The individuals must be administered three doses over a period of six months. Immunization against hepatitis B is strongly recommended to anyone coming in contact with blood or body secretions. All the health professionals—physicians, surgeons, medical laboratory technicians, nurses, dentists, besides police officers, firefighters etc., must get vaccinated against hepatitis B.

Hepatitis B vaccine in India

India is the ***fourth country*** (after USA, France and Belgium) in the world to develop an indigenous hepatitis B vaccine. It was launched in 1997, and is now being used.

Hepatitis B vaccine tomato?

Biotechnologists have been successful in inserting hepatitis B gene into the cells of the tomato plant. These genetically engineered plants produce hepatitis B antigens. The day may not be far off to get immunized against hepatitis B by having a tomato with lunch!

FOOT AND MOUTH DISEASE

Foot and mouth disease (FMD) is a highly contagious disease affecting cattle and pigs. A formalin killed foot and mouth disease virus (FMDV) was previously used to vaccinate against this disease.

The genome of FMDV is composed of a single—stranded RNA, covered by four viral proteins (VP1, VP2, VP3 and VP4). Among these, VPI is immunogenic. The nucleotide sequence encoding VPI was identified in the FMDV genome. A double-stranded complementary DNA (cDNA) from the single-stranded viral RNA (genome) was synthesized. This cDNA was then digested with restriction enzymes and the fragments were cloned by using plasmid pBR322 in *E. coli*. The recombinant vaccine for FMDV in the form of viral protein 1 was used to vaccinate animals. However, VPI vaccination was found to be less effective than that of the whole virus in protecting FMD. Further, studies are being pursued to improve the efficiency of subunit vaccine.

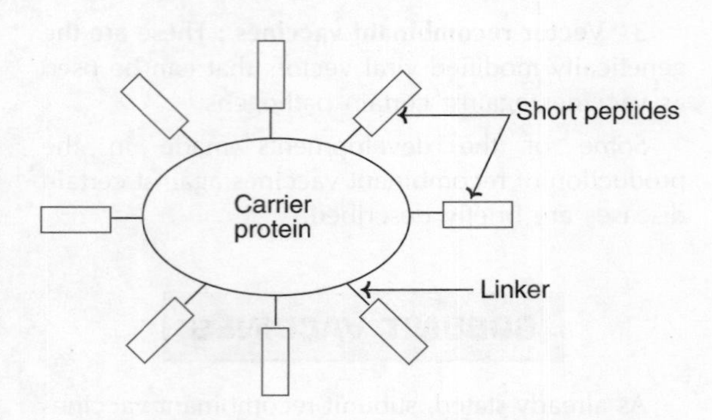

Fig. 16.2 : A general structure of a synthetic peptide vaccine.

The concept of peptide vaccines

Theoretically, it is expected that only ***small portions of a*** given ***protein*** (i.e., domains) are ***immunogenic*** and bind to antibodies. Logically, it is possible to use short peptides that are immunogenic as vaccines. These are referred to as peptide vaccines.

Peptide vaccines for foot and mouth disease

Some details on the FMD are described above. The domains of viral protein I (VPI) of FMDV were chemically synthesized. From the C-terminal end of VPI, amino acids 141 to 160, 151 to 160 and 200 to 213, and from N-terminal end, amino acids 9 to 24, 17 to 32 and 25 to 41 were synthesized. Each one of these ***short peptides*** (***domains***) was ***bound to the surface of a carrier protein*** (***Fig. 16.2***) and ***used as a vaccine***. Among the peptides used, the one corresponding to amino acids 141 to 160 was found to be effective in immunizing guinea pigs against FMD. In addition, when two peptides were joined together (amino acids 141 to 158, and amino acids 200 to 213), they served as more efficient recombinant vaccines.

The success so far to use recombinant peptides as vaccines has been very limited. This is mainly because a short peptide usually is not enough to be

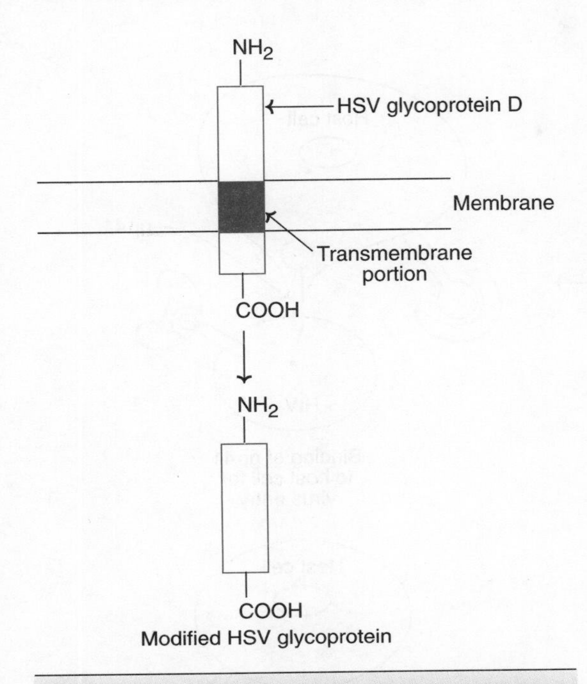

Fig. 16.3 : Modification of HSV glycoprotein D by deleting transmembrane portion. (HSV–Herpes simplex virus)

sufficienty immunogenic, since it may not have the same conformation as that of the original viral particle. However, scientists continue their search for specific, inexpensive and safe synthetic peptide vaccines for various diseases.

HERPES SIMPLEX VIRUS

Herpes simplex virus (HSV) is an oncogenic (cancer-causing) virus. In addition, it also causes sexually transmitted diseases, encephalitis and severe eye infections. Attempts have been made to produce subunit vaccines against HSV.

An envelope glycoprotein D (gD) of HSV that can elicit antibody production has been identified. This is a membrane bound protein, and difficult to isolate and purify. The ***glycoprotein D was modified by deleting the transmembrane portion of the protein*** (***Fig. 16.3***) and the gene was modified. This gene for gD was cloned in a mammalian vector and expressed in Chinese hamster ovary (CHO). The advantage here is that the protein can get glycosylated (unlike in *E. coli* system). In the experimental trials, the modified form of gD was found to be effective against HSV.

TUBERCULOSIS

Tuberculosis is caused by the bacterium *Mycobacterium tuberculosis*. It is often fatal, and as per some estimates nearly 3 million deaths occur every year due to this highly infectious disease. Antibiotics are used to treat tuberculosis. However, drug-resistant *M. tuberculosis* strains have been developed making the drug therapy some times ineffective. Vaccination for tuberculosis is therefore, advocated.

Bacillus Calmette-Guerin (BCG) vaccine

In some countries, particularly the developing ones, BCG vaccine is widely used to protect against tuberculosis. However, countries like United States have not approved BCG vaccination for various reasons. BCG vaccine itself causes tuberculosis in some individuals (AIDS victims) and the vaccinated people respond positively for laboratory diagnosis of tuberculosis.

Subunit vaccines

The secretory (extracellular proteins of *M. tuberculosis* have been purified and used for immunoprotection against tuberculosis. Of about 100 such proteins, six were found to be useful (either individually or in combination) to immunize guinea pigs.

Attempts are underway to develop recombinant subunit vaccine against tuberculosis.

MENINGITIS

Group B strain of meningococci, namely *Neisseria meningitidis* causes meningitis in adolescents and young adults. Meningitis is characterized by inflammation of the membranes covering brain and spinal cord. The symptoms include headache, photophobia, irritability, and neck stiffness.

Pizza *et al* (2000) made a novel approach to develop a vaccine against meningitis. They identified 350 proteins (potential protective antigens) and the entire sequence of genome coding for these proteins in *N. meningitidis.* All the 350 candidate antigens were expressed in *E. coli*, purified and used to immunize mice. A good bactericidal antibody response was observed in these mice.

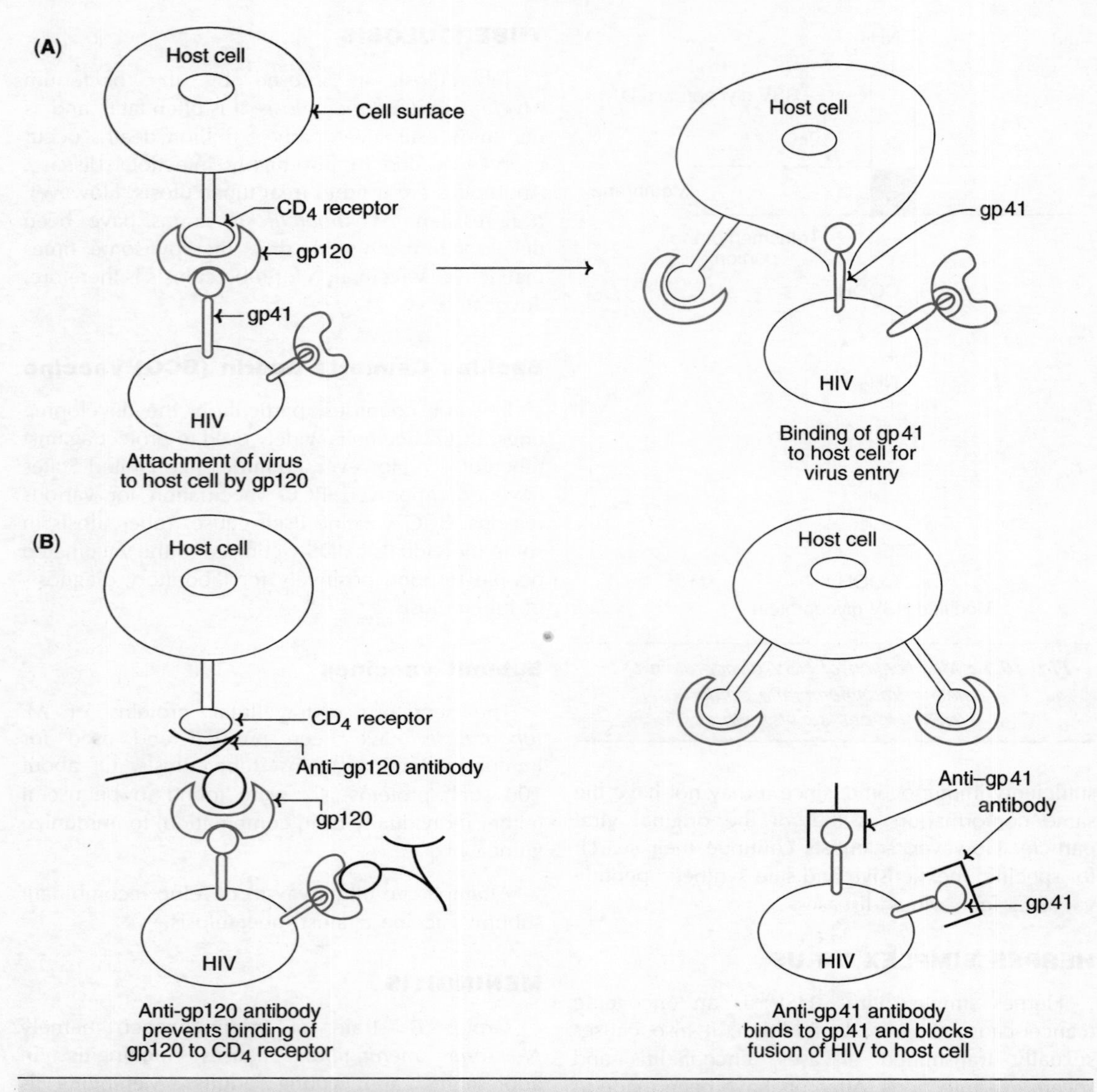

Fig. 16.4 : Subunit recombinant vaccines against AIDS. ***(A)*** *The functions of gp120 and gp41 of HIV;* ***(B)*** *The action of anti–gp120 and anti–gp41 antibodies to prevent the entry of HIV into host cell.*

AIDS (ACQUIRED IMMUNODEFICIENCY SYNDROME)

AIDS is a retroviral disease caused by ***human immunodeficiency virus (HIV)***. This disease is characterized by immunosuppression, neoplasma and neurological manifestations. AIDS is invariably fatal, since as of now there is no cure. Development of a vaccine against AIDS is a top priority by DNA technologists worldover. In fact, vaccines are being continuously developed and field tested, although there has been no success so far.

Subunit vaccines

The development of two subunit vaccines, specifically the glycoproteins of HIV envelope is described here. The functions of gp120 and gp41 of HIV are illustrated in ***Fig. 16.4A***. The glycoprotein gp120 projects out of the HIV envelope while the other glycoprotein gp41 lies beneath gp120. On entering the body, the HIV binds to the host cells (T-lymphocytes) by attaching gp120 to the CD_4 receptor sites on the cell surface. This attachment uncovers gp41 molecules and the viral envelope. Now gp41 binds to the host cell surface and opens a passage for the entry of the virus into the cell.

Biotechnologists have isolated the genes for gp120 and gp41 and inserted them into the bacterium *E. coli*. These bacterial cells produce gp120 and gp41 that can be used as recombinant vaccines against AIDS. The action of gp120 and gp41 in immunizing host T-lymphocytes is depicted in ***Fig. 16.4B***. The gp120 molecules stimulate the host immune system to produce anti- gp120 antibodies. These antibodies bind to gp120 and prevent its attachment to CD_4. In a comparable manner, gp41 molecules also result in the production of anti-gp41 antibodies. These antibodies also bind to gp41 and block the virus-host cell union. The net result of ***using gp120 and gp41 vaccines is that the entry of HIV into the host cells is prevented***.

Vaccine against AIDS— not yet a reality

The description of vaccine development against AIDS (given above), which appears attractive is not so simple. The most important limitations are that the ***HIV has high frequency of mutations***. Therefore the ***vaccines developed cannot bind to the new virus*** (i.e., mutated one). In addition, gp120 and gp41 are very poor stimulators of immune system. Despite these limitations, scientists have not lost hope, and continue their research to develop vaccines against AIDS.

DNA VACCINES (GENETIC IMMUNIZATION)

Genetic immunization by using DNA vaccines is a novel approach that came into being in 1990. The ***immune response of the body is stimulated by a DNA molecule***. A DNA vaccine consists of a gene encoding an antigenic protein, inserted onto a plasmid, and then incorported into the cells in a target animal. The plasmid carrying DNA vaccine normally contains a promoter site, cloning site for the DNA vaccine gene, origin of replication, a selectable marker sequence (e.g. a gene for ampicillin resistance) and a terminator sequence (a poly—A tail).

DNA vaccine—plasmids can be administered to the animals by one of the following delivery methods.

- Nasal spray
- Intramuscular injection
- Intravenous injection
- Intradermal injection
- Gene gun or biolistic delivery (involves pressure delivery of DNA-coated gold beads).

DNA VACCINE AND IMMUNITY

An illustration of a DNA vaccine and the mechanism of its action in developing immunity is given in ***Fig. 16.5***. The plasmid vaccine carrying the DNA (gene) for antigenic protein enters the nucleus of the inoculated target cell of the host. This DNA produces RNA, and in turn the specific antigenic protein. The antigen can act directly for developing humoral immunity or as fragments in association with major histocompatability class (MHC) molecules for developing cellular immunity.

Humoral immunity

As the antigen molecules bind to B-lymphocytes, they trigger the production of antibodies which can destroy the pathogens. Some of the B-lymphocytes become memory cells that can protect the host against future infections.

Cellular immunity

The protein fragments of the antigen bound to MHC molecules can activate the cytotoxic T-lymphocytes. They are capable of destroying the infected pathogenic cells. Some of the activated T-lymphocytes become memory cells which can kill the future infecting pathogens.

Complementary DNA vaccines

For genetic immunization, complementary DNA (cDNA) vaccines can also be used. Some workers have successfully used cDNA as vaccines e.g. immunization of mice against influenza.

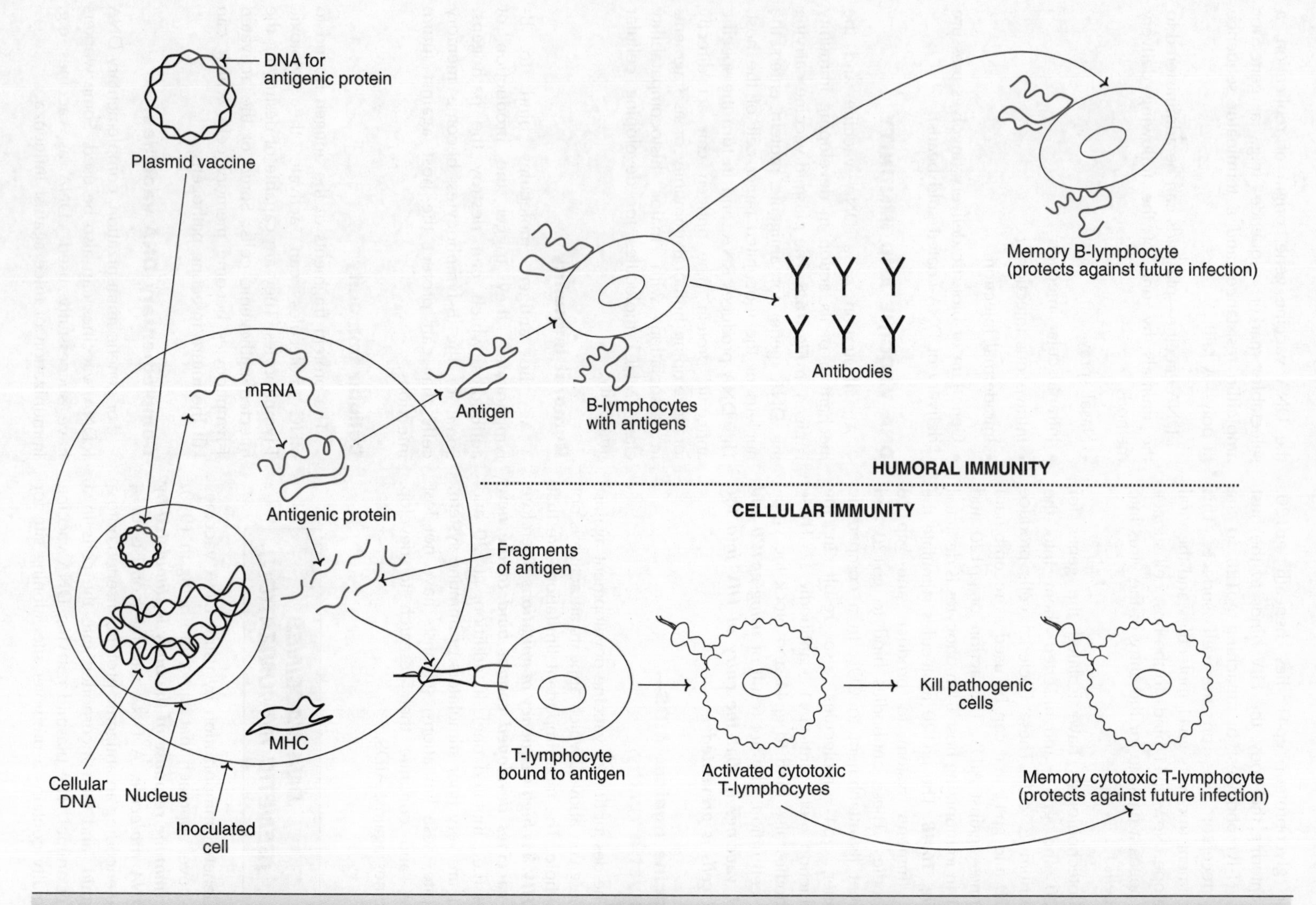

Fig. 16.5 : DNA vaccine and mechanism of its action in developing immunity (MHC–Major histocompatability complex molecule)

DNA vaccines for production of antigens and antibodies

A novel approach for the production of antigens as well as antibodies by DNA vaccine was developed in 1997. In the experiments conducted in mice, researchers ***injected plasmids containing the genes for malarial parasite and also the genes for the antibodies against malarial parasite***. The B-lymphocytes of these mice performed a double duty, and produced antigens for, and antibodies against malarial parasite. The antigens stimulate to produce more and more antibodies. The antibodies so produced react with malarial parasite. The generation of antigens and antibodies by using a DNA vaccine is a recent development in immunology, and is referred to as ***antigenic antibody approach of DNA vaccine***.

Screening of pathogenic genome for selecting DNA vaccines

The ultimate goal of scientists is to choose the right DNA fragment from the pathogen to serve as a vaccine for the strongest immune response against the invading pathogen. For this purpose, the ***pathogen's DNA can be broken into fragments and a large number of vaccine DNA—plasmids can be prepared***. The immune response for each one of the DNA vaccines can be studied by injecting the pathogen. By screening the DNA fragments of the pathogenic genome, it is possible to choose one or few DNA vaccines that can offer maximal immune protection.

Advantages of DNA vaccines

There are several advantages of using DNA vaccines in immunization.

1. The tedious and costly procedures of purifying antigens or creating recombinant vaccines are not necessary.

2. DNA vaccines are very specific in producing the target proteins (antigens or antibodies). Thus, they trigger immune response only against the specific pathogen.

3. In general, DNA vaccines elicit much higher immune response compared to other kinds of vaccines.

4. DNA vaccines are more stable for temperature variations (low or high) than the conventional vaccines. Thus, the storage and transport problems associated with vaccines are minimal.

5. The delivery methods to the host are simpler for DNA vaccines.

Disadvantages of DNA vaccines

1. The fate of the DNA vaccine in the host cells is not yet clear. There is a possibility of this DNA getting integrated into the host genome and this may interrupt the normal functions.

2. There also exists a danger of cancer due to DNA vaccines.

3. The post-translational modification of the gene (DNA vaccine) product in host cells may not be the same as that found in the native antigen.

Present status of DNA vaccines

Since 1990, several groups of workers world-over have been trying to develop DNA vaccines against various diseases in experimental animals. Genetic immunization has been done against a number of pathogenic organisms. These include influenza A virus, rabies virus, hepatitis B virus, bovine herpes virus, HIV type I, and *Plasmodium* species (malarial parasite).

It must be noted that ***DNA vaccines have not been tried in humans for*** obvious reasons. The most important being the ***unknown risks*** of these foreign DNAs in human subjects.

RNA VACCINES

Several workers are trying to use RNA molecules as vaccines. These RNAs can readily synthesize the antigenic proteins and offer immunity. But unfortunately, ***RNAs are less stable than DNAs***. This poses a big problem for RNA vaccine manufacture and distribution. Therefore, the ***progress*** in the development of RNA vaccines has been ***rather slow*** compared to DNA vaccines.

PLANTS AS EDIBLE SUBUNIT VACCINES

Plants serve as a cheap and safe production systems for subunit vaccines. The edible vaccines can be easily ingested by eating plants. This eliminates the processing and purification procedures that are otherwise needed. ***Transgenic plants*** (tomato, potato) have been ***developed for***

TABLE 16.2 A selected list of plant edible subunit vaccines

Antigen	*Host plant*
Rabies glycoprotein	Tomato
Foot and mouth virus (VPI)	*Arabidopsis*
Herpes virus B surface antigen	Tobacco
Cholera toxin B subunit	Potato
Human cytomegalovirus glycoprotein B	Tobacco

expressing antigens derived from animal viruses (rabies virus, herpes virus). A selected list of recombinant vaccines against animal viruses produced in plants is given in ***Table 16.2***.

Edible vaccine production and use

The production of vaccine potatoes is illustrated in ***Fig. 16.6***. The bacterium, *Agrobacterium tumefaciens* is commonly used to deliver the DNA (genetic material) for bacterial or viral antigens. A plasmid carrying the antigen gene and an antibiotic resistance gene are incorporated into the bacterial cells (*A. tumefaciens*). The cut pieces of potato leaves are exposed to an antibiotic which can kill the cells that lack the new genes. The surviving cells (i.e., gene altered ones) can multiply and form a callus (clump of cells). This callus is allowed to sprout shoots and roots, which are grown in soil to form plants. In about three weeks, the plants bear potatoes with antigen vaccines.

The ***first clinical trials*** in humans, using a plant-derived vaccine were conducted in 1997. This involved the ingestion ***of transgenic potatoes with a toxin of E. coli causing diarrhea***. Some success was reported. For some more details on edible vaccines, the reader must refer Chapter 51.

ATTENUATED RECOMBINANT VACCINES

In the early years of vaccine research, attenuated strains of some pathogenic organisms were prepared by prolonged cultivation — weeks, months or even years. Although the reasons are not known, the infectious organism would lose its ability to cause disease but retains its capability to act as an immunizing agent. This type of approach is almost outdated now.

It is now possible to ***genetically engineer the organisms*** (***bacteria or viruses***) ***and use them as live vaccines***, and such vaccines are referred to as attenuated recombinant vaccines. The genetic manipulations for the production of these vaccines are broadly of two types

1. Deletion or modification of virulence genes of pathogenic organisms.

2. Genetic manipulation of non-pathogenic organisms to carry and express antigen determinants from pathogenic organisms.

The advantage with attenuated vaccines is that the native conformation of the immunogenic determinants is preserved, hence the immune response is substantially high. This is in contrast to purified antigens which often elicit poor immunological response.

Some of the important attenuated vaccines developed by genetic manipulations are briefly described.

CHOLERA

Cholera is an intestinal disease characterized by diarrhea, dehydration, abdominal pain and fever. It is caused by the bacterium, *Vibrio cholerae*. This pathogenic organism is transmitted by drinking water contaminated with fecal matter. Cholera epidemics are frequently seen in developing countries where the water purification and sewage disposal systems are not well developed.

On entering the small intestine, *V. cholerae* colonizes and starts producing large amounts of a ***toxic protein***, a ***hexameric enterotoxin***. This enterotoxin stimulates the cells lining intestinal walls to release sodium, bicarbonate and other ions. Water accompanies these ions leading to severe diarrhea, dehydration, and even death.

The currently used cholera vaccine is composed of phenol-killed *V. cholerae*. The immuno-protection, lasting for 3–6 months is just moderate. Attempts are being made to develop better vaccines.

The DNA technologists have identified the gene encoding enterotoxin (toxic protein). Enterotoxin, an hexamer, consists of one A subunit and five identical B subunits. The A subunit has two functional domains-the A_1 peptide which possesses

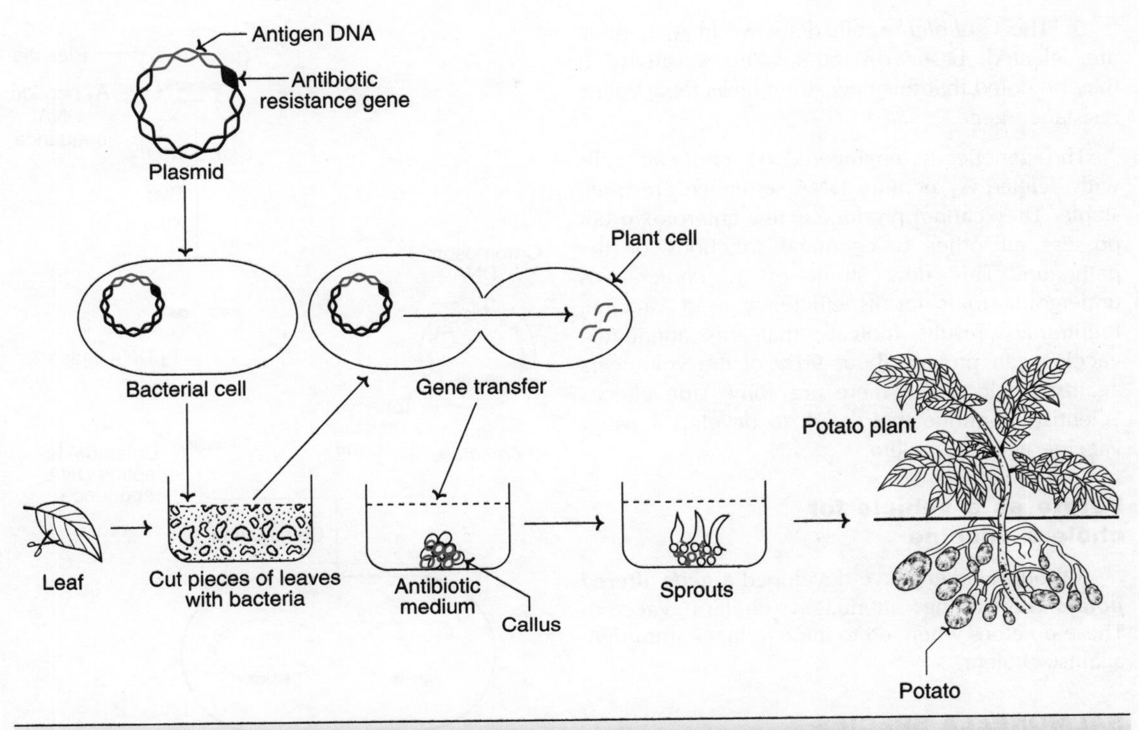

Fig. 16.6 : An illustration for edible vaccine production.

the toxic activity and A_2 peptide that joins A subunit to B subunits. By genetic engineering, it was possible to delete the DNA sequence encoding A_1 peptide and create a new strain of *V. cholerae*. This strain is non-pathogenic, since it cannot produce enterotoxin. The ***genetically engineered V. cholerae is a good candidate to serve as an attenuated vaccine***.

Creating a new strain of *V. cholerae*

The development of a new strain of *Vibrio cholerae* that can effectively serve as an attenuated recombinant vaccine is depicted in ***Fig. 16.7***, and briefly described below.

1. A tetracycline resistance gene was inserted into the A_1 peptide sequence of *V. cholerae* chromosome. This destroys the DNA sequence encoding for A_1 peptide, besides making the strain resistant to tetracycline. Unfortunately, the tetracycline resistant gene is easily lost and the enterotoxin activity is restored. Because of this, the new strain of *V. cholerae* as such cannot be used as a vaccine.

2. The DNA sequence of A_1 peptide is incorporated into a plasmid, cloned and digested with restriction enzymes (*ClaI and XbaI*). In this manner, the A_1 peptide coding sequence is deleted (the DNA encoding for 183 of the 194 amino acids of the A_1 peptide is actually removed). By using T_4 DNA ligase, the plasmid is recircularized. This plasmid contains a small portion of A_1 peptide coding sequence.

3. The plasmid, containing the deleted A_1 peptide sequence is transferred by conjugation into the *V. cholerae* strain carrying a tetracycline resistance gene.

4. Recombination can occur between the plasmid (containing a small portion of peptide A_1 coding sequence) and the chromosome of *V. cholerae* (carrying tetracycline resistance gene). The result of this double crossover is the formation of ***V. cholerae containing a chromosomal DNA lacking A_1 peptide DNA sequence***. As the bacterium, *V. cholerae* multiplies, the plasmids are lost in the next few generations.

5. The *V. cholerae* cells defective in A_1 peptide are selected, based on tetracycline sensitivity. It may be noted that this new strain lacks tetracycline resistance gene.

The genetically engineered *V. cholerae* cells with deleted A_1 peptide DNA sequence are quite stable. They cannot produce active enterotoxin but possess all other biochemical functions of the pathogen. This new strain of *V. cholerae* is undergoing trials for its efficiency as a vaccine. Preliminary results indicate that this attenuated vaccine can protect about 90% of the volunteers against cholera. But there are some side effects. Scientists continue their work to develop a better vaccine against cholera.

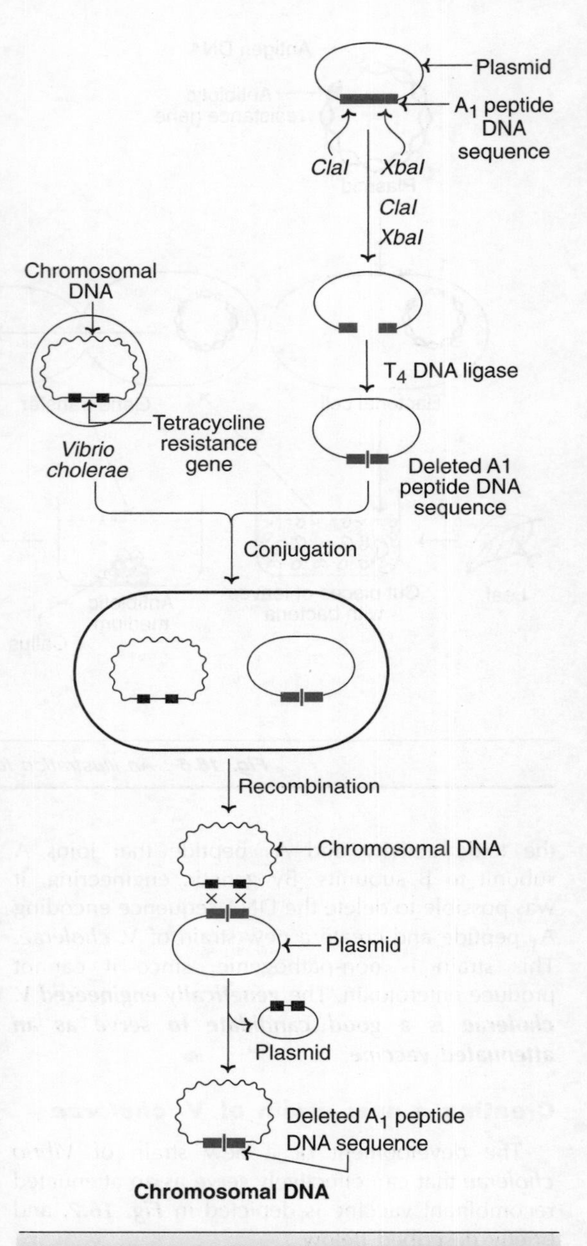

Fig. 16.7 : Development of a new strain of V. cholerae *as an attenuated recombinant vaccine (*ClaI *and* XbaI *are restriction endonucleases).*

Potato as a vehicle for cholera vaccine

A group workers have developed a ***gene altered potato*** containing attenuated cholera vaccine. These potatoes when fed to mice induced immunity against cholera.

SALMONELLA SPECIES

The different strains of Salmonella genus are responsible for causing ***typhoid***, ***enteric fever, food poisoning and infant death***. Immunoprotection against *Salmonella* pathogens is really required.

Some workers have been successful in deleting ***aro genes*** and ***pur genes*** in *Salmonella. Aro* genes encode for the enzymes responsible for the biosynthesis of aromatic compounds, while *pur* genes encode for enzymes of purine metabolism. The new strains of *Salmonella* can be grown *in vitro* on a complete medium. The ***doubly deleted strains*** have a very restricted growth *in vivo*, while they ***can stimulate immunological response***. The genetically engineered attenuated vaccines of *Salmonella* have been shown to be effective as oral vaccines in experimental animals (mice, cattle, sheep, chickens). Some workers claim that the new strain of *Salmonella* offers immunoprotection in humans also.

LEISHMANIA SPECIES

Leishmania species are flagellated protozoan parasites and are responsible for the disease ***leishmaniasis***. This disease is characterized by ***cutaneous***, ***visceral*** and ***mucosal leisons***. Leishmaniasis is transmitted by sand flies.

An ***attenuated strain of leishmania*** has been created and successfully ***used in mice to offer immunoprotection*** against leishmaniasis. In *Leishmania major*, the genes encoding dihydrofolate reductase-thymidylate synthase can be replaced by the genes encoding resistance to antibiotics G–418 and hygromycin. This new strain of *L. major* invariably requires thymidine in the medium for its growth and multiplication. The attenuated strain of *L. major* can survive only a few days when administered to mice. This short period is enough to induce immunity in mice against the lesions of leishmania. However, more experiments on animals have to be carried out before the leishmania attenuated vaccine goes for human trials.

VECTOR RECOMBINANT VACCINES

Some of vectors can be genetically modified and employed as vaccines against pathogens.

VACCINES AGAINST VIRUSES—VACCINIA VIRUS

Vaccinia viruse is basically the vaccine that was originally used by Jenner for the eradication of ***smallpox***. The molecular biology of this virus has been clearly worked out. Vaccinia virus contains a double-stranded DNA (187 kb) that encodes about 200 different proteins. The genome of this virus can accommodate stretches of foreign DNA which can be expressed along with the viral genes.

The vaccinia virus can replicate in the host cell cytoplasm (of the infected cells) rather than the nucleus. This is possible since the vaccinia virus possesses the machinery for DNA replication, transcription-DNA polymerase, RNA polymerase etc. The foreign genes inserted into the vaccinia virus can also be expressed along with the viral genome. Thus, the foreign DNA is under the control of the virus, and is expressed independently from the host cell genome.

The vaccinia viruses are generally harmless, relatively easy to cultivate and stable for years after lyophilization (freeze-drying). All these features make the vaccinia viruses strong candidates for vector vaccine. The cloned foreign genes (from a pathogenic organism) can be inserted into vaccinia virus genome for encoding antigens which in turn produces antibodies against the specific disease-causing agent. The advantage with ***vector vaccine*** is that it ***stimulates B-lymphocytes*** (to produce antibodies) ***and T-lymphocytes*** (to kill virus infected cells). This is in contrast to a subunit vaccine which can stimulate only B-lymphocytes. Thus, vaccinia virus can provide a high level of immunoprotection against pathogenic organisms. Another advantage of vaccinia virus is the ***possibility of vaccinating individuals against different diseases simultaneously***. This can be done by a recombinant vaccinia viruses which carries genes encoding different antigens.

Antigen genes for certain diseases have been successfully incorporated into vaccinia virus genome and expressed. Thus, vector vaccines have been developed against hepatitis, influenza, herpes simplex virus, rabies, angular stomatitis virus and malaria. However, none of ***these vaccines has been licensed for human use due to fear of safety***. It is argued that recombinant vaccinia virus might create life threatening complications in humans.

Production of recombinant vaccinia viruses

The development of recombinant vaccinia virus is carried out by a two-step procedure (***Fig. 16.8***).

1. **Assembly of plasmid insertion vector :** Fresh vaccinia (cow pox) viruses are processed to release their DNAs. Now genes from hepatitis B virus, herpes simplex virus and influenza virus are added one after another and inserted into vaccinia virus genome. These DNA clusters are cloned in *E. coli* for increasing their number and to produce plasmid insertion vectors. The plasmid contains the foreign subunit genes, the natural vaccinia genes, including the promoter genes. The recombinant plasmids are isolated and purified and serve as plasmid insertion vectors.

2. **Production of recombinant vaccinia viruses :** The animal cells are infected with plasmid insertion vectors and normal vaccinia viruses. As the viral replication occurs, the plasmids are taken up to produce recombinant vaccinia viruses. The plasmid insertion vector incorporates its genes into vaccinia virus genome at a place that encodes for the enzyme thymidine kinase (TK). Thus the recombinant viruses have lost their ability to produce TK. There are two advantages of loss of TK gene. One is that it is easy to select recombined vaccinia viruses that lack TK gene and the second is that these viruses are less infectious than the normal viruses.

The recombinant vaccinia viruses, released from the cultured animal cells, can be successfully used as vaccines. These live viral vaccines have some advantages over the killed or subunit vaccines.

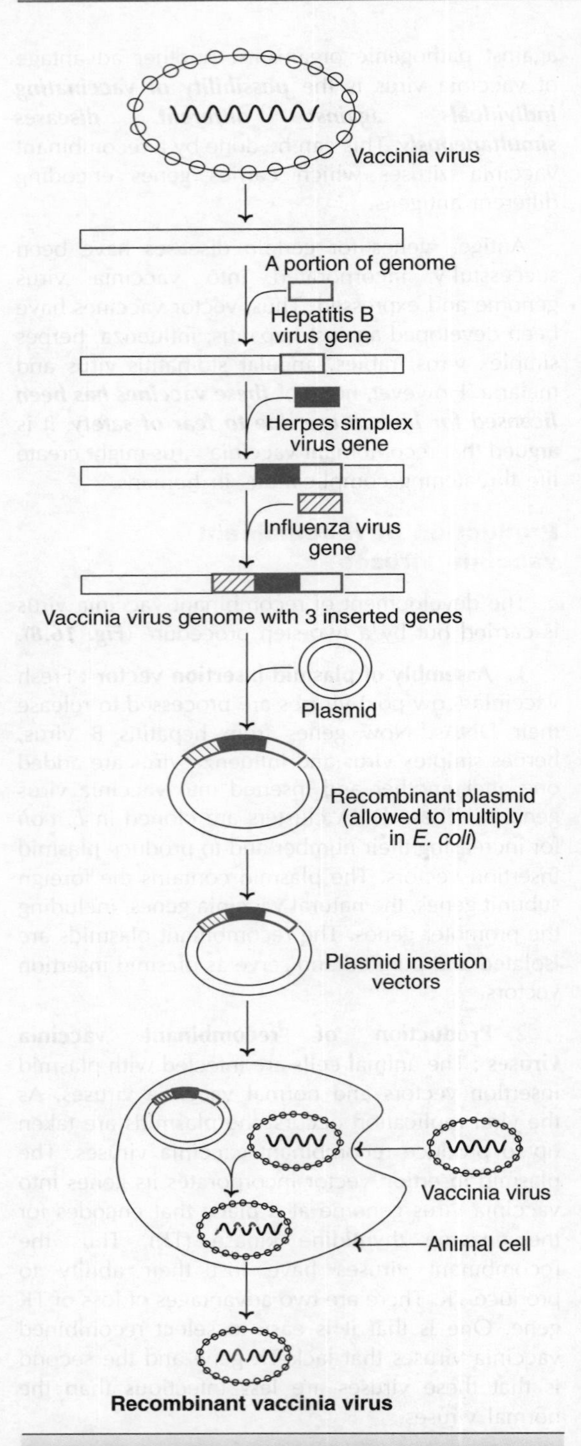

Fig. 16.8 : Production of recombinant vaccinia virus.

Advantages

1. Authenticated antigens that closely resemble natural antigens can be produced.

2. The virus can replicate in the host cells. This enables the amplification of the antigens for their action on B-lymphocytes and T-lymphocytes.

3. There is a possibility of vaccinating several diseases with one recombinant vaccinia virus.

Disadvantages

1. The most important limitation is the yet unknown risks of using these vaccines in humans.

2. There may be serious complications of using recombinant viral vaccines in immunosuppressed individuals such as AIDS patients.

Other viral recombinant vaccines

Most of the work on the development of live viral vaccines has been carried out on vaccinia virus. Other viruses such as ***adenovirus, poliovirus and varicella-zoster virus are also being tried*** as recombinant vaccines. Scientists are attracted to develop a recombinant poliovirus as it can be orally administered. It might take many more years for the recombinant viral vaccines to become a reality for human use.

DELIVERY OF ANTIGENS BY BACTERIA

It is known that the antigens located on the surface of a bacterial cell are more immunogenic than the antigens in the cytoplasm. Based on this observation, scientists have developed strategies to coat the surfaces of non-pathogenic organisms with antigens of pathogenic bacteria.

Flagellin is a protein present in the fragella (thread like filaments) of *Salmonella*. A synthetic oligonucleotide encoding the epitope of cholera toxin B subunit was inserted into *Salmonella* flagellin gene. This epitope was in fact found on the flagellum surface. These flagella-engineered bacteria, when administered to mice, raised antibodies against the cholera toxin B subunit peptide. It may be possible in future to incorporate multiple epitopes (2 or 3) into the flagellin gene to create multivalent bacterial vaccines.

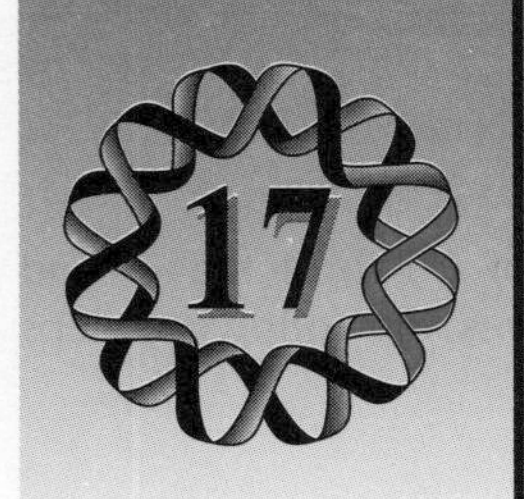

Monoclonal Antibodies (Hybridoma Technology)

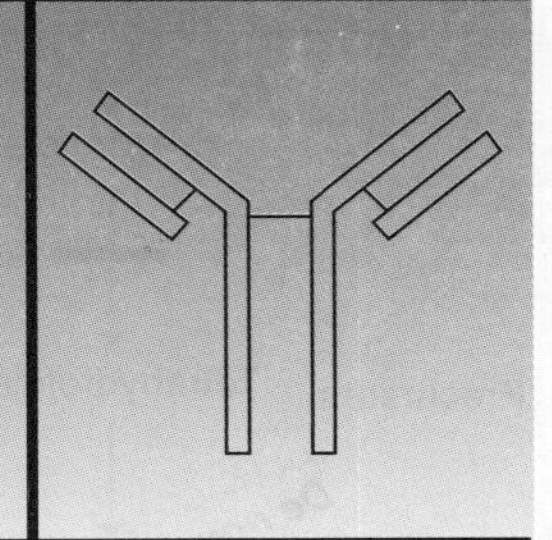

Antibodies or *immunoglobulins* are protein molecules produced by a specialized group of cells called ***B-lymphocytes*** (plasma cells) in mammals. The structures, characteristics and various other aspects of immunoglobulins (Igs) are described elsewhere (Refer Chapter 68). Antibodies are a part of the defense system to protect the body against the invading foreign substances namely ***antigens***. Each antigen has ***specific antigen determinants (epitopes)*** located on it. The antibodies have ***complementary determining regions (CDRs)*** which are mainly responsible for the antibody specificity.

In response to an antigen (with several different epitopes), B-lymphocytes gear up and produce many different antibodies. This type of antibodies which can react with the same antigen are designated as ***polyclonal antibodies***. The polyclonal antibody production is variable and is dependent on factors such as epitopes, response to immunity etc. Due to lack of specificity and heterogenic nature, there are several limitations on the utility of polyclonal antibodies for therapeutic and diagnostic purposes.

Monoclonal antibody (MAb) is a single type of antibody that is directed against a specific antigenic determinant (epitope). It was a dream of scientists to produce MAbs for different antigens. In the early years, animals were immunized against a specific antigen, B-lymphocytes were isolated and cultured *in vitro* for producing MAbs. This approach was not successful since culturing normal B-lymphocytes is difficult, and the synthesis of MAb was short-lived and very limited.

It is interesting that immortal monoclonal antibody producing cells do exist in nature. They are found in the patients suffering from a disease called ***multiple myeloma*** (a cancer of B-lymphocytes). It was in 1975. George Kohler and Cesar Milstein (Nobel Prize, 1984) achieved large scale production of MAbs. They could successfully ***hybridize*** antibody—producing ***B-lymphocytes with myeloma cells in vitro*** and create a ***hybridoma***. The result is that the artificially immortalized B-lymphocytes can multiply indefinitely *in vitro* and produce MAbs. The hybridoma cells possess the growth and multiplying properties of myeloma cells but secrete antibody of B-lymphocytes. The ***production of monoclonal antibodies by the hybrid cells is referred to as hybridoma technology***.

PRINCIPLE FOR CREATION OF HYBRIDOMA CELLS

The myeloma cells used in hybridoma technology must not be capable of synthesizing their own antibodies. The selection of hybridoma cells is based on inhibiting the nucleotide (consequently the DNA) synthesizing machinery. The mammalian cells can synthesize nucleotides by two pathways—*de novo* synthesis and salvage pathway (***Fig. 17.1***).

The ***de novo synthesis*** of nucleotides requires tetrahydrofolate which is formed from dihydro-

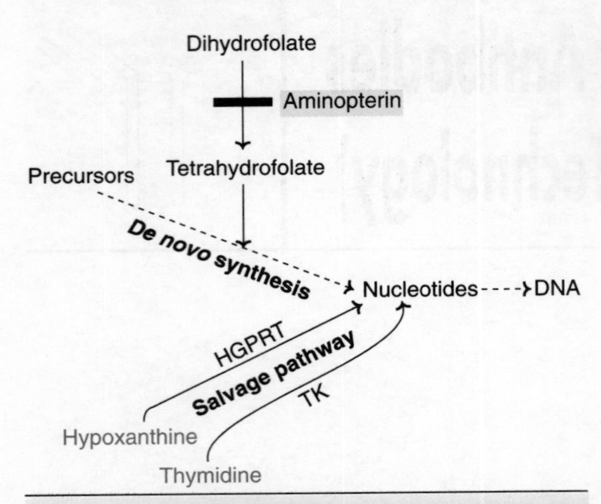

Fig. 17.1 : Pathways for the synthesis of nucleotides (HGPRT–Hypoxanthine guanine phosphoribosyl transferase; TK–Thymidine kinase)

folate. The formation of tetrahydrofolate (and therefore nucleotides) can be ***blocked by the inhibitor aminopterin***.

The ***salvage pathway*** involves the direct conversion of purines and pyrimidines into the corresponding nucleotides. Hypoxanthine guanine phosphoribosyl transferase (HGPRT) is a key enzyme in the salvage pathway of purines. It converts hypoxanthine and guanine respectively to inosine monophosphate and guanosine monophosphate. Thymidine kinase (TK), involved in the salvage pathway of pyrimidines converts thymidine to thymidine monophosphate (TMP). Any mutation in either one of the enzymes (HGPRT or TK) blocks the salvage pathway.

When cells deficient (mutated cells) in HGPRT are grown in a medium containing ***h***ypoxanthine ***a***minopterin and ***t***hymidine (***HAT*** medium), they cannot survive due to inhibition of *de novo* synthesis of purine nucleotides (**Note :** Salvage pathway is not operative due to lack of HGPRT). Thus, cells lacking HGPRT, grown in HAT medium die.

The hybridoma cells possess the ability of myeloma cells to grow *in vitro* with a functional HGPRT gene obtained from lymphocytes (with which myeloma cells are fused). Thus, only the hybridoma cells can proliferate in HAT medium, and this procedure is successfully used for their selection.

PRODUCTION OF MONOCLONAL ANTIBODIES

The establishment of hybridomas and production of MAbs involves the following steps (***Fig. 17.2***).

1. Immunization
2. Cell fusion
3. Selection of hybridomas
4. Screening the products
5. Cloning and propagation
6. Characterization and storage.

1. **Immunization :** The very first step in hybridoma technology is to immunize an animal (usually a mouse), with appropriate antigen. The antigen, along with an adjuvant like ***Freund's complete or incomplete adjuvant*** is injected subcutaneously (adjuvants are non-specific potentiators of specific immune responses). The injections at multiple sites are repeated several times. This enables increased stimulation of B-lymphocytes which are responding to the antigen. Three days prior to killing of the animal, a final dose of antigen is intravenously administered. The immune-stimulated cells for synthesis of antibodies have grown maximally by this approach. The concentration of the desired antibodies is assayed in the serum of the animal at frequent intervals during the course of immunization.

When the serum concentration of the antibodies is optimal, the animal is sacrificed. The spleen is aseptically removed and disrupted by mechanical or enzymatic methods to release the cells. The lymphocytes of the spleen are separated from the rest of the cells by density gradient centrifugation.

2. **Cell fusion :** The thoroughly washed lymphocytes are mixed with HGPRT defective myeloma cells. The mixture of cells is exposed to polyethylene glycol (PEG) for a short period (a few minutes), since it is toxic. PEG is removed by washing and the cells are kept in a fresh medium. These cells are composed of a mixture of hybridomas (fused cells), free myeloma cells and free lymphocytes.

3. **Selection of hybridomas :** When the cells are cultured in HAT medium (the principle described above), only the hybridoma cells grow, while the rest will slowly disappear. This happens in 7–10 days of culture.

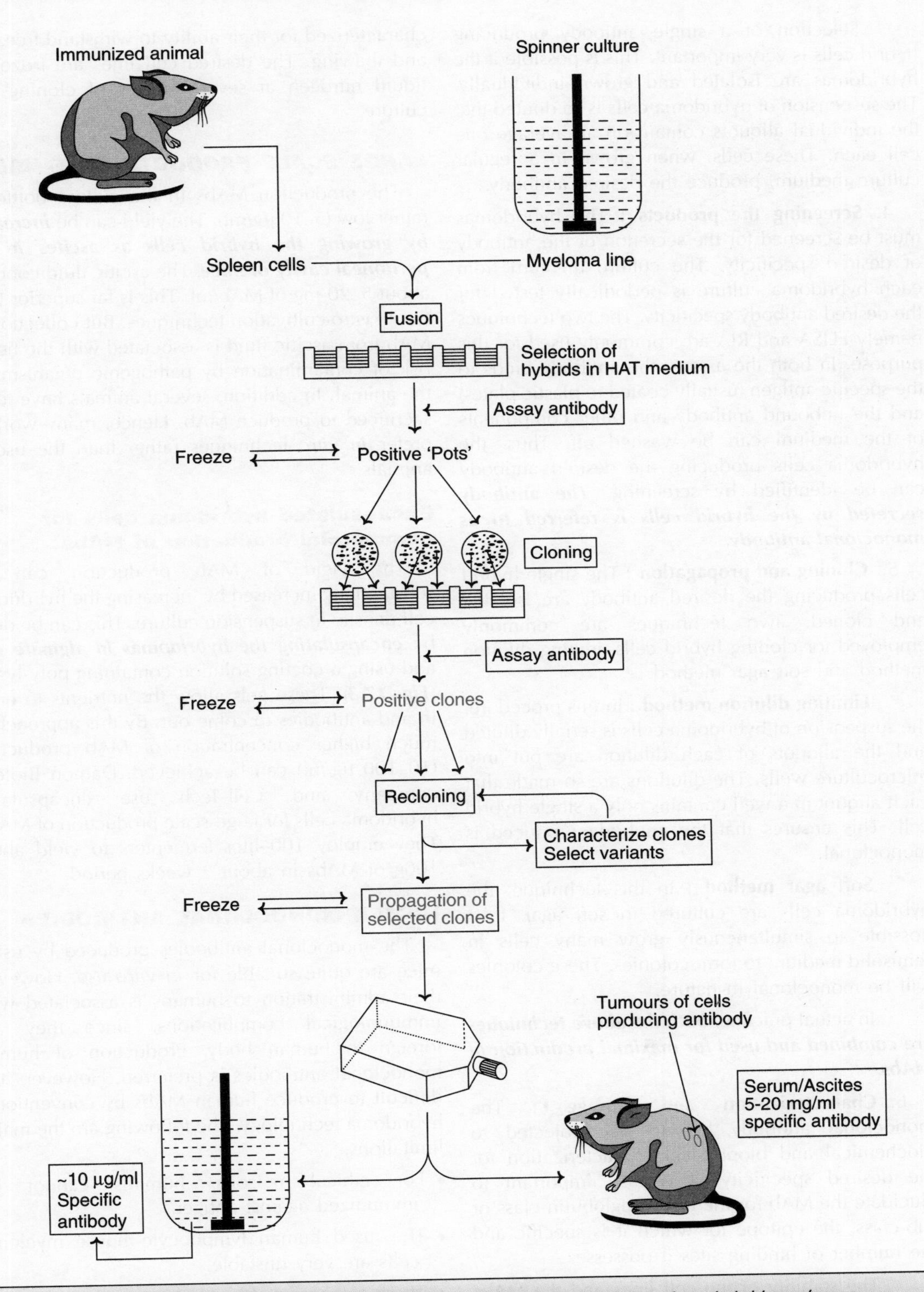

Fig. 17.2 : Basic protocol for the derivation of monoclonal antibodies from hybrid myelomas.

Selection of a single antibody producing hybrid cells is very important. This is possible if the hybridomas are isolated and grown individually. The suspension of hybridoma cells is so diluted that the individual aliquots contain on an average one cell each. These cells, when grown in a regular culture medium, produce the desired antibody.

4. **Screening the products :** The hybridomas must be screened for the secretion of the antibody of desired specificity. The culture medium from each hybridoma culture is periodically tested for the desired antibody specificity. The two techniques namely ELISA and RIA are commonly used for this purpose. In both the assays, the antibody binds to the specific antigen (usually coated to plastic plates) and the unbound antibody and other components of the medium can be washed off. Thus, the hybridoma cells producing the desired antibody can be identified by screening. ***The antibody secreted by the hybrid cells is referred to as monoclonal antibody***.

5. **Cloning and propagation :** The single hybrid cells producing the desired antibody are isolated and cloned. Two techniques are commonly employed for cloning hybrid cells-limiting dilution method and soft agar method.

Limiting dilution method : In this procedure, the suspension of hybridoma cells is serially diluted and the aliquots of each dilution are put into microculture wells. The dilutions are so made that each aliquot in a well contains only a single hybrid cell. This ensures that the antibody produced is monoclonal.

Soft agar method : In this technique, the hybridoma cells are cultured in soft agar. It is possible to simultaneously grow many cells in semisolid medium to form colonies. These colonies will be monoclonal in nature.

In actual practice, ***both the above techniques are combined and used for maximal production of MAbs***.

6. **Characterization and storage :** The monoclonal antibody has to be subjected to biochemical and biophysical characterization for the desired specificity. It is also important to elucidate the MAb for the immunoglobulin class or sub-class, the epitope for which it is specific and the number of binding sites it possesses.

The stability of the cell lines and the MAbs are important. The cells (and MAbs) must be characterized for their ability to withstand freezing, and thawing. The desired cell lines are frozen in liquid nitrogen at several stages of cloning and culture.

LARGE SCALE PRODUCTION OF MAbs

The production MAbs in the culture bottles is rather low (5–10 μg/ml). The yield can be ***increased by growing the hybrid cells as ascites in the peritoneal cavity of mice***. The ascitic fluid contains about 5–20 mg of MAb/ml. This is far superior than the *in vitro* cultivation techniques. But collection of MAb from ascitic fluid is associated with the heavy risk of contamination by pathogenic organisms of the animal. In addition, several animals have to be sacrificed to produce MAb. Hence, many workers prefer *in vitro* techniques rather than the use of animals.

Encapsulated hybridoma cells for commercial production of MAbs

The yield of MAb production can be substantially increased by increasing the hybridoma cell density in suspension culture. This can be done by ***encapsulating the hybridomas in alginate gels*** and using a coating solution containing poly-lysine (***Fig. 17.3***). These gels allow the nutrients to enter in and antibodies to come out. By this approach, a much higher concentration of MAb production (10–100 μg/ml) can be achieved. Damon Biotech company and Cell-Tech use encapsulated hybridoma cells for large-scale production of MAbs. They employ 100–liter fermenters to yield about 100g of MAbs in about 2 weeks period.

HUMAN MONOCLONAL ANTIBODIES

The monoclonal antibodies produced by using mice are quite suitable for *in vitro* use. However, their administration to humans is associated with immunological complications, since they are foreign to human body. Production of human monoclonal antibodies is preferred. However, it is difficult to produce human MAbs by conventional hybridoma technology. The following are the major limitations.

- For ethical reasons, humans cannot be immunized against antigens.
- The fused human lymphocyte-mouse myeloma cells are very unstable.
- There are no suitable myeloma cells in humans that can replace mouse myeloma cells.

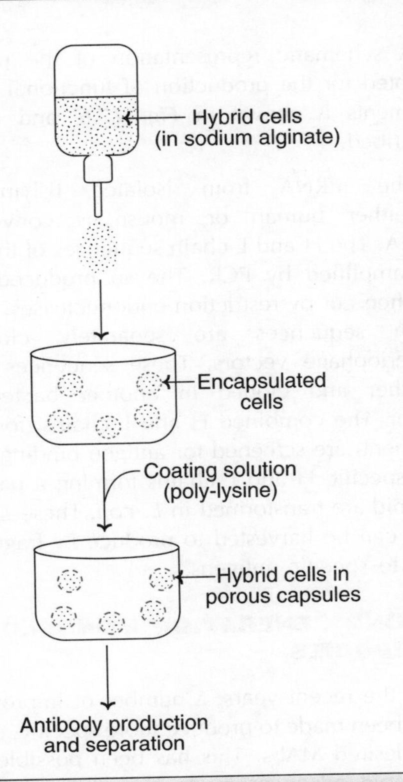

Fig. 17.3 : Production of monoclonal antibodies by microencapsulation.

For the above reasons, alternative arrangements are made to produce human MAbs. These are briefly described below.

Viral transformation of human B-lymphocytes

B-Lymphocytes, actively synthesizing antibody, are treated with fluorescent-labeled antigen. The fluorescent-activated cells are separated. However, B-cells on their own, cannot grow in culture. This limitation can be overcome by transforming B-lymphocytes with ***Epstein-Bar virus*** (EBV). Some of the EBV-transformed cells can grow in culture and produce monoclonal antibodies. Unfortunately, the yield of MAb is very low by this approach.

SCID mouse for producing human MAbs

The mouse suffering from severe combined immunodeficiency (SCID) disease lacks its natural immunological system. Such mouse can be challenged with appropriate antigens to produce human MAbs (For details, Refer Chapter 17).

Transgenic mouse for producing human MAbs

Attempts have been made in recent years to ***introduce human immunoglobulin genes into the mice*** to develop transgenic mice. Such mice are capable of synthesizing human immunoglobulins when immunized to a particular antigen. The B-lymphocytes isolated from transgenic mice can be used to produce MAbs by the standard hybridoma technology.

The above three approaches are quite laborious, and the yield of human MAbs is very low. Consequently, researchers continue their search for better alternatives.

GENETIC ENGINEERING STRATEGIES FOR THE PRODUCTION OF HUMAN-MOUSE MAbs

With the advances in genetic engineering, it is now possible to add certain human segments to a mouse antibody. This is truely a hybridized antibody and is referred to as ***humanized antibody*** or ***chimeric antibody***.

Substitution of Fv region of human Ig by mouse Fv

The DNA coding sequences for Fv regions of both L and H chains of human immunoglobulin are replaced by Fv DNA sequence (for L and H chains) from a mouse monoclonal antibody (***Fig. 17.4A***). The newly developed humanized MAb has Fc region of Ig being human. This stimulates proper immunological response.

The chimeric antibodies produced in this manner were found to be effective for the destruction of tumor cells *in vitro*.

Substitution of human Ig by mouse CDRs

Genetic engineers have been successful in developing human MAbs containing mouse complementary determining regions (CDRs). This is made possible by replacing CDRs genes (CDR_1, CDR_2, CDR_3) of humans by that of mouse. These chimeric antibodies (***Fig. 17.4B***) possess the antigen binding affinities of the mouse and they can serve as effective therapeutic agents. So far, about 50 monoclonal antibodies have been produced by this approach. However, this technique is costly and time consuming.

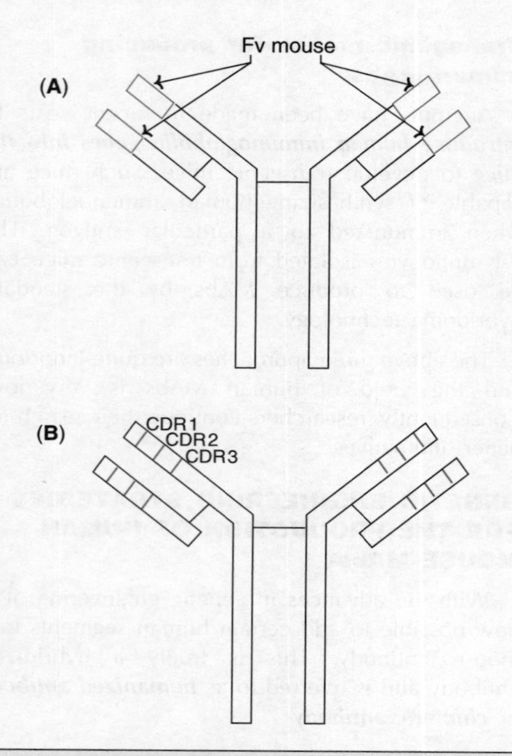

Fig. 17.4 : Genetically engineered human-mouse antibodies (A) Substitution of Fv region of human Ig by mouse Fv (B) Substitution of human Ig by mouse CDRs (CDR-Complementary determining regions).

Bispecific monoclonal antibodies

The MAbs in which the two arms of Fab (antigen-binding) have two different specificities for two different epitopes are referred to as bispecific MAbs. They may be produced by fusing two different hybridoma cell lines (***Fig. 17.5***) or by genetic engineering. Bispecific Fab MAbs theoretically, are useful for a simultaneous and combined treatment of two different diseases.

PRODUCTION OF MAbs IN *E. COLI*

The hybridoma technology is very laborious, expensive and time consuming. To overcome these limitation, researchers have been trying to genetically engineer bacteria, plants and animals. The objective is to develop ***bioreactors*** for the large scale production of monoclonal antibodies. It may be noted that the antigen binding regions of antibody (Fv or Fab fragments) are very crucial, while the Fc portion is dispensable.

A schematic representation of the procedure adopted for the production of functional antibody fragments is shown in ***Fig. 17.6***, and is briefly described.

The mRNA from isolated B-lymphocytes of either human or mouse is converted to cDNA. The H and L chain sequences of this cDNA are amplified by PCR. The so produced cDNAs are then cut by restriction endonucleases. H and L chain sequences are separately cloned in bacteriophage vectors. These sequences are put together and cloned in another bacteriophage vector. The combined H and L chains (forming Fv fragment) are screened for antigen binding activity. The specific H and L chains forming a part of the plasmid are transformed in *E. coli*. These *E. coli*, in turn, can be harvested to produce Fv fragments to bind to specific antigens.

SECOND GENERATION MONOCLONAL ANTIBODIES

In the recent years, a number of improvements have been made to produce more specific, sensitive and desired MAbs. This has been possible due to the rapid advances made in genetic engineering techniques. For instances, by employing ***site-directed mutagenesis***, it is possible to introduce cysteine residues at the predetermined positions on the MAb. These cysteine residues which facilitate the isotope labeling may be more useful in diagnostic imaging and radioimmunotherapy.

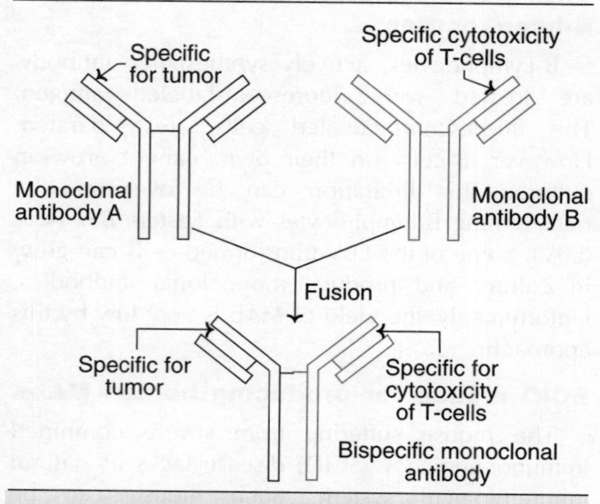

Fig. 17.5 : Production of a bispecific monoclonal antibody.

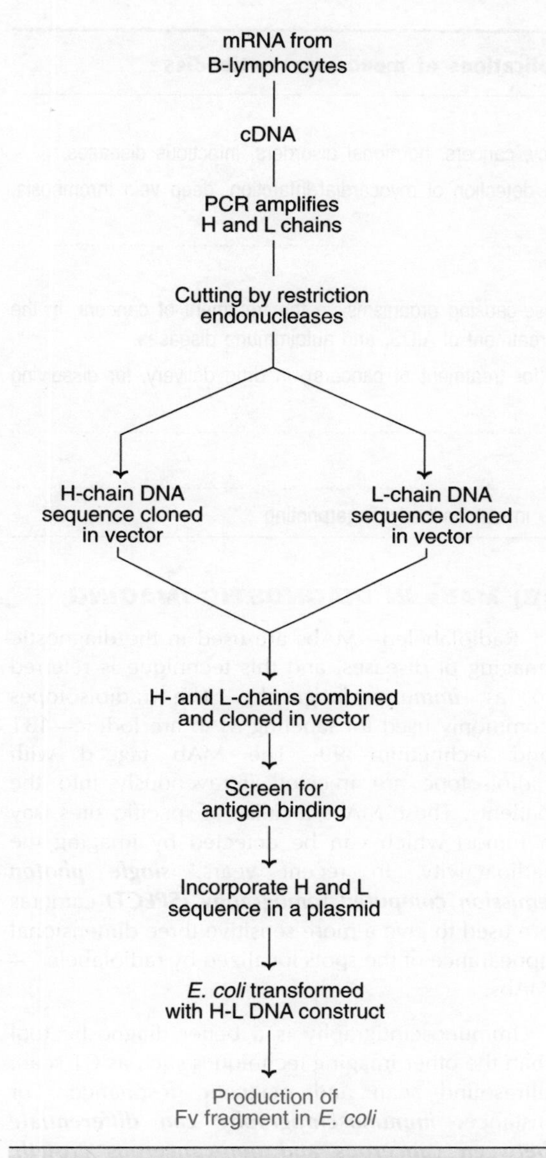

Fig. 17.6 : Production of monoclonal antibodies in E. coli.

ADVANTAGES OF MONOCLONAL ANTIBODIES

Monoclonal antibodies truely ***represent a homogeneous state of a single molecular species***. Each MAb is specific to a given antigenic determinant. This is in contrast to the conventional antiserum that contains polyclonal antibodies. The wide range of applications of MAbs are described later.

LIMITATIONS OF MONOCLONAL ANTIBODIES

Hybridoma technology is laborious and time consuming. MAbs are produced against a single antigenic determinant, therefore, they cannot differentiate the molecule as a whole. Sometimes, they may be incapable of distinguishing groups of different molecules also.

The presence of retroviruses as a part of the mammalian chromosomes is a common occurrence. Mice used in MAb production carry several viruses (adenovirus, hepatic virus, retrovirus, reovirus, cytomegalovirus, thymic virus). The presence of some of these viruses has been detected in the hybridomas. This poses a great danger, since there is no guarantee that MAb produced is totally virus-free, despite the purification. For this reason, US Food and Drug Administration insists that ***MAb for human use should be totally free from all pathogenic organisms, including viruses.***

APPLICATIONS OF MONOCLONAL ANTIBODIES

Monoclonal antibodies with specificity and high purity have a wide range of applications, which can be broadly categorized as follows.

1. Diagnostic applications
2. Therapeutic uses
3. Protein purification
4. Miscellaneous applications.

A summary of the important applications of MAbs is given in ***Table 17.1***, and briefly discussed below.

1. DIAGNOSTIC APPLICATIONS

Monoclonal antibodies have revolutionized the laboratory diagnosis of various diseases. For this purpose, MAbs may be employed as diagnostic reagents for ***biochemical analysis*** or as tools for ***diagnostic imaging of diseases.***

(A) *MAbs IN BIOCHEMICAL ANALYSIS*

Diagnostic tests based on the use of MAbs as reagents are routinely used in radioimmunoassays

TABLE 17.1 A summary of important applications of monoclonal antibodies

1. **Diagnostic applications**
   (A) ***Biochemical analysis*** for the diagnosis of pregnancy, cancers, hormonal disorders, infectious diseases.
   (B) ***Diagnositic imaging (immunoscintigraphy)*** for the detection of myocardial infarction, deep vein thrombosis, atherosclerosis, cancers, bacterial infections.
2. **Therapeutic applications**
   (A) ***Direct use as therapeutic agents*** to destroy disease-causing organisms, in the treatment of cancers, in the immunosuppression of organ transplantation, in the treatment of AIDS, and autoimmune diseases.
   (B) ***As targeting agents in therapy*** as immunotoxins (for treatment of cancers), in drug delivery, for dissolving blood clots, in radioimmunotherapy (of tumors).
3. **Protein purification** by immunoaffinity techniques.
4. **Miscellaneous applications** as catalytic agents (abzymes), in autoantibody fingerprinting.

(RIA) and enzyme-linked immunosorbent assays (ELISA) in the laboratory. These assays measure the circulating concentrations of hormones (insulin, human chorionic gonadotropin, growth hormone, progesterone, thyroxine, triiodothyronine, thyroid stimulating hormone, gastrin, renin), and several other tissue and cell products (blood group antigens, blood clotting factors, interferons, interleukins, histocompatibility antigens, tumor markers).

In recent years, a number of diagnostic kits using MAbs have become commercially available. For instance, it is now possible to do the early diagnosis of the following conditions/diseases.

Pregnancy—by detecting the urinary levels of human chorionic gonadotropin.

Cancers—estimation of plasma carcino-embryonic antigen in colorectal cancer, and prostate specific antigen for prostate cancer. Besides diagnosis, estimation of tumor markers is also useful for the prognosis of cancers. That is a gradual fall in a specific tumor marker is observed with a reduction in tumor size, following treatment.

Hormonal disorders—analysis of thyroxine, triiodothyronine and thyroid stimulating hormone for thyroid disorders.

Infectious diseases—by detecting the circulatory levels of antigens specific to the infectious agent e.g., antigens of *Neisseria gonorrhoeae* and herpes simplex virus for the diagnosis of sexually transmitted diseases.

(B) MAbs IN DIAGNOSTIC IMAGING

Radiolabeled—MAbs are used in the diagnostic imaging of diseases, and this technique is referred to as ***immunoscintigraphy***. The radioisotopes commonly used for labeling MAb are iodine—131 and technetium—99. The MAb tagged with radioisotope are injected intravenously into the patients. These MAbs localise at specific sites (say a tumor) which can be detected by imaging the radioactivity. In recent years, ***single photon emission computed tomography (SPECT)*** cameras are used to give a more sensitive three dimensional appearance of the spots localized by radiolabeled—MAbs.

Immunoscintigraphy is a better diagnostic tool than the other imaging techniques such as CT scan, ultrasound scan and magnetic resonance. For instance, ***immunoscintigraphy can differentiate between cancerous and non-cancerous growth***, since radiolabeled—MAbs are tumor specific. This is not possible with other imaging techniques.

Monoclonal antibodies are successfully used in the diagnostic imaging of cardiovascular diseases, cancers and sites of bacterial infections.

Cardiovascular diseases

Myocardial infarction : The cardiac protein myosin gets exposed wherever myocardial necrosis (death of cardiac cells) occurs. Antimyosin MAb labeled with radioisotope indium chloride (^{111} In) is used for detecting myosin and thus the site of

TABLE 17.2 Selected tumor markers along with the associated cancers used in MAb imaging

Tumor marker	*Associated cancer(s)*
Carcinoembryonic antigen (CEA)	Cancers of colon, stomach, pancreas
Alpha fetoprotein	Cancers of liver, and germ cells of testes
Human chorionic gonadotropin	Choriocarcinoma
Prostatic acid phosphatase	Prostate cancer
Epiderminal growth factor receptor	Melanoma
Tumor—associated cell surface antigens	Various cancers

myocardial infarction. Imaging of radiolabeled MAb, is usually done after 24–48 hours of intravenous administration. This is carried out either by planner gamma camera or single photon emission computed tomography (SPECT). It is possible to ***detect the location and the degree of damage to the heart by using radiolabeled antimyosin MAb***. Thus, this technique is useful for the diagnosis of heart attacks.

Deep vein thrombosis (DVT) : DVT refers to the formation of blood clots (thrombus) within the blood veins, primarily in the lower extremities. For the detection of DVT, radioisotope labeled ***MAb directed against fibrin or platelets can be used.*** The imaging is usually done after 4 hours of injection. Fibrin specific MAbs are successfully used for the detection of clots in thigh, pelvis, calf and knee regions.

Atherosclerosis : Thickening and loss of elasticity of arterial walls is referred to as atherosclerosis. Atherosclerotic plaques cause diseases of coronary and peripheral arteries. Atherosclerosis has been implicated in the development of heart diseases. ***MAb tagged with a radiolabel directed against activated platelets can be used to localize the atherosclerotic lesions by imaging technique.***

Cancers

Monoclonal antibodies against many types of human cancers are now available. A selected list of tumor markers (along with the associated cancers) that can be used for MAb imaging is given in ***Table 17.2***. Tumors can be located in patients using radioisotope labeled MAbs specific to the protein(s), particularly of membrane origin. It has been possible to detect certain cancers at early stages (lung cancer, breast cancer, ovariran cancer, malanoma, colorectal cancer) by employing MAbs. About 80 per cent specificity has been achieved for detecting cancers by this approach.

An iodine (^{131}I) labeled monoclonal antibody specific to breast cancer cells when administered to the patients detects (by imaging) the spread of cancer (metastasis) to other regions of the body. This is not possible by scanning techniques.

The imaging technique by using MAb can also be used to monitor therapeutic responses of a cancer. There are certain limitations in using MAb in cancer diagnosis and prognosis. These include the difficulty in the selection of a specific MAb and the access of MAb to the target site of the tumor which may be less vascularized.

MAbs in immunohistopathology of cancers : The pathological changes of the cancerous tissue can be detected by immunohistochemical techniques. This can be done by using MAb against a specific antigen.

MAbs in hematopoietic malignancies : Hematopoietic stem cells in bone marrow are the precursors for different blood cells, B- and T-lymphocytes which are produced in a stepwise transformation. During malignancy, transformation of lymphocytes stops at a particular stage of maturation. This can be detected by using stage-specific MAbs.

Bacterial infections

In recent years, attempts are made to detect the sites of infections by using MAbs. This is made possible by directing MAb against bacterial antigens. Further, monoclonal antibodies against inflammatory leucocytes which accumulate at infection site are also useful to specifically detect localized infections.

2. THERAPEUTIC APPLICATIONS

Monoclonal antibodies have a wide range of therapeutic applications. MAbs are used in the treatment of cancer, transplantation of bone marrow and organs, autoimmune diseases, cardiovascular diseases and infectious diseases. The therapeutic applications of MAbs are broadly grouped into 2 types.

(A) Direct use of MAbs as therapeutic agents

(B) MAbs as targeting agents.

(A) *MAbs AS DIRECT THERAPEUTIC AGENTS*

Monoclonal antibodies can be directly used for enchancing the immune function of the host. Direct use of MAbs causes minimal toxicity to the target tissues or the host.

In destroying disease-causing organisms

MAbs promote efficient opsonization of pathogenic organisms (by coating with antibody) and enhance phagocytosis. In fact, MAbs were found to protect chimpanzees against certain ***viral*** (hepatitis B-virus) and ***bacterial*** (*E. coli Haemophilus influenza, Streptococcus* sp and *Pseudomonas* sp) infections.

In the treatment of cancer

MAbs, against the antigens on the surface of cancer cells, are useful for the treatment of cancer. The antibodies bind to the cancer cells and destroy them. This is brought out by antibody—dependent cell-mediated cytotoxicity, complement-mediated cytotoxicity and phagocytosis of cancer cells (coated with MAbs) by reticuloendothelial system. The patients suffering from leukemia, colorectal cancer, lymphoma and melanoma have been treated with MAbs. However, there was a wide variation in the success rate. A monoclonal antibody specific to the cells of leukemia is used to destroy the residual leukemia cells without affecting other cells.

MAbs are used *in vitro* to remove the residual tumor cells prior to autologous bone marrow transplantation (transplantation of the patient's own bone marrow cells, due to non-availability of a suitable donor).

Limitations for direct use of MAbs in cancer

1. The MAbs produced in mice and directly used for therapeutic purposes may lead to the development of antimouse antibodies and hypersensitivity reactions.

2. All the cancer cells may not carry the same antigen for which MAb has been produced. Thus, MAbs may not be attached to some cancer cells at all.

3. The free antigens (of target cells) present in the circulation may bind to MAbs and prevent them from their action on the target cells.

In the immunosuppression of organ transplantation

In the normal medical practice, immunosuppressive drugs such as cyclosporin and prednisone are administered to overcome the rejection of organ transplantation. In recent years, MAbs specific to T-lymphocyte surface antigens are being used for this purpose. The monoclonal antibody namely ***OKT_3***, was the ***first MAb to be licensed*** by U.S. Food and Drug Adminstration ***for use as immunosuppressive agent*** after organ transplantation in humans. OKT_3 specifically directed against CD_3 antigen of T-lymphocytes is successfully used in renal and bone marrow transplantations. In the normal course, CD_3 antigen activates T-lymphocytes and plays a key role in organ transplant rejection (destroys the foreign cells in the host). This is prevented by use of MAb against CD_3 antigen.

In the treatment of AIDS

Immunosuppression is the hall mark of AIDS. This is caused by reduction in CD_4 (cluster determinant antigen 4) cells of T-lymphocytes. The human immunodeficiency virus (HIV) binds to specific receptors on CD_4 cells by using surface membrane glycoprotein (gp120). Genetic engineers have been successful to ***attach Fc portion of mouse monoclonal antibody to human CD_4 molecule***. This complex has high affinity to bind to membrane glycoprotein gp120 of virus infected cells. The ***Fc fragment induces cell-mediated destruction of HIV infected cells (Fig. 17.7)***.

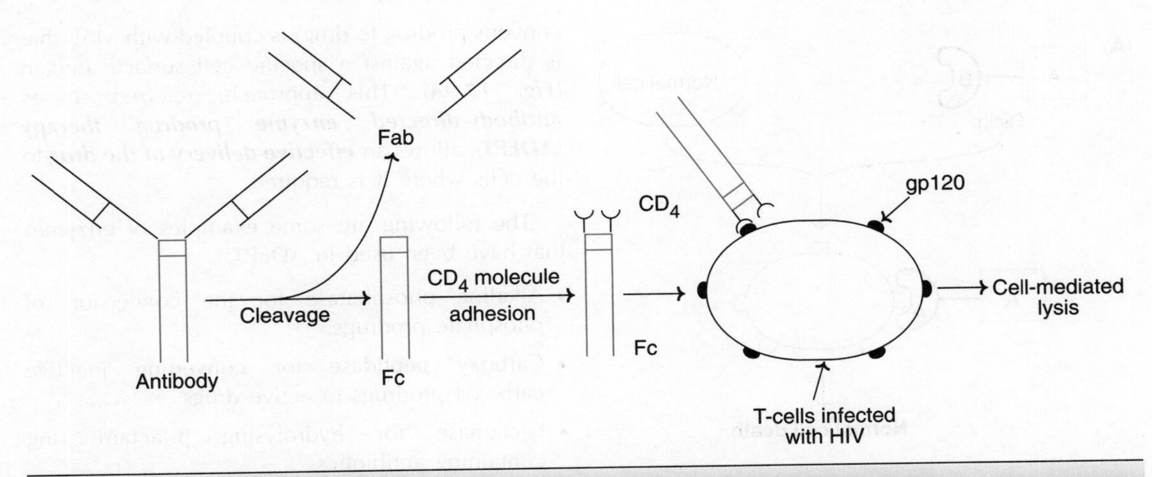

Fig. 17.7 : Modified monoclonal antibody in the treatment of AIDS.

In the treatment of autoimmune diseases

Autoimmune diseases like rheumatoid arthritis and multiple sclerosis are of great concern. Some success has been reported in the clinical trials of rheumatoid arthritis patients by using MAbs directed against T-lymphocytes and B-lymphocytes.

(B) *MAbs AS TARGETING AGENTS IN THERAPY*

Toxins, drugs, radioisotopes etc., can be attached or conjugated to the tissue-specific monoclonal antibodies and carried to target tissues for efficient action. This allows higher concentration of drugs to reach the desired site with minimal toxicity. In this way, MAbs are used for the appropriate delivery of drugs or isotopes.

MAbs in use as immunotoxins

The toxins can be coupled with MAbs to form immunotoxins and used in therapy e.g., diphtheria toxin, *Pseudomonas* exotoxin, toxins used for cancer treatment.

Anti-Tac MAb raised against IL2–R (T-cell growth factor receptor) can be conjugated with exotoxin of *Pseudomonas* sp. This immunotoxin can be used to destory the malignant T-cells in the patients suffering from T-cell leukemia (**Note :** IL2–R is expressed in abnormal T-cells with lymphoid malignancies).

Ricin is a cytotoxic protein derived from castor oil plant. It is composed of two polypeptide chains (A and B) held together by a disulfide linkage. The B-chain of ricin binds to the cell surface. This binding facilitates the A-chain of ricin to enter the cell and inhibit the function of ribosomes (i.e. biosynthesis of all proteins is blocked). This results in the death of cells (***Fig. 17.8A***). Ricin can be subjected to oxidation to separate to A and B chains. The toxic A-chain can be conjugated to MAb that is specific to cancer cells. The tumor-specific MAb bound to A-chain of ricin binds to cancer cells and not to normal cells. Once the ***A-chain*** enters the cells, it ***blocks ribosomal function, leading to the death of cancer cells (Fig. 17.8B)***.

MAbs in drug delivery

In general, the drugs are less effective *in vivo* (in the living body) when compared to *in vitro* (in laboratory when tested with cultured cells). This is mainly due to the fact that sufficient quantity of the drug does not reach the target tissue. This problem can be solved by using tissue-specific MAbs. The drugs can be coupled with MAb (directed against a cell surface antigen of the cells, say a tumor) and specifically targeted to reach the site of action (***Fig. 17.9A***).

In the treatment of certain diseases, a prodrug (an inactive form of the drug) can be used. This can be enzymatically converted to active drug in the target tissues. For this purpose, the enzyme (that

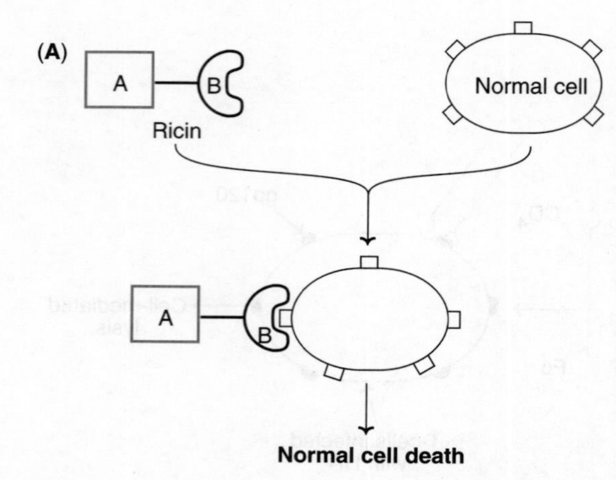

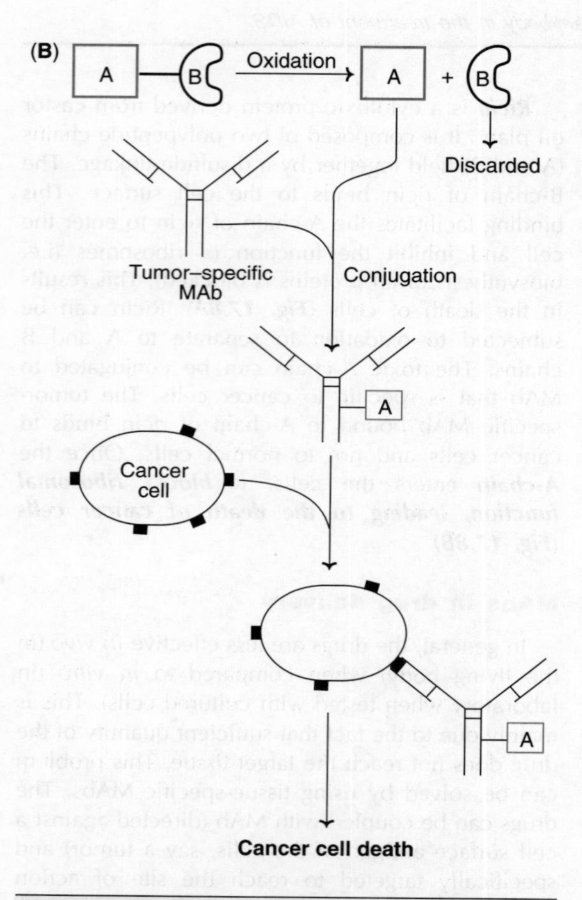

Fig. 17.8 : Use of ricin as a cytotoxic agent (A) Action of ricin on a normal cell; (B) A-chain of ricin conjugated to MAb causing cancer cell death (Note : A-chain of ricin cannot enter normal cell).

converts prodrug to drug) is coupled with MAb that is directed against a specific cell surface antigen (*Fig. 17.9A*). This approach, referred to as ***antibody-directed enzyme prodrug therapy*** (***ADEPT***), allows an ***effective delivery of the drug*** to the cells where it is required.

The following are some examples of enzymes that have been used in ADEPT.

- Alkaline phosphatase for the conversion of phosphate prodrugs.
- Carboxy peptidase for converting inactive carboxyl prodrugs to active drugs.
- Lactamase for hydrolysing β-lactam ring containing antibiotics.

MAbs in the dissolution of blood clots

A great majority of natural deaths are due to a blockage in cornary or cerebral artery by a blood

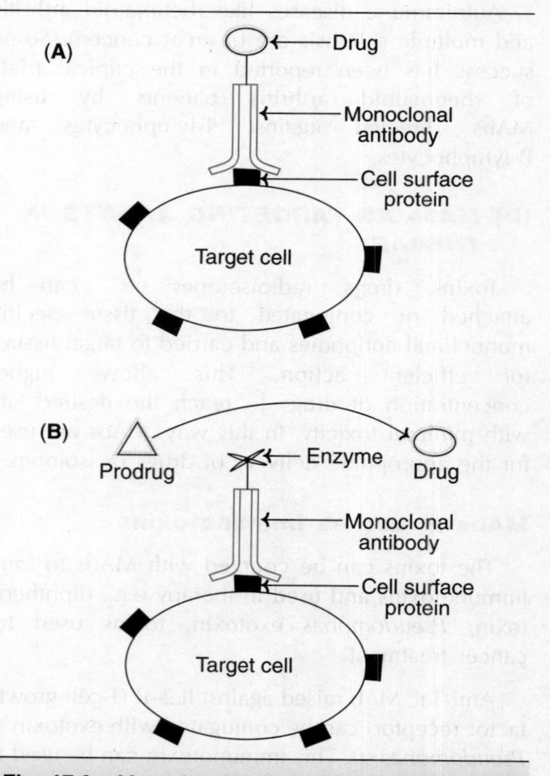

Fig. 17.9 : Monoclonal antibody based drug delivery to the target cells. (A) The drug is bound to MAb (B) The enzyme that converts prodrug to drug is bound to MAb.

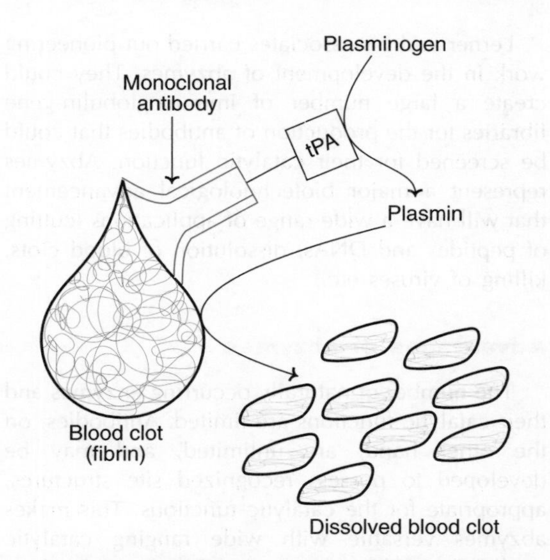

***Fig. 17.10 :** Monoclonal antibody in the dissolution of blood clot (tPA-Tissue plasminogen activator).*

clot (thrombus). Fibrin is the major constituent of blood clot which gets dissolved by plasmin. Plasmin in turn is formed by the activation of plasminogen by plasminogen activator. The blockage of arteries occurs due to inadequate dissolution of blood clots. Tissue plasminogen activator (tPA) can be used as a therapeutic agent to remove the blood clots.

A ***monoclonal antibody directed against fibrin can be coupled to tPA and used for degradation of blood clots. MAb-tPA complex due to a high affinity gets attached to fibrin (Fig. 17.10)***. Due to the concentration of tPA at the target spots, there is more efficient conversion of plasminogen to plasmin which in turn dissolves blood clot (fibrin). Good success of clot lysis has been reported by using MAb-tPA complex in experimental animals.

Drug delivery through liposomes coupled to tissue-specific MAbs

Liposomes are sacs or vesicles formed spontaneously when certain lipid molecules are exposed to aqueous environment. Drug entrapped in liposomes that are coated with MAbs directed against tissue-specific antigens are being tried for drug delivery. Unfortunately, the progress in this approach has been limited, since such liposomes do not reach the target cells. They are retained mostly in the liver and spleen (reticuloendothelial cells), and degraded.

MAbs in radioimmunotherapy (RAIT)

The ***radioisotopes can be coupled to MAbs that are directed against tumor cells***. This allows the concentration of radioactivity at the desired sites and a very efficient killing of target cells (tumor cells). The advantage with radioimmunotherapy is that conjugated complex need not penetrate the cells, as is required in immunotoxin therapy. The limitation is that the neighbouring normal cells may also get damaged or killed. This can be minimized by using radioisotopes with short half-lives. Yttrium–90 with a half-life of 64 hours is a suitable isotope to be employed in RAIT. Due to shortage in the supply of yttrium–90, indium–111 is more commonly used.

3. PROTEIN PURIFICATION

Monoclonal antibodies can be produced for any protein. And the so produced MAb can be conveniently used for the purification of the protein against which it was raised. MAbs columns can be prepared by coupling them to cyanogen bromide activated Sepharose (chromatographic matrix). The ***immobilized MAbs*** in this manner are very ***useful for the purification of proteins by immunoaffinity method***.

Advantages

There are certain advantages of using MAbs for protein purification. These include the specificity of the MAb to bind to the desired protein, very efficient elution from the chromatographic column and high degree of purification. Immunoaffinity chromatography is routinely used for the purification of recombinant interferons. The efficiency of this technique will be obvious from the fact that by a single step, it is possible to achieve more than 5,000 fold purification of interferon-α_2.

Disadvantages

It is not possible to achieve 100% puriy of the target protein by immunoaffinity. This is due to the fact that a small quantity of MAb leaks into the elution. Further, MAbs cannot distinguish between the intact target protein and a fragment of it with the antigenic site.

4. MISCELLANEOUS APPLICATIONS

CATALYTIC MAbs (ABZYMES)

Catalysis is the domain of enzymes. The most important common character between enzymes and antibodies is that both are proteins. Further, the binding of an antibody to its antigen is comparable to the binding of an enzyme to its substrate. In both instances, the binding is specific with high affinity and involves weak and non-covalent interactions (electrostatic, hydrogen and van der Waals forces). The striking difference is that the enzyme alters the substrate (to a product) while the antigen bound to antibody remains unaltered.

Certain similarities between enzyme-substrate interaction and antibody-antigen interaction have tempted researchers to explore the possibility of using antibodies in catalysis. The ***a**nti**b**ody en**zymes***, appropriately regarded as ***abzymes***, are the ***catalytic antibodies***.

There is a difference in the antibody recognition of an antigen and enzyme recognition of a substrate. While the antibodies recognize in ***ground state***, the enzymes recognize in a ***transition state*** (associated with a conformational change of protein). In fact, it is in the transition condition the catalysis occurs. If a molecule resembling the transition state and conformation (between substrate and product) could be used as a hapten the antibodies so produced should bring about catalysis. This is what precisely is done to create abzymes.

Researchers have produced a ***hapten-carrier*** complex which resembles the transition state of an ester undergoing hydrolysis. This hapten conjugate is used to generate ***anti-hapten monoclonal antibodies***. These MAbs could bring about hydrolysis of esters with great degree of specificity (to the transition state to which MAbs were raised).

Besides ester hydrolysis, there are several other types of reactions wherein antibodies can be used. These include hydrolysis of amides and carbonates, cyclization reactions, elimination reactions and biomolecular chemical reactions. Certain enzymes require cofactors for their catalytic function. MAbs incorporating metal ions have been developed to carry out catalysis.

Lerner and his associates carried out pioneering work in the development of abzymes. They could create a large number of immunoglobulin-gene libraries for the production of antibodies that could be screened for their catalytic function. Abzymes represent a major biotechnological advancement that will have a wide range of applications (cutting of peptides and DNAs, dissolution of blood clots, killing of viruses etc.)

Advantages of abzymes

The number of naturally occurring enzymes and their catalytic functions are limited. Antibodies, on the other hand, are unlimited, and may be developed to possess recognized site structures, appropriate for the catalytic functions. This makes abzymes versatile with wide ranging catalytic applications. Thus, the area of abzyme technology is very promising, although the studies are at preliminary stages.

Limitations of abzymes

Despite the progress made in the production and utility of abzymes, it is doubtful whether they will ever match the natural enzymes in their catalytic function. However, the abzymes will be certainly useful for a variety of reactions where the natural enzymes do not have the desired specificities.

AUTOANTIBODY FINGERPRINTING

The occurrence of autoantibodies and their involvement in certain diseases is well known (e.g. rheumatic arthritis). A new category of ***individual specific (IS) autoantibodies*** have been discovered in recent years. These IS-autoantibodies are produced after birth and reach maximum in number by 2 years, and then remain constant for the later part of life. Monoclonal antibodies produced against IS-autoantibodies can be used for their detection, and ***identification of individuals***. This technique referred to as ***autoantibody fingerprinting***, is particularly useful for the detection of criminals, rapists etc. The autoantibodies collected from samples such as blood, saliva, semen and tears can be used.

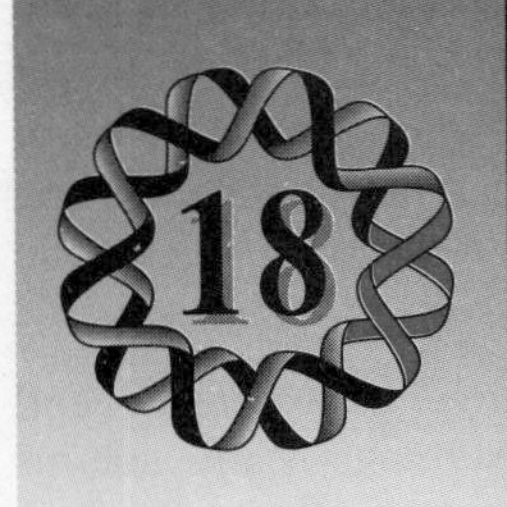

Assisted Reproductive Technology

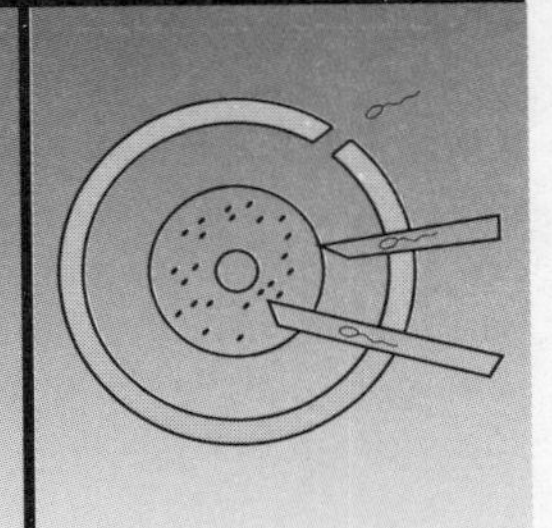

Traditional methods of breeding animals were only means of improving the genetic qualities. Despite the several advances made in biotechnology, genetic manipulations in relation to reproduction of animal and humans are very limited for obvious reasons, the most important being the unknown risks involved in the outcome.

The ***manipulations of reproduction in animals and humans*** are collectively considered under assisted reproductive technology (***ART***), and dealt with in this chapter. The objective of ART is to increase the number of progeny of the desired species.

Some of the important aspects of manipulation of reproduction in animals are first dealt with, and then the salient features of manipulations in human reproduction are described.

MANIPULATIONS OF REPRODUCTION IN ANIMALS

All the male mammals produce millions of sperms (male gametes) daily, and thus theoretically, can inseminate many females to produce a large number of offsprings. On the other hand, the female mammals produce a limited number of eggs (female gamets), usually one at a time (exception-pig), approximately at monthly intervals. The female also has the responsibility of developing the fertilized egg, besides providing nourishment to the newborn. Thus, the ruminant female mammals cannot produce more than one offspring in a year, in the normal circumstances.

The current approaches for the ***artificial breeding of animals*** with particular reference to the following are briefly described.

- Artificial insemination.
- Embryo transfer.
- *In vitro* fertilization.
- Embryo cloning.

ARTIFICIAL INSEMINATION

As the male produces millions of sperms daily, the semen can be used to produce several offsprings. This is made possible by artificial insemination (AI) of females. For an effective AI to produce the desired results, the following aspects must be considered.

Semen collection and storage

The semen ejaculate is collected, appropriately diluted and examined under microscope for the number of motile sperms. Normally, 0.2 ml of bull semen contains about 10 million motile sperms. The diluted semen can be used fresh within few days, or cryopreserved at –196°C in liquid nitrogen for long-term storage and transport.

Artificial insemination is done on standing animals through a technique, known a ***rectal***

palpation. Each semen ejaculate of a male bull, in theory, can be used to inseminate as many as 500 cows. Another advantage of AI is that the semen can be transported (in cryopreserved form) to different places/countries and used to develop superior animals.

Synchronization of ovulation

The female animals are inseminated after ovulation which can be detected by behavioural estrous. It is rather difficult to detect estrous, since it mostly occurs during night and lasts for only a few hours.

The animal breeders would like to inseminate a large number of females simultaneously, so that the management becomes easy. For this purpose, the females are induced (synchronized) to ovulate at a set time. This is achieved by administration of progesterone and/or prostaglandins, which regulate ovulation cycle. Although total synchrony of ovulation is not possible, about 80% of the females could be made to respond by this approach.

Sperm sexing

The livestock industries prefer to have animals belonging to one sex. For instance, the dairy and beef industries demand more females than males. It is possible ***to produce the animals of desired sex*** through sperm sexing.

Sperms and ova contain half of the chromosomes of a somatic cell. Thus, an ovum contains autosomes and one X chromosome while the sperm contains autosomes and one Y chromosome. Sex is determined genetically by the sex chromosomes (X and Y). X chromosome is present in all the ova, whereas half of the sperm (of a semen ejaculate) possess X and the other half Y chromosomes. The sex of the embryo is determined by the sperm (X or Y containing) that is successful in fertilization. Thus, if the embryo contains X chromosome, it is a female; while it is a male if it possesses Y chromosome. In the natural breeding, the sex ratio of progeny is close to 1:1.

It is possible to separate the sperms containing either X or Y chromosome, and use them selectively for the desired sex of the progeny.

By employing a fluorescent dye (Hoechst 33342) and an instrument namely ***fluorescent activated cell sorter (FACS),*** two populations of sperms (X or Y chromosome containing) can be separated. Using this approach and *in vitro* fertilization technique has produced pre- sexed calves.

FACS separation of sperms is expensive and time (about 24 hours)-consuming. Many sperms may die before they are actually separated. Attempts are being made to develop better separation techniques of sperms.

EMBRYO TRANSFER

As the ruminant animal produces one egg at time, it can carry one pregnancy at a time. It is possible to increase the production of female animals by increasing the number of mature eggs from a given female, fertilize them and transfer (implant) the embryos (fertilized eggs) into a ***foster mother (recipient***). The foster mother ***serves as an incubator, and does not make any genetic contribution to the offspring***.

Embryo transfer is a costly technique, and is selectively used for the production of animals of high genetic or economic valve.

Superovulation (multiple ovulation)

In the normal reproductive cycle of a non-pregnant female, one ovarian follicle (out of the 20 that develop) matures and ruptures, releasing one fertile egg at a time. The time of ovulation varies in different animals—21 days for cow and horse; 16 days for sheep and goat.

The circulating ***gonadotrophic hormone*** is closely associated with ovulation and release of egg. By increasing the concentration of this hormone, ***more ovarian follicles can be induced to ripen and produce more eggs.*** This process, known as superovulation or multiple ovulation may yield not less than 8-10 eggs at a time. Some animal breeders were successful in superovulating animals to yield as many as 60 eggs at a time. This largely depends on the breed, nutrition and health of the animal, besides the environmental factors.

By administering prostaglandin F_{2a} (PGF_{2a}) and follicle stimulating hormone (FSH), estrous can be induced. Artificial insemination is carried out in the superovulated females. AI is preferred to natural mating, since the purpose of superovulation is to genetically improve the progeny.

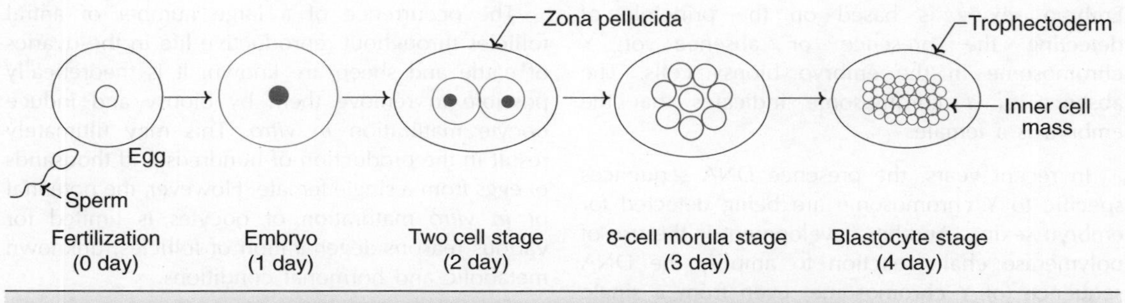

Fig. 18.1 : The early stages of embryo development.

As the eggs are fertilized, they undergo development to form embryos (***Fig. 18.1***).

Multiple ovulation with embryo transfer (MOET)

Sometimes, the process of multiple ovulation (superovulation described above) and embryo transfer are considered together which is referred to as MOET.

The embryos developed in the superovulated animals (described above) are recovered after 6-8 days of insemination. In case of cattle, the recovery process is easy and can be done by using a catheter. For certain animals with smaller reproductive tract, surgical procedures may be needed to expose the oviduct and recover the embryos. These embryos are examined microscopically and identified.

The embryos are then transferred into a synchronized recipient (i.e. the foster mother) by using a procedure, which is comparable to artificial insemination. Alternately, the embryos can be frozen and stored for use at an appropriate time and place later. About 50-60% of pregnancy could be achieved in cattle with transferred embryos. Thus, a superovulated female may result in 5-6 pregnancies.

The embryos may also be subjected to manipulations, as described below.

Embryo splitting

It is possible to increase the number of progenies (almost to double) by splitting the embryos. In addition, embryo splitting results in identical twins for various purposes (particularly genetic research).

Embryo splitting techniques have been refined, and are routinely used these days. The embryos are suspended in a hypertonic (high osmotic) sucrose and bovine serum albumin (BSA) containing culture medium. This results in shrinking of embryo cells and settling of the embryos to the bottom of the container (usually a petridish) due to increased density. Further, the embryos stick to the bottom due to electrostatic interaction of the negative charges on it (due to attachment of albumin) and the positive charges of the petridish. The inner cell mass (ICM) of the blastocyte can be bisected by using a surgical blade and a micromanipulation technique (with the help of an inverted microscope). Splitting of each embryo results in two equal halves.

As the embryos are split, each hemispherical cell mass reforms spheres. These split embryos can be transferred into the oviducts of synchronized recipients. The pregnancy rate with split embryos is about 5-10% less than the theoretical calculations. Thus, about 9 progencies (instead of only 5 in the original embryo transfer) can be developed through MOET.

By MOET, it is possible to produce at least four identical offsprings in animals at a time.

Embryo biopsy

Embryo biopsy involves the removal of a few cells from the embryo (mostly from the trophoblast cells of the trophectoderm) for analysis to determine the sex. In recent years, this technique is becoming popular for the detection of genetic diseases. By using embryo biopsy, it is possible to stop the transfer of embryos with genetic abnormalities and undesirable traits.

Embryo sexing

Before the transfer or implantation of the embryo, the progeny sex can be determined.

Embryo sexing is based on the principle of detecting the presence or absence of Y chromosome in the embryo biopsy cells. The absence of Y chromosome indicates that the embryo is a female.

In recent years, the presence DNA sequences specific to Y chromosome are being detected for embryo sexing. Another development is the use of polymerase chain reaction to amplify the DNA sequence (of Y chromosome) even from a single cell and determination the sex.

Limitations of embryo transfer

- The supply of embryo from superovulated donors is limited.
- Freezing and thawing of embryos requires a lot of care to keep them functionally intact.
- Embryo transfer requires technical skill, besides high cost factor.

IN VITRO FERTILIZATION

The limitations of embryo transfer could be successfully overcome by using *in vitro* fertilization (IVF). IVF basically involves fertilization of oocytes of a female animal in the laboratory conditions under artificial conditions. This is in contrast to the natural fertilization, which occurs in the uterus. IVF is reasonably successful as it results in 70–80% of the fertilized eggs.

Through IVF technology, a large number of offsprings can be produced from a single animal. Thus, a female animal, which normally produces 4-5 offsprings in her lifetime, can produce as many as 50–20 offsprings by employing IVF.

In vitro fertilization involves the following stages.

Oocyte recovery

During the course of estrous cycle, the ovarian follicles grow, get filled with fluid and become Graafian (antral) follicles. The oocytes from these follicls can be recovered by using laparoscopic surgery. It is possible to recover more number of oocytes from superovulated donors.

In vitro maturation (IVM) of oocytes

The immature oocytes recovered in the above step, when incubated *in vitro* will result in mature oocytes (eggs).

The occurrence of a large number of antral follicles throughout reproductive life in the ovaries of cattle and sheep are known. It is theoretically possible to remove them by biopsy and induce oocyte maturation *in vitro*. This may ultimately result in the production of hundreds and thousands of eggs from a single female. However, the potential of *in vitro* maturation of oocytes is limited for various reasons-degeneration of follicles, unknown metabolic and hormonal conditions.

Fertilization of eggs

In vitro fertilization of the eggs is carried out by using semen obtained from a superior male animal. For IVF, the eggs are carried in small droplets (microdroplets) of culture medium. Each microdroplet usually carries about 10 eggs. A dose of sperm approximately one million cells per ml is adequate for IVF. The penetration of the sperm into the egg is facilitated by supplementing the medium with certain compounds (penicillamine, epinephrine etc).

Embryo culture

The IVF embryos must be maintained in the *in vitro* conditions for a few days (about 7 days for sheep and goat, 8 days for cattle). This allows the development of embryos to blastocyte stage.

Approximately, 60% of the IVF embryos *in vitro* culture can form blastocytes.

Implantation of embryos

The 7 or 8 day old embryos from the *in vitro* culture are implanted in the reproductive tract of the recipient female which acts as a foster mother or surrogate mother.

Limitations of IVF

The pregnancy loss of IVF embryos, particularly during the first two months, is very high, although the reasons are not clearly known. The following parameters, which may be considered as limitations of IVF, may contribute to fetal losses of IVF embryos.

- Genetic defects in oocytes.
- Genetic defect in fertilizing sperms.
- Environmental mutagenesis.
- Inadequate supply of nutrients and hormones.
- Exposure to toxic agents and free radicals.

In recent years, some improvements have been made in IVF to minimize the fetal losses.

EMBRYO CLONING

A clone represents a population of cells or organisms derived from a single ancestor cell. Cloning basically means the production of identical copies of an individual.

It would be advantageous to increase the number of embryos from a particular embryo which possesses the desired characters. Two approaches are in use for embryo cloning.

1. Nuclear transfer.
2. Use of embryonic cells.

For more information on nuclear transfer and embryonic cells, the reader must refer the chapter on transgenic animals (Chapter 41).

MANIPULATIONS OF REPRODUCTION IN HUMANS

Assisted reproductive technology (ART) in humans is one of the greatest advances in reproductive medicine. ART has now become an accepted method for the treatment of infertile couple for whom there is no alternative therapy.

CAUSES OF INFERTILITY AND APPLICATION OF ART

Infertility in men and women may be due to a variety of reasons.

Male infertility

Oligospermia **:** Reduced concentration of sperms in semen (normal 15–20 million/ml).

Azoospermia : Total lack or very low concentration of motile sperm.

It is now possible to carry out ART even with a low concentration of motile sperms.

Female infertility

An outline of the female reproductive system with the essential organs is depicted in ***Fig 18.2.***

Tubal infertility : This occurs due to non-functional or damaged fallopian tubes. This can be corrected surgically or by tubal transplantation.

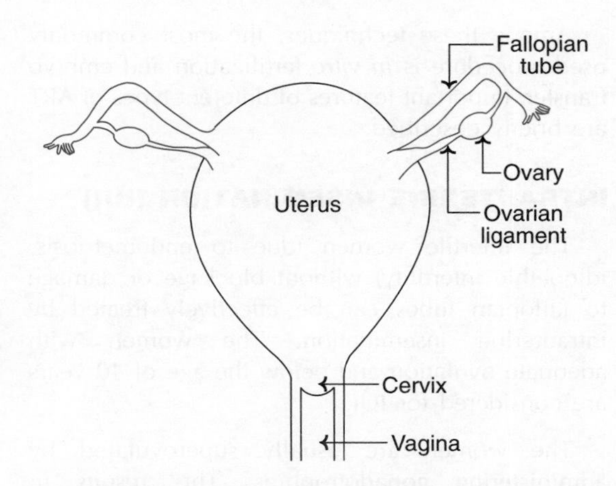

Fig. 18.2 : *An outline of the female reproduction organs.*

Non-functional ovaries : Some women may possess ovaries that are non-functional, or in some cases the ovaries may be totally absent. These women may serve as surrogate or foster mothers. The oocyte has to be obtained from a donar and ferlilized (*in vitro*) with the husbands' sperm.

Non-functional uterus : In some women, the uterus may be absent or non-functional. In such a case, the oocytes of these women can be fertilized by the husband's sperms, and then transferred into the uterus of surrogate mothers.

Idiopathic infertility : Some women may be infertile for unknown reasons which is regarded as idiopathic infertility. ART is useful for such women also.

The important ***techniques employed in assisted reproductive technology are listed*** below.

- Intrauterine insemination (IUI).
- *In vitro* fertilization and embryo transfer (IVF and ET).
- Gamete intrafallopian transfer (GIFT).
- Zygote intrafallopian transfer (ZIPT).
- Intravaginal culture (IVC).
- Cytoplasmic transfer (CT).
- Micromanipulation (Intracytoplasmic sperm injection (ICSI), subzonal insertion (SUZI).
- Cryopreservation.
- Assisted hatching (AH).

Among these techniques, the most commonly used procedure is *in vitro* fertilization and embryo transfer. Important features of different types of ART are briefly described.

INTRAUTERINE INSEMINATION (IUI)

The infertile women (due to endometriosis, idiopathic infertility) without blockage or damage to fallopian tubes can be effectively treated by intrauterine insemination. The women with adequate ovulation and below the age of 40 years are considered for IUI.

The women are usually superovulated by administering gonadotrophins. This results in multiple egg development. The IUI is timed to coincide with ovulation.

The semen is washed and the highly motile sperms are separated. By using a thin and soft catheter, the sperms are placed either in the cervix or in uterine cavity. The women subjects are advised to remain lying down for about 15-30 minutes following IUI.

Insemination should be carefully timed for good success. If it is done, a little before the expected time of ovulation, the chances for fertilization are much higher. IUI is usually successful in the first 3-4 attempts. In any case, this approach is not recommended for more than a maximum of 6 ovulation cycles.

The success rates of IUI vary considerably and are in the range of 15–30%.

IN VITRO FERTILIZATION AND EMBRYO TRANSFER (IVF and ET)

In vitro fertilization broadly deals with ***the removal of eggs from a women, fertilizing them in the laboratory, and then transferring the fertilized eggs (zygotes) into the uterus a few days later.***

Indications for IVF

Infertility due to the following causes may be considered for IVF.

- Failed ovulation induction
- Tubal diseases
- Cervical hostility
- Endometriosis
- Idiopathic infertility (in men and women).

Ideal subjects for IVF

Although it is not always possible to have a choice in the selection of subjects, the following criteria are preferred.

- Woman below 35 years.
- Presence of at least one functional ovary.
- Husband with normal motile sperm count (i.e. normal ***seminogram***).
- The couple must be negative for HIV and hepatitis.

METHODOLOGY OF IVF

The *in vitro* fertilization boardly involves the following steps.

1. Induction of superovulation.
2. Monitoring of ovarian response.
3. Oocyte retrieval.
4. Fertilization *in vitro.*
5. Embryo transfer.

Induction of superovulation

It is well known that the success rate IVF is much higher when more embryos (3-5) are transferred. This is possible only with ***controlled ovarian hyperstimulation (COH).*** The other advantages of COH include improvement in the quality of oocyte, control of ovulation timing, besides overcoming the ovulatory dysfunction. The following drug regimes are in use to induce superovulation.

- Clomiphene citrate (CC).
- CC + human menopausal gonadotrophin (hMG).
- CC + follicle stimulating hormone (FSH).
- Human menopausal gonadotrophin.
- Follicle stimulating hormone.
- Gonadotrophin releasing hormone agonists (GnRHa) + hMG (or FSH).

It is now common to use GnRH agonists to induce ovulation.

These compounds act through a process called downregulation of the physiologic hypothalamic-pituitary-ovarian feedback mechanism to effectively suppress spontaneous ovulation.

Monitoring of ovarian response

The follicular growth or ovarian response can be monitored by increase in serum estradiol level, increase in follicular diameter and thickening of endometrial bed.

Oocyte retrieval

The most common method for oocyte retrieval is carried out through vaginal route under ultrasound guidance. This method is simple and less invasive, and can be performed with analgesics only. It is easy to recognize the oocyte as a single cell surrounded by a mass of cumulus cells. The recovered oocytes are maintained *in vitro* culture for 4-6 hours.

Fertilization *in vitro*

The semen specimens are collected (just prior to oocyte retrival) via masturbation, processed, and incubated in protein-supplemented media for 3-4 hours prior to fertilization. The incubation results in sperm capacitation.

The retrieved oocytes are also cultured in protein-supplemented media for about 6-8 hours.

For the purpose of IVF, 50,000–1,00,000 capacitated sperms are placed in culture with a single oocyte. The signs of fertilization may be demonstrated 16–20 hours later by the presence of two pronuclei within the developing embryo.

There is no need to change the regime for a single failure of IVF. Many a times, success occurs in the subsequent cycles.

The two most important ***criteria for the success*** of IVF are ***sperm density and motility***.

Embryo transfer

Embryo at a stage between pronuclei and blastocyst stage are transferred. Conventionally, 4-8 cell stage embryos are transferred between 48–60 hours following insemination. The transfer procedure is carried out by use of a catheter. Not more than three embryos are transferred (per cycle) to minimize multiple pregnancies. However, in the women above the age of 40 years, higher number of embryo may be transferred. (**Note** : Excess oocytes and embryos are cryopreserved for further use. This will reduce the cost, besides the risk of ovarian hyperstimulation).

Luteal phase support is given by administration of progesterone for about two weeks. By this time, the diagnosis of pregnancy can be assessed by estimating human chorionic gonadotrophin (hCG).

SUCCESS RATES OF IVF

Success of IVF varies from programme to programme and within the same programme, the success rate is dependent on the correct diagnosis of the patient, and age.

The overall pregnancy rate in IVF is in the range of 25-35% per oocyte retrival. The ***take home baby rate is about 15-20%*** per procedure. The success rate of IVF is rather low due to the following reasons.

- Increased risk of abortion
- Multiple pregnancy
- Ectopic pregnancy
- Low birth weigh baby
- Premature delivery.

THE WORLD'S PICTURE OF TEST TUBE BABIES

By employing *in vitro* fertilization and embryo transfer, the world's ***first test tube baby*** (Louise Brown) was born in UK on 28th ***July 1978***. The world's second test tube baby (Kanupriya alias Durga) was born in Kolkata on 3rd October 1978. A team led by Subhash Mukherjee carried IVF and ET in India. Scientists responsible for the birth of test tube babies were severely criticized then.

In fact, IVF turned out to be one of the major achievements of medical sciences in the last century. It has become a novel way of treating infertility. Today, there are more than a million test tube babies born all over the world.

In 2003, the world celebrated the silver jubilee of IVF with much fanfare.

GAMETE INTRAFALLOPIAN TRANSFER (GIFT)

Gamete intrafallopian transfer involves the transfer of both sperm and unfertilized oocyte into the fallopian tube. This allows the fertilization to naturally occur *in vivo*. The prerequisite for GIFT procedure is that the woman should have at least one normal fallopian tube.

The induction of ovulation and the monitoring procedures for GIFT are almost the same as described for IVF. A couple of hours prior to oocyte retrieval, semen specimens are collected. Two oocytes along with 2-5 lakhs motile sperms for each fallopian tube are placed in a plastic tube container. It is then inserted (by laparoscopy) 4 cm into the distal end of the fallopian tube, and the oocyte sperm combination is injected.

The overall pregnancy rate is as high as 30-40%. The take home baby rate is about 25%. This is much higher when compared to IVF. But the ***major limitation*** is the requirement of ***laparoscopy*** (a major surgical procedure) to transfer oocytes and sperms into the fallopian tubes.

ZYGOTE INTRAFALLOPIAN TRANSFER (ZIFT)

ZIFT is suitable when the infertility lies in men, or in case of failure of GIFT.

The wife's oocytes are exposed to her husband's sperms in the laboratory. The fertilized eggs (zygotes) within 24 hours are transferred to the fallopian tube by using laparoscopy.

ZIPT has an advantage over GIFT with male factor infertility. Further, it can be known whether the wife's oocytes have been fertilized by her husbands' sperms.

INTRAVAGINAL CULTURE (IVC)

The ***body's own environment*** is appropriately ***utilized*** in intravaginal culture. The retrieved oocytes and sperms are placed in a culture medium inside a sealed container. This is inserted into the vagina. The container is held by a vaginal diaphragm. Thus, the oocytes and sperms are maintained at the normal body temperature (in contrast to any incubator in the laboratory). Two to 3 three days later, the container is opened, and the fertilized and dividing zygotes are transferred into the uterus.

This procedure appears simple, but the success rate is very low. Only a few centers practice this.

CYTOPLASMIC TRANSFER (CT)

Cytoplasm includes many things, the most important being mitochondria which provide energy to the cell. It is possible that deficiency in the mitochondria may leave the oocyte without the necessary power for cell division, after fertilization. This may result in abnormal cell division and poor development of embryo.

It is therefore logical to think of the transfer of cytoplasm from a donor (with active mitochondria) into the oocyte of a woman. The advantage with cytoplasmic transfer is that the ***mother's own genetic material is passed on to the offspring***.

Two methods of cytoplasmic transfer have been developed.

1. Transfer of a small amount of cytoplasm by a tiny needle from a donor to a recipient oocyte.

2. Transfer of a large amount of cytoplasm which is fused with the recipient's cytoplasm by applying electricity.

The procedure of cytoplasmic transfer is tedious and technically difficult, besides the cost factor. At least two viable pregnancies have been so far reported in literature by this approach.

MICROMANIPULATION

Micromanipulation involves *in vitro* microsurgically assisted fertilization procedures. This is required when the sperms are unable to penetrate the zona pellucida of oocyte and fertilize. Micromanipulations are usually done in severe cases of male factor infertility.

A diagrammatic representation of micro-manipulation is depicted in ***Fig 18.3.***

Intracytoplasmic sperm injection (ICSI)

Intracytoplasmic sperm injection is a new and novel infertility treatment utilizing the micromanipulation technology. Many of the previous treatment processes for male infertility have been abandoned in favour of ICSI. The male factor infertility could be due to low sperm counts, poor sperm motility, and poor quality of sperm to penetrate oocyte.

By ***partial zona dissection (PZD)***, the zona pellucida is opened using either chemical dissolution or a sharp instrument. A single

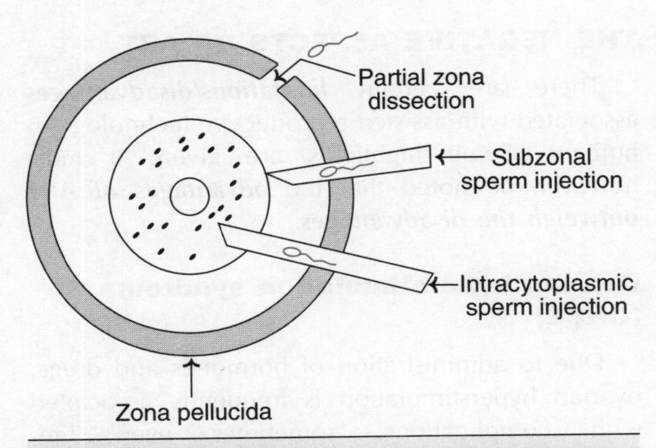

***Fig. 18.3 :** Micromanipulation for fertilization of an egg (microsurgically assisted fertilization).*

spermatozoon can be directly injected into the cytoplasm of the oocyte through the micropuncture of zona pellucida. A micropipette is used to hold the oocyte while the spermatozoon is deposited inside the ooplasm of the oocyte.

Besides using normal sperms, round-headed sperms, sperms collected directly form the epididymis and previously cryopreserved sperms can be used in ICSI.

Among the ***micromanipulation techniques ICSI*** is the ***most successful one*** with a fertilization rate of about 65%. Attempts are on to improve this further. In fact, ICSI has revolutionized assistant reproductive technology by utilizing the sperms of husbands who were once considered to be unsuitable for fertilization process.

Subzonal insertion (SUZI)

In subzonal insertion, the zona pellucida is punctured and sperms (1-30 in number) are injected into an area between the zona and the egg. It is expected that one of the sperms will fertilize the egg.

The major limitation of SUZI is polyspermy since it is not possible to control the number of sperms that enter the egg.

Round spermid nucleus injection (ROSNI)

There are a few men who cannot manufacture sperms, and therefore they have a zero sperm count. For these men, it is possible to take out the round spermatids (immature cells) directly from the testicle, isolate the nucleus (containing the genetic material) and inject it into the partner's eggs.

ROSNI is a recent exciting breakthrough to solve the problem of male infertility through micromanipulation.

CRYOPRESERVATION

Preservation in a frozen state is regarded as cryopreservation. Cryopreservation is very useful in assisted reproductive technology.

- Semen can be cryopreserved. This may be from the donors, cancer patients (before the commencement of treatment).
- Fertilized eggs after IVP or ICSI can be preserved.
- Embryos can also be preserved for transfer at a later stage.

Human embryos have been successfully preserved in the presence of cryoprotectants (1, 2-propanediol/dimethyl sulfoxide/glycerol) and stored at –196°C under liquid nitrogen. At appropriate time, the embryos are thawed, cryoprotectants removed and then transferred. Many test tube babies in fact have been born as a result of application of ***freezing technology***.

ASSISTED HATCHING (AH)

Improper implantation of the embryo in the uterus is one of the limiting factors in the success of ART in humans. Assisted hatching is a novel approach for the proper implantation of the embryo in the endrometrium.

The embryos in the uterus possess an outer coating namely zona pellucida (the shell). These embryos must be hatched to remove the shell, a step necessary for implantation. In certain women, particularly above 40 years age, natural hatching does not occur, and requires outside assistance.

Assisted hatching is carried out by using a Laser to make a small hole in the shell of the embryo. These embryos when transferred into the uterus, hatch and get implanted.

During the course of AH for 3-4 days, the women are kept on steroids (to suppress mother's immunity) and antibiotics (to counter infections). Better results are reported with this approach.

PREIMPLANTATION GENETIC DIAGNOSIS (PGD)

The genetic defects in ovum before fertilization or in the embryo before implantation can be identified by a ***new medical tool*** namely preimplantation genetic diagnosis. It is estimated that about 60% of the ART driven pregnancies are lost due to chromosomal abnormalities. This can be minimized or prevented by using PGD.

A direct determination of chromosomal abnormalities prior to implantion ensures a successful pregnancy and ultimate delivery of a healthy baby. One group of workers has reported an increase in the pregnancy rate from 15 to 30% by employing preimplantation genetic diagnosis.

DNA amplification and analysis

The latest in PGD is the direct DNA analysis. This can be carried out by removing a single cell from 6-8-cell embryo. The DNA is removed and amplified by employing polymerase chain reaction.

Direct DNA analysis is useful for the diagnosis of several genetic diseases e.g. cystic fibrosis, sickle-cell anemia, hemophilia, Duchene's muscular dystrophy, Tay-Sachs disease.

Ethical advantages of PGD

PGD is highly advantageous from the ethical point of view, since the embryos with genetic disorders can be discarded in the very stages without the formation of offsprings with undesirable characteristics.

THE NEGATIVE ASPECTS OF ART

There are certain ***limitations/disadvantages*** associated with assisted reproductive technology in humans. Some highlights are given. It must however, be noted that the ***advantages of ART outweigh the disadvantages***.

Ovarian hyperstimulation syndrome (OHSS)

Due to administration of hormones and drugs, ovarian hyperstimulation is frequently associated with complications, sometimes even life-threatening. OHSS is more severe in women who conceived in the same cycle, and received hCG as luteal support (following embryo transfer).

Risks associated with pregnancy

ART is associated with multiple pregnancy, increased risk for anemia, gestational diabetes and premature labour. Low birth weight and prematurity are closed linked with mortality and morbidity.

Premature menopause

Controlled ovarian hyperstimulation (COH) causes multiple follicular utility. There is a risk of premature menopause as COH may reduce the ovarian follicles, besides faster aging. Sometimes, a single COH may use ovarian follicles, which in the normal course are equivalent to two years of ovulation during the natural menstrual cycle.

Ovarian cancer

The use of fertility drugs and injuries to epithelium increase the risk of ovarian cancer at least by three times when compared to normal women.

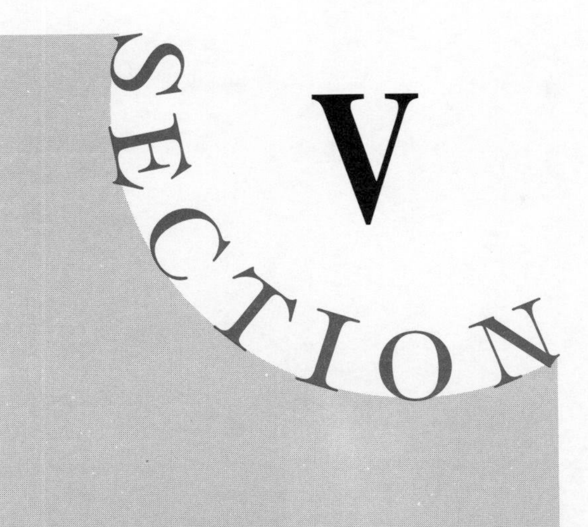

MICROBIAL/ INDUSTRIAL BIOTECHNOLOGY

CONTENTS

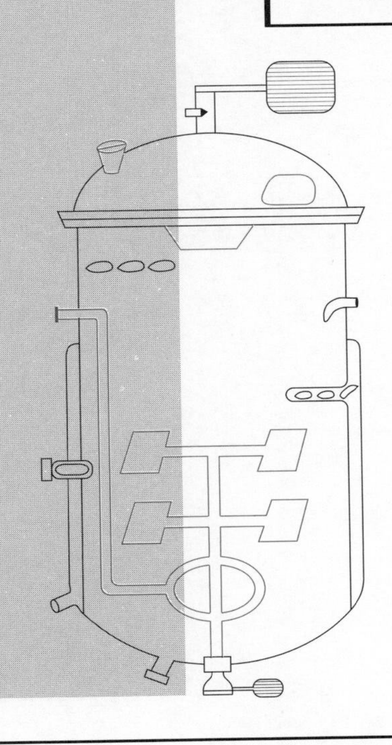

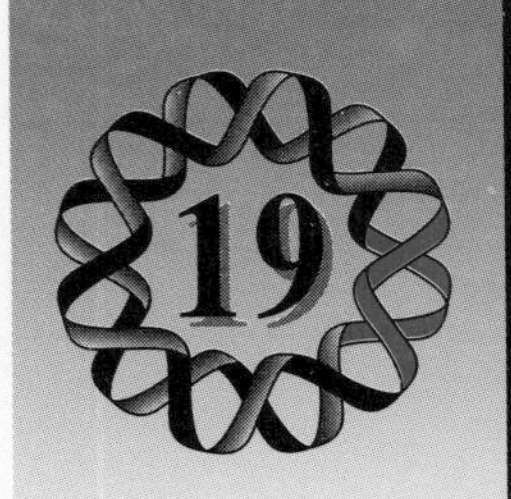

Bioprocess/Fermentation Technology

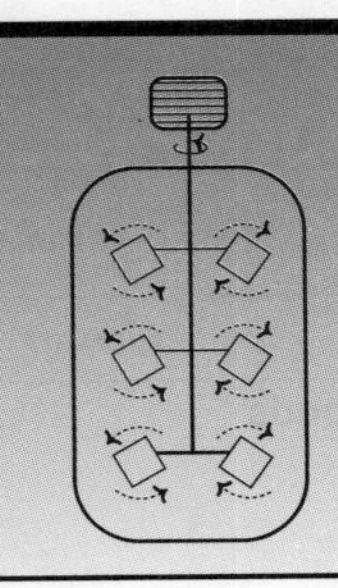

For many centuries, man has been exploiting microorganisms for the production of foods (bread, cheese, yoghurts, pickles) and beverages (beer, wine). However, the organized use of microorganism for industrial purposes is about one and a half century old.

The word ***fermentation*** originates from a *Latin* verb ***fervere*** which literally means ***to boil***. During the production of alcohol (the first truely industrialised process), the gas bubbles (of CO_2) appear at the surface of the boiling liquid. ***Fermentation in a strict sense is a biological process that occurs in the absence of oxygen (anaerobic)***. This definition however, is no more valid, since the term ***industrial fermentation*** is now used for large-scale cultivation of microorganisms, even though ***most of them are aerobic*** (use oxygen).

Bioprocess technology is a more recent usage to replace fermentation technology. Bioprocessing broadly involves a multitude of enzyme-catalysed reactions carried out by living cells (or cell-free systems) for industrial purposes. Some workers prefer to use ***bioprocess technology*** for industrial use of ***higher plant and animal cells*** while ***fermentation technology*** is confined to ***microbial use***. This demarcation is however, not very rigid.

Bioprocess/fermentation technology is very widely exploited for industrial applications. The broad range of fermentation products are listed in ***Table 19.1***.

BIOREACTORS/FERMENTERS

The heart of fermentation (or bioprocessing) technology is the fermenter (or bioreactor). *A* ***bioreactor is basically a device in which the organisms (cells) are cultivated and motivated to form the desired product(s)***. It is a ***containment system*** designed to give right environment for optimal growth and metabolic activity of the organism.

A ***fermenter*** usually refers to the containment system for the ***cultivation of prokaryotic cells*** (bacteria, fungi), while a ***bioreactor*** grows the ***eukaryotic cells*** (mammalian, insect).

Traditional fermenters are open vats made up of wood or slate. In recent years, stainless steel bioreactors are in use. A high quality stainless steel that does not corrode or leak toxic metals into the growth medium is used. The size of a bioreactor is highly variable, ranging from 20 litres to 250 million litres or even more.

TYPES OF BIOREACTORS

Based on the designs of the bioreactors, they can be grouped into the following types (***Figs. 19.1–19.4***)

1. Continuous stirred tank bioreactors
2. Bubble column bioreactors
3. Airlift bioreactors
4. Fluidized bed bioreactors

TABLE 19.1 Industrial products of fermentation (bioprocess) technology

Group	*Products*
Foods	Dairy products (cheese, yogurt) Vitamins (B_1, B_{12}) Amino acids (glutamic acid, lysine) Glucose and high fructose syrup Mushroom products Baker's yeast Food additives (antioxidants, colours, flavours) Beverages (beer, wine, whisky)
Chemicals	
Organic (bulk)	Ethanol, butanol, acetone, organic acids (citric acid, gluconic acid, lactic acid)
Organic (fine)	Enzymes, polymers (xanthan, dextran)
Inorganic	Bioaccumulation and leaching (Cu, U)
Pharmaceuticals (healthcare)	Antibiotics Vaccines Steroids Diagnostic enzymes Monoclonal antibodies Enzyme inhibitors
Agriculture	Single–cell protein Microbial pesticides Composting processes Plant cell and tissue culture

5. Packed bed bioreactors
6. Photobioreactors.

In all types of bioreactors, the ultimate aim is to ensure that all parts of the system are subjected to the same conditions.

Continuous stirred tank bioreactors

A continuous stirred tank bioreactor consists of a cylindrical vessel with motor driven central shaft that supports one or more ***agitators (impellers)***. The shaft is fitted at the bottom of the bioreactor (***Fig. 19.1A***). The number of impellers is variable and depends on the size of the bioreactor i.e., height to diameter ratio, referred to as ***aspect ratio***. The aspect ratio of a stirred tank bioreactor is usually between 3–5. However, for animal cell culture applications, the aspect ratio is less than 2. The diameter of the impeller is usually $\frac{1}{3}$rd of the vessel diameter. The distance between two impellers is approximately 1.2 impeller diameter. Different types of impellers (Rustom disc, concave bladded, marine propeller etc.) are in use.

In stirred tank bioreactors or in short ***stirred tank reactors (STRs)***, the air is added to the culture medium under pressure through a device called ***sparger***. The sparger may be a ring with many holes or a tube with a single orifice. The sparger along with impellers (agitators) enables better gas distribution system throughout the vessel. The bubbles generated by sparger are broken down to smaller ones by impellers and dispersed throughout the medium. This enables the creation of a uniform and homogeneous environment throughout the bioreactor.

Advantages of STRs : There are many advantages of STRs over other types. These include the efficient gas transfer to growing cells, good mixing of the contents and flexible operating conditions, besides the commercial availability of the bioreactors.

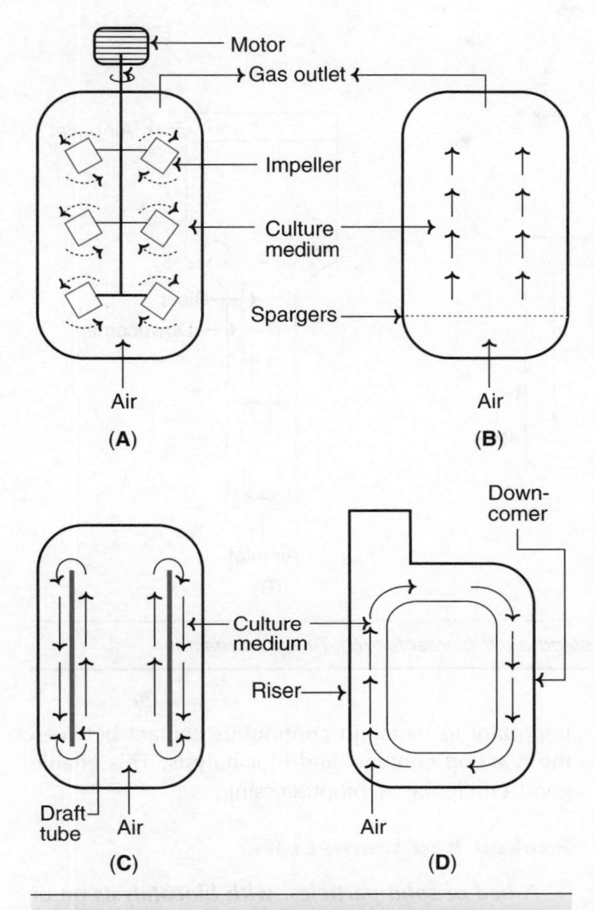

*Fig. 19.1 : Types of bioreactors **(A)** Continuous stirred tank bioreactor **(B)** Bubble column bioreactor **(C)** Internal-loop airlift bioreactor **(D)** External-loop airlift bioreactor.*

Bubble column bioreactors

In the bubble column bioreactor, the air or gas is introduced at the base of the column through perforated pipes or plates, or metal microporous ***spargers*** (***Fig. 19.1B***). The flow rate of the air/gas influences the performance factors — O_2 transfer, mixing. The bubble column bioreactors may be fitted with perforated plates to improve performance. The vessel used for bubble column bioreactors is usually cylindrical with an aspect ratio of 4-6 (i.e., height to diameter ratio).

Airlift bioreactors

In the airlift bioreactors, the medium of the vessel is divided into two interconnected zones by means of a baffle or draft tube. In one of the two zones referred to a ***riser***, the air/gas is pumped. The other zone that receives no gas is the ***downcomer***. The dispersion flows up the riser zone while the down flow occurs in the downcomer. There are two types of airlift bioreactors.

Internal-loop airlift bioreactor (***Fig. 11.1C***) has a single container with a central draft tube that creates interior liquid circulation channels. These bioreactors are simple in design, with volume and circulation at a fixed rate for fermentation.

External loop airlift bioreactor (***Fig. 19.1D***) possesses an external loop so that the liquid circulates through separate independent channels. These reactors can be suitably modified to suit the requirements of different fermentations. In general, the airlift bioreactors are more efficient than bubble columns, particularly for more denser suspensions of microorganisms. This is mainly because in these bioreactors, the mixing of the contents is better compared to bubble columns.

Airlift bioreactors are commonly ***employed for aerobic bioprocessing technology***. They ensure a controlled liquid flow in a recycle system by pumping. Due to high efficiency, airlift bioreactors are sometimes preferred e.g., methanol production, waste water treatment, single-cell protein production. In general, the performance of the airlift bioreactors is dependent on the pumping (injection) of air and the liquid circulation.

Two-stage airlift bioreactors

Two-stage airlift bioreactors are ***used for the temperature dependent formation of products***. Growing cells from one bioreactor (maintained at temperature 30°C) are pumped into another bioreactor (at temperature 42°C). There is a necessity for the two-stage airlift bioreactor, since it is very difficult to raise the temperature quickly from 30°C to 42°C in the same vessel. Each one of the bioreactors is fitted with valves and they are connected by a transfer tube and pump (***Fig. 19.2A***). The cells are grown in the first bioreactor and the bioprocess proper takes place in the second reactor.

Tower bioreactors

A ***pressure-cycle fermenter*** with large dimensions constitutes a tower bioreactor (***Fig. 19.2B***). A high hydrostatic pressure generated

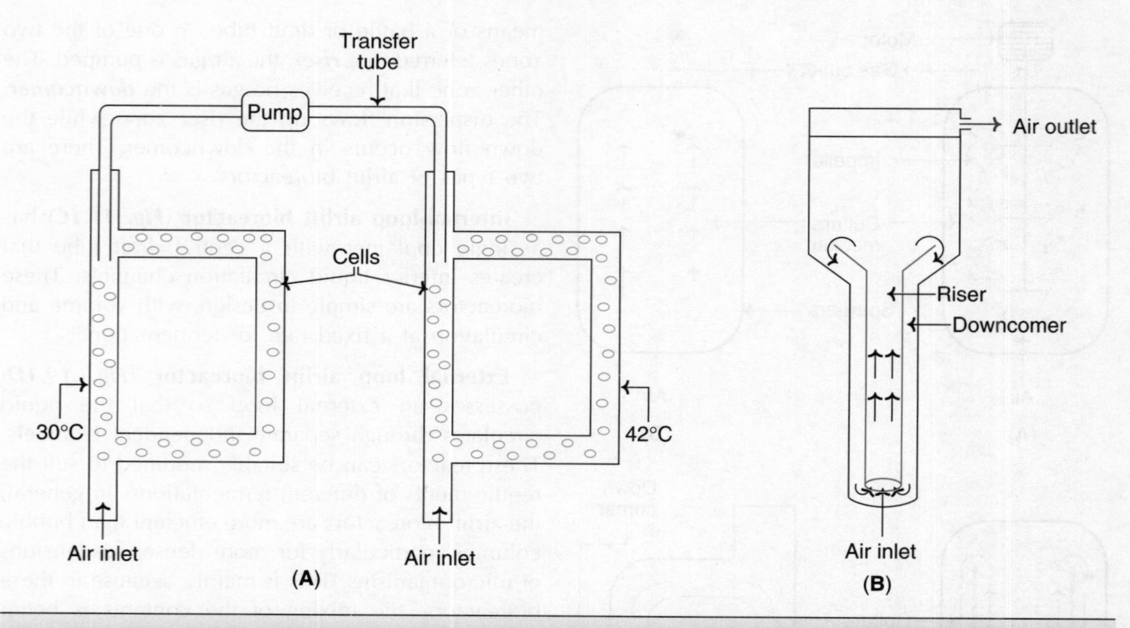

*Fig. 19.2 : Types of bioreactors (**A**) Two–stage airlift bioreactor (**B**) Tower bioreactor.*

at the bottom of the reactor increases the solubility of O_2 in the medium. At the top of the riser, (with expanded top) reduces pressure and facilitates expulsion of CO_2. The medium flows back in the downcomer and completes the cycle. The advantage with tower bioreactor is that it has high aeration capacities without having moving parts.

Fluidized bed bioreactors

Fluidized bed bioreactor is comparable to bubble column bioreactor except the top position is expanded to reduce the velocity of the fluid. The design of the fluidized bioreactors (expanded top and narrow reaction column) is such that the solids are retained in the reactor while the liquid flows out (***Fig. 19.3A***). These bioreactors are suitable for use ***to carry out reactions involving fluid suspended biocatalysts such as immobilized enzymes***, immobilized cells, microbial flocs.

For an efficient operation of fludized beds, gas is sparged to create a suitable gas-liquid-solid fluid bed. It is also necessary to ensure that the suspended solid particles are not too light or too dense (too light ones may float whereas to dense ones may settle at the bottom), and they are in a good suspended state. Recycling of the liquid is important to maintain continuous contact between the reaction contents and biocatalysts. This enable good efficiency of bioprocessing.

Packed bed bioreactors

A ***bed of solid particles, with biocatalysts*** on or within the matrix of solids, packed in a column constitutes a packed bed bioreactor (***Fig. 19.3B***). The solids used may be porous or non-porous gels, and they may be compressible or rigid in nature. A nutrient broth flows continuously over the immobilised biocatalyst. The products obtained in the packed bed bioreactor are released into the fluid and removed. While the flow of the fluid can be upward or downward, downflow under gravity is preferred.

The concentration of the nutrients (and therefore the products formed) can be increased by increasing the flow rate of the nutrient broth. Because of poor mixing, it is rather difficult to control the pH of packed bed bioreactors by the addition of acid or alkali. However, these bioreactors are preferred for bioprocessing technology involving product-inhibited reactions. The packed bed bioreactors do not allow accumulation of the products to any significant extent.

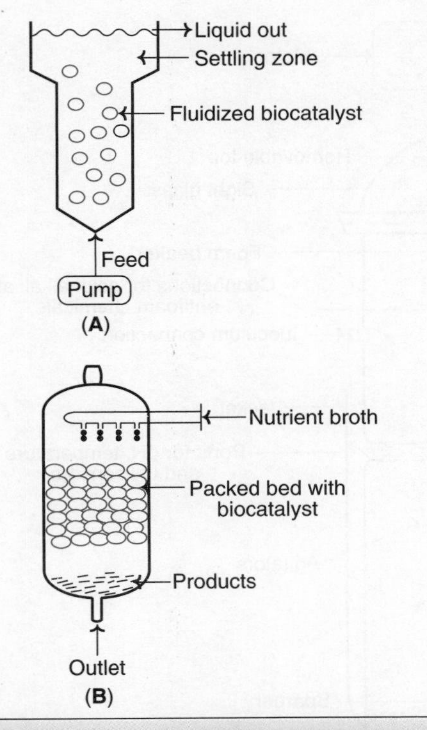

Fig. 19.3 : Types of bioreactors (A) Fluidized bed bioreactor (B) Packed bed bioreactor.

Photobioreactors

These are the bioreactors ***specialised for fermentation*** that can be carried out either ***by exposing to sunlight or artificial illumination***. Since artificial illumination is expensive, only the out door photobioreactors are preferred. Certain important compounds are produced by employing photobioreactors e.g., β-carotene, asthaxanthin.

The different types of photobioreactors are depicted in ***Fig. 19.4***. They are made up of glass or more commonly transparent plastic. The array of tubes or flat panels constitute light receiving systems (solar receivers). The culture can be circulated through the solar receivers by methods such as using centrifugal pumps or airlift pumps. It is essential that the cells are in continuous circulation without forming sediments. Further adequate penetration of sunlight should be maintained. The tubes should also be cooled to prevent rise in temperature.

Photobioreactors are usually operated in a continuous mode at a temperature in the range of

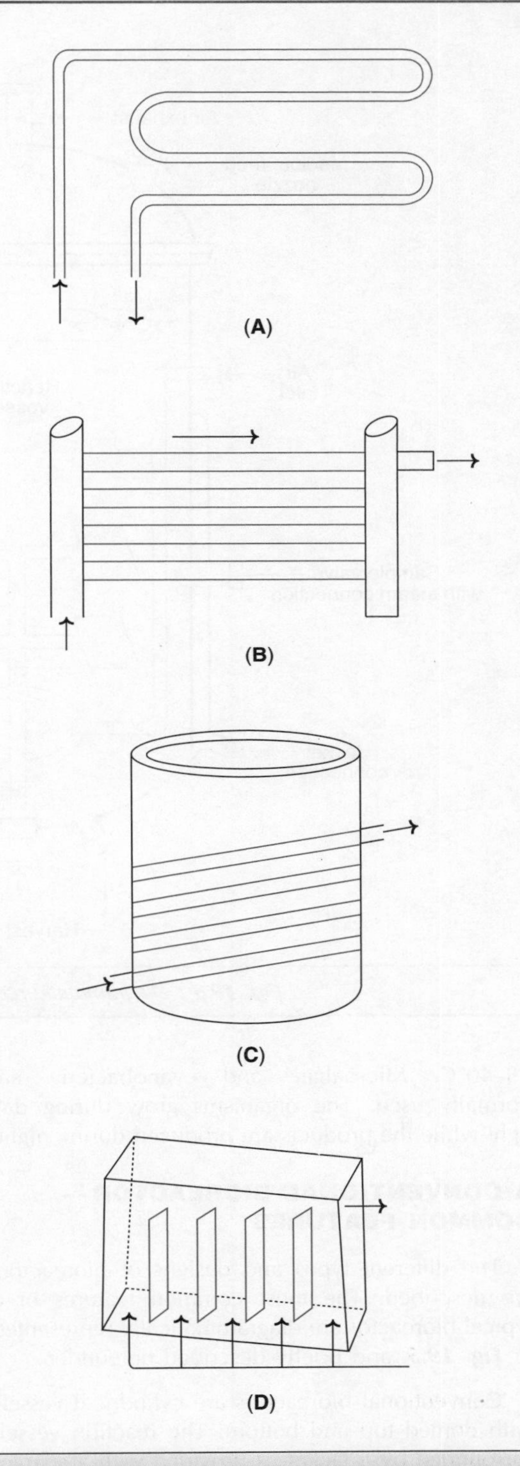

Fig. 19.4 : Types of photobioreactors (A) Continuous run tubular loop (B) Multiple parallel tube (C) Helical wound tubular loop (D) Flat panel configuration.

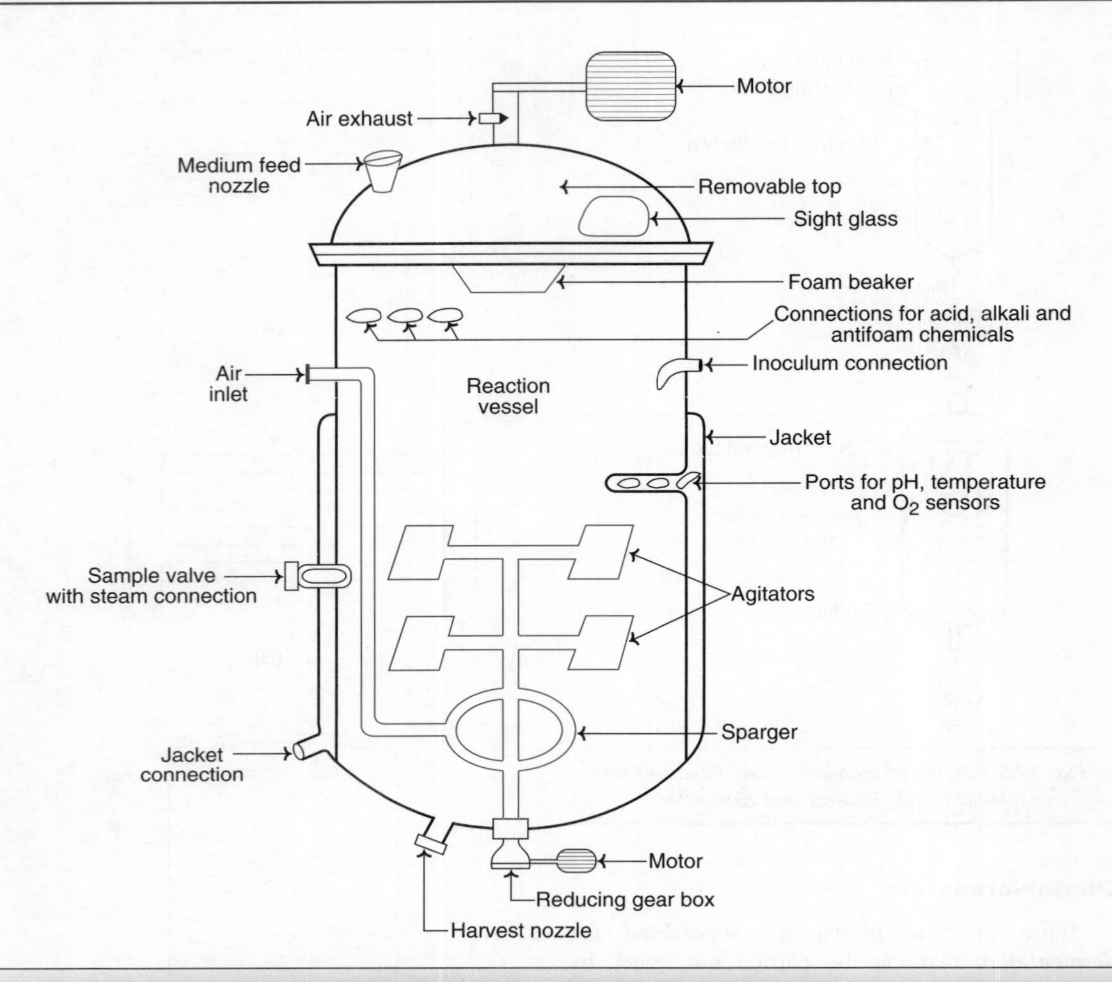

Fig. 19.5 : Diagrammatic representation of a typical bioreactor.

25–40°C. Microalgae and cyanobacteria are normally used. The organisms grow during day light while the products are produced during night.

A CONVENTIONAL BIOREACTOR — COMMON FEATURES

The different types and designs of bioreactors are described. The most common features of a typical bioreactor are diagrammatically represented in ***Fig. 19.5***, and briefly described hereunder.

Conventional bioreactors are cylindrical vessels with domed top and bottom. The reaction vessel, surrounded by a jacket, is provided with a sparger at the bottom through which air (or other gases such as CO_2 and NH_3 for pH maintenance) can be introduced. The agitator shaft is connected to a motor at the bottom. The reaction vessel has side ports for pH, temperature and dissolved O_2 sensors. Above the liquid level of the reaction vessel, connections for acid, alkali, antifoam chemicals and inoculum are located.

The bioreactor is usually designed to work at higher temperature (150–180°C), higher pressure (377-412 kPa). The reaction vessel is also designed to withstand vaccum, or else it may collapse while cooling. The materials used for the construction of bioreactor must be non-toxic and must withstand the repeated sterilization with high pressure steam.

The bioreactor vessel is usually made up of stainless steel. It should be free from crevices and stagnant areas so that no solids/liquids accumulate. Easy to clean channels and welded joints (instead of couplings) are preferred. Transparent material should be used wherever possible, since it is advantageous to inspect medium and culture frequently.

OPERATION OF A CONVENTIONAL BIOREACTOR

The operation of a bioreactor basically involves the following steps.

1. Sterilization
2. Inoculation and sampling
3. Aeration
4. Control systems
5. Cleaning.

STERILIZATION

Aseptic conditions are the basic requirements for successful fermentation. That is the bioreactor and its accessories, the growth medium and the air supplied during fermentation must be sterile.

In situ sterilization

The bioreactor filled with the required medium is injected with pressurized steam into the jacket or coil surrounding the reaction vessel. The ***whole system is heated to about 120°C*** and held at this temperature ***for about 20 minutes***. *In situ* sterilization has certain limitations. It is not energy-efficient (i.e., energy is wasted) since the bioreactor has to be heated for a long period to rise the temperature of the whole system to 120°C. Prolonged heating may destroy vitamins, besides precipitating the medium components.

Continuous heat sterilization

In this technique, empty bioreactor is first sterilized by injecting pressurised steam. The ***medium is rapidly heated to 140°C for a short period***, by injecting the pressurised steam. Alternately, the medium can be sterilized by passing through a heat exchanger heated by pressurised steam. Subjecting the medium to high temperature for a short period does not precipitate medium components. Further, there is no energy wastage in continuous heat sterilization method.

INOCULATION AND SAMPLING

The bioreactor with the growth medium under aseptic conditions is ready for inoculation with the production organism. The size of the inoculum is generally 1–10% of the total volume of the medium. A high yielding production strain of the organism taken from a stock culture (lyophilized and stored in a deep freezer or in liquid nitrogen) is used.

During the course of fermentation, samples are regularly drawn from the bioreactor. This is required to check the contamination (if any) and measurement of the product formed.

AERATION

Aeration of the fermentation medium is ***required to supply O_2 to the production organisms and remove CO_2 from the bioreactor***. The aeration system is designed for good exchange of gases. Oxygen (stored in tanks in a compressed form) is introduced at the bottom of the bioreactor through a ***sparger***. The small bubbles of the air pass through the medium and rise to the surface. The bioreactor usually has about 20% of its volume as vacant space on the upper part which is referred to as ***head space***. The bioreactor has about 80% ***working volume***. The gases released during fermentation accumulate in the headspace which pass out through an air outlet.

Air-lift system of aeration

In this type of aeration, ***sparging of air is done at the bottom of the fermenter***. This allows an upward flow of air bubbles. The more is the aeration capacity of the fermenter, the more is the dissolved O_2 in the medium. Further, the aeration capacity of the air-lift system is directly proportional to the air-flow rate and the internal pressure. Oxygen demand refers to the rate at which the growing culture requires O_2. For all the aerobic organisms, the aeration capacity should be more than the oxygen demand or else the growth of the organisms will be inhibited due to oxygen depletion (starvation).

Stirred system of aeration

The ***aeration capacity*** of the medium can be ***enhanced by stirring***. This can be done by using impellers driven by a motor. The aeration capacity of the stirred fermenter is proportional to the stirring speed, rate of air flow and the internal pressure.

Stirred fermenters are better suited than air-lift fermenters to produce better aeration capacities.

CONTROL SYSTEMS

It is essential to maintain optimal growth environment in the reaction vessel for maximum product formation. ***Maximal efficiency of the fermentation can be achieved by continuously monitoring the variables*** such as the pH, temperature, dissolved oxygen, adequate mixing, nutrient concentration and foam formation. Improved sensors are now available for continous and automated monitoring of these variables (i.e., on line measurement of pH).

Most of the microorganisms employed in fermentation grow optimally between pH 5.5 and 8.5. In the bioreactor, as the microorganisms grow, they release metabolites into the medium which change pH. Therefore, the pH of the medium should be continuously monitored and maintained at the optimal level. This can be done by the addition of acid or alkali base (as needed) and a thorough mixing of the fermentation contents. Sometimes, an acid or alkaline medium component can be used to correct pH, besides providing nutrients to the growing microorganisms.

Temperature

Temperature control is absolutely essential for a good fermentation process. Lower temperature causes reduced product formation while higher temperature adversely affects the growth of microorganisms. The bioreactors are normally equipped with heating and cooling systems that can be used as per the requirement, to maintain the reaction vessel at optimal temperature.

Dissolved oxygen

Oxygen is sparingly soluble in water (0.0084 g/1 at 25°C). Continuous supply of oxygen in the form of sterilized air is done to the culture medium. This is carried out by introducing air into the bioreactor in the form of bubbles. Continuous monitoring of dissolved oxygen concentration is done in the bioreactor for optimal product formation.

Adequate mixing

Continuous and adequate mixing of the microbial culture ensures optimal supply of nutrients and O_2, besides preventing the accumulation of toxic metabolic byproducts (if any). Good mixing (by agitation) also creates favourable environment for optimal and homogeneous growth environment, and good product formation. However, excessive agitation may damage microbial cells and increase the temperature of the medium, besides increased foam formation.

Nutrient concentration

The nutrient concentration in a bioreactor is limited so that its wastage is prevented. In addition, limiting concentrations of nutrients may be advantageous for optimal product formation, since high nutrient concentrations are often associated with inhibitory effect on microbial growth. It is now possible to do on-line monitoring of the nutrient concentration, and suitably modify as per the requirements.

Foam formation

The media used in industrial fermentation is generally rich in proteins. When agitated during aeration, it invariably results in froth or foam formation that builds in head space of the bioreactor. Antifoam chemicals are used to lower surface tension of the medium, besides causing foam bubbles to collapse. Mineral oils based on silicone or vegetable oils are commonly used as antifoam agents.

Mechanical foam control devices, referred to as mechanical foam breakers, can also be used. Such devices, fitted at the top of the bioreactor break the foam bubbles and the throw back into the fermentation medium.

CLEANING

As the fermentation is complete, the bioreactor is ***harvested*** i.e. the contents are removed for processing. The bioreactor is then prepared for the next round of fermentation after cleaning (technically called ***turn round***). The ***time taken for turn round***, referred to as ***down time***, should be as short as possible (since it is non-productive). Due to large size of the bioreactors, it is not possible to clean manually. The cleaning of the bioreactors is carried out by using high-pressure water jets from the nozzles fitted into the reaction vessel.

TABLE 19.2 A selected list of solid state fermentations

Product	*Substrate*	*Microorganism(s) involved*
Edible mushrooms	Straw manure	*Agaricus bisporus*
		Lentinula edodes
Cheeses	Milk, curd	*Penicillium roquefortii*
Soy sauce	Soy beans, wheat	*Aspergillus oryzae*
Sauekraut	Cabbage	Lactic acid bacteria
Enzymes	Wheat bran	*Aspergillus niger*
Organic acids	Cane sugar, molasses	*Aspergillus niger*
Leaching of metals	Low grade ores	*Thiobacillus sp.*
Composting	Mixed organic material	Fungi, bacteria, actinomycetes
Sewage treatment	Sewage components	Bacteria, fungi, protozoa

SOLID SUBSTRATE (SOLID STATE) FERMENTATION

There are certain fermentation processes that do not involve liquid medium. For these biotechnological processes, the ***growth of the microorganisms is carried out on solid substrates*** in the complete absence or almost complete absence of free water. The presence of some moisture (about 15%) is necessary for solid substrate (or solid state) fermentation (***SSF***). The most commonly used solid substrates for SSF are cereal grains, wheat bran, sawdust, wood shavings and several other plant and animal materials. These solid substrates are polymeric in nature, insoluble or sparingly soluble in water, and contain concentrated source of nutrients for the growth of microorganisms.

SSF is a very old traditional technique carried out in many countries. It is used for the production of ***edible mushrooms***, cheese, soy sauce and many other fermented products (including enzymes and organic acids). A selected list of solid state fermentations is given ***Table 19.2***. ***Composting is a good example of SSF***.

Solid substrate fermentation has been very popular ***for the production of fermented foods*** (idli, dosa, dhokla, bread, beverages, fermented fish, meat, yogurt, cheese, pickles). Fermentation often makes the food more nutritious, easily digestable and better in flavour.

For solid substrate fermentation, single pure cultures, mixed cultures or mixed organisms may be used. Pretreatment of substrate raw materials is sometimes done to facilitate the availability of nutrients.

Solid substrate fermentation is normally carried out as a non-aseptic process. This ***saves sterilization costs***. It is important that the substrates used in SSF have adequate spaces in between to allow good air circulation. This facilitates adequate exchange of gases, besides promoting heat elimination. Forced air circulation may be done to maintain optimal conditions in SSF.

Bioreactors for SSF

Bioreactors designed for solid state fermentation are much simpler compared to liquid-state fermentation. In the ***Fig 19.6***, ***tower reactor, drum reactor*** and ***forced aeration reactor***, used in SSF are depicted.

Advantages of SSF

- Solid substrate fermentation employs simple natural solids as the media.
- Low technology, low energy expenditure and requires less capital investment.
- No need for sterilization, less microbial contamination and easy downstream processing.
- Yield of the products is reasonably high.
- Bioreactor design, aeration process, and effluent treatment are quite simple.

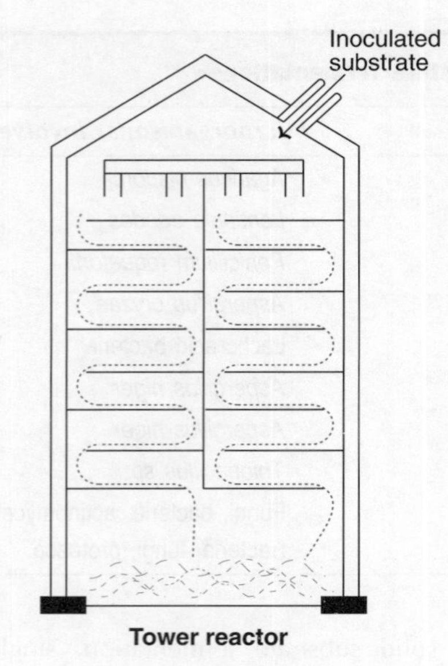

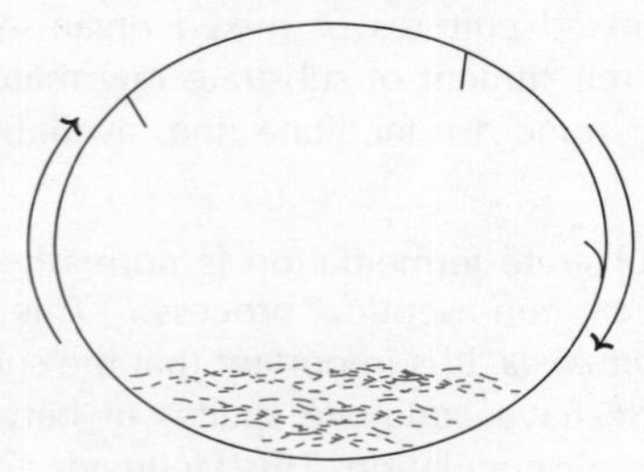

Solid substrate
Humidification temperature control
Forced air flow
Forced aeration reactor

Fig. 19.6 : Bioreactors for solid–substrate fermentation.

- Many domestic, industrial and agricultural wastes can be fruitfully used in SSF.

Limitations of SSF

- The microorganisms that tolerate only low moisture content can be used.
- Precise monitoring of SSF (e.g., O_2 and CO_2 levels, moisture content) is not possible.
- The organisms grow slowly and consequently there is a limitation in product formation.
- Heat production creates problems, and it is very difficult to regulate the growth environment.

MEDIA (SUBSTRATES) FOR INDUSTRIAL FERMENTATION

The media used for the growth of microorganisms in industrial fermentation ***must contain all the elements in a suitable form for the synthesis of cellular substances as well as the metabolic products***. While designing a medium, several factors must be taken into consideration. The most important among them is the ultimate product desired in the fermentation. For growth-linked products (primary metabolites e.g. ethanol, citric acid), the product formations is directly dependent on the growth of the organisms, hence the medium should be such that it supports good growth. On the other hand, for products which are not directly linked to the growth (secondary metabolites e.g. antibiotics, alkaloids, gibberellins), the substrate requirements for product formation must also be considered.

In the laboratory, pure defined chemicals may be used for culturing microorganisms. However, for industrial fermentations, undefined and complex substrates are frequently used for economic reasons. Cheaper substrates are advantageous since they minimize the production cost of the fermented products. Wastes from agriculture, and byproducts of other industries are generally preferred, although they are highly variable in composition. Raw materials used in fermentation largely depend on their cost at a particular time, since there are seasonal variations.

The choice of the medium is very critical for successful product formation. For industrial fermentation, the microorganisms, in general, utilize a ***luxury metabolism***. Therefore, good production yields are expected with an abundant supply of carbon and nitrogen sources, besides requisite growth factors. The media used in fermentation processes may be ***synthetic*** or ***crude***.

Synthetic media

Media with all the requisite constituents in a pure form in the desired proportion represents synthetic media. Use of this type of media in fermentations is not practicable.

Crude media

The non-synthetic media with naturally available sources are better suited for fermentation.

In practice, crude media with an addition of requisite synthetic constituents is ideal for good product yield in fermentation.

The most frequently used substrates for industrial fermentation with special reference to the supply of carbon and nitrogen sources and growth factors are briefly described below.

SUBSTRATES USED AS CARBON SOURCES

Carbohydrates constitute the most predominant source of energy in fermentation industry. Refined and pure carbohydrates such as glucose or sucrose are rarely used for economic reasons.

Molasses

Molasses is a byproduct of sugar industry and is one of the ***cheapest sources of carbohydrates***. Sugar cane molasses (sucrose around 48%) and sugar beet molasses (sucrose around 33%) are commonly used. Besides being rich in sugar, molasses also contain nitrogenous substances, vitamins and trace elements. There occurs variation in the composition of the molasses which mostly depends on the climatic conditions and production process. ***Hydrol molasses***, a byproduct in glucose production from corn, is also used as a fermentation substrate.

Malt extract

Malt extract, an aqueous extract of malted barely, contains about 80% carbohydrates (glucose, fructose, sucrose, maltose). Nitrogen compounds constitute around 4.5% (proteins, peptides, amino acids, purines, pyrimidines).

Starch, dextrin and cellulose

The polysaccharides-starch, dextrin and cellulose can be metabolised by microorganisms. They are frequently used for the industrial production of alcohol. Due to its wide availability and low cost, the use of ***cellulose for alcohol production*** is extensively studied.

Whey

Whey is a ***byproduct of dairy industry*** and is produced worldwide. Most of it is consumed by humans and animals. Whey is a reasonably good source of carbon for the production of alcohol, single-cell protein, vitamin B_{12}, lactic acid and gibberellic acid. Storage of whey is a limiting factor for its widespread use in fermentation industry.

Methanol and ethanol

Some of the microorganisms are capable of utilizing methanol and/or ethanol as carbon source. ***Methanol is the cheapest substrate for fermentation***. However, it ***can be utilized by only a few bacteria and yeasts***. Methanol is commonly used for the production of single-cell protein. Ethanol is rather expensive. However, at present it is used for the production of acetic acid.

SUBSTRATES USED AS NITROGEN SOURCES

The nitrogen supply to the fermentation microorganisms may come from inorganic or organic sources.

Inorganic nitrogen sources

Ammonium salts and free ***ammonia*** are cheap inorganic nitrogen sources, particularly in industrialised countries. However, not all the microorganisms are capable of utilising them, hence their use is limited.

Organic nitrogen sources

Urea is fairly a good source of nitrogen. However, other cheaper organic forms of nitrogen sources are preferred.

Corn steep liquor : This is formed during starch production from corn. Corn steep liquor is rich in nitrogen (about 4%) and is very efficiently utilized by microorganisms. It is rich in several amino acids (alanine, valine, methionine, arginine, threonine, glutamate).

Yeast extracts : They contain about 8% nitrogen and are rich in amino acids, peptides and vitamins.

Glucose formed from glycogen and trehalose during yeast extraction is a good carbon source. Yeast extracts are produced from baker's yeast through autolysis (at 50–55°C) or through plasmolysis (high concentration of NaCl). Yeast extracts are very good sources for many industrially important microorganisms.

Soy meal : After extracting the soy bean oil from the soy bean seeds, the left out residue is soy meal. It is rich in proteins (about 50%) as well as carbohydrates (about 30%) contents. Soy meal is often used in antibiotic production.

Peptones : The protein hydrolysates are collectively referred to as peptones, and they are good sources for many microorganisms. The sources of peptones include meat, soy meal, peanut seeds, cotton seeds and sunflower seeds. The proteins namely ***casein, gelatin and keratin can also be hydrolysed to yield peptones***. In general, peptones derived from animal sources have more nitrogen content while those from plant sources have more carbohydrate content. Peptones are relatively more expensive, hence not widely used in industries.

SOURCES OF GROWTH FACTORS

Some of the microorganisms are not capable of synthesising one or more growth factors such as vitamins. These growth factors are very expensive in pure form, hence crude sources are preferred. Yeast extract is a rich source of almost all growth factors.

Generally, the substrates derived from plant or animal sources in a crude form are reasonably rich in mineral content. Sometimes, however mineral (phosphate, sulfate) supplementation may be required.

STERILIZATION OF CULTURE MEDIA AND GASES

For successful fermentation, it is absolutely essential to ensure.

- Sterility of the media containing the nutrients.
- Sterility of incoming and outgoing air.
- Sterility of the bioreactor.
- Prevention of contamination during fermentation.

A brief account on the sterilization of the bioreactor has already been described (See p...). A bioreactor can be sterilized by destroying the organisms by heat/chemicals/radiation or sometimes by physical procedures such as filtration. Sterilization of media and air are discussed below.

STERILIZATION OF CULTURE MEDIA

The constituents of culture media, water and containers contribute to the contamination by vegetative cells and spores. The media must be free from contamination before use in fermentation. Sterilization of the media is most commonly achieved by applying heat, and to a lesser extent by other means (physical methods, chemical treatment, radiation).

Heat sterilization

Heat is the ***most widely used*** sterilization technique. The quality and quantity of contamination (i.e., the type and load of microorganisms), composition of the media and its pH and size of the suspended particles are the important factors that influence the success of heat sterilization. In general, ***vegetative cells are destroyed at lower temperature*** in a short time (around 60°C in 5–10 minutes). However, destruction of ***spores requires higher temperature*** and relatively ***longer time*** (around 80°C for 15–20 minutes). Spores of *Bacillus stearothermophilus* are the most heat resistant. In fact, this organism is exploited for testing the sterility of fermentation equipment.

Physical methods

The physical methods such as ***filtration, centrifugation,*** and ***adsorption*** (to ion-exchangers or activated carbon) are in use. Among these, filtration is most widely used. Certain constituents (vitamins, blood components, antibiotics) of culture media are heat labile and therefore, are destroyed by heat sterilization. Such components of the medium are completely dissolved (absolutely essential or else they will be removed along with microorganisms) and then subjected to filter sterilization. There are a couple of limitations of filtration technique.

1. Application of high pressure in filtration is unsuitable for industries.

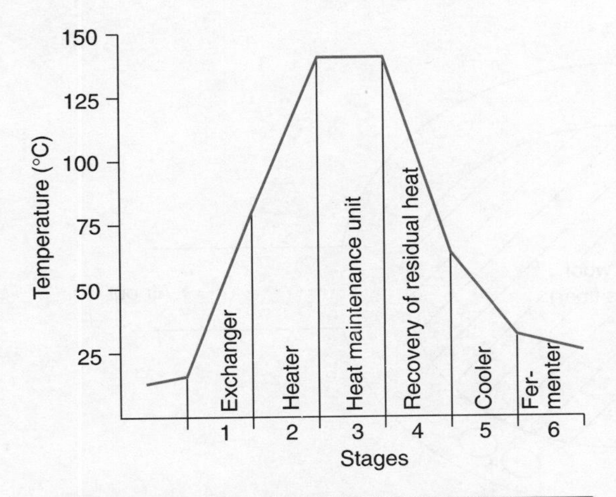

Fig. 19.7 : *Different stages in continuous sterilization process in relation to temperature.*

2. Some of the media components may be lost form the media during filtration.

Sometimes, a combination of filtration and heat sterilization are applied. For instance, the water used for media preparation is filtered while concentrated nutrient solution is subjected to heat sterilization. The filtered water is now added for appropriate dilution of the media.

The chemical methods (by using disinfectants) and ***radiation procedures*** (by using UV rays, γ rays, X-rays) are not commonly used for media sterilization.

Batch sterilization

The culture media are subjected to ***sterilization at 121°C in batch volumes, in the bioreactor***. Batch sterilization can be done by injecting the steam into the medium (direct method) or injecting the steam into interior coils (indirect method). For the direct batch sterilization, the steam should be pure, and free from all chemical additives (that usually come from steam manufacturing process). There are two disadvantages of batch sterilization.

1. **Damage to culture media :** Alteration in nutrients, change in pH and discolouration of the culture media are common.

2. **High energy consumption :** It takes a few hours (2-4 hrs) for the entire contents of the bioreactor to attain the requisite temperature (i.e. 120°C). Another 20–60 minutes for the actual process of sterilization, followed by cooling for 1-2 hours. All this process ***involves wastage of energy***, and therefore batch sterilization is quite costly.

Continuous sterilization

Continuous sterilization is ***carried out at 140°C for a very short period of time ranging from 30 to 120 seconds***. (This is in contrast to the batch fermentation done at 121°C for 20–60 minutes). This is based on the principle that the time required for killing microorganisms is much shorter at higher temperature. Continuous sterilization is carried out by directly injecting the steam or by means of heat exchangers. In either case, the temperature is very quickly raised to 140°C, and maintained for 30–120 seconds. The stages of continuous sterilization process and the corresponding temperatures are depicted in ***Fig. 19.7***. The different stages are— ***exchanger, heater, heat maintenance unit, recovery of residual heat, cooling and fermenter***.

In the continuous sterilization process, 3 types of heat exchangers are used. The first heat exchanger raises temperature to 90–120°C within 20–30 seconds. The second exchanger further raises temperature to 140°C and maintains for 30–120 seconds. The third heat exchanger brings down the temperature by cooling in the next 20–30 seconds. The actual time required for sterilization depends on the size of the suspended particles. The bigger is the size, the more is the time required.

The ***main advantage*** with continuous sterilization is that ***about 80–90% of the energy is conserved***. The limitation however, is that certain compounds in the medium precipitate (e.g., calcium phosphate, calcium oxalate) due to very high temperature differences that occur in a very short time between sterilization and cooling. The starch-containing culture media becomes viscous in continuous sterilization and therefore is not used.

STERILIZATION OF AIR

In general, the industrial fermentations are carried out under vigorous and continuous aeration. ***For an effective fermentation, the air should be completely sterile, and free from all micro-organisms*** and suspended particles. There is a wide

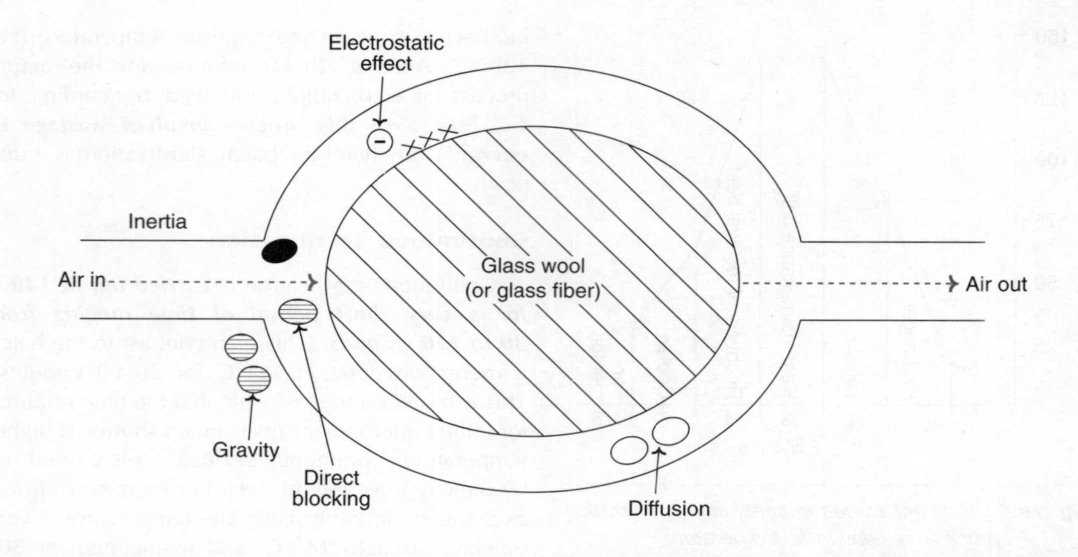

Fig. 19.8 : Use of depth filter in air sterilization.

variation in the quantity of suspended particles and microbes in the atmospheric outdoor air. The microorganisms may range from 10–2,000/m^3 while the suspended particles may be 20–100,00/m^3. Among the microorganisms present in the air, the fungal spores (50%) and Gram-negative bacteria (40%) dominate.

Air or other gases can be sterilized by filtration, heat, UV radiation and gas scrubbing. Among these, heat and filtration are most commonly used.

Air sterilization by heat

In the early years, air was passed over electrically heated elements and sterilized. But this is quite expense, hence not in use these days.

Air sterilization by filtration

Filtration of air is the most commonly used sterilization in fermentation industries.

Depth filters : When the air is passed through a glass wool containing depth filters the particles are trapped and removed (***Fig. 19.8***). This filtration technique primarily involves physical effects such as inertia, blocking, gravity, electrostatic attraction and diffusion. Glass wool filters can be subjected to steam sterilization and reused. But there is a limitation in their reuse since glass wool shrinks and solidifies on steam sterilization. In recent years, glass fiber filter cartridges (that do not have the limitations of glass wool filter) are being used.

Membrane cartridge filters : These are removable pleated membrane filters made up of cellulose ester, nylon or polysulfone. Membrane cartridge filters are smaller in size, simpler for operation and replacement.

The most important limitation of air sterilization is that there is no ***filter that can remove bacteriophages***. Bacteriophages are capable of crippling the industrial fermentation. e.g., bacteriophages interfere in the production of glutamic acid by *Corynebacterium glutamicum*.

ISOLATION OF MICROORGANISMS

There are over a million species of microorganisms widely distributed in nature. Less than 1% of the world's microorganisms have been studied. In fact, only ***a few hundred species are important for industrial use***. A selected list of organisms along with their products is given in ***Table 19.3***.

The good sources for the isolation of microorganisms are soils, lakes and river muds. It is estimated that a gram of soil contains 10^6–10^8

TABLE 19.3 A selected list of important microorganisms and their products

Microorganism	*Product*
Algae	
Chlorella sorokiniana	Single-cell protein
Spirulina maxima	Single-cell protein
Bacteria	
Acetobacter aceti	Acetic acid
Acetobacter woodii	Acetic acid
Bacillus subtilis	Bacitracin
B. brevis	Gramicidin
B. thuringiensis	Endotoxin
Clostridium aceticum	Acetic acid
Methylophilus methylotrophus	Glutamic acid
Pseudomonas denitrificans	Vitamin B_{12}
Actinomycetes	
Streptomyces aureofaciens	Tetracycline
S. griseus	Streptomycin
S. tradiae	Neomycin
Nocardia mediterranei	Rifamycin
Micromonospora purpurea	Gentamycin
Fungi	
Aspergillus niger	Citric acid
A. oryzae	Amylase, cellulase, single-cell protein
Candida lipolytica	Lipase
C. utilis	Single–cell protein
Penicillium chrysogenum	Penicillin
Saccharomyces cerevisiae	Ethanol, wine, single-cell protein
S. lipolytica	Citric acid, single-cell protein
Rhizopus nigricans	Steroids
Gibberella fujikuroi	Gibberellin
Trichoderma viride	Cellulase

bacteria, 10^4–10^6 actinomycete spores and 10^2–10^4 fungal spores. The common techniques employed for the isolation of microorganisms are given below.

1. Direct sponge of the soil
2. Soil dilution
3. Gradient plate method (pour plate and streak plate technique)
4. Aerosol dilution
5. Flotation
6. Centrifugation.

For full details on the isolation procedures, the reader must refer books on microbiology. The actual technique for the isolation of microorganisms depends on the source and the physiological properties of microorganisms. The general scheme adopted for isolating microorganisms from soil or water source is given below.

- The sample (soil or water) is diluted with sterile water to which an emulsifying agent (Tween) is added.
- Sample is throughly mixed and allowed to stand at room temperature.
- Supernatant is diluted, 10^{-1} to 10^{-10}.
- Various culture media are inoculated with diluted samples and incubated.
- Colonies from the plates are isolated and identified.
- The required pure strains are maintained and preserved.

Enrichment methods for isolation of microorganisms

The culture conditions can be appropriately modified to isolate certain types of microorganisms. The types of organisms that can be isolated by use of enrichment methods is given in ***Table 19.4***. For instance, thermophiles can be isolated by using high temperature while acidophiles can be isolated in acidic pH. Enrichment methods are certainly useful for quick isolation of specific types of organisms.

Strains of microorganisms from unusual environments

Biotechnologists often prefer to isolate microorganisms from very extreme and unusual environments. This is done with a hope that such strains may be capable of producing new products of industrial importance. The unusual environments such as ***cold habitats, high altitudes, deserts, deep sea and petroleum fields*** are constantly being tried for this purpose. The enrichment methods described above (***Table 19.4***) will be very useful for isolating unusual strains.

Table 19.4 Types of microorganisms that can be isolated by enrichment methods

Type of organisms	*Enrichment method*
Thermophiles	High temperature (42–100°C)
Psychrotrophs	Low temperature (5–15°C)
Acidophiles	Low pH (2-4)
Halophiles	High NaCl concentration
Anaerobes	N_2 atmosphere
Actinoplanes	Pollen grains
Myxobacteria	Wood bark

Screening of metabolites for isolation of microorganisms

The microorganisms can be tested directly for the product formation, and isolated. In fact, the water or soil samples can be directly used or suitably diluted for metabolite screening. Agar plates can be used for screening metabolites formed from the microorganisms. For instance, if the required product is an antibiotic, then the test system consists of the strains of organisms which inhibit the zones, on the agar plates. The inhibitory activity indicates the possible presence of some antibiotic being produced by the microorganisms. Another example is the isolation of microorganisms producing amylases. When grown on agar plates containing starch, and then stained with iodine, amylase-producing organisms can be identified and isolated.

Screening for new metabolites, and isolation of microorganisms

Industrial microbiologists continue their search for newer metabolites produced by microorganisms. Research work is particularly directed for identifying chemotherapeutically important products for the treatment of tumors, bacterial diseases (newer antibiotics against resistant strains) and viral diseases, besides several other substances (e.g. hormones, enzyme inhibitors). In addition, isolation of microorganisms for improvement of food industry, and for efficient degradation of the environmental pollutants and hazardous chemicals also assumes significance.

PRESERVATION OF MICROORGANISMS

There are distinct methods for preservation of microorganisms. The most important being storage by ***refrigeration***, ***freezing*** and ***lyophilization***.

MICROBIAL METABOLIC PRODUCTS — LOW MOLECULAR WEIGHT COMPOUNDS

The microorganisms possess tremendous capacity to produce a wide range of products that have commercial value. The primary and secondary metabolisms and bioconversions of microorganisms with special reference to their importance for the formation of biotechnologically important products are discussed hereunder (***Fig. 19.9***). Microbial growth in relation to primary and secondary metabolisms is depicted in ***Fig. 19.10***.

PRIMARY METABOLITES

Primary metabolism, also referred to as ***trophophase***, is characterized by balanced growth of microorganisms. It occurs when all the nutrients needed by the organisms are provided in the medium. Primary metabolism is essential for the very existence and reproduction of cells. In the trophophase, the cells possess optimal concentrations of almost all the macromolecules (proteins, DNA, RNA etc.).

It is during the period of trophophase, an exponential growth of microorganisms occurs. Several metabolic products, collectively referred to as ***primary metabolites***, are produced in trophophase (i.e., during the period of growth). The primary metabolites are divided into two groups.

1. **Primary essential metabolites :** These are the ***compounds*** produced in adequate quanties to ***sustain cell growth e.g. vitamins, amino acids, nucleosides***. The native microorganisms usually do not overproduce essential primary metabolites, since it is a wasteful exercise. However, for industrial overproduction, the regulatory mechanisms are suitably manipulated.

2. **Primary metabolic end products :** These are the normal and traditional ***end products of fermentation process of primary metabolism***. The end products may or may not have any significant function to perform in the microorganisms,

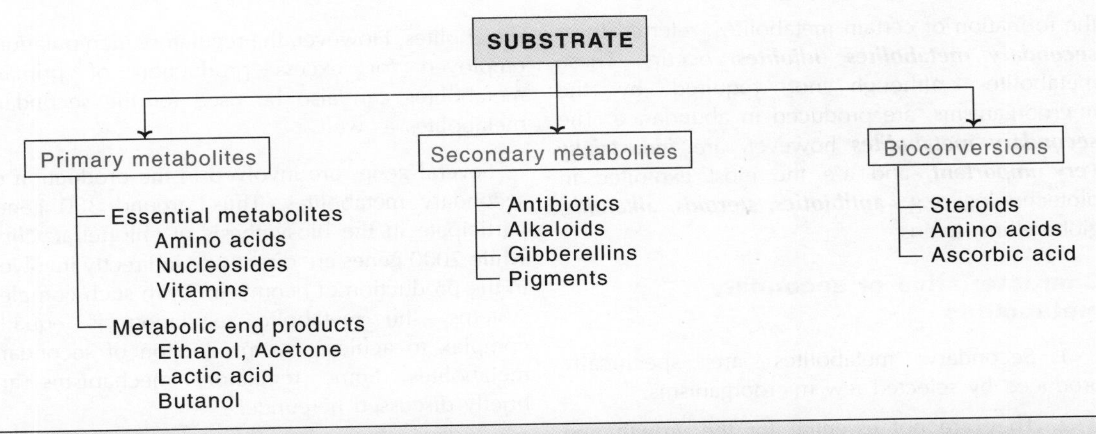

Fig. 19.9 : Different types of low–molecular weight compounds produced by microorganisms.

although they have many other industrial applications e.g. ethanol, acetone, lactic acid.

Carbon dioxide is a metabolic end product of *Saccharomyces cerevisiae*. This CO_2 is essential for leavening of dough in baking industry.

Limitations in growth : Due to insufficient/ limited supply of any nutrient (substrate or even O_2), the growth rate of microorganisms slows down. However, the metabolism does not stop. It continues as long as the cell lives, but the formation of products differs.

Overproduction of primary metabolites

Excessive production of primary metabolites is very important for their large scale use for a variety of purposes. Overproduction of several metabolites has been successfully accomplished by eliminating the feedback inhibition as briefly described below.

1. By using auxotrophic mutants with a block in one of the steps in the biosynthetic pathway concerned with the formation of primary metabolite (this should be an intermediate and not the final end product). In this manner, the end product (E) formation is blocked, hence no feedback inhibition. But overproduction of the required metabolite (C) occurs as illustrated below.

Feedback regulation :

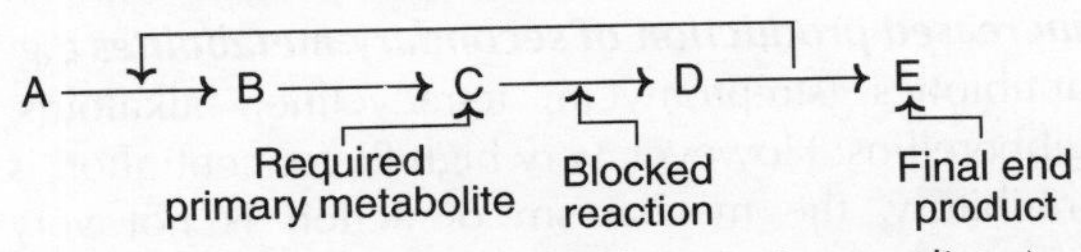

(A is starting substrate; B and D are intermediates)

In the above example, an unbranched pathway is shown. This type of manipulation for overproduction of metabolites can be done for branched metabolic pathways also.

2. Mutant microorganisms with antimetabolite resistance which exhibit a defective metabolic regulation can also overproduce primary metabolites.

SECONDARY METABOLITES

As the exponential growth of the microorganisms ceases (i.e. as the trophophase ends), they enter ***idiophase***. Idiophase is characterized by ***secondary metabolism*** wherein

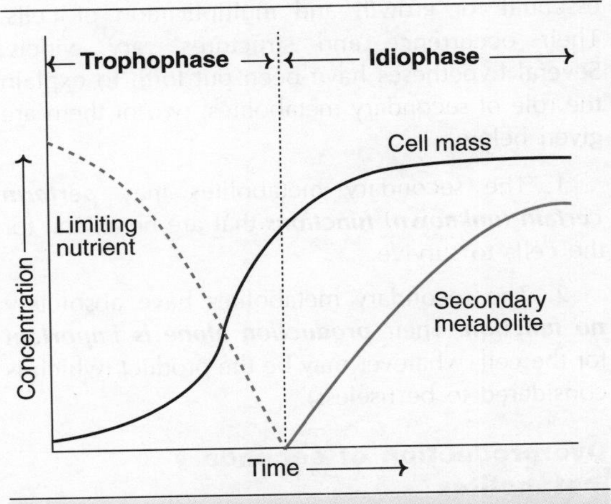

Fig. 19.10 : Microbial growth in relation to primary (trophophase) and secondary (idiophase) metabolism.

the formation of certain metabolites, referred to as ***secondary metabolites*** (***idiolites***) occurs. These metabolites, although not required by the microorganisms, are produced in abundance. The ***secondary metabolites*** however, are ***industrially very important***, and are the most exploited in biotechnology e.g., ***antibiotics, steroids, alkaloids,*** gibberellins, toxins.

Characteristics of secondary metabolites

1. Secondary metabolites are specifically produced by selected few microorganisms.

2. They are not essential for the growth and reproduction of organisms from which they are produced.

3. Environmental factors influence the production of secondary metabolites.

4. Some microorganisms produce secondary metabolites as a group of compounds (usually structurally related) instead of a single one e.g. about 35 anthracyclines are produced by a single strain of *Streptomyces*.

5. The biosynthetic pathways for most secondary metabolites are not clearly established.

6. The regulation of the formation of secondary metabolites is more complex and differs from that of primary metabolites.

Functions of secondary metabolites

As already stated, secondary metabolites are not essential for growth and multiplication of cells. Their occurrence and structures vary widely. Several hypotheses have been put forth to explain the role of secondary metabolites, two of them are given below.

1. The secondary metabolites may ***perform certain (unknown) functions*** that are beneficial for the cells to survive.

2. The secondary metabolites have absolutely ***no function***. Their ***production alone is important*** for the cell, whatever may be the product (which is considered to be useless).

Overproduction of secondary metabolites

As already stated, the production of secondary metabolites is more complex than primary metabolites. However, the regulatory manipulations employed for excess production of primary metabolites can also be used for the secondary metabolites as well.

Several genes are involved in the production of secondary metabolites. Thus, around 300 genes participate in the biosynthesis of chlortetracycline while 2000 genes are directly or indirectly involved in the production of neomycin. With such complex systems, the metabolic regulation is equally complex to achieve overproduction of secondary metabolites. Some regulatory mechanisms are briefly discussed hereunder.

Induction : Addition of methionine induces certain enzymes and ***enhances*** the production of ***cephalosporin***. Tryptophan regulates ergot alkaloid biosynthesis.

End product regulation : Some of the secondary metabolites inhibit their own biosynthesis, a phenomenon referred to as end product regulation e.g. penicillin, streptomycin, puromycin, chloramphenicol. It is possible to isolate ***mutants*** that are ***less sensitive to end product inhibition***, and in this manner the ***secondary metabolite production can be increased***.

Catabolite regulation : In this regulation process, a key enzyme involved in a catabolic pathway is inactivated, inhibited or repressed by adding a commonly used substrate. Catabolic repression can be achieved by using carbon or nitrogen sources. The mechanism of action of catabolite regulation is not very clearly understood.

The most commonly used ***carbon*** source is ***glucose***. It is found to ***inhibit the production of several antibiotics*** e.g. penicillin, streptomycin, bacitracin, chloramphenicol, puromycin.

The ***nitrogen sources*** such as ***ammonia*** also act as catabolite regulators (i.e. inhibitors) for the ***overproduction of certain antibiotics***.

Phosphate regulation : Inorganic phosphate (Pi) is required for the growth and multiplication of prokaryotes and eukaryotes. ***Increasing Pi concentration*** (up to 1mM) is associated with an ***increased production of secondary metabolites*** e.g. antibiotics (streptomycin, tetracycline), alkaloids, gibberellins. However, very high Pi concentration is inhibitory, the mechanism of action is not very clear.

Autoregulation : In some microorganisms (particularly actinomycetes), there occurs a self regulation for the production of secondary metabolites. A compound designated as ***factor A*** which is analogous to a hormone is believed to be closely involved in autoregulation for the production streptomycin by *Streptomyces griseus*. More such factors from other organisms have also been identified.

BIOCONVERSIONS

Microorganisms are also used for chemical transformation of unusual substrates to desired products. This process, also referred to as ***biotransformation***, is very important in producing several compounds e.g. conversion of ethanol to acetic acid (in vinegar), sorbitol to sorbose, synthesis of steroid hormones and certain amino acids.

In bioconversion, microorganisms convert a compound to a structurally related product in one or a few enzymatic reactions. The bioconversions can be carried out with resting cells, spores or even killed cells. Non-growing cells are preferred for bioconversions, since high substrate concentration can be used, besides washing the cells easily (to make them free from contamination).

Sometimes, mixed cultures are used for bioconversions to carry out different reactions. In recent years, the yield of bioconversion is increased by using immobilized cells at a lower cost. For more details on biotransformation, the reader must refer Chapter 22.

MICROBIAL METABOLIC PRODUCTS — HIGH MOLECULAR WEIGHT COMPOUNDS

Microorganisms are also used for the production of macromolecules i.e. high molecular weight compounds e.g. polysaccharides, proteins (including enzymes). Recombinant DNA technology has drastically improved the industrial production of various macromolecules in a cost-effective manner.

The details on the microbial production of high molecular weight compounds (pharmaceutical products) are given in Chapter 15.

GENETIC IMPROVEMENT (DEVELOPMENT) OF STRAINS

In general, the ***wild strains*** of microorganisms ***produce low quantities of commercially important metabolites***, although the yield can be increased by optimizing the fermentation conditions. The potentiality of the metabolite formation is genetically determined. Therefore, genetic improvements have to be made and new strains developed for any substantial increase in product formation in a cost-effective manner.

There are strain development programmes (mutation and recombination) to increase the product yield by 100 times or even more. The nature of the desired product determines the success associated with strain improvement. For example, if alterations in one or two genes (i.e. one or 2 key enzymes) can improve the product yield, it is simpler to achieve the target. This type of approach is sometimes possible with primary metabolites. As regards the secondary metabolites, the product formation and its regulation are quite complex. Hence, several genetic modifications have to be done to finally produce high-yielding strains. Ideally speaking, the ***improved strains*** should possess the following ***characteristics*** (as many as possible) to finally result in high product formation.

1. Shorter time of fermentation
2. Capable of metabolising low-cost substrates
3. Reduced O_2 demand
4. Decreased foam formation
5. Non-production of undesirable compounds
6. Tolerance to high concentrations of carbon or nitrogen sources
7. Resistant to infections of bacteriophages.

It is always preferable to have ***improved strains*** of microorganisms which ***can produce one metabolite*** as the main product. In this way, the production can be maximised, and its recovery becomes simpler.

Through genetic manipulations, it has been possible to develop strains for the production of modified or new metabolites which are of commercial value e.g. modified or newer antibiotics.

The ***major limitation*** of strain improvement is that for most of the industrially important microorganisms, there is lack of detailed information on the genetics, and molecular biology. This hinders the new strain development.

METHODS OF STRAIN DEVELOPMENT

There are three distinct approaches for improvement of strains-mutation, recombination and recombinant DNA technology.

MUTATION

Any change that occurs in the DNA of a gene is referred to as mutation. Thus, mutations result in a structural change in the genome. Mutations may be ***spontaneous*** (that occur naturally) or ***induced*** by mutagenic agents.

The spontaneous mutations occur at a very low frequency, and usually are not suitable for industrial purposes. Mutations may be induced by mutagenic agents such as ultraviolet light, various chemicals (nitrous oxide, nitrosoguanidine, hydroxylamine). Site-directed mutagenesis (For details Refer Chapter 10) is also important for strain improvement.

Selection of mutants

Selection and isolation of the appropriate mutant strains developed is very important for their industrial use. Two techniques commonly employed for this purpose are briefly described.

Random screening

The mutated strains are randomly selected and checked for their ability to produce the desired industrial product. This can be done with model fermentation units. The ***strains with maximum yield can be selected***. Random screening is costly and tedious procedure. But many a times, this is the only way to find the right strain of mutants developed.

Selective isolation of mutants

There are many methods for selective isolation of improved strains.

1. **Isolation of antibiotic resistant strains :** The mutated strains are grown on a selective medium containing an antibiotic. The wild strains are killed while the mutant strains with antibiotic resistance can grow. Such strains may be useful in industries.

TABLE 19.5 Antimetabolites used for screening of some common natural metabolites

Natural metabolite	*Antimetabolite(s)*
Amino acids	
Arginine	Canavanine
Histidine	2-Thiazolalanine
Valine	α-Aminobutyric acid, isoleucine
Leucine	4-Azaleucine
Methionine	α-Methylmethionine, ethionine
Phenylalanine	p-Fluorophenylalanine,
Tyrosine	p-Fluorophenylalanine
Tryptophan	5 (or 6)-Methyltryptophan
Threonine	β-Hydroxynorleucine
Proline	3, 4-Dehydroproline
Vitamins	
Thiamine	Pyrithiamine
Pyridoxine	Isoniazid
Niacin	3–Acetylpyridine
p–Aminobenzoic acid	Sulfonamide
Nitrogenous bases	
Adenine	2, 6–Diaminopurine
Guanine	8–Azaxanthine
Uracil	5–Fluorouracil

2. **Isolation of antimetabolite resistant strains :** Antimetabolites which have structural similarities with metabolites can block the normal metabolic pathways and kill the cells. The mutant strains resistant to antimetabolites can be selected for industrial purposes. In the ***Table 19.5***, a selected list antimetabolites used for screening the metabolites is given.

3. **Isolation of auxotrophic mutants :** An auxotrophic mutant is characterized by a defect in one of the biosynthetic pathways. As a result, it requires a specific compound for its normal growth. For instance, tyr mutants of *Corynebacterium glutamicus* require tyrosine for their growth while they can accumulate phenylalanine. The isolation of such mutants can be done by growing them on a complete agar medium that can specifically support the biochemically defective mutant.

GENETIC RECOMBINATION

The strain improvement can be made by combining genetic information from two genotypes, by a process called genetic recombination. The recombination can be brought out by ***transformation, transduction***, ***conjugation*** (Chapter 6) and ***protoplast fusion*** (Chapter 44). There are many advantages of genetic recombination.

1. By crossing high product yielding mutant strains with wild-type strains, the fermentation process can be further increased.

2. Different mutant strains with high-yielding properties can be combined by recombination.

3. There is gradual decline in the product yield after each stage of mutation, due to undesirable mutations. This can be prevented by using recombination.

PRINCIPLES OF MICROBIAL GROWTH AND CULTURE SYSTEMS

The growth of microorganisms is a highly complex and coordinated process, ultimately expressed by increase in cell number or cell mass. The process of growth depends on the availability of requisite nutrients and their transport into the cells, and the environmental factors such as aeration, O_2 supply, temperature and pH.

Doubling time refers to the time period required for ***doubling*** the weight of the ***biomass*** while ***generation time*** represents the period for ***doubling the cell numbers***. Doubling times normally increase with increasing cell size and complexicity as given below.

Bacteria	0.30 – 1 hour
Yeasts	1 – 2 hours
Animal cells	25 – 48 hours
Plant cells	20 – 70 hours

In general, when all other conditions are kept ideal, growth of the microorganisms is dependent on the substrate (nutrient) supply. The microorganisms can be grown in ***batch***, ***fed-batch***, ***semicontinuous*** or ***continuous culture*** systems in a bioreactor.

A diagrammatic representation of microbial cell growth in relation to substrate is depicted in ***Fig. 19.11***. In batch fermentation, the growth medium containing the substrates is inoculated with microorganisms, and the fermentation proceeds without the addition of fresh growth medium. In fed-batch fermentation, substrates are added at short time intervals during fermentation. In batch and fed-batch fermentation, the growth of the cells is quite comparable. And in both cases, growth medium is not removed until the end of fermentation process.

In case of continuous fermentation, as the fermentation proceeds, fresh growth medium is added continuously. Simultaneously, an equal volume of spent medium containing suspended microoganisms is removed. This enables the cells to grow optimally and continuously (Fig. ***19.11C***).

BATCH CULTURE OR BATCH FERMENTATION

A batch fermentation is regarded as a ***closed system***. The sterile nutrient culture medium in the bioreactor is inoculated with microorganisms. The incubation is carried out under optimal physiological conditions (pH, temperature, O_2 supply, agitation etc.). It may be necessary to add acid or alkali to maintain pH, and anti-foam agents to minimise foam. Under optimal conditions for growth, the following six typical phases of growth are observed in batch fermentation (***Fig. 19.12***).

1. Lag phase
2. Acceleration phase
3. Logarithmic (log) phase (exponential phase)
4. Deceleration phase
5. Stationary phase
6. Death phase.

1. **Lag phase :** The ***initial brief period of culturing*** after inoculation is referred to as lag phase. During the lag phase, the microorganisms adapt to the new environment—available nutrients, pH etc. There is no increase in the cell number, although the cellular weight may slightly increase. The length of the lag phase is variable and is mostly determined by the new set of physiological conditions, and the phase at which the micro-organisms were existing when inoculated. For instance, lag phase may not occur if the culture inoculated is at exponential phase (i.e., log phase), and growth may start immediately.

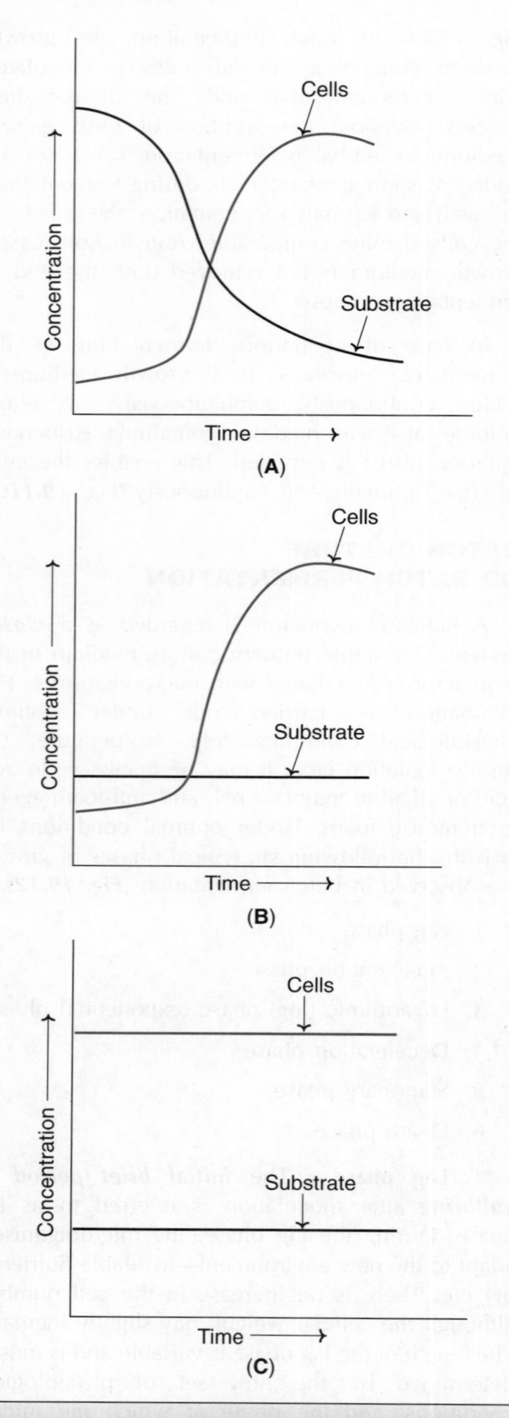

Fig. 19.11 : Diagrammatic representation of microbial cell growth in relation to substrate ***(A)*** *Batch fermentation* ***(B)*** *Fed–batch fermentation* ***(C)*** *Continuous fermentation.*

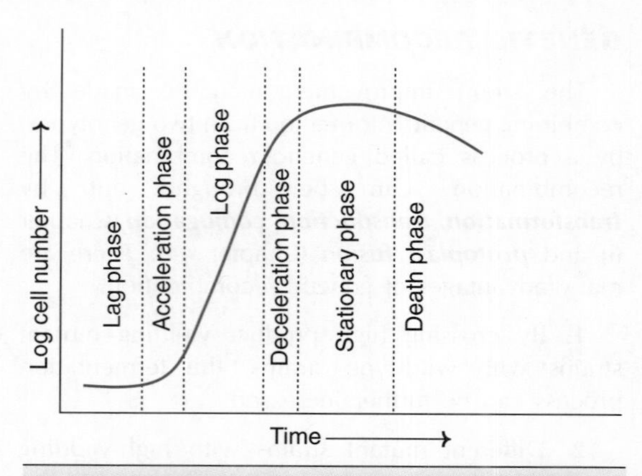

Fig. 19.12 : Pattern of microbial cell growth in batch culture or batch fermentation.

2. **Acceleration phase :** This is a brief transient period during which ***cells start growing slowly***. In fact, acceleration phase connects the lag phase and log phase.

3. **Log phase :** The most ***active growth of microorganisms and multiplication occur*** during log phase. The cells undergo several doublings and the cell mass increases. When the number of cells or biomass is plotted against time on a ***semilogarithmic graph, a straight line*** is obtained, hence the term log phase. Growth rate of microbes in log phase is independent of substrate (nutrient supply) concentration as long as excess substrate is present, and there are no growth inhibitors in the medium. In general, the specific growth rate of microorganisms for simpler substrates is greater than for long chain molecules. This is explained on the basis of extra energy needed to split long chain substrates.

Two log phases are observed when a complex nutrient medium with two substrates is used in fermentation, and this phenomenon is referred to as ***diauxy***. This happens since one of the substrates is preferentially metabolised first which represses the breakdown of second substrate. After the first substrate is completely degraded second lag phase occurs, during which period, the enzymes for the breakdown of second substrate the synthesized. Now a second log phase occurs.

More details on log phase with special reference to growth kinetics of microorganisms are discussed later.

4. **Deceleration phase :** As the growth rate of microorganisms during log phase decreases, they enter the deceleration phase. This phase is usually very short-lived and may not be observable.

5. **Stationary phase :** As the substrate in the growth medium gets depleted, and the metabolic end products that are formed inhibit the growth, the cells enter the stationary phase. The ***microbial growth may either slow down or completely stop***. The biomass may remain almost constant during stationary phase. This phase, however, is frequently associated with dramatic changes in the metabolism of the cells which may produce compounds (secondary metabolites) of biotechnological importance e.g. production of antibiotics.

6. **Death phase :** This phase is associated with ceasation of metabolic activity and depletion of energy reserves. The ***cells die at an exponential rate*** (a straight line may be obtained when the number of surviving cells are plotted against time on a semilogarithmic plot). In the commercial and industrial fermentations, the growth of the microorganisms is halted at the end of the log phase or just before the death phase begins, and the cells are harvested.

FED-BATCH CULTURE OR FED-BATCH FERMENTATION

Fed-batch fermentation (See ***Fig. 19.11***) is an improvement of batch fermentation wherein the ***substrate is added in increments at different times throughout the course of fermentation*** (**Note :** In batch culture method, substrate is added only at the beginning of the fermentation). Periodical substrate addition ***prolongs log and stationary phases*** which results in an increased biomass. Consequently, production of metabolites (e.g. antibiotics) during stationary phase is very much increased.

As it is difficult to directly measure substrate concentration in fed-batch fermentation, other indicators that correlate with substrate consumption are used. The formation of organic acids, production of CO_2 and changes in pH may be measured, and accordingly substrate addition carried out. In general, fed-batch fermentation requires more careful monitoring than batch fermentation, and is therefore not a preferred method by industrial biotechnologists.

Fed-batch fermentation for the production of recombinant proteins

In recent years, fed-batch fermentation has become popular, due to very high yield, for the production of recombinant proteins. Depending on the microorganism and the nature of recombinant protein, the fed-batch fermentation can increase the product yield from 25% to 1000% compared to batch fermentation. Careful monitoring of the fermentation reaction and appropriate addition of substrates (carbon and nitrogen sources, and trace metals) substantially increases the product yield.

Limitations : The major limitation of fed batch fermentation is that the microorganisms in the stationary phase produce proteolytic enzymes or proteases. These enzyme attack the recombinant proteins that are being produced. By carefully monitoring the fermentation, the log phase can be prolonged and the onset of stationary phase is delayed. By this way, the formation of proteases can be minimised.

Fed-batch cultures for higher organisms

Fed-batch cultures are successfully employed for mammalian and insect cells. This is very advantageous for the production of human therapeutic proteins with good yield.

SEMI-CONTINUOUS CULTURE OR SEMI-CONTINUOUS FERMENTATION

Some of the products of fermentation are growth-linked, and such products are formed at the end of the log phase e.g. ethanol production. In semi-continuous fermentation, a ***portion of the culture medium is removed from the bioreactor and replaced by fresh medium*** (identical in nutrients, pH, temperature etc.). This process of culture medium change can be repeated at appropriate intervals. In the semi-continuous fermentation, the lag phase and other non-productive phases are very much shortened. The product output is much higher compared to batch culture systems. Semi-continuous fermentation technique has been successfully used in the industrial production of alcohol.

There are however, certain disadvantages of semi-continuous fermentation. These include the technical difficulties of handling bioreactors, long culture periods that may lead to contamination, mutation and mechanical breakdown.

CONTINUOUS CULTURE OR CONTINUOUS FERMENTATION

Continuous fermentation is an ***open system.*** It involves the ***removal of culture medium continuously and replacement of this with a fresh sterile medium*** in a bioreactor. Both addition and removal are done at the same rate so that the working volume remains constant. Further, to maintain a steady state condition in continuous process, it is advisable that the cell loss as a result of outflow is balanced by growth of the organisms. The two common types of continuous fermentation and bioreactors are described below (***Fig. 19.13***).

Homogeneously mixed bioreactors

In this type, the culture solution is homogeneously mixed, and the bioreactors are of two types

Chemostat bioreactors : The concentration of any one of the substrates (carbohydrate, nitrogen source, salts, O_2) is adjusted to control the cell growth and maintain a steady state.

Turbidostat bioreactors : In this case, turbidity measurement is used to monitor the biomass concentration. The rate of addition of nutrient solution can be appropriately adjusted to maintain a constant cell growth.

Plug flow bioreactors

In plug flow bioreactors, the culture solution flows through a tubular reaction vessel without back mixing. The composition of the medium, the quantity of cells, O_2 supply and product formation vary at different locations in the bioreactor. Microorganisms along with nutrient medium are continuously added at the entrance of the bioreactor.

Industrial applications of continuous fermentation

Continuous fermentation processes have been used for the ***production of antibiotics, organic solvents, single-cell protein, beer and ethanol, besides waste-water treatment.***

Advantages of continuous fermentation

1. The size of the bioreactor and other equipment used in continuous fermentation are relatively smaller compared to batch fermentation for the production of the same quantity of product.

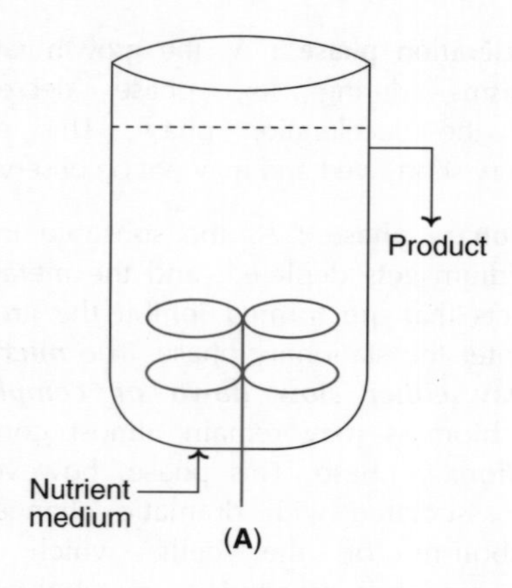

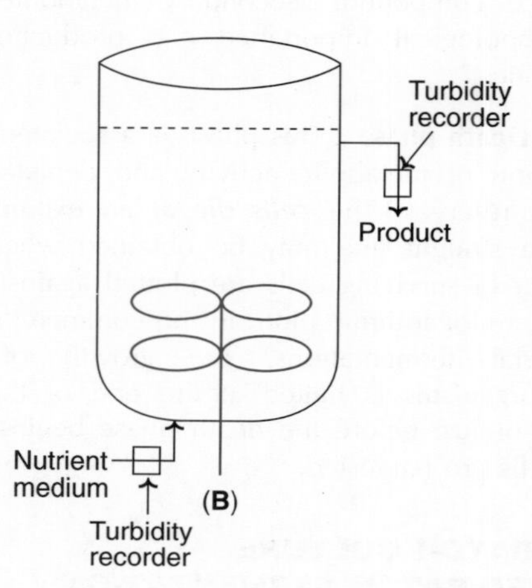

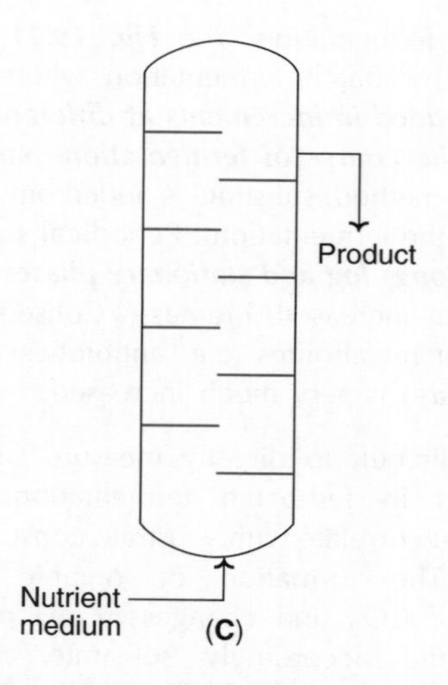

Fig. 19.13 : Continuous fermentation bioreactors (A) Chemostat bioreactor (B) Turbidostat bioreactor (C) Plug flow bioreactor.

2. The ***yield of the product is more consistent*** since the physiological state of the cells is uniform.

3. The 'down time' between two successive fermentations for cleaning and preparing the bioreactor for reuse is avoided in continuous fermentation.

4. Continuous fermentation can be run in a ***cost-effective*** manner.

Disadvantages of continuous fermentation

Despite many advantages of continuous fermentation (described above), it is not very widely used in industries. Some of the drawbacks are listed.

1. Continuous fermentation may run continuously for a period of 500 to 1,000 hours. ***Maintenance of sterile conditions for such a long period is difficult***.

2. The recombinant cells with plasmid constructs cannot function continuously and therefore the product yield decreases.

3. It is not easy to maintain the same quality of the culture medium for all the additions. Nutrient variations will alter the growth and physiology of the cells, and consequently the product yield.

In addition to the disadvantages listed above, industrial biotechnologists are rather reluctant to switch over to continuous fermentation from the batch fermentation. However, it is expected that continuous fermentation will also become, popular in due course.

GROWTH KINETICS OF MICROORGANISMS

The different types of fermentation processes-batch, fed-batch, semi-continuous and continuous are described above. The kinetics of microbial growth with special reference to log phase of batch fermentation are briefly discussed here.

After completion of lag phase, the cell enters log phase which is characterized by exponential growth (See ***Fig. 19.12***). If the initial number of cells is N_0, then

After 1st generation, the cell number will be $N_0 \times 2^1$.

After 2nd generation, the cell number will be $N_0 \times 2^2$.

After 3rd generation, $N_0 \times 2^3$, and so on. Thus, the number of cells after a given time (Nt) will be as follows :

$$Nt = N_0 \times 2^n$$

where n is the number of generations.

The term ***doubling time*** (td) or ***mean generation time*** (MGT) refers to the ***time taken for doubling the cell number or biomass***. The specific growth rate constant expressed by μ, is the direct measure of rate of growth of the organism. If N is the number of cells at a given time, then the increase in the number of cells (growth rate) with time is given by the formula.

$$\frac{dN}{dt} = \mu N \qquad (1)$$

If X is the biomass concentration at a given time, then the increase in the biomass (growth rate) with time is given by.

$$\frac{dX}{dt} = \mu X \qquad (2)$$

In general, the specific growth rate (μ) is a function of the concentration of limiting substrate (S), the maximum specific growth rate (μ_{max}) and a substrate specific constant (K_s). Their relationship was expressed by ***Monond*** by the following ***equation***

$$\mu = \mu_{max} \frac{S}{K_s + S} \qquad (3)$$

Both S and K_s are expressed as concentrations e.g., in moles or grams per liter.

The growth rate (μ) of an organism is not fixed but it is variable depending on the environmental conditions such as concentration of substrate and temperature. At a low concentration, the substrate is the limiting factor for growth (***Fig. 19.14A***). The ***Fig. 19.14B*** represents the growth rate for a given substrate concentration (by plotting μ against S).

In batch culture, the substrate is initially present at a higher concentration i.e. (S) > K_s, hence the equation (3) is approximately 1.

$$\frac{S}{K_s + S} = 1$$

Thus, $\mu = \mu_{max}$.

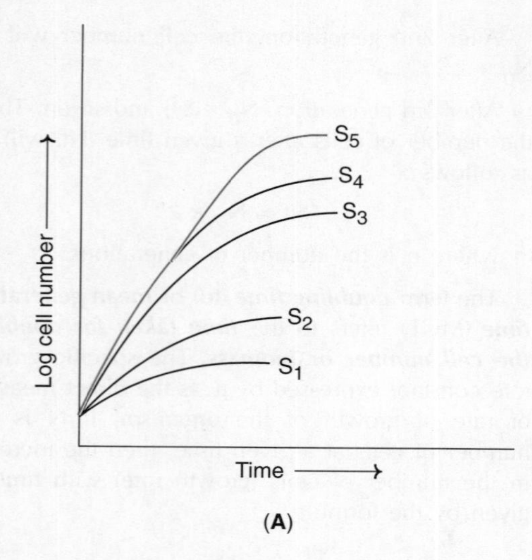

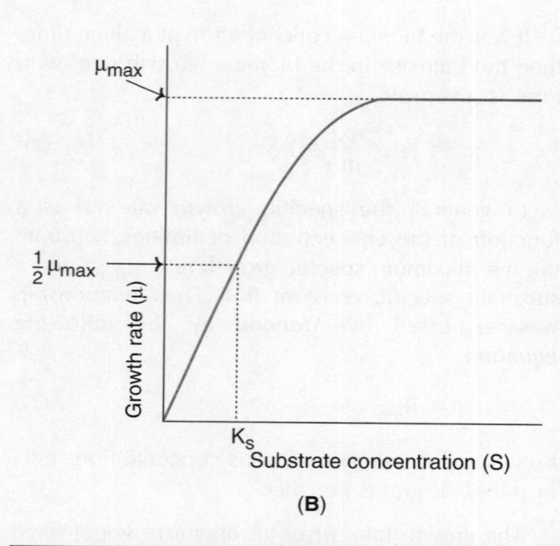

*Fig. 19.14 : Growth curves for unicellular organism in batch culture **(A)** With increasing concentrations of a substrate ($S_1<S_2<S_3<S_4<S_5$) **(B)** The effect of a given substrate concentration on growth rate (K_s = substrate concentration to produce half–maximal growth rate)*

When the substrate concentration is low, as usually occurs at the end of growth phase, then,

$$\frac{S}{K_s + S} < 1$$

Hence $\mu < \mu_{max}$.

CLASSIFICATION OF FERMENTATION PROCESSES

There are different ways of classifying the fermentation processes. The major classification as batch, fed-batch, semi-continuous and continuous fermentation processes are already described in some detail (See p. 259). Another classification, based on the product formation in relation to energy metabolism is briefly discussed below (***Fig. 19.15***).

Type I fermentation

When the ***product*** is formed directly ***from the primary metabolism*** used for energy production, it is referred to as type I and may be represented as.

Substrate A ⟶ Product

Substrate A ⟶ B ⟶ C ⟶ D ⟶ Product

Growth, energy metabolism and product formation almost run in a parallel manner (***Fig. 19.15A***). In this type, trophophase and iodophase are not separated from each other e.g. production of ethanol, gluconic acid and single-cell protein.

Type II fermentation

In type II category, the product is also formed from the substrate used for primary energy metabolism. However, the ***product is produced in the secondary pathway***, as illustrated below.

Substrate A → B → C → D···Primary metabolism

↳ E → F → G → Product

At the beginning, the growth of the microorganisms is accompanied by high substrate utilization with little or no product formation. Now the growth is slowed down but the substrate consumption is high, and this is coupled with product formation. As is evident from ***Fig. 19.15B***, in type II fermentation, the trophophase and idiophase are separate. Production of some amino acids, citric acid and itaconic acid are good examples of type II fermentation.

Type III fermentation

There is a clear distinction between the primary metabolism and product formation in type III fermentation (***Fig. 19.15C***) as they occur at separate times. Substrate consumption and ***rapid growth occur in the first phase and the product formation***

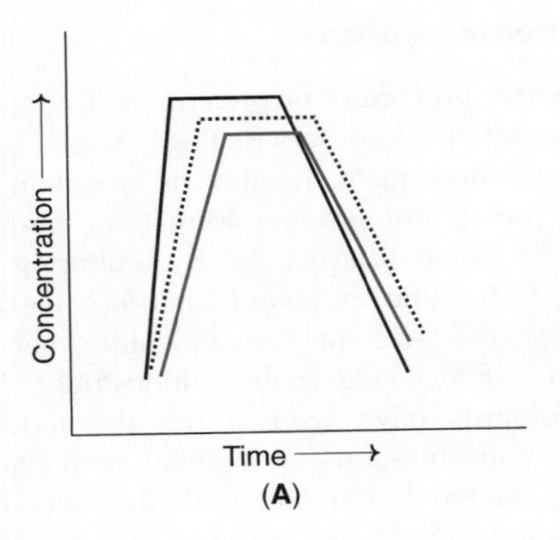

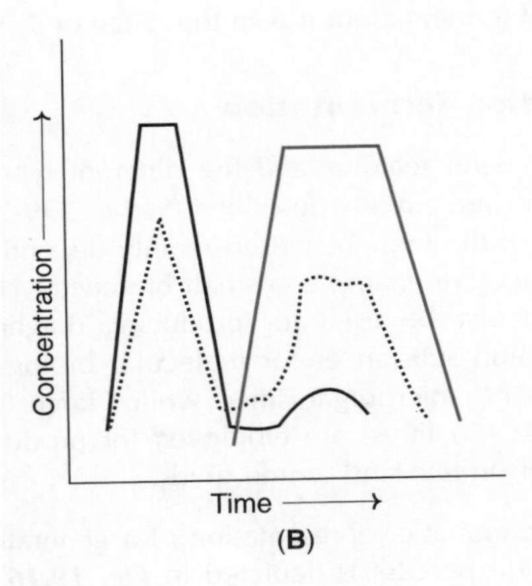

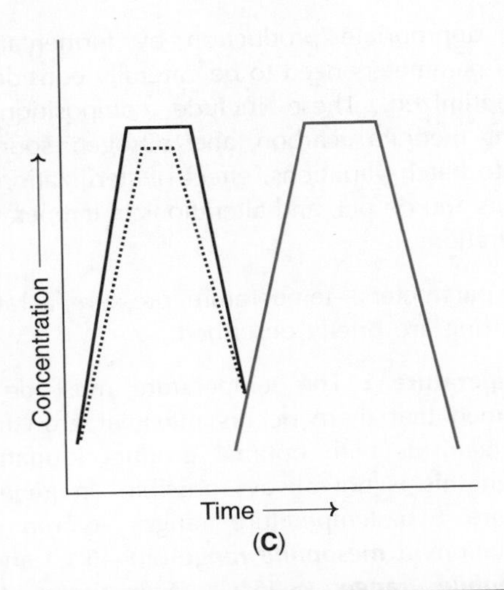

Fig. 19.15 : Types of fermentations in relation to product formation (A) Type I fermentation (B) Type II fermentation (C) Type III fermentation (— represents growth rate; .... correspond to substrate consumption; — indicates product formation).

occurs in the second phase. The product is formed from amphibolic metabolic pathways and not from primary metabolism e.g. production of vitamins and antibiotics.

Overlap of different types of fermentations

Types I, II and III fermentations, originally categorized by Garden (in 1959) are not very rigid. There are intermediate forms based on the composition of the nutrient culture medium, strain of the microorganism used and product formation. For instance, industrial production of lactic acid falls between type I and II, while production of the antibiotic amyloglycoside is intermediate between types II and III.

It is sometimes difficult to categorize the industrial fermentations under any one of these types (I, II, III) due to complex nature of the process e.g. mycelium producing microorganisms in relation to antibiotic production.

THE FERMENTATION PROCESS

The fermentation process basically ***consists of inoculum preservation, inoculum build-up, prefermenter culture*** and finally ***production fermentation***. A brief account of the four stages of fermentation is given below.

Inoculum preservation (culture maintenance)

The preservation of high-yielding strains of microorganisms for fermentation is very important for product formation in substantial amounts. The ultimate purpose of preservation is to maintain the strains, as long as possible, without cell division. There are different methods of preservation.

Storage at low (2-6°C) temperature : In this method, the microorganisms can be stored in a refrigerator in liquid culture or as stab culture. Although this is the easiest method of preservation, there is a high risk of contamination.

Storage by freezing : The microbial cultures can be frozen and preserved for several years. In the freezers, the preservation can be done at –18°C or, at –80°C. For preservation at –196°C, liquid nitrogen must be used. It is very important that the freezing (and later thawing when required) is done slowly (usually with a change of 1°C/min) to prevent damage and killing of the microorganisms. If proper care is not taken, as many as 95% of the cells may be killed by freezing and thawing.

Storage by lyophilization : Preservation of microorganisms by lyophilization (i.e., freeze drying) is the best method, although, it requires special equipment. In fact, ***lyophilization is the method of choice*** by many fermentation biotechnologists.

The storage of microorganisms can be done by any one of the three techniques described above. However, for each method, optimal conditions for preservation must be worked out for each strain separately. In general, the preserved ***master strains*** are cultivated once in two years for checking of their activity. When needed for use, the ***working strains*** can be obtained from the master strains.

Inoculum build up

The preserved cultures have to be revived for their industrial use. This can be done by growing the cultures in liquid or on solid media. The actual process and the conditions used for inoculum build-up largely depend on the preservation technique used. There are wide variations in the growth times which depend on the type of preservation and the organisms used as given below.

Refrigerated cultures (2-6°C) :

Bacteria 6–24 hours

Actinomycetes 1-3 days

Fungi 1-5 days

Frozen cultures (18°C, –80°C, –196°C) :

Bacteria 6–48 hours

Actinomycetes 1-5 days

Fungi 1-7 days

Lyophilized cultures :

For all organisms 4–10 days

For proper growth, and to obtain sufficient quantity of inoculum, a series of cultures are prepared. For good fermentation yield, the number of cells and spores, nutrient medium, temperature and age of the inoculum are important.

The inoculum build-up is suspended in a surface-active agent such as Tween 80 and transferred to the bioreactor for fermentation.

Prefermenter culture

Fermenter preculture or prefermenter culture is often required for inoculating large sized bioreactors. Inadequate quantity of inoculum will not only delay the product formation, but also reduce the yield drastically. By culturing the microorganisms (the inoculum build-up) in small fermenters, the size of the inoculum can be increased for large-scale industrial use. Biotechnologists have worked out the requisite inoculum concentrations for optimal fermentation e.g., for bacterial fermentation, the inoculum concentration should be between 0.2 to 3.0%; for fungal fermentation, it is in the range of 5–10%.

Production fermentation

The general features and the different types of bioreactors are already described (See p. 239-244). The size of the fermenter used mainly depends on the product. For example, a small bioreactor (1–20 litre size) can be used for producing diagnostic enzymes and substances for molecular biology by recombinant microorganisms, while large bio-reactors (≥ 450 litres) are employed for producing single-cell protein and amino acids.

A diagrammatic representation of a generalized fermentation process is depicted in ***Fig. 19.16***.

For appropriate production by fermentation, several parameters need to be carefully considered and optimized. These include composition of nutrient medium, carbon and nitrogen sources, batch to batch variations, effect of sterilization on nutrients and on pH, and alterations in temperature and aeration.

The parameters—temperature, pressure, aeration and stirring are briefly described.

Temperature : The temperature must be so maintained that there occurs maximal growth of microorganisms with optimal product formation, although this is not always possible. In general, there are two temperature ranges to run the fermentations a ***mesophile range*** (20–45°C) and a ***thermophile range*** (> 45°C). Sometimes, two different temperatures are used for the same fermentation process—a higher temperature is employed for good growth (in trophophase), and then the temperature is decreased for optimizing product formation (in idiophase).

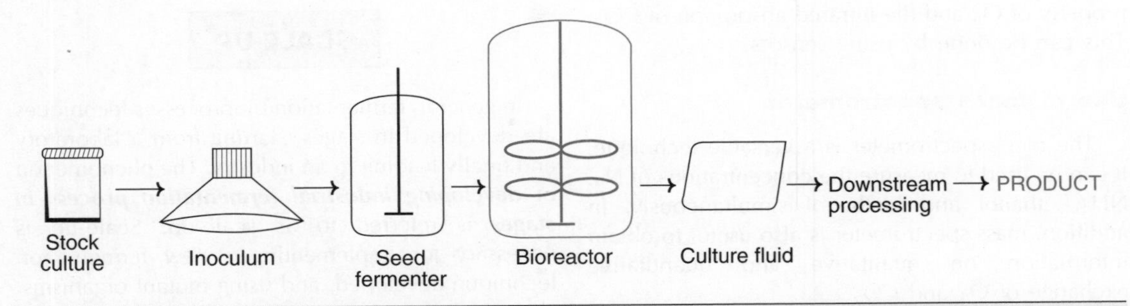

Fig. 19.16 : Diagrammatic representation of a generalized fermentation process.

Pressure : Appropriate maintenance of hydrostatic pressure, particularly in large sized bioreactors is very important. This is because pressure influences the solubility of O_2 and CO_2 in the culture medium. An overpressure in the range 0.2–0.5 bar is generally used.

Aeration : A bioreactor gets aerated by the supply of O_2 and therefore, adjustment must be made to furnish required amount of O_2 to the microorganisms. Usually, the aeration rate is in the range of 0.25–1.25 *vvm* (*v*olume of air/*v*olume of liquid/*m*inute).

Stirring : The type and the speed of impellers determines the stirring rate in a fermenter. In general, the impeller speed decreases as the size of the fermenter increases. Thus, for a small bioreactor (size 1–20 litres), the impeller speed is in the range of 250–350 rpm, while for a large bioreactor (size around 450 litres, the impeller speed is 60–120 rpm.

MEASUREMENT AND CONTROL OF BIOPROCESS PARAMETERS

There are a large number of physical, chemical and biological parameters that can be measured during fermentation/bioprocessing (***Table 19.6***) for data analysis and appropriate control. Some ***special sensors*** have been developed to carry out measurements in the bioreactors. The basic requirement of all the sensors is that they must be sterilizable. The measurements of the parameters (listed in Table) can be done either directly in the bioreactor or in the laboratory.

pH measurement : There are pH electrodes that can withstand high temperature (sterilization) pressure and mechanical stresses, and yet measure the pH accurately. Combination electrodes (reference electrode, glass electrode) are being used. In fact, electrodes are also available for measuring several other inorganic ions.

O_2 and CO_2 measurement : Oxygen electrodes and CO_2 electrodes can be used to measure O_2 and CO_2 concentrations respectively. The electrodes are amperometric in nature. They are however, susceptible for damage on sterilization.

In a commonly used technique, O_2 and CO_2 respectively can be measured by the magnetic

TABLE 19.6 Important parameters that can be measured during bioprocessing

Physical parameters
Temperature
Pressure
Flow rates
Viscosity
Turbidity
Power consumption
Chemical parameters
pH
Substrate concentration
Product concentration
O_2 concentration (dissolved)
Waste gases concentration (e.g. CO_2)
Ionic strength
Biological parameters
Activities of specific enzymes
Protein concentration
Energetics (ATP concentration)
DNA/RNA content

property of O_2 and the infrared absorption of CO_2. This can be done by using sensors.

Use of mass spectrometer

The mass spectrometer is a versatile technique. It can be used to measure the concentrations of N_2, NH_3, ethanol and methanol simultaneously. In addition, mass spectrometer is also useful to obtain information on qualitative and quantitative exchange of O_2 and CO_2.

Use of gas-permeable membranes

The measurement of dissolved gases, up to 8 simultaneously, can be done almost accurately by using gas-permeable membranes. The advantage is that such measurement is possible to carry out in the nutrient medium.

Use of computers

Computers are used in industrial biotechnology for data acquisition, data analysis and developing fermentation models.

Data acquisition : By employing ***on-line sensors*** and computers in fermentation system, data can be obtained with regard to the concentration of O_2 and CO_2, pH, temperature, pressure, viscosity, turbidity, aeration rate etc. Certain other parameters (e.g. nutrient concentration, product formation, biomass concentration) can be measured in the laboratory i.e. ***off-line measurements***. The information collected from on-line and off-line measurements can be entered into a computer. In this fashion, the entire data regarding a fermentation can be processed, stored and retrieved.

Data analysis : The data collected on a computer can be used for various calculations e.g. rate of substrate utilization, rate of product formation, rates of O_2 uptake and CO_2 formation, heat balance, respiratory quotient. Through computer data analysis, it is possible to arrive at the optimal productivity for a given fermentation system.

Development of fermentation models : The computer can be used to develop mathematical models of fermentation processes. These models in turn will be useful to have a better control over fermentation systems with high productivity in a cost-effective manner.

SCALE-UP

In general, fermentation/bioprocesses techniques are developed in stages, starting from a laboratory and finally leading to an industry. The phenomenon of ***developing industrial fermentation process in stages*** is referred to as scale-up. Scale-up is necessary for implementing a new fermentation technique developed, and using mutant organisms.

The very purpose of scale-up is ***to develop optimal environmental and operating conditions at different levels for a successful fermentation industry***. The conditions that need to be studied include substrate concentration, agitation and mixing, aeration, power consumption and rate of O_2 transfer.

In a conventional scale-up, a fermentation technique is developed in 3-4 stages (i.e., scales). The initial stage involves a screening process using petri dishes or Erlenmeyer flasks. The next stage is a pilot project to determine the optimal operating conditions for a fermentation process with a capacity of 5–200 litres. The final stage involves the ***transfer of technology developed in the laboratory to industry***.

It has to be continuously noted that a fermentation process that works well at the ***laboratory scale*** may work poorly or may not work at all on ***industrial scale***. Therefore, it is not always possible to blindly apply the laboratory conditions of a fermentation technique developed to industry. At the laboratory scale, one is interested in the maximum yield of the product for unit time. At the industry level, besides the product yield, minimal operating cost is another important factor for consideration. An industrial biotechnologist has to apply his/her intellect and technical skill for establishing a successful fermentation set up in a cost-effective manner.

FOOD TECHNOLOGY

Food technology is a vast field. The salient features of food processing which has some relevance to bioprocess engineering and technology are given here. In general, the food processing is carried out to acheive the following objectives.

- For the purpose of storage and transport.
- To protect from contamination
- To increase the shelf-life
- To make it attractive for the consumers.

For appropriate processing of food, many criteria need to be taken into account. These include the ability of the microorganisms and pests to invade and grow on foods, and the chemical instability and biological activity of foods.

FOOD PRESERVATION

Among the many food processing techniques, food preservation is the most important one. Selected food preservation processes are briefly described.

Drying

Exposure of foods to sunlight and drying is a natural, and an earliest method of food preservation. Drying involves the removal of water. Consequently, the moisture content of the food falls, and the invading microorganisms cannot grow.

Hot air is most frequently used to remove moisture. In actual practice, foods are dried by using different types of equipment.

- ***Shallow-bed dryers*** (drying is carried out in perforated conveyor beds).
- ***Deep-bed dryers*** (drying occurs in bins).
- ***Spray dryers*** (to dry liquid foods and food slurries).
- ***Freeze dryers*** (to dry soup ingradients, beverage extracts).

Chilling

The technique of chilling is commonly used to preserve foods without freezing. The process of chilling is carried out around 0°C with humidity between 85–95%. The shelf–life of fresh foods like meat, fish and dairy products can be extended by chilling (usually less than a month). It is reported that the if chilling is done under low oxygen conditions, the shelf-life of foods increases.

Chilling is frequently used for long distance shipping of meat, apples, vegetables etc.

Freezing

Foods can be preserved in a frozen state (–30° to –10°C). At a very low temperatures, the water activity and reactant mobility are low, hence the chemical reactions are reduced.

Foods can be frozen by using a stream of refrigerated air, or by passing inert refrigerant or cryogenic gas. Rapid freezing is advocated to minimize the adverse effects on the texture of foods.

Thermal processing

By applying heat (comparable to sterilization), majority of the microorganisms and spores present in the foods can be killed. Thermal processing is carried out in sealed containers devoid of oxygen, and thus aerobic organisms cannot grow. Further, higher temperature also leads to inactivation of enzymes, and consequently microbial growth will be retarded.

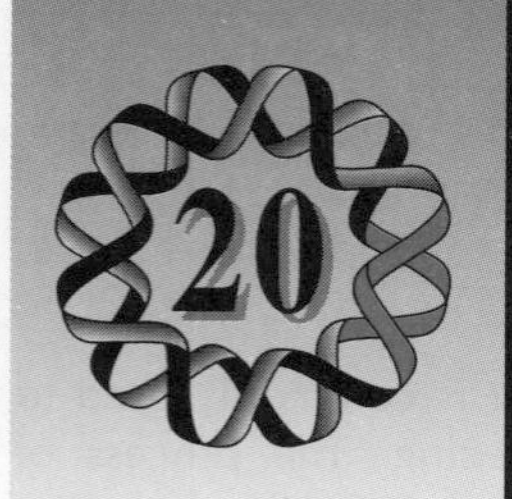

Downstream Processing

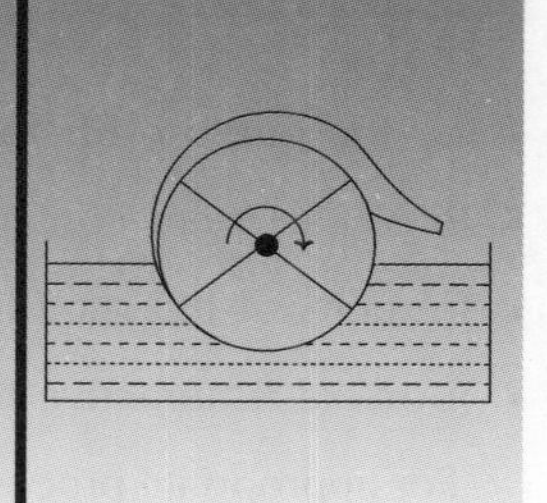

As the fermentation is complete (described in Chapter 19), it is necessary to recover the desired end product. The end products include antibiotics, amino acids, vitamins, organic acids, industrial enzymes, and vaccines. The ***extraction and purification of a biotechnological product from fermentation is*** referred to as ***downstream processing (DSP) or product recovery***. DSP is as complex and important as fermentation process. It often requires the expertise and technical skills of chemists, process engineers, besides bioscientists.

In the present day biotechnology, the fermentation and downstream processing are considered as an integrated system. The methodology adopted for downstream processing depends on the nature of the end product, its concentration, stability and the degree of purification required, besides the presence of other products. The product recovery yield in general is expected to be higher, if the number of steps in DSP is lower.

The desired products for isolation by DSP are most frequently metabolites which may be present as follows.

1. **Intracellular metabolites :** These products are located within the cells e.g. vitamins, enzymes.

2. **Extracellular metabolites :** They are present outside the cells (culture fluids) e.g. most antibiotics (penicillin, streptomycin), amino acids, alcohol, citric acid, some enzymes (amylases, proteases).

3. **Both intracellular and extracellular** e.g. vitamin B_{12}, flavomycin.

Sometimes, the microorganism may itself be the desired end product for isolation e.g. single-cell protein. The product recovery as a biomass is simpler. When subjected to heat, the cells aggregate and form clumps which can be separated by sedimentation.

STAGES IN DOWNSTREAM PROCESSING

Downstream processing of metabolites is a ***multistage operation***, and may be broadly divided into the following stages.

1. Solid-liquid separation
2. Release of intracellular products
3. Concentration
4. Purification
5. Formulation.

In ***Fig. 20.1***, an outline of the major steps in downstream processing is given, and they are described in some detail in the following pages.

SOLID-LIQUID SEPARATION

The first step in product recovery is the separation of whole cells (cell biomass) and other insoluble ingradients from the culture broth (**Note :** If the desired product is an intracellular metabolite, it must be released from the cells before

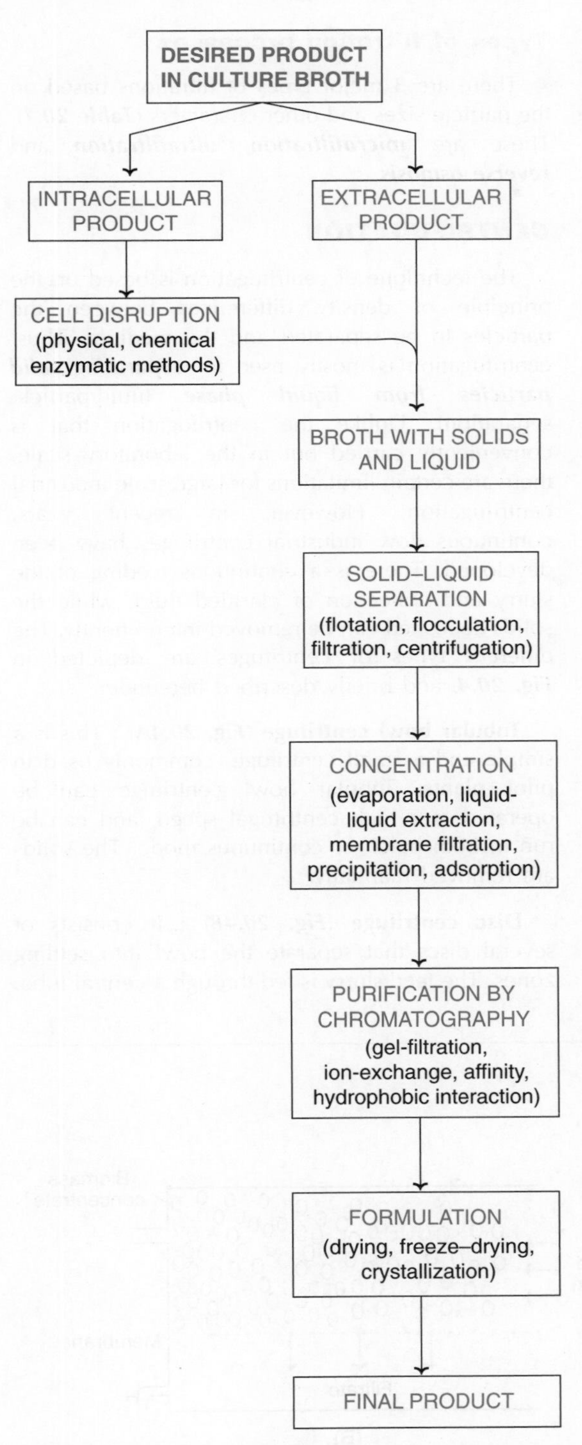

Fig. 20.1 : A summary of the major steps in downstream processing.

subjecting to solid-liquid separation. Details of cell disruption are described later). Some authors use the term ***harvesting of microbial cells*** for the separation of cells from the culture medium.

Several methods are in use for solid-liquid separation. These include flotation, flocculation, filtration and centrifugation.

FLOTATION

When a gas is introduced into the liquid broth, it forms bubbles. The cells and other solid particles get adsorbed on gas bubbles. These bubbles rise to the foam layer which can be collected and removed. The presence of certain substances, referred to as ***collector substances***, facilitates stable foam formation e.g., long chain fatty acids, amines.

FLOCCULATION

In flocculation, the cells (or cell debris) form large aggregates to settle down for easy removal. The process of flocculation depends on the nature of cells and the ionic constituents of the medium. Addition of flocculating agents (inorganic salt, organic polyelectrolyte, mineral hydrocolloid) is often necessary to achieve appropriate flocculation.

FILTRATION

Filtration is the most commonly used technique for separating the biomass and culture filtrate. The efficiency of filtration depends on many factors—the size of the organism, presence of other organisms, viscosity of the medium, and temperature. Several filters such as depth filters, absolute filters, rotary drum vacuum filters and membrane filters are in use.

Depth filters : They are composed of a filamentous matrix such as glass wool, asbestos or filter paper. The particles are trapped within the matrix and the fluid passes out. Filamentous fungi can be removed by using depth filters.

Absolute filters : These filters are with specific pore sizes that are smaller than the particles to be removed. Bacteria from culture medium can be removed by absolute filters.

Rotary drum vacuum filters : These filters are frequently used for separation of broth containing 10–40% solids (by volume) and particles in the size of 0.5–10μm. Rotary drum vacuum filters have been successfully used for filtration of yeast cells

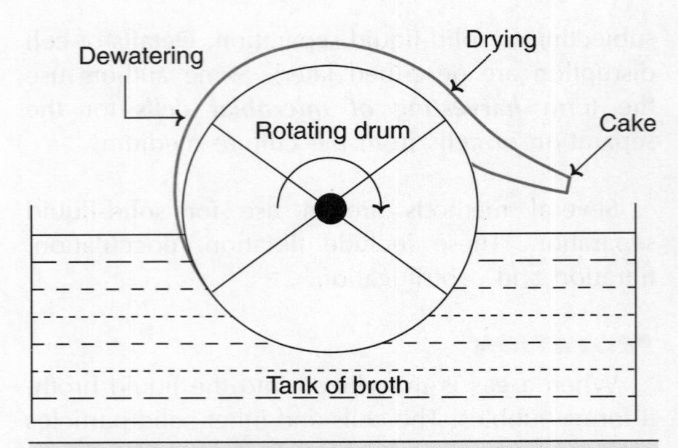

Fig. 20.2 : Diagrammatic representation of a rotary drum vacuum filter.

and filamentous fungi. The equipment is simple with low power consumption and is easy to operate. The filtration unit consists of a rotating drum partially immersed in a tank of broth (***Fig. 20.2***). As the drum rotates, it picks up the biomass which gets deposited as a cake on the drum surface. This filter cake can be easily removed.

Membrane filters : In this type of filtration, membranes with specific pore sizes can be used. However, clogging of filters is a major limitation. There are two types of membrane filtrations—***static filtration*** and ***cross-flow filtration*** (***Fig. 20.3***). In cross-flow filtration, the culture broth is pumped in a crosswise fashion across the membrane. This reduces the clogging process and hence better than the static filtration.

Types of filtration processes

There are 3 major types of filtrations based on the particle sizes and other characters (***Table 20.1***). These are ***microfiltration***, ***ultrafiltration*** and ***reverse osmosis***.

CENTRIFUGATION

The technique of centrifugation is based on the principle of density differences between the particles to be separated and the medium. Thus, centrifugation is mostly used for ***separating solid particles from liquid phase*** (fluid/particle separation). Unlike the centrifugation that is conveniently carried out in the laboratory scale, there are certain limitations for large scale industrial centrifugation. However, in recent years, continuous flow industrial centrifuges have been developed. There is a continuous feeding of the slurry and collection of clarified fluid, while the solids deposited can be removed intermittently. The different types of centrifuges are depicted in ***Fig. 20.4***, and briefly described hereunder.

Tubular bowl centrifuge (***Fig. 20.4A***) **:** This is a simple and a small centrifuge, commonly used in pilot plants. Tubular bowl centrifuge can be operated at a high centrifugal speed, and can be run in both batch or continuous mode. The solids are removed manually.

Disc centrifuge (***Fig. 20.4B***) **:** It consists of several discs that separate the bowl into settling zones. The feed/slurry is fed through a central tube.

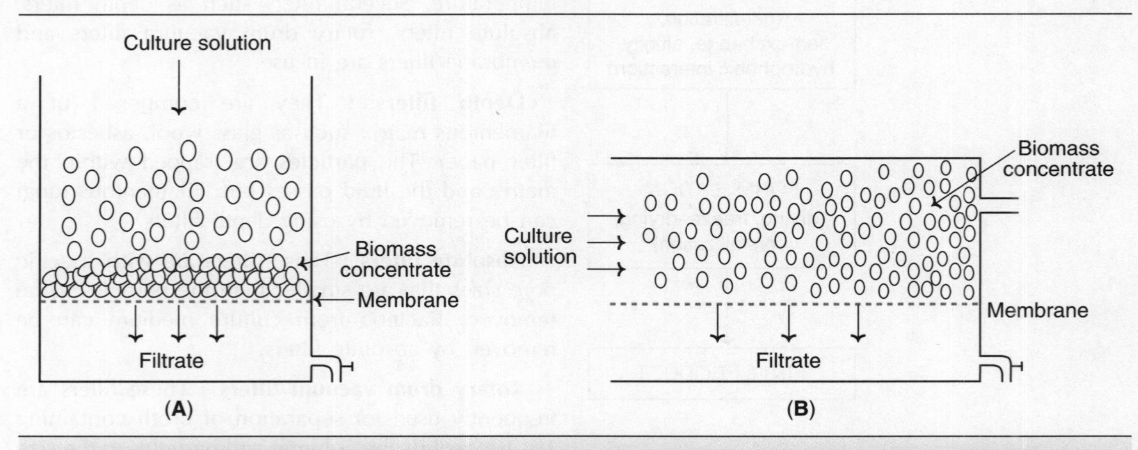

Fig. 20.3 : Filter systems for separation of biomass and culture filtrate (A) Static–flow filtration (B) Cross–flow filtration.

TABLE 20.1 Major types of filtration processes with characteristic features

Type	*Sizes of particles separated*	*Compound or particle separated*
1. Microfiltration	0.1–10 μm	Cells or cell fractions, viruses.
2. Ultrafiltration	0.001–0.1 μm	Compounds with molecular weights greater than 1000 (e.g. enzymes).
3. Reverse osmosis (hyperfiltration)	0.0001–0.001 μm	Compounds with molecular weights less than 1000 (e.g. lactose).

The clarified fluid moves upwards while the solids settle at the lower surface.

Multichamber centrifuge (*Fig. 20.4C*) **:** This is basically a modification of tubular bowl type of centrifuge. It consists of several chambers connected in such a way that the feed flows in a zigzag fashion. There is a variation in the centrifugal force in different chambers. The force is much higher in the periphery chambers, as a result smallest particles settle down in the outermost chamber.

Scroll centrifuge or decanter (*Fig. 20.4D*) **:** It is composed of a rotating horizontal bowl tapered at one end. The decanter is generally used to concentrate fluids with high solid concentration (biomass content 5–80%). The solids are deposited on the wall of the bowl which can be scrapped and removed from the narrow end.

RELEASE OF INTRACELLULAR PRODUCTS

As already stated, there are several biotechnological products (vitamins, enzymes) which are located within the cells. Such compounds have to be first released (maximally and in an active form) for their further processing and final isolation. The microorganisms or other cells can be disintegrated or disrupted by ***physical, chemical*** or ***enzymatic methods***. The outline of different techniques used for breakage of cells is given in ***Fig. 20.5***. The selection of a particular method depends on the nature of the cells, since there is a wide variation in the property of cell disruption or breakage. For instance, Gram-negative bacteria and filamentous fungi can be more easily broken compared to Gram-positive bacteria and yeasts.

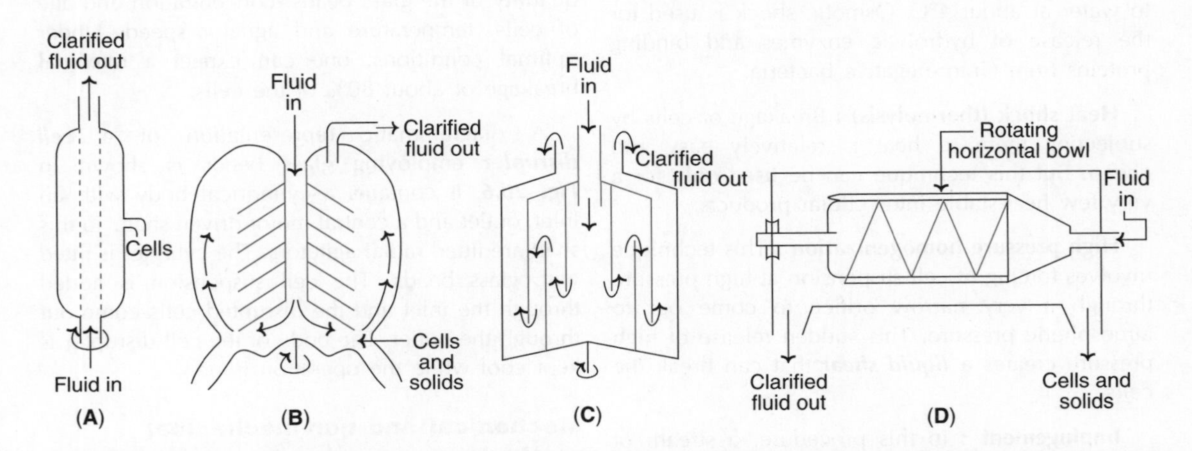

Fig. 20.4 : Centrifuges commonly used in downstream processing (A) Tubular bowl centrifuge (B) Disc centrifuge (C) Multichamber centrifuge (D) Scroll centrifuge (decanter).

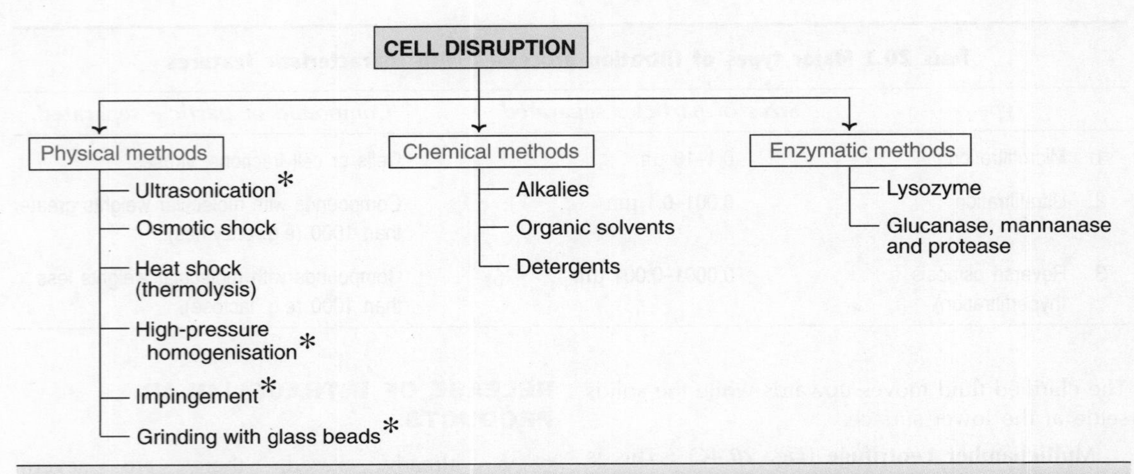

Fig. 20.5 : Major methods for cell disruption to release the intracellular products (indicate mechanical methods while all the remaining are non-mechanical).*

CELL DISRUPTION

Physical methods of cell disruption

The microorganisms or cells can be disrupted by certain physical methods to release the intracellular products.

Ultrasonication : Ultrasonic disintegration is widely employed in the laboratory. However, due to high cost, it is not suitable for large-scale use in industries.

Osmotic shock : This method involves the suspension of cells (free from growth medium) in 20% buffered sucrose. The cells are then transferred to water at about 4°C. Osmotic shock is used for the release of hydrolytic enzymes and binding proteins from Gram-negative bacteria.

Heat shock (thermolysis) : Breakage of cells by subjecting them to heat is relatively easy and cheap. But this technique can be used only for a very few heat-stable intracellular products.

High pressure homogenization : This technique involves forcing of cell suspension at high pressure through a very narrow orifice to come out to atmospheric pressure. This sudden release of high pressure creates a ***liquid shear*** that can break the cells.

Impingement : In this procedure, a stream of suspended cells at high velocity and pressure are forced to hit either a stationary surface or a second stream of suspended cells (impinge literally means to strike or hit). The cells are disrupted by the forces created at the point of contact. ***Microfluidizer*** is a device developed based on the principle of impingement. It has been successfully used for breaking *E. coli* cells. The advantage with impingement technique is that it can be effectively used for disrupting cells even at a low concentration.

Grinding with glass beads : The cells mixed with glass beads are subjected to a very high speed in a reaction vessel. The cells break as they are forced against the wall of the vessel by the beads. Several factors influence the cell breakage-size and quantity of the glass beads, concentration and age of cells, temperature and agitator speed. Under optimal conditions, one can expect a maximal breakage of about 80% of the cells.

A diagrammatic representation of a ***cell disrupter*** employing glass beeds is shown in ***Fig. 20.6***. It contains a cylindrical body with an inlet, outlet and a central motor-driven shaft. To this shaft are fitted radial agitators. The cylinder is fitted with glass beads. The cell suspension is added through the inlet and the disrupted cells come out through the outlet. The body of the cell disrupter is kept cool while the operation is on.

Mechanical and non-mechanical methods

Among the ***physical methods of cell disruption*** described above, ultrasonication, high-pressure

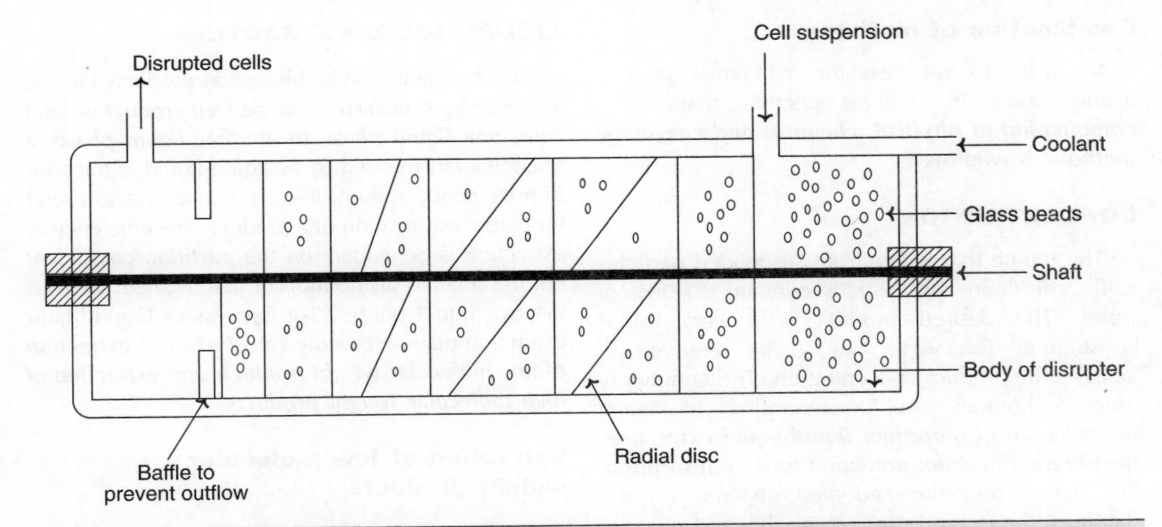

Fig. 20.6 : Diagrammatic representation of a cell disrupter.

homogenisation, impigement and grinding with glass beads are ***mechanical*** while osmotic shock and heat shock are non-mechanical. The ***chemical and enzymatic methods*** (described below) ***are non-mechanical in nature***.

Chemical methods of cell disruption

Treatment with alkalies, organic solvents and detergents can lyse the cells to release the contents.

Alkalies : Alkali treatment has been used for the extraction of some bacterial proteins. However, the alkali stability of the desired product is very crucial for the success of this method e.g., recombinant growth hormone can be efficiently released from *E. coli* by treatment with sodium hydroxide at pH 11.

Organic solvents : Several water miscible organic solvents can be used to disrupt the cells e.g., methanol, ethanol, isopropanol, butanol. These compounds are inflammable, hence require specialised equipment for fire safety. The organic solvent toluene is frequently used. It is believed that toluene dissolves membrane phospholipids and creates membrane pores for release of intracellular contents.

Detergents : Detergents that are ionic in nature, ***cationic***-cetyl trimethyl ammonium bromide or ***anionic***-sodium lauryl sulfate can denature membrane proteins and lyse the cells. Non-ionic detergents (although less reactive than ionic ones) are also used to some extent e.g., Triton X-100 or Tween. The problem with the use of detergents is that they affect purification steps, particularly the salt precipitation. This limitation can be overcome by using ultrafiltration or ion-exchange chromatography for purification.

Enzymatic methods of cell disruption

Cell disruption by enzymatic methods has certain advantages i.e., lysis of cells occurs under mild conditions in a selective manner. This is quite ***advantageous for product recovery***.

Lysozyme is the most frequently used enzyme and is commercially available (produced from hen egg white). It hydrolyses β-1, 4-glycosidic bonds of the mucopeptide in bacterial cell walls. The ***Gram-positive bacteria*** (with high content of cell wall mucopeptides) are more susceptible for the action of lysozyme. For Gram-negative bacteria, lysozyme in association with EDTA can break the cells. As the cell wall gets digested by lysozyme, the osmotic effects break the periplasmic membrane to release the intracellular contents.

Certain other enzymes are also used, although less frequently, for cell disruption. For the lysis of yeast cell walls, glucanase and mannanase in combination with proteases are used.

Combination of methods

In order to increase the efficiency of cell disintegration in a cost-effective manner, a ***combination of physical, chemical and enzymatic methods is employed***.

CONCENTRATION

The filtrate that is free from suspended particles (cells, cell debris etc.) usually contains 80–98% of water. The desired product is a very minor constituent. The water has to be removed to achieve the product concentration. The commonly used techniques for concentrating biological products are ***evaporation, liquid-liquid extraction, membrane filtration, precipitation*** and ***adsorption***. The actual procedure adopted depends on the nature of the desired product (quality and quantity to be retained as far as possible) and the cost factor.

EVAPORATION

Water in the broth filtrate can be removed by a simple evaporation process. The evaporators, in general, have a heating device for supply of steam, and unit for the separation of concentrated product and vapour, a condenser for condensing vapour, accessories and control equipment. The capacity of the equipment is variable that may range from small laboratory scale to industrial scale. Some of the important types of evaporators in common use are briefly described.

Plate evaporators : The liquid to be concentrated flows over plates. As the steam is supplied, the liquid gets concentrated and becomes viscous.

Falling film evaporators : In this case, the liquid flows down long tubes which gets distributed as a thin film over the heating surface. Falling film evaporators are suitable for removing water from viscous products of fermentation.

Forced film evaporators : The liquid films are mechanically driven and these devices are suitable for producing dry product concentrates.

Centrifugal forced film evaporators : These equipment evaporate the liquid very quickly (in seconds), hence suitable for concentrating even heat-labile substances. In these evaporators, a centrifugal force is used to pass on the liquid over heated plates or conical surfaces for instantaneous evaporation.

LIQUID-LIQUID EXTRACTION

The concentration of biological products can be achieved by ***transferring the desired product*** (solute) ***from one liquid phase to another liquid phase***, a phenomenon referred to as liquid-liquid extraction. Besides concentration, this technique is also useful for partial purification of a product. The efficiency of extraction is dependent on the ***partition coefficient*** i.e. the relative distribution of a substance between the two liquid phases. The process of liquid-liquid extraction may be broadly categorized as ***extraction of low molecular weight products*** and ***extraction of high molecular weight products***.

Extraction of low molecular weight products

By using organic solvents, the lipophilic compounds can be conveniently extracted. However, it is quite difficult to extract hydrophilic compounds. Extraction of lipophilic products can be done by the following techniques.

Physical extraction : The compound gets itself distributed between two liquid phases based on the physical properties. This technique is used for extraction of non-ionising compounds.

Dissociation extraction : This technique is suitable for the extraction of ionisable compounds. Certain antibiotics can be extracted by this procedure.

Reactive extraction : In this case, the desired product is made to react with a carrier molecule (e.g., phosphorus compound, aliphatic amine) and extracted into organic solvent. Reactive extraction procedure is quite useful for the extraction of certain compounds that are highly soluble in water (aqueous phase) e.g., organic acids.

Supercritical fluid (SCF) extraction : This technique differs from the above procedures, since the materials used for extraction are supercritical fluids (SCFs). ***SCFs are intermediates between gases and liquids*** and exist as fluids above their critical temperature and pressure. Supercritical CO_2, with a low critical temperature and pressure is commonly used in the extraction. Supercritical fluid extraction is rather expensive, hence not widely used (SCF has been used for the extraction of caffeine from coffee beans, and pigments and flavor ingradients from biological materials).

Extraction of high molecular weight compounds

Proteins are the most predominant high molecular weight products produced in fermentation industries. Organic solvents cannot be used for protein extraction, as they lose their biological activities. They are extracted by using an aqueous ***two-phase systems*** or ***reverse micelles formation***.

Aqueous two-phase systems (ATPS) : They can be prepared by mixing a polymer (e.g., polyethylene glycol) and a salt solution (ammonium sulfate) or two different polymers. Water is the main component in ATPS, but the two phases are not miscible. Cells and other solids remain in one phase while the proteins are transferred to other phase. The distribution of the desired product is based on its surface and ionic character and the nature of phases. Th separation takes much longer time by ATPS.

Reverse miceller systems : Reverse micelles are stable aggregates of surfactant molecules and water in organic solvents. The proteins can be extracted from the aqueous medium by forming reverse micelles. In fact, the enzymes can be extracted by this procedure without loss of biological activity.

MEMBRANE FILTRATION

Membrane filtration has become a common separation technique in industrial biotechnology. It can be conveniently used for the separation of biomolecules and particles, and for the concentration of fluids. The membrane filtration technique basically involves the use of a semi-permeable membrane that selectively retains the particles/molecules that are bigger than the pore size while the smaller molecules pass through the membrane pores.

Membranes used in filtration are made up of polymeric materials such as polyethersulfone and polyvinyl difluoride. It is rather difficult to sterilize membrane filters. In recent years, microfilters and ultrafilters composed of ceramics and steel are available. Cleaning and sterilization of such filters are easy.

The filtration techniques namely ***microfiltration, ultrafiltration,*** and ***hyperfiltration*** (reverse osmosis) have already been described (Refer ***Table 20.1***). The other types of membrane filtration techniques are discribed briefly.

Membrane adsorbers : They are micro- or macroporous membranes with ion exchange groups and/or affinity ligands. Membrane adsorbers can bind to proteins and retain them. Such proteins can be eluted by employing solutions in chromatography.

Pervaporation : This is a technique in which volatile products can be separated by a ***process of permeation through a membrane coupled with evaporation***. Pervaporation is quite useful for the extraction, recovery and concentration of volatile products. However, this procedure has a limitation since it cannot be used for large scale separation of volatile products due to cost factor.

Perstraction : This is an advanced technique working on the principle of membrane filtration coupled with solvent extraction. The hydrophobic compounds can be recovered/concentrated by this method.

PRECIPITATION

Precipitation is the most commonly used technique in industry for the concentration of macromolecules such as proteins and polysaccharides. Further, precipitation technique can also be employed for the removal of certain unwanted byproducts e.g. nucleic acids, pigments. Neutral salts, organic solvents, high molecular weight polymers (ionic or non-ionic), besides alteration in temperature and pH are used in precipitation. In addition to these non-specific protein precipitation reactions (i.e. the nature of the protein is unimportant), there are some protein specific precipitations e.g., affinity precipitation, ligand precipitation.

Neutral salts : The most commonly used salt is ***ammonium sulfate***, since it is highly soluble, non-toxic to proteins and low-priced. Ammonium sulfate ***increases hydrophobic interactions*** between protein molecules that result in their precipitation. The precipitation of proteins is dependent on several factors such as protein concentration, pH and temperature.

Organic solvents : ***Ethanol, acetone*** and ***propanol*** are the commonly used organic solvents for protein precipitation. They ***reduce the dielectric constant*** of the medium and enhance electrostatic interaction between protein molecules that lead to precipitation. Since proteins are denatured by organic solvents, the precipitation process has to be carried out below 0°C.

Non-ionic polymers : ***Polyethylene glycol*** **(*PEG*)** is a high molecular weight non-ionic polymer that can precipitate proteins. It ***reduces*** the quantity of water available for ***protein solvation*** and precipitates protein. PEG does not denature proteins, besides being non-toxic.

Ionic polymers : The charged polymers such as ***polyacrylic acid*** and ***polyethyleneimine*** are used. They form complexes with oppositely charged protein molecules that causes charge neutralisation and precepitation.

Increase in temperature : The heat sensitive proteins can be precipitated by increasing the temperature.

Change in pH : Alterations in pH can also lead to protein precipitation.

Affinity precipitation : The affinity interaction (e.g., between antigen and antibody) is exploited for precipitation of proteins.

Precipitation by ligands : Ligands with specific binding sites for proteins have been successfully used for selective precipitation.

ADSORPTION

The biological products of fermentation can be concentrated by using solid adsorbent particles. In the early days, activated charcoal was used as the adsorbent material. In recent years, cellulose-based adsorbents are employed for protein concentration. And for concentration of low molecular weight compounds (vitamins, antibiotics, peptides) polystyrene, methacrylate and acrylate based matrices are used. The process of adsorption can be carried out by making a bed of adsorbent column and passing the culture broth through it. The desired product, held by the adsorbent, can be eluted.

PURIFICATION BY CHROMATOGRAPHY

The biological products of fermentation (proteins, pharmaceuticals, diagnostic compounds and research materials) are very effectively purified by chromatography. It is basically an analytical technique dealing with the separation of closely related compounds from a mixture. Chromatography usually consists of a ***stationary phase*** and ***mobile phase***. The stationary phase is the porous solid matrix packed in a column (equilibrated with a suitable solvent) on to which the mixture of compounds to be separated is loaded. The compounds are eluted by a mobile phase. A single mobile phase may be used continuously or it may be changed appropriately to facilitate the release of desired compounds. The eluate from the column can be monitored continuously (e.g. protein elution can be monitored by ultraviolet adsorption at 280 nm), and collected in fractions of definite volumes.

TABLE 20.2 Chromatographic techniques along with the principles for separation of proteins

Chromatography	*Principle*
Gel-filtration (size exclusion)	Size and shape
Ion-exchange	Net charge
Chromatofocussing	Net charge
Affinity	Biological affinity and molecular recognition
Hydrophobic interaction	Polarity (hydrophobicity of molecules)
Immobilized metal-ion affinity	Metal ion binding

The different types of chromatography techniques used for separation (mainly proteins) along with the principles are given in ***Table 20.2***. A large number of matrices are commercially available for purification of proteins e.g., agarose, cellulose, polyacrylamide, porous silica, cross-linked dextran, polystyrene. Some of the important features of selected chromatographic techniques are briefly described.

Gel-filtration chromatography : This is also referred to as ***size-exclusion chromatography***. In this technique, the separation of molecules is based on the size, shape and molecular weight. The sponge-like gel beads with pores serve as molecular sieves for separation of smaller and bigger molecules. A solution mixture containing molecules of different sizes (e.g. different proteins) is applied to the column and eluted. The smaller molecules enter the gel beads through their pores and get

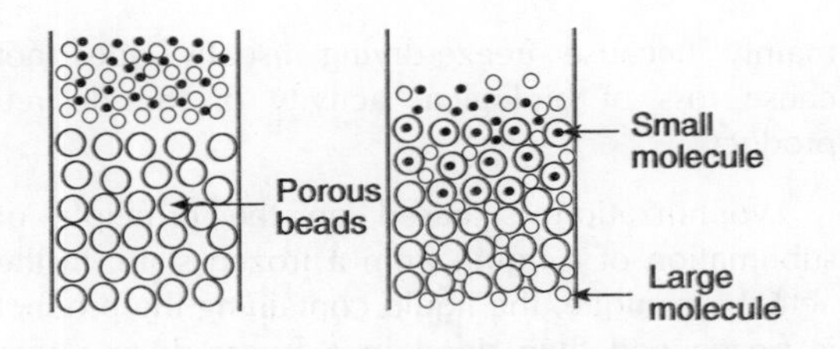

Fig. 20.7 : The principle of gel-filtration chromatography.

trapped. On the other hand, the larger molecules cannot pass through the pores and therefore come out first with the mobile liquid (***Fig. 20.7***). At the industrial scale, gel-filtration is particularly useful to remove salts and low molecular weight compounds from high molecular weight products.

Ion-exchange chromatography : It involves the separation of molecules based on their surface charges. Ion-exchangers are of two types (***cation-exchangers*** which have negatively charged groups like carboxymethyl and sulfonate, and ***anion-exchangers*** with positively charged groups like diethylaminoethyl (DEAE). The most commonly used cation-exchangers are Dowex HCR and Amberlite IR, the anion-exchangers are Dowex SAR and Amberlite IRA.

In ion-exchange chromatography, the pH of the medium is very crucial, since the net charge varies with pH. In other words, the pH determines the effective charge on both the target molecule and the ion-exchanger. The ionic bound molecules can be eluted from the matrix by changing the pH of the eluant or by increasing the concentration of salt solution. Ion-exchange chromatography is useful for the purification of antibiotics, besides the purification of proteins.

Affinity chromatography : This is an elegant method for the purification of proteins from a complex mixture. Affinity chromatography is based on an interaction of a protein with an immobilized ligand. The ligand can be a specific antibody, substrate, substrate analogue or an inhibitor. The immobilized ligand on a solid matrix can be effectively used to fish out complementary structures. In ***Table 20.3***, some examples of ligands used for the purification of proteins are given. The protein bound to the ligand can be eluted by reducing their interaction. This can be achieved by changing the pH of the buffer, altering the ionic strength or by using another free ligand molecule. The fresh ligand used has to be removed in the subsequent steps.

Hydrophobic interaction chromatography (HIC) : This is based on the principle of weak hydrophobic interactions between the hydrophobic ligands (alkyl, aryl side chains on matrix) and hydrophobic amino acids of proteins. The differences in the composition of hydrophobic amino acids in proteins can be used for their separation. The elution of proteins can be done by lowering the salt concentration, decreasing the polarity of the medium or reducing the temperature.

FORMULATION

Formulation broadly refers to the maintenance of activity and stability of a biotechnological products during storage and distribution. The formulation of low molecular weight products (solvents, organic acids) can be achieved by concentrating them with removal of most of the water. For certain small molecules, (antibiotics, citric acid), formulation can be done by crystallization by adding salts.

Proteins are highly susceptible for loss of biological activity, hence their formulation requires special care. Certain stabilizing additives are added to prolong the shelf life of protein. The ***stabilizers of protein formulation*** include ***sugars*** (sucrose, lactose), ***salts*** (sodium chloride, ammonium sulfate), ***polymers*** (polyethylene glycol) and ***polyhydric alcohols*** (glycerol). Proteins may be formulated in the form of solutions, suspensions or dry powders.

TABLE 20.3 Some examples of ligands used for separation of proteins by affinity chromatography

Ligand	*Type of protein*
Antibody	Antigen
Cofactor	Enzyme
Receptor	Hormone
Hapten	Antibody
Inhibitor	Enzyme
Lectins	Glycoproteins
Heparin	Coagulation factors
Metal ions	Metal ion binding proteins

Drying

Drying is an essential component of product formulation. It basically involves the transfer of heat to a wet product for removal of moisture. Most of the biological products of fermentation are sensitive to heat, and therefore require gentle drying methods.

Based on the method of heat transfer, drying devices may be categorized as ***contact***-, ***convection***-, ***radiation dryers***. These three types of dryers are commercially available.

Spray drying

Spray drying is used for drying large volumes of liquids. In spray drying, small droplets of liquid containing the product are passed through a nozzle directing it over a stream of hot gas. The water evaporates and the solid particles are left behind.

Freeze-drying

Freeze-drying or ***lyophilization*** is the most preferred method for drying and formulation of a wide-range of products—pharmaceuticals, foodstuffs, diagnostics, bacteria, viruses. This is mainly because freeze-drying usually does not cause loss of biological activity of the desired product.

Lyophilization is based on the principle of sublimation of a liquid from a frozen state. In the actual technique, the liquid containing the product is frozen and then dried in a freeze-dryer under vacuum. The vacuum can now be released and the product containing vials can be sealed e.g., penicillin can be freeze dried directly in ampules.

INTEGRATION OF DIFFERENT PROCESSES

It is ideal to ***integrate the fermentation and downstream processing to finally get the desired product***. However, this has not been practicable for various reasons.

Integration of certain stages in downstream processing for purification of product has met with some success. For instance, protein concentration by extraction into two phase systems combined with clarification and purification can be done together.

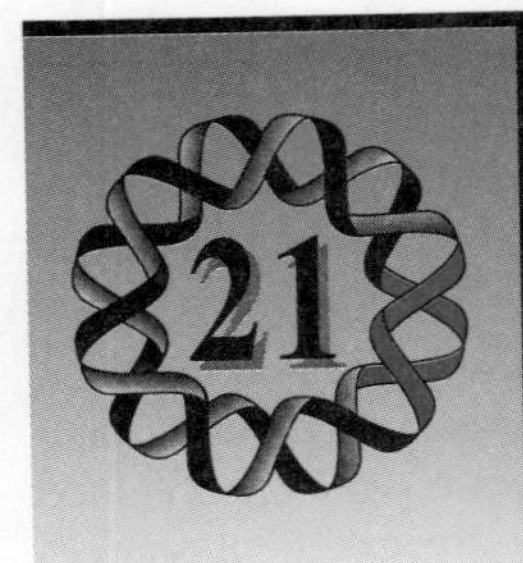

Enzyme Technology

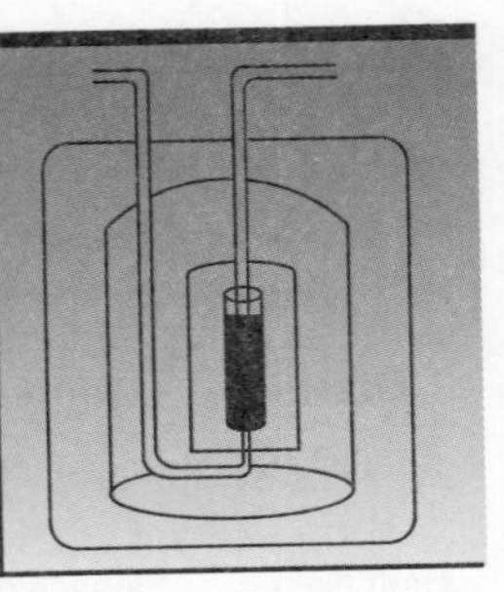

Enzymes are the biocatalysts synthesized by living cells. They are complex protein molecules that bring about chemical reactions concerned with life. The general features of enzymes are given in Chapter 66.

It is fortunate that enzymes continue to function (bring out catalysis) when they are separated from the cells i.e. *in vitro*. Basically, enzymes are non-toxic and biodegradable. They can be produced in large amounts by microorganisms for industrial applications.

Enzyme technology broadly involves production, isolation, purification and use of enzymes (in soluble or immobilized form) for the ultimate benefit of humankind. In addition, recombinant DNA technology and protein engineering involved in the production of more efficient and useful enzymes are also a part of enzyme technology. The commercial production and use of enzymes is a major part of biotechnology industry. The specialities like microbiology, chemistry and process engineering, besides biochemistry have largely contributed for the growth of enzyme technology.

APPLICATIONS OF ENZYMES

Enzymes have wide range of applications. These include their use in food production, food processing and preservation, washing powders, textile manufacture, leather industry, paper industry, medical applications, improvement of environment and in scientific research. As per recent estimates, a great majority of ***industrially produced enzymes are useful in processes related to foods*** (45%), ***detergents*** (35%), ***textiles*** (10%) and ***leather*** (3%). For details on the applications of individual enzymes, ***Tables 21.1–21.3*** (given later) must be referred.

COMMERCIAL PRODUCTION OF ENZYMES

Microbial enzymes have been utilized for many centuries without knowing them fully. The ***first enzyme produced industrially was takadiastase*** (a fungal amylase) in 1896, in United States. It was used as a pharmaceutical agent to cure digestive disorders.

In Europe, there existed a centuries old practice of softening the hides by using feces of dogs and pigeons before tanning. A German scientist (Otto Rohm) demonstrated in 1905 that extracts from animal organs (pancreases from pig and cow) could be used as the source of enzymes-proteases, for leather softening.

The utilization of enzymes (chiefly proteases) for laundry purposes started in 1915. However, it was not continued due to allergic reactions of impurities in enzymes. Now special techniques are available for manufacture, and use of enzymes in washing powders (without allergic reactions).

Table 21.1 Commercially produced enzymes from plant sources and their applications

Enzyme	*Source(s)*	*Application(s)*
β–Amylase	Barley, soy bean	Baking, preparation of maltose syrup
Bromelain	Pineapple	Baking
Esterase	Wheat	Ester hydrolysis
Ficin	Fig	Meat tenderiser
Papain	Papaya	Meat tenderiser, tanning, baking
Peroxidase	Horse radish	Diagnostic
Urease	Jack bean	Diagnostic

Commercial enzymes can be produced from a wide range of biological sources. At present, a great ***majority*** (80%) of them are ***from microbial sources.***

The different organisms and their relative contribution for the production of commercial enzymes are given below.

- Fungi – 60%
- Bacteria – 24%
- Yeast – 4%
- Streptomyces – 2%
- Higher animals – 6%
- Higher plants – 4%

A real breakthrough for large scale industrial production of enzymes from microorganisms occurred after 1950s.

Enzymes from animal and plant sources

In the early days, animal and plant sources largely contributed to enzymes. Even now, for certain enzymes they are the major sources. A selected list of plant (***Table 21.1***) and animal (***Table 21.2***) enzymes with their sources and applications are given.

Animal organs and tissues are very good sources for enzymes such as lipases, esterases and proteases. The enzyme lysozyme is mostly obtained from hen eggs. Some plants are excellent sources for certain enzymes-papain (papaya), bromelain (pineapple).

Limitations : There are several drawbacks associated with the manufacture of enzymes from animal and plant sources. The quantities are limited and there is a wide variation in their distribution. The most important limitations are the difficulties in isolating, purifying the enzymes, and the cost factor. As regards extraction of industrial enzymes from bovine sources, there is a heavy risk of contamination with bovine spongiform encephalopathy (BSE is prion disease caused by ingestion of abnormal proteins). For these reasons, ***microbial production of enzymes is preferred.***

Enzymes from mammalian cell cultures

There exists a possibility of producing commercial enzymes directly by mammalian cell cultures. But the main constraint will the cost factor which will be extremely high. However, certain therapeutic enzymes such as ***tissue plasminogen activator are produced by cell cultures.***

Enzymes from microbial sources

Microorganisms are the most significant and convenient sources of commercial enzymes. They can be made to produce abundant quantities of enzymes under suitable growth conditions. Microorganisms can be cultivated by using inexpensive media and production can take place in a short period. In addition, it is easy to manipulate microorganisms in genetic engineering

Table 21.2 Commercially produced enzymes from animal sources and their applications

Enzyme(s)	*Source(s)*	*Application(s)*
Amylase, esterase pepsin, trypsin, lipase, rennin (chymosin), phospholipase, phytase	Lamb, calf, bovine, porcine	Digestive aids, preparation of cheese
Lysozyme	Hen eggs	Cell wall breakage in bacteria
Human urine	Urokinase	For dissolution of blood clots

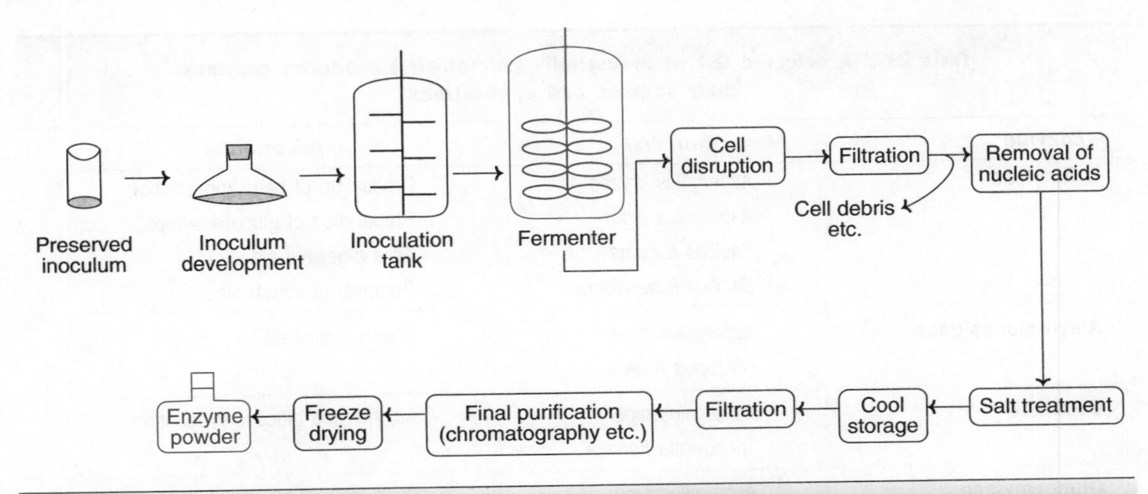

Fig. 21.1 : An outline of the flow chart for the production of enzymes by microorganisms.

techniques to increase the production of desired enzymes. Recovery, isolation and purification processes are easy with microbial enzymes than that with animal or plant sources.

In fact, most enzymes of industrial applications have been successfully produced by microorganisms. Various fungi, bacteria and yeasts are employed for this purpose. A selected list of enzymes, microbial sources and the applications are given in ***Table 21.3***.

Aspergillus niger—A unique organism for production of bulk enzymes

Among the microorganisms, *A. niger* (a fungus) occupies a special position for the manufacture of a large number of enzymes in good quantities. There are well over 40 commercial enzymes that are conveniently produced by *A. niger*. These include α-amylase, cellulase, protease, lipase, pectinase, phytase, catalase and insulinase.

THE TECHNOLOGY OF ENZYME PRODUCTION—GENERAL CONSIDERATIONS

In general, the techniques employed for microbial production of enzymes are comparable to the methods used for manufacture of other industrial products (Refer Chapter 15). The salient features are briefly described.

1. Selection of organisms
2. Formulation of medium
3. Production process
4. Recovery and purification of enzymes.

An outline of the flow chart for enzyme production by microorganisms is depicted in ***Fig. 21.1***.

Selection of organism

The most important criteria for selecting the microorganism are that the organism should produce the maximum quantities of desired enzyme in a short time while the amounts of other metabolite produced are minimal. Once the organism is selected, strain improvement for optimising the enzyme production can be done by appropriate methods (mutagens, UV rays). From the organism chosen, inoculum can be prepared in a liquid medium.

Formulation of medium

The culture medium chosen should contain all the nutrients to support adequate growth of microorganisms, that will ultimately result in good quantities of enzyme production. The ingradients of the medium should be readily available at low cost and are nutritionally safe. Some of the commonly used substrates for the medium are starch hydrolysate, molasses, corn steep liquor, yeast extract, whey, and soy bean meal. Some cereals (wheat) and pulses (peanut) have also been used. The pH of the medium should be kept optimal for good microbial growth and enzyme production.

Table 21.3 A selected list of industrially (microbially) produced enzymes, their sources and applications

Enzyme	*Source(s)*	*Application(s)*
α-Amylase	*Aspergillus oryzae* *Aspergillus niger* *Bacillus subtilus* *Bacillus licheniforms*	Production of beer and alcohol, Preparation of glucose syrups, As a digestive aid Removal of starch sizes
Amyloglucosidase	*Aspergillus niger* *Rhizopus niveus*	Starch hydrolysis
Cellulase	*Aspergillus niger* *Tricoderma koningi*	Alcohol and glucose production
Glucoamylase	*Aspergillus niger* *Bacillus amyloliquefaciens*	Production of beer and alcohol Starch hydrolysis
Glucose isomerase	*Arthrobacter sp* *Bacillus sp*	Manufacture of high fructose syrups
Glucose oxidase	*Aspergillus niger*	Antioxidant in prepared foods
Invertase	*Saccharomyces cerevisiae*	Surcose inversion Preparation of aritficial honey, confectionaries
Keratinase	*Streptomyces fradiae*	Removal of hair from hides
Lactase	*Kluyveromyus sp* *Saccharomyces fragilis*	Lactose hydrolysis Removal of lactose from whey
Lipase	*Candida lipolytica* *Asperigillus niger*	Preparation of cheese Flavour production
Pectinase	*Aspergillus sp* *Sclerotina libertina*	Clarification of fruit juices and wines Alcohol production, coffee concentration
Penicillin acylase	*Escherichia coli*	Production of 6-aminopenicillanic acid
Penicillanase	*Bacillus subtilis*	Removal of penicillin
Protease, acid	*Aspergillus niger*	Digestive aid Substitute for calf rennet
Protease, neutral	*Bacillus amyloliquefaciens*	Fish and meat tenderiser
Protease, alkaline	*Aspergillus oryzae* *Streptomyces griseus* *Bacillus sp*	Meat tenderiser Detergent additive Beer stabilizer
Pollulanase	*Klebsiella aerogens*	Hydrolysis of starch
Takadiastase	*Aspergillus oryzae*	Supplement to bread, Digestive aid

Production process

Industrial production of enzymes is mostly carried out by ***submerged liquid conditions***, and to a lesser extent by ***solid-substrate fermentation***. In submerged culture technique, the yields are more and the chances of infection are less. Hence, this is a preferred method. However, solid substrate fermentation is historically important and still in use for the production of fungal enzymes e.g. amylases, cellulases, proteases and pectinases.

The medium can be sterilized by employing batch or continuous sterilization techniques. The fermentation is started by inoculating the medium. The growth conditions (pH, temperature, O_2 supply, nutrient addition) are maintained at optimal levels. The froth formation can be minimised by adding antifoam agents.

The ***production of enzymes*** is mostly carried out ***by batch fermentation***, and to a lesser extent by continuous process. The bioreactor system must be maintained sterile throughout the fermentation process. The duration of fermentation is variable around 2-7 days, in most production processes. Besides the desired enzyme(s), several other metabolites are also produced. The enzyme(s) have to be recovered and purified.

Recovery and purification of enzymes

The desired enzyme produced may be excreted into the culture medium (extracellular enzymes) or may be present within the cells (intracellular enzymes). Depending on the requirement, the commercial enzyme may be crude or highly purified. Further, it may be in the solid or liquid form. The steps involved in ***downstream processing*** i.e. recovery and purification steps employed will depend on the nature of the enzyme and the degree of purity desired.

In general, recovery of an extracellular enzyme which is present in the broth is relatively simpler compared to an intracellular enzyme. For the release of intracellular enzymes, special techniques are needed for cell disruption. The ***physical, chemical and enzymatic methods adopted to break the cells and release their contents are described elsewhere*** (Chapter 20). The reader must invariably refer them now and learn all the details, as they form part of enzyme technology. Microbial cells can be broken down by physical means (sonication, high pressure, glass beads). The cell walls of bacteria can be lysed by the enzyme lysozyme. For yeasts, the enzyme β-glucanase is used. However, enzymatic methods are expensive.

The ***recovery and purification*** (briefly described below) steps will be the same for both intracellular and extracellular enzymes, once the cells are disrupted and intracellular enzymes are released. The most important consideration is to minimise the loss of desired enzyme activity.

Removal of cell debris : Filtration or centrifugation can be used to remove cell debris.

Removal of nucleic acids : Nucleic acids interfere with the recovery and purification of enzymes. They can be precipitated and removed by adding polycations such as polyamines, streptomycin and polyethyleneimine.

Enzyme precipitation : Enzymes can be precipitated by using salts (ammonium sulfate) organic solvents (isopropanol, ethanol, acetone). Precipitation is advantageous since the precipitated enzyme can be dissolved in a minimal volume to concentrate the enzyme.

Liquid-liquid partition : Further concentration of desired enzymes can be achieved by liquid-liquid extraction using polyethylene glycol or polyamines.

Separation by chromatography : There are several chromatographic techniques for separation and purification of enzymes. These include ***ion-exchange***, ***size exclusion***, ***affinity***, ***hydrophobic interaction*** and ***dye ligand chromatography*** (Refer Chapters 20 and 64). Among these, ion-exchange chromatography is the most commonly used for enzyme purification.

Drying and packing : The concentrated form of the enzyme can be obtained by drying. This can be done by film evaporators or freeze dryers (lyophilizers). The dried enzyme can be packed and marketed. For certain enzymes, stability can be achieved by keeping them in ammonium sulfate suspensions.

All the ***enzymes used in foods or medical treatments must be of high grade purity***, and must meet the required specifications by the regulatory bodies. These enzymes should be totally ***free from toxic materials, harmful microorganisms and should not cause allergic reactions***.

REGULATION OF MICROBIAL ENZYME PRODUCTION —GENERAL CONSIDERATIONS

A maximal production of microbial enzymes can be achieved by optimising the fermentation conditions (nutrients, pH, O_2, temperature etc.). For this purpose, a clear understanding of the genetic regulation of enzyme synthesis is required. Some of the general aspects of microbial enzyme regulation are briefly described.

Induction

Several enzymes are inducible i.e. they are synthesized only in the presence of inducers. The inducer may be the substrate (sucrose, starch, galactosides) or product or intermediate (fatty acid, phenylacetate, xylobiose). A selected list of inducible enzymes and the respective inducers is given in ***Table 21.4***.

The inducer compounds are expensive and their handling (sterilization, addition at specific time) also is quite difficult. In recent years, attempts are being made to develop mutants of microorganisms in which inducer dependence is eliminated.

Feedback repression

Feedback regulation by the end product (usually a small molecule) significantly influences the enzyme synthesis. This occurs when the end product accumulates in large quantities. Large scale production of feedback regulated enzymes is rather difficult. However, mutants that lack feedback repression have been developed to overcome this problem.

Nutrient repression

The native metabolism of microorganism is so devised that there occurs no production of unnecessary enzymes. In other words, the microorgnaisms do not synthesize enzymes that are not required by them, since this is a wasteful exercise. The inhibition of unwanted enzyme production is done by nutrient repression. The nutrients may be carbon, nitrogen, phosphate or sulfate suppliers in the growth medium. For large scale production of enzymes, nutrient repression must be overcome.

Glucose repression is a classical example of nutrient (more appropriately ***catabolite*** *)* ***repression***.

TABLE 21.4 Selected examples of inducible enzymes along with the inducers

Enzyme	*Inducer*
Invertase	Sucrose
Amylase	Starch
Lipase	Fatty acids
β-Galactosidase	Galactosides
Penicillin G amidase	Phenylacetate
Xylanase	Xylobiose

That is in the presence of glucose, the enzymes needed for the metabolism of rest of the compounds are not synthesized. Glucose repression can be overcome by feeding of carbohydrate to the fermentation medium in such a way that the concentration of glucose is almost zero at any given time. In recent years, attempts are being made to select mutants that are resistant to catabolite repression by glucose.

For certain microorganisms, other carbon sources such as pyruvate, lactate, citrate and succinate also act as catabolite repressors.

Nitrogen source repression is also observed in microorganisms. This may be due to ammonium ions or amino acids. Most commonly inexpensive ammonium salts are used as nitrogen sources. The repression by ammonium salts can be overcome by developing mutants resistant to this nitrogen source.

GENETIC ENGINEERING FOR MICROBIAL ENZYME PRODUCTION

Enzymes are the functional products of genes. Therefore, theoretically, enzymes are good candidates for improved production through genetic engineering.

During the past 15 years, the advances in the recombinant DNA technology have certainly helped for increasing the microbial production of commercial enzymes. It is now possible to transfer the desired enzyme genes from one organism to the other. Once an enzyme with a potential use in industry is identified, the relevant gene can be cloned and inserted into a suitable production host.

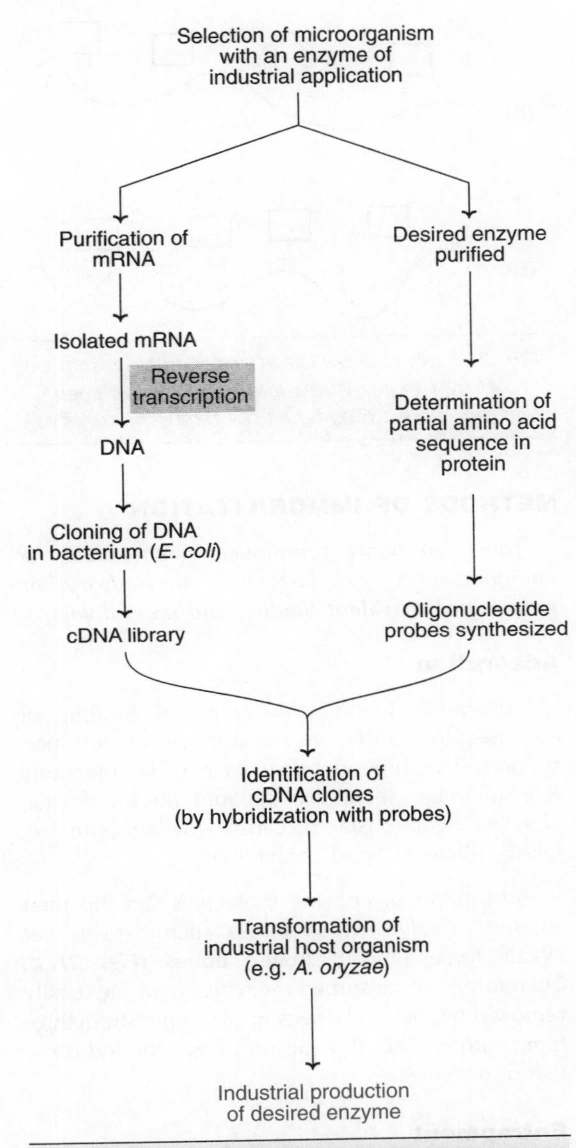

Fig. 21.2 : Schematic representation of a cloning strategy for industrial production of enzymes.

Cloning strategies

A diagrammatic representation of a cloning strategy for industrial production of enzymes is given in ***Fig. 21.2***. This involves the development of cDNA library for the mRNA, and creation of oligonucleotide probes for the desired enzyme. On hybridization with oligonucleotide probes, the specific cDNA clones can be identified. The next step is the transformation of industrially important host organism (e.g. *Aspergillus oryzae*) for the production of the desired enzyme. By this approach, it is possible to manufacture high quality industrial enzymes. A couple of enzymes produced by employing cloning strategies are described below.

1. The enzyme ***lipolase***, found in the fungus *Humicola languinosa* is very effective to remove fat stains in fabrics. However, industrial production of lipolase by this organism is not possible due to a very low level of synthesis. The gene responsible for lipolase was isolated, cloned and inserted into *Aspergillus oryzae*. Thus, large scale production of this enzyme was successfully achieved. Lipolase is very stable and resistant to degradation by proteases that are commonly used in detergents. All these properties make lipolase a strong candidate for its use fabric washing.

2. ***Rennet*** (***chymosin***) is an enzyme widely used in making cheese. It is mainly obtained from the stomachs of young calves. Consequently, there is a shortage in its supply. The gene for the synthesis of chymosin has been cloned for its large scale production.

Protein engineering for modification of industrial enzymes

It is now possible to alter the structure of a protein/enzyme by ***protein engineering and site-directed mutagenesis*** (For full details Refer Chapter 10). The changes in the enzymes are carried out with the objectives of increased enzyme stability and its catalytic function, resistance to oxidation, changed substrate preference and increased tolerance to alkali and organic solvents. By site-directed mutagenesis, selected amino acids at specific positions (in enzyme) can be changed to produce an enzyme with desired properties. For instance, protein engineering has been used to structurally modify ***phospholipase*** A_2 that can resist high concentration of acid. The modified enzyme is more efficiently used as a food emulsifier.

Genetic engineering has tremendous impact on the industrial production of enzymes with desired properties in a cost-effective manner.

IMMOBILIZATION OF ENZYMES AND CELLS

Traditionally, enzymes in free solutions (i.e. in soluble or free form) react with substrates to result in products. Such use of enzymes is wasteful, particularly for industrial purposes, since enzymes are not stable, and they cannot be recovered for reuse.

Immobilization of enzymes (or cells) refers to the ***technique of confining/anchoring the enzymes (or cells) in or on an inert support for their stability and functional reuse***. By employing this technique, enzymes are made more efficient and cost-effective for their industrial use. Some workers regard immobilization as a goose with a golden egg in enzyme technology.

Immobilized enzymes retain their structural conformation necessary for catalysis. There are several ***advantages of immobilized enzymes***.

- Stable and more efficient in function.
- Can be reused again and again.
- Products are enzyme-free.
- Ideal for multi-enzyme reaction systems.
- Control of enzyme function is easy.
- Suitable for industrial and medical use.
- Minimize effluent disposal problems.

There are however, certain ***disadvantages*** also associated with immobilization.

- The possibility of loss of biological activity of an enzyme during immobilization or while it is in use.
- Immobilization is an expensive affair often requiring sophisticated equipment.

Immobilized enzymes are generally preferred over immobilized cells due to specificity to yield the products in pure form. However, there are several advantages of using immobilized multienzyme systems such as organelles and whole cells over immobilized enzymes. The immobilized cells possess the natural environment with cofactor availability (and also its regeneration capability) and are particularly suitable for multiple enzymatic reactions.

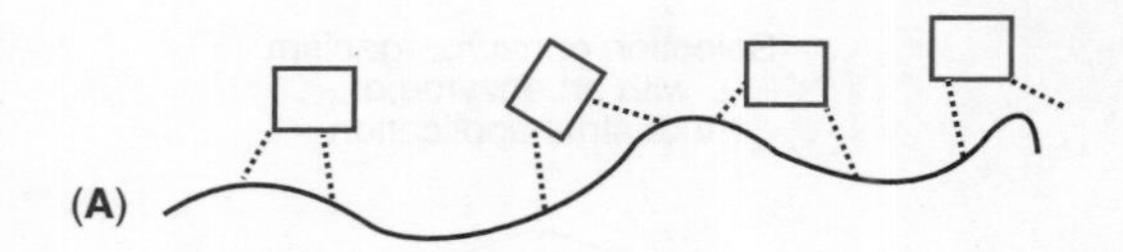

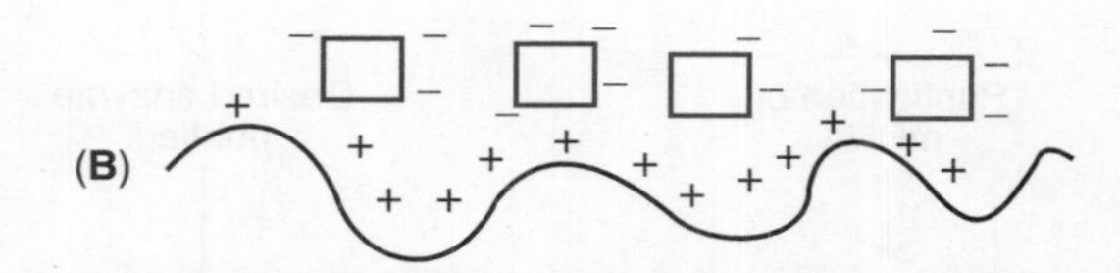

Fig. 21.3 *: Immobilization of enzymes by adsorption* ***(A)*** *By van der Waals forces* ***(B)*** *By hydrogen bonding (****Note*** *: Cloured blocks represent enzymes)*

METHODS OF IMMOBILIZATION

The commonly employed techniques for immobilization of enzymes are—***adsorption, entrapment, covalent binding and cross-linking***.

Adsorption

Adsorption involves the physical binding of enzymes (or cells) on the surface of an inert support. The support materials may be inorganic (e.g. alumina, silica gel, calcium phosphate gel, glass) or organic (starch, carboxymethyl cellulose, DEAE-cellulose, DEAE-sephadex).

Adsorption of enzyme molecules (on the inert support) involves weak forces such as van der Waals forces and hydrogen bonds (***Fig. 21.3***). Therefore, the adsorbed enzymes can be easily removed by minor changes in pH, ionic strength or temperature. This is a disadvantage for industrial use of enzymes.

Entrapment

Enzymes can be immobilized by physical entrapment inside a polymer or a gel matrix. The size of the matrix pores is such that the enzyme is retained while the substrate and product molecules pass through. In this technique, commonly referred to as ***lattice entrapment***, the enzyme (or cell) is not subjected to strong binding forces and structural distortions. Some deactivation may however, occur during immobilization process due to changes in pH or temperature or addition of solvents. The matrices used for entrapping of enzymes include polyacrylamide gel, collagen, gelatin, starch,

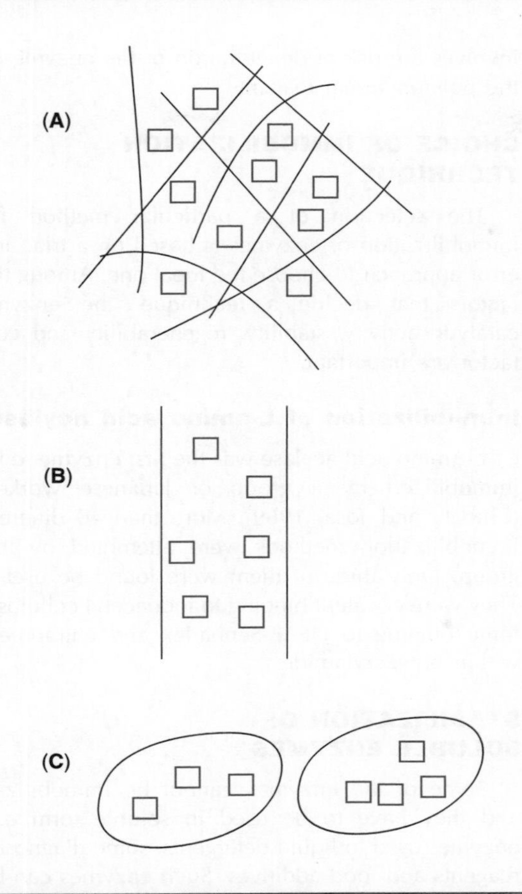

*Fig. 21.4 : Immobilization of enzymes by entrapment (A) Inclusion in gels (B) Inclusion in fibres (C) Inclusion in microcapsules (**Note** : Coloured blocks represent enzymes)*

cellulose, silicone and rubber. Enzymes can be entrapped by several ways.

1. **Enzyme inclusion in gels :** This is an entrapment of enzymes inside the gels (***Fig. 21.4A***).

2. **Enzyme inclusion in fibres :** The enzymes are trapped in a fibre format of the matrix (***Fig. 21.4B***).

3. **Enzyme inclusion in microcapsules :** In this case, the enzymes are trapped inside a microcapsule matrix (***Fig. 21.4C***). The hydrophobic and hydrophilic forms of the matrix polymerise to form a microcapsule containing enzyme molecules inside.

The major limitation for entrapment of enzymes is their leakage from the matrix. Most workers prefer to use the technique of entrapment for immobilization of whole cells. Entrapped cells are in use for industrial production of amino acids (L-isoleucine, L-aspartic acid), L-malic acid and hydroquinone.

Microencapsulation

Microencapsulation is a type of entrapment. It refers to the process of spherical particle formation wherein a liquid or suspension is enclosed in a semipermeable membrane. The membrane may be polymeric, lipoidal, lipoprotein-based or non-ionic in nature. There are three distinct ways of microencapsulation.

1. Building of special membrane reactors.
2. Formation of emulsions.
3. Stabilization of emulsions to form microcapsules.

Microencapsulation is recently being used for immobilization of enzymes and mammalian cells. For instance, pancreatic cells grown in cultures can be immobilized by microencapsulation. Hybridoma cells have also been immobilized successfully by this technique.

Covalent binding

Immobilization of the enzymes can be achieved by creation of covalent bonds between the chemical groups of enzymes and the chemical groups of the support (***Fig. 21.5***). This technique is widely used. However, covalent binding is often associated with loss of some enzyme activity. The inert support usually requires pretreatment (to form pre-activated support) before it binds to enzyme. The following are the common methods of covalent binding.

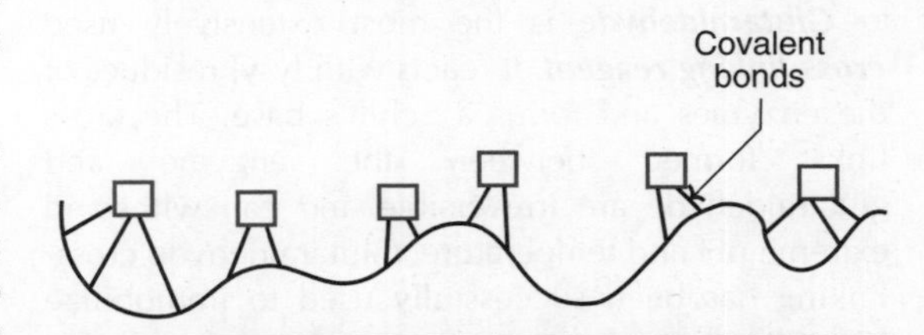

*Fig. 21.5 : A general representation of immobilization of enzymes by covalent binding (**Note** : coloured blocks represent enzymes).*

1. **Cyanogen bromide activation :** The inert support materials (cellulose, sepharose, sephadex) containing glycol groups are activated by CNBr, which then bind to enzymes and immobilize them (***Fig. 21.6A***).

2. **Diazotation :** Some of the support materials (aminobenzyl cellulose, amino derivatives of polystyrene, aminosilanized porous glass) are subjected to diazotation on treatment with $NaNO_2$ and HCl. They, in turn, bind covalently to tyrosyl or histidyl groups of enzymes (***Fig. 21.6B***).

3. **Peptide bond formation :** Enzyme immobilization can also be achieved by the formation of peptide bonds between the amino (or carboxyl) groups of the support and the carboxyl (or amino) groups of enzymes (***Fig. 21.6C***). The support material is first chemically treated to form active functional groups.

4. **Activation by bi- or polyfunctional reagents :** Some of the reagents such as ***glutaraldehyde*** can be used to create bonds between amino groups of enzymes and amino groups of support (e.g. aminoethylcellulose, albumin, amino alkylated porous glass). This is depicted in ***Fig. 21.6D***.

Cross-linking

The absence of a solid support is a characteristic feature of immobilization of enzymes by cross-linking. The enzyme molecules are immobilized by creating cross-links between them, through the involvement of polyfunctional reagents. These reagents in fact react with the enzyme molecules and create bridges which form the backbone to hold enzyme molecules (***Fig. 21.7***). There are several reagents in use for cross-linking. These include glutaraldehyde, diazobenzidine, hexamethylene diisocyanate and toluene di-isothiocyanate.

Glutaraldehyde is the most extensively used ***cross-linking reagent.*** It reacts with lysyl residues of the enzymes and forms a Schiff's base. The cross links formed between the enzyme and glutaraldehyde are irreversible and can withstand extreme pH and temperature. Glutaraldehyde cross-linking has been successfully used to immobilize several industrial enzymes e.g. glucose isomerase, penicillin amidase.

The technique of cross-linking is quite simple and cost-effective. But the disadvantage is that it involves the risk of denaturation of the enzyme by the polyfunctional reagent.

CHOICE OF IMMOBILIZATION TECHNIQUE

The selection of a particular method for immobilization of enzymes is based on a trial and error approach to choose the ideal one. Among the factors that decide a technique, the enzyme catalytic activity, stability, regenerability and cost factor are important.

Immobilization of L-amino acid acylase

L-Amino acid acylase was the first enzyme to be immobilized by a group of Japanese workers (Chibata and Tosa, 1969). More than 40 different immobilization methods were attempted by this group. Only three of them were found be useful. They were covalent binding to iodoacetyl cellulose, ionic binding to DEAE-Sephadex and entrapment within polyacrylamide.

STABILIZATION OF SOLUBLE ENZYMES

Some of the enzymes cannot be immobilized and they have to be used in soluble form e.g. enzymes used in liquid detergents, some diagnostic reagents and food additives. Such enzymes can be stabilized by using certain additives or by chemical modifications. The stabilized enzymes have longer half-lives, although they cannot be recycled. Some important methods of enzyme stabilization are briefly described.

Solvent stabilization

Certain solvents at low concentrations, stabilize the enzymes, while at high concentrations the enzymes get denatured e.g. acetone (5%) and ethanol (5%) can stabilize benzyl alcohol dehydrogenase.

Substrate stabilization

The active site of an enzyme can be stabilized by adding substrates e.g. starch stabilizes α-amylase; glucose stabilizes glucose isomerase.

Stabilization by polymers

Enzymes can be stabilized, particularly against increased temperature, by addition of polymers such as gelatin, albumin and polyethylene glycol.

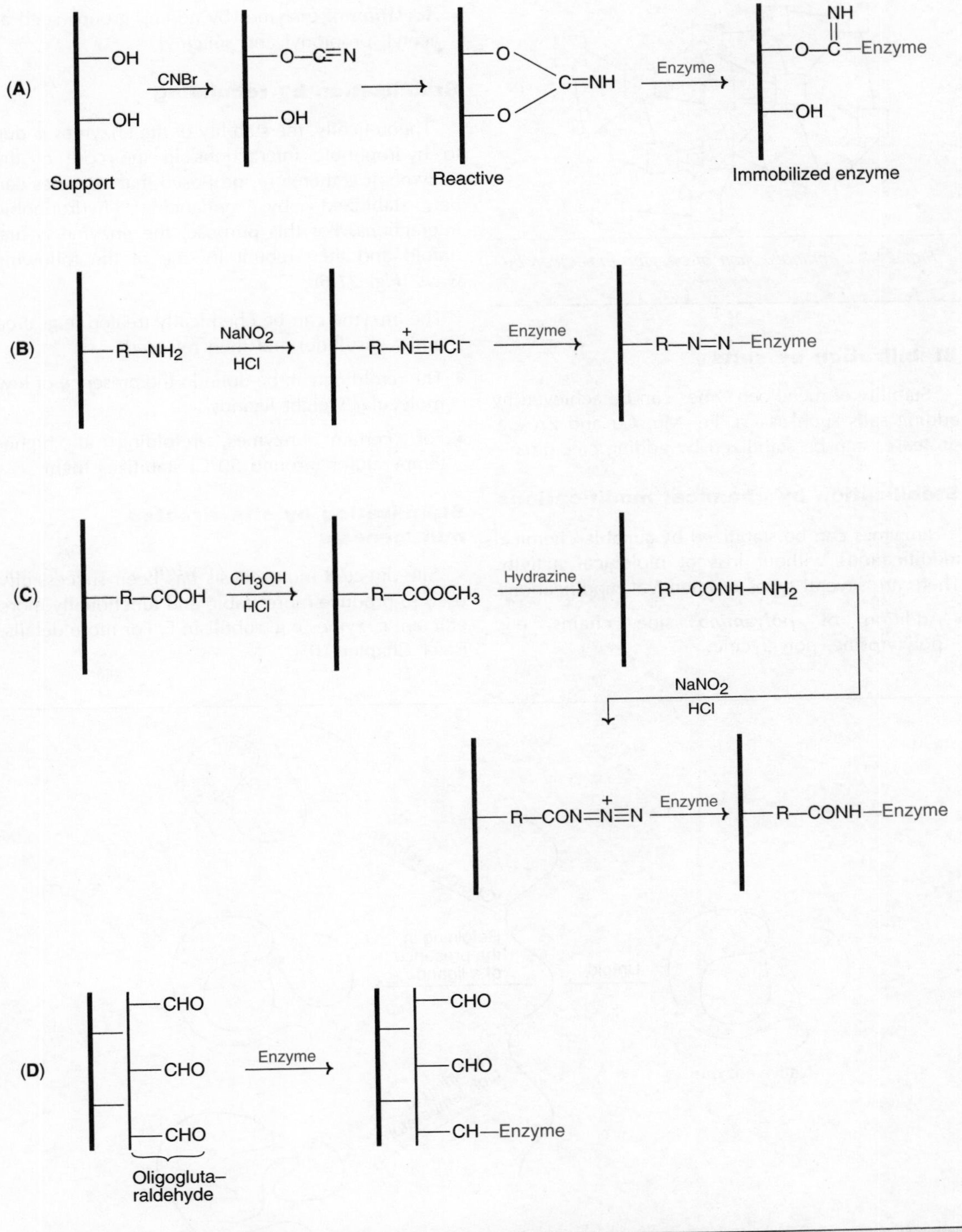

(A)
Support —OH —OH $\xrightarrow{CNBr}$ —O—C≡N —OH → Reactive (—O, —O)C=NH $\xrightarrow{Enzyme}$ —O—C(=NH)—Enzyme —OH
Immobilized enzyme

(B)
—R—NH_2 $\xrightarrow[HCl]{NaNO_2}$ —R—$\overset{+}{N}$≡HCl^- $\xrightarrow{Enzyme}$ —R—N=N—Enzyme

(C)
—R—COOH $\xrightarrow[HCl]{CH_3OH}$ —R—$COOCH_3$ $\xrightarrow{Hydrazine}$ —R—CONH—NH_2 $\xrightarrow[HCl]{NaNO_2}$ —R—CON=$\overset{+}{N}$≡N $\xrightarrow{Enzyme}$ —R—CONH—Enzyme

(D)
—CHO —CHO —CHO (Oligoglutaraldehyde) $\xrightarrow{Enzyme}$ —CHO —CHO —CH—Enzyme

Oligogluta–
raldehyde

*Fig. 21.6 : Immobilization of enzymes by covalent binding **(A)** Cyanogen bromide activation, **(B)** Diazotation, **(C)** Peptide bond formation, **(D)** Activation by bifunctional agent.*

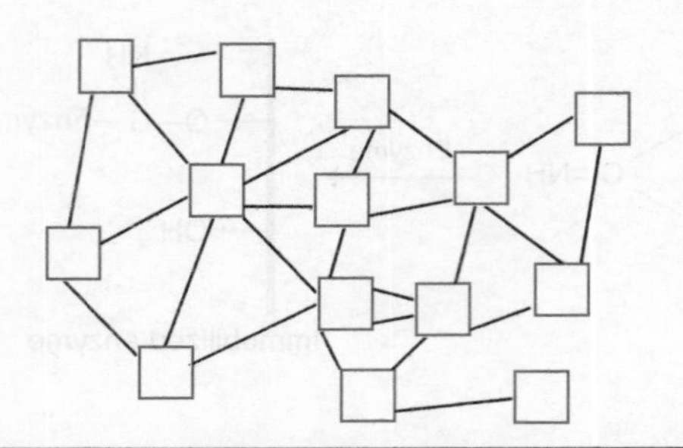

Fig. 21.7 : Immobilization of enzyme molecules by cross linking.

Stabilization by salts

Stability of metalloenzymes can be achieved by adding salts such as Ca, Fe, Mn, Cu and Zn e.g. proteases can be stabilized by adding calcium.

Stabilization by chemical modifications

Enzymes can be stabilized by suitable chemical modifications without loss of biological activity. There are several types of chemical modifications.

- Addition of ***polyamino*** side chains e.g. polytyrosine, polyglycine.
- ***Acylation*** of enzymes by adding groups such as acetyl, propionyl and succinyl.

Stabilization by rebuilding

Theoretically, the stability of the enzymes is due to hydrophobic interactions in the core of the enzyme. It is therefore, proposed that enzymes can be stabilized by enhancing hydrophobic interactions. For this purpose, the enzyme is first unfold and then rebuilt in one of the following ways (***Fig. 21.8***).

- The enzyme can be chemically treated (e.g. urea and a disulfide) and then refolded.
- The refolding can be done in the presence of low molecular weight ligands.
- For certain enzymes, refolding at higher temperatures (around 50°C) stabilizes them.

Stabilization by site-directed mutagenesis

Site-directed mutagenesis has been successfully used to produce more stable and functionally more efficient enzymes e.g. subtilisin E. For more details, Refer Chapter 10.

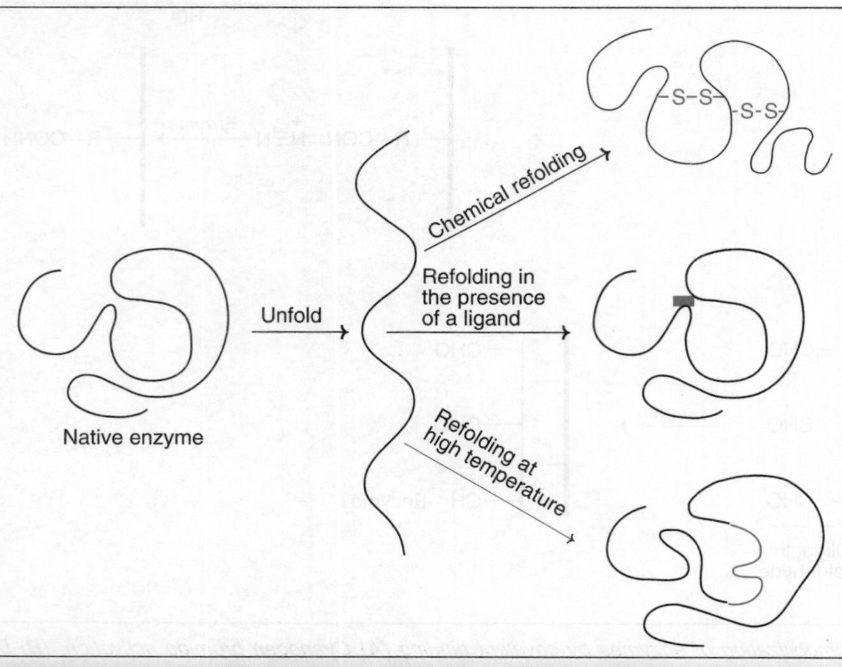

Fig. 21.8 : Stabilization of an enzyme by refolding.

TABLE 21.5 Selected examples of immobilized cells (to bring out one or two enzyme reactions) in industrial applications

Immobilized microorganism (microbial biocatalyst)	*Application(s)*
Escherichia coli	For the synthesis of L-aspartic acid from fumaric acid and NH_3
Escherichia coli	For the production of L-tryptophan from indole and serine
Pseudomonas sp	Production of L-serine from glycine and methanol
Saccharomyces cerevisiae	Hydrolysis of sucrose
Saccharomyces sp	Large scale production of alcohol
Zymomonas mobilis	Synthesis of sorbitol and gluconic acid from glucose and fructose
Anthrobacter simplex	Synthesis of prednisolone from hydrocortisone
Pseudomonas chlororaphis	Production of acrylamide from acrylonitrile
Humicola sp	For the conversion of rifamycin B to rifamycin S
Bacteria and yeasts (several sp)	In biosensors

IMMOBILIZATION OF CELLS

Immobilized individual enzymes can be successfully used for single-step reactions. They are, however, not suitable for multienzyme reactions and for the reactions requiring cofactors. The whole cells or cellular organelles can be immobilized to serve as multienzyme systems. In addition, immobilized cells rather than enzymes are sometimes preferred even for single reactions, due to cost factor in isolating enzymes. For the enzymes which depend on the spacial arrangement of the membrane, cell immobilization is preferred.

Immobilized cells have been traditionally ***used for the treatment of sewage.***

The techniques employed for immobilization of cells are almost the same as that used for immobilization of enzymes (discussed already) with appropriate modifications. ***Entrapment and surface attachment techniques are commonly used***. Gels, and to some extent membranes, are also employed.

Immobilized viable cells

The viability of the cells can be preserved by mild immobilization. Such immobilized cells are particularly useful for fermentations. Sometimes mammalian cell cultures are made to function as immobilized viable cells.

Immobilized non-viable cells

In many instances, immobilized non-viable cells are preferred over the enzymes or even the viable cells. This is mainly because of the costly isolation and purification processes. The best example is the immobilization of cells containing glucose isomerase for the industrial production of high fructose syrup. Other important examples of microbial biocatalysts and their applications are given in ***Table 21.5***.

Limitations of immobilizing eukaryotic cells

Prokaryotic cells (particularly bacterial) are mainly used for immobilization. It is also possible to immobilize eukaryotic plant and animal cells. Due to the presence of cellular organelles, the metabolism of eukaryotic cells is slow. Thus, for the industrial production of biochemicals, prokaryotic cells are preferred. However, for the ***production of complex proteins*** (e.g. immunoglobulins) and for the proteins ***that undergo post-translational modifications, eukaryotic cells may be used***.

EFFECT OF IMMOBILIZATION ON ENZYME PROPERTIES

Enzyme immobilization is frequently associated with alterations in enzyme properties, particularly

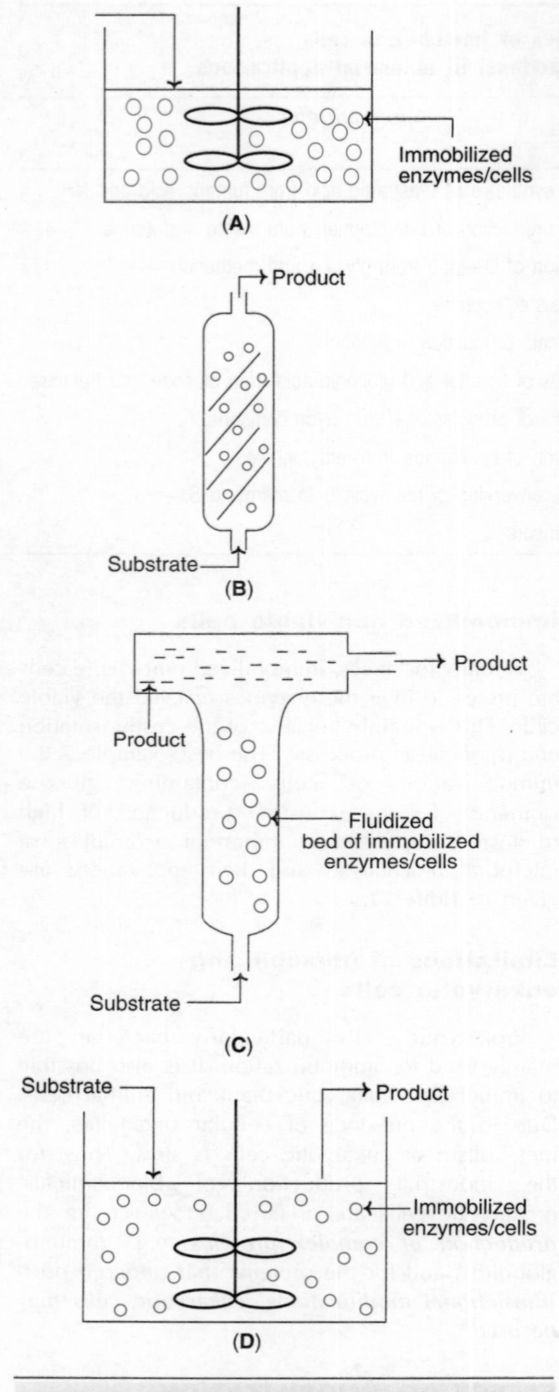

*Fig. 21.9 : Immobilized enzyme (cell) reactors (**A**) Batch stirred tank reactor, (**B**) Packed bed reactor, (**C**) Fluidized bed reactor, (**D**) Continuous stirred tank reactor.*

the kinetic properties of enzymes. Some of them are listed below.

1. There is a substantial decrease in the enzyme specificity. This may be due to conformational changes that occur when the enzyme gets immobilized.

2. The kinetic constants K_m and V_{max} of an immobilized enzyme differ from that of the native enzyme. This is because the conformational change of the enzyme will affect the affinity between enzyme and substrate.

IMMOBILIZED ENZYME REACTORS

The immobilized enzymes cells are utilized in the industrial processes in the form of enzyme reactors. They are broadly of two types — batch reactors and continuous reactors. The frequently used enzyme reactors are shown in ***Fig. 21.9***.

Batch reactors

In batch reactors, the immobilized enzymes and substrates are placed, and the reaction is allowed to take place under constant stirring. As the reaction is completed, the product is separated from the enzyme (usually by denaturation).

Soluble enzymes are commonly used in batch reactors. It is rather difficult to separate the soluble enzymes from the products, hence there is a limitation of their reuse. However, special techniques have been developed for recovery of soluble enzymes, although this may result in loss of enzyme activity.

Stirred tank reactors : The simplest form of batch reactor is the ***stirred tank reactor*** (***Fig. 21.9A***). It is composed of a reactor fitted with a stirrer that allows good mixing, and appropriate temperature and pH control. However, there may occur loss of some enzyme activity. A modification of stirred tank reactor is ***basket reactor***. In this system, the enzyme is retained over the impeller blades. Both stirred tank reactor and basket reactor have a ***well mixed flow pattern***.

Plug flow type reactors : These reactors are alternatives to flow pattern type of reactors. The flow rate of fluids controlled by a plug system. The plug flow type reactors may be in the form of ***packed bed or fluidized bed*** (***Fig. 21.9B*** and ***21.9C***). These reactors are particularly useful when

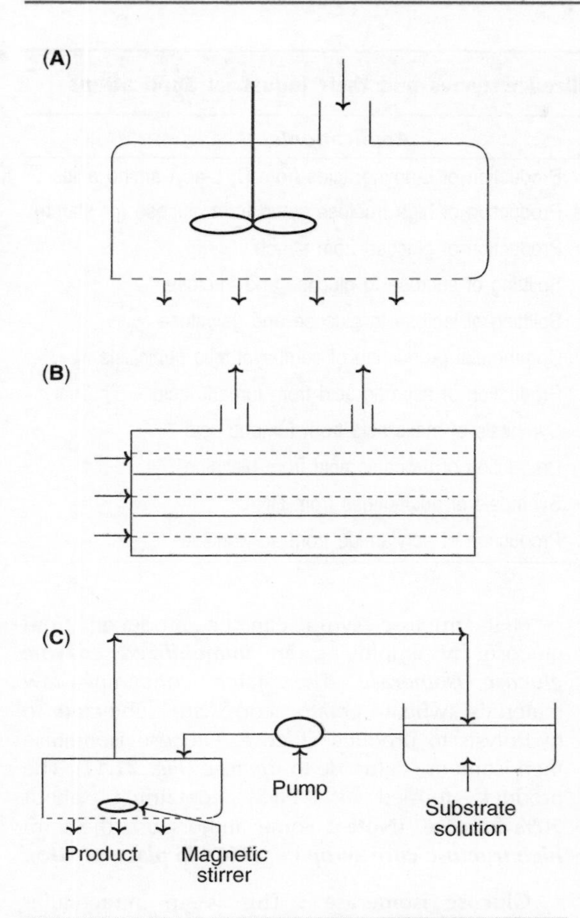

*Fig. 21.10 : Membrane reactors (**A**) Batch membrane reactor, (**B**) Continuous membrane reactor, (**C**) Recycle membrane reactor (Coloured lines indicate membranes).*

there occurs inadequate product formation in flow type reactors. Further, plug flow reactors are also useful for obtaining kinetic data on the reaction systems.

Continuous reactors

In continuous enzyme reactors, the substrate is added continuously while the product is removed simultaneously. Immobilized enzymes can also be used for continuous operation. Continuous reactors have certain advantages over batch reactors. These include control over the product formation, convenient operation of the system and easy automation of the entire process. There are mainly two types of continuous reactors-***continuous stirred tank reactor*** (***CSTR***) and ***plug reactor*** (***PR***). A diagrammatic representation of CSTR is depicted in ***Fig. 21.9D***. CSTR is ideal for good product formation.

Membrane reactors

Several membranes with a variety of chemical compositions can be used. The commonly used membrane materials include polysulfone, polyamide and cellulose acetate. The biocatalysts (enzymes or cells) are normally retained on the membranes of the reactor. The substrate is introduced into reactor while the product passes out. Good mixing in the reactor can be achieved by using ***stirrer*** (***Fig. 21.10A***). In a ***continuous membrane reactor***, the biocatalysts are held over membrane layers on to which substrate molecules are passed (***Fig. 21.10B***).

In a ***recycle model membrane reactor***, the contents (i.e. the solution containing enzymes, cofactors, and substrates along with freshly released product are recycled by using a pump (***Fig. 21.10C***). The product passes out which can be recovered.

APPLICATIONS OF IMMOBILIZED ENZYMES AND CELLS

Immobilized enzymes and cells are very widely used for ***industrial***, ***analytical*** and ***therapeutic purpose***, besides their involvement in ***food production*** and exploring the knowledge of biochemistry, microbiology and other allied specialities. A brief account of the industrial applications of immobilized cells is given in ***Table 21.5***.

MANUFACTURE OF COMMERCIAL PRODUCTS

A selected list of important immobilized enzymes and their industrial applications is given in ***Table 21.6***. Some details on the manufacture of L-amino acids and high fructose syrup are given hereunder.

Production of L-amino acids

L-Amino acids (and not D-amino acids) are very important for use in food and feed supplements and medical purposes. The chemical methods employed for their production result in a racemic mixture of D- and L-amino acids. They can be

TABLE 21.6 A selected list of important immobilized enzymes and their industrial applications

Immobilized enzyme	*Application(s)*
Aminoacylase	Production of L-amino acids from D, L-acyl amino acids
Glucose isomerase	Production of high fructose syrup from glucose (or starch)
Amylase	Production of glucose from starch
Invertase	Splitting of sucrose to glucose and fructose
β-Galactosidase	Splitting of lactose to glucose and galactose
Penicillin acylase	Commercial production of semi-synthetic penicillins
Aspartase	Production of aspartic acid from fumaric acid
Fumarase	Synthesis of malic acid from fumaric acid
Histidine ammonia lyase	Production of urocanic acid from histidine
Ribonuclease	Synthesis of nucleotides from RNA
Nitrilase	Production of acrylamide from acrylonitrile

acylated to form D, L-acyl amino acids. The immobilized enzyme ***aminoacylase*** (frequently immobilized on DEAE sephadex) can selectively hydrolyse D, L-acyl amino acids to produce L-amino acids.

$$\text{D, L-Acyl amino acids} \xrightarrow{\text{Aminoacylase}} \text{L-Amino acids + D, L-Acyl amino acids}$$

The free L-amino acids can separated from the unhydrolysed D-acyl amino acids. The latter can be recemized to D, L-acyl amino acids and recycled through the enzyme reactor containing immobilized aminoacylase. Huge quantities of L-methionine, L-phenylalanine L-tryptophan and L-valine are produced worldwide by this approach.

Production of high fructose syrup

Fructose is the sweetest among the monosaccharides, and has twice the sweetening strength of sucrose. Glucose is about 75% as sweet as sucrose. Therefore, glucose (the most abundant monosaccharide) cannot be a good substitute for sucrose for sweetening. Thus, there is a great demand for fructose which is very sweet, but has the same calorific value as that of glucose or sucrose.

High fructose syrup (HFS) contains approximately equivalent amounts of glucose and fructose. HFS is almost similar to sucrose from nutritional point of view. HFS is a good substitute for sugar in the preparation of soft drinks, processed foods and baking.

High fructose syrup can be produced from glucose by employing an ***immobilized enzyme glucose isomerase***. The starch containing raw materials (wheat, potato, corn) are subjected to hydrolysis to produce glucose. Glucose isomerase then isomerises glucose to fructose (***Fig. 21.11***). The product formed is HFS containing about 50% fructose. (**Note :** Some authors use the term ***high fructose corn syrup*** i.e. ***HFCS in place of HFS***).

Glucose isomerase : This is an intracellular enzyme produced by a number of microorganisms. The species of *Arthrobacter, Bacillus* and *Streptomyces* are the preferred sources. Being an intracellular enzyme, the isolation of glucose isomerase without loss of biological activity requires special and costly techniques. Many a times, whole cells or partly broken cells are immobilized and used.

IMMOBILIZED ENZYMES AND CELLS-ANALYTICAL APPLICATIONS

In biochemical analysis

Immobilized enzymes (or cells) can be used for the development of precise and specific analytical techniques for the estimation of several biochemical compounds. The principle of analytical assay primarily involves the action of the immobilized enzyme on the substrate. A decrease in the substrate concentration or an increase in the product level or an alteration in the cofactor concentration can be used for the assay. A selected list of examples of

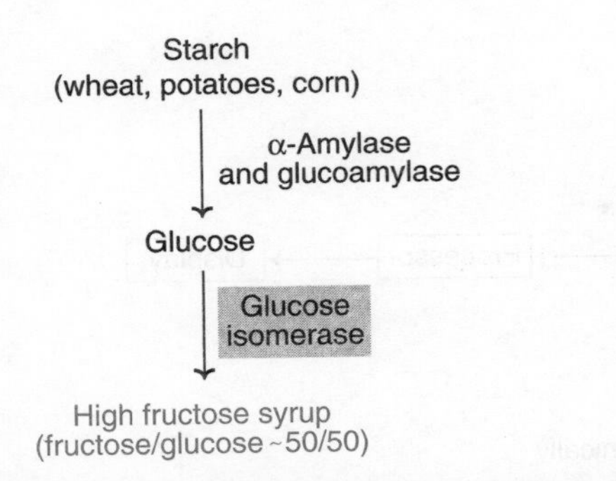

Fig. 21.11 : Production of high fructose syrup from starch (glucose isomerase is the immobilized enzyme).

immobilized enzymes used in the assay of some substances is given in ***Table 21.7***. Two types of detector systems are commonly employed.

Thermistors are heat measuring devices which can record the heat generated in an enzyme catalysed reaction. ***Electrode*** devices are used for measuring potential differences in the reaction system. In the ***Fig. 21.12***, an ***enzyme thermistor*** and an ***enzyme electrode***, along with a specific ***urease electrode*** are depicted.

In affinity chromatography and purification

Immobilized enzymes can be used in affinity chromatography. Based on the property of affinity, it is possible to purify several compounds e.g. antigens, antibodies, cofactors.

TABLE 21.7 Selected examples of immobilized enzymes used in analytical biochemistry

Immobilized enzyme	*Substance assayed*
Glucose oxidase	Glucose
Urease	Urea
Cholesterol oxidase	Cholesterol
Lactate dehydrogenase	Lactate
Alcohol oxidase	Alcohol
Hexokinase	ATP
Galactose oxidase	Galactose
Penicillinase	Penicillin
Ascorbic acid oxidase	Ascorbic acid
L-Amino acid oxidase	L-Amino acids
Cephalosporinase	Cephalosporin
Monoamine oxidase	Monoamine

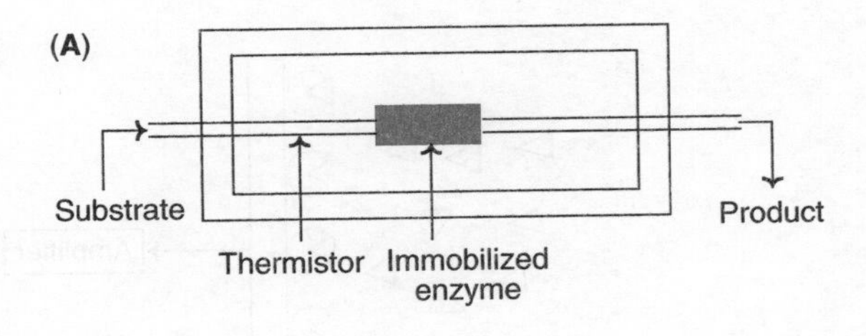

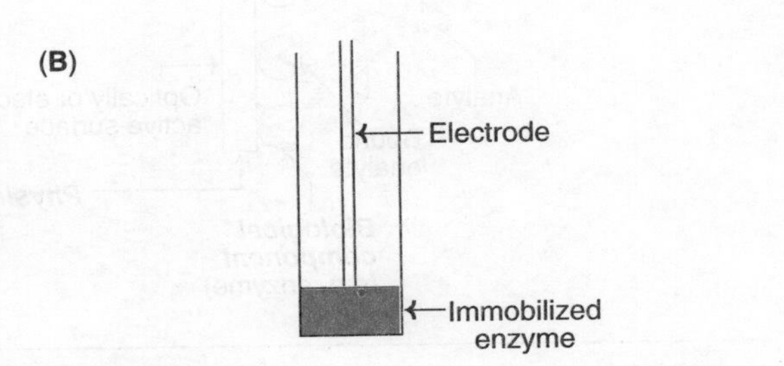

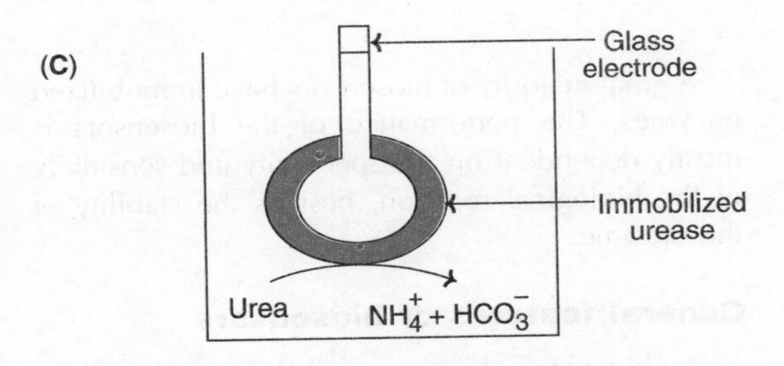

Fig. 21.12 : Immobilized enzymes or cells in analytical biochemistry (A) Enzyme thermistor, (B) Enzyme electrode, (C) Urease electrode.

BIOSENSORS

A biosensor is an analytical device containing an ***immobilized biological material*** (enzyme, antibody, nucleic acid, hormone, organelle or whole cell) which can specifically ***interact with an analyte and produce physical, chemical or electrical signals that can be measured***. An analyte is a compound (e.g. glucose, urea, drug, pesticide) whose concentration has to be measured. Biosensors basically involve the quantitative analysis of various substances by converting their biological actions into measurable signals.

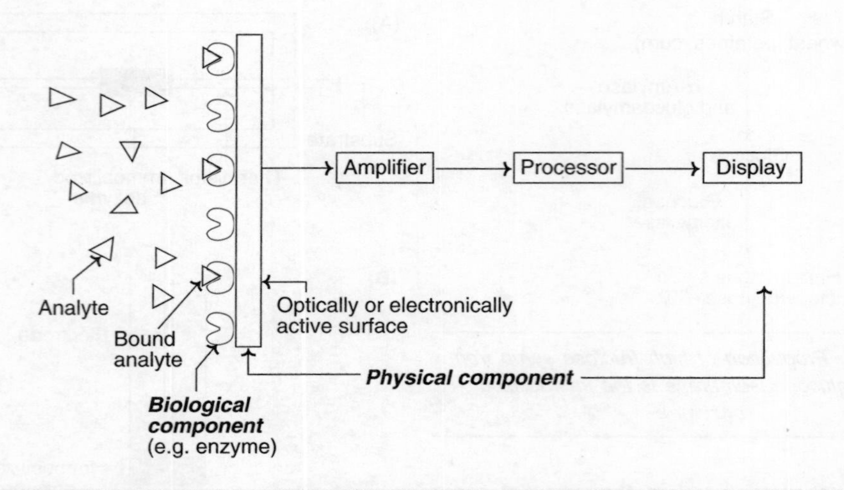

Fig. 21.13 : A diagrammatic representation of a biosensor.

A great majority of biosensors have immobilized enzymes. The performance of the biosensors is mostly dependent on the specificity and sensitivity of the biological reaction, besides the stability of the enzyme.

General features of biosensors

A biosensor has two distinct components (***Fig. 21.13***).

1. Biological component—enzyme, cell etc.
2. Physical component—transducer, amplifier etc.

The biological component recognises and interacts with the analyte to produce a physical change (a signal) that can be detected by the transducer. In practice, the biological material is appropriately immobilized on to the transducer and the so prepared biosensors can be repeatedly used several times (may be around 10,000 times) for a long period (many months).

Principle of a biosensor

The desired biological material (usually a specific enzyme) is immobilized by conventional methods (physical or membrane entrapment, non-covalent or covalent binding). This immobilized biological material is in intimate contact with the transducer. The analyte binds to the biological material to form a bound analyte which in turn produces the electronic response that can be measured.

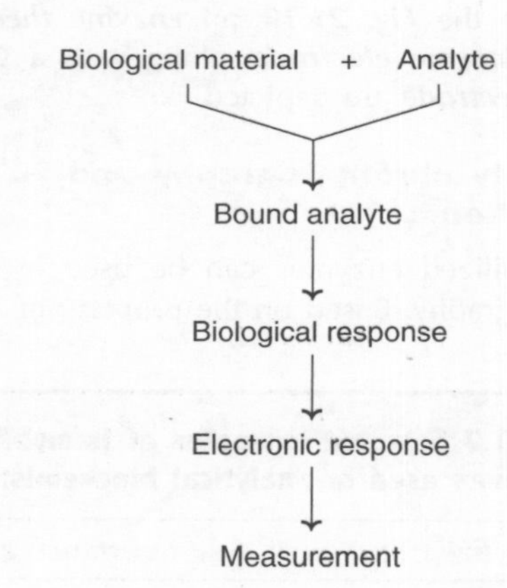

In some instances, the analyte is converted to a product which may be associated with the release of heat, gas (oxygen), electrons or hydrogen ions. The transducer can convert the product linked changes into electrical signals which can be amplified and measured.

TYPES OF BIOSENSORS

There are several types of biosensors based on the sensor devices and the type of biological materials used. A selected few of them are discussed below.

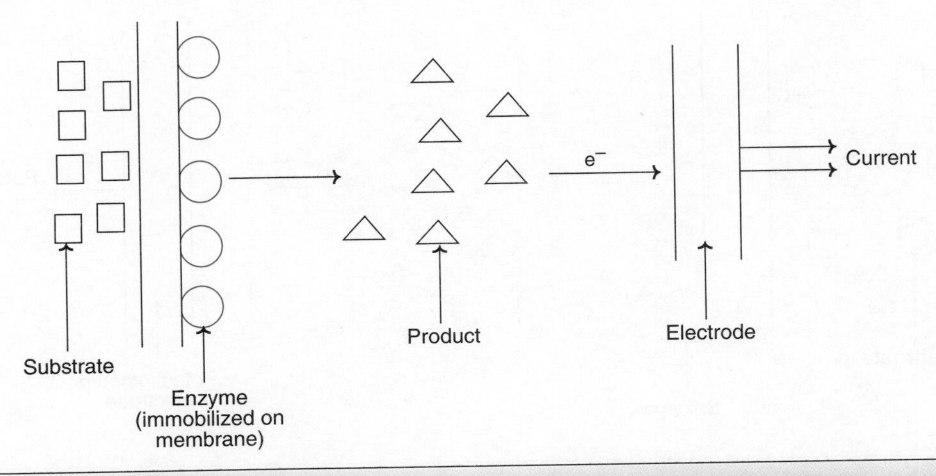

Fig. 21.14 : A diagrammatic representation of an amperometric biosensor.

ELECTROCHEMICAL BIOSENSORS

Electrochemical biosensors are simple devices based on the ***measurements of electric current***, ionic or conductance changes carried out by ***bioelectrodes***.

Amperometric biosensors

These biosensors are ***based on the movement of electrons*** (i.e. determination of electric current) as a result of enzyme-catalysed redox reactions. Normally, a constant voltage passes between the electrodes which can be determined. In an enzymatic reaction that occurs, the substrate or product can transfer an electron with the electrode surface to be oxidised or reduced (***Fig. 21.14***). This results in an altered current flow that can be measured. The magnitude of the current is proportional to the substrate concentration. Clark oxygen electrode which determines reduction of O_2, is the simplest form of amperometric biosensor. ***Determination of glucose by glucose oxidase*** is a good example.

In the ***first generation amperometric biosensors*** (described above), there is a direct transfer of the electrons released to the electrode which may pose some practical difficulties. A ***second generation amperometric biosensors*** have been developed wherein a mediator (e.g. ferrocenes) takes up the electrons and then transfers them to electrode. These biosensors however, are yet to become popular.

Blood-glucose biosensor : It is a good example of amperometric biosensors, widely used throughout the world by diabetic patients. Blood-glucose biosensor looks like a watch pen and has a single use disposable electrode (consisting of a Ag/AgCl reference electrode and a carbon working electrode) with glucose oxidase and a derivative of ferrocene (as a mediator). The electrodes are covered with hydrophilic mesh guaze for even spreading of a blood drop. The disposable test strips, sealed in aluminium foil have a shelf-life of around six months.

An ***amperometric biosensor for assessing the freshness of fish has been developed.*** The accumulation of ionosine and hypoxanthine in relation to the other nucleotides indicates freshness of fish-how long dead and stored. A biosensor utilizing immobilized nucleoside phosphorylase and xanthine oxidase over an electrode has been developed for this purpose.

Potentiometric biosensors

In these biosensors, changes in ionic concentrations are determined by use of ion-selective electrodes (***Fig. 21.15***). pH electrode is the most commonly used ion-selective electrode, since many enzymatic reactions involve the release or absorption of hydrogen ions. The other important electrodes are ammonia-selective and CO_2 selective electrodes. The potential difference obtained between the potentiometric electrode and

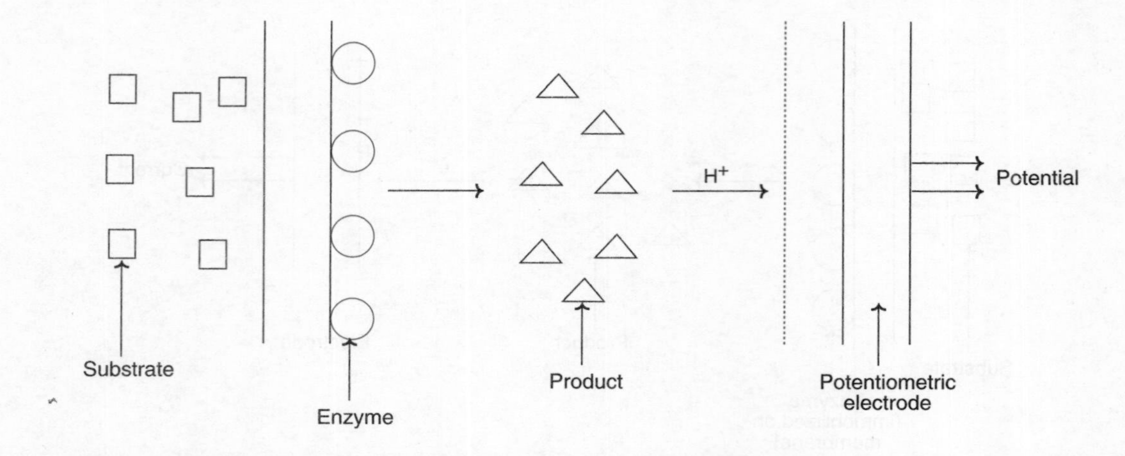

Fig. 21.15 : A diagrammatic representation of a potentiometric biosensor.

the reference electrode can be measured. It is proportional to the concentration of the substrate. The major limitation of potentiometric biosensors is the sensitivity of enzymes to ionic concentrations such as H^+ and NH_4^+.

Ion-selective field effect transistors (ISFET) are the low cost devices that can be used for miniaturization of potentiometric biosensors. A good example is an ISFET biosensor used to monitor intramyocardial pH during open-heart surgery.

Conductimetric biosensors

There are several reactions in the biological systems that bring about changes in the ionic species. These ionic species alter the electrical conductivity which can be measured. A good example of conductimetric biosensor is the ***urea biosensor*** utilizing immobilized urease. Urease catalyses the following reaction.

$$(H_2N)_2C{=}O + 3H_2O \xrightarrow{\text{Urease}} 2NH_4^+ + HCO_3^- + OH^-$$

The above reaction is associated with drastic alteration in ionic concentration which can be used for monitoring urea concentration. In fact, urea biosensors are very successfully used during dialysis and renal surgery.

THERMOMETRIC BIOSENSORS

Several biological reactions are associated with the ***production of heat*** and this forms the basis of thermometric biosensors. They are more commonly referred to as ***thermal biosensors*** or ***calorimetric biosensors***. A diagrammatic representation of a thermal biosensor is depicted in ***Fig. 21.16***. It consists of a heat insulated box fitted with heat exchanger (aluminium cylinder). The reaction takes place in a small enzyme packed bed reactor. As the substrate enters the bed, it gets converted to a product and heat is generated. The difference in the temperature between the substrate and product is measured by thermistors. Even a small change in

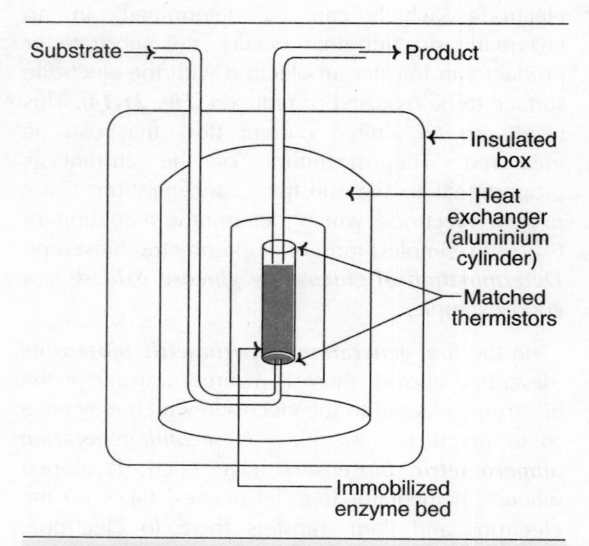

Fig. 21.16 : A diagrammatic representation of thermometric biosensor.

the temperature can be detected by thermal biosensors.

Thermometric biosensors are in use for the estimation of ***serum cholesterol***. When cholesterol gets oxidized by the enzyme cholesterol oxidase, heat is generated which can be measured. Likewise, estimations of ***glucose*** (enzyme-glucose oxidase), ***urea*** (enzyme-urease), ***uric acid*** (enzyme-uricase) and ***penicillin G*** (enzyme-β lactamase) can be done by these biosensors. In general, their utility is however, limited.

Thermometric biosensors can be used as a part of enzyme-linked immunoassay (ELISA) and the new technique is referred to as ***thermometric ELISA*** (***TELISA***).

OPTICAL BIOSENSORS

Optical biosensors are the devices that utilize the principle of ***optical measurements*** (absorbance, fluorescence, chemiluminescence etc.). They employ the use of fibre optics and optoelectronic transducers. The word ***optrode***, representing a condensation of the words ***op***tical and elec***trode***, is commonly used. Optical biosensors primarily involve enzymes and antibodies as the transducing elements.

Optical biosensors allow a safe non-electrical remote sensing of materials. Another advantage is that these biosensors usually do not require reference sensors, as the comparative signal can be generated using the same source of light as the sampling sensor. Some of the important optical biosensors are briefly described hereunder.

Fibre optic lactate biosensor

Fig. 21.17 represents the fibre optic lactate biosensor. Its working is based on the measurement of changes in molecular O_2 concentration by determining the quenching effect of O_2 on a fluorescent dye. The following reaction is catalysed by the enzyme lactate monooxygenase.

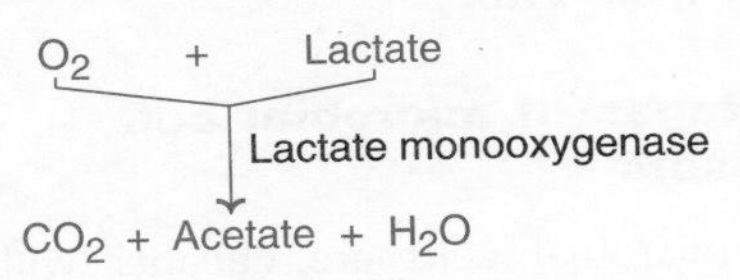

The amount of fluorescence generated by the dyed film is dependent on the O_2. This is because O_2 has a quenching (reducing) effect on the fluorescence. As the concentration of lactate in the reaction mixture increases, O_2 is utilized, and consequently there is a proportionate decrease in the quenching effect. The result is that there is an increase in the fluorescent output which can be measured.

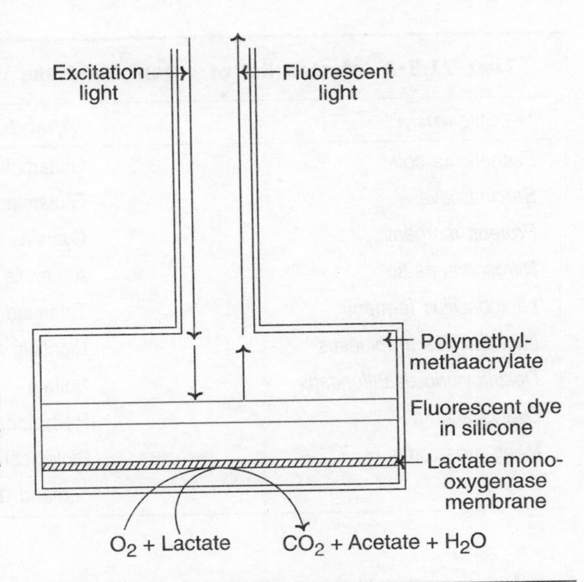

Fig. 21.17 : *Diagrammatic representation of a fibre optic lactate biosensor.*

Optical biosensors for blood glucose

Estimation of blood glucose is very important for monitoring of diabetes. A simple technique involving paper strips impregnated with reagents is used for this purpose. The strips contain glucose oxidase, horse radish peroxidase and a chromogen (e.g. toluidine). The following reactions occur.

$$\text{Glucose} \xrightarrow[\text{oxidase}]{\text{Glucose}} \text{Gluconic acid} + H_2O_2$$

$$\text{Chromogen} + 2H_2O_2 \xrightarrow{\text{Peroxidase}} \text{Colour dye} + 2H_2O$$

The intensity of the colour of the dye can be measured by using a portable reflectance meter. Glucose strip production is a very big industry worldwide.

Colorimetric test strips of cellulose coated with appropriate enzymes and reagents are in use for the estimation of several blood and urine parameters.

Table 21.8 A selected list of organisms along with the analytes and the types of biosensors

Organism	*Analyte*	*Type of biosensor*
Escherichia coli	Glutamate	Potentiometric (CO_2)
Sarcina flava	Glutamine	Potentiometric (NH_3)
Proteus morganii	Cysteine	Potentiometric (H_2S)
Nitrosomanas sp	Ammonia	Amperometric (O_2)
Lactobacillus fermenti	Thiamine	Amperometric (mediated)
Lactobacillus arabinosus	Nicotinic acid	Potentiometric (H^+)
Desulfovibrio desulfuricans	Sulfate	Potentiometric (SO_3^-)
Cyanobacteria	Herbicides	Amperometric (mediated)
Many organisms	Biological oxygen demand (BOD)	Amperometric (O_2)

Luminescent biosensors to detect urinary infections

The microorganisms in the urine, causing urinary tract infections, can be detected by employing luminescent biosensors. For this purpose, the immobilized (or even free) enzyme namely ***luciferase*** is used. The microorganisms, on lysis release ATP which can be detected by the following reaction. The quantity of light output can be measured by electronic devices.

$$\text{Leuciferin} + \text{ATP} + O_2 \xrightarrow{\text{Luciferase}} \text{Oxyluciferin} + CO_2 + \text{AMP} + \text{Pyrophosphate} + \text{Light}$$

Other optical biosensors

Optical fibre sensing devices are in use for measuring pH, pCO_2 and pO_2 in critical care, and surgical monitoring.

PIEZOELECTRIC BIOSENSORS

Piezoelectric biosensors are based on the ***principle of acoustics*** (sound vibrations), hence they are also called as ***acoustic biosensors***. Piezoelectric crystals form the basis of these biosensors. The crystals with positive and negative charges vibrate with characteristic frequencies. Adsorption of certain molecules on the crystal surface alters the resonance frequencies which can be measured by electronic devices. Enzymes with gaseous substrates or inhibitors can also be attached to these crystals.

A piezoelectric biosensor for organophosphorus insecticide has been developed incorporating acetylcholine esterase. Likewise, a biosensor for formaldehyde has been developed by incorporating formaldehyde dehydrogenase. A biosensor for cocaine in gas phase has been created by attaching cocaine antibodies to the surface of piezoelectric crystal.

Limitations of piezoelectric biosensors

It is very difficult to use these biosensors to determine substances in solution. This is because the crystals may cease to oscillate completely in viscous liquids.

WHOLE CELL BIOSENSORS

Whole cell biosensors are particularly useful for multi-step or cofactor requiring reactions. These biosensors may ***employ live or dead microbial cells***. A selected list of some organisms along with the analytes and the types of biosensors used is given in ***Table 21.8***.

Advantages of microbial cell biosensors

The microbial cells are cheaper with longer half-lives. Further, they are less sensitive to variations in pH and temperature compared to isolated enzymes.

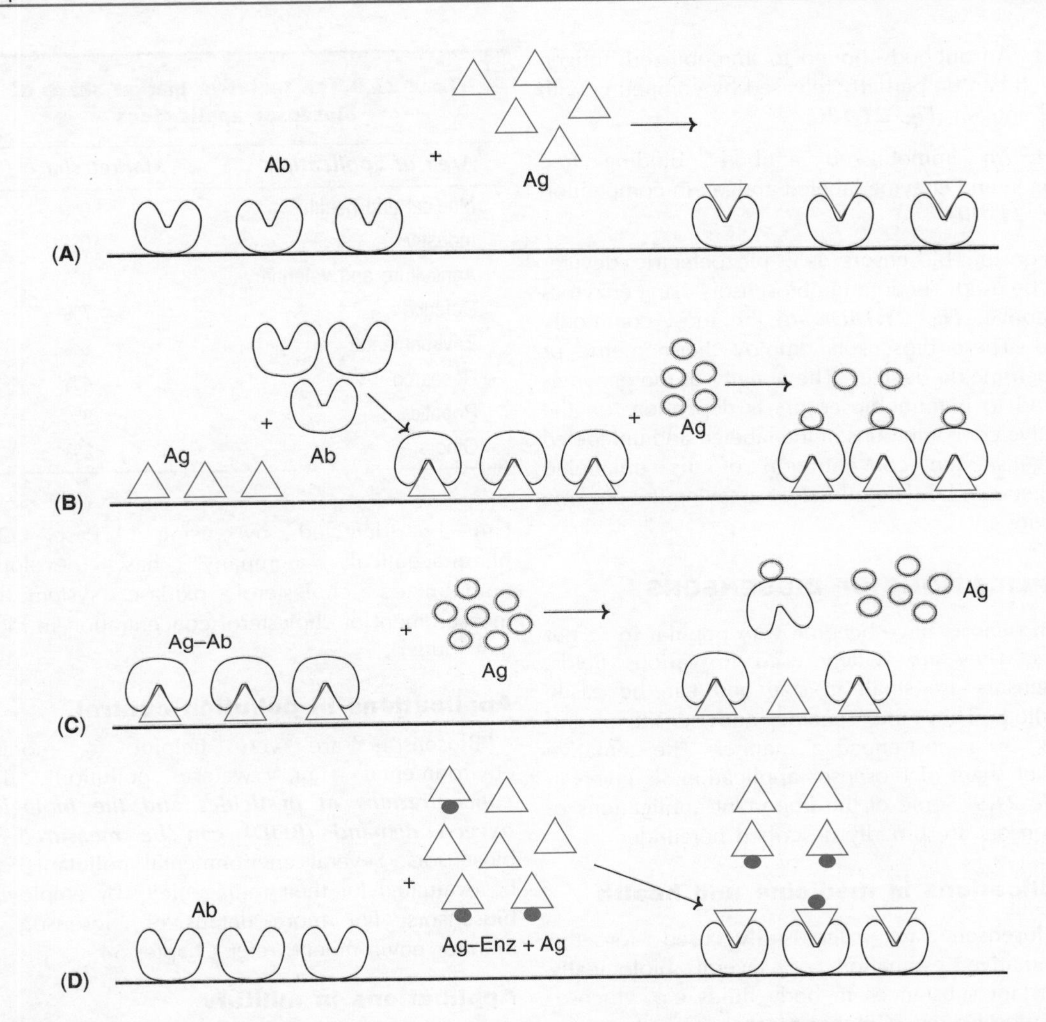

***Fig. 21.18 :** Diagrammatic representation of selected immunobiosensors **(A)** Direct binding of antigen to immobilized antibody, **(B)** Antigen–antibody sandwiches (immobilized antigen binds to antibody and then to a second antigen), **(C)** Antibody binds to immobilized antigen which gets partially released by a competitive free antigen, **(D)** Immobilized antibody binds to free antigen and enzyme labeled antigen (in competition).*

Limitations of microbial cell biosensors

The whole cells, in general, require longer periods for catalysis. In addition, the specificity and sensitivity of whole cell biosensors may be lower compared to that of enzymes.

IMMUNOBIOSENSORS

Immunobiosensors or ***immunochemical biosensors*** work on the principle of immunological specificity, coupled with measurement (mostly) based on amperometric or potentiometric biosensors. There are several possible configurations for immunobiosensors and some of them are depicted in ***Fig. 21.18***, and briefly described hereunder.

1. An immobilized antibody to which antigen can directly bind (***Fig. 21.18A***).

2. An immobilized antigen that binds to antibody which in turn can bind to a free second antigen (***Fig. 21.18B***).

3. An antibody bound to immobilized antigen which can be partially released by competing with free antigen (***Fig. 21.18C***).

4. An immobilized antibody binding free antigen and enzyme labeled antigen in competition (***Fig. 21.18D***).

For the biosensors 1-3, piezoelectric devices can be used. The immunobiosensors using enzymes (4 above, ***Fig. 21.18D***) are the most commonly used. These biosensors employ thermometric or amperometric devices. The activity of the enzymes bound to immunobiosensors is dependent on the relative concentrations of the labeled and unlabeled antigens. The concentration of the unlabeled antigen can be determined by assaying the enzyme activity.

APPLICATIONS OF BIOSENSORS

Biosensors have become very popular in recent years. They are widely used in various fields. Biosensors are small in size and can be easily handled. They are specific and sensitive, and work in a cost-effective manner. The tentative market share of biosensor applications is given in ***Table 21.9***. Some of the important applications of biosensors are broadly described hereunder.

TABLE 21.9 The tentative market share of biosensor applications

Area of application	*Market share (%)*
Medical and health	60%
Industry	10%
Agriculture and veterinary	8%
Defence	7%
Environmental	6%
Research	4%
Robotics	3%
Others	2%

Applications in medicine and health

Biosensors are successfully used for the quantitative estimation of several biologically important substances in body fluids e.g. glucose, cholesterol, urea. ***Glucose biosensor*** is a boon for diabetic patients for regular monitoring of blood glucose. ***Blood gas monitoring*** for pH, pCO_2 and pO_2 is carried out during critical care and surgical monitoring of patients. Mutagenicity of several chemicals can be determined by using biosensors. Several toxic compounds produced in the body can also be detected.

Applications in industry

Biosensors can be used for ***monitoring of fermentation products*** and estimation of various ions. Thus, biosensors help for improving the fermentation conditions for a better yield.

Now a days, biosensors are employed to ***measure the odour and freshness of foods***. For instance, freshness of stored fish can be detected by ATPase. ATP is not found in spoiled fish and this can be detected by using ATPase. One pharmaceutical company has developed immobilized cholesterol oxidase system for measurement of cholesterol concentration in foods (e.g. butter).

Applications in pollution control

Biosensors are very helpful to monitor environmental (air, water) pollution. The ***concentrations of pesticides and the biological oxygen demand (BOD) can be measured*** by biosensors. Several environmental pollutants can be evaluated for their mutagenicity by employing biosensors. For more details or biosensors to monitor environment, refer Chapter 54.

Applications in military

Biosensors have been developed to detect the toxic gases and other chemical agents used during war.

IMMOBILIZED ENZYMES AND CELLS-THERAPEUTIC APPLICATIONS

The industrial and analytical applications of immobilized enzymes have been described in the preceeding pages. The therapeutic applications are dealt with here.

There are several limitations for the direct use of enzymes for therapeutic purposes. These include the poor availability of the enzyme at the site of action, sensitivity to natural inhibitors, degradation by endogenous proteases and immunogenicity of certain enzymes.

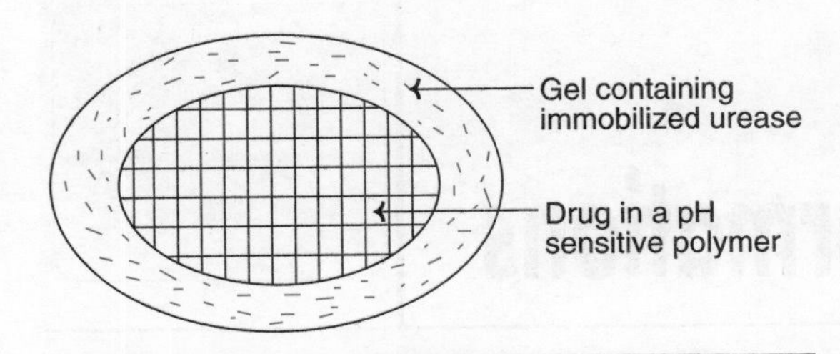

Fig. 21.19 : A diagrammatic representation of immobilized urease for drug delivery.

Some of these limitations can be overcome by employing immobilized enzymes for therapeutic applications. A few examples are listed below.

1. Immobilized streptokinase and urokinase (on Sephadex) can be used ***for the treatment of thromboses***.

2. Some success has been reported in the ***treatment of inborn errors*** by employing immobilized enzymes e.g. phenylalanine hydroxylase to treat phenylketonuria, lysosomal α 1, 4-glucosidase to correct type II glycogen storage disease (Pompe's disease).

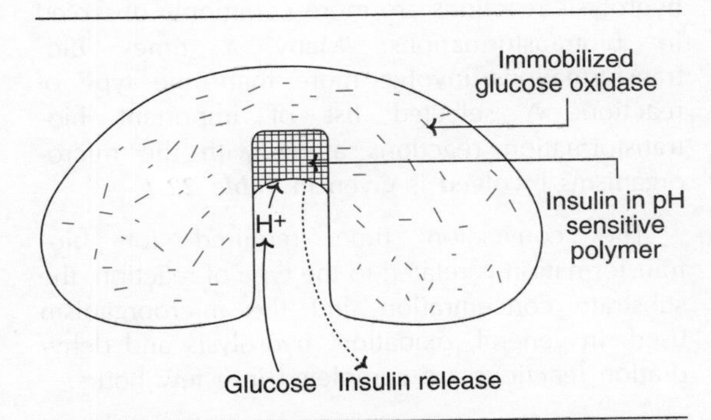

Fig. 21.20 : A diagrammatic representation of immobilized glucose oxidase for insulin delivery.

Some other important therapeutic applications of immobilized enzymes and cells are briefly described.

Improved drug delivery by using immobilized enzymes

Urea-urease modulated system : By using immobilized urease enzyme along with the substrate urea, the drug delivery can be enhanced. As urease splits urea, there is an increase in the pH due to the formation of ammonium hydroxide. The drug located in a pH sensitive bioerodible polymer can be effectively released for its action (***Fig. 21.19***).

Glucose oxidase-glucose modulated system : For insulin delivery to the human body, a bioerodible polymeric system containing insulin has been developed. The delivery of insulin can be modulated by immobilized glucose oxidase enzyme (***Fig. 21.20***). As glucose oxidase acts on glucose, gluconic acid is produced which lowers the pH. The low pH in turn, causes the release of insulin from the bioerodible polymeric system.

Immobilization of artificial cells

An artificial cell primarily consists of a spherical semipermeable membrane with comparable dimensions of a living cell. The biological materials such as enzymes enclosed within the artificial cells can be immobilized. The so immobilized compact artificial cells can function as artificial organs. The important artifical organs constructed include artificial kidney, artificial liver, blood detoxifiers and immunosorbents. Their functioning is however, very limited.

Multienzyme system can be immobilized in the form of artificial cells for the conversion of a substrate to a product, through a series of reactions.

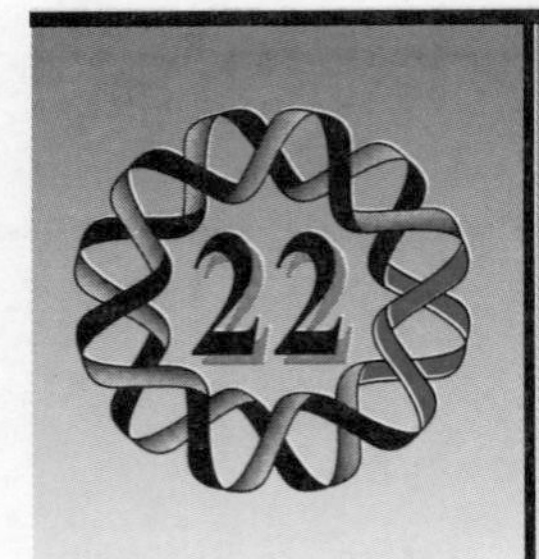

Biotransformations

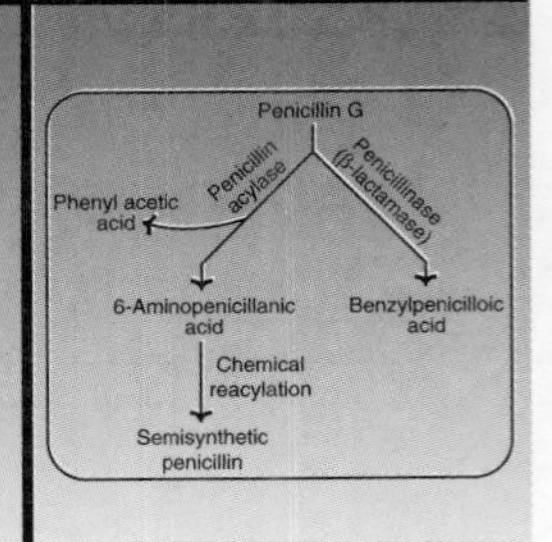

Microorganisms possess the capability to enzymatically modify a wide range of organic compounds. Biotransformations (***biconversions*** or ***microbial transformations***) broadly refer to the ***processes in which microorganisms convert organic compounds into structurally related products***. In other words, biotransformation deals with microbial (enzymatic) conversion of a substrate into a product with a limited number (one or a few) enzymatic reactions. This is in contrast to ***fermentation*** which ***involves a large number reactions*** (often complex in nature).

Although there are hundreds of biotransformations known, only a selected few of them are useful for the synthesis of commercially important products. The significance of bioconversion reactions becomes obvious when the production of a particular compound is either difficult or costly by chemical methods. Further, biotransformations are generally preferred to chemical reactions because of substrate specificity, stereospecificity and mixed reaction conditions (pH, temperature, pressure). The environmental pollution due to biotransformation is almost insignificant or negligible. In addition, it is easy to apply recombinant DNA technology to make desired improvements in biotransformations. Another practical advantage of biotransformations is that it is easy to scale-up the processes due to limited number of reactions.

TYPES OF BIOTRANSFORMATION REACTIONS

Many types of chemical reactions occur in biotransformations. These include ***oxidation, reduction, hydrolysis, condensation, isomerization, formation of new C—C bonds, synthesis of chiral compounds*** and ***reversal of hydrolytic reactions***. Among these, oxidation, isomerization and hydrolysis reactions are more commonly observed in biotransformations. Many a times biotransformations involve more than one type of reaction. A selected list of important biotransformation reactions along with the microorganisms involved is given in ***Table 22.1***.

The conversion time required for biotransformation is related to the type of reaction, the substrate concentration and the microorganism used. In general, oxidation, hydrolysis and dehydration reactions are completed in a few hours.

SOURCES OF BIOCATALYSTS AND TECHNIQUES FOR BIOTRANSFORMATION

A wide variety of biological catalysts can be used for biotransformation reactions. These include ***growing cells, resting cells, killed cells, immobilized cells***, cell-free extracts, enzymes and ***immobilized enzymes***. The most important sources of biocatalysts and the procedures employed for biotransformation are briefly described.

TABLE 22.1 A selected list of important biotransformation reactions

Type of reaction	*Example*	*Commonly used microorganism*
Oxidation	Tryptophan ⟶ 5–Hydroxytryptophan	*Bacillus subtitis*
	Naphthalene ⟶ Salicylic acid	*Corynebacterium* sp
Reduction	Benzaldehyde ⟶ Benzyl alcohol	*Saccharomyces cerevisiae*
	Nitropentachlorobenzol ⟶ Pentachloroaniline	*Streptomyces aureofaciens*
Hydrolysis	Anhydrotetracycline ⟶ Tetracycline	*Streptomyces aureofaciens*
	Menthyl laureate ⟶ Menthol	*Mycobacterium phlei*
Condensation	Streptomycin ⟶ Streptomycin-phosphate	*Streptomyces griseus*

Growing cells

The desired cells are cultivated in a suitable medium. As the growth of the cells occurs (6–24 hours), a concentrated substrate is added to the culture. Sometimes, addition of emulsifiers (Tween, organic solvents) is required to solubilize substrates and/or products e.g. steroid biotransformation. The substrate conversion to product can be monitored by spectroscopic or chromatographic techniques. Biotransformation can be terminated when the product formation is optimum.

Non-growing cells

The non-growing cells are preferred for biotransformation reactions for the following reasons.

- Very high concentration of substrate can be used (with high substrate concentration, growing cells stop their growth).
- Cells can be washed and used and thus there will be no contaminating substances.
- ***Conversion efficiency of substrate to product is high***.
- Biotransformation can be optimized by creating suitable environmental conditions (pH, temperature etc.).
- Product isolation and its recovery are easy.

Immobilized cells

Biotransformations can be carried out continuously by employing immobilized cells. Further, the same cells can be used again and again. Several bioconversions with single or multistage reactions are in fact carried out by using immobilized cells e.g. commercial production of L-alanine and malic acid (for details Refer Chapter 21).

Immobilized enzymes

Cell-free enzyme systems in the form of immobilized enzymes are ***most commonly used in biotransformations***, due to the following advantages.

- ***No occurrence of undesirable side reactions***.
- The desired products are not degraded.
- There is no transport barrier across the cell membrane for the substrate or product.
- The isolation and recovery of the product is simpler and easier.

Several immobilized enzyme systems have been developed for biotransformations e.g. glucose isomerase, penicillin acylase (For details, Refer Chapter 21).

PRODUCT RECOVERY IN BIOTRANSFORMATIONS

In most biotransformation reactions, the desired end products are extracellular. The product may be either in a soluble or suspended state. When whole cells are used, they have to be separated and repeatedly washed (with water or organic solvent) as required. The extracted product can be recovered by employing the commonly used techniques-precipitation by salts, extraction with solvents, adsorption to ion-exchangers etc. The volatile poducts can be recovered by direct distillation from the medium.

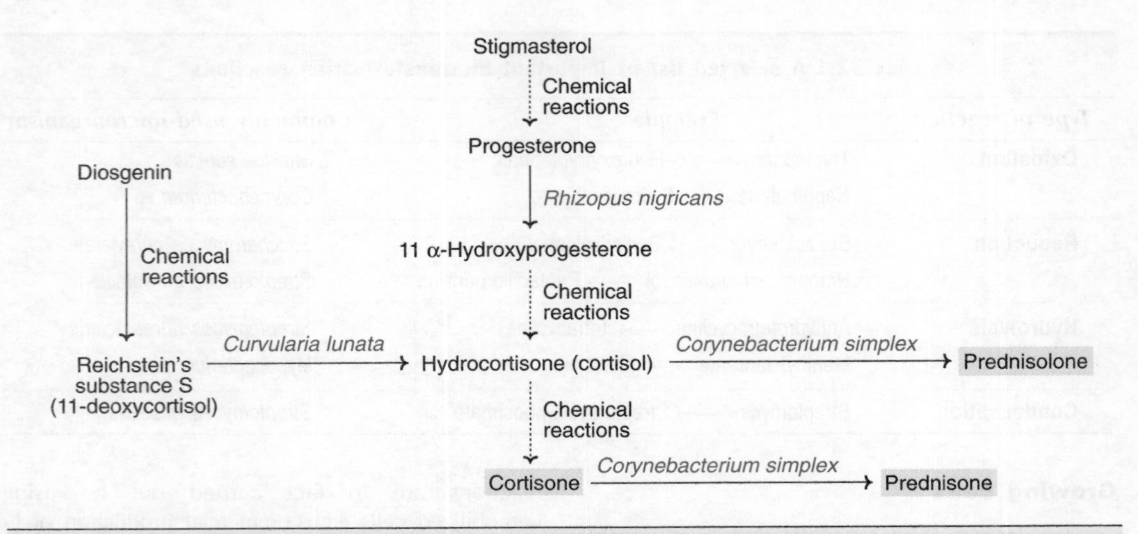

Fig. 22.1 : Biotransformation of commercially important steroids.

EXAMPLES OF BIOTRANSFORMATIONS

A large number of biotransformations are described in literature. Of these, only a selected few are important for industrial and commercial purposes. The major limitations with some of the biotransformations are that either yields are low or the process is expensive or the market itself is very limited.

BIOTRANSFORMATION TO PRODUCE COMMERCIAL PRODUCTS

As already stated, among the large number and a wide range of biotransformations, only a selected few are commercially important. Some of these are briefly described hereunder.

BIOTRANSFORMATION OF STEROIDS

All the ***steroids possess the basic structure*** namely ***cyclopentanoperhydrophenanthrene***. Steroids as hormones (glucocorticoids, mineralocorticoids, androgens, estrogens) perform a wide range of functions. They are very useful therapeutically. For instance, cortisone, due to its anti-inflammatory action is used in the treatment of rheumatoid arthritis and skin diseases; derivatives of progesterone and estrogens are employed as contraceptives. Certain derivatives of cortisone (e.g. prednisolone) are more effective in their therapeutic action.

Commercial production of steroids is very important. Earlier, cortisone was chemically synthesized, and this process involved as many as 37 reactions. The cost of the so obtained product was around $200/g (in 1950). With the introduction of biotransformation reactions, the number of steps (microbial and chemical put together) was reduced to II, and cost of the product was reduced to just $1/g in 1980! The credit obviously goes to the developments in biotransformation.

Types of reactions in biotransformation of steroids

The microbial transformation of steroids broadly involves ***oxidation*** (introduction of hydroxyl groups, splitting of side chains, production of epoxides etc.) ***reduction*** (conversion of aldehydes or ketones to alcohols, hydration of double bonds), ***hydrolysis*** and ***ester formation***.

Production process of steroids

The production of steroids, entirely by biotransformation reactions is not practicable. Therefore, microbial transformation along with chemical reactions is carried out. The major steps involved in the biotransformation of steroids are depicted in ***Fig. 22.1***. ***Stigmasterol*** extracted from soybeans or ***diosgenin*** isolated from the roots of the Mexican barbasco plant can serve as the starting material. Stigmasterol can be chemically converted to progesterone which is subjected to biotransformation to form 11α-hydroxyprogesterone by the microorganism, *Rhizopus nigricans*. Cortisol (hydrocortisone), produced from 11α-hydroxyprogesterone by chemical reactions, undergoes microbial transformation (organism-*Corynebacterium simplex*) to form prednisolone. Further, cortisone formed from cortisol can be subjected to biotransformation by *Corynebacterium simplex* to produce prednisone. When diosgenin is used as the starting compound, substance S can be produced by chemical reactions which can be converted to cortisol by biotransformation with the help of the microorganism *Curvularia lunata*.

Biotransformation of steroids is usually carried out by ***batch fermentation***. Use of immobilized cells or immobilized enzymes is gaining importance in recent years. This is advantageous since the biotransformation is more efficient with high substrate concentration, short conversion time and good product recovery. Since the steroids are not water soluble, the microbial transformation reactions have to be carried out in organic solvent (water-immiscible) system. However, the organic solvents are toxic to micro-organisms or enzymes. It is ideal to use an aqueous two phase system for biotransformation of steroids.

Biotransformation of cholesterol

Certain commercially important steroids (e.g. androstendione, androstadiendione) can be produced directly from cholesterol by biotransformation (***Fig. 22.2***).

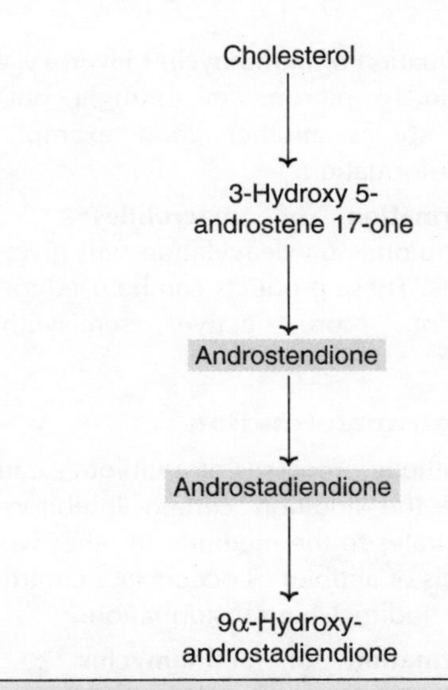

Fig. 22.2 : Biotransformation of cholesterol by mycobacteria to commercial products.

BIOTRANSFORMATION OF ANTIBIOTICS

Production of new antibiotics or modifications in the existing ones for more effective treatment of the diseases is always on the priority of the pharmaceutical industry. Further, antibiotics with wider antimicrobial spectrum, reduced toxicity, low allergic reactions and decreased resistance are highly advantageous. Biotransformation reactions significantly contribute for improving the pharmaceutical products.

Direct biotransformation

Acylation and deacylation, phosphorylation, adenylation and hydrolysis are some of the reactions involved in the microbial transformation of antibiotics.

Biotransformation of penicillin G : Microbial transformation, in association with chemical synthesis, is routinely used for the commercial production of semisynthetic penicillins and cephalosporins. The enzymatic cleavage of penicillin by ***penicillin acylase*** into 6-aminopenicillanic acid is a very important reaction (***Fig. 22.3***). Penicillin G gets inactivated by its conversion to benzylpenicilloic acid by the enzyme ***penicillinase*** (β-lactamase).

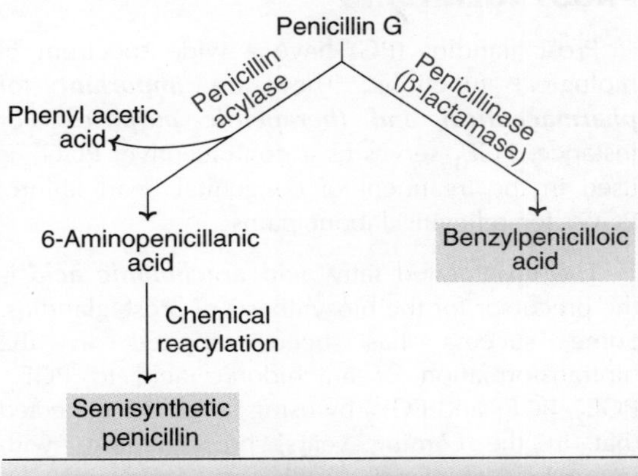

Fig. 22.3 : Biotransformation of penicillin G.

Biotransformation of narbomycin : Hydroxylation of narbomycin to picromycin (brought out by *Streptomyces* sp) is another good example of microbial transformation.

Biotransformation of macrolides : The macrolide antibiotics on deacylation will give less active products. These products can be used for the production of more active semisynthetic macrolides.

Indirect biotransformation

The biosynthetic processes of antibiotics can be controlled by the addition certain inhibitors or modified substrates to the medium. In other words, the biosynthesis of antibiotics occurs in a controlled fashion in the indirect biotransformation.

Biotransformation of actinomycins : The microorganism *Streptomyces parvulus* produces new actinomycins in the presence of 4-methyl-proline (proline analog) in the medium. The new antibiotics will have 4-methylproline in place of proline and these actinomycins are more efficient in their function.

Biotransformation of ribostamycin : In the biosynthesis of neomycin, ribostamycin is an intermediate. By employing mutant strains of *Streptomyces fradiae*, ribostamycin can be produced in large quantities.

Several other mutant strains of microorganisms have been created by recombinant DNA technology for the production of modified antibiotics of aminoglycosides and rifamycins.

BIOTRANSFORMATION OF ARACHIDONIC ACID TO PROSTAGLANDINS

Prostaglandins (PG) have a wide spectrum of biological functions. They are ***important for pharmaceutical and therapeutic purposes***. For instance, PGE_1 serves as a contraceptive; PGG_1 is used in the treatment of congenital heart failure; PGG_2 for relieving labour pains.

The unsaturated fatty acid ***arachidonic acid*** is the precursor for the biosynthesis of prostaglandins. Some success has been reported in the biotransformation of arachidonic acid to PGE_1, PGE_2, PGF_1 and PGF_2 by using fungi. It is expected that in the coming years, prostaglandins with improved efficiency will be produced by biotransformations.

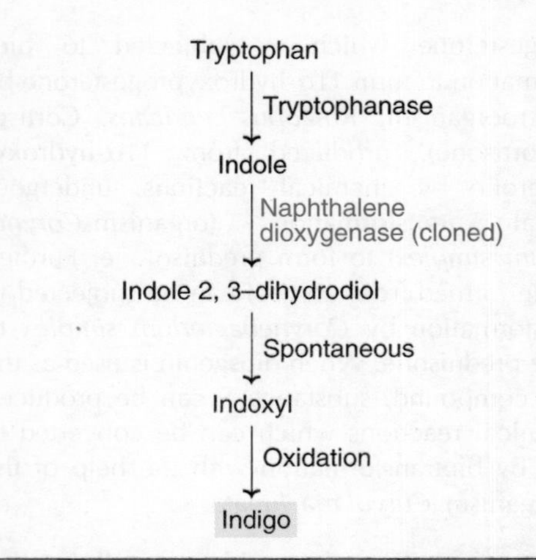

Fig. 22.4 : Microbial production of indigo.

BIOTRANSFORMATION FOR THE PRODUCTION OF ASCORBIC ACID

Ascorbic acid (vitamin C) can be commercially produced by a combination of chemical and microbial transformation processes. For full details, the reader must refer Chapter 24.

BIOTRANSFORMATION OF GLYCEROL TO DIHYDROXYACETONE

Dihydroxyacetone is used in cosmotics and suntan lotions. Certain acetic acid bacteria can convert glycerol to dihydroxyacetone through the process of biotransformation.

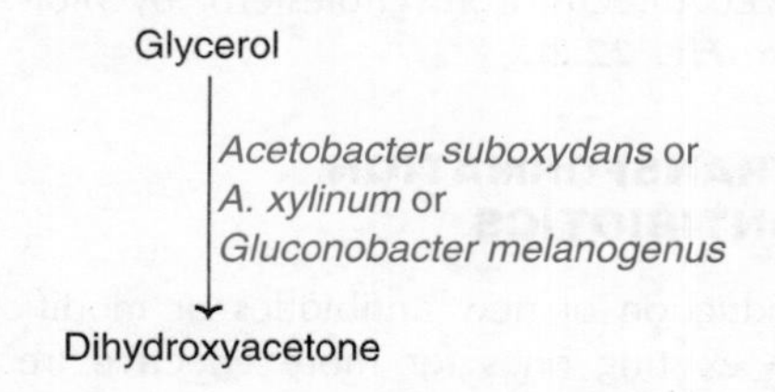

Good oxygen supply, temperature 26–28°C and pH 6.0 are ideal for the optimal biotransformation.

BIOTRANSFORMATION FOR THE PRODUCTION OF INDIGO

Indigo can be synthesized by microbial transformation. This has been made possible by cloning a single *Pseudomonas* gene that encodes naphthalene dioxygenase in the creation of *E. coli*. The relevant reactions of biotransformation for the production of indigo are depicted in ***Fig. 22.4***.

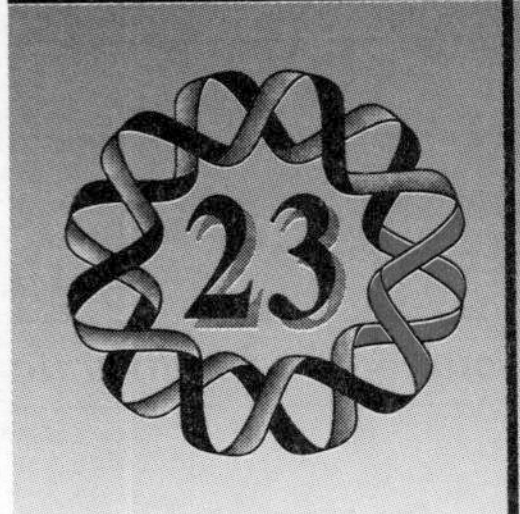

Microbial Production of Organic Solvents

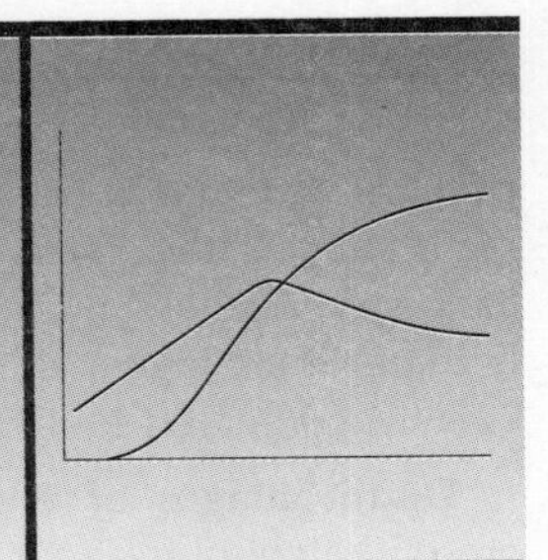

The commercially important organic solvents are ***ethanol*, *acetone, butanol and glycerol*.** These compounds were mostly being produced in petrochemical industries and little attention was paid for their microbial production. It was in mid 1970, due to economic and political reasons, petroleum and natural gas became scarce. Since then, scientists have started looking for suitable alternatives for commercial production of organic solvents. Microbial production of organic solvents utilizing low cost raw materials (e.g. wood, cellulose, starch), is considered to be an ideal alternative.

ALCOHOL

Alcohol, chemically ethanol (C_2H_5OH) has been produced by fermentation for thousands of years. However, this was mostly associated with brewer and distiller industries. At present, most developed countries produce industrial alcohol by chemical means. The petrochemical ethanol is manufactured by hydration of ethylene (C_2H_4).

In the developing countries, microbial fermentation processes are preferred for the production of alcohol. This is mainly because of the cheap raw materials available. At the current rate of oil price, it is cheaper to produce alcohol by petrochemical means rather than fermentation. However, large scale production of alcohol in a given country depends on the political and economic considerations, besides the availability of raw materials. With increasing oil prices, many countries now realise the potential of alcohol production by fermentation.

Ethanol as a motor fuel

Prior to Second World War, ethanol was extensively used as a motor fuel. In fact, some motor companies (e.g. Henry Ford) designed some vehicles to run on alcohol or petrol or a mixture of both.

Brazil was the first country to produce ethanol in large scale by yeast fermentation, utilizing sugarcane and cassava. This ***alcohol used as motor fuel is referred to as green petrol***. Brazil started growing ***alcohol-producing plants*** in a vast area, and installed several fermentation and distillation plants. By 1988, about 90% of the new cars in Brazil had engines that run on alcohol as a fuel. Excited by the success of Brazil, many other countries have also started large scale production of alcohol by fermentation.

Advantages of ethanol as motor fuel : There are distinct advantages of using ethanol in place of petrol for motor vehicles. Ethanol powered engines cause less environmental pollution. They produce 60% less carbon dioxide, 65% less hydrocarbons and 15% less nitric oxide when compared to petrol-run vehicles. Thus, vehicles run on ethanol or ethanol-petrol mix cause comparatively less global warming, and are considered to be ***environmental-***

friendly. Another advantage of ethanol use as a motor fuel is the ***safety***. The flash point (i.e. the temperature at which a substance ignites) of ethanol is three times higher than that of petrol (45°C for ethanol compared to 13°C for petrol).

Disadvantages of ethanol as motor fuel : At present, alcohol is about twice ***costilier than petrol*** in most countries (This may not however, be a limitation in the long run with the availability of cheap substrates and large scale industrial production of alcohol). Since the flash point for ethanol is higher, starting of engines in cold will be difficult. Ethanol may react with alloys containing aluminium and magnesium and may ***damage the containers***. The alcohol used in motor vehicles should be of high purity, and should not be allowed to pick up water from the air. A mixture of ethanol with water does not burn readily, and further it also causes corrosion of engines and tanks.

Gasohol as a fuel : ***A mixture of about 20% ethanol with 80% petrol***, known as gasohol is now being used as a motor fuel some countries like USA. The ethanol used for this purpose should of 100% purity, otherwise petrol and ethanol do not form a uniform mixture.

PRODUCTION OF ETHANOL BY FERMENTATION

As already stated, in recent years many countries have started production of ethanol by fermentation process. The organisms and the raw materials used, along with the biosynthetic pathway, the production and recovery processes for alcohol are briefly described.

Microorganisms

Certain yeasts and bacteria are employed for alcohol fermentation. The type of the organism chosen mostly depends on the nature of the substrate used (***Table 23.1***). Among the yeasts, *Saccharomyces cerevisiae* is the most commonly used, while among the bacteria, *Zymomonas mobilis* is the most frequently employed for alcohol production.

Table 23.1 Microorganisms used in alcohol fermentation

Microorganism	*Source of carbohydrate*
Yeasts	
Saccharomyces cerevisiae	Starch, sugar
S. ellipsoideus	Starch, sugar
Kluyveromyces fragilis	Starch, sugar
Bacteria	
Zymomonas mobilis	Starch
Candida pseudotropicalis	Lactose, whey
C. utilis	Sulfite waste liquor

Raw materials

There are a large number of raw materials that can serve as substrates for alcohol fermentation. They may be broadly categorized as ***sugary materials*** (e.g. molasses, whey, glucose, sucrose), ***starchy materials*** (wheat, rice, maize, potato) and ***cellulosic materials*** (wood, agricultural wastes). Some more examples of potential raw materials are given in ***Table 23.2***. The biomass (starchy and cellulosic materials) significantly contributes for the production of alcohol. For more details on biomass, refer Chapter 31.

Pretreatment of raw materials : Most of the raw materials of alcohol fermentation require some degree of pretreatment. The actual process depends on the chemical composition of the raw material. In general, the sugary raw materials require mild or no pretreatment while the ***cellulosic materials need***

Table 23.2 Potential raw materials for alcohol production

Sugary materials	*Starchy materials*	*Cellulosic materials*
Molasses	**Cereals**	Wood
Sugar cane	Wheat	Saw dust
Sugar beet	Maize	Agricultural wastes
Sweet potato	Barley	Paper wastes
Sweet sorghum	Sorghum	Municipal solid wastes
Whey	Corn	
Sulfite waste	Rice	
Sucrose	**Starchy roots**	
Lactose	Potato	
Glucose	Tapioca	
	Milled products	
	Wheat flour	
	Corn feed	

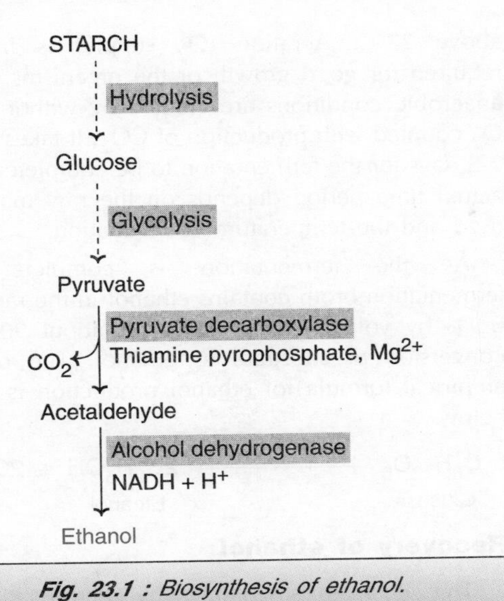

Fig. 23.1 : Biosynthesis of ethanol.

extensive pretreatment. This is because the cellulosic substances have to be subjected to acidic or enzyme hydrolysis to release monosaccharide units that are needed for alcohol production.

Biosynthesis of ethanol

The pathway for the biosynthesis of ethanol is depicted in ***Fig. 23.1***. Glucose gets broken down to pyruvate by glycolysis. Under anaerobic conditions (i.e. in the absence of O_2), pyruvate is converted to acetaldehyde by the enzyme pyruvate decarboxylase. Acetaldehyde is then reduced by alcohol dehydrogenase to form ethanol.

It is observed that under aerobic conditions (adequate O_2 supply) with excess glucose content in the medium, the microorganisms (e.g. *S. cerevisiae*) grow well without producing alcohol. However, ***under anaerobic conditions, growth slows down and alcohol production occurs.***

Regulation of synthesis : ***Ethanol at high*** concentration in the medium ***inhibits its own biosynthesis***. This is particularly observed when yeasts are the fermentation organisms. It is generally seen that growth of yeasts ceases at 5% ethanol concentration (volume/volume in water). It is striking to note that yeasts are sensitive to inhibition by endogenously synthesized ethanol and not to the ethanol added to the medium. Some biotechnologists prefer to use the bacterium *Zymononas mobilis,* since it can tolerate a high concentration of alcohol (up to 13% by some strains against 5% by yeasts).

Glucose to alcohol-conversion profile : Theoretically, one gram of glucose can be converted to 0.511 grams of ethanol. In fact, a conversion yield of 95% was observed when pure substrates (glucose, lactose, sucrose) are used. For industrial grade raw materials (corn starch) the yield is around 90%. It is estimated that ***for 100 g pure glucose, 48.5 g of ethanol is produced***, along with 46.5 g of CO_2, 3.3 g glycerol and 1.3 g of biomass (yeast cells).

Production process of ethanol

Ethanol production can be carried out in three stages-preparation of nutrient solution and inoculum, fermentation proper and recovery. A flow diagram for alcohol production is depicted in ***Fig. 23.2***.

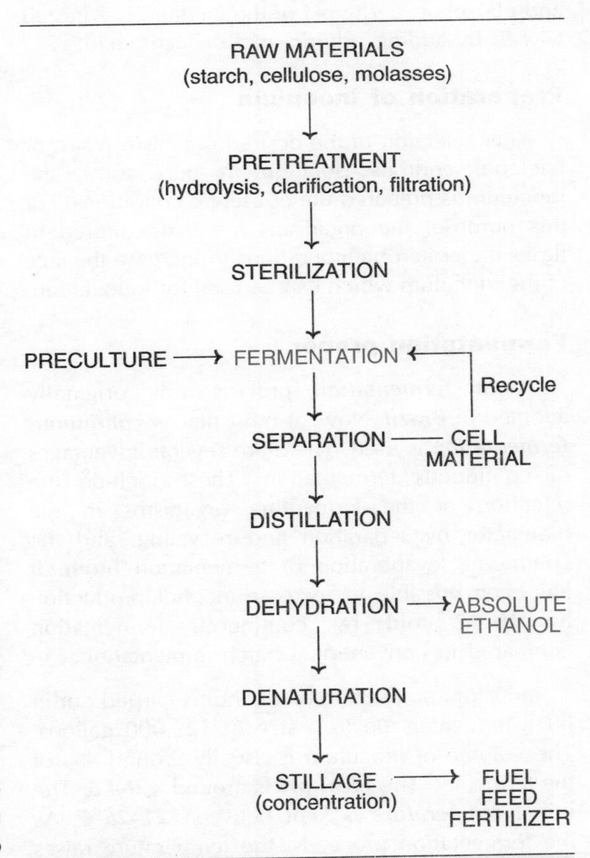

Fig. 23.2 : A schematic representation of ethanol production by fermentation.

Preparation of nutrient solution (media)

The various raw materials for alcohol production have already been described (Refer ***Table 23.1***). The most commonly used raw materials are molasses, whey, grains, potatoes and wood wastes.

When molasses is used for fermentation, it is diluted with water so that the sugar concentration is in the range of 10–18%. A concentration higher than this is detrimental to the yeast. When starchy materials (corn, barely) are used, they have to be first hydrolysed by pretreatment for use as nutrients. This may be done by barley malt, dilute acids or fungal amylases (e.g. *Aspergillus* sp, *Rhizopus* sp). Most frequently mashing with barely malt is used.

Molasses contains most of the nutrients required for alcohol fermentation. However, ammonium salts such as ammonium sulfate or phosphate are added to the nutrient solution to supply nitrogen and phosphorus. The pH of the medium is adjusted to 4-5, by adding sulfuric acid or lactic acid.

Preparation of inoculum

After selection of the desired organism (yeast or bacteria) and its isolation in pure form, the inoculum is prepared under aseptic conditions. For this purpose, the organisms are first cultured in flasks under aerobic conditions to increase the size of the inoculum which can be used for inoculation.

Fermentation proper

Batch fermentation process was originally adopted in ***Brazil***. Now, at most places ***continuous fermentation*** is used. There are several advantages of continuous fermentation. These include the retention of the fermenting organisms in the bioreactor by separation and recycling, and the continuous evaporation of fermentation broth. It has been possible to increase alcohol production by 10–12 fold by continuous fermentation compared to conventional batch fermentation.

Industrial production of alcohol is carried out in huge fermenters up to a size of 125,000 gallons. The volume of inoculum is usually around 4% of the fermenter. The ***ideal pH*** is around ***4.0-4.5***. The initial ***temperature*** is kept between ***21–26°C***. As the fermentation proceeds, the temperature raises to around 30°C. It is necessary to use cooling devices and bring down the temperature to less than 27°C. Ethanol gets evaporated at temperature above 27°C. Aeration (O_2 supply) is initially required for good growth of the organisms. Later, anaerobic conditions are created by withdrawl of O_2 coupled with production of CO_2. It takes about 2-3 days for the fermentation to be completed. The actual time period depends on the raw materials used and the temperature of incubation.

As the fermentation is complete, the fermentation broth contains ethanol in the range of 6-9% by volume. This represents about 90–95% conversion of substrate to ethanol. The overall empirical formula for ethanol production is given below.

$$\underset{\text{Glucose}}{C_6H_{12}O_6} \xrightarrow{\text{Fermentation}} \underset{\text{Ethanol}}{2C_2H_5OH} + 2CO_2$$

Recovery of ethanol

The cell mass is separated by centrifugation or sedimentation. Ethanol from the fermentation broth can be recovered by successive distillations. By this processes, it is easy to obtain ethanol of around 95%. For a concentration above 95%, special techniques of distillation have to be adopted. For preparation of absolute (100%) alcohol, an ***azeotropic mixture*** of benzene, water and alcohol is first prepared. This mixture is then distilled by gradually increasing the temperature. By this technique, it is possible to first remove benzene-ethanol-water mixture, and then ethanol-benzene mixture. Thus, absolute alcohol is left out.

Stillages in alcohol production

Large volumes of ***wastes*** which are technically referred to stillages are formed during the course of alcohol fermentation. Attempts are made to fruitfully utilize stillages for various purposes.

- To use as feed or fertilizers.
- For converting to single-cell protein.
- To use a fuel.
- For production of methanol.

Genetic engineering for improved alcohol production

With the advent of recombinant DNA technology, attempts are being made worldwide to develop new strains of organisms for increasing alcohol production. Some success has been achieved in creating more efficient microorganisms with the desired characteristics.

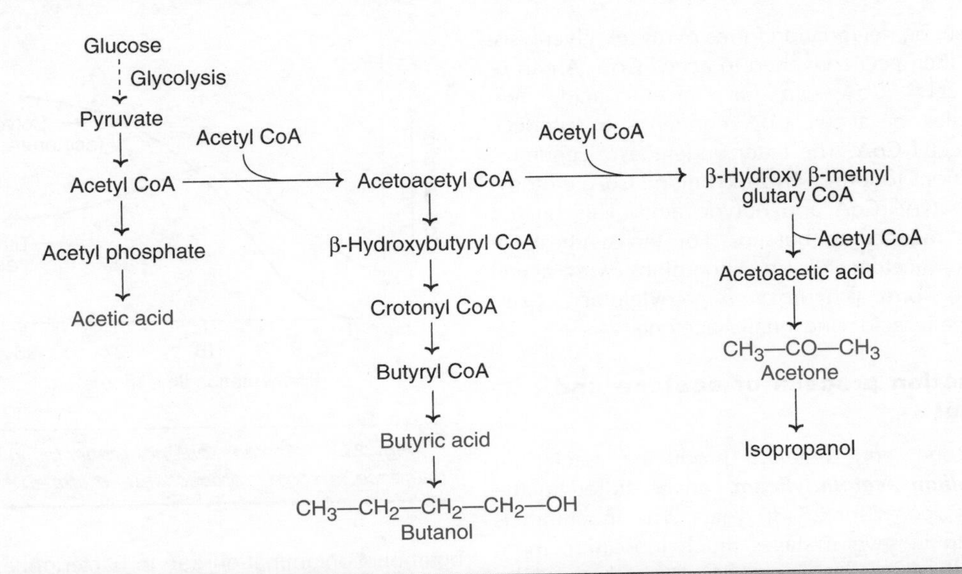

*Fig. 23.3 : Biosynthesis of acetone and butanol (**Note** : Acetic acid and butyric acid can also be produced by this pathway)*

- Improved production of alcohol.
- Resistance to high alcohol concentration.
- Resistance to high temperature.
- Rapid conversion of substrate to alcohol.

It has also been possible to improve alcohol production by using immobilized enzymes in reactor systems.

ACETONE AND BUTANOL

Both acetone and butanol are good ***organic solvents***. Decades ago, acetone was used as a gelatinizing agent for nitrocellulose in the manufacture of explosives. It is also used in dyestuff industry. Butanol is required for the synthesis of butadiene to produce synthetic rubber. At present, butanol is extensively used in break fluids, for antibiotic recovery, as amines for gasoline additives and as ester in protective-coating industry.

The production of acetone and butanol by ***anaerobic fermentation*** is almost a century old. This process was carried out by using starch or sugar-rich raw materials (potato, molasses) and the organism *Clostridium acetobutylicum*. After World War II, acetone and butanol became readily available from the byproducts of the petroleum industry. The production of acetone and butanol by fermentation is ***almost discontinued in many countries***. It is however, said that being a very simple process, developing countries (with cheap raw materials) may soon opt for fermentation rather than petroleum-based products due to economic reasons.

Production of acetone and butanol

Certain bacteria of *Clostridium* species are capable of producing acetone, butanol, butyric acid and isopropanol through fermentation of molasses, wood hydrolysates, starch, sucrose and pentoses. Depending on the strain of the bacterium and the fermentation conditions employed, the relative production of the four compounds varies.

For *Clostridium acetobutylicum*, the fermentation products are acetone and butanol. Butanol-isopropanol or butyric acid-acetic acid can be produced by *Clostridium butyricum*.

Biosynthesis of acetone and butanol

The sequence of reactions leading to the formation of acetone and butanol, along with acetic acid and butyric acid is depicted in ***Fig. 23.3***.

Glucose, on degradation forms pyruvate (glycolysis) which then gets converted to acetyl CoA. A part of this acetyl CoA can form acetic acid. Two molecules of acetyl CoA condense to produce acetoacetyl CoA. The latter undergoes a sequence of reactions to form β-hydroxybutyryl CoA, crotonyl CoA, butyryl CoA and butyric acid. This butyric acid is reduced to butanol. For the synthesis of acetone, acetoacetyl CoA combines with acetyl CoA to form β-hydroxy β-methylglutaryl CoA, acetoacetic acid, and finally acetone.

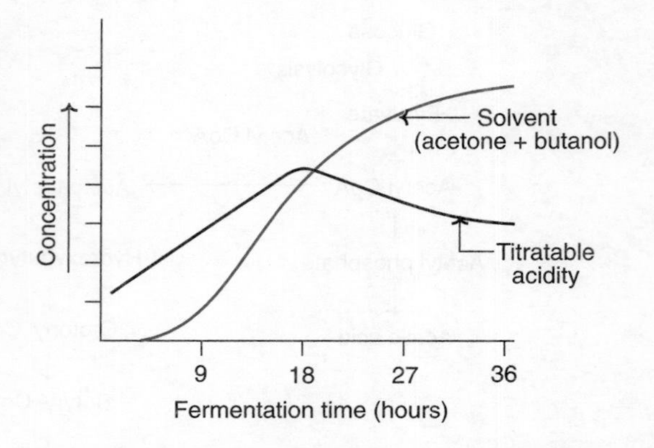

Fig. 23.4 : Acetone–butanol fermentation with reference to solvent production and titratable acidity.

Production process of acetone and butanol

Acetone and butanol producing bacterium ***Clostridium acetobutylicum*** can be stored in the form of spores for 25–30 years. The inoculum is build up in several stages. Such inoculum, more efficiently ferments sugars to give a high yield. These organisms are also resistant to contamination.

The fermentation is usually carried out in corn or molasses based medium. The molasses medium contains molasses, ammonium sulfate, calcium carbonate and sometimes corn steep liquor.

The fermenters after sterilization are gased with CO_2. After the addition of the medium and inoculum (approximately 2-4% by volume), the fermenter contents are again stirred with CO_2. The fermentation is carried out with a starting pH 5.8-6.0, and temperature 34°C. The actual process of fermentation, spread over 36 hours, occurs in three phases.

Phase I is characterized by rapid growth of the organism and production acetic acid and butyric acid. There is an increase in titratable acidity. The pH of the medium drops to around 5.2.

In phase 2, an increased production of acetone and butanol (solvents) coupled with a decrease in titratable acidity (the latter phenomenon is referred to as ***acid break***).

During the ***third phase***, there is a decrease in the solvent production with a slight or no increase in pH.

In ***Fig. 23.4***, the fermentation processes with reference to solvent production and titratable acidity are depicted.

Contamination : Absolute sterile conditions are required for good production of acetone and butanol. Contamination due to bacteriophages and lactobacilli (particularly *Lactobacillus leichmannii*) is a major problem that hinders the yield.

Product yield : Approximately, 30% of the carbohydrate gets converted to neutral solvents in the fermentation. In molasses medium, the ratio of butanol and acetone is 7 : 3, while in corn medium it is 6 : 3. The actual production of butanol is influenced by its toxicity to the organism. Butanol is toxic at a concentration higher than 13.5% in the medium.

Product recovery : Acetone and butanol are recovered through continuous distillation and fractionation. The left over residue after distillation can be dried and used as animal feed.

GLYCEROL

Glycerol is widely used in industry and commerce. It is particularly important as a ***starting material for the manufacture of explosives***. Glycerol is commercially ***produced by the saponification of fats and oils***. It can also be chemically synthesized from propylene or propane. As such, glycerol is not usually produced by fermentation.

During the First World War, the Germans could not import vegetable oils to produce glycerol, due to British naval blockade. And for this reason, Germans were forced to produce glycerol by microbial fermentation. At present, glycerol

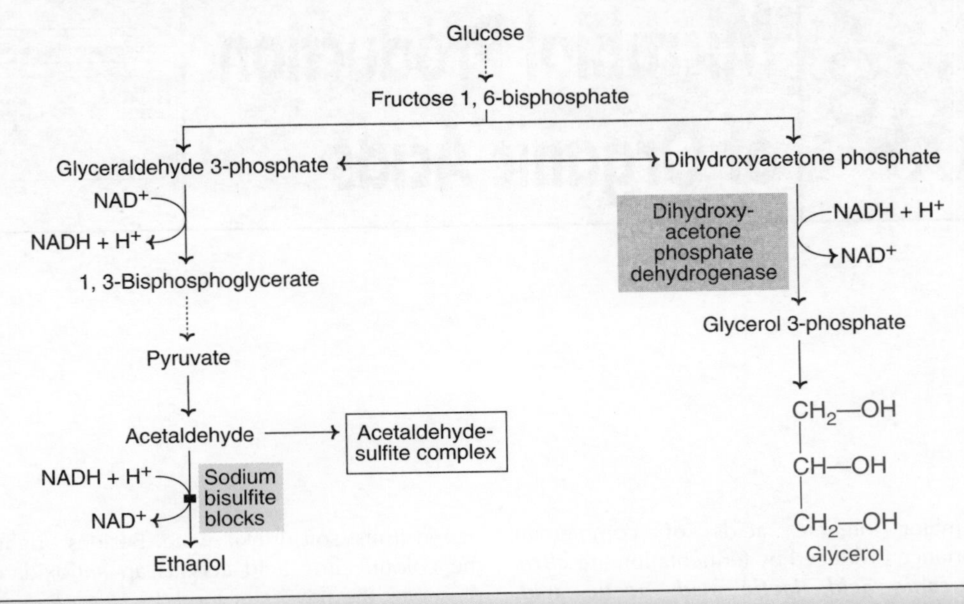

Fig. 23.5 : Biosynthesis of glycerol.

fermentation is of no significance except theoretical and historical importance. In addition, this fermentation process also demonstrates how a modification in the fermentation condition leads to a modification in the product formed.

Production process of glycerol

Basically, glycerol is produced by yeast during the course of alcohol fermentation. However, in the normal process, the quantity of glycerol formed is very low. Addition of sodium sulfite blocks alcohol production and diverts the pathway for the large scale production of glycerol (***Fig. 23.5***). Sodium sulfite reacts with CO_2 in the medium and gets converted to sodium bisulfite. The latter combines with acetaldehyde (an intermediate in ethanol formation) to form acetaldehyde-sulfite complex and thus blocks alcohol synthesis. NADH, generated in one of the early reactions of glycolysis is utilized for glycerol production (instead of ethanol formation due to inhibition).

The fermentation is run for 2-3 days. The yield of glycerol is in the range of 20–30% of the sugar used. This yield is about half of the theoretical value (~ 50%) due to the fact that ethanol fermentation cannot be completely inhibited. Further, the recovery of glycerol from the fermentation broth also is incomplete.

Glycerol production by alga

A novel fermentation process for glycerol production by the alga *Dunaliella salina* has been developed in Israel. This organism, commonly found in salty (hypersaline) lakes synthesizes glycerol within the cells to balance the high osmotic pressure in the surroundings (due to salts). Thus, the higher is the salt concentration in the surroundings, the more is the intracellular glycerol production. However, when the surrounding salt concentration is suddenly reduced, glycerol is excreted into the medium. This principle is successfully exploited for the production glycerol by *D. salina*.

Glycerol production by *Bacillus subtilis*

Bacillus subtilis is normally an aerobic microorganism. It is capable of converting glucose to glycerol, ethanol, lactic acid, butanediol etc. But the production of glycerol under aerobic conditions is very low. However, under anaerobic conditions, the production of glycerol by *B. subtilis* is quite high. And the yield of glycerol comparable to that obtained by yeast fermentation.

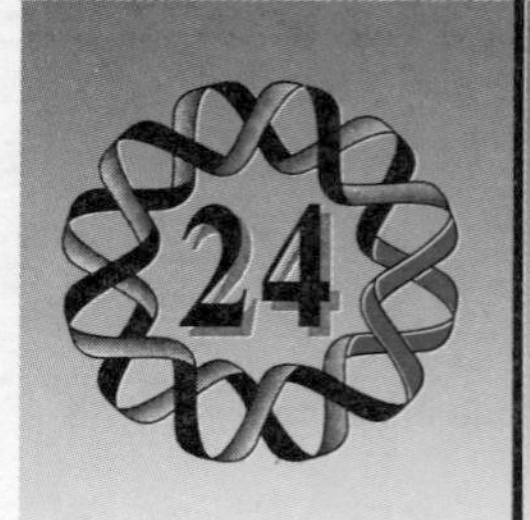

Microbial Production of Organic Acids

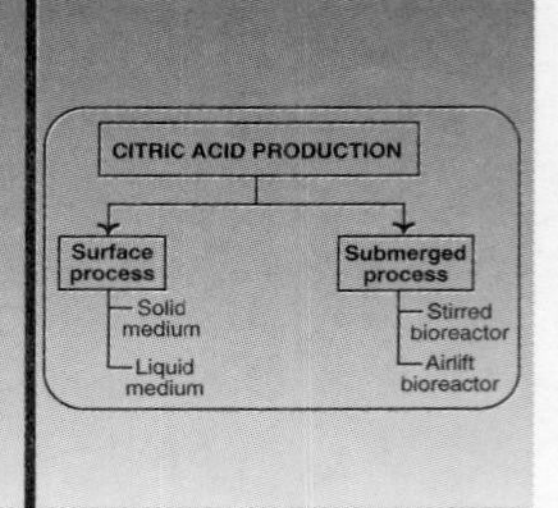

The major organic acids of commercial importance produced by fermentation are ***citric acid***, ***gluconic acid***, ***lactic acid***, ***acetic acid***, ***ascorbic acid*** and ***itaconic acid***. These compounds may be produced directly from glucose (e.g., gluconic acid) or formed as end products from pyruvate or ethanol (e.g., lactic acid and acetic acid). The production of most of the organic acids is directly or indirectly linked with Krebs cycle.

Besides microbiological production by fermentation, some organic acids are also produced by chemical methods e.g. acetic acid and lactic acid. Some details on the production of important organic acids by fermentation are given in the following pages.

CITRIC ACID

Citric acid was first discovered as a constituent of lemon. Today, we know citric acid as an intermediate of ubiquitous Krebs cycle (citric acid cycle), and therefore, it is present in every living organism. In the early days, citric acid was isolated from lemons (that contain 7-9% citric acid), and today about 99% of the world's citric acid comes from microbial fermentation.

Applications of citric acid

1. Citric acid, due to its pleasant taste and palatability, is used as a ***flavouring agent*** in foods and beverages e.g., jams, jellies, candies, desserts, frozen fruits, soft drinks, wine. Besides brightening the colour, citric acid acts as an antioxidant and preserves the flavors of foods.

2. It is used in the ***chemical industry*** as an antifoam agent, and for the treatment of textiles. In metal industry, pure metals are complexed with citrate and produced as metal citrates.

3. In ***pharmaceutical industry***, as trisodium citrate, it is used as a blood preservative. Citric acid is also used for preservation of ointments and cosmotic preparations. As iron citrate, it serve as a good source of iron.

4. Citric acid can be utilized as an ***agent for stabilization*** of fats, oils or ascorbic acid. It forms a complex with metal ions (iron, copper) and prevents metal catalysed reactions. Citric acid is also used as a stabiliser of emulsions in the preparation of cheese.

5. In ***detergent/cleaning*** industry, citric acid has slowly replaced polyphosphates.

Microbial strains for citric acid production

Many microorganisms can produce citric acid. The ***fungus Aspergillus niger*** is most ***commonly used*** for industrial production of citric acid. The other organisms (although less important) include *A. clavatus, A. wentii, Penicillium luteum, Candida catenula, C. guilliermondii* and *Corynebacterium* sp.

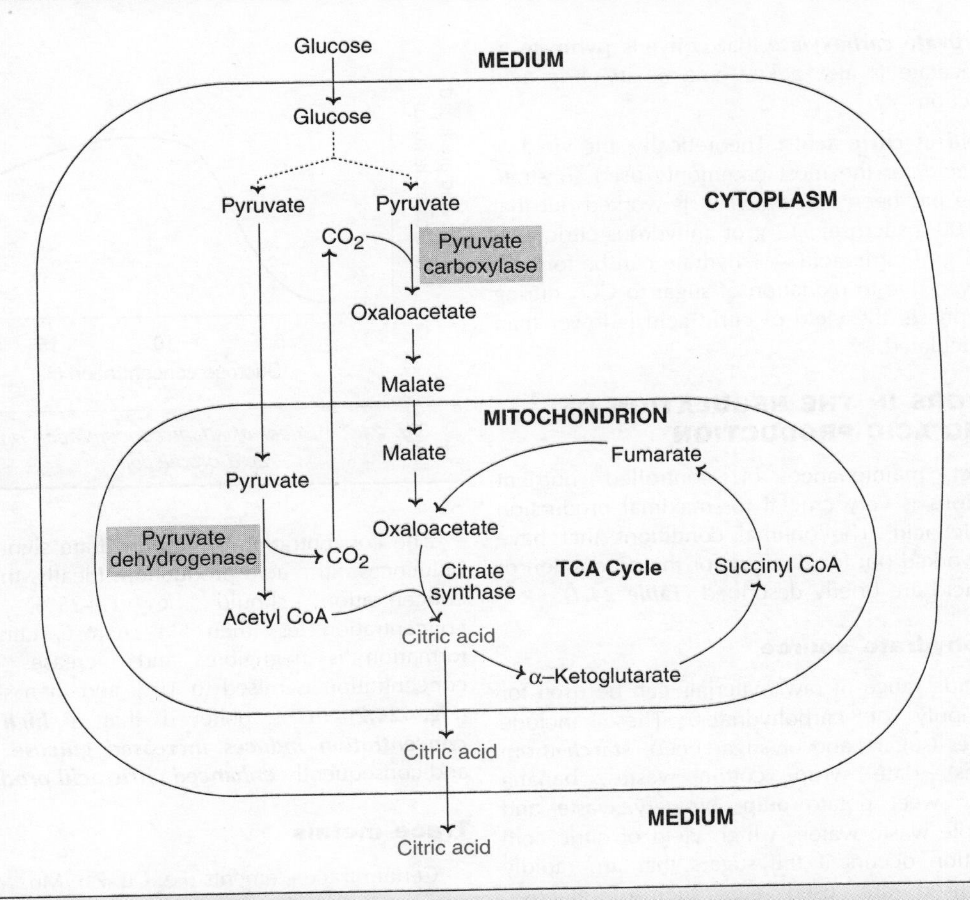

Fig. 24.1 : An outline of metabolic pathway for the biosynthesis of citric acid (TCA cycle-Tricarboxylic acid cycle).

For improved industrial production of citric acid, mutant strains of *A. niger* have been developed. The strains that can tolerate high sugar concentration and low pH with reduced synthesis of undersirable byproducts (oxalic acid, isocitric acid and gluconic acid) are industrially important.

Microbial biosynthesis of citric acid

Citric acid is a ***primary metabolic product*** (of primary metabolism) formed in the tricarboxylic acid (Krebs) cycle. Glucose is the predominant carbon source for citric acid production. The biosynthetic pathway for citric acid production involves ***glycolysis*** wherein ***glucose*** is converted ***to two molecules of pyruvate.*** Pyruvate in turn forms acetyl CoA and oxaloacetate which condense to finally give citrate. The major steps in the biosynthesis of citric acid are depicted in ***Fig. 24.1***.

Enzymatic regulation of citric acid production : During the synthesis of citric acid, there is a tenfold increase in the activity of the enzyme ***citrate synthase*** while the activities of other enzymes (aconitase, isocitrate dehydrogenase) that degrade citric acid are reduced. However, recent evidence does not support the theory that reduction in the operation of tricarboxylic acid (i.e. degradation of citric acid) contributes to accumulation of citric acid. Increased citric acid is more likely due to enhanced biosynthesis rather than inhibited degradation. Further, there are anaplerotic reactions that replenish the TCA cycle intermediates to keep the cycle continuously in operation.

Pyruvate carboxylase that converts pyruvate to oxaloacetate is also a key enzyme in citric acid production.

Yield of citric acid : Theoretically, the yield of citric acid for the most commonly used substrate sucrose has been calculated. It is worked out that from 100 g sucrose, 112 g of anhydrous citric acid or 123 g of citric acid — 1 hydrate can be formed. However, due to oxidation of sugar to CO_2 during trophophase, the yield of citric acid is lower than the calculated.

FACTORS IN THE REGULATION OF CITRIC ACID PRODUCTION

Strict maintenance of controlled nutrient conditions is very crucial for maximal production of citric acid. The optimal conditions that have been worked out for *A. niger* for the production of citric acid are briefly described (***Table 24.1***).

Carbohydrate source

A wide range of raw materials can be used for the supply of carbohydrates. These include ***molasses*** (sugar cane or sugar beet), ***starch*** (from potatoes), date syrup, cotton wastes, banana extract, sweet potato pulp, brewery waste and pineapple waste water. A high yield of citric acid production occurs if the sugars that are rapidly metabolised are used e.g. sucrose, glucose, maltose. At present, cane molasses and beet molasses are commonly used. The variations in the composition of molasses (seasonal and production level), have to be carefully considered for optimising citric acid production.

TABLE 24.1 Optimal parameters/conditions for citric acid production

Condition/parameter	*Optimum*
Sugar concentration	10–25%
Trace metal concentration	
Manganese	$<10^{-8}$ M
Zinc	$<10^{-7}$ M
Iron	$<10^{-4}$ M
pH	1.5–2.5
Dissolved O_2 tension	150 mbr
Ammonium salts concentration	>0.2%
Time	150–250 hours

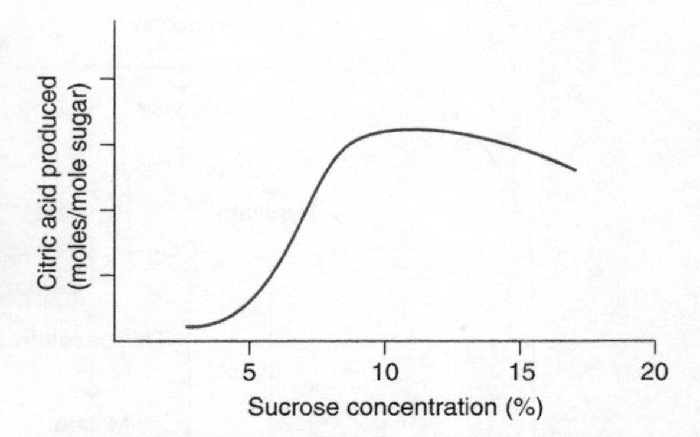

Fig. 24.2 : Effect of sugar concentration on citric acid production.

The concentration of carbohydrate significantly influences citric acid production. Ideally, the sugar concentration should be 12–25%. At a concentration less than 5% sucrose, citric acid formation is negligible, and increases as the concentration is raised to 10% and then stablises (***Fig. 24.2***). It is believed that a ***high sugar concentration induces increased glucose uptake*** and consequently ***enhanced citric acid production***.

Trace metals

Certain trace elements (Fe, Cu, Zn, Mn, Mg, Co) are essential for the growth of *A. niger*. Some of the trace metals particularly Mn^{2+}, Fe^{3+} ***and*** Zn^{2+} ***increase the yield of citric acid***.

The effect of manganese ions has been investigated to some extent. These ions promote glycolysis and reduce respiration, both these processes promote citric acid production.

As regards iron, it is a cofactor for the enzyme aconitase (of TCA cycle). It is estimated that an Fe concentration of 0.05-0.5 ppm is ideal for optimal citric acid production. At higher Fe concentration, the yield is lower which can be reversed to some extent by adding copper.

pH

The pH of the medium influences the yield of citric acid, and it is ***maximal when pH is below 2.5***. At this pH, the production of oxalic acid and gluconic acid is suppressed. Further, at low pH, transport of citric acid is much higher. If the pH is above 4, gluconic acid accumulates at the expense of citric acid. And when the pH goes beyond 6, oxalic acid accumulates.

Another advantage with low pH is that the risk of contamination is very minimal, since many organisms cannot grow at this pH.

Dissolved O_2

The yield of ***citric acid production*** substantially ***increases when the dissolved O_2 tension is higher***. This can be achieved by strong aeration or by sparging with pure O_2. It has been observed that sudden interruptions in O_2 supply (as occurs during power breakdowns) cause drastic reduction in citric acid production without harming the growth of the organism.

Nitrogen source

Ammonium salts, nitrates and urea are the nitrogen sources used in the media for citric acid production. All the three compounds are equally good sources, as long as they do not adversely effect the pH of the medium. If molasses are used for nutrient supply, addition of extra nitrogen source is not required. However, some workers have shown that exogenous ***addition of ammonium ions stimulates citric acid production***.

PRODUCTION PROCESSES FOR CITRIC ACID

There are two processes by which citric acid can be industrially produced — the surface process and submerged process (***Fig. 24.3***).

The surface process : This is characterized by growing the ***microorganisms*** as a layer or a film ***on a surface*** in contact with the nutrient medium, which may be ***solid or liquid*** in nature. Thus, the surface process has supported-growth systems.

The submerged process : In this case, the ***organisms*** are immersed in or ***dispersed throughout*** the nutrient ***medium***. There are two types of submerged fermenters (bioreactors) ***stirred bioreactors*** and ***airlift bioreactors***.

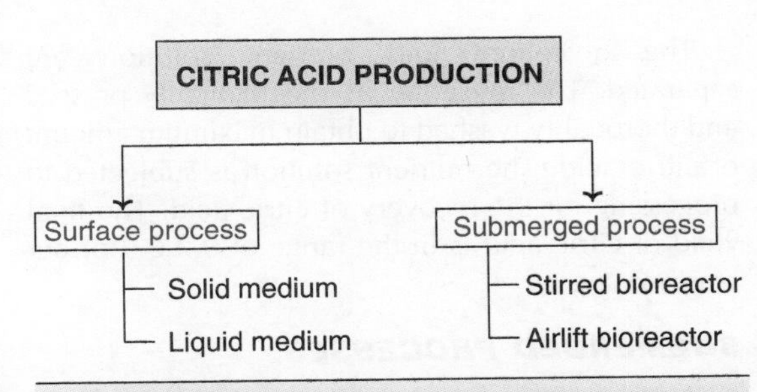

Fig. 24.3 : The industrial processes for the production of citric acid.

SURFACE PROCESSES

Solid surface fermentation

Surface processes using solid substrates are particularly carried out in less developed areas of some Asian countries. The solid substrates such as wheat bran or pulp from sweet potato starch are used, as culture media. The pH of the medium is adjusted to 4-5, and then sterilized. Now the inoculum in the form of spores of *A. niger* is spread as layers (3-6 cm thickness) and incubated at 28°C. The growth of the organisms can be accelerated by the addition of α-amylase. Solid-state fermentation takes about 80 to 100 hours for maximal production of citric acid. At the end of the process, citric acid can be extracted into hot water and isolated.

Liquid surface fermentation

Surface fermentation using liquid as nutrient medium is the oldest method for citric acid production. It is still in use due to a simple technology, low energy costs and higher reproducibility. Further, the interference of trace metals and dissolved O_2 tension are minimal. The labour costs are however, higher since the manpower requirements are more for cleaning the systems. About 20% of the citric acid in the world is produced by surface processes.

The nutrient supply for surface fermentation normally comes from beet molasses. The fermentation is usually carried out in aluminium trays filled with sterile nutrient medium. The inoculum in the form of spores is sprayed over the medium. A sterile air is passed for supplying O_2 as well as cooling. The temperature is maintained around 30°C during fermentation. As the spores germinate (that occurs within 24 hours of inoculation), a layer of mycelium is formed over the medium. The pH of the nutrient medium falls to less than 2, as the mycelium grows in size and forms a thick layer on the surface of the nutrient solution. The fermentation is stopped after 7–15 days.

The mycelium and nutrient solution are separated. The mycelium is mechanically pressed and thoroughly washed to obtain maximum amount of citric acid. The nutrient solution is subjected to processing for the recovery of citric acid. The final yield of citric acid is in the range of 0.7-0.9 of per gram of sugar.

SUBMERGED PROCESSES

Around 80% of the world's supply of citric acid is produced by submerged processes. This is the most preferred method due to its high efficiency and easy automation. The disadvantages of submerged fermentation are — adverse influence of trace metals and other impurities, variations in O_2 tension, and advanced control technology that requires highly trained personnel.

Two types of bioreactors are in use — ***stirred tanks*** and ***aerated towers***. The vessels of the bioreactors are made up of high-quality stainless steel. The sparging of air occurs from the base of the fermenter.

The success and yield of citric acid production mainly depend on the structure of mycelium. The mycelium with forked and bulbous hyphae and branches which aggregate into pellets is ideal for citric acid formation. On the other hand, no citric acid production occurs if the mycelium is loose and filamentous with limited branches. An adequate supply of O_2 (20–25% of saturation value) is required for good production of citric acid. The ideal aeration rate is in the range of 0.2-1 vvm (volume/volume/minute).

The submerged fermenters have the problem of foam formation which may occupy about 1/3rd of the bioreactor. Antifoam agents (e.g. lard oil) and mechanical antifoam devices are used to prevent foaming.

Nutrient concentration is very important in the industrial production of citric acid. A diagrammatic representation of sucrose, citric acid and biomass concentration with respect to cultivation time is shown in ***Fig. 24.4***. It is estimated that under optimal conditions, in about 250–280 hours, 100–110 g/l of citric acid is obtained from 140 g/l of sucrose with a biomass (dry weight) of 8–12 g/l.

PRODUCTION OF CITRIC ACID FROM ALKANES

Both yeasts and bacteria can be used for citric acid production from n-alkanes (C_9–C_{23} hydrocarbons). The citric acid yield is better from hydrocarbons compared to sugars i.e. 145% of citric acid from paraffin. The most commonly used organism is *Candida lipolytica*. The fermentation can be carried out in batch, semi-continuous or continuous modes. The pH should be kept above 5.

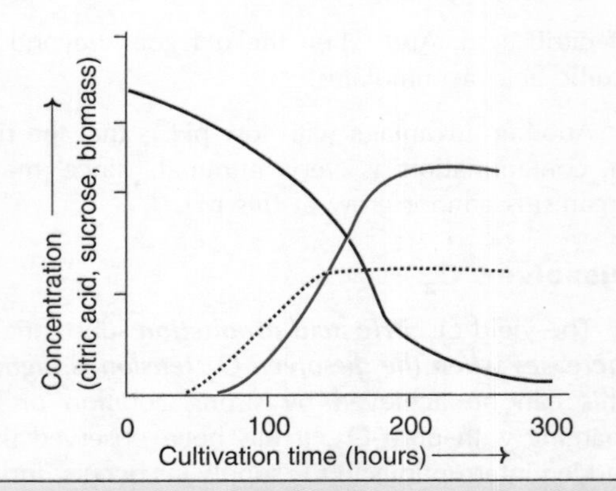

***Fig. 24.4 :** A diagrammatic representation of citric acid (—) production along with sucrose (—) and biomass (- - -) concentration in relation to time.*

The major limitations of citric acid production from alkanes are—very low solubility of alkanes and increased production of unwanted isocitric acid.

RECOVERY OF CITRIC ACID

The steps for the recovery of citric acid either from surface process or submerged process are comparable (***Fig. 24.5***). The recovery starts with the filtration of the culture broth and washing of mycelium (which may contain about 10% of citric acid produced). Oxalic acid is an unwanted byproduct and it can be removed by precipitation by adding lime at pH < 3. The culture broth is then subjected to pH 7.2 and temperature 70–90°C for precipitating citric acid. For further purification, citric acid is dissolved in sulfuric acid (calcium sulfate precipitate separates). The final steps for ***citric acid recovery*** are — ***treatment with activated charcoal, cation and anion-exchangers and crystallization***. Citric acid monohydrate formed below 36°C is the main commercial product. Above 40°C, citric acid crystallizes in an anhydrous form. The degree of purity of citric acid produced depends on the purpose for which it is required. For instance, pure forms of citric acid are needed for use in food preparations, while for industrial use it can be crude form.

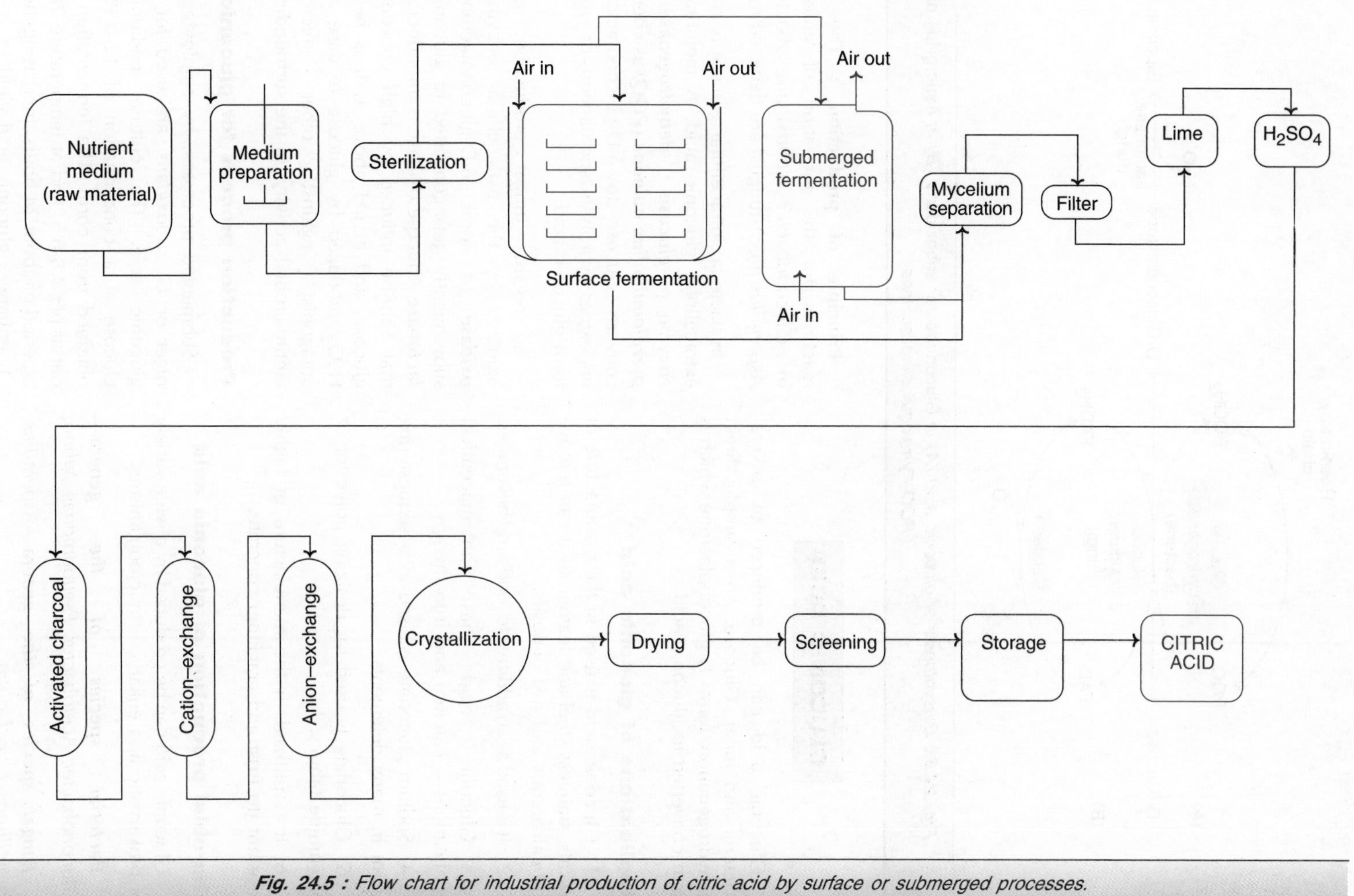

Fig. 24.5 : Flow chart for industrial production of citric acid by surface or submerged processes.

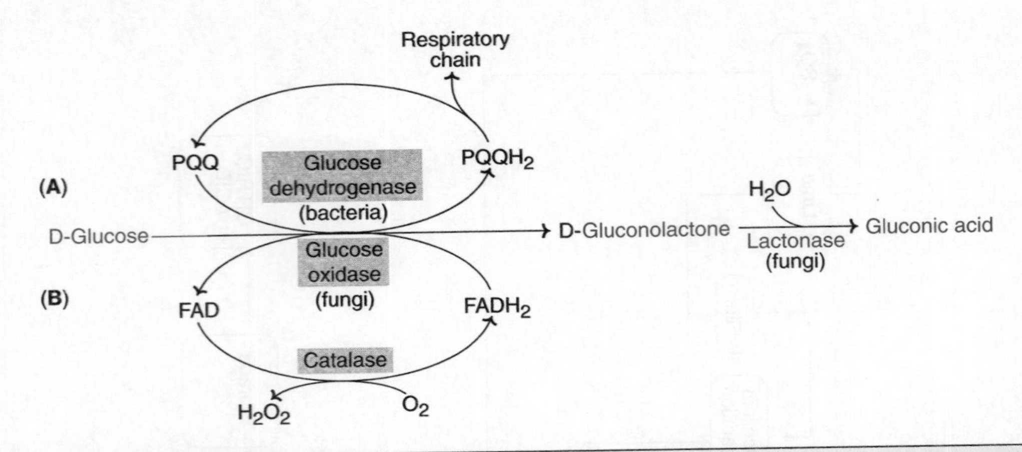

Fig. 24.6 : Biosynthesis of gluconic acid (A) in Gluconobacter suboxidans *(B) in* Aspergillus niger. *(PQQ-Pyrroloquinoline quinone)*

GLUCONIC ACID

Gluconic acid can be produced by several bacteria and fungi. Glucose, on a simple direct dehydrogenation, forms D-gluconolactone which is then converted to gluconic acid.

Applications of gluconic acid

1. Gluconic acid is used in the manufacture of metals, stainless steel and leather, as it can remove the calcareous and rust deposits.

2. It is used as an additive to foods and beverages.

3. Gluconic acid has pharmaceutical applications — calcium and iron therapy.

4. Sodium gluconate is used as a sequestering agent in many detergents.

5. Gluconate is used for desizing polyester or polyamide fabrics.

6. It is utilized in the manufacture of highly resistant (to frost and cracking) concrete.

Microbial production of gluconic acid

Gluconic acid can be produced by a wide variety of prokaryotic and eukaryotic microorganisms.

Bacterial species of the genera—*Gluconobacter, Acetobacter, Pseudomonas, Vibrio.*

Fungal species of the genera—*Aspergillus, Penicillium, Gliocladium.*

Principle of production : The enzymatic reactions for the formation of gluconic acid in *Gluconobacter suboxidans* (bacteria) and *Aspergillus niger* (fungus) are depicted in **Fig. 24.6**.

In bacteria, intracellular glucose is converted to extracellular gluconic acid. A membrane bound enzyme, ***glucose dehydrogenase*** utilizes ***pyrroloquinoline quinone (PQQ)*** as coenzyme and converts glucose to δ-D-gluconolactone which undergoes hydrolysis (spontaneous or enzymatic) to form gluconic acid.

As regards fungal production, glucose is oxidized by the extracellular enzyme ***glucose oxidase*** to form δ-D-gluconolactone, which subsequently gets converted to gluconic acid by ***lactonase***. Glucose oxidase is an inducible enzyme that can be induced by high concentrations of glucose, and at pH above 4. It is believed that H_2O_2 produced by glucose oxidase acts as an antagonist against other microorganisms (antimicrobial activity) in the surroundings.

Production process for gluconic acid

Submerged processes, by employing either *A. niger* or *G. suboxidans,* are used for producing gluconic acid. The culture medium contains glucose at a concentration of 12–15% (usually obtained from corn). The fermentation is carried out at pH 4.5-6.5, and at temperature 28–30°C for a period of about 24 hours. Increasing the supply of O_2 enhances gluconic acid yield.

Biotechnologists exploit the fermentation process of gluconic acid for the production of the enzyme glucose oxidase, besides producing calcium gluconate and sodium gluconate.

Chemical synthesis of gluconic acid : By employing the immobilized enzyme glucose oxidase, gluconic acid can also be produced.

LACTIC ACID

Lactic acid occurs in two isomeric forms i.e. L(+) and D(–) isomers, and as a racemic mixture (DL-lactic acid). The isolation of lactic acid from milk was done in 1798. It was the first organic acid produced by microorganisms in 1880. Today, lactic acid is competitively produced both by microbiological and chemical methods.

Applications of lactic acid

There are different grades of lactic acid mainly based on the percentage of lactic acid. The grades and their applications are given in ***Table 24.2***.

Microorganisms for production of lactic acid

Lactic acid producing bacteria are broadly categorized into two types.

Heterofermentative bacteria—produce other byproducts, besides lactic acid, and therefore are not useful for industrial production of lactic acid. These bacteria are employed in food or feed preservation.

Homofermentative bacteria—specialised for exclusive production of lactic acid and therefore are suitable for industrial purpose.

TABLE 24.2 Commercial grades of lactic acid along with their applications

Grade (% lactic acid)	*Application(s)*
Technical grade (20–50%)	Ester manufacture, textile industry
Food grade (>80%)	Food additive (sour flour and dough)
Pharmaceutical grade (>90%)	Intestinal treatment (metal ion lactates)

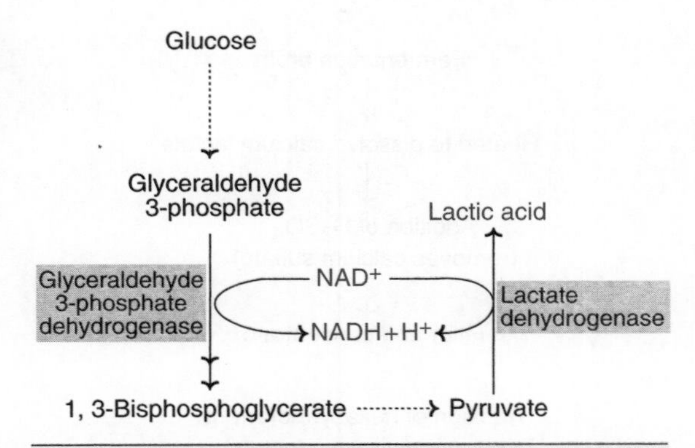

***Fig. 24.7 :** An outline of the pathway (glycolysis) for the biosynthesis of lactic acid.*

Lactobacillus sp are used for lactic acid production. However, there are variations in the substrates utilised as indicated below.

L. delbrueckii, *L. leichamanni* } Glucose

L. bulgaricus, *L. helvetii* } Whey (lactose)

L. lactis — Maltose

L. amylophilus — Starch

L. pentosus — Sulfite waste liquor

Biosynthesis of lactic acid : The synthesis of lactic acid occurs through glucose oxidation by glycolysis to produce pyruvate which on reduction gives lactic acid. The reducing equivalents ($NADH^+ + H^+$) produced during the oxidation of glyceraldelyde 3-phosphate are utilised by the enzyme lactate dehydrogenase to form lactate (***Fig. 24.7***). Most of the lactic acid producing microorganisms normally produce only one isomer of lactic acid L(+) or D(–). However, some bacteria which usually occur as infection can form racemic mixture.

Production process for lactic acid

The fermentation medium contains 12–15% of glucose, nitrogen and phosphate containing salts and micronutrients. The process is carried out at pH 5.5-6.5 and temperature 45–50°C for about 75 hours. Generally, the strains operating at higher temperature (45–60°C) are preferred, since it reduces the need for medium sterilization. As the lactic acid is produced, it has to be removed since

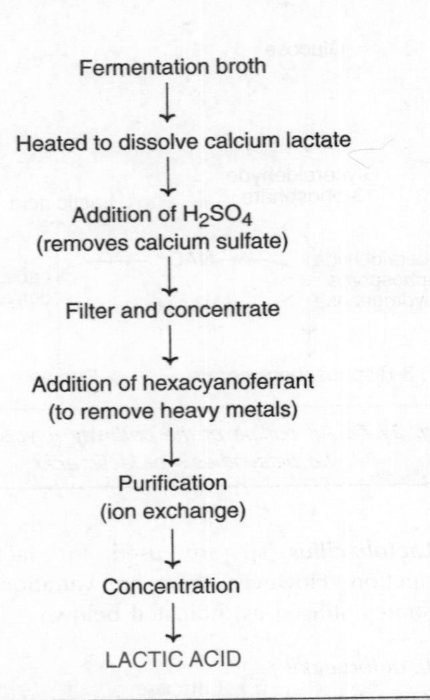

Fig. 24.8 : Flow chart for recovery of lactic acid from fermentation broth.

it is toxic to the organisms. This can achieved either by a continuous culture technique or by removal of lactic acid by electrodialysis. Theoretically, every molecule of glucose forms two molecules of lactic acid. About 90% of theoretical yield is possible in fermentation industry. L(+) Lactic acid is predominantly produced. The outline of the steps involved in the recovery lactic acid is depicted in ***Fig. 24.8.***

ACETIC ACID

The production of acetic acid, in the form of vinegar (used as a refreshing drink), from alcoholic liquids has been known for centuries.

Microorganisms used for production of acetic acid

The commercial production of acetic acid is carried out by a special group of ***acetic acid bacteria***, which are divided into two genera.

Gluconobacter that oxidizes ethanol exclusively to acetic acid.

Acetobacter that oxidizes ethanol first to acetic acid, and then to CO_2 and H_2O. These ***over-oxidizers*** are Gram-negative and acid tolerant e.g. *A. aceti, A. peroxidans, A. pasteurianus.*

Biosynthesis of acetic acid : Acetic acid is a product of incomplete oxidation of ethanol. Ethanol is first oxidized by alcohol dehydrogenase to acetaldehyde which then gets hydrated to form acetaldehyde hydrate. The latter is then acted upon by acetaldehyde dehydrogenase to form acetic acid (***Fig. 24.9***).

Production process for acetic acid

For every molecule of ethanol oxidised, one molecule of acetic acid is produced. Thus, high-yielding strains can produce 11–12% acetic acid from 12% alcohol. For optimal production, adequate supply of oxygen is very essential. Insufficient O_2, coupled with high concentration of alcohol and acetic acid result in the death of microorganisms.

Surface fermentation or submerged fermentation processes can be carried out to produce acetic acid. ***Trickling generation*** process, a type of surface fermentation, is very commonly used.

Recovery : The acetic acid produced is clarified by filtration and then subjected to decolourization by $K_4(FeCN)_6$.

Production of vinegar

Vinegar is an aqueous solution containing ***about 4%*** by volume ***acetic acid*** and small quantities of alcohol, salts, sugars and esters. It is widely used as a ***flavouring agent*** for processed liquid foods such as sauces and ketchups.

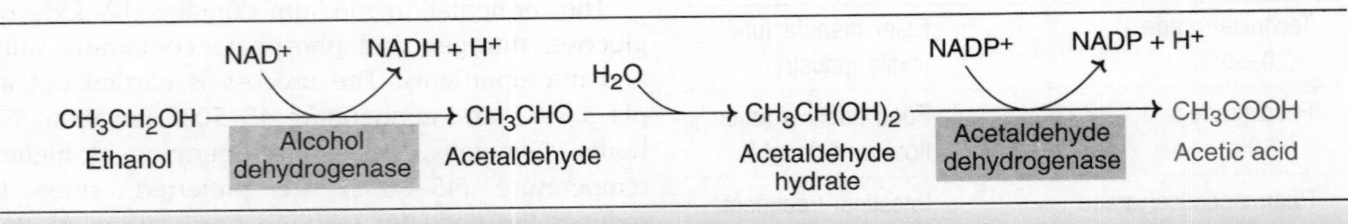

Fig. 24.9 : Biosynthesis of acetic acid from ethanol.

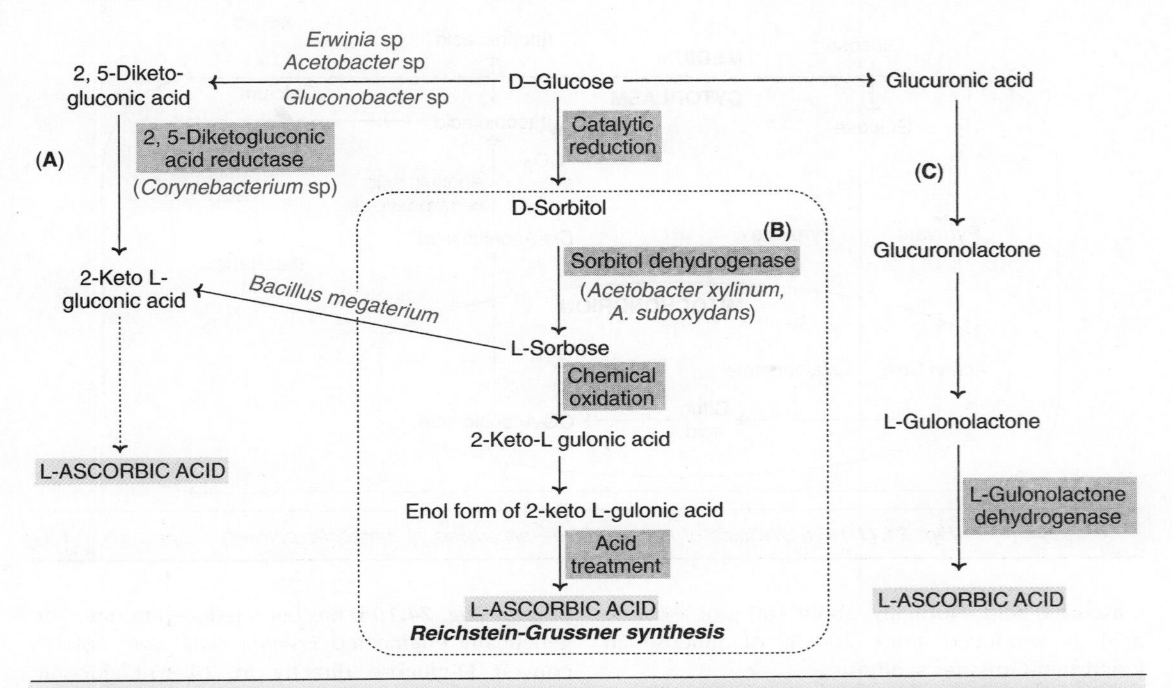

***Fig. 24.10 :** Pathways for the commercial production of ascorbic acid. **(A)** Two-step fermentation process **(B)** Reichstein-Grussner synthesis **(C)** Production via L-gulonolactone.*

The starting materials for vinegar production are wine, whey, malt (with low alcohol content). Vinegar production can be carried out either by ***surface process*** (trickling generator) or by ***submerged process***.

Surface process : The fermentation material is sprayed over the surface which trickles through the shavings that contain the acetic acid producing bacteria. The temperature is around 30°C on the upper part while it is around 35°C on the lower part. Vinegar is produced in about 3 days.

Submerged process : The fermentation bioreactors are made up of stainless steel. Aeration is done by a suction pump from the top. The production rate in the submerged process is about 10 times higher than the surface process.

L-ASCORBIC ACID

L-Ascorbic acid is the commonly used chemical name for the water soluble ***vitamin C***. This vitamin forms a redox system and participates in several biological processes. It is intimately involved in the biosynthesis of collagen, the most abundant protein in the human body. Vitamin C also protects the body against carcinogenic nitrosamines and free radicals. The deficiency of ascorbic acid causes ***scurvy***.

Applications of ascorbic acid

Because of the wide range of physiological and beneficial functions of ascorbic acid, its commercial production assumes significance. Vitamin C is mainly used in ***food and pharmaceutical industries***.

Industrial production of ascorbic acid

Ascorbic acid is commercially produced by a combination of several chemical steps, and one reaction of ***biotransformation*** brought out by microorganisms. This process is referred to as ***Reichstein-Grussner synthesis*** (***Fig. 24.10B***). D-Glucose is first converted to D-sorbitol. Oxidation of D-sorbitol to L-sorbose is carried out by *Acetobacter xylinum* or *A. suboxydans* (The enzyme being sorbitol dehydrogenase). A submerged bioreactor fermentation process is ideal for this reaction. It takes about 24 hours at temperature 30–35°C. Sorbose by a couple of chemical reactions can be finally converted to

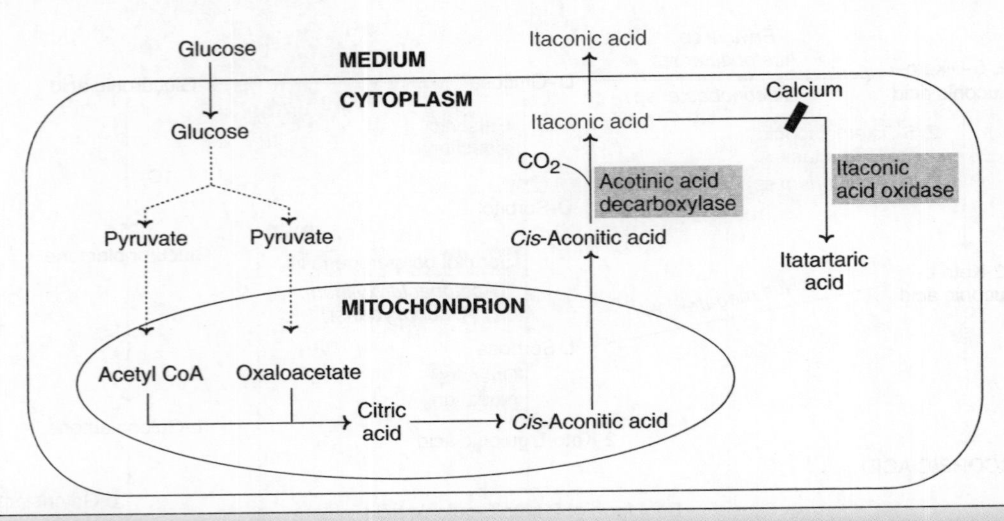

Fig. 24.11 : Biosynthesis of itaconic acid—an outline of metabolic pathway.

L-ascorbic acid. Normally, about 100 g of ascorbic acid is produced from 200 g of glucose in Reichstein-Grussner synthesis.

Two-step fermentation process : In this, D-glucose is converted to 2, 5-diketogluconic acid by *Erwinia, Acetobacter* or *Gluconobacter* sp. In the second step, *Corynebacterium* sp converts 2, 5-diketogluconic acid to 2-keto-L-gluconic acid, (***Fig. 24.10A***). It is also possible to involve ***Bacillus megaterium*** for converting L-sorbose to 2-keto-L-gluconic acid. The latter, by chemical reactions, can be converted to ascorbic acid.

Production via L-gulonolactone

Ascorbic acid can also be synthesized via-gulonolactone which can be directly converted to L-ascorbic acid by the enzyme L-gulonolactone dehydrogenase (***Fig. 24.10C***).

Direct production of ascorbic acid by fermentation

Several workers are trying to produce ascorbic acid directly from glucose. Microalgae of *Chlorella* have shown some promising results, although the yield is very low.

Genetic engineering for ascorbic acid production

Biotechnologists have been successful in ***cloning*** and expressing the gene for ***2, 5-diketogluconic acid reductase*** of *Corynebacterium* sp into *Erwinia herbicola*. By cloing this, the two step fermentation process (***Fig. 24.10A***) has been reduced to one. The genetically engineered *Erwinia* cells were able to convert D-glucose directly to 2-keto-L-gluconic acid. This is certainly advantageous since the metabolic capabilities of two different micro-organisms could be combined into one organism. However, the yield of ascorbic acid by the hybrid strain was very low. Scientists are now trying to alter certain amino acids in 2-5 diketogluconic acid reductase and increase the catalytic activity of this enzyme.

ITACONIC ACID

Itaconic acid is used in plastic industry, paper industry and in the manufacture of adhesives.

Itaconic acid can be commercially produced by *Aspergillus itoconicus* and *A. terreus*. The biosynthesis of itaconic acid occurs by way of Krebs cycle. The metabolite *cis*-aconitic acid (formed from citric acid) undergoes decarboxylation catalysed by the enzyme *cis*-aconitic decarboxylase (***Fig. 24.11***). Itaconic acid is oxidised to itatartaric acid by itaconic acid oxidase. This enzyme has to be inhibited for a maximum yield of itaconic acid. This can be achieved by adding calcium.

Batch submerged fermentation process is commonly used for itaconic acid production. The yield is around 75% of the theoretical calculation when the medium contains 15% sucrose.

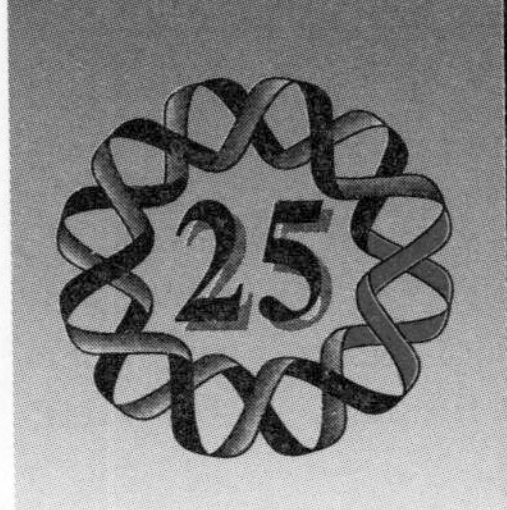

Microbial Production of Antibiotics

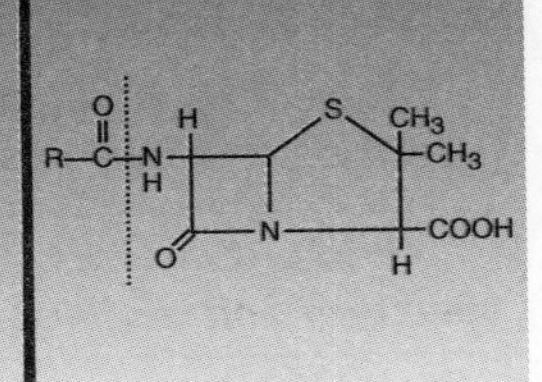

Antibiotics are the ***chemical substances that can kill microorganisms or inhibit their growth***, and are therefore used to fight infections in humans or animals. Most of the antibiotics are produced by microorganisms (i.e. product of one organism that can kill other organism). Certain semi-synthetic antibiotics are the chemically modified natural antibiotics.

Antibiotics have undoubtedly changed the world we live in, and have certainly contributed to the increase in the human life-span. This is mainly due to the fact that several life-threatening infectious diseases could be conveniently cured by administration of antibiotics.

ANTIBIOTICS — GENERAL

A brief history of antibiotics along with the microorganisms producing them, and their applications are given hereunder.

History of antibiotic discovery

It was in 1928, Alexander Fleming made an accidental discovery that the fungus *Penicillium notatum* produced a compound (penicillin) that selectively killed a wide range of bacteria without adversely affecting the host cells. There are records that in some parts of Europe (in 1908) extracts of moldy bread were applied to wounds or abrasions to prevent infections, although the biochemical basis was not known. The ***penicillin discovery of Fleming has revolutionised antibiotic research.***

Wide range of antibiotics

Antibiotics are the most important class of pharmaceuticals produced by microbial biotechnological processes. They are the ***products of secondary metabolism***.

Around 10,000 different antibiotics are known, and 200–300 new ones are being added each year. Most of these antibiotics are not of commercial importance due to various reasons—toxicity, ineffectiveness or high cost of production. There are around 50 antibiotics which are most widely used.

In ***Table 25.1***, a selected list of important antibiotics, their properties and the producing organisms is given.

Broad spectrum antibiotics : They can control the growth of several unrelated organisms e.g. tetracyclines, chloramphenicol.

Narrow spectrum antibiotics : They are effective against selected species of bacteria e.g. penicillin, streptomycin.

Microorganisms producing antibiotics

A great majority of antibiotics are produced by ***actinomycetes*** particularly of the genus ***Streptomyces*** e.g. tetracyclines, actinomycin D.

Table 25.1 A selected list of important antibiotics along with producing organisms

Antibiotic activity spectrum and antibiotic	*Producing microorganism*
Antibacterial	
Penicillin G	*Penicillium* sp
Cephalosporin	*Acremonium* sp
Streptomycin	*Streptomyces* sp
Tetracycline	*Streptomyces* sp
Chloramphenicol	*Cephalosporium* sp
Bacitracin	*Bacillus* sp
Antitumor	
Actinomycin D	*Streptomyces* sp
Mitomycin C	*Streptomyces* sp
Bleomycin	*Streptomyces* sp
Adriamycin	*Streptomyces* sp
Daunomycin	*Streptomyces* sp
Antifungal	
Griseofulvin	*Penicillium* sp
Food preservative	
Natamycin	*Streptomyces* sp
Nisin	*Streptomyces* sp
Antiprotozoal	
Daunorubicin	*Steptomyces* sp
Antituberculosis	
Refamycin	*Nocardia* sp
Antiamoebic	
Tetracycline	*Streptomyces* sp
Fumagillin	*Aspergillus* sp

The bacteria other than actinomyces also produce certain antibiotics e.g. bacitracin.

Among the ***fungi***, the two groups ***Aspergillaceae*** and ***Moniliales*** are important for antibiotic production e.g. penicillin, cephalosporin, griseofulvin.

APPLICATIONS OF ANTIBIOTICS

Antibiotics are particularly important ***as antimicrobial agents for chemotherapy***. A large number of bacterial diseases have been brought under control by use of antibiotics. These include pneumonia, cholera, tuberculosis and leprosy. The antifungal antibiotic griseofulvin has controlled the debilitating fungal skin diseases such as ring worm.

Besides serving as antimicrobial agents, there are several other applications of antibiotics.

Antitumor antibiotics : There are a selected few antibiotics that are in use for control of cancer growth, although with a limited success e.g. actinomycin D, mitomycin C.

Food preservative antibiotics : Certain antibiotics are used in canning industry (e.g. chlortetracycline), and for preservation of fish, meat and poultry (e.g. pimaricin, nisin). The use of antibiotics in food preservation is usually under the control of the Governments.

Antibiotics used in animal feed and veterinary medicine : Till some time ago, antibiotics (penicillins, tetracyclines, erythromycins) were very widely used in processing of animal feeds. Such an indiscriminate use resulted in the development of antibiotic resistance in animals and humans. A new class of antibiotics have been developed for specific use in animal feed e.g. enduracidin, tylosin. Likewise, specific antibiotics have been developed for exclusive use in veterinary medicine e.g. hygromycin B, theostrepton, salinomycin.

Antibiotics for control of plant diseases : In recent years, several antibiotics have been developed for exclusive use to control plant diseases e.g. blasticidin, tetranactin, polyoxin.

Antibiotics as tools in molecular biology : Some of the antibiotics can selectively inhibit certain biological reactions at the molecular level. These antibiotics do in fact serve as tools for exploring the knowledge of life sciences. Thus, certain antibiotics have been used to obtain some important information on DNA replication, transcription and translation.

PRODUCTION OF ANTIBIOTICS — A MAJOR PHARMACEUTICAL INDUSTRY

The commercial production of antibiotics is a highly profitable industry worldover. Annual sales of antibiotics will run into several billions of dollars with an annual growth potential of about 10%.

Antibiotics may be ***produced by microbial fermentation***, or ***chemical synthesis***, or a ***combination of both***. For certain antibiotics, the basic molecule is produced by fermentation and its therapeutic value can be increased by chemical modifications. The cost involved in production and chemical modifications, besides the efficacy of the antibiotic is very important in its manufacture.

Biotechnologists continue their efforts to increase the fermentation yield and recovery processes to produce pure antibiotics.

The industrial production of selected antibiotics is briefly described in the following pages.

PENICILLINS

Penicillins are a group of β-lactam containing bactericidal antibiotics. Being the first among the antibiotics to be discovered, penicillins are historically important. The structures of important synthetic and semi-synthetic penicillins are depicted in ***Fig. 25.1***. The basic structure of all the penicillins consists of a lactam ring and a thizolidine ring fused together to form 6-aminopenicillanic acid.

Action of penicillins

Natural penicillins (penicillins V and G) are ***effective against several Gram-positive bacteria***. They inhibit the bacterial cell wall (i.e. peptoglycan) synthesis and cause cell death. Some persons (approximately 0.5-2% of population) are allergic to penicillin.

Natural penicillins are ***ineffective against microorganisms that produce β-lactamase***, since this enzyme can hydrolyse penicillins e.g. *Staphylococcus aureus.* Several semi-synthetic penicillins that are resistant to β-lactamase have been developed and successfully used against a large number of Gram-negative bacteria. Cloxacillin, ampicillin, floxacillin and azlocillin are some examples of semi-synthetic penicillins. These are quite comparable in action to cephalosporins.

From the huge quantities of penicillins produced by fermentation, about 40% are used for human healthcare, 15% for animal healthcare and 45% for the preparation of semi-synthetic penlcillins.

Organisms for penicillin production

In the early days, ***Penicillium notatum*** was used for the large-scale production of penicillins.

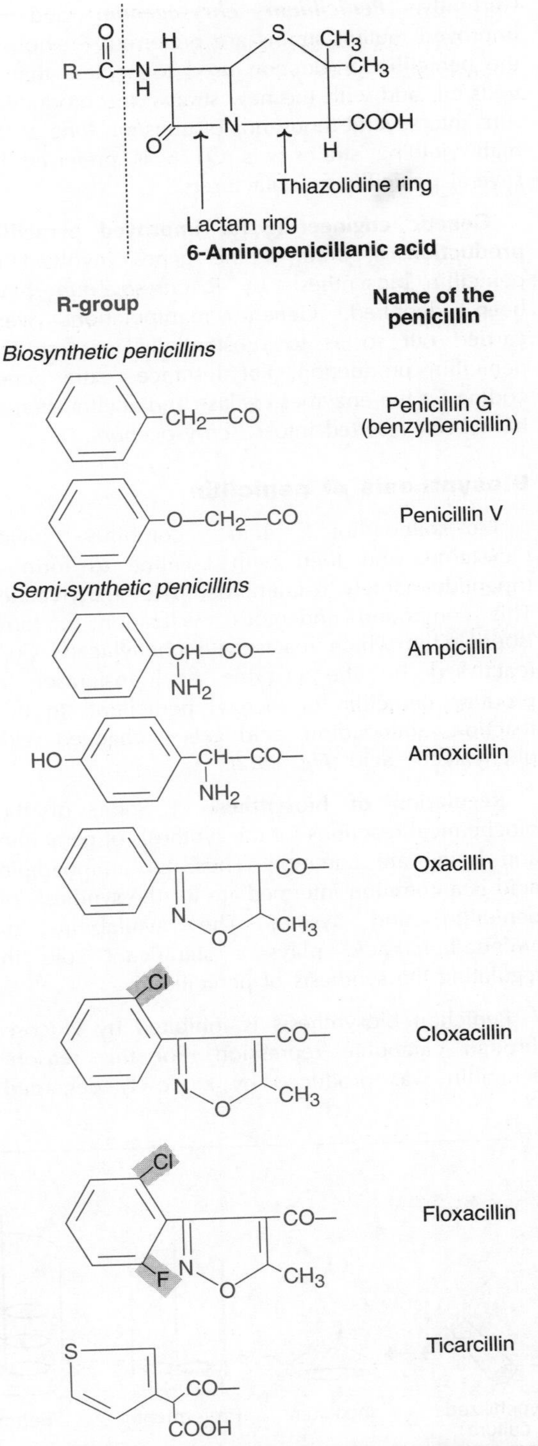

Thiazolidine ring
Lactam ring
6-Aminopenicillanic acid

R-group	**Name of the penicillin**
Biosynthetic penicillins	
$-CH_2-CO$	Penicillin G (benzylpenicillin)
$-O-CH_2-CO$	Penicillin V
Semi-synthetic penicillins	
$-CH(NH_2)-CO-$	Ampicillin
$HO-$ ... $-CH(NH_2)-CO-$	Amoxicillin
$-CO-$, CH_3	Oxacillin
Cl, $-CO-$, CH_3	Cloxacillin
Cl, F, $-CO-$, CH_3	Floxacillin
S, $-CO-$, COOH	Ticarcillin

Fig. 25.1 : *Structures of important penicillins.*

Currently, ***Penicillium chrysogenum*** and its improved mutant strains are preferred. Previously, the penicillin production used to be less than 2 units/ml, and with the new strains, the production runs into several thousands of units/ml. One of the high yielding strains wis Q176 is preferred by several penicillin manufacturers.

Genetic engineering for improved penicillin production : Some of the genes involved in penicillin biosynthesis by *P. chrysogenum* have been identified. Genetic manipulations were carried out so as to substantially increase the penicillin production. For instance, extra genes coding for the enzymes cyclase and acyltransferase have been inserted into *C. chrysogenum*.

Biosynthesis of penicillin

L-α-Aminoadipic acid combines with L-cysteine, and then with L-valine to form a tripeptide namely α-L-aminoadipylcysteinylvaline. This compound undergoes cyclization to form isopenicillin which reacts with phenylacetyl CoA (catalysed by the enzyme acyltransferase) to produce penicillin G (benzyl penicillin). In this reaction, aminoadipic acid gets exchanged with phenylacetic acid (***Fig. 25.2***).

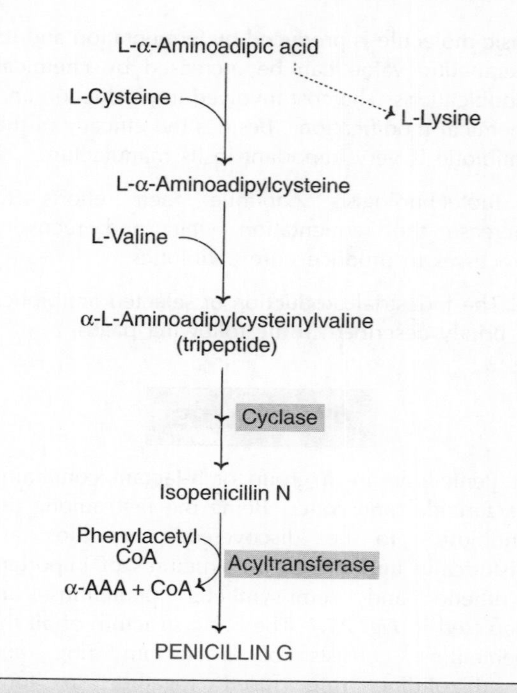

Fig. 25.2 : *Biosynthesis of penicillin by* Penicillium chrysogenum *(α-AAA — α-Amino adipic acid; CoA–Coenzyme A.*

Regulation of biosynthesis : Some of the biochemical reactions for the synthesis of penicillin and lysine are common. Thus, L-α-aminoadipic acid is a common intermediate for the synthesis of penicillin and lysine. The availability of aminoadipic acid plays a significant role in regulating the synthesis of penicillin.

Penicillin biosynthesis is inhibited by glucose through catabolite repression. For this reason, penicillin was produced by a slowly degraded sugar like lactose. The concentrations of phosphate and ammonia also influence penicillin synthesis.

PRODUCTION PROCESS OF PENICILLIN

An outline of the flow chart for the industrial production of penicillin is depicted in ***Fig. 25.3.*** The lyophilized culture of spores is cultivated for inoculum development which is transferred to prefermenter, and then to fermenter.

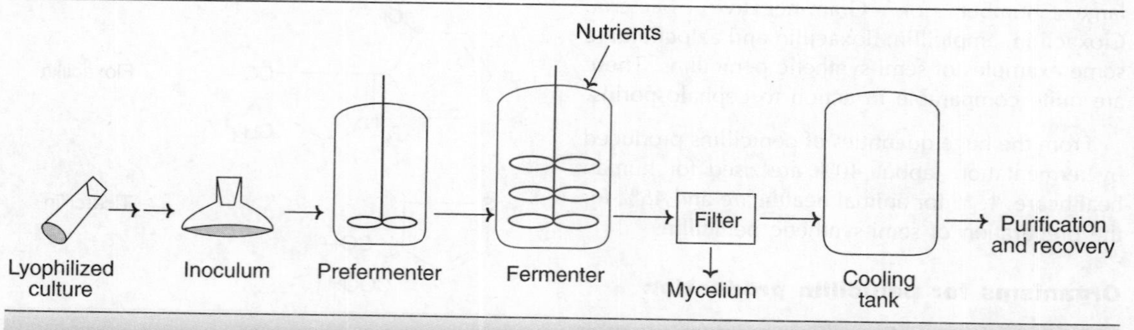

Fig. 25.3 : *An outline of the flow chart for penicillin fermentation.*

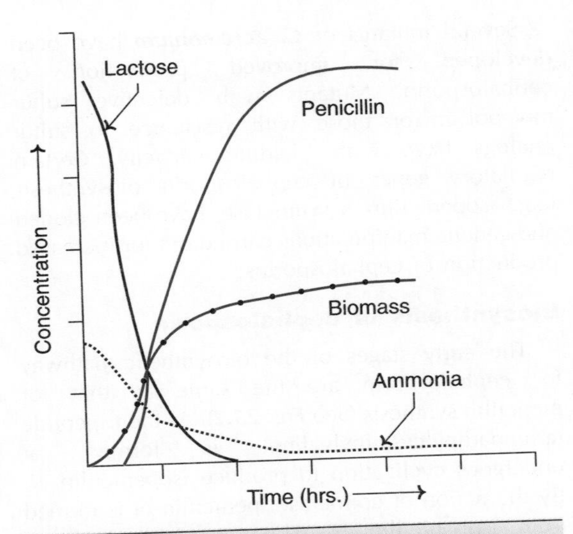

Fig. 25.4 : Penicillin production in relation to substrates utilization and biomass formation.

Penicillin production is an ***aerobic process*** and therefore, a continuous supply of O_2 to the growing culture is very essential. The required aeration rate is 0.5-1.0 vvm. The pH is maintained around 6.5, and the optimal temperature is in the range of 25–27°C. Pencillin production is usually carried out by ***submerged processes.***

The medium used for fermentation consists of corn steep liquor (4-5% dry weight) and carbon source (usually lactose). An addition of yeast extract, soy meal or whey is done for a good supply of nitrogen. Sometimes, ammonium sulfate is added for the supply of nitrogen. Phenylacetic acid (or phenoxyacetic acid) which serves as a precursor for penicillin biosynthesis is continuously fed. Further, continuous feeding of sugar is advantageous for a good yield of penicillin. The penicillin production profiles are depicted in ***Figs. 25.4*** and ***Fig. 25.5.***

It is estimated that approximately 10% of the metabolised carbon contributes to penicillin production, while 65% is utilised towards energy supply and 25% for growth of the organisms. The efficiency of penicillin production can be optimized by adequate supply of carbon source. Thus, by adding glucose and acetic acid, the yield can be increased by about 25%.

For efficient synthesis of penicillin, the growth of the organism from spores must be in a loose form and not as pellets. The growth phase is around 40 hours with a doubling time of 6-8 hours. After the growth phase is stabilized, the penicillin production exponentially increases with appropriate culture conditions. The penicillin production phase can be extended to 150–180 hours.

Recovery of penicillin

As the fermentation is complete, the broth containing about 1% penicillin is processed for extraction. The mycelium is removed by filtration. Penicillin is recovered by solvent (n-butylacetate or methylketone) extraction at low temperature (<10°C) and acidic pH (<3.0). By this way, the chemical and enzymatic (bacterial penicillinase) degradations of penicillin can be minimized.

The penicillin containing solvent is treated with activated carbon to remove impurities and pigments. Penicillin can be recovered by adding potassium or sodium acetate. The potassium or sodium salts of penicillin can be further processed (in dry solvents such as n-butanol or isopropanol) to remove impurities. The yield of penicillin is around 90%.

As the water is totally removed, penicillin salts can be crystallized and dried under required pressure. This can be then processed to finally produce the pharmaceutical dosage forms.

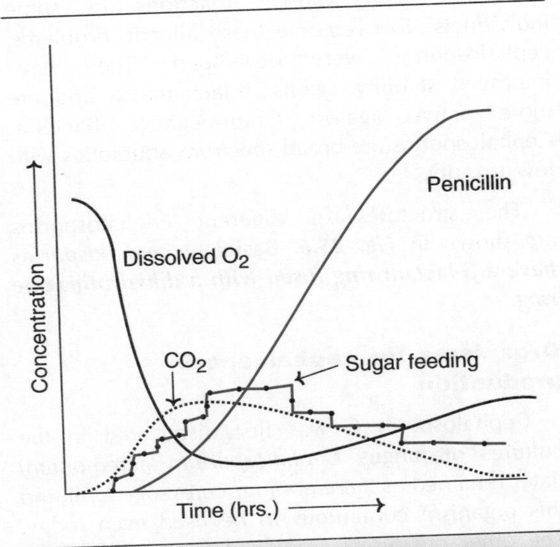

Fig. 25.5 : Penicillin production in relation to continuous feeding of sugar, O_2 utilization, and CO_2 formation.

Penicillins G and H are the fermented products obtained from the fungus *Penicillium chrysogenum.*

PRODUCTION OF 6-AMINO PENICILLANIC ACID

The penicillins G and H are mostly used as the starting materials for the production of several ***synthetic penicillins containing the basic nucleus namely 6-amino penicillanic acid*** (***6-APA***). About 10 years ago, only chemical methods were available for hydrolysis of penicillins to produce 6-APA. Now a days, enzymatic methods are preferred.

Immobilized penicillin amidases enzymes have been developed for specific hydrolysis of penicillin G and penicillin V. Penicillin salt of either G or V can be used for hydrolysis by immobilized enzyme system. The pH during hydrolysis is kept around 7-8, and the product 6-APA can be recovered by bringing down the pH to 4. At pH 4, 6-amino penicillanic acid gets precipitated almost completely in the presence of a water immiscible solvent.

In general, the enzymatic hydrolysis is more efficient for penicillin V than for penicillin G. However, penicillin G is a more versatile compound, as it is required for ring expansions.

CEPHALOSPORINS

The pharmaceutical uses of penicillins are associated with allergic reactions in some individuals. To overcome these allergic problems, cephalosporins were developed. They have improved stability against β-lactamases, and are more active against Gram-negative bacteria. Cephalosporins are broad spectrum antibiotics with low toxicity.

The structures of different cephalosporins are shown in ***Fig. 25.6***. Basically ***cephalosporins have a β-lactam ring fused with a dihydrothiazine ring***.

Organisms for cephalosporin production

Cephalosporin C was first discovered in the cultures of fungus *Cephalosporium acremonium* (later renamed as *Acremonium chreysogenum*) and this organism continuous to be used even today. The other organisms employed for cephalosporin production are *Emericellopsis* sp, *Paecilomyces* sp and *Streptomyces* sp.

Several mutants of ***C. acremonium*** have been developed for improved production of cephalosporin. Mutants with defective sulfur metabolism or those with resistance to sulfur analogs have high yielding capacity. Certain regulatory genes of cephalosporin biosynthesis (e.g., isopenicillin N synthetase) have been cloned and genetic manipulations carried out for increased production of cephalosporins.

Biosynthesis of cephalosporin

The early stages of the biosynthetic pathway for cephalosporin are the same as that for penicillin synthesis (See ***Fig. 25.2***). As the tripeptide (aminoadipylcysteinylvaline) is formed, it undergoes cyclization to produce isopenicillin N. By the action of epimerase, penicillin N is formed from isopenicillin N. Then, penicillin N gets converted to cephalosporin C by a three stage reaction catalysed by three distinct enzymes namely expandase, hydroxylase and acetyl transferase (***Fig. 25.7***).

Regulation of biosynthesis : A low concentration of lysine promotes cephalosporin synthesis. The inhibitory effect of lysine at a higher concentration can be overcome by adding L-aminoadipic acid. The carbon sources that get rapidly degraded (e.g. glucose, glycerol) reduce cephalosporin production. Methionine promotes cephalosporin synthesis in *C. acremonium*, but has no influence on *Streptomycetes*.

PRODUCTION PROCESS OF CEPHALOSPORIN

The fermentation process concerned with the production of cephalosporin is similar to that of penicillin. The culture media consists of corn steep liquor and soy flour-based media in a continuous feeding system. The other ingradients of the medium include sucrose, glucose and ammonium salts. Methionine is added as a source of sulfur.

The fermentation is carried out at temperature 25–28°C and pH 6-7. The growth of micro-organisms substantially increases with good O_2 supply, although during production phase, O_2 consumption declines.

Cephalosporin C from the culture broth can be recovered by ion-exchange resins, and by using column chromatography. Cephalosporin C can be precipitated as zinc, sodium or potassium salt, and isolated.

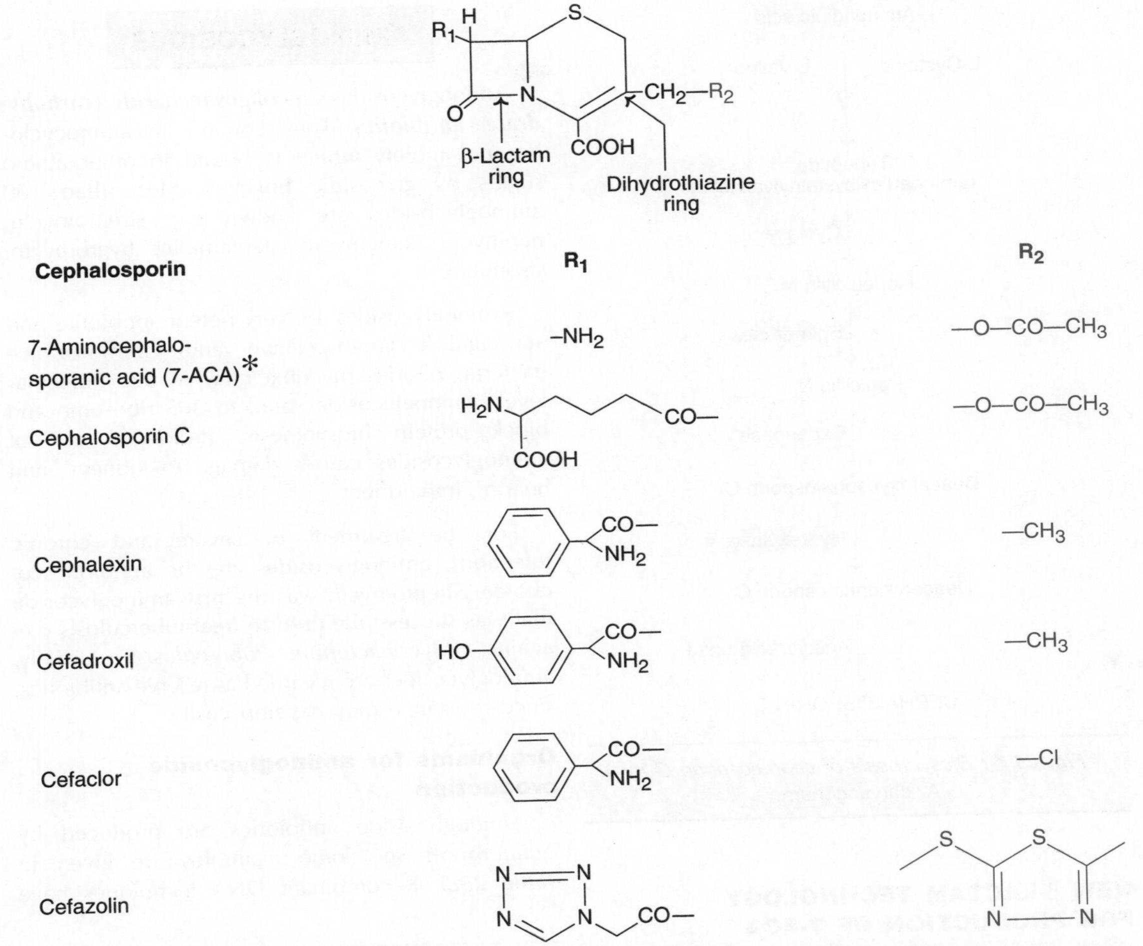

Cephalosporin	R_1	R_2
7-Aminocephalosporanic acid (7-ACA)*	$-NH_2$	$-O-CO-CH_3$
Cephalosporin C	$H_2N-CH(COOH)-CH_2-CH_2-CH_2-CO-$	$-O-CO-CH_3$
Cephalexin	$C_6H_5-CH(NH_2)-CO-$	$-CH_3$
Cefadroxil	$HO-C_6H_4-CH(NH_2)-CO-$	$-CH_3$
Cefaclor	$C_6H_5-CH(NH_2)-CO-$	$-Cl$
Cefazolin	tetrazolyl$-CH_2-CO-$	methylthiadiazolylthio

Structure labels: R_1, H, S, N, O, CH_2-R_2, COOH, β-Lactam ring, Dihydrothiazine ring

Fig. 25.6 : A selected list of cephalosporins (–Active nucleus of cephalosporins).*

Chemical synthesis of cephalosporin

In recent years, by using penicillin V as the starting material, chemical synthesis of cephalosporin has become possible. This is being done due to low cost of production of penicillin.

PRODUCTION OF 7-AMINOCEPHALOSPORANIC ACID

7-Aminocephalosporonic acid (7-ACA) is the nucleus structure present in all the cephalosporins. Cephalosporin C, produced by fermentation, can be subjected to chemical hydrolysis to form 7-ACA. This is tedious, and is associated with several drawbacks.

Recently, enzymatic hydrolysis of cephalosporin C to 7-ACA has been developed. This is mainly carried out by two enzymes-*D-**amino acid oxidase*** (isolated from *Trigonopsis variabilis*) and ***glutaryl amidase*** (source-*Pseudomonas* sp). Biotechnologists have been successful in immobilizing these two enzymes for efficient and large scale manufacture of 7-ACA.

Cephalosporin C
↓ D–Amino acid oxidase
↓ Glutaryl amidase
7–Aminocephalosporanic acid

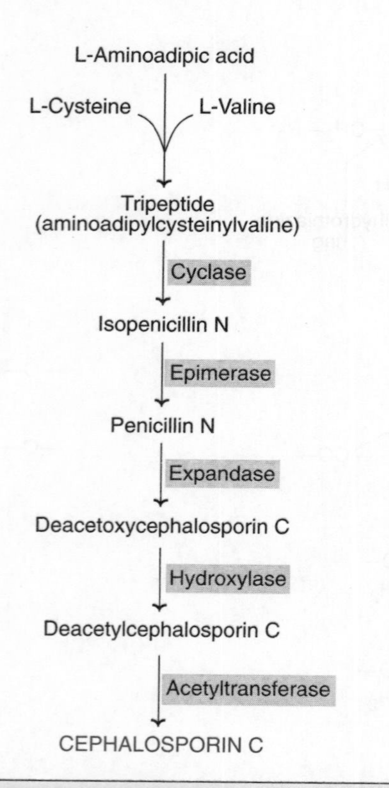

***Fig. 25.7 :** Biosynthesis of cephalosporin C by* A. chrysogenum.

NEW β-LACTAM TECHNOLOGY FOR PRODUCTION OF 7-ACA

Scientists have been successful in producing 7-aminocephalosporanic acid by *P. chrysogenum* fermentation. This is possible through genetic manipulations. As already described in cephalosporin biosynthesis (***Fig. 25.7***), penicillin N is the substrate for the enzyme expandase. Adipyl-6-aminopenicillanic acid (produced by *P. chrysogenum* on adding adipic acid) which resembles in structure with penicillin N, can also serve as a substrate for expandase. By inserting expandase and hydroxylase gene (*cefEF*), and acetyl transferase gene (*cefG*) from *S. clavuligerus* into *P. chrysogenum*, the production of adipyl-7-ACA has become possible (***Fig. 25.8***). Further, the genes responsible for the enzymes D-amino acid oxidase (from *Pseudomonas diminuta*) have also been inserted into *P. chrysogenum*. Both these enzymes act on adipyl-7-ACA to produce 7-amino-cephalosporanic acid.

AMINOGLYCOSIDES

Aminoglycosides are ***oligosaccharide*** (***carbohydrate***) ***antibiotics***. They contain an aminocyclo-hexanol moiety which is bound to other amino sugars by glycosidic linkages. More than 100 aminoglycosides are known e.g. streptomycin, neomycin, kanamycin, gentamicin, hygromycin, sisomicin.

Aminoglycosides are very potent antibiotics and act against Gram-positive and Gram-negative bacteria, besides mycobacteria. At the molecular level, aminoglycosides bind to 30S ribosome and block protein biosynthesis. Prolonged use of aminoglycosides causes damage to kidneys, and hearing impairment.

For the treatment of severe and chronic infections, aminoglycosides are the antibiotics of choice. Streptomycin was the first aminoglycoside that was successfully used to treat tuberculosis (i.e. against *Mycobacterium tuberculosis*). Usually, aminoglycosides are regarded as reserve antibiotics, since resistance may develop easily.

Organisms for aminoglycoside production

Aminoglycoside antibiotics are produced by *Actinomyces* sp. Some examples are given in ***Table 25.2***. Recombinant DNA techniques have

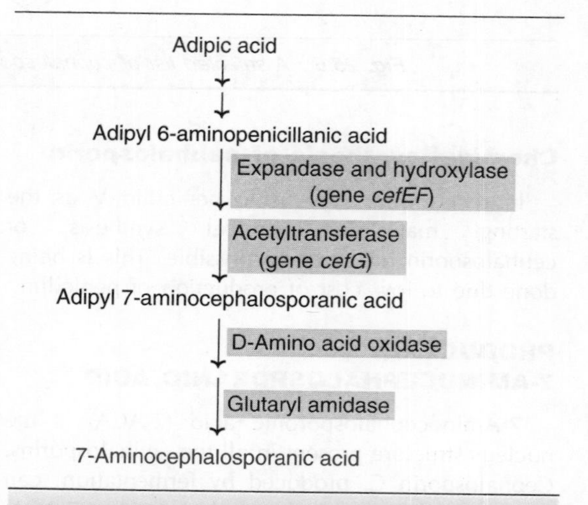

***Fig. 25.8 :** Biosynthesis of 7-aminocephalosporanic acid by* P. chrysogenum *transformants (after suitable gene insertions).*

TABLE 25.2 Selected examples of aminoglycosides with the organisms responsible for their production

Aminoglycoside	*Organism*
Streptomycin	*Streptomyces griseus*
Neomycin B and C	*S. fradiae*
Kanamycin A, B and C	*S. kanamyceticus*
Hygromycin B	*S. hygroscopicus*
Gentamicin	*Micromonospora purpurea*
Sisomicin	*M. inyoensis*

been used to produce hybrid aminoglycosides, and for increasing the fermentation yield.

Biosynthesis of aminoglycosides

All the ring structures in the molecules of aminoglycosides are ultimately derived from glucose. Most of the biosynthetic pathways concerned with the formation of at least some aminoglycosides have been elucidated.

Biosynthesis of streptomycin

The outline of the pathway for the synthesis of streptomycin is depicted in ***Fig. 25.9***. More than 30 enzymatic steps have been identified. ***Glucose 6-phosphate*** obtained from glucose takes three independent routes to respectively produce streptidine 6-phosphate, L-dehydrostreptose and N-methylglucosamine. The former two compounds condense to form an intermediate which later combines with methylglucosamine to produce dihydrostreptomycin-6-phosphate. This compound, in the next of couple of reactions, gets converted to streptomycin.

Regulation of biosynthesis : Very little is known about the regulation of streptomycin synthesis. A compound named as ***factor A*** (chemically isocapryloyl-hydroxymethyl-γ-butyrate) has been isolated from streptomycin-producing strains of *S. griseus*. Factor A promotes streptomycin production. In fact, factor A^- mutants that cannot synthesize streptomycin have been isolated. They can synthesize streptomycin on adding factor A. The nutrient sources-carbohydrates (glucose), ammonia and phosphate also regulate (by feedback mechanism) streptomycin production.

PRODUCTION PROCESS OF STREPTOMYCIN

The medium used for streptomycin usually consists of soy meal or soy flour or corn syrup that can supply glucose at a slow rate (amylase activity is poor in *Streptomyces* sp). The initial supply of nitrogen (NH_3) and phosphate is also obtained from soy meal. This is required since glucose, ammonia and phosphate in high quantities inhibit streptomycin synthesis.

The fermentation conditions for optimal production of streptomycin are — temperature 27–30°C, pH 6.5-7.5, aeration rate 0.5-1.0 vvm. The duration of fermentation process depends on the strain used, and is between 6 to 8 days.

Recovery of streptomycin

Streptomycin or other aminoglycosides are basic in nature. They can be recovered

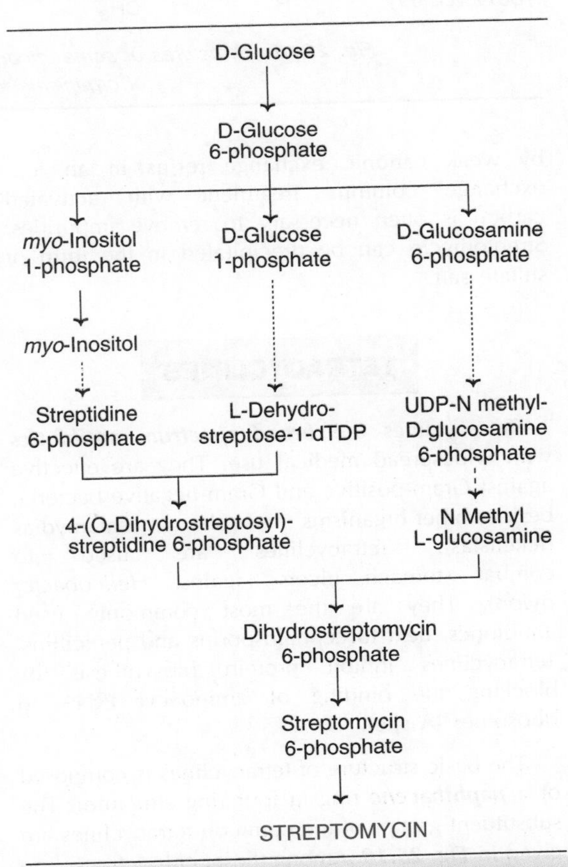

***Fig. 25.9** : An outline of streptomycin biosynthesis.*

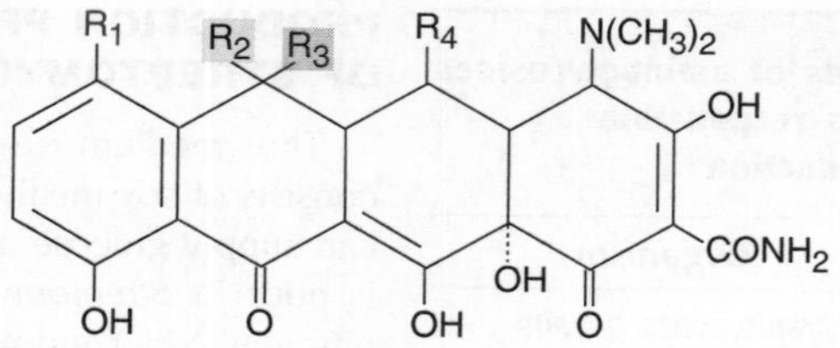

Tetracycline	R_1	R_2	R_3	R_4	Examples of producing organisms
Tetracycline	H	CH_3	OH	H	*Streptomyces aureus, S. flavus, S. antibioticus*
Chlortetracycline	Cl	CH_3	OH	H	*S. aureofaciciens, S. viridifaciens, S. flavus*
Oxytetracycline	H	CH_3	OH	OH	*S. antibioticus, S. cellulosae S. parvus, S. rimosus*
Minocycline	$N(CH_3)_2$	H	H	H	Semisynthetic
Doxycycline	H	CH_3	H	OH	Semisynthetic

Fig. 25.10 : Structures of some important tetracyclines along with the examples of organisms for their production.

by weak cationic exchange resins in an ion-exchange column. Treatment with activated carbon is often necessary to remove impurities. Streptomycin can be precipitated in the form of sulfate salt.

TETRACYCLINES

Tetracyclines are ***broad spectrum antibiotics*** with widespread medical use. They are effective against Gram-positive and Gram-negative bacteria, besides other organisms (mycoplasmas, chlamydias rickettsias). Tetracyclines are used to combat stomach ulcers (against *Helicobacter pylori*). They are the most commonly used antibiotics, next to cephalosporins and penicillins. Tetracyclines inhibit protein biosynthesis by blocking the binding of aminoacyl tRNA to ribosomes (A site).

The basic structure of tetracyclines is composed of a ***naphthacene*** ring (a four ring structure). The substituent groups of the common tetracyclines are given in ***Fig. 25.10***. Among these, chlortetracycline and oxytetracycline are most commonly used in the treatment of human and veterinary deseases, besides in the preservation of fish, meat and poultry (in some countries).

Organisms for tetracycline production

The first tetracycline antibiotic that was isolated was chlortetracycline from the cultures of *Streptomyces aureofaciens* (in 1945). There are at least 20 streptomycetes identified now that usually produce a mixture of tetracyclines. In the ***Fig. 25.10***, a selected list of these organisms for producing tetracyclines is also given.

High-yielding strains of *S. aureofaciens* and *S. rimosus* have been developed by using ultraviolet radiation and/or other mutagens (nitrosoguanidine). Such strains are very efficient for the production of chlortetracycline. Further, genetically engineered strains of *S. rimosus* have been developed for increased synthesis of oxytetracycline.

Biosynthesis of tetracyclines

The pathway for the biosynthesis of tetracyclines is very complex. An outline of the synthesis of chlortetracycline by *S. aureofaciens* is given in

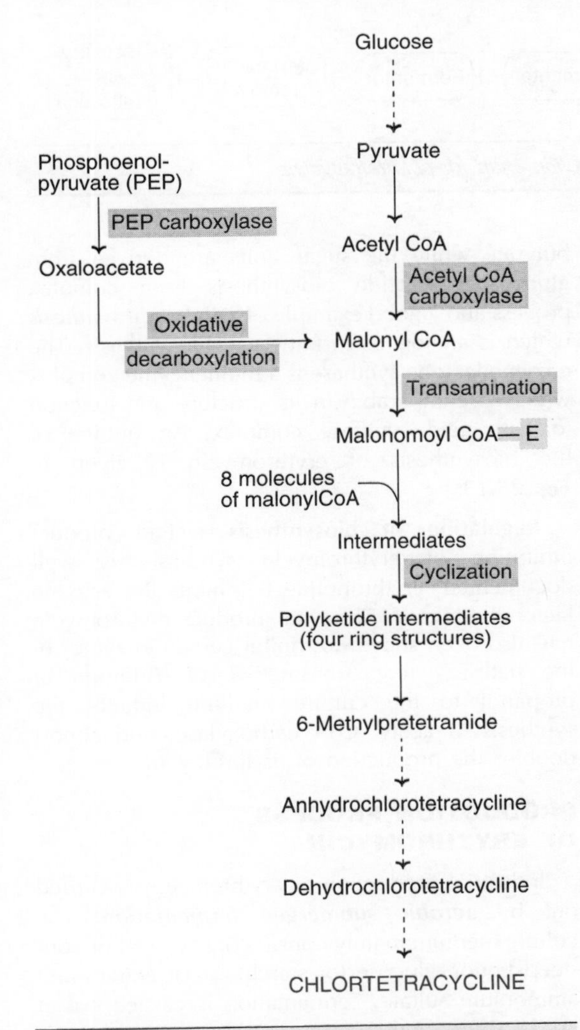

Fig. 25.11 : An outline of the biosynthesis of chlortetracycline by S. aureofaciens (E *—Anthracene synthase enzyme complex)*

Fig. 25.11. There are at least 72 intermediates formed during the course of chlortetracycline biosynthesis, some of them have not been fully characterized.

Polyketide antibiotic synthesis : The term polyketide refers to a group of ***antibiotics*** that are ***synthesized*** by ***successive condensation of small carboxylic acids*** such as acetate, butyrate, propionate and malonate. The synthesis of polyketide antibiotics is comparable to that of long chain fatty acids. That is the carbon chain grows by cyclic condensation process. The synthesis of tetracyclines is a good example of polyketide antibiotic synthesis.

As glucose gets oxidised, it forms acetyl CoA and then malonyl CoA. On transamination, the later gives malonomoyl CoA. The enzyme anthracene synthase complex binds to malonomoyl CoA and brings out the condensation of 8 molecules of malonyl CoA to form a polyketide intermediates (four ring structures). These intermediates undergo a series of reactions to finally produce chlortetracycline.

Regulation of biosynthesis : Carbohydrate metabolism (particularly glycolysis) controls chlortetracycline synthesis. For more efficient synthesis of the antibiotic, glycolysis has to be substantially low. The addition of phosphate reduces chlortetracycline production.

PRODUCTION PROCESS OF CHLORTETRACYCLINE

The fermentation medium consists of corn steep liquor, soy flour or peanut meal for the supply of nitrogen and carbon sources. Continuous feeding of carbohydrate is desirable for good growth of the organism and production of the antibiotic. This can be done either by addition of crude carbon sources (as given above) or by supplying glucose or starch. For more efficient production of chlortetracycline, the supply of ammonium and phosphate has to be maintained at a low concentration.

An outline of the production process for chlortetracycline is depicted in ***Fig. 25.12***. The ideal fermentation conditions are — temperature 27–30°C, pH-6.5-7.5, aeration 0.8-1.0 vvm. The duration of fermentation is around 4 days.

Recovery of chlortetracycline

At the end of the fermentation, the culture broth is filtered to remove the mycelium. The filtrate is treated with n-butanol or methylisobutylketone in acidic or alkaline condition for extracting the antibiotic. It is then absorbed to activated charcoal to remove other impurities. Chlortetraycline is eluted and crystallized.

PRODUCTION OF TETRACYCLINE —DIFFERENT PROCESSES

The production of tetracycline can be achieved by one or more of the following ways.

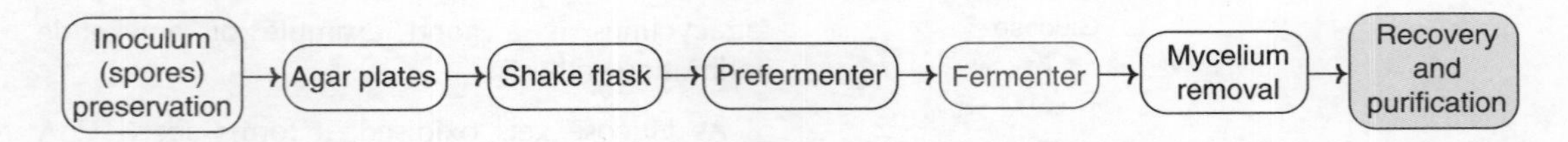

Fig. 25.12 : An outline of production chart for chlortetracycline.

- By chemical treatment of chlortetracycline.
- By carrying out fermentation in a chloride-free culture medium.
- By employing mutants in which chlorination reaction does not occur.
- By blocking chlorination reaction by the addition of inhibitors e.g. thiourea, 2-thiouracil.

MACROLIDES

Macrolides are a group of ***antibiotics with large lactone rings*** (i.e. macrocylic lactone rings). They consist of 12-, 14-, or 16-membered lactone rings with 1-3 sugars linked by glycosidic bonds. The sugars may be 6-deoxyhexoses or aminosugars. ***Erythromycin*** and ***oleandomycin*** are 14-membered (lactone ring containing) macrolides while leucomycin and tylosin are examples for 16-membered microlides.

Erythromycin and its derivative clarithromycin are the most commonly prescribed microlides. They are effective against Gram-positive bacteria, and are frequently used to kill penicillin-resistant organisms. Clarithromycin is currently used to combat stomach ulcers caused by *H. pylori*. The macrolides inhibit the protein biosynthesis by binding to 50S ribosome.

Polyene macrolides is the term applied for very large ring macrolides that many contain lactone rings in the range of 26–28. e.g. nystatin, amphotericin. These polyene macrolides are ***antifungal***.

Production of macrolides

Macrolides are produced ***by actinomycetes***. The major macrolide antibiotics and the corresponding organisms synthesizing them are given in ***Table 25.3***.

Biosynthesis of erythromycin

In the biosynthesis of erythromycin, the lactone rings are contributed by acetate, propionate or butyrate while the sugar units are derived from glucose. Macrolide biosynthesis is a complex process and a good example of ***polyketide synthesis*** which is analogous to fatty acid biosynthesis. The enzyme lactone synthase is a multienzyme complex which is comparable in its structure and function to fatty acid synthase complex. An outline of the biosynthesis of erythromycin is given in ***Fig. 25.13***.

Regulation of biosynthesis : End product inhibition of erythromycin synthesis is well documented. Erythronolide B inhibits the enzyme lactone synthase. The final product erythromycin has also been shown to inhibit certain enzymes of the pathway (e.g. transmethylase). Addition of propanol to the culture medium induces the synthesis of acetyl CoA carboxylase, and almost doubles the production of erythromycin.

PRODUCTION PROCESS OF ERYTHROMYCIN

Industrial production of erythromycin is carried out by ***aerobic submerged fermentation***. The culture medium mainly consists of soy meal or corn steep liquor, glucose (or starch), yeast extract and ammonium sulfate. Fermentation is carried out at 30–34°C for about 3-7 days. Conventional methods are used for the recovery and purification of erythromycin.

TABLE 25.3 Important macrolide antibiotics with the organisms producing them

Macrolid antibiotic	*Producing organism*
Erythromycin	*Streptomyces erythreus*
Oleandomycin	*S. antibiotics*
Pikromycin	*S. felleus*
Megalomicin	*Micromonospora inositola*
Tylosin	*S. fradiae*
Carbomycin A	*S. halstedii*
Leucomycins	*Streptoverticillium kitasatoensis*

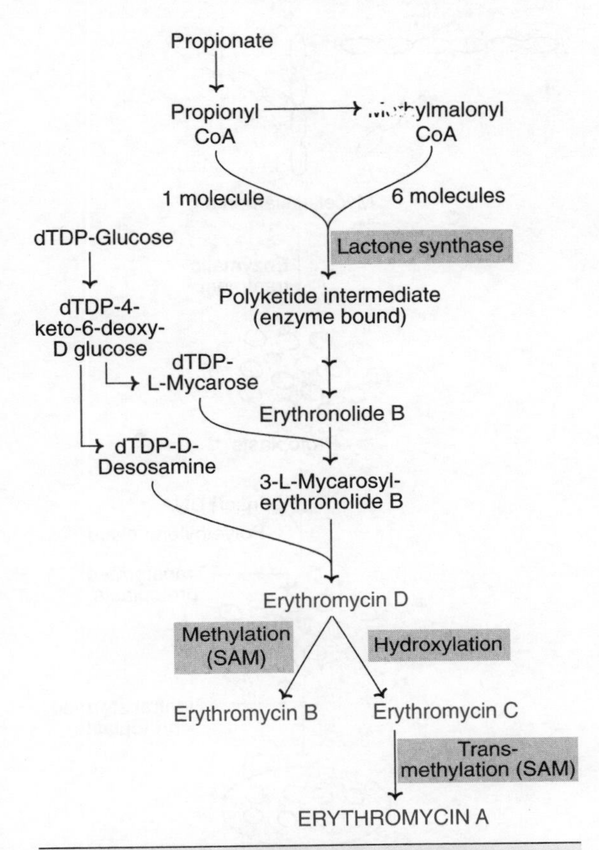

Fig. 25.13 : An outline of the biosynthesis of erythromycin by Streptomyces erythreus *(SAM — S-adenosylmethionine)*

AROMATIC ANTIBIOTICS

The antibiotics with aromatic rings in their structure are regarded as aromatic antibiotics. In a strict since, all the antibiotics containing aromatic nuclei should be considered in this group. However, most authors prefer to treat the three important antibiotics namely chloramphenicol, griseofulvin (***Fig. 25.14***) and novobiocin in the category of aromatic antibiotics, and the same is done in this book also.

CHLORAMPHENICOL

Chloramphenicol is a ***broad spectrum antibiotic*** that can act against Gram-positive and Gram-negative bacteria, besides rickettsias, actinomycetes and chlamydias. However, administration of chloramphenicol is associated with side effects, the most significant being damage to bone-marrow. As such, chloramphenicol is treated as a reserve antibiotic and selectively used.

Chloramphenicol binds to 50S ribosmal subunit and blocks (peptidyltransferase reaction) protein biosynthesis.

Production of chloramphenicol

Chloramphenicol can be produced by ***Streptomyces venezuelae*** and *S. omiyanesis.* However, chemical synthesis is mostly preferred for the commercial production of chloramphenicol.

GRISEOFULVIN

Griseofulvin is an antibiotic that acts specifically on fungi with chitinous cell walls. It is used in the ***treatment*** of various ***fungal skin infections***. Further, griseofulvin is also employed in the treatment of plant diseases caused by *Biotrytis* and *Alternaria solani.*

Although the exact mechanism of action of griseofulvin is not known, it is believed that chitin biosynthesis is adversely affected.

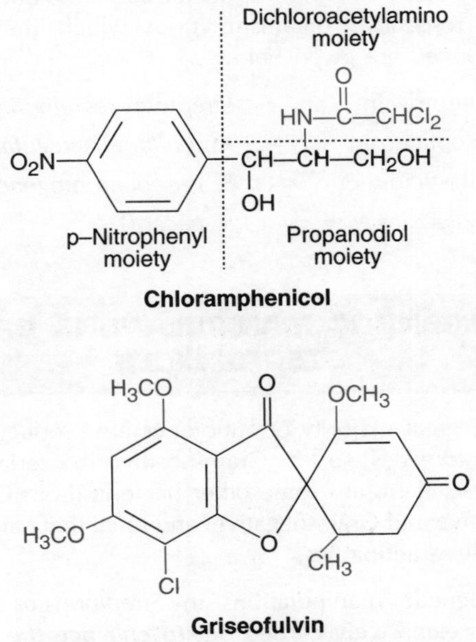

Dichloroacetylamino moiety

p–Nitrophenyl moiety

Propanodiol moiety

Chloramphenicol

Griseofulvin

Fig. 25.14 : Structures of chloramphenicol and griseofulvin.

Production of griseofulvin

Commercial production of griseofulvin is carried out by employing ***Penicillium patulum***. The chemical synthesis is less frequently used due to high cost.

The fermentation is carried out by an ***aerobic submerged process*** with a glucose rich medium. Nitrogen is supplied by sodium nitrate. The optimal conditions for fermentation are—temperature 23–26°C, pH 6.8-7.3, aeration 0.8-1 vvm, and the period is 7–10 days.

NUCLEOSIDE ANTIBIOTICS

There are several antibiotics (more than 200 or so) which have nucleoside like structures e.g. puromycin, blasticidin S. Nucleoside antibiotics have diverse structures and biological activities.

Puromycin is used to understand the ribosomal function in protein biosynthesis. Neplanosin possesses antiviral activity. Blasticidin S is a fungicide antibiotic used in plant pathology.

Production of nucleoside antibiotics

Selected examples of nucleoside antibiotics and the respective organisms from which they are produced are given below.

Puromycin — *Streptomyces alboniger*
Neplamosin A — *Ampullariella regularis*
Blasticidin S — *S. griseochromogenes*
Polyoxins — *S. cacaoi*

GENETIC MANIPULATIONS OF *STEPTOMYCES*

A great majority of antibiotics are produced by *Streptomyces* sp, a Gram-positive bacteria. Of course, there are some other bacteria (both Gram-positive and Gram-negative) and fungi that can also produce antibiotics.

Genetic manipulations in *Streptomyces* have been extensively carried out ***to enhance the yield of antibiotics and reduce cost of production***, besides developing newer and more effective antibiotics.

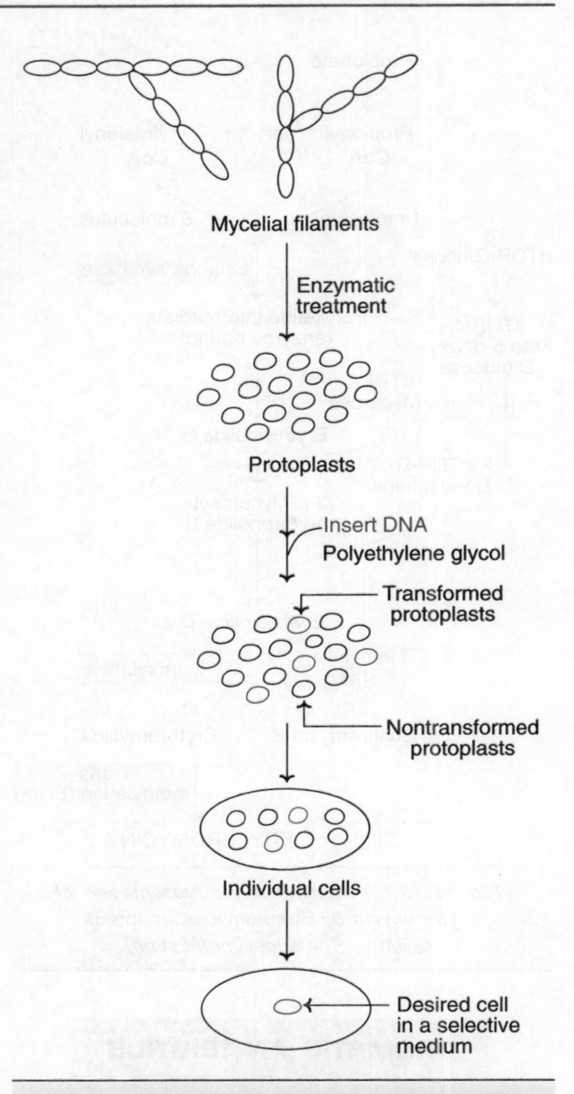

Fig. 25.15 : A diagrammatic representation of transformation in Streptomyces *sp.*

Transformation of streptomyces

Streptomyces strains exist as aggregates of mycelial filaments and not as individual cells. This is in contrast to *E. coli*. It is therefore essential that the cell walls of *Streptomyces* are broken to release protoplasts for transformation (***Fig. 25.15***). By adding the desired DNA (in plasmids) and polyethylene glycol, the cells can be transformed. These protoplasts are grown on a solid medium to regenerate the cell walls. The transformed cells with desired properties can be isolated for further use.

Cloning of antibiotic biosynthesis genes

In general, biosynthesis of antibiotics involves several reactions and participation of a large number of enzymes (and of course, several genes). It is rather difficult to clone so many genes. Mutant strains of *Streptomyces* that totally lack the synthesizing machinery for a particular antibiotic are very useful. Genes from a clone bank can be incorported into such mutants and screened for the desired properties. This is a lengthy and tedious procedure but has been successfully used for the improved production of certain antibiotics e.g. undeylprodigiosin.

Direct strategies of gene cloning : It is often possible to identify one or a few important enzymes in the synthesis of antibiotics. From the sequence of amino acids in the enzyme, gene can be constructed, and cloned. For instance, the gene for isopenicillin N synthase from *P. chrysogenum* has been successfully constructed in this fashion and used for increased production of penicillins and cephalosporins.

Genetic engineering for the production of novel antibiotics

Genetic manipulations can be done in the antibiotic synthesizing organisms to ultimately produce totally new and novel antibiotics.

Wild-type *Streptomyces coelicolor* genes encode the enzymes to produce the antibiotic actinorhodine. *S. violaceoruber* produces a related antibiotic namely granaticin. Genetic manipulations can be done between these organisms to produce novel hybrid antibiotics such as medarrhodine A and dihydrogranatirhodine.

The newly synthesized antibiotics are in fact structural variants of the existing antibiotics. As the biosynthetic pathways for antibiotic production and their corresponding genes are better understood, it becomes possible to design newer antibiotics with more efficient action.

Genetic engineering for improving antibiotic production

For aerobic microorganisms (e.g. *Streptomyces* sp), there is often the limitation of oxygen supply that hinders antibiotic production. Some workers have isolated a hemoglobin-like protein produced by the bacterium *Vitreoscilla* sp. The gene synthesizing this protein was isolated and cloned in a plasmid vector. The hemoglobin gene of *Vitroscilla* sp was finally incorporated into *Streptomyces.* These newly transformed strains have better capacity to take O_2 from the medium even at a low concentration.

The new strain of *S. coelicolor* (with hemoglobin gene) was found to produce 10 times more antibiotic actinorhodine than the wild strain, even at a low concentration of oxygen.

GOOD ANTIBIOTIC MANUFACTURING PRACTICES

Manufacture of antibiotics is highly commercialised due to a heavy demand worldwide. It is mandatory that detailed clinical trials are carried out before considering the manufacture of any antibiotic. More than half of the antibiotics produced are for human use. If is therefore ***absolutely essential that each antibiotic produced is safe, consistent and poses no health complications.*** Government authorities play a predominant role in regulating the production of antibiotics. These guidelines ensure that correct procedures are followed at each stage of manufacturing the antibiotics. The product produced should be of consistently high quality. Quality of the products should be checked at different stages of manufacture.

It is expected that the antibiotic manufactured should be in the purest form, although 100% purity is not practicable. It is mandatory that the impurities (if any), their quantities, and their ill effects should be made known.

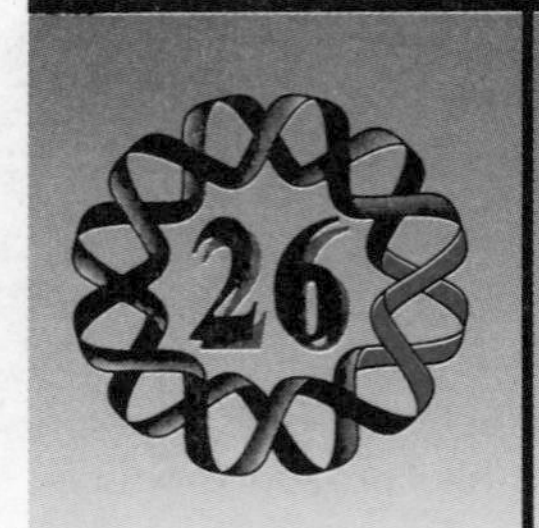

Microbial Production of Amino Acids

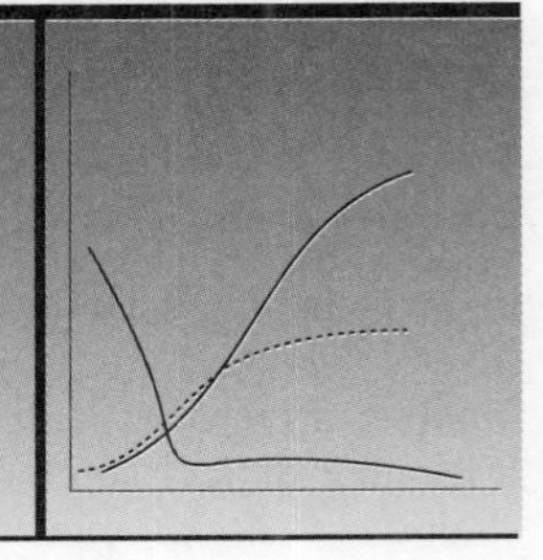

The first commercial production of the amino acid, glutamic acids, was started in Japan in as early as 1908. It was Ikeda (of Japan) who first identified that glutamic acid (in the form of monosodium glutamate) possesses taste-enchancing properties. In the early days, monosodium glutamate (MSG) was extracted from the vegetable proteins (wheat and soy). It was only in 1957, the large scale industrial production of MSG by using microorganisms commenced. Today, commercial production of amino acids is one of the biggest industries worldover with an annual increase in the demand by about 10%.

Glutamic acid continues to be ***largest producer*** among the amino acids, followed by lysine, methionine, threonine and aspartic acid.

AMINO ACID PRODUCTION — GENERAL CONSIDERATIONS

Some general considerations on the commercial applications of amino acids, their production methods, and the development of strains of microorganisms for improved amino acid production are briefly described.

COMMERCIAL APPLICATIONS OF AMINO ACIDS

Amino acids have a wide range of applications. The proportionate use of amino acids is given in the next column.

Food industry — 65%
Feed additives — 30%
Pharmaceutical — 5%

The individual L-amino acids (except glycine) along with their production methods and uses are given in ***Table 26.1***. The applications are broadly discussed hereunder.

Food industry

Amino acids are used either alone or in combination, as flavour enhancers. ***Monosodium glutamate is the most frequently*** used in food industry. Glycine and alanine also enhance taste and flavour. Tryptophan, in association with histidine, acts as an antioxidant to preserve milk powder. For the preservation of fruit juices, cysteine serves as an antioxidant.

Aspartame, a dipeptide (aspartyl-phenylalanine methyl ester) produced by a ***combination of aspartic acid and phenylalanine***, is about 200 times sweeter than sucrose. It is used as a low-calorie artificial sweetener in soft-drink industry.

There are certain essential amino acids that are deficient or limiting in plant proteins. These include lysine, methionine, threonine and tryptophan. Addition of the deficient amino acid(s) improves the nutritional quality of human foods as well as animal feeds. Thus, bread enriched with lysine, soy products supplemented with methionine are of better nutritional value. Methionine added soy bean meal is a better feed for pigs and other animals.

Pharmaceutical industry

The amino acids can be used as medicines. Essential amino acids are useful as ingradients of infusion fluids, for administration to patients in post-operative treatment.

Chemical industry

Amino acids serve as starting materials for producing several compounds. Glycine is used as a precursor for the synthesis of ***glyphosate*** (a herbicide), while threonine is the starting material for the production of azthreonam (another herbicide). Poly-methylglutamate is utilised for manufacturing synthetic leather. Some amino acids in the form of N-acyl derivatives are useful for the preparation of cosmotics.

METHODS FOR PRODUCTION OF AMINO ACIDS

The industrial production of amino acids is carried out by one or more of the following three processes.

1. **Extraction :** Amino acids are the building blocks in protein structure. The proteins can be subjected to hydrolysis, and the requisite amino acids can be isolated e.g. cysteine, tyrosine, leucine.

2. **Chemical synthesis :** Chemical synthesis results in a mixture of D- and L-amino acids. Most of the amino acids required for commercial

TABLE 26.1 Amino acids along with their production methods and applications

*Amino acid**	*Preferred production method*	*Application(s)*
Glutamic acid	Fermentation	Flavour enhancer
Lysine	Fermentation	Feed additive, infusion solution
Methionine	Chemical synthesis	Feed additive
Threonine	Fermentation	Feed additive
Phenylalanine	Fermentation	Aspartame production
Aspartate	Enzymatic synthesis, extraction	Aspartame production
Glycine	Chemical synthesis	Sweetener, food additive
Arginine	Fermentation, extraction	Infusions, therapy for liver diseases, cosmotics
Valine	Fermentation, extraction	Infusions, pesticides
Tryptophan	Extraction, immobilized cells	Infusions, antioxidant
Isoleucine	Extraction, fermentation	Infusions
Alanine	Extraction, enzymatic	Flavour enhancer
Leucine	Extraction, enzymatic	Infusions
Proline	Extraction	Infusions
Serine	Extraction, chemical synthesis	Cosmotics
Histidine	Extraction, fermentation	Therapy for ulcers
Asparagine	Extraction, chemical synthesis	Diuretic
Glutamine	Fermentation	Therapy for ulcers
Cysteine	Extraction	Infusion
Tyrosine	Extraction, enzymatic	Infusion
Ornithine	Extraction, enzymatic	Therapy for liver diseases

* *The order of amino acids is approximately in the decreasing order of their annual production; Extraction refers to the extraction of the specific amino acid from protein hydrolysates.*

applications are of L-category. However, for the synthesis of glycine (optically inactive) and some other amino acids which can be used in L- or D-form (D, L-alanine, D, L-methionine) for certain purposes, chemical methods are employed.

3. **Microbiological production : *For the large-scale production of amino acids***, microbiological methods are employed. There are three different approaches.

(a) **Direct fermentation methods :** Amino acids can be produced by microorganisms by utilising several carbon sources e.g. glucose, fructose, alkanes, ethanol, glycerol, propionate. Certain industrial byproducts like molasses and starch hydrolysate can also be used. Methanol, being a cheap carbon source, is tried for amino acid production, but with limited success.

(b) **Conversion of metabolic intermediates into amino acids :** In this approach, the microorganisms are used to carry out selected reactions for amino acid production e.g. conversion of glycine to serine.

(c) **Direct use of microbial enzymes or immobilized cells :** Sometimes resting cells, immobilized cells, crude cell extracts or enzyme-membrane reactors can be used for the production of amino acids. Some examples are given below.

Amino acid dehydrogenases from certain bacteria (e.g. *Bacillus megaterium*) can be used for the amination of α-keto acids to produce L-amino acids e.g. alanine (from pyruvate), leucine (from α-ketoisocaproic acid) and phenylalanine (from phenylpyruvate). Immobilized cells or enzyme-membrane reactors can be used.

Enzymes or immobilised cells are also employed for the production of several other amino acids e.g. tryptophan, tyrosine, lysine, valine.

STRAIN DEVELOPMENT FOR AMINO ACID PRODUCTION

The metabolic pathways, for the synthesis of amino acids by microorganisms, are tightly controlled and they operate in an economical way. Therefore, a natural overproduction of amino acids is a rare occurrence. Some strains that excrete certain amino acids have been isolated e.g. glutamic acid, alanine, valine.

In order to achieve an overproduction of any amino acid by a microorganism, methods have to be devised for the elimination of the metabolic regulatory/control processes. In fact, several amino acid-producing ***microorganisms have been developed by mutagenesis and screening programmes***.

The following are the major ways of strain development. In fact, several methods are combined to successfully develop a new strain for producing amino acids.

Auxotrophic mutation : These mutants are characterized by a lack of the formation of regulatory end product (i.e. repressor or regulatory effector). The intermediates of the metabolic pathways accumulate and get excreted.

Genetic recombination : Mutants can be developed by genetic recombination for over-production of amino acids. Protoplast fusion in certain bacteria is used for development of hybrids e.g. *Corynebacterium glutamicum* and *Bacillus flavum*.

Recombinant DNA technology : The classical techniques of genetic engineering can be used for strain development. Strains with increasing activities of rate-limiting enzymes have been developed. In one of the techniques, *E. coli* and cloning vector pBR322 were used to increase the genes for the production of amino acids e.g. glutamic acid, lysine, phenylalanine, valine.

Functional genomics : a new approach

Analysis of genomes from the wild and mutant strains of microorganisms will help in creating improved strains. Once the entire sequence of the chromosomes in the organisms (e.g. *C. glutamicum*, *E. coli*) is established, efforts can be made to carry out genetic manipulations for efficient overproduction of desired amino acids. ***Chip technology*** can be used to detect new mutations and consequently the fermentation processes.

L-GLUTAMIC ACID

L-Glutamic acid was the ***first amino acid to be produced by microorganisms***. The original

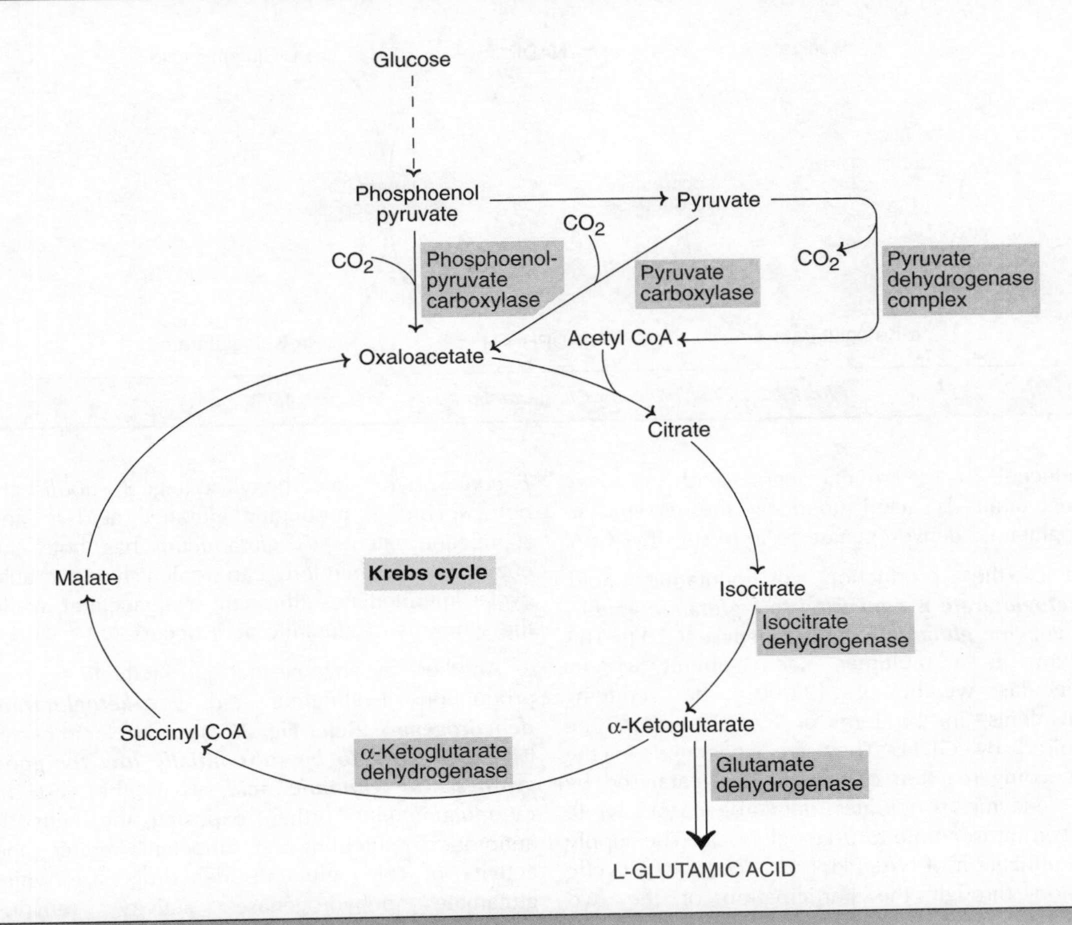

Fig. 26.1 : Biosynthesis of L-glutamic acid in Corynebacterium glutamicum.

bacterium, ***Corynebacterium glutamicum***, that was first used for large scale manufacture of glutamic acid continues to be successfully used even today. The other important organisms (although used to a lesser extent due to low yield) employed for glutamic acid production belong to genera *Microbacterium*, *Brevibacterium* and *Arthrobacter*. All these organisms have certain morphological and physiological characters comparable to *C. glutamicum*. Biochemically, ***glutamic acid-producing bacteria have a high activity of glutamate dehydrogenase and a low activity of α-ketoglutarate dehydrogenase***. They also require the vitamin biotin.

Improved production strains

Several improvements have been made, particularly in *C. glutamicum*, for improving the strains to produce and excrete more and more of glutamic acid. These include the strains that can tolerate high concentrations of biotin, and lysozyme-sensitive mutants with high yield.

Biosynthesis of L-glutamic acid

The pathway for the synthesis of glutamic acid with glucose as the carbon source is depicted in ***Fig. 26.1***. Glucose is broken down to phosphoenol pyruvate and then to pyruvate. Pyruvate is converted to acetyl CoA. Phosphoenol pyruvate (by the enzyme phosphoenol pyruvate carboxylase) can be independently converted to oxaloacetate. Both these carboxylation reactions are quite critical, and require biotin as the cofactor.

The next series of reactions that follow are the familiar citric acid (Krebs) cycle reactions wherein the key metabolite namely α-ketoglutarate is

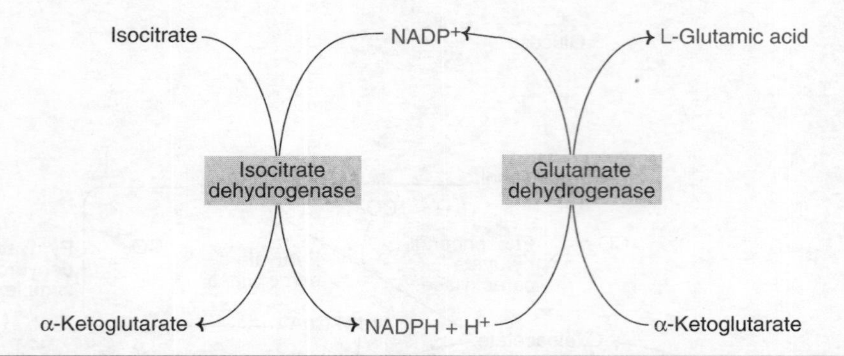

Fig. 26.2 : Biosynthesis of L. glutamic acid — role of NADP+.

produced. In the routine citric acid cycle, α-ketoglutarate is acted upon by the enzyme α-ketoglutarate dehydrogenase to form succinyl CoA.

For the production of glutamic acid, ***α-ketoglutarate is converted to L-glutamic acid*** by the enzyme ***glutamate dehydrogenase*** (GDH). This enzyme is a multimer, each subunit with a molecular weight of 49,000. The reducing equivalents, in the form of NADPH + H^+, are required by GDH. They are generated in the preceeding reaction of Krebs cycle (catalysed by the enzyme isocitrate dehydrogenase) while converting isocitrate to α-ketoglutarate. The supply and utilization of NADPH + H^+ occurs in a cyclic fashion through the participation of the two enzymes, namely isocitrate dehydrogenase and glutamate dehydrogenase (***Fig. 26.2***).

Theoretically, one molecule of glutamic acid can be formed from one molecule of glucose. In practice, the conversion efficiency of glucose to glutamic acid was found to be around 70%.

Regulation of glutamic acid biosynthesis

The essential requirement for glutamic acid production is the high capability for the supply of the citric acid cycle metabolites. This is made possible by an efficient conversion of phosphoenol pyruvate as well as pyruvate to oxaloacetate (Refer ***Fig. 26.1***). Thus, there are two enzymes (phosphoenol pyruvate carboxylase and pyruvate carboxylase) to efficiently produce oxaloacetate, while there is only one enzyme (pyruvate dehydrogenase) for the formation of acetyl CoA. Certain microorganisms which have either phosphoenol pyruvate carboxylase (e.g., *E. coli*) or pyruvate carboxylase (e.g. *B. subtilis*) are not capable of producing glutamic acid to any significant extent. *C. glutamicum* has both the enzymes and therefore can replenish citric acid cycle intermediates (through oxaloacetate) while the synthesis of glutamic acid occurs.

Another key enzyme that can facilitate optimal production of glutamic acid is ***α-ketoglutarate dehydrogenase*** (Refer ***Fig. 26.1***) of citric acid cycle. Its ***activity has to be substantially low for good synthesis of glutamic acid***, as is the case in *C. glutamicum*. Further, exposing the cells to antibiotics (penicillin) and surfactants reduces the activity of α-ketoglutarate dehydrogenase while glutamate dehydrogenase activity remains unaltered. By this way, oxidation of α-ketoglutarate via citric acid cycle can be minimised, while the formation of glutamic acid is made maximum possible.

Release of glutamic acid

Glutamic acid is ***synthesized intracellularly***, and therefore ***its release or export is*** equally important. It now appears that there is a ***carrier-mediated energy-dependent active process*** involved for the export of glutamic acid. There are several ways of increasing the membrane permeability for exporting glutamic acid.

- Biotin limitation
- Addition of saturated fatty acids
- Addition of penicillin
- Use of oleic acid auxotrophs
- Use of glycerol auxotrophs
- Addition of local anesthetics
- Addition of surfactants (Tween 40).

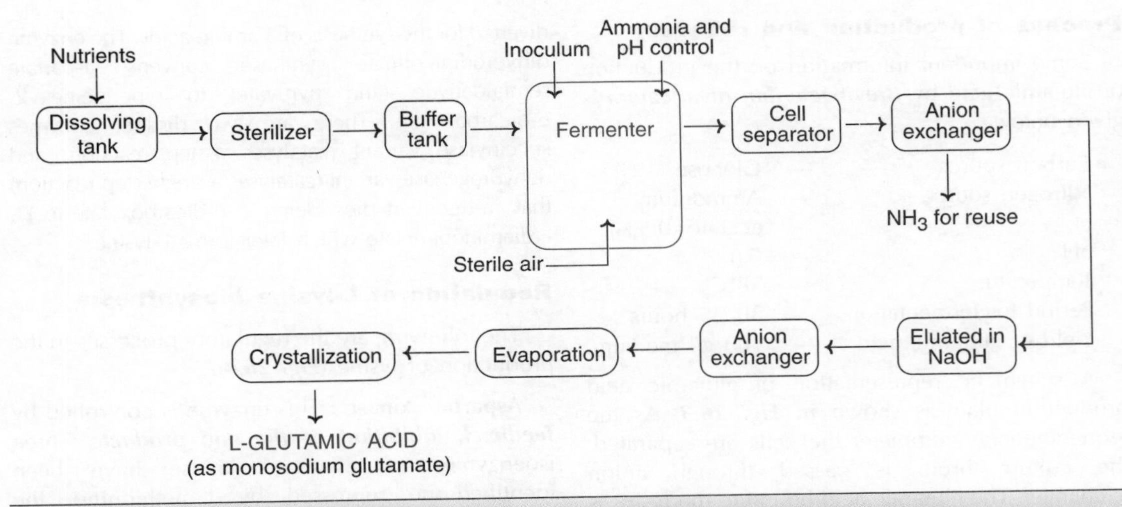

Fig. 26.3 : Diagrammatic representation of glutamic acid production plant.

The effect of biotin deficiency in facilitating the release of intracellular glutamic acid has been worked out. Biotin is an essential cofactor (required by the enzyme acetyl CoA carboxylase) for the biosynthesis of fatty acids. Due to a limited supply or deficiency of biotin, fatty acid biosynthesis and consequently phospholipid synthesis is drastically reduced. As a result, membrane formation (protein-phospholipid complex) is defective which alters permeability for an increased export of intracellular glutamic acid.

It is found that there is an alteration in the membrane composition of phospholipids in oleic acid and glycerol auxotroph mutants. This facilitates release of intracellular glutamic acid.

The knowledge on the membrane permeability of glutamic acid is successfully exploited for increased industrial production of glutamic acid.

Production of glutamic acid-requirements and influencing factors

The industrial production of glutamic acid is influenced by carbon sources, nitrogen sources, growth factors, pH and O_2 supply. The relevant aspects are briefly described.

Carbon sources : Either ***refined*** (glucose, sucrose, fructose, maltose) ***or unrefined*** (sugar beet molasses, sugar cane molasses) ***carbon sources*** are used. In countries like Japan, acetate (inexpensive) is utilized. Other substrates like alkanes, ethanol and methanol are less frequently used.

Nitrogen sources : The concentration of ***ammonia is very crucial for converting carbon source to glutamic acid***. However, high concentration of ammonia inhibits the growth of the organisms. In the beginning of fermentation, ammonium salts and a low concentration of ammonia are added. During the course of fermentation, ammonia in aqueous solution is continuously fed. In this way, pH can be controlled, besides continuous supply of nitrogen source. Sometimes, urea is also used as a nitrogen source, since glutamic acid-producing bacteria possess urease that can split urea and release ammonia.

Growth factors : ***Biotin*** is an important growth factor and its concentration in the medium is influenced by the carbon source. For instance, a supply 5 μg of biotin per liter medium is recommended if the carbon source is 10% glucose, while for acetate as the carbon source, the biotin requirement is much lower (0.1-1.0 μg/l). Addition of L-cysteine in the medium is recommended for certain strains.

Supply of O_2 : O_2 supply should be adequately and continuously maintained. It is observed that a high O_2 concentration inhibits growth of the organisms while a low O_2 supply leads to the production of lactic acid and succinic acid. In both instances, glutamic acid formation is low.

Process of production and recovery

Some important information on the production of glutamic acid by *Brevibacterium divaricatum* is given below.

Carbon source	—	Glucose (12%)
Nitrogen source	—	Ammonium acetate (0.5%)
pH	—	7.8
Temperature	—	38°C
Period for fermentation	—	30–35 hours
Yield of glutamic acid	—	100 g/l medium.

A schematic representation of glutamic acid production plant is shown in ***Fig. 26.3***. As the fermentation is complete, the cells are separated, the culture broth is passed through anion exchanger. The glutamic acid bound to the resins is eluted in NaOH, while the ammonia released can be reused. With NaOH, glutamic acid forms monosodium glutamate (MSG) which can be purified by passing through anion exchanger. MSG can be subjected to evaporation and crystallization.

L-LYSINE

Lysine is present at a low concentration in most of the plant proteins. Being an essential amino acid, supplementation of plant foods with lysine increases their nutritional quality.

L-Lysine is predominantly produced by ***Corynebacterium glutamicum*** and to some extent by *Brevibacterium flavum* or *B. lactofermentum*.

Biosynthesis of L-lysine

The pathway for the synthesis of L-lysine is complex, and an outline of it is depicted in ***Fig. 26.4***. This metabolic pathway is also involved in the formation of 3 other amino acids, namely methionine, threonine and isoleucine.

As the glucose gets oxidised by glycolysis, phosphoenol pyruvate and pyruvate are formed. Both these metabolites can be converted to oxaloacetate, a key component of citric acid cycle. On transamination, oxaloacetate forms aspartate. The enzyme aspartate kinase converts aspartate to aspartyl phosphate which later forms aspartate semialdehyde. Aspartate semialdehyde has two fates—the biosynthesis of lysine and formation of 3 other amino acids (methionine, threonine and isoleucine). When homoserine dehydrogenase acts on aspartate semialdehyde, it is diverted for the synthesis of 3 amino acids. The enzyme dihydrodipicolinate synthase converts aspartate semialdehyde (and pyruvate) to piperideine 2, 6-dicarboxylate. There are two distinct enzymes succinylase variant (catalyses 4-step reaction) and dehydrogenase variant (catalyses a single step reaction) that can convert piperideine 2, 6-dicarboxylate to D, L-diaminopimelate which later forms L-lysine.

Regulation of L-lysine biosynthesis

The following are the regulatory processes in the production of lysine (***Fig. 26.4***).

Aspartate kinase : This enzyme is controlled by ***feedback inhibition of the end products***. Three isoenzymes of aspartate kinase have been identified-one repressed by L-methionine, the second one repressed by L-threonine and L-isoleucine, and the third one being inhibited and repressed by L-lysine. The amino acid sequence and structure of aspartate kinase have been elucidated. And by genetic manipulations, it has been possible to create mutants (of aspartate kinase) that are insensitive to feedback regulation by L-lysine.

Dihydrodipicolinate synthase : This enzyme competes with homoserine dehydrogenase to act on aspartate semialdehyde. Overexpression of dihydrodipicolinate synthase has been shown to increase the production of L-lysine.

Succinylase and dehydrogenase variants : The conversion of piperideine 2, 6-dicarboxylate to D, L-diaminopimelate is carried out by these two enzymes. At the start of the fermentation, dehydrogenase variant predominantly acts, and later succinylase variant comes into picture for the biosynthesis of L-lysine.

Role of D, L-diaminopimelate : This amino acid, an immediate precursor for the synthesis of L-lysine, is also required for the synthesis of a tripeptide (L-Ala-γ-D-Glu-D, L-Dap) which is part of the peptidoglycan of cell wall. The activities of both the enzymes (succinylase and dehydrogenase) that form diaminopimelate (Dap) are important for the production of L-lysine and for the proper formation of cell wall structure.

Improved production strains

Based on the biosynthetic pathway and the regulatory steps (discussed above), certain improvements have been made in the strains of

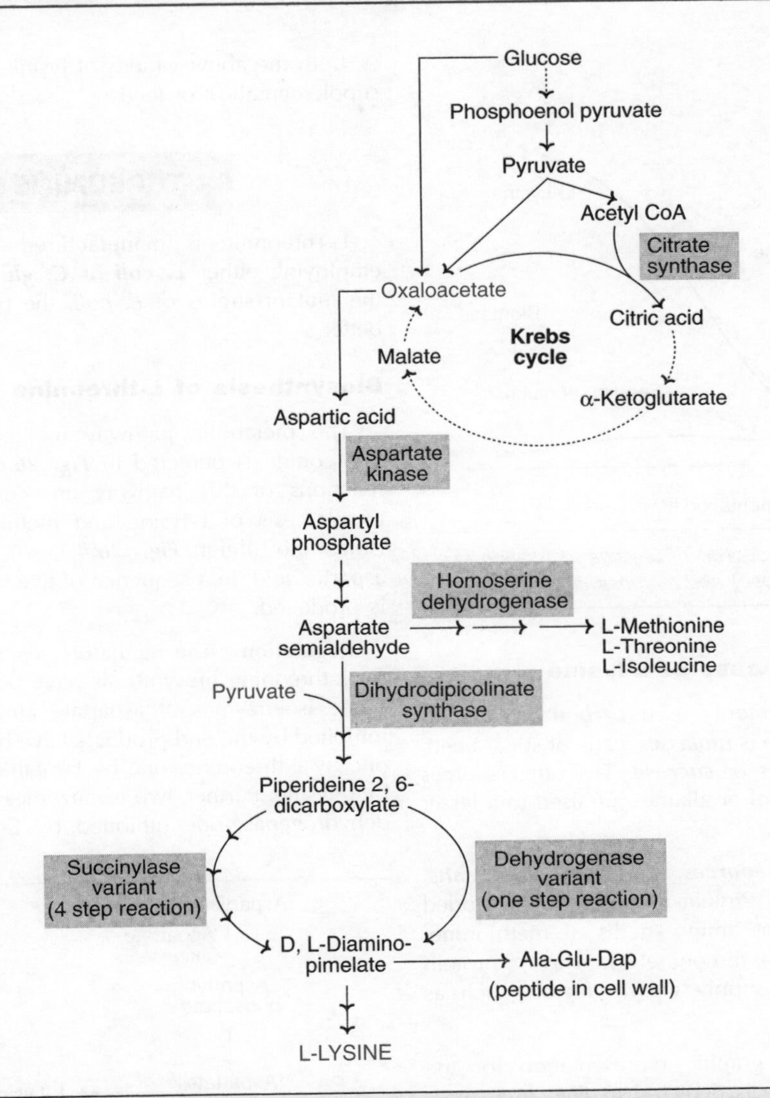

Fig. 26.4 : Biosynthesis of L-lysine in C. glutamicum
(Ala-Glu-Dap — Alanyl-glutamyl-diaminopimelate, a tripeptide)

C. glutamicum and *B. flavum* for overproduction of lysine.

- Mutant organisms resistant to lysine antimetabolites (e.g. b-aminoethyl-L-lysine).
- A mutant strain with an altered enzyme aspartokinase, so that it is not regulated by end product inhibition.
- A strain with a decreased homoserine dehydrogenase activity (so that diversion for the synthesis of methionine, threonine and isoleucine is minimised).
- A strain with reduced citrate synthase activity (to lower the occurrence of citric acid cycle).

Release of L-lysine

The export or release of L-lysine from the cells into the surrounding medium occurs through a ***lysine-export (LysE)*** carrier protein. It is a trans-membrane protein (mol. wt-25,400) with six segments that participate in lysine transport. The exporter system is very efficient active process to export large quantities of intracellular lysine.

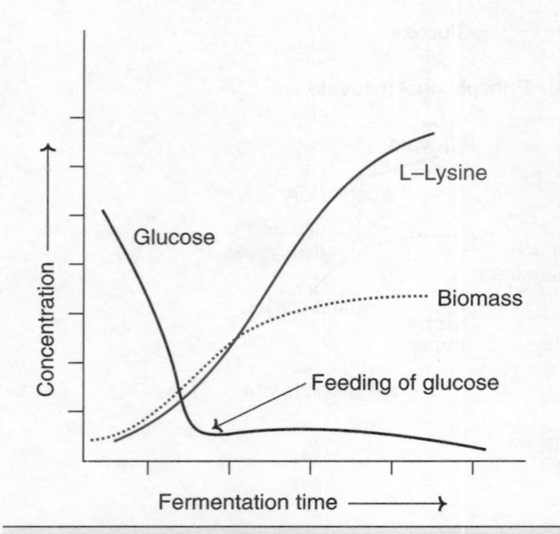

Fig. 26.5 : Production of L-lysine in relation to substrate (glucose) and biomass concentration.

Production process of L-lysine

The most commonly used ***carbon sources*** for lysine manufacture is ***molasses*** (cane or sugar beet), starch hydrolysates or ***sucrose***. The other sources like acetate, ethanol or alkanes are used to a lesser extent.

The ***nitrogen sources*** are ***ammonium salts***, gaseous ***ammonia***. Protein hydrolysates are added to supply certain amino acids (L-methionine, L-homoserine, L-threonine). The protein hydrolysates also supply growth factors such as biotin.

A time-course graphic representation for the formation of lysine is depicted in ***Fig. 26.5***. As is evident, a continuous supply of glucose (or other sugar) is required for sustained production of lysine. Under optimal fermentation conditions, the yield of lysine (in the form of L-lysine HCl) is 40–50 g per 100 g carbon source.

There are different recovery processes for lysine depending on its application.

- An alkaline solution containing about 50% L-lysine can be obtained after biomass separation, evaporation and filtration.
- A crystalline preparation with 98–99% L-lysine (as L-lysine HCl) can be obtained by subjecting the culture broth to ion-exchange chromatography, evaporation and crystallization.

Both the above grades of lysine are suitable for supplementation of feeds.

L-THREONINE

L-Threonine is manufactured industrially by employing either ***E. coli*** or ***C. glutamicum***. With the mutant strains of *E. coli*, the product yield is better.

Biosynthesis of L-threonine

The metabolic pathway for the synthesis of L-threonine is depicted in ***Fig. 26.6***. Some of the reactions of this pathway are common for the biosynthesis of L-lysine and methionine, besides isoleucine (Refer ***Fig. 26.4*** also). Starting with aspartic acid, in a sequence of five steps, threonine is produced.

Regulation : The regulatory reactions in *E. coli* for L-threonine biosynthesis have been elucidated. Three isoenzymes of aspartate kinase, separately inhibited by the end products have been identified-one by L-threonine, one by L-methionine and one by L-lysine. Further, two isoenzymes of homoserine dehydrogenase-one inhibited by L-threonine and

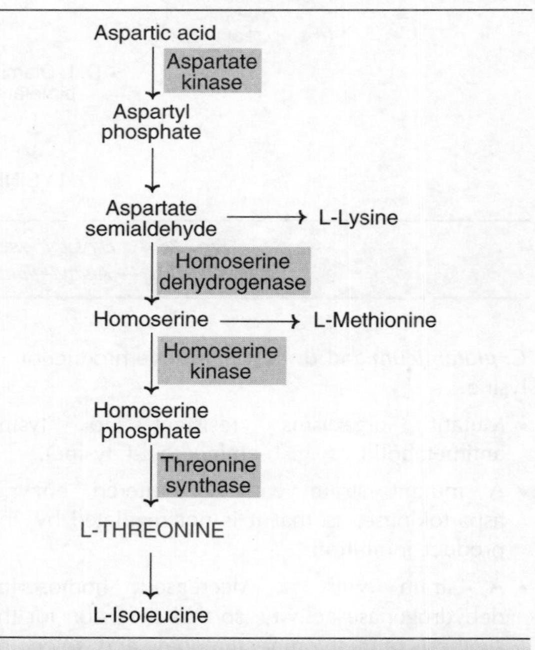

Fig. 26.6 : Biosynthesis of L-threonine in E. coli.

other by L-methionine are also known. A gene *thrABC* that encodes three polypeptides (one polypeptide possesses the activity of kinase and homoserine dehydrogenase, the second homoserine kinase and the third threonine synthase) in *E. coli* has been identified.

Improved production strains : The efficiency of the producer strains can be increased by creating *E. coli* mutants with high-level expression of the gene *thrABC*. Further, mutants with minimal production of L-isoleucine also result is high yield of L-threonine.

Production process of L-threonine

The culture medium containing glucose or sucrose, yeast extract and ammonium salts is adequate for L-threonine production. The sugar feeding has to be continued for good yield (about 60% of the carbon source).

The downstream processing for the isolation of L-threonine consists of coagulation of the cell mass (by heat), filtration, concentration by evaporation, and crystallization.

L-PHENYLALANINE

Both ***E. coli*** and ***C. glutamicum*** can be used for the production of L-phenylalanine. The biosynthetic pathway is quite complex and an outline is shown in ***Fig. 26.7***. An interesting feature is that the same pathway is responsible for the synthesis of all the three aromatic amino acids-tyrosine and tryptophan, besides phenylalanine.

The synthetic pathway commences with the condensation of erythrose 4-phosphate with phosphoenol pyruvate to form deoxy-arabinoheptulosonate phosphate (DAHP). DAHP in the next series of reactions is converted to chorismate which can form L-tryptophan. Chorismate mutase converts chorismate to prephenate which forms L-phenylalanine through the participation of prephenate dehydrogenase. Prephenate also serves as a precursor for the synthesis of tyrosine.

The genes responsible for the formation of the regulatory enzymes of L-phenylalanine have been identified. By employing genetic manipulations, strains for improved production of L-phenylalanine have been developed.

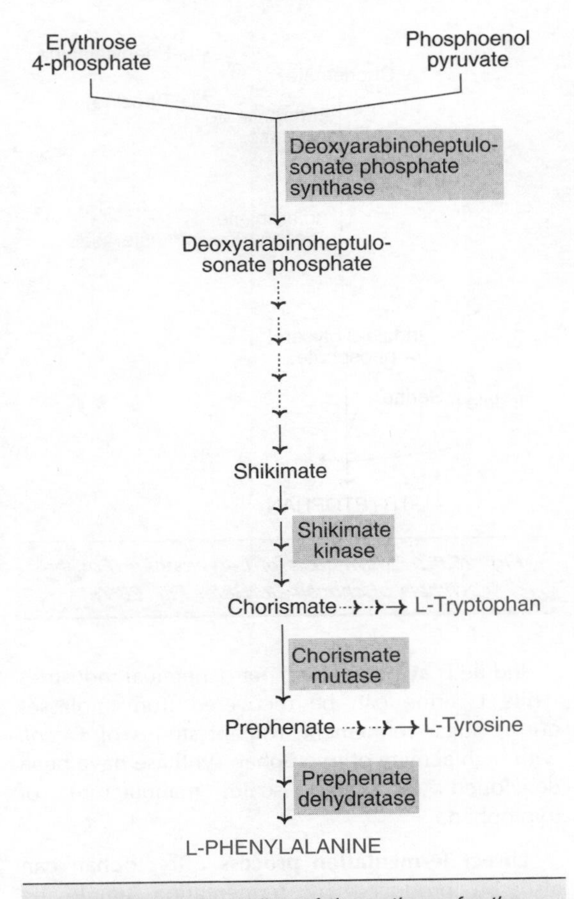

***Fig. 26.7 :** An outline of the pathway for the synthesis of L-phenylalanine, L-tyrosine and L-tryptophan.*

L-TRYPTOPHAN

There are different ways of synthesizing L-tryptophan-chemical, enzymatic and fermentation methods. At present, large scale manufacture of tryptophan is carried out by using the enzyme ***tryptophan synthase*** of ***E. coli***. Tryptophan synthase combines indole with L-serine to form tryptophan.

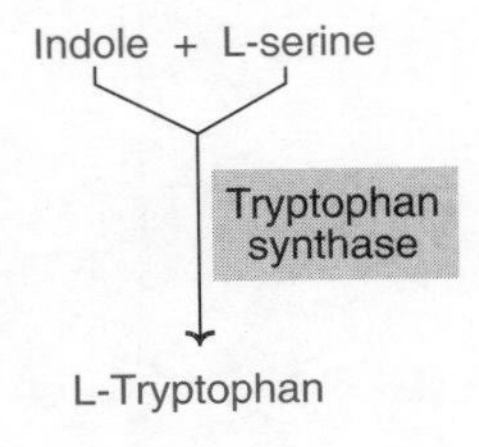

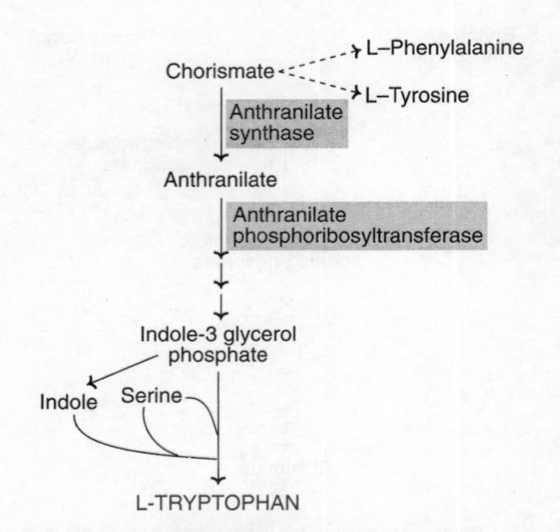

Fig. 26.8 : Biosynthesis of L-tryptophan (For the syntheis of chorismate Refer Fig. 26.7).

Indole is available from petrochemical industries while L-serine can be recovered from molasses during sugar refinement. Mutant strains of *E. coli* with high activity of tryptophan synthase have been developed for large scale manufacture of tryptophan.

Direct fermentation process : Tryptophan can also be produced by fermentation employing *C. glutamicum,* or *E. coli*. For the biosynthetic pathway, refer ***Fig. 26.7***. Mutant strains of both these organisms have been developed for increased yield of tryptophan.

Mutant strains for overproduction L-tryptophan

The production of tryptophan by *C. glutamicum* was increased by introducing a second gene encoding ***anthranilate synthase***, a key enzyme in its biosynthesis (***Fig. 26.8***). Further, genes encoding other important enzymes (deoxyarabino-heptulosonate phosphate synthase, anthranilate phosphoribosyltransferase) were also be modified. The result is that the pathway becomes insensitive to feedback inhibition by end products, leading to an overproduction of L-tryptophan.

L-ASPARTIC ACID

There is a growing demand for aspartate, as it is a ***component of aspartame*** (an artificial sweetener), besides its use as a food additive, and in pharmaceutical preparations.

The preferred method for aspartate production is enzymatic in nature. The enzyme aspartase converts fumarate and ammonia to aspartate. Although this reaction is reversible, aspartate formation is favoured.

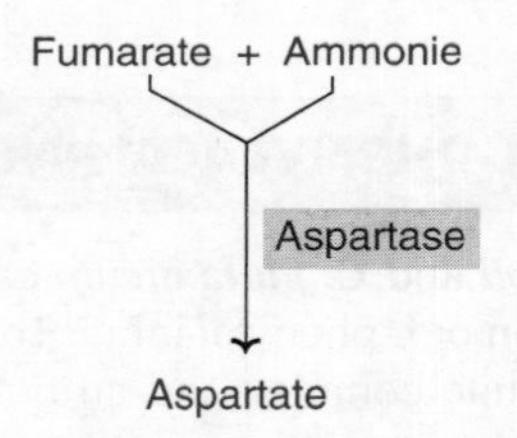

The aspartase of *E. coli* is used. It is a tetramer with a molecular weight 196,000. This enzyme is quite unstable. Immobilization of aspartase in polyacrylamide or carrageenan that enhances the stability of the enzyme is commonly used.

Immobilized *E. coli* cells with good activity of aspartase are also used for aspartate production.

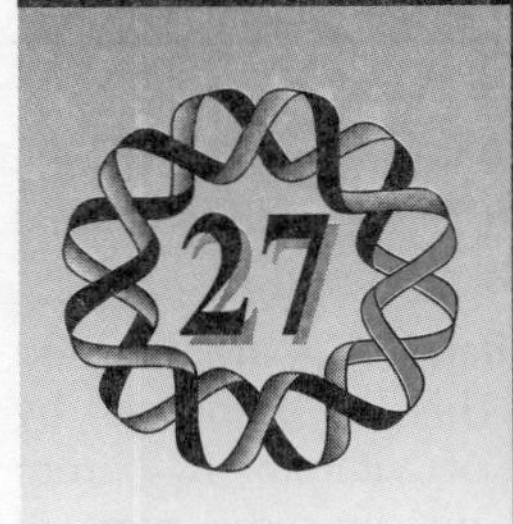

Microbial Production of Vitamins

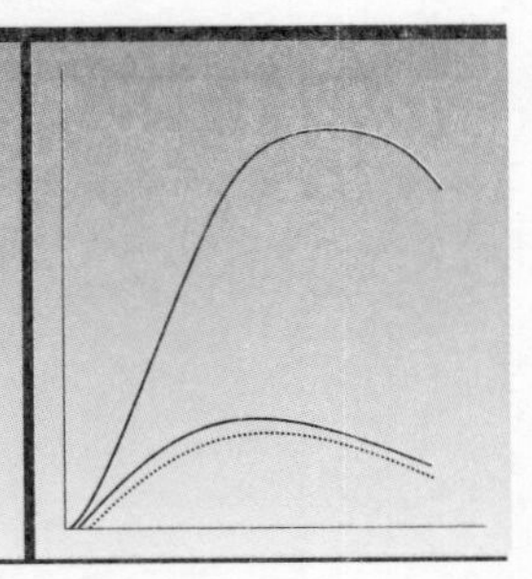

Vitamins are organic compounds that perform specific biological functions for normal maintenance and optimal growth of an organism. These ***vitamins cannot be synthesized by the higher organisms***, including man, and therefore they have to be supplied in small amounts in the diet.

Microorganisms are capable of synthesizing the vitamins. In fact, the bacteria in the gut of humans can produce some of the vitamins, which if appropriately absorbed can partially meet the body's requirements. It is an accepted fact that after administration of strong antibiotics to humans (which kill bacteria in gut), additional consumption of vitamins is recommended.

Microorganisms can be successfully used for the commercial production of many of the vitamins e.g. thiamine, riboflavin, pyridoxine, folic acid, pantothenic acid, biotin, vitamin B_{12}, ascorbic acid, β-carotene (provitamin A), ergosterol (provitamin D). However, from economic point of view, it is feasible to produce vitamin B_{12}, riboflavin, ascorbic acid and β-carotene by microorganisms. ***For the production of ascorbic acid (vitamin C), the reader must refer Chapter 24.***

VITAMIN B_{12}

The disease, ***pernicious anemia***, characterized by low levels of hemoglobin, decreased number of erythrocytes and neurological manifestations, has been known for several decades. It was in 1926 some workers reported the liver extracts could cure pernicious anemia. The active principle was later identified as vitamin B_{12}, a water soluble B-complex vitamin.

Occurrence

Vitamin B_{12} is present in animal tissue at a very low concentration (e.g. 1 ppm in the liver). It occurs mostly in the coenzyme forms-methylcobalamin and deoxyadenosylcobalamin. Isolation of vitamin B_{12} from animal tissues is very expensive and tedious.

Chemistry

Vitamin B_{12} (cyanocobalamin) is a water soluble vitamin with complex structure. The empirical formula of cyanocobalamin is $C_{63}H_{90}N_{14}O_{14}PCO$. The structure of vitamin B_{12} consists of a corrin ring with a central cobalt atom. The corrin ring is almost similar to the tetrapyrrole ring structure found in other porphyrin compounds e.g. heme (with Fe) and chlorophyll (with Mg).

The corrin ring has four pyrrole units. Cobalt present at the centre of the corrin ring is bonded to the four pyrrole nitrogens. Cobalt also binds to dimethylbenzimidazole and aminoisopropanol. Thus, cobalt atom present in vitamin B_{12} is in a coordination state of six.

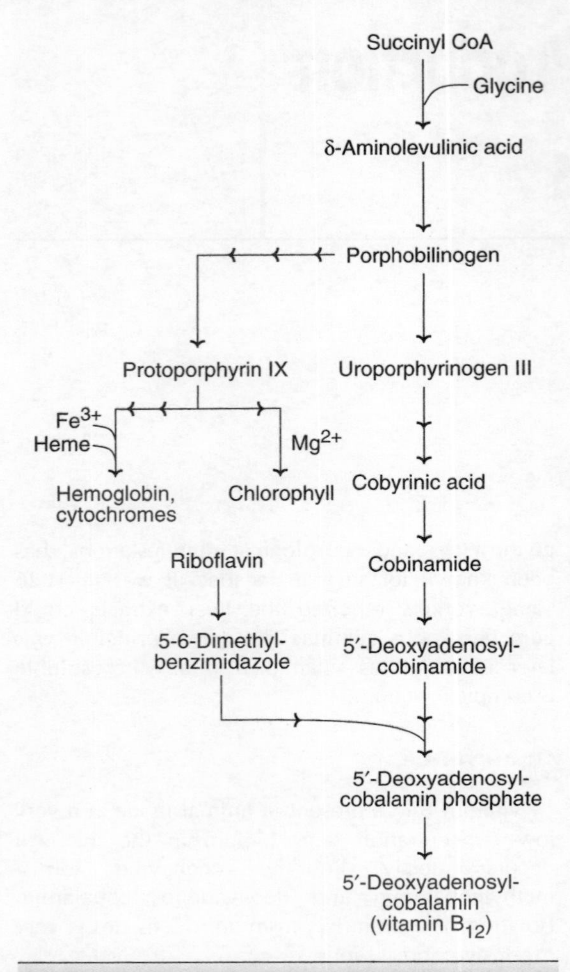

Fig. 27.1 : An outline of the biosynthesis of vitamin B_{12}

Biosynthesis

Vitamin B_{12} is ***exclusively synthesized*** in nature ***by microorganisms***. An outline of the pathway is depicted in ***Fig. 27.1***. The biosynthesis of B_{12} is comparable with that of chlorophyll and hemoglobin. Many of the reactions in the synthesis of vitamin B_{12} are not yet fully understood.

COMMERCIAL PRODUCTION OF VITAMIN B_{12}

Vitamin B_{12} is commercially produced by fermentation. It was first obtained as a byproduct of *Streptomyces* fermentation in the production of certain antibiotics (streptomycin, chloramphenicol, or neomycin). But the yield was very low. Later, high-yielding strains were developed. And at present, vitamin B_{12} is entirely produced by fermentation. It is estimated that the world's annual production of vitamin B_{12} is around 15,000 kg.

High concentrations of vitamin B_{12} are detected in sewage-sludge solids. This is produced by microorganisms. Recovery of vitamin B_{12} from sewage-sludge was carried out in some parts of United States.

Unlike most other vitamins, the chemical synthesis of vitamin B_{12} is not practicable, since about 20 complicated reaction steps need to be carried out. ***Fermentation of vitamin B_{12} is the only choice.***

Microorganisms and yields of vitamin B_{12}

Several microorganisms can be employed for the production of vitamin B_{12}, with varying yields. Glucose is the most commonly used carbon source. Some examples of microbes and their corresponding yields are given in ***Table 27.1***. The most commonly used microorganisms are — *Propionibacterium freudenreichii, Pseudomonas denitrificans, Bacillus megaterium* and *Streptomyces olivaceus.*

Genetically engineered strains for vitamin B_{12} production : By employing modern techniques of genetic engineering, vitamin B_{12} production can be enhanced. A protoplast fusion technique between *Protaminobacter rubber* and *Rhodopseudomonas spheroides* resulted in a hybrid strain called *Rhodopseudomonas protamicus*. This new strain can produce as high as 135 mg/l of vitamin B_{12} utilizing carbon source.

TABLE 27.1 Microorganisms with corresponding yields of vitamin B_{12}

Microorganism	*Yield (mg/l)*
Bacillus megaterium	0.51
Streptomyces olivaceus	3.31
Butyribacterium rettgeri	5.0
Micromonospora sp	11.5
Propionibacterium freudenreichii	19.0
Propionibacterium shermanii	35.0
Pseudomonas denitrificans	60.0
Hybrid strain	
Rhodopseudomonas protamicus	135.0

Production of vitamin B_{12} using *Propionibacterium* sp

Propionibacterium freudenreichii and *P. shermanii*, and their mutant strains are commonly used for vitamin B_{12} production. The process is carried out by adding cobalt in two phases.

Anaerobic phase : This is a preliminary phase that may take 2-4 days. In the anaerobic phase 5′-deoxyadenosylcobinamide is predominantly produced.

Aerobic phase : In this phase, 5, 6-dimethyl-benzimidazole is produced from riboflavin which gets incorporated to finally form coenzyme of vitamin B_{12} namely 5′-deoxyadenosylcobalamin.

In recent years, some fermentation technologists have successfully clubbed both an anaerobic and aerobic phases to carry out the operation continuously in two reaction tanks.

The ***bulk production of vitamin B_{12}*** is mostly done ***by submerged bacterial fermentation with beet molasses medium supplemented with cobalt chloride***. The specific details of the process are kept as a guarded secret by the companies.

Recovery of vitamin B_{12} : The cobalamins produced by fermentation are mostly bound to the cells. They can be solubilized by heat treatment at 80–120°C for about 30 minutes at pH 6.5-8.5. The solids and mycelium are filtered or centrifiged and the fermentation broth collected. The cobalamins can be converted to more stable cyanocobalamins. This vitamin B_{12} is around 80% purity and can be directly used as a feed additive. However, for medical use (particularly for treatment of pernicious anemia), vitamin B_{12} should be further purified (95–98% purity).

Production of vitamin B_{12} using *Pseudomonas* sp

Pseudomonas denitrificans is also used for large scale production of vitamin B_{12} in a cost-effective manner. Starting with a low yield (0.6 mg/l) two decades ago, several improvements have been made in the strains of *P. denitrificans* for a tremendous improvement in the yield (60 mg/l).

Addition of cobalt and 5, 6-dimethyl benzimidazole to the medium is essential. The yield of vitamin B_{12} increases when the medium is supplemented with betaine (usual source being sugar beet molasses).

Carbon sources for vitamin B_{12} production

Glucose is the most commonly used carbon source for large scale manufacture of vitamin B_{12}. Other carbon sources like ***alcohols*** (methanol, ethanol, isopropanol) and ***hydrocarbons*** (alkanes, decane, hexadecane) with varying yields can also be used.

A yield of 42 mg/l of vitamin B_{12} was reported using methanol as the carbon source by the microorganism *Methanosarcina barkeri*, in fed-batch culture system.

RIBOFLAVIN

Riboflavin (vitamin B_{12}) is a water soluble vitamin, essential for growth and reproduction in man and animals. Deficiency of riboflavin in rats causes growth retardation, dermatitis and eye lesions. In humans, ***vitamin B_2 deficiency*** results in ***cheilosis*** (fissures at the corner of mouth), ***glossitis*** (purplish tounge) and ***dermatitis***. Riboflavin exerts its biochemical functions through the coenzymes namely ***flavin adenine dinucleotide (FAD)*** and ***flavin mononucleotide (FMN)***.

Occurrence

Riboflavin occurs in milk and milk products, meat, eggs, liver and kidney. While in milk and eggs, it is present in free form, in other foods it is found in the form of flavoproteins (i.e. coenzymes of riboflavin bound to proteins).

Chemistry

Riboflavin contains **6, 7-*dimethyl isoalloxazine*** (a heterocyclic 3 ring structure) attached to ***D-ribitol*** by a nitrogen atom. The isoalloxazine ring participates in the oxidation-reduction reactions brought out by the coenzymes (FAD and FMN).

Biosynthesis

The biosynthetic pathway of riboflavin, elucidated for the microorganisms *Ashbya gossypii* and *Eremothecium ashbyii* is depicted in ***Fig. 27.2***. The overproduction of riboflavin in these organisms takes place mainly due to the constitutive nature of the riboflavin synthesizing enzymes. Iron which inhibits the production of vitamin B_{12} in clostridia and yeasts, has no effect on *A. gossypii* and *E. ashbyii*.

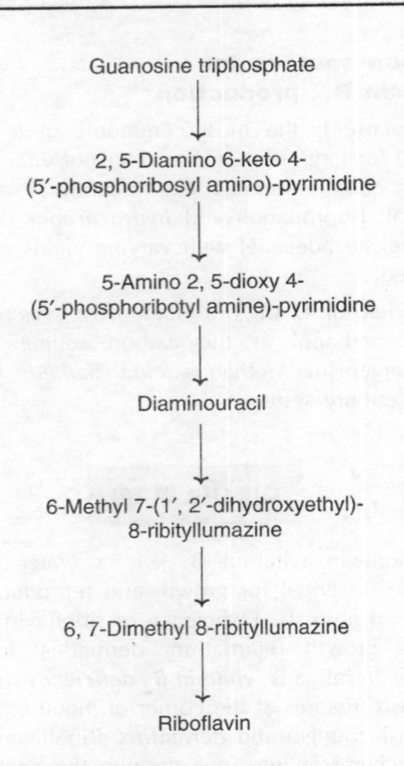

Fig. 27.2 : Biosynthesis of riboflavin.

COMMERCIAL PRODUCTION OF RIBOFLAVIN

There are three processes employed for the large scale production of riboflavin. The worldwide requirement of riboflavin is estimated to be around 2,500 tones per year.

1. **Biotransformation** : About 50% of the world's requirement of riboflavin is produced by biotransformation, followed by chemical synthesis. For this purpose, glucose is first converted to D-ribose by mutant strains of *Bacillus pumilus.* The D-ribose so produced is converted to riboflavin by chemical reactions.

2. **Chemical synthesis :** Approximately 20% of the world's riboflavin is produced by direct chemical synthesis.

3. **Fermentation :** At least one third of world's riboflavin requirements are met by direct fermentation processes.

Microorganisms and yields of riboflavin

Several microorganisms (bacteria, yeasts and fungi) can be employed for the production of riboflavin. In the acetone-butanol fermentation, employing the organisms *Clostridium acetobutylicum* and *Clostridium butylicum,* riboflavin is formed as a byproduct.

Commercial production of riboflavin is predominantly carried out by direct fermentation using the ascomycetes. The different organisms used and the corresponding yields of riboflavin are given in ***Table 27.2***. The two plant pathogens namely *Ashbya gossypii* and *Eremothecium ashbyii* are most commonly employed due to high yield. Among these two organisms, *A. gossypii* is preferred as it is more stable with a high producing capacity of riboflavin.

Genetically engineered strains for riboflavin production : High yielding strains of *Ashbya gossypii* have been developed by genetic manipulations. Such strains can yield as high as 15 g/l riboflavin.

Production process of riboflavin

Industrial production of riboflavin is mostly carried out with the organism, ***Ashbya gossypii*** by using simple sugars such as glucose and corn steep liquor. Glucose can be replaced by sucrose or maltose for the supply of carbon source. In recent years, lipids such as corn oil, when added to the medium for energy purpose, have a profound influence on riboflavin production. Further, supplementation of the medium with yeast extract, peptones, glycine, inositol, purines (not pyrimidines) also increase the yield of riboflavin.

It is essential to carefully sterilize the medium for good yield of riboflavin. The initial pH of the culture medium is adjusted to around 6-7.5. The

TABLE 27.2 Microorganisms with corresponding yields of riboflavin

Microorganism	*Yield (mg/l)*
Clostridium acetobutylicum	0.097
Clostridium butylicum	0.120
Mycobacterium smegmatis	0.060
Mycocandida riboflavina	0.200
Candida flareri	0.575
Eremothecium ashbyii	2.500
Ashbya gossypii	7.500

fermentation is conducted at temperature 26–28°C with an aeration rate 0.3 vvm. The process is carried out for about 5-7 days by submerged aerated fermentation.

Riboflavin fermentation by *Eremothecium ashbyii* is comparable to that described above for *Ashbya gossypii*. *Candida* sp can also produce riboflavin, but this fermentation process is extremely sensitive to the presence of iron. Consequently, iron or steel equipment cannot be used. Such equipment have to be lined with plastic material.

Fermentation through phases

Some studies have been carried out to understand the process of fermentation of riboflavin particularly by ascomycetes. It is now accepted that the fermentation occurs through ***three phases***.

Phase I : This phase is characterized by rapid growth of the organism utilizing glucose. As pyruvic acid accumulates, pH becomes acidic. The growth of the organism stops as glucose gets exhausted. In phase I, there is no production of riboflavin.

Phase II : Sporulation occurs in this phase, and pyruvate concentration decreases. Simultaneously, there is an accumulation of ammonia (due to enhanced deaminase activity) which makes the medium alkaline. Phase II is characterized by a maximal production of riboflavin. But this is mostly in the form of FAD and a small portion of it as FMN.

Phase III : In this last phase, cells get disrupted by a process of autolysis. This allows release of FAD, FMN and free riboflavin into the medium.

Recovery : Riboflavin is found in fermentation broth and in a bound form to the cells. The latter can be released by heat treatment i.e. 120°C for about 1 hour. The cells can be discarded after filtration or centrifugation. The filtrate can be further purified and dried, as per the requirements.

Other carbon sources for riboflavin production

Besides ***sugars***, other carbon sources have also been used for riboflavin production. A pure grade of riboflavin can be prepared by using *Saccharomyces* sp, utilizing ***acetate*** as sole carbon source. Methanol-utilizing organism *Hansenula polymorpha* was found to produce riboflavin. The other carbon sources used with limited success for riboflavin production are aliphatic hydrocarbons (organism *Pichia guilliermoudii*) and n-hexadecane (organisms — *Pichia miso*).

β-CAROTENE

β-Carotene is the ***provitamin A***. When ingested, it gets converted to vitamin A in the intestine. Vitamin A is a fat soluble vitamin required for vision, proper growth and reproduction. The ***deficiency of vitamin A causes night blindness***, changes in the skin and mucosal membranes.

Occurrence and chemistry

β-Carotene is found in many animal and plant tissues. However, it originates exclusively from plants or microorganisms. Yellow and dark green vegetables and fruits are rich in β-carotene e.g. carrots, spinach, amaranthus, mango, papaya.

Carotenoids are isoprene derivatives. Chemically, they are tetraterpenoids with eight isoprene residues. There are around 400 naturally occurring carotenoids. The most important carotenoids are β-carotene, α-carotene, δ-carotene, lycopene and zeaxanthin.

Carotenoids are mainly used as colouring agents e.g., β-carotene, lycopene, xanthophylls. Several foods (cheese, meat, egg products) can be made attractive by coloration. It may be noted that the demand for β-carotene as the provitamin A is comparatively less.

Biosynthesis

The pathway for the biosynthesis of β-carotene and some other important carotenoids, elucidated in plants and fungi, is shown in ***Fig. 27.3***.

COMMERCIAL PRODUCTION OF β-CAROTENE

β-Carotene can be produced by microbial fermentation. However, for economic reasons, direct chemical synthesis of vitamin A is preferred rather than using its provitamin (β-carotene).

Microorganisms

The organisms *Blakeslea trispora, Phycomyces blakesleeanus* and *Choanephora cucurbitarum* are most frequently used for the production of

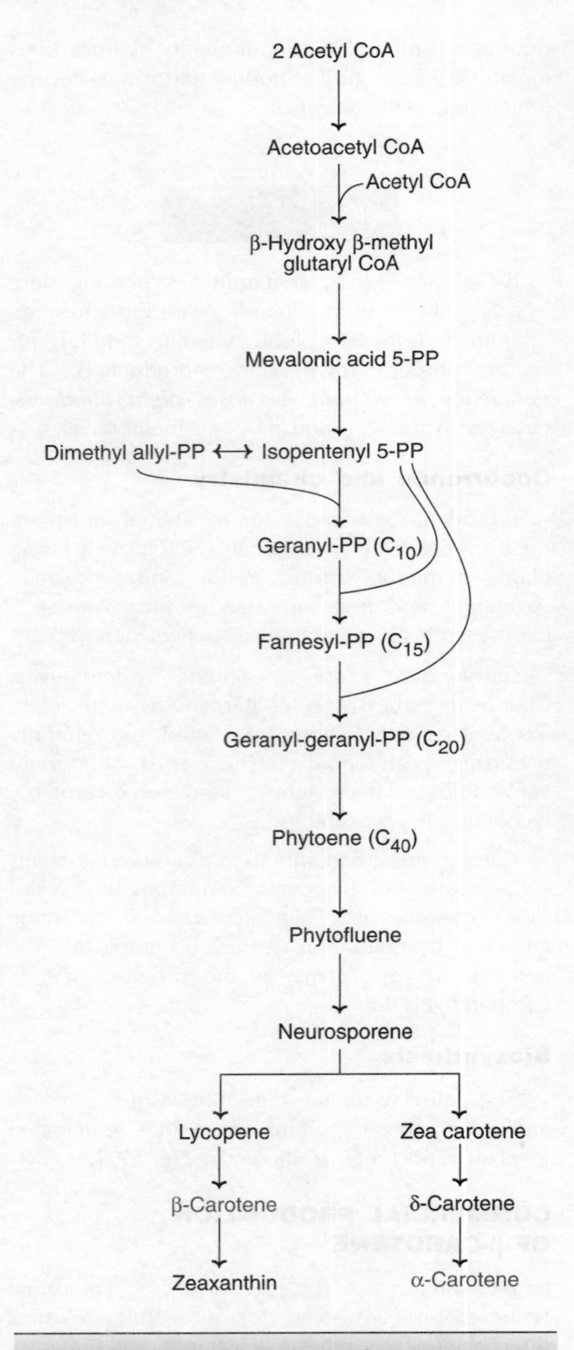

Fig. 27.3 : Biosynthesis of carotenes.

β-carotene. Among these, *Blakeslea trispora* is preferred due to high yield. In the ***Table 27.3***, some important carotenoids, the organisms and the production yields are given.

TABLE 27.3 Microbial production of important carotenoids

Carotenoid	*Organism*	*Production yield (g/l)*
β-Carotene	*Blakeslea trispora* (mixed cultures of + and – sexual forms)	3.0
Lycopene	*Blakeshlea trispora* (mixed culture)	0.4
	Streptomyces chrestomyceticus	0.5
Zeaxanthin	*Flavobacterium* sp	0.4

Production process of β-carotene

As already stated, the industrial production of β-carotene is mostly carried out by *Blakeslea trispora*. The fermentation medium contains corn starch, soybean meal, β-ionone, antioxidants etc. Addition of antioxidants improves the stability of β-carotene with in the cells. The ***fermentation is carried out by submerged process***.

The fermentation is usually started by mixing the cultures of both sexual forms, (+) and (–) strains of *B. trispora*. The yield of β-carotene is significantly higher with mixed cultures, compared to + or – strains (***Fig. 27.4***). This is due to the fact that

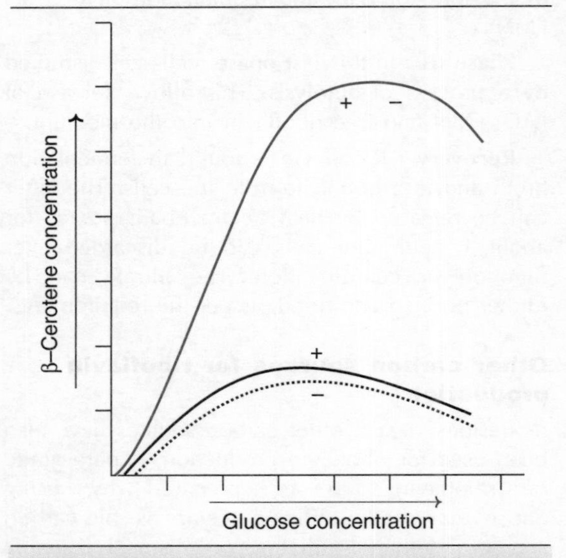

Fig. 27.4 : Yield of β–carotene by +, – and mixed (+ –) cultures of Blakesba trispora.

β-carotene production predominantly occurs during the process of zygospore formation. It may be stated here that the use of mixed strains does not improve the yield for other microorganisms (as observed in case of *Blakeslea trispora*).

Factors affecting production : Trisporic acid which can act as a microbial sexual hormone improves production yield of β-carotene. β-Ionones enhance β-carotene synthesis by increasing the activity of enzymes, and not by their direct incorporation into β-carotene. When the fermentation medium is supplemented with purified kerosene, β-carotene production is almost doubled. Kerosene increases the solubility of hydrophobic substrates.

Recovery : The mycelium rich in β-carotene can be directly used as a feed additive. For purification, mycelium is removed, subjected to dehydration (by methanol) and extracted in methylene chloride. This product is of 70–85% purity which can be further purified as per the requirements.

GIBBERELLINS — PLANT GROWTH STIMULANTS

Gibberellins are plant hormones that stimulate plant growth. They promote growth by cell enlargement and cell division. The observable effects of gibberellins include stimulus to seed germination, flowering and lengthening of stems.

MICROBIAL PRODUCTION OF GIBBERELLINS

So far only one microorganism, ***the fungus*** namely ***Gibberella fujikuroi has been found to produce gibberellins***. This is actually a pathogenic fungus of rice seedlings.

Gibberellin production can be carried out by using a glucose-salt medium at pH 7.5 and temperature 25°C for 2-3 days. The fermentation process is conducted in aerated submerged process. After the growth of the fungus is maximum, the production of gibberellins commences.

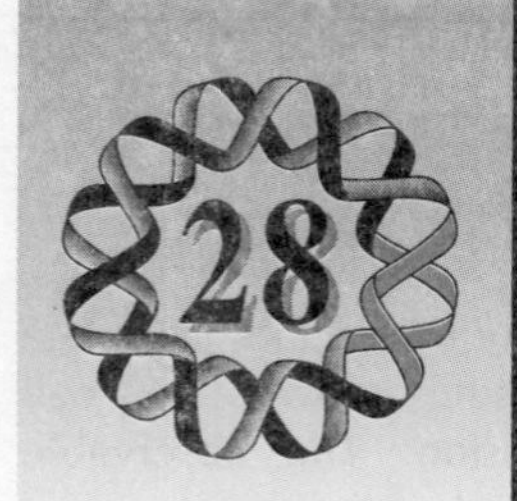

Microbial Production of Foods and Beverages

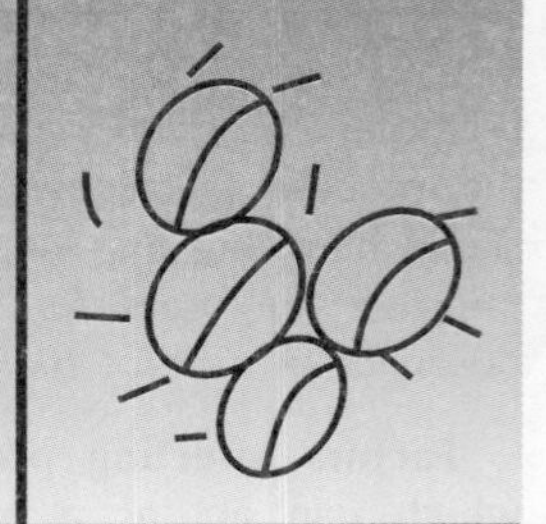

It is estimated that about 20–30% of the household budget is spent towards foods in the developed countries. This may be a little less in the developing nations. Therefore, food and beverage biotechnology occupies a prominent place world-over.

There are records that man was making bread, wine, curd etc., as early as 4000 BC. These processes, collectively referred to as ***traditional*** or ***old biotechnology***, mostly employed for the preparation of foods and beverages, were ***based on the natural capabilities of the microorganisms*** (although their existence was unknown at that time).

With the advances made in microbiology and recently biotechnology, food and beverage production is a major industry. Food biotechnology is also concerned with the improved quality, nutrition, consistency, colour, safety and preservation of foods, besides making them available round the year (**Note :** Most foods are seasonal in nature and therefore as such are not available throughout the year). In addition, modern biotechnological processes also take into account the health aspects of the people.

FERMENTED FOODS

The production of fermented foods is variable. This depends on geographical region, availability of raw materials, traditions and food habits of the people. A selected list of fermented foods along with raw materials and fermenting microorganisms is given in ***Table 28.1***.

Advantages of fermented foods

- Enhanced nutritive value.
- Increased digestibility.
- Improved flavour and texture.
- Serve as supplements in preparing several dishes.

Besides the list given in ***Table 28.1***, there are many other compounds that are directly or indirectly used as food supplements which must also be referred by the reader. These include vitamins (Chapter 27), amino acids (Chapter 26), organic acids (Chapter 23), enzymes (Chapter 21), biopolymers (Chapter 30), single-cell proteins and mushrooms (Chapter 29).

A selected few of the fermented foods with special reference to their production are described briefly in this chapter.

CHEESE

Cheese production is the largest dairy industry in the world. There are around 1,000 types of different cheeses. They are broadly of two types — ***unripened cheeses*** (cottage cheese with low fat, cream cheese with high fat) and ***ripened cheeses*** (hard cheese e.g. chedder, blue cheese; soft cheese e.g. limburger, camembert). Irrespective of the type of the cheese, all of them are invariably ***made from the casein of milk***, that is produced after separating

TABLE 28.1 A selected list of fermented foods along with the raw materials and fermenting organisms

Fermented food/food product (country)	*Raw material (substrate)*	*Fermenting organism(s)*
Dairy products		
Cheese (worldwide)	Milk	*Streptococcus* sp *Penicillium roquefortii, P. camembertii*
Yogurt (worldwide)	Milk	*Streptococcus thermophilus* *Lactobacillus bulgaricus*
Kefir (Russia)	Milk	*Lactobacillus* sp, *Candida* sp
Vegetarian products		
Cocoa beans (worldwide)	Cocoa fruit	*Candida krusei, Geotrichum* sp
Coffee beans (worldwide)	Coffee cherries	*Edwinia dissolvens, Saccharomyces* sp
Tempeh (Indonesia)	Soy beans	*Rhizopus oryzae, Lactobacillus delbrueckiia*
Soy sauce (worldwide)	Soy beans	*Aspergillus orzyae, A. soyae*
Sauekraut (Europe)	Cabbage	*Leuconostoc mesenteroides, L. plantarum*
Breads (worldwide)	Wheat flour	*Saccharomyces cerevisiae*
Rolls, cakes (worldwide)	Wheat flour	*Saccharomyces cerevisiae*
Idli (India)	Rice and black gram	*Leuconotoc mesenteroides*
Non-vegetarian products		
Dry sausages (worldwide)	Beef, pork	*Pedicoccus cerevisiae*
Fish sauces (worldwide)	Small fish	*Halophilic* sp, *Bacillus* sp
Country-cured hams (worldwide)	Pork, hams	*Aspergillus* sp, *Penicillium* sp

the whey (liquid portion of milk). Milk from different animals can be used e.g. sheep, cow, goat, buffalo.

Historical perspective

The use of animal stomachs for carrying liquids is centuries old. When milk was transported in this fashion, the formation of solids (that were tasty) was observed. The solids were concentrated after draining liquids. These solids were salted and consumed later. A good example of food preservation, long long ago! We now know that this solid portion is the cheese. It is produced by the combined action of enzymes (rennet) of the stomach living and the bacterial contamination.

Production process

As already stated, cheese is produced from milk. This is carried out by a process of dehydration wherein casein (milk protein) and fats are concentrated 5–15 fold. Cheese production is very complicated, and broadly involves four stages- acidification of milk, coagulum formation, separation of curd from whey and ripening of cheese.

1. **Acidification of milk :** By employing lactic acid bacteria (*Streptococcus lactis, Lactobacillus lactis*) the sugar of milk (lactose) can be converted to lactic acid. This lowers the pH to around 4.6, and thus acidifies milk.

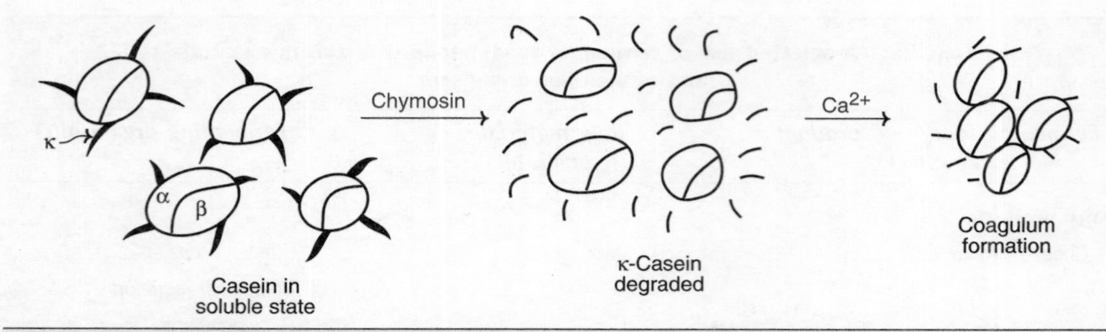

Fig. 28.1 : Formation of coagulum (curd) in the production of cheese.

2. **Coagulum formation :** When the acidified milk is treated with **rennet** (i.e. the enzyme chymosin of animal or fungal origin), casein gets coagulated. Casein mainly consists of three components-insoluble α and β caseins and a κ-casein that keeps them in soluble state. By the action of chymosin, κ-casein is degraded. Consequently, α and β caseins and the degraded products of κ casein combine to form a coagulum (curd) (***Fig. 28.1***). This process of coagulation is dependent on calcium ions.

3. **Separation of curd from whey :** When the temperature of the coagulum is raised to around 40°C; the coagulum (curd) and whey (fluid portion) get separated. The separated curd is cut into blocks, drained and pressed into different shapes.

4. **Ripening of cheese :** The flavour of raw cheese (with rubber texture) such as ***cheddar*** is bland. Ripening imparts flavours, besides making changes in its texture. The procedures adopted for ripening (or maturation) are highly variable depending on the type of cheese to be prepared. The blocks of curd separated are subjected to the action of proteases and/or lipases. Alternatively, they may be inoculated with certain fungi (e.g. *Penicillium roquefortii*). The hydrolysis of proteins and fats (either by enzymes or microorganisms) results in certain compounds which imparts flavour to the cheese. Mild hydrolysis of fats (or cheese), usually carried out by lipases or *Aspergillus niger* or *Mucor maihai* results in butyric acid formation with characteristic flavour.

A diagrammatic representation of cheese production is depicted in ***Fig. 28.2***.

Sources of chymosin for cheese production

There are several sources of rennet (chymosin enzyme) for cheese production. These include calves, adult cows, pigs and fungal sources. Fortunately, the fungal (e.g. *Mucor meihei*) sources of chymosin are almost comparable to the animal sources and are widely used in some countries. However, some people always prefer animal rennet used cheese due to its slight superior flavour.

Genetically engineered microorganisms for chymosin : Some workers could successfully clone the genes of animal chymosin and transfer the same into microorganisms. The chymosin so produced by genetic manipulation is very widely used these

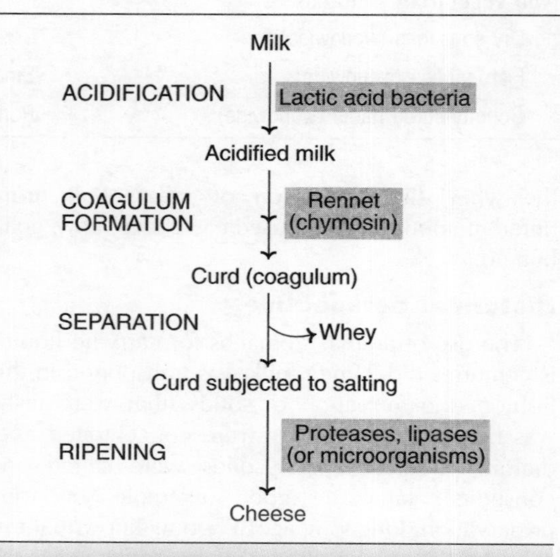

Fig. 28.2 : A diagrammatic representation of cheese production.

days in some countries. The taste of cheese manufactured by microbial chymosin (i.e. genetically engineered) and the animal chymosin are identical. Public as well as the vegetarian societies in some countries have accepted the cheese produced by the genetic manipulation of the enzyme, chymosin.

YOGHURT

Yoghurt is produced ***by fermenting whole milk*** by employing a mixed culture of *Lactobacillus bulgaricus* and *Streptococcus thermophilus*. While *L. bulgaricus* produces acetaldehyde that imparts a characteristic taste, *S. thermophilus* results in the formation of lactic acid to give acid flavour. In addition, both these bacteria produce extracellular polymers that increase the viscosity of the fermented milk. Yoghurt is very delicious and in fact frozen yoghurt is becoming popular as an alternative to ice cream.

SAUEKRAUT

Sauekraut is prepared in most western countries. It is a ***fermented and preserved form of cabbage***. The shredded cabbage is mixed with salt (approximately at 2.5% concentration) and packed anaerobically. High salt concentration promotes leakage of sugars from the cabbage while reducing the water activity. As the growth of the lactic acid bacteria occurs, the pH is lowered. At this low pH, the putrifying bacteria cannot grow. In this way, sauekraut can be preserved for long. Sauekraut is nutritious as well as delicious.

The traditional pickles (mango, lemon, etc.) in India are also good examples of fermentation and preservation, based on the principles of biotechnology.

BREAD

Bread making from the dough by employing microorganisms is one of the oldest examples of fermentation processes known to mankind. There is evidence that bread was prepared in Egypt in 3000 BC.

Primarily, bread is a ***fermented product of cereal flours such as wheat and rye***. The cereal flour mixed with water, salt, sugar, fat and other ingradients (as desired for enrichment of bread) is subjected to fermentation by yeast, *Saccharomyces cerevisiae* (top fermenting strain). The main reaction that occurs during bread formation is the fermentation of hexoses to CO_2 and ethanol.

$$C_6H_{12}O_6 \longrightarrow 2C_2H_5OH + 2CO_2$$

The ethanol produced either gets evaporated or forms esters. The CO_2 gets entrapped in the dough resulting in its expansion. The expansion and stretching of the dough, particularly with wheat is due to the unique ***elastic protein*** namely ***gluten***. Gluten is mainly responsible for retaining the shape of bread.

Besides yeast enzymes, the enzymes (e.g. amylases) of other microorganisms also help in fermentation and baking of bread. The texture of bread is influenced by fats and emulsifiers added to the dough. The bread making is carried out with three objectives :

- Good leavening due to CO_2 formation.
- Flavour development.
- Good texture.

The yeast fermented bread has the above characteristics. This is in contrast to the bread produced with baking powder which also produces CO_2. But this does not have the same flavour and texture as that produced by yeast. Thus the yeast, which is appropriately referred to as ***baker's yeast*** is a package of enzymes to give a desired product.

In recent years, some workers have reported the development of ***genetically engineered strains*** of ***Saccharomyces cerevisiae*** with improved fermentation properties. Such organisms, when used in baking industry, are believed to further enhance the quality of bread with regard to flavour, texture etc.

Sour-dough breads : In some parts of the world, sour breads are prepared by using the yeast, *Candida milleri* and bacterium, *Lactobacillus sanfrancisco*.

BAKER'S YEAST

The living cells of aerobically grown Saccharomyces cerevisiae are collectively referred to as baker's yeast. Baker's yeast is commercially available either as a dried powder i.e. dry yeast with about 95% dry weight or in the form of cakes (about 25–30% dry weight). These commercially available yeast preparations can be used in bread making.

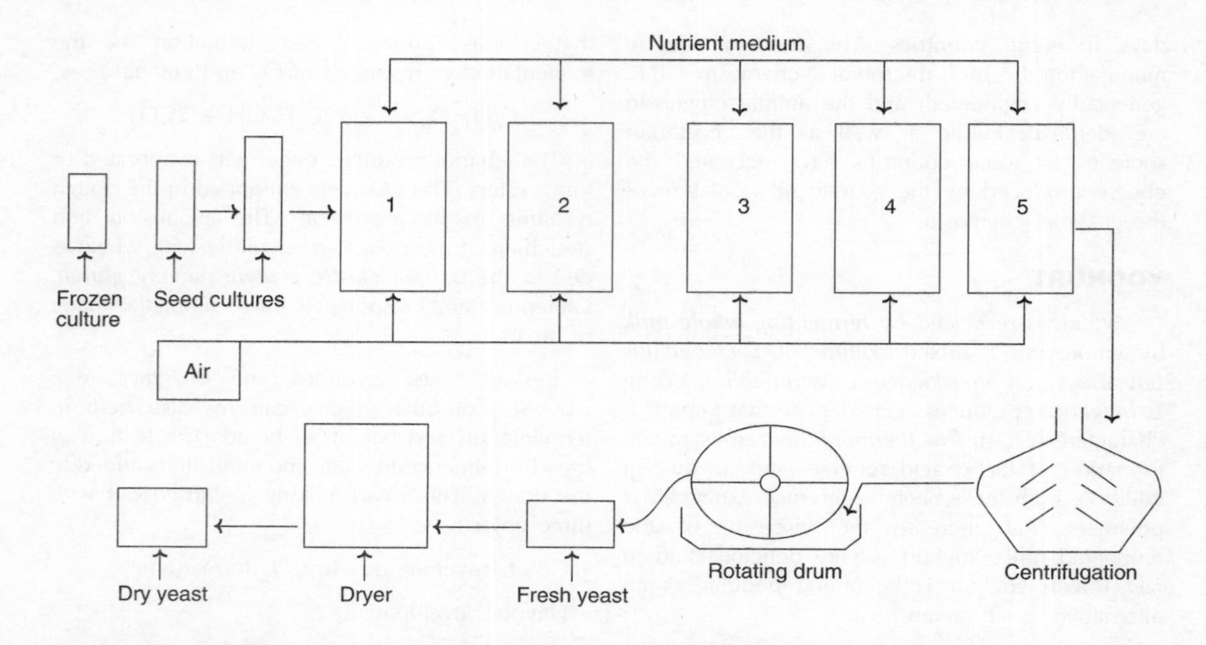

Fig. 28.3 : Flow chart for the production of baker's yeast (1 is the inoculation reactor, 2–5 are production reactors).

Production of baker's yeast : The medium for baker's yeast production contains molasses, ammonium salts (or ammonia), vitamins, phosphates and antifoam agents. Sugar cane or sugar beet molasses can be used. A commercially available molasses with a sugar concentration of 45–50% is usually preferred. Baker's yeast production is carried out by an ***aerobic fed-batch process***.

The flow chart for the production of baker's yeast is depicted in ***Fig. 28.3***. The actual production process and the strain of *Saccharomyces cerevisiae* used depends on the company. The desired strain is maintained in a frozen state. The inoculum is prepared in stages so that large volumes are finally obtained. From the inoculation reactor (fermenter), the culture is transferred to production reactors. The process is carried out in air-lift or bubble column type reactors at pH 4-5, temperature 28–30°C for about 12–18 hours. The yeast cells are washed, centrifuged and then dewatered on a rotating drum. The fresh yeast obtained can be either directly used or dried and stored.

The yeast cells may be mixed with plasticizer (e.g. vegetable oil) and prepared in a block form. This block can be cut into small pieces, wraped and stored (at –4°C) until used. The samples of yeast are usually tested for baking properties before they are put in use.

OTHER VEGETARIAN PRODUCTS

Besides the bread which is consumed worldwide, there are several other vegetarian fermented foods. These include ***rolls*** and ***cakes*** (worldwide) ***soy sauce*** (worldwide) ***idli*** (India) and ***tempeh*** (Indonesia).

Coffee, tea and cocoa

Coffee, tea and cocoa are very popular non-alcoholic fermented beverages, and extensively consumed throughout the world.

When the tea leaves are crushed, the chemical components of tea are released by enzymatic activity. For coffee and cocoa, a natural fermentation process (by bacteria, yeast and fungi) on the pulp surrounding beans results in the development of flavour and aroma. The exact nature of the fermentation processes involved in tea, coffee and cocoa are not fully known.

The dried products namely tea leaves, and coffee and cocoa beans are commercially available for beverage preparation.

SWEETENERS

Sweeteners occupy a prominent place in food consumption, by all the people. The most predominantly used ***natural sweetener*** is ***sucrose*** (obtained from sugar cane or beet). Sweeteners are invariably required for the preparation of soft drinks, ice creams, jams, jellies, sauces, bread, confectionery, pickles etc. Hence there is a continuous search for low calorie sweeteners.

Saccharin, a chemically synthesized sweetener (300 times sweeter than sucrose) was used for several years, and its use is now being restricted due to certain adverse health effects. ***High fructose corn syrup*** (***HFCS***), produced from sucrose is sweeter (1.5 times) than sucrose. ***Aspartame*** (aspartyl phenylalanine) is a product of innovative biotechnology. It is about ***200 times sweeter than sucrose*** and is truely a ***low calorie sweetener***. Aspartame is approved for human consumption and is widely used in soft drink and other industries.

THAUMATIN-A SWEET PROTEIN

Thaumatin is a protein extracted from the berries of the *Thaumatococcus daniellii*, a native plant in Africa. Thaumatin is about ***3000 times sweeter than sucrose***. Thaumatin certainly appears to be a good sugar substitute and a low-calorie sweetener. It is in fact being used as a sweetener and flavour enhancer of various foods. At least five different forms of thaumatins with a molecular weights in the range of 20,000–22,000 have been isolated and characterized.

Genetic engineering to produce thaumatin

Natural production of thaumatin is very limited and therefore can never meet the demands of consumption. Biotechnological production of this sweetener is the method of choice for its large scale manufacture.

Thaumatin-encoding mRNA species have been isolated, identified and converted to cDNA and finally to double-stranded DNA. These DNAs were cloned and transferred to *E. coli*. But the yield of thaumatin production was very low. Attempts were also made to express thaumatin genes in yeasts such as *S. cerevisiae* and *Kluyveromyces lactis*. Some success has been reported in this direction.

MONELLIN-A CANDIDATE FOR SUGAR SUBSTITUTE

Monellin is a ***protein*** found in the fruit of an African plant *Discorephyllum cumminsii*. It is about ***100,000 times sweeter than sucrose*** (on molar basis). Monellin is dimer composed of an A-chain (45 amino acids) and a B-chain (50 amino acids). This protein is optimally sweet when both the chains are held together and not when they are separated.

It has been possible to chemically synthesize a gene that encodes both A and B chains as a single polypeptide. This gene was in fact introduced and expressed in tomatoes for the production of monellin. However, the success has been very limited.

FLAVOUR ENHANCERS

Taste and flavour are very important for the acceptability of foods. ***Monosodium glutamate is the most commonly used flavour enhancer***. Its production and other aspects are described elsewhere (Chapter 26). The degraded products of proteins and RNAs also impart flavour. Thaumatin and monellin (described above) are also flavour enhancing agents, besides sweetening.

The other flavouring agents are citric acid (produced by *Aspergillus niger*), acetone and butanol (produced by *Clostridium acetobutylicum*). The lactones formed by some microbial fermentations also enhance flavour e.g. γ-butyrolactone produced in yeast fermentation of wine and beer. Mention must be made about alcohol also which can increase flavour and taste when added at appropriate concentrations e.g. certain medicinal syrups.

ALCOHOLIC BEVERAGES

Alcoholic beverages are produced throughout the world. The type of the beverage and the substrate used for its production mostly depends on the crops grown in the region. For instance, in

TABLE 28.2 Alcoholic beverages along with the common substrates used for their production

Beverage	*Alcohol (%)*	*Substrate(s)*
Beer (ale, lager)	4–8	Barley and other cereals
Wine (red, white)	10–16	Grapes
Sake	10–14	Rice
Champagne	10–12	Grapes
Cidar	7–12	Apple juice
Brandy	35–45	Grapes or other fruits
Whisky	40–55	Cereals (barley, rye, corn)
Rum	50–60	Molasses
Gin, vodka	40–50	Potato, wheat, rye
Chinese brandy	30–40	Rice
Toddy	5–15	Palmyra juice
Arrack	60–75	Rice, jaggery, waste carbohydrates

Poland, Russia and Scandinavia, beers manufactured from barely are consumed while in France, Italy and Greece, wines obtained from palmyra juice are mostly consumed by rural people.

The common types of alcoholic beverages with their alcoholic contents and substrates used for their production are given in ***Table 28.2***.

Historical perspective

Archaelogical evidence indicates that there existed fermentation of grains as early as 4000 B.C. Production of alcoholic beverages is considered to be a part of human civilization. The biological and chemical principles underlying alcoholic beverage production were elucidated by Louis Pasteur in the second half of nineteenth century.

Saccharomyces cerevisiae—the key organism for the production of alcoholic beverages

The most commonly used organism for the production of beverages is the yeast, *Saccharomyces cerevisiae*. This organism is capable of utilizing simple sugars (glucose, fructose) and converting them to ethanol. It is fortunate that *S. cerevisiae* is a unique organism that can ***tolerate*** and grow even at a ***high concentration of alcohol***. This is advantageous for good production yield of alcoholic beverages.

There are two types of *S. cerevisiae* strains—***bottom yeast*** and ***top yeast***. The bottom yeast settles to the bottom whereas the top yeast raises to the top while carrying out fermentation. Top yeast are frequently used for the production of beer while bottom yeast are employed for wine production. However, both strains can be used for beverage production.

Genetically engineered strains of *S. cerevisiae* : By employing recombinant DNA technology, new strains of *Saccharomyces cerevisiàe* are constantly being developed. Some of these strains with ***improved production yields of alcoholic beverages***, are in fact approved for use in beverage industries.

ALCOHOLIC BEVERAGE PRODUCTION —GENERAL ASPECTS

The starting materials for beverage production are sugary or starchy materials.

Sugary materials : Fruit juice (or fruits), plant sap and honey that can be directly used.

Starchy materials—various grains and roots : They have to be subjected to hydrolysis to yield simple fermentable sugars. This process, referred to as ***saccharification***, is carried out either by plant materials (barley malt, rye malt or millet malt) or microorganisms (*Aspergillus* sp, *Rhizopus* sp. *Mucor sp*) rich in starch hydrolytic enzymes.

Fermentation process : When subjected to fermentation under ideal conditions, alcohol production ranging from 2 to 16% is usually observed. These alcoholic beverages may be appropriately processed and drunk. e.g. beers. However, for the production of beverages with higher concentration of alcohol (brandy, whisky, rum, gin etc.), distillation has to be carried out to increase the alcohol content.

Brewing is the technical term used for the ***production of malt beverages***. Besides *S. cerevisiae* (described already), *S. carlsbergensis* is also used in brewing industry. The finished products in brewing namely the alcoholic beverages differ from the other industrial fermented products. This is because besides the alcohol content, several other factors are important in finished beverages. These include flavour, aroma, colour, clarity, foam production and stability, and satiety. These factors decide the consumer acceptance and the commercial value of alcoholic beverages. All these beverages can be consumed when freshly produced. However, they are normally kept for storing or aging before consumption. Aging certainly improves flavour, aroma etc.

The commercial production processes employed for the manufacture of beer and wine are briefly described hereunder.

BEER

Beer is an ***undistilled alcoholic beverage*** with alcohol content in the range of 4-8%. It is produced by fermentation of barley or other cereals, by employing the yeasts (most frequently) *S. cerevisiae* or (sometimes) *S. carlsbergensis*.

It is often necessary to add starch — rich materials (wheat, maize, rice) known as ***adjuncts***, to enhance fermentation, besides reducing the cost of raw materials. There are four major steps involved in the production of beer (***Fig. 28.4***).

1. **Malting :** Dried barely are cleaned and soaked in water for a period of two days. The excess water is drained and the soaked barley are incubated for 4-6 days to germinate. Germination process is associated with the formation of enzymes-***amylases*** (starch hydrolysing) and ***proteases*** (protein degrading). The germinated seeds are slowly subjected to increased temperature (up to 80°C) so that the germination process is halted, but the enzymes retain their activities. Malt is prepared by powdering the seeds.

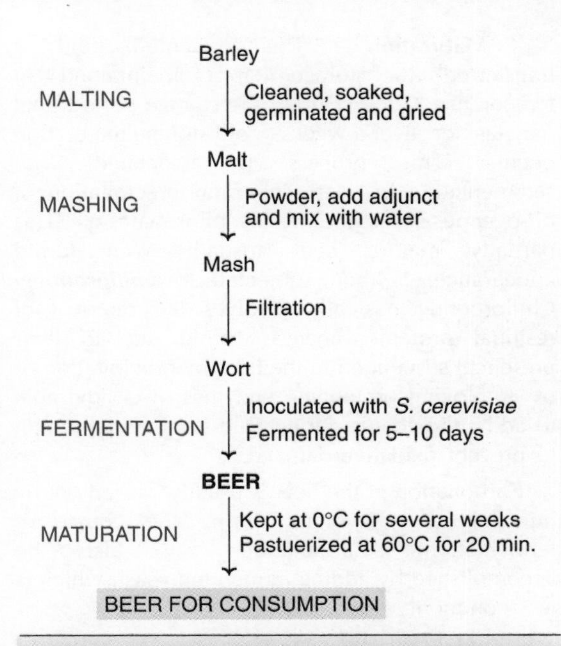

***Fig. 28.4 :** Flow chart representing an outline of beer production.*

2. **Mashing :** The powdered malt is mixed with hot water (55–65°C). During the course of mashing, the soluble materials from malt and malt adjuncts are extracted. Mashing is also associated with degradation of starches (by amylases) to produce dextrins, maltose and glucose and hydrolysis of protein (by proteases) to peptones, peptides and amino acids. The temperature and pH influence the activities of enzymes. At the end of mashing, the medium for fermentation which is referred to as ***beer wort*** is developed. This is rich in sugars, amino acids, minerals and vitamins.

Hops are the dried female flowers obtained from hop plant. Addition of hops to wort is often done to provide characteristic flavour, aroma and stabilizing effect to the beer. Besides providing a mild antibacterial activity.

3. **Fermentation :** The beer wort, kept in open or closed bioreactors, is inoculated with pure strains of yeast. *S. cerevisiae* (usually top fermenting strains). The fermentation is carried out at temperature 20–28°C for 5–10 days. In some countries, the bottom fermenting yeast *S. uvarum* is used. For this organism, the ideal temperature for optimal fermentation is 10–15°C.

4. **Maturation** : The fermented fluid is transferred to storage tanks maintained at temperature 0-3°C. During the storage period (that may last for several weeks), cold storage maturation occurs. This process is associated with sedimentation of yeast cells and precipitation of nitrogenous substances, resins, phosphates etc. This partially mature beer (usually with turbid appearance) is then subjected to ***chillproofing***. Chillproofing basically involves the removal of residual proteins (beer is turbid due to their presence) suspended in the beer by precipitation or by employing proteolytic enzymes. It is advisable to add antioxidants during cold-storage maturation to prevent oxidative damage.

Carbonation of the beer is usually carried out by injecting CO_2 (evolved during the course of fermentation). Carbonation can also be accomplished by adding fermenting yeast, which is less commonly done.

The matured and carbonated beer is bottled or canned, and then pasteurized at 60°C for about 20 minutes.

As already stated, there is variation in the raw materials used for beer production. For instance, in Africa it is ***sorghum beer*** that are commonly produced. This is in contrast to the ***barley beer*** produced in most Western countries.

WINES

Wines are originally Middle East and European drinks, although almost every country now produces them. Large scale production of wines is carried out by using ***grapes*** of species *Vitis vinifera*. Grape juice is a good source for wine production because of its high concentration of sugar and other nutrients, natural acidity (that can inhibit unwanted growth of microorganisms) and the capability to produce pleasant aroma and flavour.

Louis Pasteur often used to state ***'wine is the most healthy and most hygienic of beverages'***. There is some recent scientific evidence also in support of this view, since moderate wine consumption reduces the risk for coronary heart disease (CHD).

Production of wines

Quality of the grapes is very important for the production of wines. The grapes are crushed (mechanically or by treading of feet) and the juice extracted. This ***grape juice ready for fermentation*** process is technically referred to as ***must***. It is a practice to add sulfur dioxide to must to inhibit the growth of non-wine yeast and contaminating bacteria. Sulfur dioxide which can kill other organisms can be tolerated by wine-fermenting yeasts. Sometimes, the must may also be subjected to partial or complete sterilization. The must in suitable bioreactors is inoculated with desired strains of the yeast *Saccharomyces cerevisiae*. Initially, oxygen is bubbled through the fermentation medium to promote good growth of yeast cells and gradually anaerobic conditions are established. The wine production normally takes a few days (2-5 days). The fermentation conditions (temperature, time etc.) are actually dependent on the type of wine produced. At the end of fermentation, wines are transferred to storage tanks (or vats) and allowed to age, which may take some months or years. ***Ageing*** of wine is very important ***for the development of characteristic flavour and aroma***. The alcohol content of wines is in the range of 10–16%.

Types of wines

There are hundreds of different types of wines produced in different parts of the world.

Red wine : The red colour of this wine is due the colour extracted from the black grape skins (when crushed totally). Red wines are commonly drunk, by many people in the west, along with lunch and dinner.

White wine : Black grapes after removal of skins or white grapes are used for the production of white wine.

Rose wine : This can be produced with a limited contact to the skins of grapes during fermentation.

Dry wine : It contain relatively higher alcohol content and produced when sugars are completely fermented.

Sweet wine : This is sweet to taste since it contains some residual sugars after fermentation.

Fortified wines : The normal concentration of alcohol in wines is less than 16%. The wines can be fortified with addition of alcohol (usually done by adding brandy or other distilled spirits) to the desired concentration. Some examples of fortified wines are sherry, port and vermouth.

TABLE 28.3 Enzymes used in various food and beverage industries

Industry	*Enzymes*
Dairy	Chymosins (animal/microbial), lipase, lactase, lysozyme
Baking	α–Amylase, protease, phospholipases, xylanase
Starch and sugar	Amylases (α– and β–), glucoamylase, pollulanase, invertase, glucose isomerase, xylanase
Fruit and vegetable processing	Pectin esterase, pectin lyase, hemicellulases, polygalacturanase
Meat processing	Proteases, papain
Animal and fish bone processing	Alkaline phosphatase
Egg white processing	Glucose oxidase, catalase
Brewing production of beer and alcoholic beverage	Amylases (α– and β–), proteases, cellulases, papain, aminoglucosidases, xylanase

OTHER MICROBIALLY-DERIVED FOOD PRODUCTS

There are a large number food products or their ingradients, produced by microorganisms. For full details on them, the reader must refer the corresponding Chapters — single-cell protein and mushrooms (Chapter 29), vitamins (Chapter 27), amino acids (Chapter 26), organic acids (Chapter 24), polysaccharides (Chapter 30), and vinegar (Chapter 24).

ENZYMES IN FOOD AND BEVERAGE INDUSTRIES

Food and beverage biotechnology is very closely linked with the use of enzymes. While a majority of enzymes are microbial in nature, some other sources of enzymes can also be used. In ***Table 28.3***, a selected list of enzymes employed in food processing and beverage industries is given. Some of the aspects of enzymes in dairy, baking and brewing industries are described in the foregoing pages. A few more important ones are described hereunder.

Proteases in food industry

Proteases (proteolytic enzymes) are used ***for tenderisation of meat*** which flavours the meat, besides easy digestion. Proteases are employed for removal of meal attached to bones in the form of a slurry. This can be used for the preparation of soups and canned meats. Partial hydrolysis of certain vegetable proteins also increases their flavour e.g. proteins of soy bean; protein (gluten) of dough in preparing bread.

Lactase in dairy industry

Milk and whey contain about 4-5% lactose. ***Lactose intolerance***, due to a defect in the intestinal enzyme lactase, is ***very common in humans***. It is estimated that half of the world's population suffers from lactose intolerance. These individuals when consume milk and milk products containing lactose (particularly in large quantities) suffer from diarrhea and flatulance (abdominal cramps and increased intestinal motility). Obviously, lactose intolerant persons require milk products with a low lactose concentration.

The enzyme lactase cleaves lactose to glucose and galactose which can be easily assimilated by the body. The lactase enzyme may be obtained from microbial sources e.g. *Kluyveromyces fragilis, Aspergillus niger*. Sometimes, immobilized lactase can also be used to degrade lactose.

For the preparation of flavoured and condensed milks and ice creams, lactase is widely used.

ENZYMES IN THE PREPARATION OF FRUIT JUICES

The turbidity and cloudiness, commonly seen in fruit juices, is due to the presence of pectins and cell debris. Enzyme preparation containing ***pectin esterase, polygalacturonase, pectin lyase*** and hemicellulase is added to the fruit pulp ***for the removal of pectins and other turbid-causing materials***.

Removal of glucose and oxygen from foodstuffs

The presence of glucose and oxygen in the foods is often associated with certain amount of damage. Their removal enhances the storability of foods. Glucose from the foodstuffs can be removed by the combined action of glucose oxidase and catalase, as illustrated below.

$$\text{Glucose} + O_2 \xrightarrow{\text{Glucose oxidase}} \text{Gluconic acid} + H_2O_2$$

$$2H_2O_2 \xrightarrow{\text{Catalase}} 2H_2O + O_2$$

The egg white used in baking industry is made free from glucose by the enzymatic treatment, given above. This pair of enzymes (glucose oxidase + catalase) is also useful for the removal of O_2 present in the head space of bottled and canned foods and drinks.

DIAGNOSTICS IN FOOD BIOTECHNOLOGY

It is essential to ensure that the foods produced by biotechnological processes are free from disease-causing organisms and toxins. Then only the foods are suitable for human consumption. The most common pathogens present in foods are *Salmonella* sp, *Campylobacter* sp and *Listeria* sp. The food toxins are derived from bacterial (endototoxins) and fungal (mycotoxins) sources.

Several novel and innovative techniques have been developed in recent years for testing the safety of foods. For instance, the presence of *Salmonella* in foods can be detected by an immunoassy on the same day (This is in contrast to the traditional methods that take 5-7 days).

In fact, ***kits are available for the detection of concentrations of several undesirable compounds in the foods*** e.g. endotoxins, mycotoxins, antibiotics, hormones.

FOOD BIOTECHNOLOGY-PUBLIC ACCEPTANCE

In general, the public have a ***negative attitude towards*** the biotechnology based foods, particularly involving ***genetic manipulations***. For this reason, the application of genetic engineering techniques for food biotechnology is rather slow. Several factors influence the public acceptance. These include the type of biotechnology adopted, the regulatory procedures, economics of the people and consumer acceptance. For more details on this aspect, refer Chapter 61.

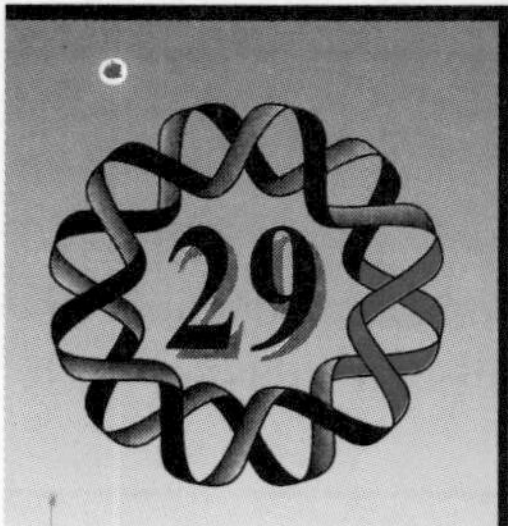

Single-Cell Protein, and Mushrooms

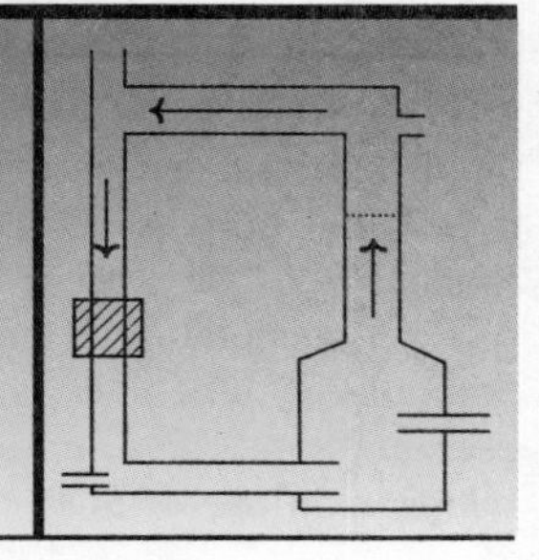

Single-cell protein (SCP) refers to the microbial cells or total protein extracted from pure microbial cell culture (monoculture) which can be used as protein supplement for humans or animals. The word SCP is considered to be appropriate, since most of the microorganisms grow as single or filamentious individuals. This is in contrast to complete multicellular plants and animals. If the ***SCP*** is suitable for human consumption, it is considered as ***food grade***. SCP is regarded as ***feed grade***, when it is used as animal feed supplement, but not suitable for human consumption.

Single-cell protein broadly refers to the ***microbial biomass*** or ***protein extract used as food or feed additive***. Besides high protein content (about 60–80% of dry cell weight), SCP also contains fats, carbohydrates, nucleic acids, vitamins and minerals. Another advantage with SCP is that it is rich in certain essential amino acids (lysine, methionine) which are usually limiting in most plant and animal foods. Thus, SCP is of high nutritional value for human or animal consumption.

It is estimated that about 25% of the world's population currently suffers from hunger and malnutrition. Most of these people live in developing countries. Therefore, SCP deserves a serious consideration for its use as food or feed supplement. In addition to its utility as a nutritional supplement, SCP can also be used for the isolation of several compounds e.g. carbohydrates, fats, vitamins, minerals.

Advantages of using microorganisms for SCP production

The protein-producing capabilities of a 250 kg cow and 250 g of microorganisms are often compared. The cow can produce about 200 g protein per day. On the other hand, microorganisms, theoretically, when grown under ideal conditions, could produce about 20–25 tonnes of protein. There are many advantages of using microorganisms for SCP production.

1. Microorganisms grow at a very rapid rate under optimal culture conditions. Some microbes double their mass in less than 30 minutes.

2. The ***quality and quantity of protein content in microorganisms is better compared to higher plants and animals***.

3. A ***wide range of raw materials***, which are otherwise wasted, ***can be fruitfully used*** for SCP production.

4. The culture conditions and the fermentation processes are very simple.

5. Microorganisms can be easily handled, and subjected to genetic manipulations.

Safety, acceptability and toxicology of SCP

There are many non-technological factors that influence the production of SCP. These include the geographical, social, political and psychological factors. In many countries, there are social and psychological barriers to use microorganisms as food sources. It is desirable to first consider the safety, acceptability and toxicology of SCP, particularly when it is considered for human consumption. There are several ***limitations for the widespread use of SCP***.

1. The ***nucleic acid content*** of microbial biomass is ***very high*** (4-6% in algae; 10–15% in bacteria; 5–10% in yeast). This is highly hazardous, since humans have a limited capacity to degrade nucleic acids.

2. The presence of ***carcinogenic and other toxic substances*** is often observed in association with SCP. These include the hydrocarbons, heavy metals, mycotoxins and some contaminants. The nature and production of these compounds depends on the raw materials, and the type of organism used.

3. There is a possibility of contamination of pathogenic microorganisms in the SCP.

4. The digestion of microbial cells is rather slow. This is frequently ***associated with indigestion and allergic reactions*** in individuals.

5. Food grade production of SCP is more expensive than some other sources of proteins e.g. soy meal. Of course, this mainly depends on the cost of raw materials. In general, SCP for human consumption is 10 times more expensive than SCP for animal feed.

For the above said reasons, many countries give low priority for the use of SCP for human consumption. In fact, mass production of SCP using costly raw materials has been discontinued in some countries e.g. Japan, Britain, Italy. However, these countries continue their efforts to produce SCP from cheap raw materials such as organic wastes.

MICROORGANISMS AND SUBSTRATES USED FOR PRODUCTION OF SCP

Several microorganisms that include bacteria, yeasts, fungi, algae and actiomycetes utilizing a wide range of substrates are used for the production of SCP. A selected list is given in ***Table 29.1***.

The selection of microorganisms for SCP production is based on several criteria. These include their nutritive value, non-pathogenic nature, production cost, raw materials used and growth pattern.

Substrates

The nature of the raw materials supplying substrates is very crucial for SCP production. The cost of raw material significantly influences the

TABLE 29.1 A selected list of microorganisms and substrates used for single-cell protein production

Microorganism	*Substrate(s)*
Bacteria	
Methylophilus methylotrophus	Methane, methanol
Methylomonas sp	Methanol
Pseudomonas sp	Alkanes
Brevibacterium sp	C_1–C_4 hydrocarbons
Yeasts	
Saccharomycopsis lipolytica (previous name—*Candida lipolytica*)	Alkanes
Candida utilis	Sulfite liquor
Kluyveromyces fragilis	Whey
Saccharomyces cerevisiae (baker's yeast)	Molasses
Lactobacillus bulgaricus	Whey
Tosulopsis sp	Methanol
Fungi	
Chaetomium cellulolyticum	Cellulosic wastes
Paecilomyces varioti	Sulfite liquor
Aspergillus niger	Molasses
Trichoderma viride	Straw, starch
Algae	
Spirulina maxima	Carbon dioxide
Chlorella pyrenoidosa	Carbon dioxide
Scenedesmus acutus	Carbon dioxide
Actinomycetes	
Nocardia sp	Alkanes
Thermomonospora fusca	Cellulose
Mushrooms (a type of fungi)	
Agaricus biosporus	Compost, rice straw
Morchella crassipes	Whey, sulfite liquor
Auricularia sp	Saw dust, rice bran
Lentinus edodes	Saw dust, rice bran
Volvariella volvaceae	Cotton, straw

final cost of SCP. The most commonly used raw materials may be grouped in the following categories.

1. **High-energy sources** e.g. alkanes, methane, methanol, ethanol, gas oil.

2. **Waste products** e.g. molasses, whey, sewage, animal manures, straw, begasse.

3. **Agricultural and foresty sources** e.g. cellulose, lignin.

4. **Carbon dioxide**, the simplest carbon source.

Some details on the production of SCP from most important raw materials are briefly described.

PRODUCTION OF SCP FROM HIGH ENERGY SOURCES

There are a large number of energy-rich carbon compounds or their derivatives which serve as raw materials for SCP production. These include ***alkanes, methane, methanol, ethanol and gas oil***. Bacteria and yeasts are mostly employed for SCP production from high energy sources. Some scientists question the wisdom of using (rather misusing) high-energy compounds for the production of food, since they regard it as a wasteful exercise.

Production of SCP from alkanes

Alkanes can be degraded by many yeasts, certain bacteria and fungi. The major limitation of alkanes is that they are not easily soluble, hence they cannot enter the cells rapidly. It is believed that the cells produce emulsifying substances which convert insoluble alkanes into small droplets (0.01-0.5 μm) that can enter the cells by passive diffusion. It is observed that when cells are grown on a medium of alkanes enriched with lipids, the diffusion of alkanes into the cells is enhanced.

Certain yeasts have been successfully used for producing SCP from alkanes e.g. *Saccharomycopsis lipolytica, Candida tropicalis, Candida oleophila.*

Petroleum products for SCP production : Several oil companies have developed fermentation systems, employing petroleum products for large scale manufacture of SCP by yeasts. Two types of petroleum products are mainly used for this purpose.

1. ***Gas oil*** or ***diesel oil*** containing 10-25% of alkanes with carbon length C_{15}–C_{30} (i.e. long chain alkanes).

2. ***Short chain alkanes*** with carbon length in the range of C_{10}–C_{17}, isolated from gas oil by use of molecular sieves.

Airlift bioreactor system with continuous operation was once used (in France and Britain) to produce SCP from gas oil employing the organism *Saccharomycopsis lipolytica*. But this is now discontinued for political reasons.

Degradation of alkanes : Alkanes have to be first broken down to appropriate metabolites for their utilization to form SCP. The most important step in this direction is the introduction of oxygen into alkanes which can be brought out by two pathways-terminal oxidation and subterminal oxidation (***Fig. 29.1***).

In ***terminal oxidation***, the terminal carbon gets oxidized to the corresponding monocarboxylic acid. The latter then undergoes β-oxidation to form acetic acid. In some microorganisms, the oxidation may occur at both the terminal carbon atoms (by a process referred to as ω-oxidation) to form a dicarboxylic acid. This can be further broken down to acetate and succinate by β-oxidation. Terminal oxidation is the predominant pathway occurring in majority of yeasts and bacteria.

Subterminal oxidation involves the oxidation of interminal carbon atoms (any carbon other than terminal i.e. C_2, C_3, C_4, and so on). The corresponding ketone produced undergoes α-oxidation, decarboxylation, and finally β-oxidation to form acetate and propionate.

The individual enzymes responsible for terminal oxidation or subterminal oxidation have not been fully identified.

Limitations of SCP production from alkanes

The production of SCP from alkanes is a very complex biotechnological process and has been extensively studied. The major drawback of alkanes as substrates is the formation of carcinogens, along with SCP which are highly harmful. For this reason, many countries have discontinued alkane-based production of SCP.

Production of SCP from methane

Methane is the chief constituent of natural gas in many regions. Although methane can be isolated in pure gas form, it cannot be liquified. The handling

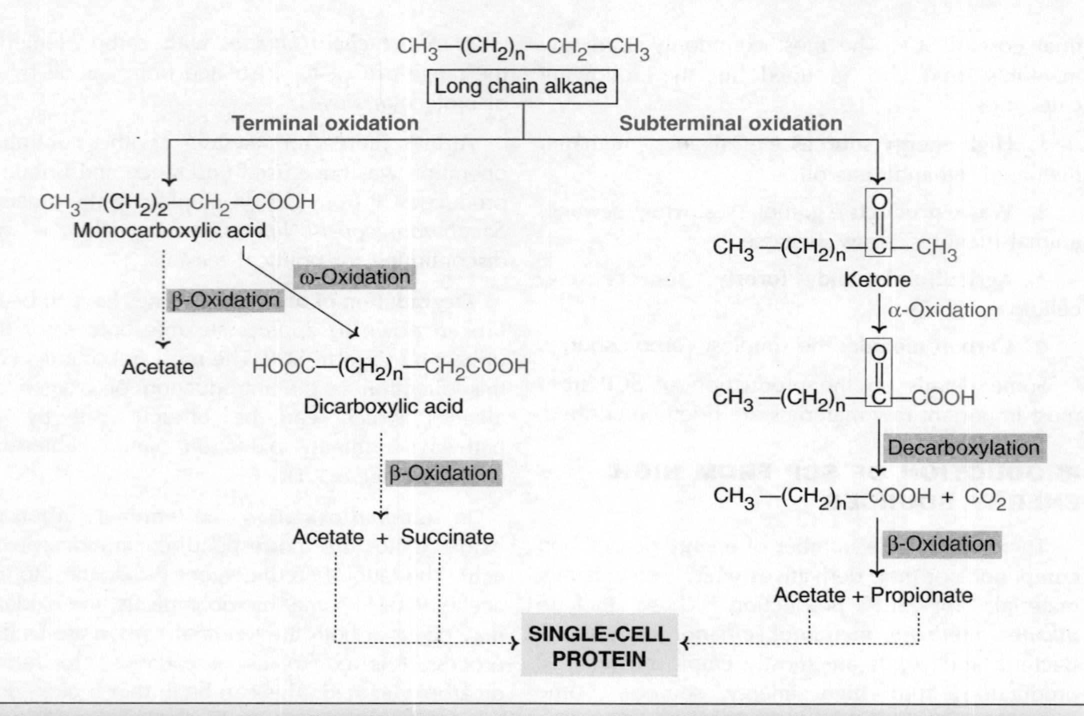

Fig. 29.1 : Oxidation of alkanes by yeasts (e.g. Saccharomycopsis lipolytica*) to produce single-cell protein.*

and transportation of methane (an explosive gas) are very difficult and expensive.

Certain bacteria that can utilize methane for SCP production have been identified e.g. *Methylococcus capsulatus, Methylomonas methanica, Methylovibrio soehngenii*. So far, yeasts that can utilize methane have not been identified.

The bacterial enzyme ***methane oxygenase*** oxidizes methane to methanol, which can be converted to formaldehyde and then to formic acid.

Although methane was extensively researched for its use as a source of SCP, it is not widely used due to technical difficulties.

Production of SCP from methanol

Methanol is a good substrate for producing SCP. Methanol as a carbon source for SCP has several advantages over alkanes and methane. Methanol is easily soluble in aqueous phase at all concentrations, and no residue of it remains in the harvested biomass. Technically, methanol can be easily handled. The sources for methanol are natural gas, coal, oil and methane. Many species of ***bacteria*** (*Methylobacter, Arthrobacter, Bacillus, Pseudomonas, Vibrio*) ***yeasts*** (*Candida biodinii, Hansenula* sp, *Torulopsis* sp) and ***fungi*** (*Trichoderma lignorum, Gliocladium delinquescens*) are capable of producing SCP from methanol. Bacteria are mostly preferred because they require simple fermentation conditions, grow rapidly and possess high content of protein.

Oxidation of methanol : Methanol gets oxidized to formaldehyde, then to formic acid and finally to carbon dioxide, as depicted in ***Fig. 29.2***.

The products obtained from methanol have to form C_3 compounds (such as pyruvate) for final production of SCP. Carbon dioxide formed from methanol can be utilized by photosynthetic organisms for the formation of ribulose diphosphate. Alternately, formaldehyde may condense with ribulose 5-phosphate to form 3-keto 6-phosphohexulose which then gives fructose 6-phosphate and finally pyruvate. This pathway is referred to as ***ribulose monophosphate*** (or ***Quayle***) ***cycle***.

Formaldehyde can condense with glycine to form serine which in a series of reactions forms phosphoenol pyruvate. This is referred to as ***serine pathway***.

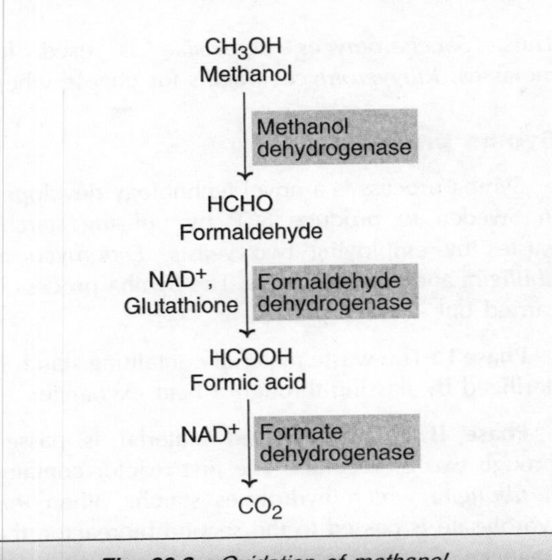

Fig. 29.2 : Oxidation of methanol.

Production process : Imperial Chemical Industries (ICI), U.K. was the first company to develop a process for continuous methanol fermentation for large scale production of SCP. Later, Hoechst (Germany) and Mistubishi (Japan) also developed similar fermentation systems.

ICI employed *Methylophilus methylotrophus* (formerly called *Pseudomonas methylotrophus*) for producing SCP from methanol. A bioreactor, referred to as ***ICI pressure cycle fermenter*** was used for this purpose (***Fig. 29.3***). This fermenter has three components-airlift column, down-flow tube and gas release space. The operation was carried out at temperature 35–37°C and pH 6.5-7.0. The cells were subjected to disruption by heat or acid treatment. The nutrient solution can be clarified by decanting.

ICI pruteen

The ***single-cell protein*** produced by ICI ***from methanol and ammonia*** using *M. methylotrophus* was referred to as ICI pruteen. This SCP was exclusively used for animal feeding. ICI invested a huge amount (around £40 million) in 1979 and installed a continuous culture system for SCP production. This was the world's largest continuous airlift fermenter. Unfortunately, the plant could not be operated for long due to economic reasons. For instance, in 1984 the cost of soy meal was around $125–200 per ton while ICI pruteen was sold at $600 per ton! This is mainly because of the high cost of methanol which represents approximately half of the production cost expenses. In the Middle East, due to high availability and low cost of methanol, the production of SCP appeared to be attractive. In the erstwhile Russia, there were several plants producing SCP from methanol which were later closed.

Genetic engineering for improved SCP production from methanol

The efficiency of SCP production has been improved by using genetic engineering. The assimilation of ammonia by *M. methylotrophus* is an essential step for cellular growth. This organism lacks glutamate dehydrogenase. It possesses glutamine synthase and glutamine ketoglutarate transaminase to utilize ammonia for the formation of glutamate (***Fig. 29.4A***). This is an energy (ATP) dependent reaction. By employing recombinant DNA technology, the gene for the enzyme glutamate dehydrogenase from *E. coli* was cloned and expressed in *M. methylotrophus*. These genetically transformed organisms were more efficient in assimilating ammonia. They could grow rapidly and convert more methanol to SCP. However, the overall increase in the production of SCP did not exceed 10%.

Production of SCP from ethanol

Ethanol is a good substrate for the production of SCP for human consumption (feed grade SCP).

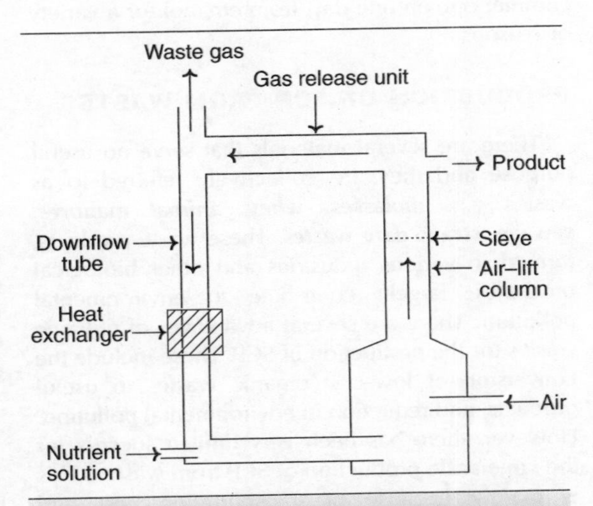

Fig. 29.3 : A diagrammatic representation of ICI pressure cycle fermenter to produce SCP from methanol.

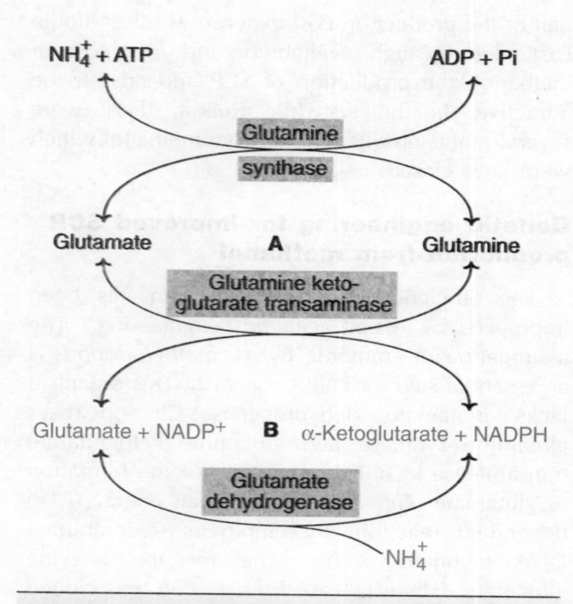

Fig. 29.4 : Assimilation of ammonia by Methylophilus methylotrophus *(A) Normal pathway, (B) Genetically engineered pathway.*

However, this process, as such, is not economically feasible. However, several factors-local raw materials, innovative fermentation technology, political decisions and foreign trade balances influence production of SCP. It may not be surprising if large scale production of SCP commences, on one day, from ethanol for a variety of reasons.

PRODUCTION OF SCP FROM WASTES

There are several materials that serve no useful purpose and they are collectively referred to as wastes e.g. ***molasses, whey, animal manures, sewage, straw, date wastes***. These waste products, formed in various industries and other biological processes, largely contribute to environmental pollution. There are several advantages of utilizing wastes for the production of SCP. These include the conversion of low-cost organic wastes to useful products, and reduction in environmental pollution. However, there has been very limited success for the large scale production of SCP from wastes. This is mainly because of transportation cost and technical difficulties. The technology adopted and the organism employed for SCP production depends on the waste being used as the substrate. Thus, *Saccharomyces cerevisiae* is used for molasses, *Kluyveromyces fragilis* for cheese whey.

Symba process

Symba process is a novel technology developed in Sweden to produce SCP by utilising starchy wastes by employing two yeasts, *Endomycopsis fibuligira* and *Candida utilis*. The Symba process is carried out in three phases.

Phase I : The waste material containing starch is sterilized by passing through a heat exchanger.

Phase II : The sterilized material is passed through two bioreactors. The first reactor contains *E. fibuligira* which hydrolyses starch. When this hydrolysate is passed to the second bioreactor, the organism, *C. utilis* grows to form biomass.

Phase III : The microbial biomass can be separated by centrifugation. The samples of SCP can be dried, packaged and stored.

Applications of Symba product : The yeast biomass produced in Symba process is of good nutritive value. It is widely used as an animal feed for pigs, calves and chicken. The animals grow quite well and no adverse effects have been reported.

Pekilo — a fungal protein rich product

A filamentous fungus, *Paecilomyces variotii*, with good fibrous structure was used for the production of Pekilo. This protein, rich in fungal biomass, was produced by fermentation of wastes such as molasses, whey, sulfite liquor and agricultural wastes. It can be produced by a continuous fermentation process. Pekilo is ***rich in proteins*** (containing essential amino acids), ***vitamins and minerals***. It was used as an animal feed in supplementing the diets of calves, pigs, chickens and hens without any adverse effects. It is unfortunate that the production of Pekilo has been discontinued at most places due to economic and commercial considerations.

Quorn-the mycoprotein for humans

The protein Quorn is the mycoprotein produced by the fungus *Fusarium graminearum*. Many companies in the developed countries are engaged in the production of fungal proteins for human consumption. Quorn is the trade name for ***Fusarium***

TABLE 29.2 Nutritional composition (in percentage) of mycoprotein in comparison to beef

Nutrient	*Mycoprotein*	*Beef (raw lean beefstreak)*
Protein	4	68
Lipid	15	30
Carbohydrate	10	0
Fiber	25	Traces
Ash (minerals etc.)	3	2
RNA	1	Traces

mycoprotein produced in Britain by Marlow Foods (ICI in association with Bank-Hovis-McDougall).

The fungus *Fusarium* can be grown continuously on simple carbohydrate sources (like glucose). Ammonium ions supply nitrogen. Mineral salts and vitamins are also added. The fermentation is carried out at pH 6.0 and temperature 30°C. At the end of fermentation, the culture is heated to 65°C to activate RNases. This is necessary to degrade RNA and reduce the content from 10% to around 1%. The breakdown products of RNA namely the nucleotides diffuse out from the cells and can be easily removed. (Reduction in RNA content is desirable to make the product acceptable for human consumption. This is because humans have a very limited capacity to digest nucleic acids). It is possible to produce 1 kg of fungal biomass with a protein content of about 135 g from 1 kg glucose utilized in the culture medium.

The dried *Fusarium* product is artificially flavoured and marketed in pieces that resemble beef, pork and chicken. The nutritional composition of mycoprotein when compared to beef is given in ***Table 29.2***. Besides being ***rich in essential nutrients***, mycoprotein has a ***good content of dietary fiber***. There are several advantages of fiber consumption-prevents constipation, decreases intestinal cancers, improves glucose tolerance and reduces serum cholesterol.

PRODUCTION OF SCP FROM WOOD

The natural waste wood sources containing ***cellulose, hemicellulose*** and ***lignin*** are attractive natural sources for the production of SCP. It is however, essential to breakdown these cellulosic compounds into fermentable sugars. For this purpose, extracellular cellulases can be used. Certain bacteria (*Cellulomonas* sp) and fungi (*Trichoderma* sp, *Penicillium* sp) are good sources for cellulases.

Techniques for the production of cellulases have been well standardized from several organisms. The cost of production of cellulases is a critical factor in determining the ultimate production cost of SCP.

In some instances, the cellulosic materials can be directly used for biomass production. The resultant SCP is used as animal feed.

PRODUCTION OF SCP FROM CO_2

Certain algae grown in open ponds require only CO_2 as the carbon source. In the presence of sunlight, they can effectively carry out photosynthesis, and produce SCP. The examples of these algae are *Chlorella* sp, *Senedesmus* sp and *Spirulina* sp. *Chlorella* is used as a protein and vitamin supplement for enriching ice-creams, breads and yoghurts in some countries.

In some parts of the world, the algae in ponds are used for the removal of organic pollutants. The resultant algae biomass can be harvested, dried and powdered. Algae SCP are very useful as animal supplements.

Nutritive value of *Spirulina* SCP : Traditionally *Spirulina* sp have been eaten by people in some parts of Africa and Mexico. SCP of *Spirulina* is of high nutritive value (protein-65%, carbohydrate-20%, fat-4%, fibre-3%, chlorophyll-5%, ash-3%). Spirulina is a good source of protein for human consumption, particularly in developing countries.

PRODUCTION OF SCP FROM SEWAGE

Domestic sewage is normally used for large scale production of methane, which in turn may be utilized for the production of SCP. The sewage obtained from industrial wastes in cellulose processing, starch production and food processing can be utilized for the production of SCP. The organism *Candida utilis* is used to produce SCP by using effluent formed during the course of paper manufacture. Other microorganisms namely *Candida tropicalis, Paecilomyces varioti* are

Table 29.3 A selected list of the edible mushrooms cultivated on commercial scale

Mushroom species	*Common name*	*Substrate(s)*
Agaricus bisporus	Button mushroom	Straw, horse manure, compost
Leutinule edodes	Oak or shiitake mushroom	Saw dust, wooden logs, rice bran
Pleurotus ostreatus	Oyster mushroom	Straw, saw dust, paper
Volvariella volvacea	Chinese mushroom or padi–straw mushroom	Straw, cotton
Auricularia sp	Wood–ear mushroom	Saw dust, rice bran
Coprinus sp	— — —	Straw

employed to use sulfite waste liquor for the production of SCP.

GENETICALLY ENGINEERED ARTIFICIAL PROTEIN AS ANIMAL FEED

Rumen bacteria can synthesize amino acids. Some workers have developed genetically engineered strains of rumen bacteria that can produce a protein rich in methionine, threonine, lysine and leucine. This artificial protein has a total of 100 amino acids, of which 57 are essential.

The gene for artificial protein was synthesized by 14 overlapping oligonucleotides held to maltose binding protein gene. This gene was expressed in *E. coli* under the transcriptional control of *tac* promoter. The production of this artificial protein accounts to around 12% of the intracellular proteins.

However, the large scale production of artificial protein by rumen bacteria is yet to be clearly established and commercialised.

MUSHROOMS

Mushrooms are fungi belonging to the classes basidiomycetes (*Agaricus* sp, *Auricularia* sp, *Tremella* sp) and ascomycetes (*Morchella* sp, *Tuber* sp). Majority of edible mushrooms are the species of basidomyces. It is estimated that there are around 4,000 species of basidiomyces. Of these, around 200 are edible, and a dozen of them are cultivated on large scale. Some of the most important edible mushrooms, their common names and the substrates used are given in ***Table 29.3***.

The cultivation of edible mushrooms is one of the rare examples of a microbial culture wherein the cultivated macroscopic organism itself is directly used as ***human food***. Mushroom growing is one of the fastest developing biotechnological industries worldover. Further growth of mushroom industry is expected ***for the production of enzymes, and pharmaceutical compounds, including antitumor agents and antibiotics***.

Poisonous mushrooms

There are certain poisonous mushrooms also. They usually possess unpleasant taste and odour. These mushrooms produce some poisonous substances like ***phallin*** and ***muscarine***. The examples of poisonous mushrooms are *Amanita phalloides, A. muscaria, A. viraosa, Lepiota morgani* and *Boletus satanas*.

Nutritive value of edible mushrooms

Some people regard ***edible mushrooms as vegetable meat***. Mushrooms contain 80–90% water, depending on the growth conditions (temperature, humidity). Edible mushrooms are rich sources of protein (35–45% of dry weight). However, all these proteins are not easily digestible by humans. Mushrooms also contain fats and free fatty acids (7–10%), carbohydrates (5–15%) and minerals in good concentration. Certain undesirable substances may also be present in edible mushrooms e.g. cadmium, chromium.

Many delicious recipes of edible mushrooms can be prepared. This actually depends on the dietary habits of the people. Some of the common recipes are mushroom soup, mushroom paneer, mushroom pulao, and mushroom omelette.

Advantages of edible mushroom biotechnology

1. Mushrooms can be produced by utilizing cheap and often waste substrates (industrial and wood wastes).

2. They are of high nutritive value being rich in proteins, vitamins and minerals.

3. Many delicious recipes can be prepared from mushrooms.

4. Due to low carbohydrate content, consumption of mushrooms is advocated to diabetic patients.

PRODUCTION OF EDIBLE MUSHROOMS

Mushroom production is basically a fermentation process. This is mostly carried out by ***solid-substrate fermentation***. A wide range of substrates (straw, saw dust, compost, wooden logs) depending the organism can be used (Refer ***Table 29.3***). Mushroom production is a good example of a low technology utilization in an otherwise sophisticated modern biotechnology.

The most common edible mushroom cultivated worldover (that may constitute about 20% world mushroom produce) is the ***white button mushroom, Agaricus bisporus. Lentinula edodes*** is the second most cultivated mushroom in the world. The substrates straw, compost or horse manure can be used. The substrate selection depends on the local factors.

A schematic representation of mushroom production is depicted in ***Fig. 29.5***. The compost with desired formulation is prepared and sterilized. It is spread into the trays which are then transferred to production room and inoculated with ***spawn***. Spawn is the term used for the ***mushroom inoculum containing spores*** and/or small pieces of fruiting body. After inoculation (spawning), the culture is maintained at optimal growth conditions. The trays are regularly watered to maintain 70–80% humidity. The ideal temperature is about 15°C, and pH about 7.0. It takes about 7–10 days for each crop of mushroom production. It is possible to have 3-4 crops, before terminating the production process. The mushrooms can be harvested and marketed.

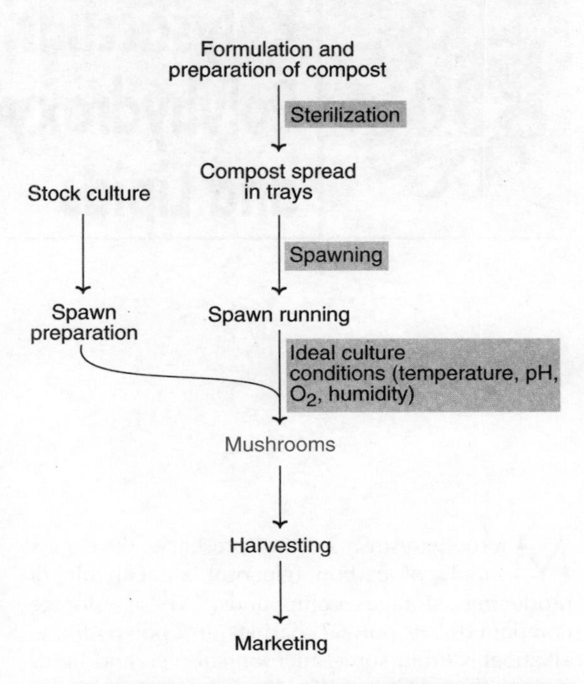

Fig. 29.5 : An overview of edible mushroom production.

Mushrooms have a very short life 8–12 hours, unless stored at low temperature (refrigerator 2-5°C). Therefore, they should be immediately consumed, stored or canned.

Variations in culturing mushrooms : The production of mushrooms is highly variable and mostly depends on the organism and the substrate used, besides several other local factors. There are distinct differences in the mushroom cultivation methods between different countries. For instance, ***garden and field cultivation*** methods are used in Europe, while in USA, ***cave and house cultivation*** techniques are employed.

Some mushrooms (e.g. *Volirariella* sp) are suitable for cultivation in summer and rainy reason while others grow well in winter (*Agaricus bisporus, Pleurotus* sp). It is however, possible to grow these mushrooms any time in a year with appropriate temperature and humidity control arrangements.

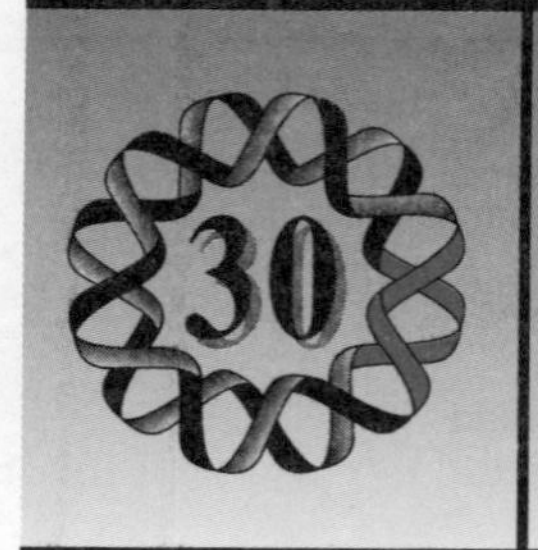

Polysaccharides, Polyhydroxyalkanoates, and Lipids

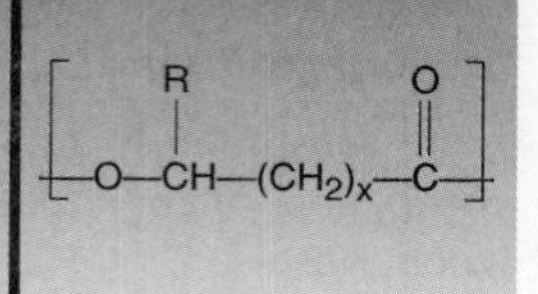

Microorganisms, in the presence of excess supply of carbon (glucose) are capable of producing storage compounds. These storage compounds are polysaccharides and polyhydroxyalkanoates (from some microorganisms), and lipids (from some yeasts and fungi).

In general, the synthesis of storage compounds by microorganisms is higher on restricting their growth, by limiting the supply of one or more essential nutrients (other than carbon source).

POLYSACCHARIDES

The microorganisms can produce large amounts of polysaccharides in the presence of surplus carbon source. Some of these polysaccharides (e.g. glycogen) serve as storage compounds. The polysaccharides excreted by the cells, referred to as ***exopolysaccharides***, are of commercial importance. The exopolysaccharides may be found in association with the cells or may remain in the medium.

The microbial polysaccharides may be neutral (e.g. dextran, scleroglucan) or acidic (xanthan, gellan) in nature. Acidic polysaccharides possessing ionized groups such as carboxyl, which can function as polyelectrolytes, are commercially more important.

Applications of microbial polysaccharides

Microbial polysaccharides have immense commercial importance. They are employed in the stabilization of foods, and production of several industrial and pharmaceutical compounds. The ***commercial value of a polysaccharide is based on its ability to modify the flow characteristics of solutions*** (technically known as ***rheology***). Polysaccharides can increase the viscosity and, are therefore useful as thickening and gelling agents.

Microbial polysaccharides are of great importance in ***oil industry***. By conventional methods, only 50% of the oil can be extracted. And the rest is either trapped in the rock or too viscous to be pumped out. It is now possible to recover such oils also by a technique called ***microbial enhanced oil recovery (MEOR)***. This can be done by injecting surfactants and viscosity decreasing biological agents (i.e. the microbial polysaccharides e.g. xanthan and emulsan).

Production of microbial polysaccharides

The synthesis of polysaccharides favourably occurs in the excess supply of carbon substrate in the growth medium while limiting nitrogen supply. A carbon/nitrogen ratio of around 10 : 1 is considered to be favourable for optimal polysaccharide synthesis. The production process is mostly carried out by ***batch culture fermentation***. By manipulating the nutrient supply, differential synthesis of polysaccharides can be achieved. By limiting nitrogen supply in the medium, mostly neutral polysaccharides are produced. When metal ions are limited, acidic polysaccharides are mainly synthesized. Molecular oxygen supply of around 90% saturation is ideal for good growth and polysaccharide synthesis.

Biosynthesis of polysaccharides : Microorganisms are capable of producing a large number of polysaccharides. The pathways for their biosynthesis are comparable to the processess that occur for the formation bacterial cell wall. It is estimated that there are well over 100 enzymatic reactions, directly or indirectly involved in the synthesis of polysaccharides. ***Starting with glucose, appropriate sugars*** (by transforming glucose to others) ***are incorporated in the formation of polysaccharides.***

Recovery of polysaccharides : As the polysaccharide production increases, there occurs a marked increase in viscosity of the culture broth. The polysaccharides can be precipitated by salts, acids or organic solvents, and recovered by employing appropriate techniques.

Microbial polysaccharides versus plant polysaccharides

There is a lot of competition between microbial and plant polysaccharides for industrial applications. Production of plant polysaccharides is relatively cheap, although it is uncontrolled and occurs for a short period in a year. In contrast, production of microbial polysaccharides is well controlled and can be ***continued throughout the year***. However, fermentation processes for manufacture of cheap (from plant sources) polysaccharides is not advisable.

GENERAL FEATURES OF MICROBIAL POLYSACCHARIDES

Of the several microbial polysaccharides, around 20 are of industrial importance. As already stated, the ***commercial value*** of a polysaccharide is mostly dependent on its ***rheological properties*** i.e. its ability to modify the flow characteristics of solutions.

A selected list of commercially important polysaccharides, the microorganisms used for their production, and their applications are given in the ***Table 30.1***. Some of the important features of individual microbial polysaccharides are briefly described hereunder.

XANTHAN

Xanthan or more frequently referred to as ***xanthan gum*** was the first polysaccharide available commercially. It is a well studied and most widely used ***hexopolysaccharide***.

Chemistry : Xanthan has a molecular weight in the range of 2–15 × 10^4 daltons. The basic repeating unit of xanthan is a pentasaccharide containing glucose (Glc), mannose (Man) and glucuronic acid (GlcA) with acetate (Ac) and pyruvate (Pyr) as depicted below.

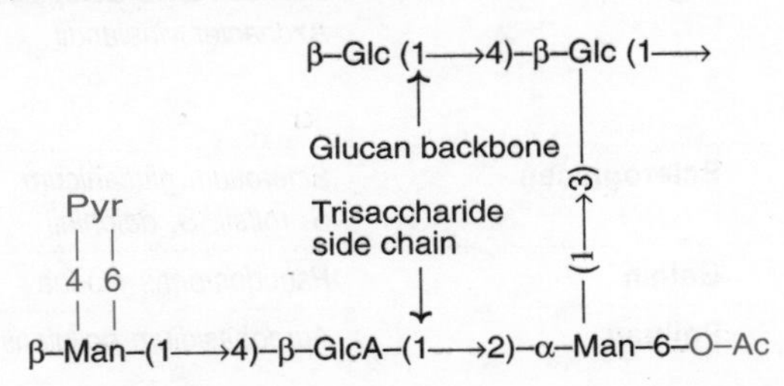

Basically, xanthan is a branched polymer with β (1→4) linked glucan (glucose polymer) backbone bound to a trisaccharide (Man, GlcA, Man) side chain on alternate glucose residues. The mannose has either acetate or pyruvate groups. The number of acetate or pyruvate molecules in xanthan is variable and is dependent on the bacterial strain used. The culture conditions and the recovery processes also influence the quantities of pyruvate and acetate residues. It is believed that the viscosity of xanthan gum is influenced by the contents of pyruvate and acetate.

Applications : Xanthan gum is used as a ***food additive for the preparation of soft foods*** (ice cream, cheese). It is also used in oil industry for enhancing oil recovery. Further, xanthan is useful for the preparation of tooth pastes and water based paints.

Biosynthesis : For the biosynthesis of xanthan, the monomers are bound to a carrier lipid molecule and then transferred to a growing polymer chain. The activated monosaccharide nucleotides (e.g. uridine diphosphate glucose, UDP-glucose) supply energy for the formation of glycosidic bonds

TABLE 30.1 Commercially important microbial polysaccharides and their applications

Polysaccharide	*Producing organism(s)*	*Application(s)*
Xanthan	*Xanthomonas campestris*	As a food additive for stabilization, gelling and viscosity control, i.e. for the preparation of soft foods e.g. ice cream, cheese. In oil industry for enhanced oil recovery. In the preparation of toothpastes, and water based paints.
Dextran	*Leuconostoc mesenteroides, Acetobacter* sp, *Streptococcus mutans*	Blood plasma expander. Used in the preventionn of thrombosis, and in wound dressing (as adsorbent). In the laboratory for chromatographic and other techniques involved in purification. As a foodstuff.
Alginate	*Pseudomonas aeruginosa* *Azobacter vinelandii*	In food industry as thickening and gelling agent. Alginate beads are employed in immobilization of cells and enzymes. Used as ion-exchange agent.
Scleroglucan	*Sclerotium glucanicum* *S. rolfsii, S. delphinii*	Used for stabilizing latex paints, printing inks, and drilling muds.
Gellan	*Pseudomonas elodea*	In food industry as a thickner and solidifying agent.
Polluan	*Aureobasidium pollulans*	Being a biodegradable polysaccharide, it is used in food coating and packaging.
Curdlan	*Alcaligenes faecalis*	As a gelling agent in cooked foods (forms a strong gel above 55°C) Useful for immobilization of enzymes.
Emulsan	*Acinetobacter calcoaceticus* *Arthrobacter* sp	In oil industry for enhanced recovery. For cleaning of oil spills.

between adjacent units. The biosynthesis of other exopolysaccharides is comparable with that of xanthan. Dextran synthesis, however is much simpler as described later.

Production : Xanthan is commercially produced by the Gram-negative bacterium, *Xanthomonas campestris*. The culture medium usually consists of 4-5% carbohydrate (glucose, sucrose, corn starch hydrolysate), 0.05-0.1% nitrogen (ammonium nitrate, urea, yeast extract) and salts. The pH is maintained around 7.0, and the fermentation is carried out by batch culture for 2-3 days. Xanthan in the culture broth is precipitated by isopropanol or methanol. These agents also kill the microorganisms. The precipitated xanthan can be dried and used for commercial purposes.

Genetic engineering of *Xanthomonas campestris* for xanthan production

The wild type *X. campestris* can efficiently utilize glucose, sucrose or starch as a carbon source. They are however, unable to use lactose as a carbon substrate.

Whey is a byproduct obtained in the manufacture of cheese. Disposal of large quantities of whey is a major problem in dairy industry. Fortunately, whey is rich in lactose, besides containing small quantities of proteins, vitamins and minerals. Atempts are made to use whey in fermentation industries.

Genetically engineered *X. campestris* have been developed ***that can utilize lactose (from whey)*** for the production of xanthan. For this purpose, the *E. coli* ***laczy*** genes (encoding the enzyme β-galactosidase and lactose permease respectively) were cloned under the transcriptional control of *X. campestris* bacteriophage promoter. This construct was first introduced into *E. coli*, and then transferred to *X. campestris*. The genetically engineered strains of *X. campestris* expressed the genes and produced high quantities of the enzymes β-galactosidase and lactose permease. These new strains utilize lactose or whey very efficiently for the industrial production of xanthan. This is a good example of successfully ***converting a waste product*** (***whey***) ***into a commercially important and valuable product*** (***a biopolymer namely xanthan gum***).

DEXTRAN

Chemically, dextrans are ***glucans*** (polymers of glucose) containing 1 → 6 glycosidic linkages. Some dextrans also have α 1→2, α 1→3 and α 1→4 linkages. The molecular weights of dextrans are in the range of 15,000–500,000.

Applications : Dextrans are used as ***blood plasma expanders***, ***for the prevention of thrombosis*** and in wound dressing. In addition, dextrans are useful in the laboratory analytical techniques for purification of biomolecules.

Production : Dextrans can be produced by a wide range of Gram-positive and Gram-negative bacteria e.g. *Leuconostoc mesenteroides* and *Streptococcus mutans*. In contrast to other exopolysaccharides (which are synthesized within the cells), dextrans are produced ***by extracellular enzyme*** in the medium. The enzyme is ***dextransucrase*** (a transglucosidase) which acts on sucrose and brings about polymerisation of glucose residues, and simultaneously liberates free fructose into the medium.

The commercial production is carried out by using lactic acid bacterium, *L. mesenteroides* by a ***batch fermentation process***. Besides sucrose, the culture medium contains organic nitrogen source and inorganic phosphate. The crude dextran produced is precipitated by alcohol and then subjected to acid hydrolysis. In recent years, the alcohol precipitated polymeric dextran is subjected to enzymatic hydrolysis by using ***exo-*** or ***endo-α dextranases*** to get dextrans of desired molecular weight. The resultant dextrans can be fractionated and dried.

It is also possible to use a cell free system for the production of dextrans. The extracellular enzyme dextrasucrase can transform sucrose into dextran in a cell-free nutrient solution. This reaction is optimum at pH 5.0-5.5 and temperature 25–30°C.

ALGINATE

Alginate is a linear ***polymer composed of mannuronic acid and glucuronic acid*** (both of them being uronic acids) in a proportion ranging from 4 : 1 to 20 : 1. Some of the mannuronic acid residues are acetylated. Alginate is commercially produced by Gram-negative bacteria, *Pseudomonas aeruginosa* and *Azobacter vinelandii*.

The type of organism used and the culture conditions determine the relative proportion of mannuronic acid and glucuronic acid residues and the degree of acetylation in alginate. Alginates with high contents of mannuronic acid are elastic in nature while those with high concentration of glucuronic acid are strong and brittle.

Algal (seaweed) alginates are also polymers of mannuronic acid and glucuronic acid, and comparable in structure with bacterial alginates. However, algal alginates lack acetylation.

For commercial purposes, seaweed alginates are more commonly used than bacterial alginates. This is mainly because bacterial alginates are relatively unstable and get easily degraded. Alginates are ***useful as thickening agents in food industry***, and for immobilization of cells and enzymes.

SCLEROGLUCAN

Scleroglucan is a ***glucose polymer*** (***glucomer***). It is a neutral polysaccharide with β 1→3 glucan backbone and single glucose (Glc) residue branches (β 1→6 linkage). The branching occurs at a regular sequence at every third glucose unit in the polymer backbone chain.

$$\longrightarrow 3)\text{-}\beta\text{-Glc}\,(1\longrightarrow 3)\text{-}\beta\text{-Glc}\,(1\longrightarrow 3)\text{-}\beta\text{-Glc}\,(1\longrightarrow$$

(branch from the middle Glc: (1→6) — β-Glc)

Scleroglucan is a fungal heoxpolysaccharide. It is commercially produced by *Sclerotium glucanicum*, *S. rolfsii* and *S. delphinii*. Scleroglucan is ***useful for stabilizing latex paints***, printing inks and drilling muds.

GELLAN

Gellan is ***a linear heteropolysaccharide***. The repeating unit of gellan is composed of two glucose, one glucuronic acid and one rhamnose molecules. Gellan is produced by *Pseudomonas elodea*.

A deacetylated gellan which forms firm and brittle gels under the trade name ***Gelrite*** has been developed by a reputed company in USA (Kalco Inc).

Gellan is used in food industry. Even at a low concentration, it is a thickner.

POLLULAN

Pollulan is an α-glucose polymer (α-glucan) with α 1→4, and a few α, 1→6 glycosidic bonds. Pollulan is produced by using the fungus, *Aureobasidium pollulans*. It is estimated that about 70% of glucose (the substrate) is converted to pollulan during fermentation, although the time taken is rather long (5-7 days).

Pollulan is mainly used in food coating and packaging.

CURDLAN

Curdlan is a β-glucose polymer (β-glucan). The glucose residues are held together by β 1→3 glycosidic bonds. The exopolysaccharide curdlan is commercially produced by employing *Alcaligenes faecalis*. Curdlan-like polysaccharides are also produced by other microorganisms such as *Agrobacterium rhizogenes* and *Rhizobium trifolii*.

Curdlan forms strong gels when heated to above 55°C. Therefore, it is used as a gelling agent for cooked foods. In addition, curdlan is also employed for immobilization of enzymes.

POLYHYDROXYALKANOATES

Polyhydroxyalkanoates (***PHA***) are ***intracellular carbon and energy storage compounds***, produced by many microorganisms. They are ***biodegradable polymers***, and are elastic in nature depending on the polymer composition. PHA are well suited for the synthesis of plastics, the biodegradable packing materials.

The conventional plastics, made from coal or oil, are not biodegradable. They survive hundreds

$$\left[-O-\underset{}{\overset{R}{\overset{|}{C}}}H-(CH_2)_x-\overset{O}{\overset{\|}{C}}-\right]$$

(A) General structure of a monomer in PHA

$$\left[-O-\overset{CH_3}{\overset{|}{C}}H-CH_2-\overset{O}{\overset{\|}{C}}-\right]_n$$

(B) Polyhydroxybutyrate

$$\left[-O-\overset{CH_3-CH_2-CH_2-CH_2-CH_2}{\overset{|}{C}}H-CH_2-\overset{O}{\overset{\|}{C}}-\right]_n$$

(C) PHA with 3-hydroxyoctanoate

$$\left[-O-\overset{CH_3}{\overset{|}{C}}H-CH_2-\overset{O}{\overset{\|}{C}}-\right]\left[-O-\overset{CH_3-CH_2}{\overset{|}{C}}H-CH_2-\overset{O}{\overset{\|}{C}}-\right]$$

(D) 3-Hydroxybutyrate-co-3-hydroxyvalerate

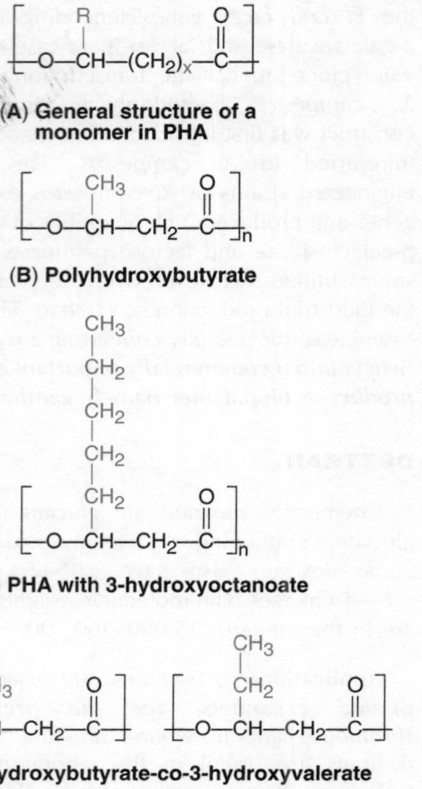

Fig. 30.1 : Structures of polyhydroxyalkanoates (PHA).

of years and are a major source of environmental pollution, often resulting in ecological imbalance. A heavy demand for biodegradable plastic materials exists. There are some attempts to chemically synthesize biodegradable polyesters e.g. polylactic acid and polyglycolic acid. The production of polyhydroxyalkanoates by fermentation is preferred for use as ***biodegradable plastics***.

PHA-CHEMISTRY AND PROPERTIES

PHA serve as ***lipid reserve materials in bacteria***. Their function in bacteria is comparable to that of fats and oils in yeasts and fungi. The granules of PHA, stored within the cells are clearly visible under electron microscope. Some bacteria may accumulate huge quantities (upto 80% of dry weight) of PHA.

Polyhydroxyalkanoates are linear polyester polymers composed of hydroxyacid monomers (***Fig. 30.1A***). The most commonly found monomers are 3 hydroxy acids with a carbon length ranging from C_3 to C_{14}.

Homopolymer PHA-polyhydroxybutyrate

The most common PHA is ***polyhydroxybutyrate*** which is frequently referred to as ***PHB***. It is a polyester with 3-hydroxybutyrate as the repeating unit (***Fig. 30.1B***). PHB is the homopolymer PHA. PHB, as such, is rather hard and inflexible.

Being a high molecular weight compound, the accumulation of PHB in huge quantities also does not significantly effect the osmotic pressure within the cell. The reserve carbon compound PHB can be oxidized to carbon dioxide and water, releasing large amount of energy. Bacteria require energy, although they are not growing, to maintain pH gradient and concentration gradient of several compounds. This energy, referred to as ***maintenance energy*** essential for the survival of the cells, is met by the reserve material PHB.

Heteropolymers of PHA

Majority of polyhydroxyalkanoates, with the exception of PHB, contain two or more different monomers and are referred to as heteropolymers. These heteropolymers are usually composed of a random sequence of monomers, and not different monomers, in different chains. Besides 3-hydroxy acids, several other hydroxy acids are found in the structure of PHA. e.g. 4-hydroxybutyrate (4HB). In fact, it has been found that the bacteria are capable of incorporating more than 100 different hydroxylated monomers into PHA. This depends on the organism and the nature of the carbon source supplied during the accumulation of the polymer.

The properties of PHA mostly depend on the nature of the monomers it contains. In general, PHA with longer side chains (e.g. 3-hydroxy-octanoate containing PHA) and heteropolymeric PHA are more flexible and soft.

3-Hydroxybutyrate-*co*-3-hydroxyvalerate

As already stated, by selecting a specific organism and by manipulating the composition of the medium, the chemical construction of the PHA can be altered. Thus, when the medium contains glucose and propionic acid, the organism *Ralstonia*

Glucose

CH_3—CO—SCoA
Acetyl CoA

CH_3—CO—SCoA
CoA
3-Ketothiolase

CH_3—C(=O)—CH_2—C(=O)—SCoA
Acetoacetyl CoA

NADPH
$NADP^+$
Acetoacetyl CoA reductase

CH_3—CH(OH)—CH_2—C(=O)—SCoA
3-Hydroxybutyryl CoA

CoA
Poly (3-hydroxybutyric acid) synthase

[—O—CH(CH_3)—CH_2—C(=O)—]
Poly 3-hydroxybutyric acid

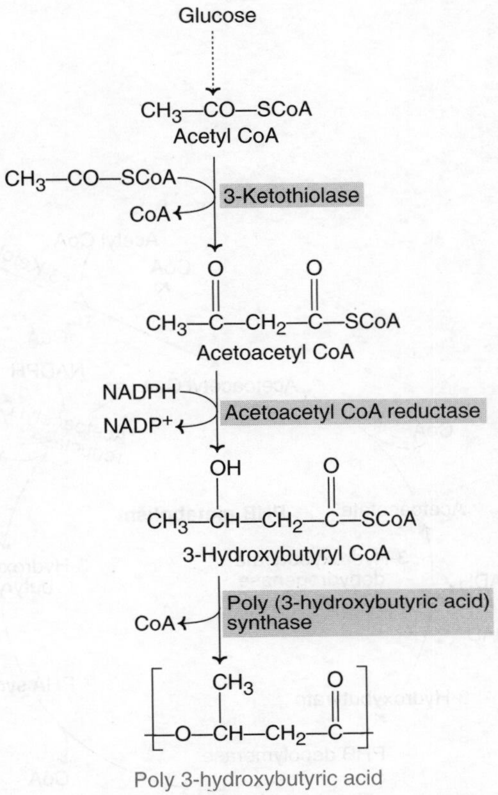

Fig. 30.2 : *Biosynthesis of polyhydroxybutyric acid (PHB).*

eutrophia produces a copolymer of ***3-hydroxybutyrate*** and ***3-hydroxyvalerate*** (abbreviated PHB/V). PHB as such is hard and brittle but the presence 3-hydroxyvalerate monomers makes PHB/V flexible and stronger. The properties of PHB/V are similar to those of polypropylene, and therefore it is commercially more useful.

POLYHYDROXYBUTYRATE (PHB)

Biosynthesis of PHB

Among the several PHA, the pathway for the biosynthesis of polyhydroxybutyrate (PHB) has been thoroughly investigated. Starting with ***acetyl CoA***, PHB is synthesized in three reaction steps (***Fig. 30.2***). Acetyl CoA is converted acetoacetyl CoA by the enzyme 3-ketothiolase which is then reduced to 3-hydroxybutyryl CoA by acetoacetyl CoA reductase. The reducing equivalents are

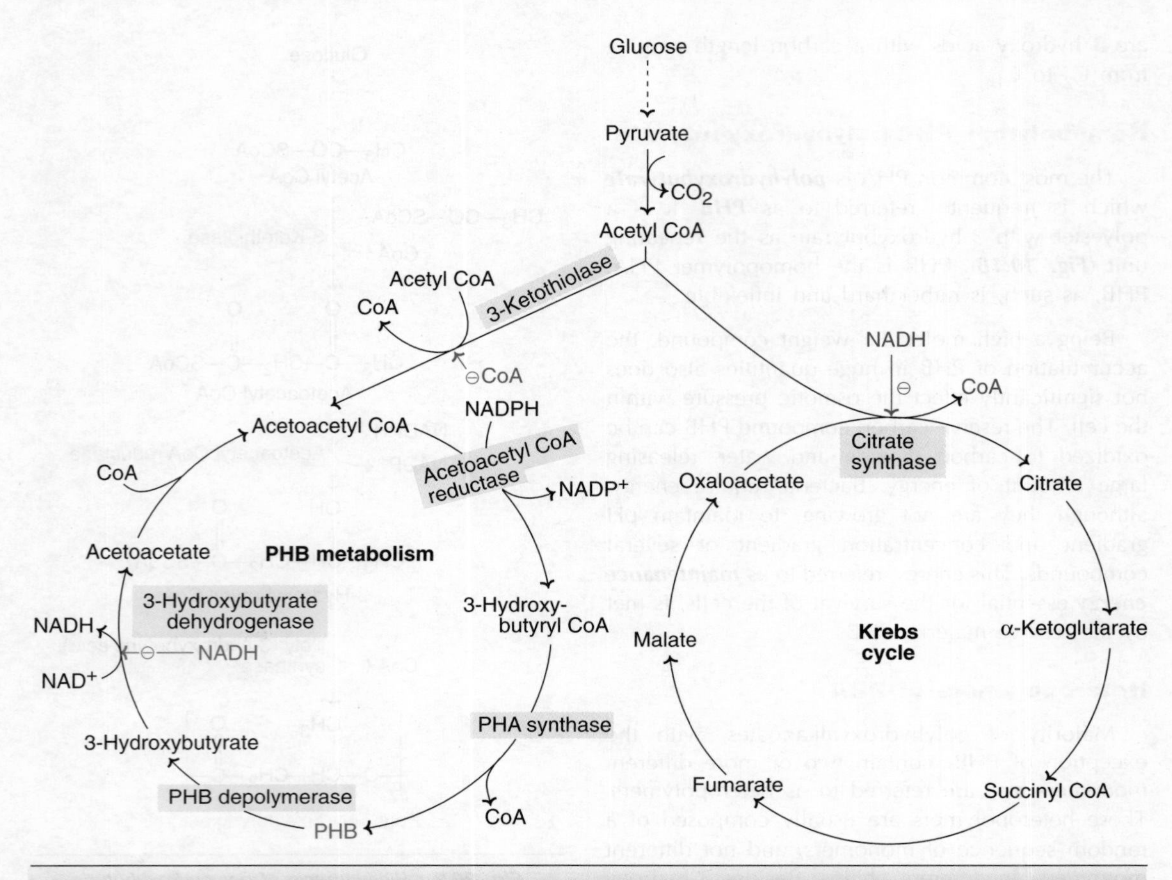

Fig. 30.3 : Regulation of polyhydroxybutyrate (PHB) metabolism.

supplied by NADPH. The enzyme PHA synthase is responsible for the addition of 3-hydroxybutyrate residues to the growing PHB chain.

Regulation of PHB biosynthesis

The outline pathways concerned with the biosynthesis and degradation of PHB in *Ralstonia eutrophia* are depicted in ***Fig. 30.3***. The ***enzymes of PHB biosynthesis*** are ***constitutive*** in nature. Thus the enzyme machinery for PHB synthesis is present all the time in the cell. When the growth of the microorganism is restricted by limiting an essential nutrient, PHB synthesis rapidly occurs.

During the active growth phase, acetyl CoA gets oxidized through the Krebs cycle. Further, free coenzyme A inhibits 3-ketothiolase and therefore very little PHB is synthesized. When the growth ceases or is restricted by limiting a nutrient, the operation of Krebs cycle (i.e. oxidation of acetyl CoA) decreases. This is mainly due to the inhibition of citrate synthase by NADH. A decrease in the concentration of coenzyme A (as citrate is not formed from acetyl CoA, CoA is low) relieves the inhibition of 3-ketothiolase. This enables the diversion of acetyl CoA for the production of PHB. The supply of reducing equivalents (NADPH) required by the enzyme acetoacetyl CoA reductase also regulates the synthesis of PHB.

PHB, the storage energy reserve compound, can be degraded to acetyl CoA and metabolised via Krebs cycle. This occurs when the organism is deprived of energy supplying carbon sources. PHB is degraded by PHB depolymerase to form 3-hydroxybutyrate. NADH is the inhibitor of the subsequent reaction, catalysed by the enzyme 3-hydroxybutyrate dehydrogenase i.e. formation of acetoacetate from 3-hydroxybutyrate. The biosynthesis and breakdown of PHB form a cyclic process, as depicted in ***Fig. 30.3***.

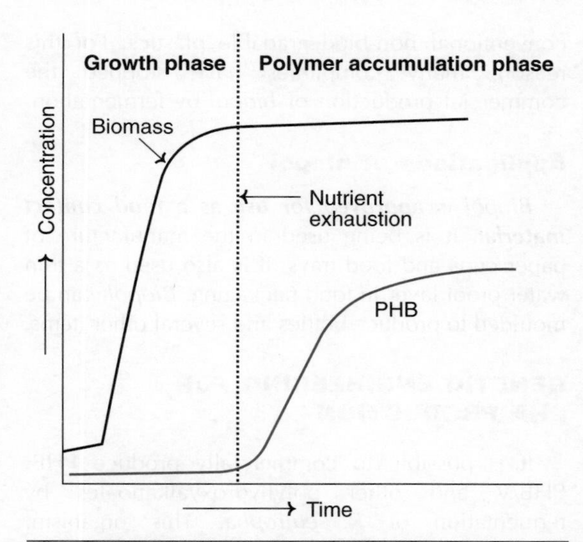

Fig. 30.4 : Production of polyhydroxybutyrate (PHB).

Production of PHB

Polyhydroxybutyrate is mostly manufactured by ***batch culture***. PHB production occurs when there is an excess supply of carbon source, and limitation of some other essential nutrient such as nitrogen, phosphorus or sulfur source. The production/accumulation of PHB is depicted in ***Fig. 30.4***. There are two distinct phases—a ***growth phase*** and a ***polymer accumulation phase***. As the growth phase ceases, due to nutrient exhaustion, synthesis of polymer (PHB) commences. It is also possible to produce PHB by restricting the oxygen supply to aerobic bacteria.

Applications of PHB

PHB can be implanted in the human body without rejection. This is because PHB does not produce any immune response and thus it is ***biocompatible***. PHB has several medical applications e.g. as durable bone implants, for wound dressings. Attempts to use PHB as degradable sutures and other implants has not met with success due to very slow degradation of PHB.

BIOSYNTHESIS OF OTHER PHA

The biosynthesis of other PHA is quite comparable to that described for PHB. Some important features with regard to the synthesis of two important PHA are described.

Biosynthesis of PHB/V

Some strains of *Ralstonia eutropha* (formerly known as *Alcaligenes eutrophus*) are capable of synthesizing poly (hydroxybutyrate-*co*-hydroxyvalerate) (PHB/V). For the formation of PHB/V, ***glucose and propionic acid are required as substrates***. Propionic acid as propionyl CoA is responsible for the synthesis of 3-hydroxyvalerate. The three enzymes involved in the synthesis of 3-hydroxybutyrate (3-HB) also participate in the formation of 3-hydroxyvalerate (3-HV). The polymer PHB/V contains 3-HB and 3-HV monomers in a random sequence (no individual polymers of 3-HB or 3-HV exist). The relative concentrations of glucose (precursor for 3-HB) and propionic acid (precursor for 3-HV) in the culture medium determine the chemical composition of PHB/V.

The biosynthetic pathway for the formation of PHB/V is depicted in ***Fig. 30.5***.

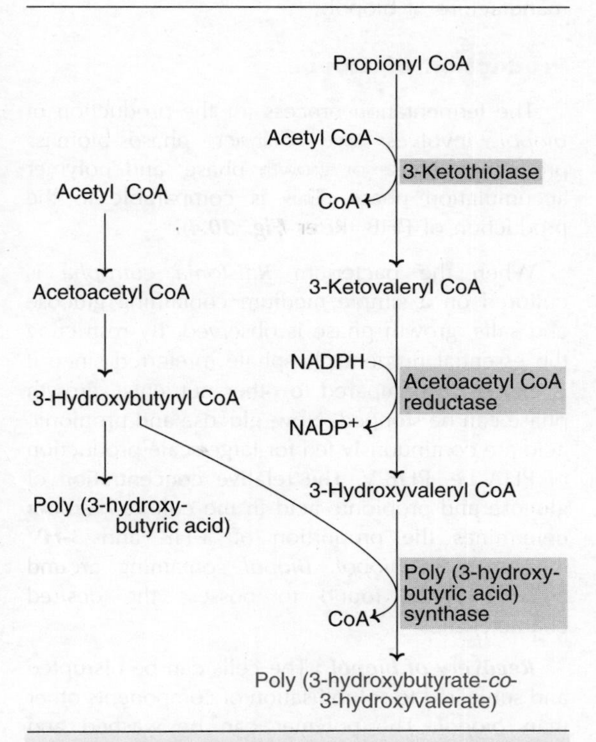

*Fig. 30.5 : Biosynthesis of poly (3-hydroxybutyrate-co-3-hydroxyvalerate) (**Note** : The same 3 enzymes are required for the synthesis of poly 3-hydroxybutyric acid; For details refer Fig. 30.2).*

Biosynthesis of PHA with long side chains

It is generally observed that when a PHA producing organism is grown on a carbon source containing ***n*** carbons, 3-hydroxy monomers with ***n-2*** or ***n + 2*** carbons are produced. This suggests the involvement of β-oxidation of fatty acids (which sequentially removes 2-carbon fragment) in the biosynthesis of PHA.

The organism *Pseudomonas oleovorans* can synthesize PHA when organic acids and alkanes are supplied in the medium as carbon sources. For instance, PHA with high content of 3-hydroxyoctanoate can be produced from *n*-octane or *n*-octanoic acid.

BIOPOL-A BIODEGRADABLE PLASTIC

Biopol was the trade name used by ICI plc in UK for the biodegradable plastics composed of PHB and PHB/V. The Gram-negative soil bacterium, ***Ralstonia eutropha*** was employed for the manufacture of biopol.

Production of biopol

The fermentation process for the production of *biopol* involves two distinct phases-biomass production phase or growth phase, and polymer accumulation phase. This is comparable to the production of PHB (Refer ***Fig. 30.4***).

When the bacterium *Ralstonia eutropha* is cultured on a simple medium containing glucose and salts, growth phase is observed. By restricting the essential nutrient phosphate (preferred since it is expensive compared to other nutrients), growth phase can be stopped. Now, glucose and propionic acid are continuously fed for large scale production of PHA i.e. PHB/V. The relative concentration of glucose and propionic acid in the culture medium determines the proportion of 3-HB and 3-HV monomers in *biopol*. *Biopol* containing around 10% 3-HV is found to possess the desired characteristics.

Recovery of biopol **:** The cells can be disrupted and subjected to solubilisation of components other than *biopol*. The polymer can be washed and recovered by centrifugation.

Limitations in the production of biopol : The manufacture of *biopol* by fermentation is very expensive when compared to the production of conventional non-biodegradable plastics. For this reason, many companies have stopped the commercial production of *biopol* by fermentation.

Applications of biopol

Biopol is ***approved for use as a food contact material***. It is being used in the manufacture of paper cups and food trays. It is also used as a thin water proof layer in food packaging. *Biopol*, can be moulded to produce bottles and several other items.

GENETIC ENGINEERING FOR PHA PRODUCTION

It is possible to commercially produce PHB, PHB/V and other polyhydroxyalkanoates by fermentation of *R. eutropha*. This organism, however, grows very slowly and utilizes only a limited number of carbon sources for growth. For these reasons, the production of PHA by *R. eutropha* is expensive.

Fortunately, the genes responsible for the synthesis of important types of PHA by *R. eutropha* have been characterized and cloned. These ***genes have been transferred to E. coli*** (a bacterium that does not normally synthesize PHA). The resultant transformants, *E. coli* cells, grow rapidly and produced large quantities of PHB. But the major limitation is that about half of the *E. coli* cells lose the plasmid constructs in about 50 generations. This poses a big problem, particularly for large scale continuous cultures. In recent years, some workers have tried to genetically manipulate and produce stable plasmids with some success.

Recombinant strains of *E. coli* have been used for the production of PHB, PHB/V and other types of PHA. There are some other ***advantages of producing PHA by E. coli*** instead of *R. eutropha*. The polymers are produced in a crystalline state by *E. coli* (they are in amorphous state in *R. eutropha*), and their ***extraction and recovery are much easier***.

PHA production by plants

The major limitation of producing PHA by fermentation is the cost factor. Approximately, it is ten times more expensive to produce PHA by bacteria compared to the manufacture of petrochemical plastics.

Plants are attractive sources for a less expensive production of PHA. A ***transgenic plant of Arabidopsis thaliana, containing the bacterial genes for PHB genes, was developed*** in 1992. However, the ***yield of PHB*** was rather ***low***.

Oil seed plants which have plenty of acetyl CoA (for oil biosynthesis) are attractive sources for PHA production. This is because the acetyl CoA is the key substrate for PHA synthesis. No significant success has been achieved so far for PHA production by oil seed plants.

MICROBIAL LIPIDS

Among the microorganisms, the eukaryotes can accumulate triacylglycerols. In contrast, prokaryotes predominantly accumulate polyhydroxyalkanoates (as described above).

Microorganisms as oil factories

In general, commercial oils (and fats) used in foodstuffs and cosmotics are obtained from plants and animals. Thus, the traditional sources of oils are plants and animals. In recent years, microbial production of oils is gaining importance. There is a trend to use ***microorganisms as oil factories*** for the following reasons.

1. Plant oils contain residues of pesticides and herbicides that are used in the cultivation of oil seed plants.

2. Fats and fatty acids from animal sources are unacceptable by some sections of the society on moral and/or religious grounds. Further, animal fats have the risk of transfer of disease-causing agents (e.g. prions) to humans.

3. The eukaryotic microorganisms are capable of producing a wide range of polyunsaturated fatty acids. Certain microorganisms can synthesize huge quantities of a single fatty acid which is quite advantageous for large scale production and easy recovery of a particular fatty acid.

4. Microbially produced oils which are devoid of harmful contaminants will be acceptable to the public on moral and ethical grounds also.

PRODUCTION OF SINGLE-CELL OILS

Oils rich in a particular fatty acid are regarded as single-cell oils. So far, researchers have been successful in producing single-cell oils rich in three polyunsaturated fatty acids. These developments have occurred due to the interest taken by multinational pharmaceutical companies.

Linolenic acid : Single-cell oil rich in linolenic acid was the first oil produced by the fungus *Mucor circinelloides*. Its production however, was later discontinued due to cost factor.

Arachidonic acid : The soil fungus, *Mortierella alpina* has been used for the production of oils rich in arachidonic acid.

Docosahexaenoic acid : The marine alga, *Crypthecodinium cohnii* has been employed for commercial production of decosahexaenoic acid (DHA). Microbial DHA is used for inclusion, in baby foods.

Limitations in the production of single-cell oils

The fermentation technology used for the production of single-cell oils is very expensive.

It is visualised that the day may not be far off to transfer the genes producing single cell oils from microorganisms to plants. These transgenic plants can produce large quantities of single-cell oils more cheaply. But these oils will be genetically engineered, and therefore, it is doubtful whether they will have wide-spread public acceptance.

MICROBIAL RUBBER

Natural rubber is produced by a large number of plants. Chemically, it is a ***biopolymer composed of cis-1, 4-polyisoprene***. The biosynthetic pathway for rubber has been worked out. About 17 enzymatic reactions occur for the formation of rubber. The substrates are simple sugars. The final step involves the polymerisation of isopentenyl pyrophosphate on to allylic pyrophosphate, catalysed by the enzyme rubber polymerase.

Attempts are on to ***synthesize rubber in genetically engineered microorgnaisms***. For this purpose, the rubber producing plant *Hevea brasiliensis* was selected and a cDNA library by using mRNA was contructed. It may be possible in the near future, to synthesize rubber from genetically manipulated microorganisms.

MICROBIAL ADHESIVE BIOPOLYMER

The biopolymer, adhesive protein produced by the blue mussel *Mytilus edulis* is very strong and water proof. It is useful for the mussel to attach itself to different surfaces. As the adhesive is secreted, it gets randomly cross-linked, hence it cannot be sequenced. Fortunately, the immediate precursor for the formation of adhesive protein has been isolated and characterized. It is a 130-kDa protein rich in certain amino acids like serine threonine, tyrosine, lysine and proline. Most of the proline and tyrosine residues are hydroxylated. Further, biochemical analysis revealed that this precursor protein contains repeating units of a decapeptide.

The cDNA for the precursor adhesive protein has been constructed by using mRNA. This cDNA was introduced into yeast cells and ***adhesive protein molecules were synthesized by the recombinant yeast***.

The gene encoding the repeating unit of decapeptide has been identified and chemically synthesized. This gene was incorporated into *E. coli* cells for synthesizing adhesive protein. But there is a limitation-*E. coli* cannot carry out post-translational reactions i.e. hydroxylation of the adhesive protein. This deficiency can be overcome by carrying out *in vitro* hydroxylation. It is possible to hydroxylate amino acids by employing bacterial enzymes (e.g. tyrosinase) in the presence of vitamin C.

It is expected that adhesive biopolymers will be soon produced for widespread use in dentistry and medicine.

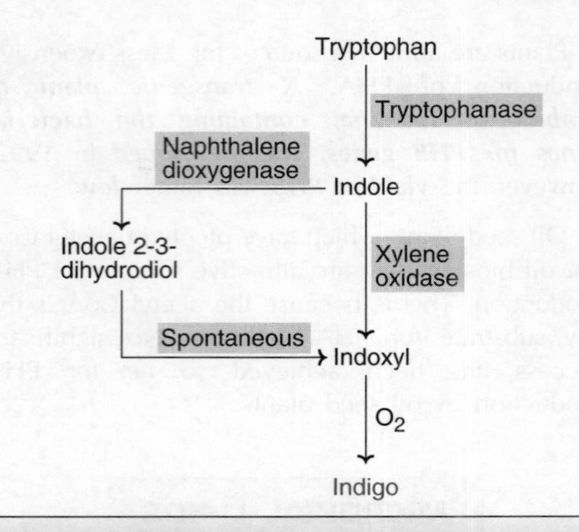

***Fig. 30.6 :** Biosynthesis of indigo from tryptophan by genetically engineered* E. coli.

MICROBIAL PRODUCTION OF INDIGO

Indigo is a ***blue pigment***, extensively used ***to dye cotton and wool***. There is a heavy demand for indigo worldover, and it is at present the largest selling dye in the world. Originally, indigo was isolated from plants. Now, it is being synthesized by using the hazardous compounds such a aniline, formaldehyde and cyanide.

In the recent years, it has been possible to synthesize indigo from tryptophan, by genetically engineered *E. coli*. The biosynthetic pathway for the production of indigo is given in ***Fig. 30.6***. However, a large scale commercial manufacture of indigo by genetically engineered *E. coli* is yet to commence.

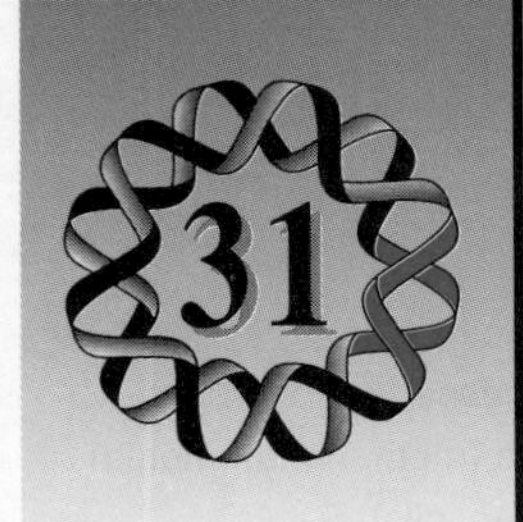

Biomass and Bioenergy

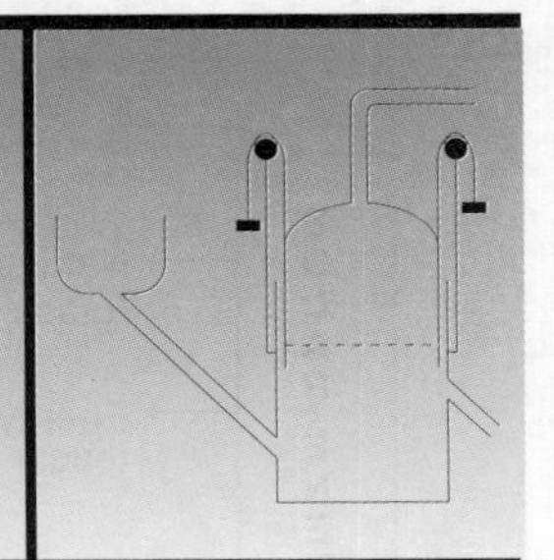

The capacity to do work is referred to as energy. Energy may be considered as a form of matter which is interconvertible. The modern man is mostly dependent on three sources for his energy needs—***coal, natural gas and oils***, collectively referred to as ***fossil fuels*** or ***fossil energy sources***. The fear of depletion of global fossil fuels has forced man to look for suitable alternative energy sources such as solar, hydro, tidal and wind power, and more recently nuclear energy. In addition to these, advances in biotechnology have helped to fruitfully utilize the ***energy from biological systems***.

BIOMASS

Biomass is the ***total cellular and organic mass, produced by the living organisms***. It is the ***primary product of photosynthesis*** and is a ***good source of energy*** i.e. bioenergy. Broadly speaking, biomass represents all forms of matter derived from biological activities. These include plants and agricultural products, microorganisms, animal wastes and manure. The term biomass is also used to collectively describe the waste materials produced in food and agricultural industries. Besides being a good source of energy, biomass is important for the production of several commercially important products. Thus, biomass is appropriately regarded as a renewable source of energy which can be directly converted to energy or energy carrier compounds by various means.

In most developed countries, biomass is utilized for the production of industrial and commercial products (ethanol, oils, methane, single-cell protein). In contrast, in the developing countries (India, Latin America, Africa), a major part of the biomass is directly used as a source of energy (as firewood).

It is estimated that the annual net yield of plant biomass is around 175 billion tons of dry matter (125 billion tons on land and 50 billion tons on oceans). Forests significantly contribute to the production of land based biomass (around 45%). Agricultural crops on the cultivated land account for about 6% of the plant biomass. The agricultural biomass products (cereals, pulses, oils, animal feed etc.) adequately meet requirements of foods for humans and animals, besides other basic needs (fuels, chemicals etc.). From the chemical point of view, about ***50% of the land produced biomass*** is in the complex form of ***lignocellulose***.

Fossil fuels-derivatives of biomass

The modern society is dependent of on the non-renewable sources of energy namely oil, gas and coal. These fossil fuels are actually derivatives of ancient biomass. It took millions of years for the fossil fuels to be deposited beneath the earth and oceans. However, in just within a century of exploration, the major fuel reserves (particularly gas and oil) are depleted, and at the present rate, they are not likely to last long. As such, there exists

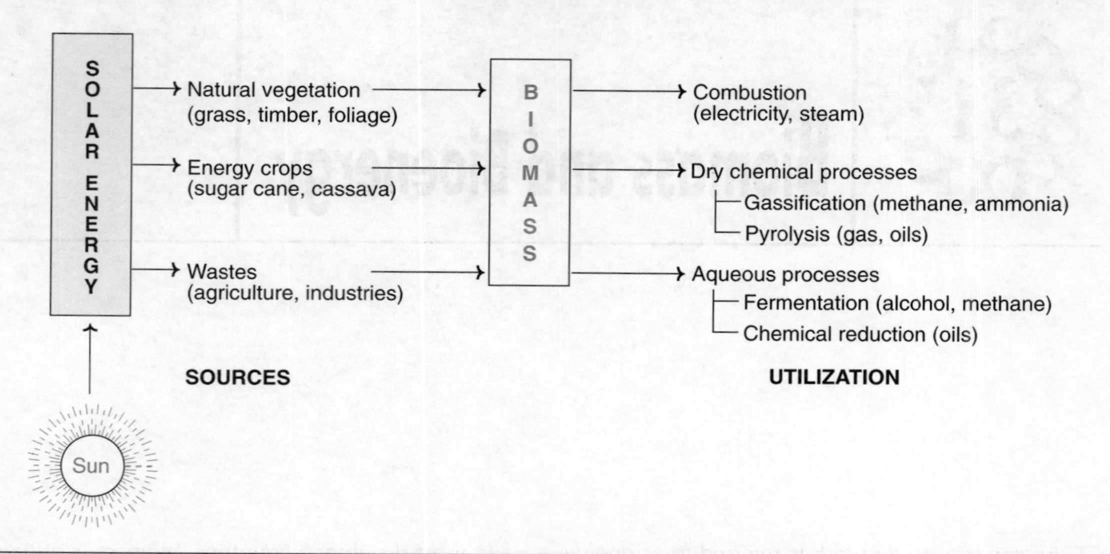

Fig. 31.1 : An overview of the sources and utilization of biomass.

an ***energy crisis*** throughout the world. Consequently, researchers continue their search for alternate and renewable sources of energy.

Photosynthesis-the ultimate source of energy

Photosynthetic organisms are the ultimate sources for trapping the solar energy. In the presence of photosynthetic pigment chlorophyll, carbon dioxide is converted into complex carbohydrates with the evolution of oxygen.

$$CO_2 + H_2O \xrightarrow[\text{Light}]{\text{Chlorophyll}} (CH_2O) + O_2$$

In the reactions that follow later, solar energy is trapped into molecules such as fat and proteins, besides other complex carbohydrates (cellulose, hemicellulose, lignin).

Photosynthetic organisms are the true solar energy converters. It is estimated that at present more than 10 times more energy is generated by photosynthesis annually than consumed by the world's population. Unfortunately, the role of photosynthesis is not well recognized to solve the present day problem of energy crisis. This, despite the fact that it is only the photosynthetically produced biomass that is available today in the form of fossil fuels.

The biomass produced by photosynthesis can be appropriately utilized for the production of fuels (alcohol, methane) and various other commercial products.

Chemical nature of biomass

The plant biomass is mainly composed of ***cellulose, hemicellulose, lignin, starch,*** proteins, water soluble (sugars, amino acids) and fat soluble (oils, pigments) compounds. In fact, majority of these constituents are present in the plant cell walls. There is a wide variation in the chemical composition of the biomass, depending on the source. For instance, the biomass obtained from sugar cane and beet sugar is rich in sugars while the biomass of potato and topioca is rich in starch. On the other hand, cotton has high content of cellulose.

The chemical nature of biomass derived from industrial and municipal wastes is highly variable which mostly depends on the sources that contribute to the biomass.

SOURCES AND UTILIZATION OF BIOMASS

The major sources of biomass are natural vegetation, energy crops, and agricultural, industrial and urban organic wastes (***Fig. 31.1***). Their production in turn is dependent on the solar energy.

The natural vegetation (growing natural forests and aquatic weeds) significantly contributes to biomass. Wood-rich plants are grown in many countries (particularly developing countries) to generate fire for cooking and other purposes. In recent years, well planned and organized plantations are carried out in some countries to produce biomass to meet energy demands. For instance, sugar cane and cassava plantations in Brazil and Australia are used for ethanol production. Plants rich in lignocellulose are grown in America and Sweden which are useful for the production of liquid fuels (ethanol, methanol).

Agricultural, industrial and municipal wastes were earlier considered as useless and discarded. But in the recent past, many countries have developed methods for converting these ***wastes into biofuels and commercially important products***. The successfully used agricultural wastes include straw, bagasse, bran, cotton wastes. Among the industrial wastes, molasses, whey, distillery wastes and sewage are the important ones.

As already stated, the biomass is utilized for the production of biofuels and various other compounds. The technique mainly depends on the chemical nature and moisture content of biomass.

Combustion : Low moisture containing biomass (wood, straw, bran) can be ***directly burnt*** by a process referred to as ***combustion*** to generate electricity.

Dry chemical processes : The biomass with little moisture content can be subjected to various dry chemical processes-pyrolysis, gassification to produce methanol, oil and ammonia biomass.

Aqueous processes : The biomass with high water content is used in aqueous processes such as fermentation to produce ethanol, oils and methane.

An overview of the sources and utilization of biomass is depicted in ***Fig. 31.1***. The biotechnological strategies for the production of biofuels (alcohol, hydrogen) from biomass are briefly described in the following pages.

PRODUCTION OF ALCOHOL FROM BIOMASS

Alcohol, chemically ethanol (C_2H_5OH) has been produced by fermentation for thousands of years. Although the developed countries these days prefer to manufacture ethanol by chemical means, the developing countries continue to produce it by microbial fermentation. ***Alcohol is the liquid fuel*** which is mostly ***produced from the biomass***. The ***raw materials*** (biomass) used for alcohol production include ***starchy materials*** (wheat, rice, maize, potato) and ***cellulosic materials*** (wood, agricultural wastes).

The reader must refer the Chapter 23 for full details on alcohol fermentation.

PRODUCTION OF BIOGAS FROM BIOMASS

Biogas is a mixture of gases composed of ***methane*** (50–80%), ***carbon dioxide*** (15–40%), ***nitrogen*** (4%) and hydrogen sulfide (1%) with traces of hydrogen, oxygen and carbon monoxide. There are many other common names for biogas—***gobar gas***, ***sewage gas***, ***klar gas*** and ***sludge gas***. Biogas is a ***gaseous fuel*** and serves as a good source of energy for various purposes.

1. It can be ***used for cooking purposes*** (on combustion).

2. Gobar gas can generate electricity.

3. It can be purified to yield good grade methane. Methane gas is extensively used as a fuel for domestic and industrial purposes. It is employed for the generation of electrical, mechanical and heat energy.

It is estimated that under ideal conditions, 10 kg of biomass can produce 3 m^3 of biogas. This biogas can provide 3 hour cooking, 3 hour lighting or 24 hour refrigeration (with suitable equipment). The calorific value of biogas (with 80% methane) is around 8,500 cal/m^3.

Biogas production in different countries

Biogas production significantly contributes to world's energy source. China has the largest number of biogas or gobar gas systems, with an estimated 7 million units. Government of China encourages and offers subsidies for construction of biogas units. As a result, the cost of a biogas plant is cheaper than a bicycle in China!

Governments in many developing countries also encourage installation of biogas plants. In India, Government provides 25% subsidy, besides encouraging banks to offer loans for construction of biogas plants. They are becoming popular in rural areas. Pakistan also has a good number of gobar gas plants.

Substrates for biogas

The usual substrates for biogas production are the waste products of animal husbandry, industries, agriculture and municipalities. In India and other developing countries, ***cattle dung (gobar) is most commonly used***. The major raw material for biogas in China is pig dung.

The concentration of organic dry matter or total solids (TS) is useful for grading the industrial, agricultural and municipal wastes. Thus, low grade (< 1% TS), medium grade (1-5% TS), high grade (5–20% TS) and solid (20–40% TS) wastes are available. Solid or high grade wastes are preferred as substrates for biogas production.

In general, most of the substrates used in biogas plants contain adequate quantities of almost all the essential nutrients required for microbial growth. If necessary, nitrogen, phosphorus and trace elements are added. A carbon nitrogen ratio (C/N) less than 40 : 1 is preferred for optimal biogas formation.

Water hyacinth (*Eichornia crasipes*) an aquatic weed with huge biomass is a good source (raw material) for methane production. With high C/N ratio and low lignin content, the yield of methane is high. Another aquatic weed ***Azolla*** is equally important for methane generation.

Microbial production of methane (biogas)

Methane is the most abundant constituent of biogas. It can also be directly used for various domestic and industrial purposes. The microbial generation of methane, appropriately referred to as ***methanogenesis*** from biomass occurs in four phases (***Fig. 31.2***).

1. **Hydrolytic phase** : Certain facultative anaerobic bacteria hydrolyse the complex organic materials of the biomass (cellulose, starch, proteins, lipids) to low molecular weight soluble products and some organic acids.

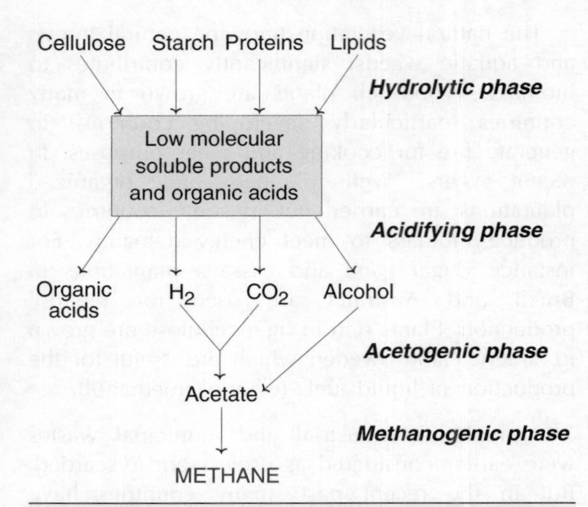

Fig. 31.2 : Microbial production of methane (methanogenesis from biomass).

2. **Acidifying phase** : This phase is characterized by more formation of organic acids, besides H_2, CO_2, and alcohol.

3. **Acetogenic phase** : Acetogenic bacteria convert alcohol into acetate. These bacteria also generate acetate from H_2 and CO_2.

4. **Methanogenic phase** : This is the actual phase of methane gas formation. The methanogenic bacteria (e.g. *Methanobacterium omelianskii, M. formicicum, M. bryantii, Methanosarcina barkeri*) convert acetate, and CO_2 and H_2 into methane.

$$CH_3COOH \longrightarrow CH_4 + CO_2$$

$$4H_2 + CO_2 \longrightarrow CH_4 + 2H_2O$$

Some other substrates like formate and methanol can also be converted to methane.

$$4HCOOH \longrightarrow CH_4 + 3CO_2 + 2H_2O$$

$$4CH_3OH \longrightarrow 3CH_4 + CO_2 + 2H_2O$$

The overall reaction of methane formation from glucose as the starting material may be represented as follows.

$$C_6H_{12}O_6 \longrightarrow 3CH_4 + 3CO_2$$

The complex polysaccharides particularly lignin and cellulose due to their inefficient conversion, limit methane production. In the normal process of methanogenesis, approximately 50% of the complex polysaccharides contribute to methanogenesis.

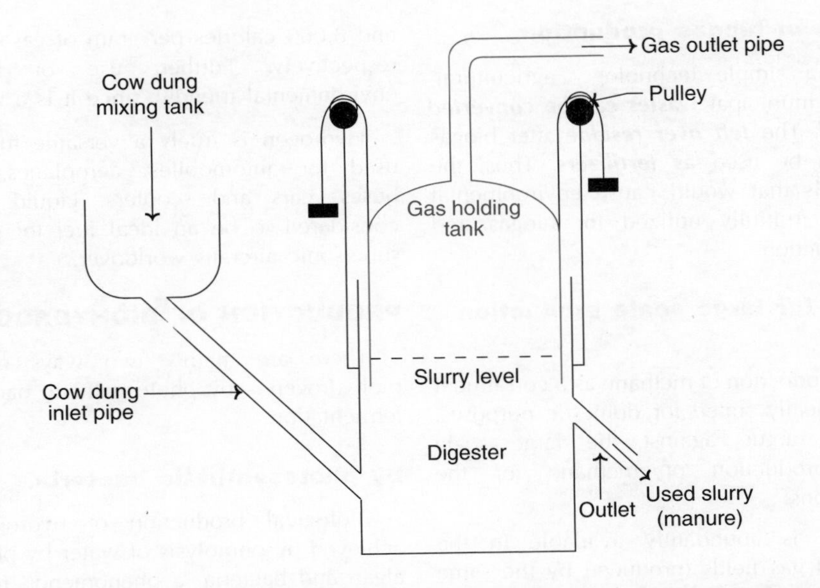

Fig. 31.3 : Diagrammatic representation of a biogas plant (gobar gas plant).

PROCESS OF BIOGAS PRODUCTION (BIOGAS PLANT)

Biogas poduction from biomass is an ***anaerobic process***. The anaerobic digestion is usually carried out by using air tight cylindrical tanks which are referred to as ***anaerobic digesters***. A digester may be made up of concrete bricks and cement or steel, usually built underground. The digester has an inlet attached to a mixing tank for feeding cow dung (***Fig. 31.3***). The methanogenic bacteria from another digester are also added with cow dung. The digester is attached to a movable gas holding or storage tank with a gas outlet. The ***used slurry*** (spent cow dung) comes out from the digester through an outlet. This can be used ***as a manure***. The anaerobic digester described above, is a low technology gobar gas plant, commonly used for domestic purposes in rural areas in India. The process of digestion usually takes about 2-3 weeks when cow dung is used as the substrate.

Landfill sites for methane production

Landfill sites are low cost ***digesters built underground for the digestion of solid wastes*** (of industries and municipalities). As the anaerobic digestion of solid organic material occurs, methane gas is generated. It can be recovered by boring gas wells into the top of the landfill. (For more details Refer Chapter 58).

Factors affecting biogas (methane) production

The factors affecting methane production, with special reference to biogas plant, are briefly described.

1. **Temperature and pH :** The ideal temperature is 30–40°C, while the pH is 6-8, for good yield.

2. **Slurry composition :** The ratio between solid and water composition in the slurry should be around 1 : 1. A carbon nitrogen ratio of 30 : 1 in the slurry results in optimal methane production. Good mixing and solubilization of the organic constituents is required.

3. **Anaerobic conditions :** The digester should be completely airtight, so as to create suitable anaerobic conditions.

4. **Presence of inhibitors :** Ammonium sulfate and antibiotics inhibit methane production. Agricultural wastes, pig and chicken manure (generating ammonia) and wastes from paper (rich in sulfate) inhibit biogas production.

Advantages of biogas production

By using a simple technology, agricultural, industrial and municipal ***wastes can be converted into a biofuel***. The ***left over residue*** after biogas formation can be used ***as fertilizers***. Thus, the waste materials that would cause environmental pollution are fruitfully utilized for biogas and fertilizer production.

Limitations for large scale production of methane

Although production of methane as a constituent of biogas is ideally suited for domestic purposes. Many people argue against the large scale commercial production of methane for the following reasons.

1. Methane is abundantly available in the natural oil and gas fields (produced by the same mechanism of methanogenesis, over a period of years).

2. Microbial production of methane is more expensive than its isolation from the natural gas.

3. Methane production by gassification of coal is more economical than its production from biomass.

4. Being a gaseous fuel, it is quite difficult as well as expensive to store, transport and distribute methane.

5. Methane is unsuitable for use as a fuel in automobiles. This is because it is very difficult to convert the gaseous methane into liquid state.

Despite the limitations listed above, production of methane from a wide range of biodegradable materials (particularly the wastes) is still attractive. This is due to the fact that the biomass used for methane generation is renewable, in contrast to the permanent depletion of naturally produced methane (in the gas and oil fields).

HYDROGEN — A NEW BIOFUEL

Hydrogen is a simple molecule which can be easily collected, stored (as a gas or liquid) and transported. It is highly combustible and can be ***used as a fuel or for the production of electricity***. Hydrogen, on mixing with oxygen, provides around 30,000 calories per gram as compared to 11,000 and 8,000 calories per gram of gasoline and coal respectively. Further, use of hydrogen is environmental friendly, since it is a non-pollutant.

Hydrogen is truely a versatile fuel. It can be used for automobiles, aeroplanes, helicopters, buses, cars and scooters. Liquid hydrogen is considered to be an ideal fuel for subsonic and supersonic aircrafts worldover.

PRODUCTION OF BIOHYDROGEN

There are mainly two ways of generating biohydrogen — by photosynthetic bacteria and by fermentation.

By photosynthetic bacteria

Biological production of hydrogen can be achieved by photolysis of water by photosynthetic algae and bacteria, a phenomenon referred to as ***biophotolysis***. Certain microalgae, and cyanobacteria (e.g. *Chlorella, Chlamydomonas, Scenedesmus, Microcystis, Oscillatoria, Aneboena*) can generate molecular hydrogen. Water is the source of raw material.

$$H_2O \xrightarrow{\text{Photolysis}} O_2 + H^+ + e^-$$

$$H^+ + H^+ \xrightarrow{\text{Hydrogenase}} H_2$$

The action of hydrogenase can be inhibited by creating oxygen pressure. This condition favours release of free hydrogen.

Isolated chloroplasts along with the bacterial enzyme hydrogenase have also been used for production of hydrogen.

By fermentation

It is possible to produce hydrogen from glucose, by bacterial action. However, the yield is less and uneconomical. Hydrogen can also be generated by anaerobic fermentation, by a process comparable to that of methane production. This is also not economical, besides being low in efficiency. Photosynthetic bacterium *Rhodospirillium* can be used to produce hydrogen from organic wastes.

By legume crops

The leguminous plants convert N_2 to NH_3 and H_2. This reaction is catalysed by the enzyme ***nitrogenase***. In the normal circumstances, this H_2

gas, a byproduct of nitrogen metabolism is lost in the soil. It is estimated that from a soybean crop in one hectare field, about 30 billion m^3 hydrogen is generated and lost annually. As such, there are no methods available to trap such huge quantities of hydrogen produced in agricultural fields.

ENERGY-RICH CROPS

Some of the plants are ***very efficient in converting CO_2 into biomass*** and such plants are collectively referred to as energy-rich crops.

Sugar and starch crops

Certain plants like sugar cane, sugar beet, cereals and tuber crops produce high quantities of starch and fermentation sugars. These crops supply energy-rich foods and feeds. Such plants are useful for production of ***biofuels***, particularly ethanol often referred to as ***bioethanol***.

Wood-rich plants

Some plants grow very fast and they serve as good suppliers of wood. e.g. *Eucalyptus, Butea, Melia, Casurina*. These plants are important sources of firewood. It is estimated that approximately 50% of the total wood harvested annually is utilized for the purpose of firewood. Wood is also useful for the supply of pulp for paper manufacture.

Petroleum plants

There are certain plants which can ***accumulate high molecular weight hydrocarbons***. They are referred to as ***petro-crops*** or ***gasoline plantations***. The products of these hydrocarbon-rich plants can serve as good ***substitutes of conventional petroleum*** and petroleum products.

The ***rubber plant*** (*Hevea rubber*), grown in South-East Asia is the principal source of rubber. Rubber is collected in the form of latex from the stems of trees. This plant meets about one third of the total world's demand of rubber. However, the rubber produced from petroleum is preferred for use in automobiles and planes, due to low-cost and high elasticity. Besides *Hevea rubber*, there are some other plants for the production of natural rubber e.g. *Parthenium agrentatum* (guayule) *Taraxacum koksaghyz* (Russian dandelion) grown in Mexico and some parts of USA.

Euphorbia lathyrus and *E. terucalli* contain high contents of terpenoids (complex hydrocarbons) that can be directly converted to gasoline/petrol. It is estimated that *E. terucelli* can yield about 5–10 barrels of oil/acre/year.

Aak plant (*Calotropis procera*) secretes latex which is very rich in hydrocarbons. These hydrocarbons, and the yield are comparable to *Euphorbia lathyrus*, and they also serve as good substitutes of petroleum.

For obvious reasons, the cultivation of petroleum plants is encouraged throughout the world.

THE FUTURE OF BIOMASS

Besides its utility for the generation biofuels (alcohol, methane), biomass is also used for the ***production of butanol, acetone, single-cell protein and many other products*** (Chapter 29).

As such, the contribution of biomass to the world's requirements of energy is very low. It is around 5% in the U.S.A., and may be a little higher in the developing countries. However, ***being a renewable source of energy, biomass will have immense value in future***. This is particularly true as the world's non-renewable fuels (gas and oil) get depleted. There is a growing realisation on the fuel value of biomass. In the coming years, biomass production and utilization strategies will be fully exploited. In addition, further improvements in the biotechnological processes for better management and utilization of industrial, agricultural and domestic wastes will also solve the problem of world energy crisis.

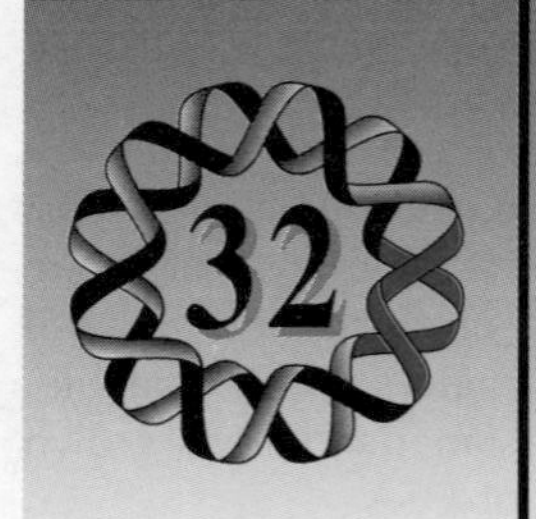

Microbial Mining and Metal Biotechnology

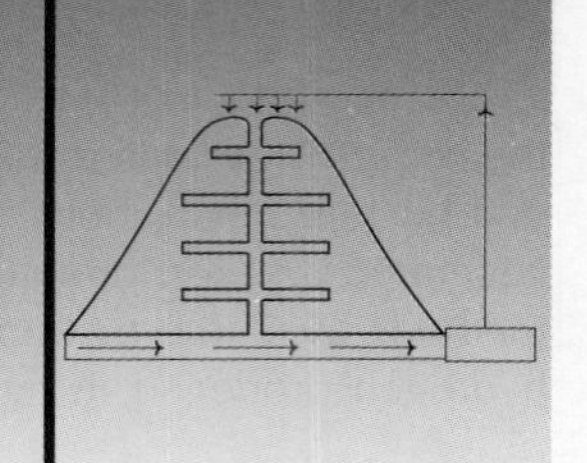

Soil microorganisms are very closely involved as catalytic agents in many geological processes. These include mineral formation, mineral degradation, sedimentation and geochemical cycling.

In recent years, a new discipline of mineral science namely ***biohydrometallurgy*** or ***microbial mining*** (***mining with microbes***) is rapidly growing. Broadly speaking, biohydrometallurgy deals with the ***application of biotechnology in mining industry***. In fact, microorganisms can be successfully used for the extraction of metals (e.g., copper, zinc, cobalt, lead, uranium) from low grade ores. Mining with microbes is both economical and environmental friendly.

The term metal is used to any substance that is hard, possessing silvery lusture, and is a good conductor of heat and electricity. Some of the metals, however, are relatively soft, malleable and ductile e.g. sulfur. An ore is a naturally occurring solid mineral aggregate from which one or more minerals can be recovered by processing.

Majority of microorganisms can interact with metals. The metals can be recovered by the microorganisms by two processes.

1. **Bioleaching or microbial leaching :** This broadly involves the extraction or solubilization of minerals from the ores by the microorganisms.

2. **Biosorption :** It deals with the microbial cell surface adsorption of metals from the mine wastes or dilute mixtures.

BIOLEACHING

In ***microbial leaching*** (bioleaching), metals can be extracted from large quantities of low grade ores. Although recovery of metals (e.g. copper) from the drainage water of mines has been known for centuries, the involvement of microbes in this process was recognized about 40 years ago.

The bacteria which are naturally associated with the rocks can lead to bioleaching by one of the following ways.

1. ***Direct action*** of bacteria on the ore to extract metal.

2. Bacteria produce certain substances such as sulfuric acid and ferric iron which extract the metal (***indirect action***).

In practice, ***both the methods may work together*** for efficient recovery of metals.

Organisms for bioleaching

The ***most commonly used*** microorganisms for bioleaching are ***Thiobacillus ferrooxidans*** and ***Thiobacillus thiooxidans***.

Thiobacillus ferrooxidans is a rod-shaped, motile, non-spore forming, Gram-negative bacterium. It derives energy for growth from the oxidation of iron or sulfur. This bacterium is capable of oxidising ferrous iron (Fe^{2+}) to ferric form (Fe^{3+}), and converting sulfur (soluble or insoluble sulfides, thiosulfate, elemental sulfur) to sulfate (SO_4^{2-}). *Thiobacillus thiooxidans* is comparable with *T. ferrooxidams*, and grows mostly on sulfur compounds.

Several studies indicate that the two bacteria *T. ferrooxidans* and *T. thiooxidans*, when put together, work synergistically and improve the extraction of metals from the ores.

Besides the above two bacteria, there are other microorganisms involved in the process of bioleaching. A selected few of them are briefly described below.

Sulfolobus acidocaldarius and ***S. brierlevi*** are thermophilic and acidophilic bacteria which can grow in acidic hot springs (>60°C). These bacteria can be used to extract copper and molybdenum respectively from chalcopyrite ($CuFeS_2$) and molybdenite (MoS_2).

A combination of two bacteria *Leptospirillum ferrooxidans* and *Thiobacillus organoparpus* can effectively degrade pyrite (FeS_2) and chalcopyrite ($CuFeS_2$). The individual organisms alone are of no use in extracting metals.

Pseudomonas aeruginosa can be employed in mining low grade uranium (0.02%) ore. This organism has been shown to accumulate about 100 mg uranium per one liter solution in less than ten seconds. Another organism, *Rhizopus arrhizus* is also effective for extracting uranium from waste water.

Certain ***fungi*** have also found use in bioleaching. Thus, ***Aspergillus niger*** can extract copper and nickel while *Aspergillus oryzae* is used for extracting gold.

As already stated, among the various microorganisms, *T. ferrooxidans* and *T. thiooxidans* are the most widely used in bioleaching. The utilization of many of the other organisms is still at the experimental stage.

Mechanism of bioleaching

The mechanism of bioleaching is rather complex and not well understood. The chemical transformation of metals by microorganisms may occur by direct or indirect bioleaching.

Direct bioleaching : In this process, there is a ***direct enzymatic attack on the minerals*** (which are susceptible to oxidation) by the microorganisms. For instance, certain bacteria (e.g., *T. ferrooxidans*) can transfer electrons (coupled with ATP production) from iron or sulfur to oxygen. That is these organisms can obtain energy from the oxidation of Fe^{2+} to Fe^{3+} or from the oxidation of sulfur and reduced sulfur compounds to sulfate as illustrated below.

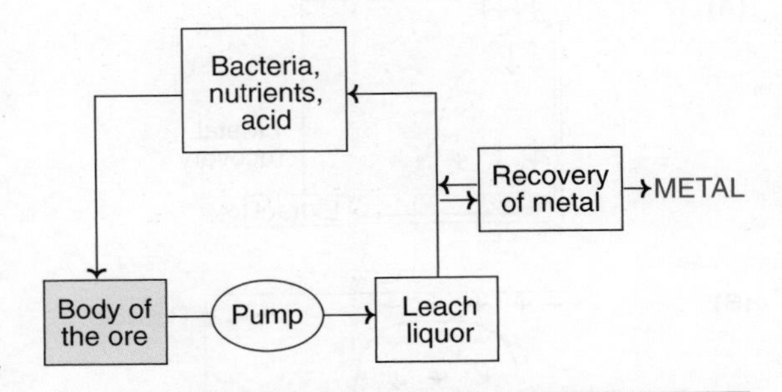

Fig. 32.1 : A flow diagram for microbial bioleaching– a general picture.

$$4FeSO_4 + 2H_2SO_4 + O_2 \longrightarrow 2Fe_2(SO_4)_3 + 2H_2O$$

$$2S^0 + 3O_2 + 2H_2O \longrightarrow 2H_2SO_4$$

$$2FeS_2 + 7O_2 + 2H_2O \longrightarrow 2FeSO_4 + 2H_2SO_4$$

As is evident from the third reaction given above, iron is extracted in the soluble form the iron ore pyrite (FeS_2).

Indirect bioleaching : In this indirect method, the ***bacteria produce strong oxidizing agents*** such as ferric iron and sulfuric acid on oxidation of soluble iron or soluble sulfur respectively. Ferric iron or sulfuric acid, being powerful oxidizing agents ***react with metals and extract them***. For indirect bioleaching, acidic environment is absolutely essential in order to keep ferric iron and other metals in solution. It is possible to continuously maintain acidic environment by the oxidation of iron, sulfur, metal sulfides or by dissolution of carbonate ions.

COMMERCIAL PROCESS OF BIOLEACHING

The naturally occurring mineral leaching is very slow. The microbial bioleaching process can be optimized by creating ideal conditions—temperature, pH, and nutrient, O_2 and CO_2 supply etc. A diagrammatic representation of general bioleaching process is depicted in ***Fig. 32.1***. The desired microorganisms with nutrients, acid etc, are pumped into the ore bed. The microorganisms

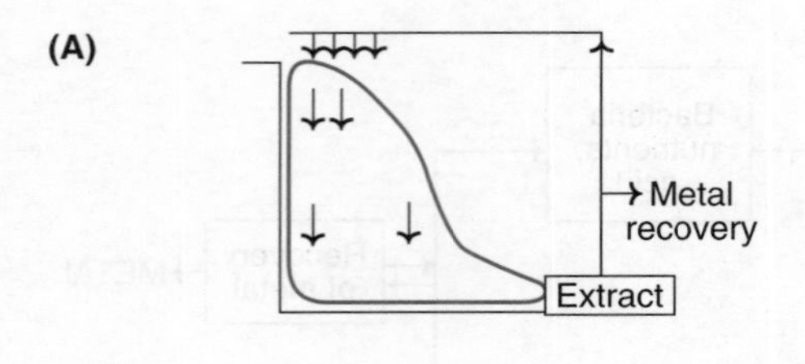

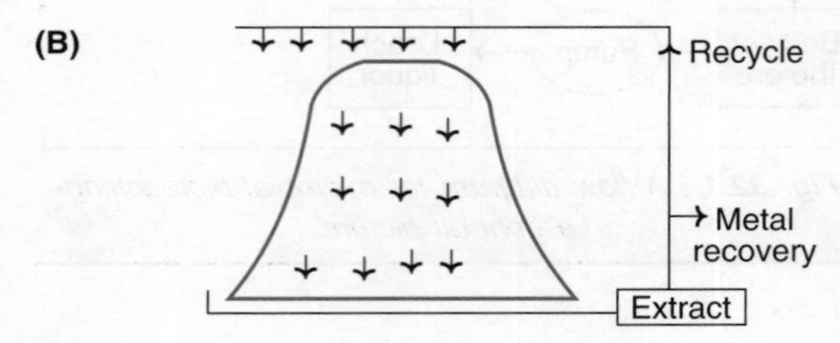

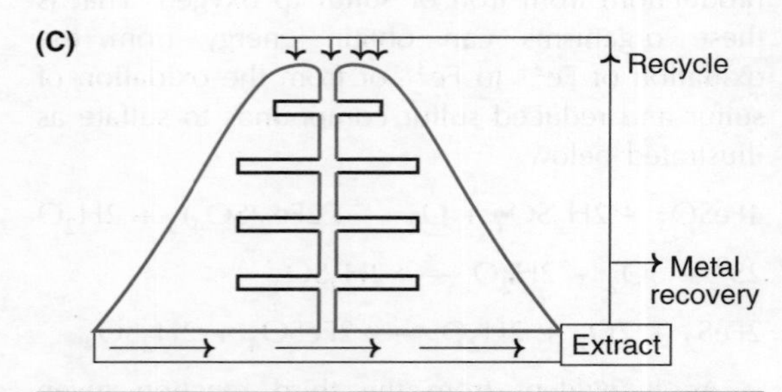

Fig. 32.2 : Commercial bioleaching processes (A) Slope leaching (B) Heap leaching (C) In situ *leaching.*

grow and produce more acid. The extracted ***leach liquor*** is processed for the metal recovery. The leach liquor can be recycled again and again for further metal extraction.

In commercial bioleaching, three methods are commonly used-slope leaching, heap leaching and *in situ* leaching (***Fig. 32.2***).

Slope leaching : The ore is finally ground and dumped in large piles down a mountainside (***Fig. 32.2A***). This ore is then subjected to continuous sprinkling of water containing the desired microorganism (*T. ferrooxidans*). The water collected at the bottom is used for metal extraction. The water can be recycled for regeneration of bacteria.

Heap leaching : In this case, the ore is arranged in large heaps (***Fig. 32.2B***) and subjected to treatments as in slope leaching.

In situ* leaching :** The ore, in its original natural place is subjected to leaching (Fig. 32.2C***). Water containing the microorganisms is pumped through drilled passages. In most cases, the permeability of rock is increased by subsurface blasting of the rock. As the acidic water seeps through the rock, it collects at the bottom which is used for metal extraction. This water can be recycled and reused.

Selected examples of microbial bioleaching are briefly described below.

BIOLEACHING OF COPPER

Copper ores (chalcopyrite, covellite and chalcocite) are mostly composed of other metals, besides copper. For instance, chalcopyrite mainly contains 26% copper, 26% iron, 33% sulfur and 2.5% zinc.

Bioleaching of copper ore (chalcopyrite) is widely used in many countries. This is ***carried out by the microorganism Thiobacillus ferrooxidans*** which oxidises insoluble chalcopyrite ($CuFeS_2$) and converts it into soluble copper sulfate ($CuSO_4$). Sulfuric acid, a byproduct formed in this reaction, maintains acidic environment (low pH) required for growth of the microorganisms.

Copper leaching is usually carried out by ***heap*** and ***in situ process*** (details given above). As the copper-containing solution (i.e., copper in the dissolved state) comes out, copper can be precipitated and the water is recycled, after adjusting the pH to around 2.

Extraction of copper by bioleaching is very common since the technique is efficient, besides being economical. It is estimated that about 5% of the world's copper production is obtained via microbial leaching. In the USA alone, at least 10% of the copper is produced by bioleaching process.

BIOLEACHING OF URANIUM

Bioleaching is the method of choice ***for the large-scale production uranium from its ores***. Uranium bioleaching is widely used in India, USA, Canada and several other countries. It is possible to recover uranium from low grade ores (0.01 to 0.5% uranium) and low grade nuclear wastes.

In situ bioleaching technique is commonly used for extracting uranium. In the technique employed, the insoluble tetravalent uranium is oxidized (in the presence of hot H_2SO_4/Fe^{3+} solution) to soluble hexavalent uranium sulfate.

$$UO_2 + Fe_2(SO_4)_3 \longrightarrow UO_2SO_4 + 2FeSO_4$$

Bioleaching of uranium is an indirect process since the microbial action is on the iron oxidant, and not directly on the uranium. The organism *Thiobacillus ferrooxidans* is capable of producing sulfuric acid and ferric sulfate from the pyrite (FeS_2) within the uranium ore.

For optimal extraction of uranium by bioleaching, the ideal conditions are temperature 45–50°C, pH 1.5-3.5, and CO_2 around 0.2% of the incoming air.

The soluble form of uranium from the leach liquor can be extracted into organic solvents (e.g., tributyl phosphate) which can be precipitated and then recovered.

Heap leaching process is sometimes preferred instead of the ***in situ*** technique. This is because the ***recovery of uranium in much higher*** with heap leaching.

BIOLEACHING OF OTHER METALS

Besides copper and uranium, bioleaching technique is also used for extraction of other metals such as ***nickel, gold, silver, cobalt, molybdenum*** and antimony. It may be noted that removal of iron is desirable prior to the actual process of leaching for other metals. This can be done by using the organism *Thiobacillus ferrooxidans* which can precipitate iron under aerobic conditions.

Bioleaching is also useful for the removal of certain impurities from the metal rich ores. For instance, the microorganisms such as *Rhizobium* sp and *Bradyrhizobium* sp can remove silica from bauxite (aluminium ore).

Bioleaching in desulfurization of coal

The process of ***removal of sulfur containing pyrite*** (FeS_2) ***from high sulfur coal*** by microorganisms is referred to as ***biodesulfurization***. High sulfur coal, when used in thermal power stations, emits sulfur dioxide (SO_2) that causes environmental pollution.

By using the microorganisms *Thiobacillus ferrooxidans* and *T. thiooxidans*, the pyrite which contains most of the sulfur (80–90%) can be removed. Thus, by employing bioleaching, high sulfur coal can be fruitfully utilized in an environment friendly manner. In addition, this approach is quite economical also.

ADVANTAGES OF BIOLEACHING

When compared to conventional mining techniques, bioleaching offers several advantages. Some of them are listed below.

1. Bioleaching can ***recover metals from low grade ores*** in a cost-effective manner.

2. It can be successfully employed for concentrating metals from wastes or dilute mixtures.

3. Bioleaching is ***environmental friendly***, since it does not cause any pollution (which is the case with conventional mining techniques).

4. It can be used to produce refined and expensive metals which otherwise may not be possible.

5. Bioleaching is a simple process with low cost technology.

6. It is ideally suited for the developing countries.

The major ***limitation*** or disadvantage ***of bioleaching*** is the ***slowness of the biological process***. This problem can, however, be solved by undertaking an in depth research to make the process faster, besides increasing the efficiency.

BIOSORPTION

Biosorption primarily deals with the ***microbial cell surface adsorption of metals*** from the mine wastes or dilute mixtures. The microorganisms can be used as ***biosorbents*** or ***bioaccumulators*** of metals. The process of biosorption performs two important functions.

1. Removal of toxic metals from the industrial effluents.

2. Recovery of valuable but toxic metals.

Both the above processes are concerned with a reduction in environmental poisoning/pollution.

A wide range of microorganisms (bacteria, algae, yeasts, moulds) are employed in biosorption. In fact, some workers have developed ***biosorbent-based granules for waste water/industrial effluent treatment, and metal recovery***.

In general, the microbial cell membranes are negatively charged due to the presence of carboxyl

(COO⁻), hydroxyl (OH⁻) phosphoryl (PO_4^{3-}) and sulfhydryl (HS⁻) groups. This enables the positively charged metal ions (from solutions) to be adsorbed on to the microbial surfaces.

The different groups of microorganisms used in biosorption processes are briefly described below.

Bacteria

Several bacteria and actinomycetes ***adsorb and accumulate metals*** such as mercury, cadmium, lead, zinc, nickel, cobalt and uranium. For example, *Rhodospirullum* sp can accumulate Cd, Pb and Hg. *Bacillus circulans* can adsorb metals such as Cu, Cd, Co, and Zn. By use of electron microscopy, deposition of metals on the bacterial cell walls was recorded. It appears that the cell wall composition plays a key role in the metal adsorption.

Fungi

There is a large scale production of fungal biomass in many fermentation industries. This biomass can be utilized ***for metal biosorption from industrial effluents***. Immobilized fungal biomass is more effective in biosorption due to increased density, mechanical strength and resistance to chemical environment. Further, immobilized biomass can be reused after suitable processing.

The fungus *Rhizopus arrhizus* can adsorb several metallic cations e.g. uranium, thorium. *Pencillium lapidorum, P. spimulosum* are useful for the biosorption of metals such as Hg, Zn, Pb, Cu. Several fungi were tried with some degree of success to selectively adsorb uranium e.g. *Aspergillus niger, A. oryzae, Mucor haemalis, Penicillium chrysogenum*.

Edible mushrooms were also found to adsorb certain metals. For instance, fruit bodies of *Agaricus bisporus* can take up mercury while *Pleurotus sajor-caju can* adsorb lead and cadmium.

Many yeasts, commonly used in fermentation industries, are capable of adsorbing and accumulating metals. For instance, *Saccharomyces cerevisae* and *Sporobolomyces salmonicolour* can respectively adsorb mercury and zinc.

Algae

Several species of algae (fresh water or marine) can ***serve as bioaccumulators of metals***. For instance, *Chlorella vulgaris* and *C. regularis* can accumulate certain metals like Pb, Hg, Cu, Mo and U. The green algae *Hydrodictyon reticulatum* adsorbs and accumulates high quantities of Pb, Fe and Mn.

Some workers are in fact trying to use marine algae (e.g., *Luminaria, Ulva, Codium* sp) as bioaccumulators to reduce the metal pollution in rivers.

Higher plants in control of metal pollution

Besides the microorganisms described above, there are some higher aquatic plants (i.e., aquatic macrophytes) that can accumulate potential toxic wastes including many metals. ***Water hyacinth*** (*Eichornia crassipes*), ***duck weeds*** (*Spirodel* sp), ***water lettuce*** (*Pistia stratiotes*) and certain ferns (*Salvinia* sp) are important in the control of metal pollution. For more details, the reader must refer Chapter 54.

MICROBIAL RECOVERY OF PETROLEUM

By the conventional technique used in the oil fields, approximately one-third of the oil can be recovered. However, the oil recovery can be enhanced by using solvents, and surfactants. ***Certain polymers produced by microorganisms*** (e.g., ***xanthan gum***), ***when added to oil wells are capable of increasing oil recovery***. Xanthan gum can pass through small pore spaces and promote the release of more trapped oil.

In recent years, oil technologists are trying to directly use microorganisms *in situ* for increasing the oil recovery. In this process, there is no formalised use of a bioreactor. The natural geological site itself is the bioreactor. This allows the water and microorganisms to flow over the ore which are collected after seepage and outflow. The microorganisms, through surfactant production, gas formation or by other microbial activities reduce the viscosity of the oil so as to enhance its recovery. However, the success in this direction is not very commendable.

Continued further research may one day help to use microbes for commercial release of oil from oil wells or tar sands.

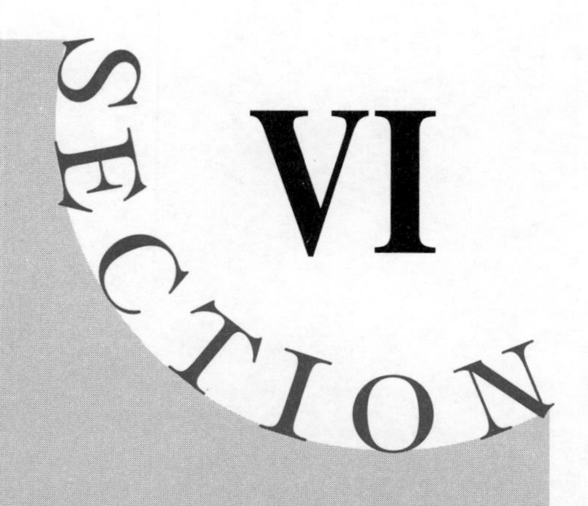

ANIMAL CELL/ ANIMAL BIOTECHNOLOGY

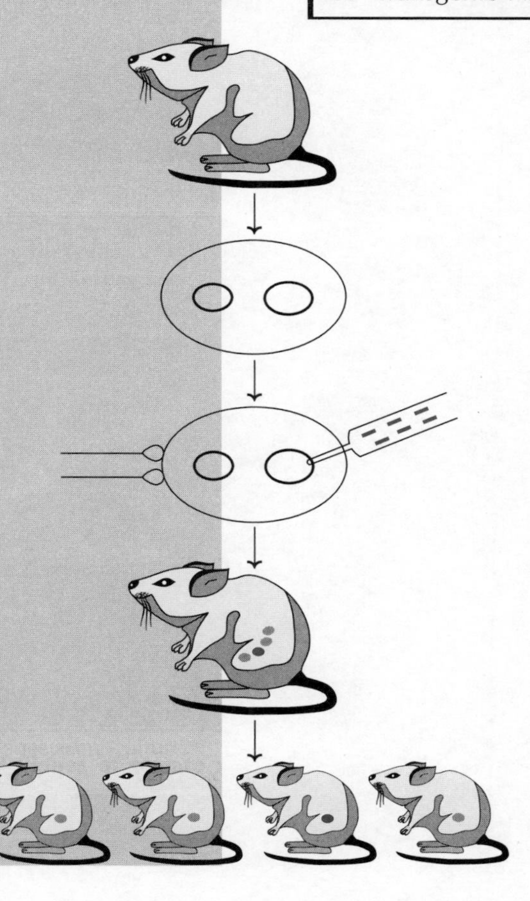

CONTENTS

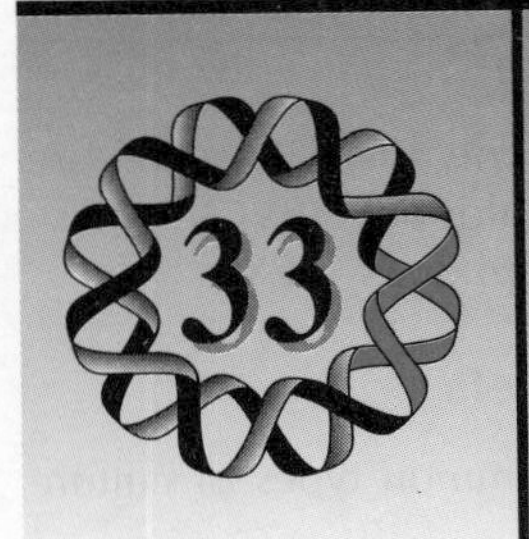

Animal Cell Culture — Fundamentals, Facilities and Applications

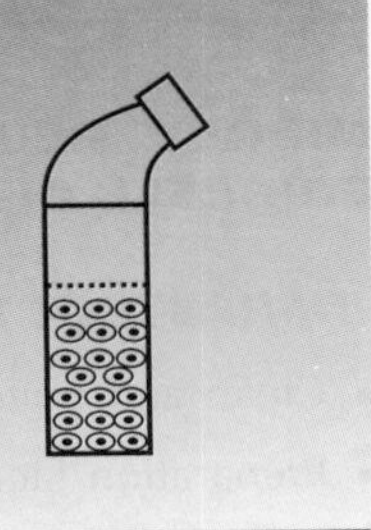

Animal cell culture basically involves the *in vitro* (in the laboratory) maintenance and propagation of animal cells in a suitable nutrient media. Thus, ***culturing is a process of growing cells artificially***. Cell culture has become an indispensible technology in various branches of life sciences.

Historical background

It was in 1907, Ross Harrison first developed a frog tissue culture technique. He probably chose frog for two reasons—being a cold-blooded animal, no incubation is required and tissue regeneration is fast in frog. In 1940's chick embryo tissue became a favourite for culture techniques. Interest in culturing human tissues started in 1950's after it was demonstrated (by HeLa; Gey) that human tumor cells could give rise to continuous cell lines. Among the various animal cell cultures, mouse cell cultures are the most commonly used in the laboratory.

Terminology in cell culture

The term ***tissue culture*** is commonly used to include both organ culture and cell culture.

Organ culture : The culture of native tissue (i.e. undisaggregated tissue) that retains most of the *in vivo* histological features is regarded as organ culture.

Cell culture : This refers to the culture of dispersed (or disaggregated) cells obtained from the original tissue, or from a cell line.

Histotypic culture : The culturing of the cells for their reaggregation to form a tissue—like structure represents histotypic culture.

Organotypic culture : This culture technique involves the recombination of different cell types to form a more defined tissue or an organ.

Primary culture : The culture produced by the freshly isolated cells or tissues taken from an organism is the primary culture. These cell are heterogenous and slow growing, and represent the tissue of their origin with regard to their properties.

Cell line : The subculturing of the primary culture gives rise to cell lines. The term ***continuous cell lines*** implies the ***indefinite growth of the cells*** in the subsequent subculturing. On the other hand, ***finite cell lines*** represent the death of cells after several subcultures.

FACILITIES FOR ANIMAL CELL CULTURE

While designing the laboratory for animal cell culture technology, utmost care should be taken with regard to the maintenance of aspetic conditions. The facilities required with regard to infrastructure and equipment are listed in the next page.

MINIMAL REQUIREMENTS FOR CELL CULTURE

INFRASTRUCTURE

- Clean and quite sterile area
- Preparation facilities
- Animal house
- Microbiology laboratory
- Storage facilities (for glassware, chemicals, liquids, small equipment).

EQUIPMENT

Laminar-flow, sterilizer, incubator, refrigerator and freezer (–20°C), balance, CO_2 cylinder, centrifuge, inverted microscope, water purifier, hemocytometer, liquid nitrogen freezer, slow-cooling device (for freezing cells), pipette washer, deep washing sink.

Besides the basic and minimal requirements listed above, there are many more facilities that may be beneficial or useful for tissue cultures. These include air-conditioned rooms, containment room for biohazard work, phase-contrast microscope, fluorescence microscope, confocal microscope, osmometer, high capacity centrifuge and time lapse video equipment.

CULTURE VESSELS

In the tissue culture technology, the cells attach to the surface of a vessel which ***serves as the substrate***, and grow. Hence there is a lot of importance attached to the nature of the materials used and the quality of the culture vessels.

The term ***anchorage dependent cells*** is used when the cells require an attachment for their growth. On the other hand, some cells undergo transformation, and become ***anchorage independent***.

Materials used for culture vessels

Glass : Although glass was the original substrate used for culturing, its use is almost discontinued now. This is mainly because of the availability of more suitable and alternate substrates.

Disposable plastics : Synthetic plastic materials with good consistency and optical properties are now in use to provide uniform and reproducible cultures. The most commonly used plastics are polystyrene, polyvinyl chloride (PVC), poly-carbonate, metinex and thermonex (TPX).

Types of culture vessels

The following are the common types of culture vessels.

- Multiwell plates
- Petridishes
- Flasks
- Stirrer bottles.

The actual choice of selecting a culture vessel depends on several factors.

1. The way cells grow in culture—monolayer or suspension.
2. The quantity of the cells required.
3. The frequency of sampling for the desired work.
4. The purpose for which the cells are grown.
5. The cost factor.

In general, for ***monolayer cultures***, the cell yield is almost proportional to the surface area of the culture vessel. The flasks are usually employed for this purpose.

Any type of culture vessel can be used to grow suspension cultures. It is necessary to slowly and continuously agitate the suspended cells in the vessel.

Treatment of culture vessel surfaces

For improving the attachment of cells to the surfaces, and for efficient growth, some devices have been developed. It is a common observation that the growth of the culture cells is better on the surfaces for second seeding. This is attributed to ***matrix coating of the surfaces*** due to the accumulation of certain compounds like collagen and fibronectin released by the cells of the previous culture.

There are now commercially available matrices (e.g. matrigel, pronectin, cell-tak).

Feeder layers : Some of the tissue cultures require the support of metabolic products from living cells e.g. mouse embryo fibroblasts. In this case, the growing fibroblasts release certain products which when fed to new cells enhance their growth.

Alternate substrates as substitutes of culture vessels

In recent years, certain alternatives for culture vessels have been developed. The important alternative artificial substrates are microcarriers and metallic substrates.

Microcarriers : They are in bead form and are made up of collagen, gelatin, polyacrylamide and polystyrene. Microcarriers are mostly used for the propagation of anchorage-dependent cells in suspension.

Metallic substrates : Certain types of cells could be successfully grown on some metallic surfaces or even on the stainless steel discs. For instance, fibroblasts were grown on palledium.

USE OF NON-ADHESIVE SUBSTRATES IN TISSUE CULTURE

The growth of anchorage independent cells can be carried out by plating cells on non-adhesive substrate like ***agar, agarose and methyl cellulose***. In this situation, as the cell growth occurs, the parent and daughter cells get immobilized and form a colony, although they are non-adhesive.

CONTAMINATION, ASEPTIC CONDITIONS, AND STERILIZATION

There are several ***routes of contamination*** in the tissue culture laboratory (***Table 33.1***). These include the various ***materials*** (glassware, pipettes), ***equipment*** (incubators, refrigerators, laminar-flow hoods), ***reagents*** (media, solutions), ***contaminated cell lines*** and ***poor techniques***.

The routes of contamination are mostly associated with the laboratory environment, and operating techniques.

Types of microbial contamination

Several species of bacteria, yeasts, fungi, molds and mycoplasmas, besides viruses are responsible for contamination. Major problems of contamination are linked to the repeated recurrence of a single species. Despite utmost care taken, no laboratory can claim to be totally free from contamination. It is necessary to continuously monitor for contamination and eliminate the same at the earliest.

TABLE 33.1 Major routes of contamination in a tissue culture laboratory

Equipment and facilities
Laminar-flow hoods
Dry incubators
CO_2 incubators
Humidified incubators
Wooden furniture, benches
Other instruments
Glassware and reagents
Pipettes
Screw caps
Culture glasses
Media bottles
Media and various solutions
Biological materials
Infected tissue samples
Cell lines
Operating techniques
Operator hands, hair, clothing, breathing
Work spaces
Pipetting, dispensing
Operating manipulations

ASEPTIC CONDITIONS

Maintenance of proper aseptic conditions is necessary ***to eliminate various contaminants (due to different microorganisms and viruses)***. The following measures are suggested for minimizing contamination, and maintenance of aseptic conditions.

- Strict adherence to standard sterile techniques and code of practices.

- Checking of reagents and media for sterility before use.
- Checking of cultures by eyes, and microscopes (phase contrast) every time they are used.
- Use of media and separate bottles for each cell line is advised.
- Maintenance of clean and tidy conditions at work places.
- Personal hygiene of the staff is very important.

STERILIZATION

The sterilization procedures are designed to kill the microorganisms, besides destroying the spores. There are three major devices for sterilization.

1. Dry heat
2. Moist heat (autoclave)
3. Filters.

In the ***Table 33.2***, the sterilization of major equipment, apparatus and liquids is given.

Sterilization by dry heat : This is carried out at a minimum temperature of 160°C for about one hour.

Sterilization by moist heat : Certain fluids and perishable items can be sterilized in an autoclave at 121°C for 15–20 minutes. For effective moist heat sterilization, it is necessary that the steam penetrates to all the parts of the sterilizing materials.

Sterilization by filters : The use of filters for sterilization of liquids often becomes necessary, since the constituents of these liquids may get destroyed at higher temperatures (dry heat or moist heat).

Sterile filtration is a novel technique for heat-labile solutions. The size of micropores of the filters is 0.1-0.2 μm. Filters, made from several materials are in use. These materials include nylon, cellulose acetate, cellulose nitrate, polycarbonate, polyethersulfone (PES) and ceramics. The filters are made in different designs-disc filters, cartridges and hollow fiber.

In fact, many commercial companies (e.g. Millipore, Durapore) supply ***reusable*** and ***disposable filters***, designed for different purposes of sterilization.

TABLE 33.2 Sterilization of major equipment, apparatus and liquids used in tissue culture

Sterilization device	*Items sterilized*
I *For equipment and apparatus*	
Dry heat	Glass slides Pipettes Ampoules (glass) Pasteur pipettes Instruments Test tubes
Autoclave	Ampoules (plastic) Apparatus with silicone tubing Filters (reusable) Glass bottles with screw caps Glass syringes Magnetic stirrer bases Screw caps Stoppers (rubber silicone)
II *For liquids and nutrients*	
Autoclave	Salt solutions Glucose–20% Agar Bacto–peptone Glycerol Lactalbumin hydrolysate Phenol red Tryptose HEPES EDTA Water
Filter	Serum Amino acids Vitamins Antibiotics Bovine serum albumin Collagenase Glutamine Drugs NaOH Trypsin Transferrin

ADVANTAGES AND LIMITATIONS OF TISSUE CULTURE

ADVANTAGES OF TISSUE CULTURE

Tissue culture technique has a wide range of applications. The most important advantages of this technique are listed below.

1. Control of physico-chemical environment-pH, temperature, dissolved gases (O_2 and CO_2), osmolarity.

2. ***Regulation of physiological conditions***-nutrient concentration, cell to cell interactions, hormonal control.

3. The cultured cell lines become homogenous (i.e. cells are identical) after one or two subcultures. This is in contrast to the heterogenous cells of tissue samples. ***The homogenous cells are highly useful for a wide range of purposes***.

4. It is easy to characterize cells for cytological and immunological studies.

5. Cultured cells can be stored in liquid nitrogen for several years.

6. Due to direct access and contact to the cells, biological studies can be carried out more conveniently. The main advantage is the low quantities of the reagents required in contrast to *in vivo* studies where most of the reagents (more than 90% in some cases) are lost by distribution to various tissues, and excretion.

7. Utility of tissue cultures will drastically reduce the use of animals for various experiments.

Limitations of tissue culture

There are several limitations of tissue culture, some of them are given below.

1. Need of expertise and technical skill for the development, and regular use of tissue culture.

2. ***Cost factor*** is a major limitation. Establishment of infrastructure, equipment and other facilites are expensive.

3. It is estimated that the cost of production of cells is about 10 times higher than direct use of animal tissues.

4. Control of the environmental factors (pH, temperature, dissolved gases, disposal of biohazards) is not easy.

5. The native *in vivo* cells exist in a three-dimensional geometry while in *in vitro* tissue culture, the propagation of cells occurs on a two dimensional substrate. Due to this, the ***cell to cell interactive characters are lost***.

6. The cell lines may represent one or two types of cells from the native tissue while others may go unrepresented.

7. Tissue culture techniques are associated with the differentiation i.e. loss of the characters of the tissue cells from which they were originally isolated.

8. This happens due to adaptation and selection processes while culturing.

9. Continuous cell lines may result in genetic instability of the cells. This may ultimately lead to heterogeneity of cells.

10. The components of homeostatic *in vivo* regulation (nervous system, endocrine system, metabolic integration) are lacking in *in vitro* cultures. Addition of hormones and growth factors has been started recently.

APPLICATIONS OF ANIMAL CELL CULTURES

There is a widespread concern that extensive use of animals for laboratory experiments is not morally and ethically justifiable. ***Animal welfare groups worldover are increasingly criticising the use of animals***. Some research workers these days prefer to ***utilize animal cell cultures wherever possible*** for various studies. The major applications of laboratory animal cell cultures are given in ***Table 33.3***, and listed below.

- Studies on intracellular activity e.g. cell cycle and differentiation, metabolisms.
- Elucidation of intracellular flux e.g. hormonal receptors, signal transduction.
- Studies related to cell to cell interaction e.g. cell adhesion and motility, metabolic cooperation.
- Evalution of environmental interactions e.g. cytotoxicity, mutagenesis.

TABLE 33.3 Summary of the applications of animal cell cultures

Category	*Applications*
Intracellular activity	Studies related to cell cycle and differentiation, transcription, translation, energy metabolism, drug metabolism.
Intracellular flux	Studies involving hormonal receptors, metabolites, signal transduction, membrane trafficking.
Cell to cell interaction	Studies dealing with cell adhesion and motility, matrix interaction, morphogenesis, paracrine control, metabolic cooperation.
Environmental interaction	Studies related to drug actions, infections, cytotoxicity, mutagenesis, carcinogenesis.
Genetics	Studies dealing with genetic analysis, transfection, transformation, immortalization, senescence.
Cell products	Wide range of applications of the cellular products formed (Refer ***Table 33.4***) e.g. vaccines, hormones, interferons etc.

- Studies dealing with genetics e.g. genetic analysis, immortalization, senescence.
- Laboratory production of medical/pharmaceutical compounds for wide range of applications e.g. vaccines, interferons, hormones.

There are however, several limitations on the use of animal cell cultures. This is mostly due to the differences that exist between the *in vivo* and *in vitro* systems, and the validity of the studies conducted in the laboratory.

MEDICAL / PHARMACEUTICAL PRODUCTS OF ANIMAL CELL CULTURES

The most important application of animal cell cultures is the production of a wide range of commercial compounds for medical and pharmaceutical use. The commercial production of several biological compounds by the microorganisms is described in Chapters 23–30.

A selected list of animal cell culture products of commercial importance is given in ***Table 33.4***.

Production of vaccines

Monkey kidney or chick embryo cells, or recently human diploid cells are in use for the production of vaccines. The vaccine manufacture in animal cell cultures is rather complex with risk of contamination, and safety aspect. For these reasons, production of vaccines by recombinant DNA technology employing bacteria or yeasts is preferred (Refer Chapter 16).

Production of high value therapeutics

Many human proteins with high therapeutic potential are often in short supply e.g. tissue plasminogen activator, clotting factors (VIII and IX), erythropoietin. There is a major limitation to produce human proteins that undergo post-translational modifications (glycosylation, carboxylation etc.) in bacteria and yeasts. This is due to the fact that these organisms do not possess the machinery to perform post-translational changes. However, pharmaceutical proteins that do not require post-translational modifications can be produced by bacteria or yeasts e.g. insulin, albumin, growth hormone.

Animal cell cultures (particularly mammalian cell cultures) are useful for the production of many pharmaceutically/medically important proteins (***Table 33.4***). These include the following.

- Plasminogen
- Interferons
- Blood clotting factors
- Hormones
- Monoclonal antibodies
- Erythropoietin.

Purification of pharmaceutical products

As the desired product is produced in the cell culture medium, its purification, isolation and storage (collectively referred to as downstream processing) assumes significance. The final product for therapeutic applications is expected to satisfy the following criteria.

- The product should have a stable structure with optimal activity.

TABLE 33.4 Selected examples of animal cell culture products (proteins) of medical/pharmaceutical importance

Product(s)	*Application(s)*
Vaccines	
Polio vaccines	Poliomyelitis prophylaxis
Measles vaccine	Measles prophylaxis
Rabies vaccine	Rabies prophylaxis
Malaria vaccines	Malaria prophylaxis
HIV vaccine	AIDS prophylaxis and treatment
Plasminogen activators	
Tissue-type plasminogen activator	Acute myocardial infarction, pulmonary embolism, deep vein thrombosis, acute stroke.
Urokinase-type plasminogen activator	
Recombinant plasminogen activator	
Interferons	
Interferon-α	Anticancer, immunomodulator
Interferon-β	Anticancer, antiviral
Interferon-γ	Anticancer, immunomodulator
Blood clotting factors	
Factors VII, VIII, IX and X	Hemophilia, as blood clotting agents.
Hormones	
Human growth hormone	Growth retardation in children
Somatotropin	Chronic renal insufficiency
Follicle stimulating hormone	Treatment of infertility
Human chorionic gonadotropin	Treatment of infertility
Monoclonal antibodies	
Anti-lipopolysaccharide	Treatment of sepsis
Human B-cell Lymphomas	Treatment of B-cell lymphoma
Anti-fibrin 99	Diagnosis of blood clot by imaging
Tcm-FAb (breast)	Diagnosis of breast cancer
Others	
Erythropoietin	Antianaemic agent
Interleukin-2	Anticancer, HIV treatment
Tumor necrosis factor	Anticancer
Granulocyte stimulating factor	Anticancer
Carcinoembryonic antigen	Diagnosis and monitoring of cancer patients.

- The product should be free from other biomolecules that may interfere with its activity and/or cause immunological complications.
- It should be free from all pathogens including viruses.

GENETIC ENGINEERING OF ANIMAL CELLS AND THEIR APPLICATIONS

It is now possible to genetically modify the animal (mammalian) cells to introduce the genes needed for the production of a specific protein or improve the characteristics of a cell line. The following methods are used to introduce foreign DNA into mammalian cells.

1. Electroporation
2. Lipofection
3. Microinjection
4. Fusion of mammalian cells with bacteria or viruses.

As the foreign DNA gets integrated into the mammalian cellular genome, the gene expresses to produce the desired protein. It is however, necessary to select the best producing recombinant cells by conventional methods using selectable marker genes. The following selectable markers are used for choosing the transfected cells.

- Viral thymidine kinase
- Bacterial dihydrofolate reductase
- Bacterial neomycin phosphotransferase

It has been possible to overproduce several proteins in mammalian cells through genetic manipulations e.g., tissue plasminogen activator, erythropoietin, interleukin-2, interferon-β, clotting factors VIII and IX, tumor necrosis factors.

The ***recombinant mammalian cells are conveniently used for the production of monoclonal antibodies*** which have wide range of applications (Refer Chapter 17).

RISKS IN A TISSUE CULTURE LABORATORY AND SAFETY

There are several risks associated with tissue culture technology. Most of the accidents that occur in culture laboratories are ***due to negligence and casual approach while dealing with biological and radiological samples***, besides improper maintenance

TABLE 33.5 Risks in a tissue culture laboratory

Category	*Contributing factor(s)*
Maintenance risks	Age and condition of various equipment, leakage of disposals.
Personnel risks	Inadequate training, lack of concentration and interest.
Physical risks	Electric shocks, fire, intense cold.
Chemical risks	Toxicity due to poisons, carcinogens, mutagens, irritants, allergens.
Biohazards	Pathogenic organisms, viruses, genetic manipulations, culture cells and DNA (quality and quantity).
Radioisotope risks	Energy emission and its penetration, ionization.

of the laboratory. A broad categorization of risks and the contributory factors is given in ***Table 33.5***.

Safety regulations

Some of the developed countries have formulated general safety regulations ***to minimize the risks associated with tissue culture laboratories***. Selected examples :

1. "Biosafety in microbiological and biomedical laboratories", U. S. Department of Health and Human Sciences (1993).

2. "Safe working and the prevention of infection in clinical laboratories" U.K. Health Services Advisory Committee (1991).

Some of the general precautions for the safety of a tissue culture laboratory are listed here.

- Strict adherence to recommendations of regulatory bodies.
- Periodical meetings and discussions of local safety committees.
- Regular monitoring of the laboratories.
- Periodical training of the personnel through seminars and workshops.
- Print and make the standard operating procedures (SOPs) available to all staff.
- Good record keeping.
- Limited access to the laboratory (only for the trained personnel and selected visitors).
- Appropriate waste disposal system for biohazards, radioactive wastes, toxins and corrosives.

BIOHAZARDS

The accidents or the risks associated with the biological materials are regarded as biohazards or ***biological hazards***. There are two main systems that contribute to the occurrence of biohazards (***Table 33.6***).

1. The direct sources of the biological materials.

2. The processes or operations involved in their handling.

Control of biohazards

Biohazards can be controlled to a large extent by strict adherence to the regulatory guidelines and maintenance programmes. Some important aspects are listed.

- Microbiological safety cabinet or biohazard wood with pathogen trap filters have been developed.
- Vertical laminar-flow hood (instead of horizontal laminor-flow hood) is recently in use. This minimizes the direct exposure of the operator to the samples/processes.
- Pathogen containing samples are treated in separate rooms with separate facilities (centrifuge, incubator, cell counting etc.).
- Sterilization of all wastes, solid glassware etc. and their proper disposal.
- Facilities for change of clothing while entering and leaving the rooms.
- Strict adherence to the access of designated personnel to the culture rooms.

TABLE 33.6 Sources that contribute to biohazards

Biological material(s)
Tissue samples and cultures with human pathogens.
Human cells infected with viruses (including retroviruses)
Cells subjected to various genetic manipulations.
Operating processes
Preparation of the media.
Development of primary cultures, cell lines and other laboratory works.

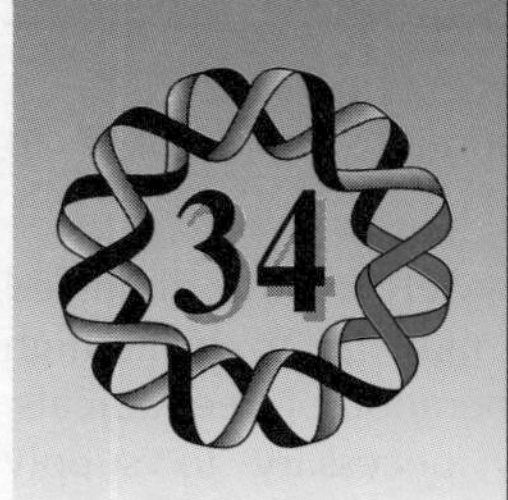

Culture Media for Animal Cells

MCDB 202
MCDB 402
MCDB 110
MCDB 131
MCDB 170
WAJC 404
LHC 9
MCDB 202
MCDB 402

The selection of an appropriate growth medium for the *in vitro* cultivation of cells is an important and essential step. The mammalian cells of an organ in the body receive nutrients from blood circulation. For culturing these cells *in vitro*, ***it is expected that they should be provided with the components similar to those present in blood***. In general, the choice of the medium mostly depends on the type of the cells to be cultured, and the purpose of the culture (growth, differentiation, production of desired products). The culture media may be natural or artificial.

NATURAL MEDIA

In the early years, the natural media obtained from various biological sources were used.

Body fluids : Plasma, serum, lymph, amniotic fluid, ascitic and pleural fluids, aqueous humour from eyes and insect hemolymph were in common use. These fluids were tested for sterility and toxicity before their utility.

Tissue extracts : Among the tissue extracts, ***chick embryo extract*** was the most commonly employed. The extracts of liver, spleen, bone marrow and leucocytes were also used as culture media.

Some workers still prefer natural media for organ culture.

ARTIFICIAL MEDIA

The artificial media (containing partly defined components) have been in use for cell culture since 1950. The minimal criteria needed for choosing a medium for animal cell cultures are listed below.

- The medium should provide all the nutrients to the cells.
- Maintain the physiological pH around 7.0 with adequate buffering.
- The medium must be sterile, and isotonic to the cells.

The basis for the cell culture media was the ***balanced salt solution*** which was originally ***used to create a physiological pH and osmolarity*** required to maintain cells *in vitro*. For promoting growth and proliferation of cells, various constituents (glucose, amino acids, vitamins, growth factors, antibiotics etc.) were added, and several media developed. Addition of serum to the various media is a common practice. However, some workers in recent years have started using serum-free media.

The physicochemical properties of media required for tissue cultures are briefly described. This is followed by a brief account on balanced salt solutions, commonly used culture media and the serum-free media.

PHYSICOCHEMICAL PROPERTIES OF CULTURE MEDIA

The culture media is expected to possess certain physicochemical properties (pH, O_2, CO_2, buffering, osmolarity, viscosity, temperature etc.) to support good growth and proliferation of the cultured cells.

pH

Most of the cells can grow at a pH ***in the range of 7.0-7.4***, although there are slight variations depending on the type of cells (i.e. cell lines). The indicator ***phenol red*** is most commonly used for visible detection of pH of the media. Its colouration at the different pH is shown below.

At pH 7.4 — Red
At pH 7.0 — Orange
At pH 6.5 — Yellow
At pH 7.8 — Purple

CO_2, bicarbonate and buffering

Carbon dioxide in the medium is in a dissolved state, the concentration of which depends on the atmospheric CO_2 tension and temperature. CO_2 in the medium exists as carbonic acid (H_2CO_3), and bicarbonate (HCO_3^-) and H^+ ions as shown below.

$$CO_2 + H_2O \longleftrightarrow H_2CO_3 \longleftrightarrow H^+ + HCO_3^-$$

As is evident from the above equation, the concentrations of CO_2, HCO_3^- and pH are interrelated. By increasing the atmospheric CO_2, the pH will be reduced making the medium acidic.

Addition of sodium bicarbonate (as a component of bicarbonate buffer) neutralizes bicarbonate ions.

$$NaHCO_3 \longleftrightarrow Na^+ + HCO_3^-$$

In fact, the commercially available media contain a recommended concentration of bicarbonate, and CO_2 tension for the required pH. ***In recent years HEPES*** (hydroxyethyl piperazine 2-sulfonic acid) ***buffer which is more efficient than bicarbonate buffer is being used in the culture media***. However, bicarbonate buffer is preferred by most workers because of the low cost, less toxicity and nutritional benefit to the medium. This is in contrast to HEPES which is expensive, besides being toxic to the cells.

The presence of pyruvate in the medium results in the increased endogenous production of CO_2 by the cells. This is advantageous since the dependence on the exogenous supply of CO_2 and HCO_3^- will be less. In such a case, the buffering can be achieved by high concentration of amino acids.

Oxygen

A great majority of cells *in vivo* are dependent on the O_2 supply for aerobic respiration. This is in fact made possible by a continuous supply of O_2 to the tissues by hemoglobin.

The cultured cells mostly rely on the dissolved O_2 in the medium which may be toxic at high concentration due to the generation of free radicals. Therefore, it is absolutely necessary to supply adequate quantities of O_2 so that the cellular requirements are met, avoiding toxic effects. Some workers add free-radical scavengers (glutathione, mercaptoethanol) to nullify the toxicity. Addition of selenium to the medium is also advocated to reduce O_2 toxicity. This is because selenium is a cofactor for the synthesis of glutathione.

In general, the glycolysis occurring in cultured cells is more anaerobic when compared to *in vivo* cells. Since the depth of the culture medium influences the rate of O_2 diffusion, it is advisable to keep the depth of the medium in the range 2-5 mm.

Temperature

In general, the optimal temperature for a given cell culture is ***dependent on the body temperature of the organism, serving as the source of the cells***. Accordingly, for cells obtained from humans and warm blooded animals, the optimal temperature is 37°C. *In vitro* cells cannot tolerate higher temperature and most of them die if the temperature goes beyond 40°C. It is therefore absolutely necessary to maintain a constant temperature (± 0.5°C) for reproducible results.

If the cells are obtained from birds, the optimal temperature is slightly higher (38.5°C) for culturing. For cold blooded animals (poikiltherms) that do not regulate their body heat (e.g. cold-water fish), the culture temperature may be in the range of 15–25°C.

Besides directly influencing growth of cells, temperature also affects the solubility of CO_2 i.e. higher temperature enhances solubility.

Osmolality

In general, the osmolality for most of the cultured cells (from different organisms) is in the range of 260–320 mosm/kg. This is ***comparable to the osmolality of human plasma*** (290 mosm/kg). Once an osmolality is selected for a culture medium, it should be maintained at that level (with an allowance of ± 10 mosm/kg).

TABLE 34.1 Composition (g/l) of balanced salt solutions (BSS)

Ingradient	*Earle's BSS*	*Hank's BSS*
NaCl	6.68	8.0
KCl	0.4	0.4
$CaCl_2$ (anhydrous)	0.02	0.14
$MgSO_4.7H_2O$	0.2	0.1
$NaHCO_3$	2.2	0.35
$NaH_3PO_4.H_2O$	0.14	—
$Na_2HPO_4.7H_2O$	—	0.09
KH_2PO_4	—	0.06
D-Glucose	1.0	1.0
Phenol red	0.01	0.01
HEPES, Na salt (buffer)	13.02	2.08

Whenever there is an addition of acids, bases, drugs etc. to the medium, the osmolality gets affected. The instrument osmometer is employed for measuring osmolalities in the laboratory.

BALANCED SALT SOLUTIONS

The balanced salt solutions (***BSS***) are ***primarily composed of inorganic salts***. Sometimes, sodium bicarbonate, glucose and HEPES buffer may also be added to BSS. ***Phenol red serves as a pH indicator***. The important functions of balanced salt solutions are listed hereunder.

- Supply essential inorganic ions.
- Provide the requisite pH.
- Maintain the desired osmolality.
- Supply energy from glucose.

In fact, balanced salt solutions form the basis for the preparation of complete media with the requisite additions. Further, BSS is also useful for a short period (up to 4 hours) incubation of cells.

The composition of two most widely used BSS namely Earle's BSS and Hank's BSS is given in ***Table 34.1***.

COMPLETE CULTURE MEDIA

In the early years, balanced salt solutions were supplemented with various nutrients (amino acids, vitamins, serum etc.) to promote proliferation of cells in culture. Eagle was a pioneer in media formulation. He determined (during 1950–60) the nutrient requirements for mammalian cell cultures. Many developments in media preparation have occurred since then. There are more than a dozen media now available for different types of cultures. Some of them are stated below.

EMEM—Eagle's minimal essential medium

DMEM—Dulbecco's modification of Eagle's medium

GMEM—Glasgow's modification of Eagle's medium

RPMI 1630 and RPMI 1640—Media from Rosewell Park Memorial Institute.

The other important culture media are Ham's F10, and F12, TC 199 and CMRL 1060.

The detailed composition of three commonly used media namely Eagle's MEM, RPMI 1640 and Ham's F12 is given in ***Table 34.2***. The ***complete media, in general, contains*** a large number of components ***amino acids, vitamins, salts, glucose, other organic supplements, growth factors and hormones, and antibiotics, besides serum***. Depending on the medium, the quality and quantity of the ingradients vary. Some important aspects of the media ingradients are briefly described.

Amino acids

All the ***essential amino acids*** (which cannot be synthesized by the cells) have to be added to the medium. In addition, even the ***non-essential amino acids*** (that can be synthesized by the cells) are also usually added to avoid any limitation of their cellular synthesis. Among the non-essential amino acids, glutamine and/or glutamate are frequently added in good quantities to the media since these amino acids serve as good sources of energy and carbon.

Vitamins

The quality and quantity of vitamins depends on the medium. For instance, Eagle's MEM contains only water soluble vitamins (e.g. B-complex, choline, inositol). The other vitamins are obtained from the serum added. The medium M 199 contains all the fat soluble vitamins (A, D, E and K) also. In general, ***for the media without serum,***

Table 34.2 Composition of three commonly used culture media

Component	Eagle's MEM	RPMI 1640	Ham's F 12
Amino acids			
L-Alanine			8.91
L-Arginine HCl	105	200	211
L-Asparagine H_2O		50	15.0
L-Aspartic acid		20	13.3
L-Cystine	24	50	24.0
L-Glutamic acid		20	14.7
L-Glutamine	292	300	146.2
Glycine		10	7.51
L-Histidine HCl H_2O	31	15	21.0
L-Isoleucine	52	50	3.94
L-Leucine	52	50	13.12
L-Lysine	58	40	36.54
L-Methionine	15	15	4.48
L-Phenylalanine	32	15	4.96
L-Proline		20	34.5
L-Serine		30	10.51
L-Threonine	48	20	11.91
L-Tryptophan	10	5	2.042
L-Tyrosine	36	20	5.43
L-Valine	46	20	11.7
Glutathione (red)		1	
L-Hydroxyproline		20	
Vitamins			
D-Biotin		0.2	0.007
Ca D-pantothenate	1	0.25	0.26
Choline chloride	1	3.0	13.96
Folic acid	1	1.0	1.32
i-Inositol	2		18.02
Nicotinamide	1	35	0.037
p-Aminobenzoic acid		1.0	
Pyridoxine HCl		1	0.062
Pyridoxal HCl	1		
Riboflavin	0.1	0.2	0.038
Thiamine HCl	1	1.0	0.34
Vitamin B_{12}		0.005	1.36
Inorganic salts			
$CaCl_2.2H_2O$	200		44.1
$CaNO_3.4H_2O$		100	
$CuSO_4.5H_2O$			0.0025
$FeSO_4.7H_2O$			0.83
KCl	400	400	223
$MgSO_4.7H_2O$	220	100	133
NaCl	6800	6000	7599
$NaHCO_3$	2000	2000	1176
$Na_2HPO_4.7H_2O$		1512	268
$NaH_2PO_4.2H_2O$	150		
Other components			
D-Glucose	1000	2000	1801
Phenol red		5.0	1.2
Sodium pyruvate			110
Lipoic acid			0.21
Linoleic acid			0.084
Hypoxanthine			4.08
Putrescine 2HCl			0.16

Table 34.2 contd. next column

more vitamins in higher concentrations are required.

Salts

The salts present in the various media are basically those found in ***balanced salt solutions*** (Eagle's BSS and Hank's BSS). The salts contribute to cations (Na^+, K^+, Mg^{2+}, Ca^{2+} etc.) and anions (Cl^-, HCO_3^-, SO_4^{2-}, PO_4^{3-}), and are mainly responsible for the maintenance of osmolality. There are some other important functions of certain ions contributed by the salts.

- Ca^{2+} ions are required for cell adhesion, in signal transduction, besides their involvement in cell proliferation and differentiation.
- Na^+, K^+ and Cl^- ions regulate membrane potential.

- PO_4^{3-}, SO_4^{2-} and HCO_3^- ions are involved in the maintenance of intracellular charge, besides serving as precursors for the production of certain important compounds e.g. PO_4^{3-} is required for ATP synthesis.

Glucose

Majority of culture media contain glucose which ***serves as an important source of energy***. Glucose is degraded in glycolysis to form pyruvate/lactate. These compounds on their further metabolism enter citric acid cycle and get oxidized to CO_2. However, experimental evidence indicates that the contribution of glucose for the operation of citric acid cycle is very low *in vitro* (in culture cells) compared to *in vivo* situation. ***Glutamine*** rather than glucose ***supplies carbon for the operation of citric acid cycle***. And for this reason, the cultured cells require very high content of glutamine.

Hormones and growth factors

For the media with serum, addition of hormones and growth factors is usually not required. They are frequently added to serum-free media.

Other organic supplements

Several additional organic compounds are usually added to the media to support cultures. These include certain proteins, peptides, lipids, nucleosides and citric acid cycle intermediates. For serum-free media, supplementation with these compounds is very useful.

Antibiotics

In the early years, culture media invariably contained antibiotics. The most commonly used antibiotics were ampicillin, penicillin, gentamycin, erythromycin, kanamycin, neomycin and tetracycline. Antibiotics were added to reduce contamination. However, ***with improved aseptic conditions in the present day tissue culture laboratories, the addition of antibiotics is not required.*** In fact, the use of antibiotics is associated with several disadvantages.

- Possibility of developing antibiotic-resistant cells in culture.
- May cause antimetabolic effects and hamper proliferation.
- Possibility of hiding several infections temporarily.
- May encourage poor aseptic conditions.

The present recommendation is that for the routine culture of cells, antibiotics should not be added. However, they may be used for the development of primary cultures.

SERUM

Serum is a natural biological fluid, and is rich in various components to support cell proliferation. The major constituents found in different types of sera are listed in ***Table 34.3***. The most commonly used sera are ***calf serum*** (CS), ***fetal bovine serum*** (FBS), ***horse serum*** and human serum. While using human serum, it must be screened for viral diseases (hepatitis B, HIV).

Approximately 5–20% (v/v) of serum is mostly used for supplementing several media. Some of the important features of the serum constituents are briefly described.

Proteins

The *in vitro* functions of serum protein are not very clear. Some of them are involved in promoting cell attachment and growth e.g. fetuin, fibronectin. Proteins ***increase the viscosity*** of the culture medium, besides ***contributing to buffering action***.

Nutrients and metabolites

Serum contains several amino acids, glucose, phospholipids, fatty acids, nucleosides and metabolic intermediates (pyruvic acid, lactic acid etc.). These constituents do contribute to some extent for the nutritional requirements of cells. This may however, be insignificant in complex media with well supplemented nutrients.

Growth factors

There are certain growth factors in the serum that stimulate the proliferation of cells in the culture.

- Platelet-derived growth factor (PDGF).
- Fibroblast growth factor (FGF).
- Epidermal growth factor (EGF).
- Vascular endothelial growth factor (VEGF).
- Insulin-like growth factors (IGF-1, IGF-2).

In fact, almost all these growth factors are commercially available for use in tissue culture.

Table 34.3 Major constituents of serum

Proteins
Albumin
Globulins
Fetuin
Fibronectin
Transferrin
Protease inhibitors
(α_1-antitrypsin)
Amino acids
Almost all the 20
Lipids
Cholesterol
Phospholipids
Fatty acids
Carbohydrates
Glucose
Hexosamine
Other organic compounds
Lactic acid
Pyruvic acid
Polyamines
Urea
Vitamins
Vitamin A
Folic acid
Growth factors
Epidermal growth factor
Platelet-derived growth factor
Fibroblast growth factor
Hormones
Hydrocortisone
Thyroxine
Triiodothyronine
Insulin
Inorganics
Calcium
Sodium
Potassium
Chlorides
Iron
Phosphates
Zinc
Selenium

Hormones

Hydrocortisone promotes cell attachment, while insulin facilitates glucose uptake by cells. Growth hormone, in association with somatomedins (IGFs), promotes cell proliferation.

Inhibitors

Serum may also contain cellular growth inhibiting factors. Majority of them are artefacts e.g. bacterial toxins, antibodies. The natural serum also contains a physiological growth inhibitor namely ***transforming growth factor β (TGF-β)***. Most of these growth inhibitory factors may be removed by heat inactivation (at 56°C for 30 minutes).

SELECTION OF MEDIUM AND SERUM

As already stated, there are around a dozen media for the cell cultures. The selection of a particular medium is based on the cell line and the purpose of culturing. For instance, for chick embryo fibroblasts and HeLa cells, EMEM is used. The medium DMEM can be used for the cultivation of neurons. A selected list of cells and cell lines along with the media and sera used is given in ***Table 34.4***. In fact, information on the selection of appropriate medium for a particular cell line is available from literature.

The selection of serum is also based on the type of cells being cultured. The following criteria are taken into consideration while choosing serum.

- Batch to batch variations.
- Quality control.
- Efficiency to promote growth and preservation of cells.
- Sterility.
- Heat inactivation.

In recent years, there is a tendency to discontinue the use of serum, and switch over to more clearly defined media (described later).

SUPPLEMENTATION OF THE MEDIUM WITH TISSUE EXTRACTS

Besides serum, the culture media can also be supplemented with certain tissue extracts and microbial culture extracts. The examples are—chick embryo extract, proteolytic digests of beef heart, bactopeptone, lactalbumin hydrolysate, tryptose.

The ***chick embryo extract*** was found to contain both high molecular weight and low molecular weight compounds that ***support growth and proliferation of cells***.

SERUM-FREE MEDIA

Addition of serum to the culture media has been an age-old practice. However, in recent years, certain serum-free media have been developed. It is worthwhile to know the disadvantages associated with the the use of serum, and the advantages and disadvantages of serum-free media.

Disadvantages of serum in media

Variable composition : There is no uniformity in the composition of the serum. It is highly variable (source, batch, season, collection method, processing). Such differences in the composition significantly influence the cells in culture.

Quality control : To maintain a uniform quality of the serum, special tests have to be performed with each batch of serum, before its use.

Table 34.4 A selected list of the cells or cell lines along with the media and serum used for their culture

Cells or cell line	*Medium*	*Serum*
Chick embryo fibroblasts	EMEM	CS
Chinese hamster ovary (CHO)	EMEM, Ham's F12	CS
HeLa cells	EMEM	CS
Human leukemia	RPMI 1640	FB
Mouse leukemia	Fischer's medium, RPMI 1640	FB, HoS
Neurons	DMEM	FB
Mammary epithelium	RPMI 1640, DMEM	FB
Hematopoietic cells	RPMI 1640, Fischer's medium	FB
Skeletal muscle	DMEM, F 12	FB, HoS
Glial cells	MEM, F 12, DMEM	FB
3T3 cells	MEM, DMEM	CS

(EMEM—Eagle's minimal essential medium; RPMI 1640–Medium from to Rosewell Park Memorial Institute; DMEM–Dulbecco's modification of Eagle's medium; CS–Calf serum; FB–Fetal bovine serum; HoS–Horse serum)

Contamination : It is rather difficult to get serum totally free from all pathogens, particularly viruses.

Presence of growth inhibitors : In general, the concentration of growth promoters in the serum is much higher than the inhibitors. But sometimes, the growth inhibitors such as TGF-β may dominate and inhibit cell proliferation.

Availability and cost : There is a dependence on the cattle for the supply of serum. Hence the availability may be restricted on several occasions for political and economic reasons. Further, cost also is another factor for discouraging the use of serum.

Downstream processing : The presence of serum in the culture medium ***interferes with the isolation and purification of cell culture products***. For this reason, several additional steps may be required for the isolation of the desired product.

ADVANTAGES AND DISADVANTAGES OF SERUM-FREE MEDIA

Advantages

The limitations associated with the use of serum in the media (described above) are eliminated in the serum-free media. In addition, there are two more distinct advantages.

Selection of media with defined composition : The main advantage of serum-free medium is to ***control growth of the cells as desired, with a well defined medium***. This is in contrast to the use of serum wherein the growth frequently proceeds in an uncontrolled fashion.

Regulation of differentiation : It is possible to use a factor or a set of factors to achieve differentiation of cells with the desired and specialised functions.

Disadvantages

Slow cell proliferation : Most of the serum-free media are not as efficient as serum added media in the growth promotion of cells.

Need for multiple media : A large number of serum-free media need to be developed for different cell lines. This may create some practical difficulties in a laboratory simultaneously handling several cell lines. Another limitation of serum-free medium is that a given medium may not be able to support the different stages of development even for a given cell line. Hence, sometimes separate media may be required even for the same cell line.

Purity of reagents : The native serum does possess some amount of protective and detoxifying machinary that can offer a cleansing effect on the apparatus and reagents. And therefore, in the absence of serum, pure grade reagents and completely sterile apparatus should be used.

Availability and cost : In general, the serum-free media are costlier than the serum added media. This is mainly due to the fact that many of the pure chemicals added to the serum-free media are themselves expensive. Further, the availability of serum-free media is also another limitation.

DEVELOPMENT OF SERUM-FREE MEDIA

While designing serum-free media, it is desirable to identify the various serum constituents (Refer ***Table 34.3***) and their quantities. The most important constituents of natural serum with reference to their use in cell cultures may be categorized as follows.

- Growth regulatory factors e.g. PDGF, TGF-β.
- Cell adhesion factors e.g. vitamins.
- Essential nutrients e.g. vitamins, metabolites, minerals, fatty acids.
- Hormones e.g. insulin, hydrocortisone.

For replacing the serum and development of serum-free media, several constituents should supplement the media. Some highlights are given below.

Growth factors

A large number of growth factors (nearly 100) that promote *in vitro* cell proliferation and differentiation have been idenfitied. Besides the factors described already (above), some others are listed below.

- Erythropoietin (EPO).
- Eye-derived growth factors (EDGF 1 and EDGF 2).
- Interleukins (IL-1, IL-2).
- Hepatocyte growth factor (HGF).
- Brain-derived neurotrophic factor (BDNF).
- Phytohemagglutinin (PHA).
- Lipopolysaccharide (LPS).

The growth factors may act synergistically or additively with each other or with other factors (e.g. hormones, prostaglandins).

TABLE 34.5 A selected list of cell lines along with serum-free media

Cell line	*Medium*
Chick embryo fibroblasts	MCDB 202
Chinese hamster ovary (CHO)	MCDB 402
Human lung fibroblasts	MCDB 110
Human vascular endothelium	MCDB 131
Mammary epithelium	MCDB 170
Prostatic epithelium	WAJC 404
Bronchial epithelium	LHC 9
Fibroblasts	MCDB 202
3T3 cells	MCDB 402

Almost all the growth factors are now commercially available for the preparation of serum-free media.

Hormones

Growth hormone, insulin and hydrocortisone are the most commonly added hormones into the serum-free media. A combination of steroid hormones-hydrocortisone, estrogen, androgen and progesterone are used in formulating serum-free media for the maintenance of mammary epithelium.

Nutrients

Addition of certain nutrients-choline, ethanolamine, linoleic acid, iron, copper, selenium etc., are added in most of the serum-free media.

Proteins

Bovine serum albumin (BSA) is the most commonly added protein. It promotes cell survival and growth.

Polyamines

Putrescine is the most widely added polyamine to the serum-free media. Polyamines promote cellular growth and differentiation.

Protease inhibitors

Addition of protease inhibitors (e.g. soy bean trypsin inhibitor) is done to the serum-free media for the trypsin-mediated subcultures.

COMMONLY USED SERUM-FREE MEDIA

Several types of serum-free media have been developed for different cell lines. A selected list of cell lines and the media is given in the ***Table 34.5***.

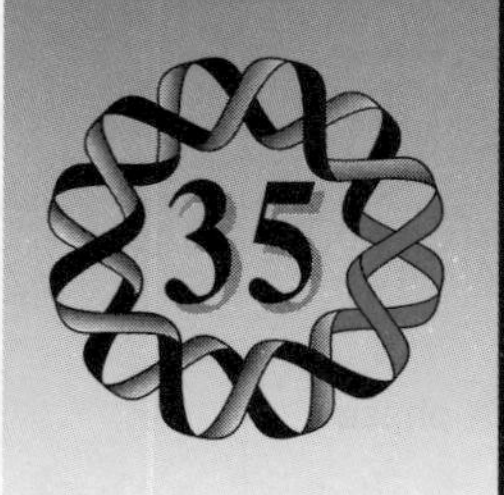

Cultured Cells — Biology and Characterization

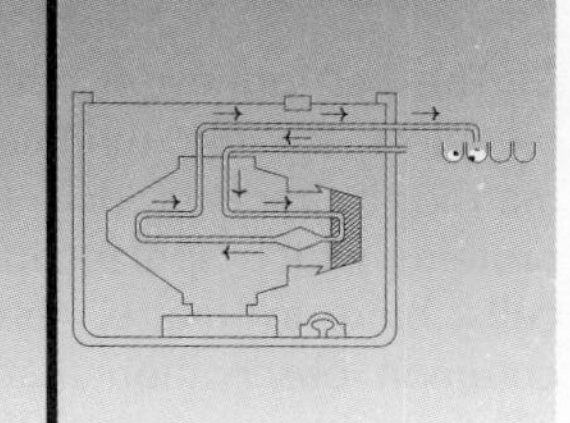

It is an accepted fact that the *in vitro* cultured cells do not possess the same characteristics as the *in vivo* cells. This is mostly due to the changes in the cellular environment.

CHARACTERISTICS OF CULTURED CELLS

Some of the important ***distinguishing properties of cultured cells*** are given below.

1. Cells which do not normally proliferate *in vivo* can be grown and proliferated in cultures.

2. ***Cell to cell interactions*** in the cultured cells are very ***much low***.

3. The three dimensional architecture of the *in vivo* cells is not found in cultured cells.

4. The hormonal and nutritional influence on the cultured cells differs from that on the *in vivo* cells.

5. Cultured cells ***cannot perform*** differentiated and ***specialized functions***.

6. The environment of the cultured cells favours proliferation and spreading of unspecialized cells.

Environmental influence on cultured cells

The environmental factors strongly influence the cells in culture. The major routes through which environmental influence occurs are listed.

- The nature of the substrate or phase in which cells grow. For monolayer cultures, the substrate is a solid (e.g. plastic) while for suspension cultures, it is a liquid.
- The composition of the medium used for culture-nutrients and physicochemical properties.
- Addition of hormones and growth factors.
- The composition of the gas phase.
- The temperature of culture incubation.

The ***biological and other aspects of cultured cells*** with special reference to the following parameters are briefly described.

1. Cell adhesion.
2. Cell proliferation.
3. Cell differentiation.
4. Metabolism of cultured cells.
5. Initiation of cell culture.
6. Evolution and development of cell lines.

CELL ADHESION

Most of the cells obtained from solid tissues grow as adherent monolayers in cultures. The cells, derived from tissue aggregation or subculture, attach to the substrate and then start proliferating. In the early days of culture techniques, slightly negatively charged glasses were used as substrates. In recent years, plastics such as polystyrene, after treatment with electric ion discharge, are in use.

The cell adhesion occurs through cell surface receptors for the molecules in the extracellular matrix. It appears that the cells secrete matrix proteins which spread on the substrate. Then the cells bind to matrix through receptors. It is a common observation that the substrates (glass or plastic) with previous cell culture are conditioned to provide better surface area for adhesion.

Cell adhesion molecules

Three groups of proteins collectively referred to as cell adhesion molecules (***CAMs***) are involved in the cell-cell adhesion and cell-substrate adhesion.

Cell-cell adhesion molecules: These proteins are primarily involved in cell-to-cell interaction between the homologous cells. CAMs are of two types — calcium-dependent ones ***(cadherins)*** and calcium-independent CAMs.

Integrins : These molecules mediate the cell substrate interactions. Integrins possess receptors for matrix molecules such as fibronectin and collagen.

Proteoglycans : These are low affinity transmembrane receptors. Proteoglycans can bind to matrix collagen and growth factors.

Cell adhesion molecules are attached to the cytoskeletons of the cultured cells.

CELL PROLIFERATION

Proliferation of cultured cells occurs through the ***cell cycle***, which has four distinct phases (***Fig. 35.1***)

M phase : In this phase (***M = mitosis***), the two chromatids, which constitute the chromosomes, segregate to daughter cells.

G_1 phase : This ***gap 1 phase*** is highly susceptible to various control processes that determine whether cell should proceed towards DNA synthesis, re-enter the cycle or take the course towards differentiation.

S phase : This phase is characterized by ***DNA synthesis*** wherein DNA replication occurs.

G_2 phase : This is ***gap 2 phase*** that prepares the cell for reentry into mitosis.

The integrity of the DNA, its repair or entry into ***apoptosis*** (programmed cell death) if repair is not possible is determined by two check points-at the beginning of DNA synthesis and in G_2 phase.

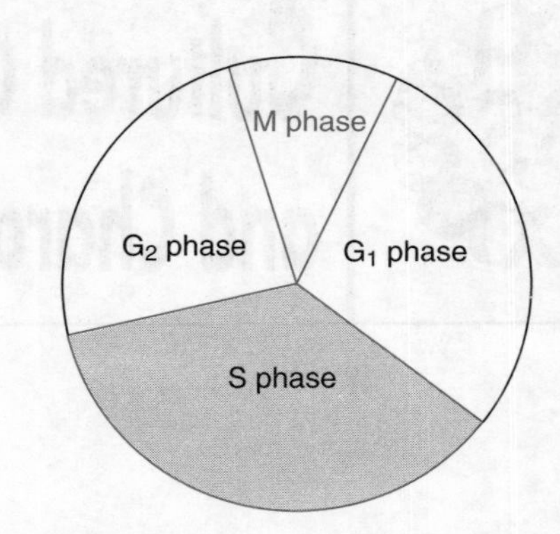

Fig. 35.1 : *The cell cycle.*

Control of cell proliferation

For the cells in culture, the environmental signals regulate the cell cycle, and thereby the cell proliferation. Low density of the cells in a medium coupled with the presence certain growth factors (e.g. epidermal growth factor, platelet-derived growth factor) allows the cells to enter the cell cycle. On the other hand, high cell density and crowding of cells inhibits the cell cycle and thereby proliferation.

Besides the influence of the environmental factors, certain intracellular factors also regulate the cell cycle. For instance, ***cyclins promote while p53 and Rb gene products inhibit cell cycle.***

CELL DIFFERENTIATION

The various cell culture conditions favour maximum cell proliferation and propagation of cell lines. Among the factors that promote cell proliferation, the following are important.

- Low cell density
- Low Ca^{2+} concentration
- Presence of growth factors

For the process of cell differentiation to occur, the proliferation of cells has to be severely limited or completely abolished. Cell differentiation can be promoted (or induced) by the following factors.

- High cell density.
- High Ca^{2+} concentration.
- Presence of differentiation inducers (e.g. hydrocortisone, nerve growth factor).

As is evident from the above, different and almost opposing conditions are required for cell proliferation, and for cell differentiation. Therefore if cell differentiation is required two distinct sets of conditions are necessary.

1. To optimize cell proliferation.
2. To optimize cell differentiation.

Maintenance of differentiation

It is now recognized that the ***cells retain their native and original functions for long when their three dimensional structures are retained***. This is possible with organ cultures. However, organ cultures cannot be propagated. In recent years, some workers are trying to create three dimensional structures by perfusing monolayer cultures. Further, *in vitro* culturing of cells on or in special matrices (e.g. cellulose, collagen gel, matrix of glycoproteins) also results in cells with three dimensional structures.

Dedifferentiation

Dedifferentiation refers to the ***irreversible loss of specialized properties of cells when they are cultured in vitro***. This happens when the differentiated *in vitro* cells lose their properties (***Fig. 35.2***).

In the ***in vivo situation, a small group of stem cells give rise to progenitor cells that are capable of producing differentiated cell pool*** (***Fig. 35.2A***). On the other hand, in the *in vitro* culture system, progenitor cells are predominantly produced which go on proliferating. Very few of the newly formed cells can form differentiated cells (***Fig. 35.2B***). The net result is a blocked differentiation.

As already described, dedifferentiation implies an irreversible loss of specialized properties of the cells. On the other hand, ***deadaptation*** refers to the reinduction of specialized properties of the cells by creating appropriate conditions.

METABOLISM OF CULTURED CELLS

The metabolism of mammalian cultured cells with special reference to energy aspects is depicted in ***Fig. 35.3***. The cultured cells can use ***glucose or glutamine as the source of energy***. These two compounds also generate important anabolic precursors.

As glucose gets degraded by glycolysis, lactate is mainly produced. This is because oxygen is in limited supply in the normal culture conditions (i.e. atmospheric oxygen and a submerged culture) creating an anaerobic situation. Lactate, secreted into the medium, accumulates. Some amount of pyruvate produced in glycolysis gets oxidized through Krebs cycle. ***A small fraction of glucose*** (4-9%) ***enters pentose phosphate pathway*** to supply ribose 5-phosphate and reducing equivalents (NADPH) for biosynthetic pathways e.g. synthesis of nucleotides.

Glutamine is an important source of energy for the cultured cells. By the action of the enzyme glutaminase, glutamine undergoes deamination to produce glutamate and ammonium ions. Glutamate, on transamination (or oxidative deamination) forms α-ketoglutarate which enters the Krebs cycle. Pyruvate predominantly participates in transamination reaction to produce alanine, which is easily excreted into the medium. In the rapidly growing cultured cells, transamination reaction is a dominant route of glutamine metabolism.

Deamination of glutamine releases free ammonium ions, which are toxic to the cultured cells, limiting their growth. In recent years, dipeptides ***glutamyl-alanine*** or ***glutamyl-glycine*** are being used to minimize the production of ammonia. Further, these dipeptides are more stable in the medium.

As already stated, α-ketoglutarate obtained from glutamine (via glutamate) enters the Krebs cycle and gets oxidized to carbon dioxide and water. For proper operation of Kerbs cycle, balancing of the intermediates of the cycle is required. Two metabolites of Kerbs cycle namely malate and oxaloacetate leave the cycle and get converted respectively to pyruvate and phosphoenol pyruvate. The latter two compounds can reenter the Krebs cycle in the form of acetyl CoA. Thus, the continuity of Kerbs cycle is maintained.

Glucose as well as glutamine gets metabolised by the cultured cells to supply energy in the form of ATP.

INITIATION OF CELL CULTURE

The cell culture can be initiated by the cells derived from a tissue through enzymatic or mechanical treatments. For details on primary culture, the reader must refer Chapter 36. Primary culture is a selective process that finally results in a relatively uniform cell line. The selection occurs by virtue of the capacity of the cells to survive as

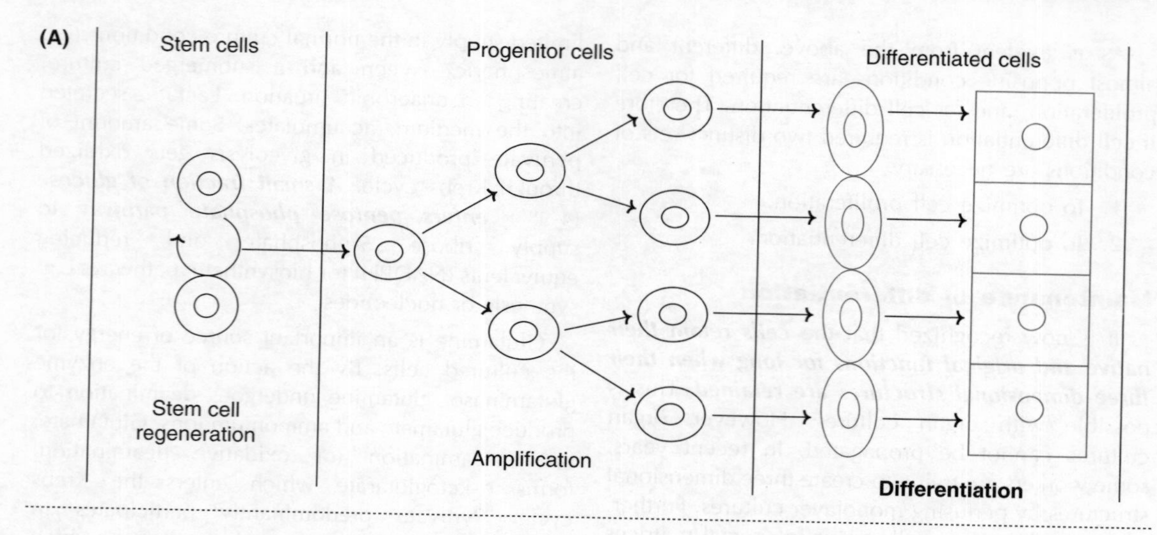

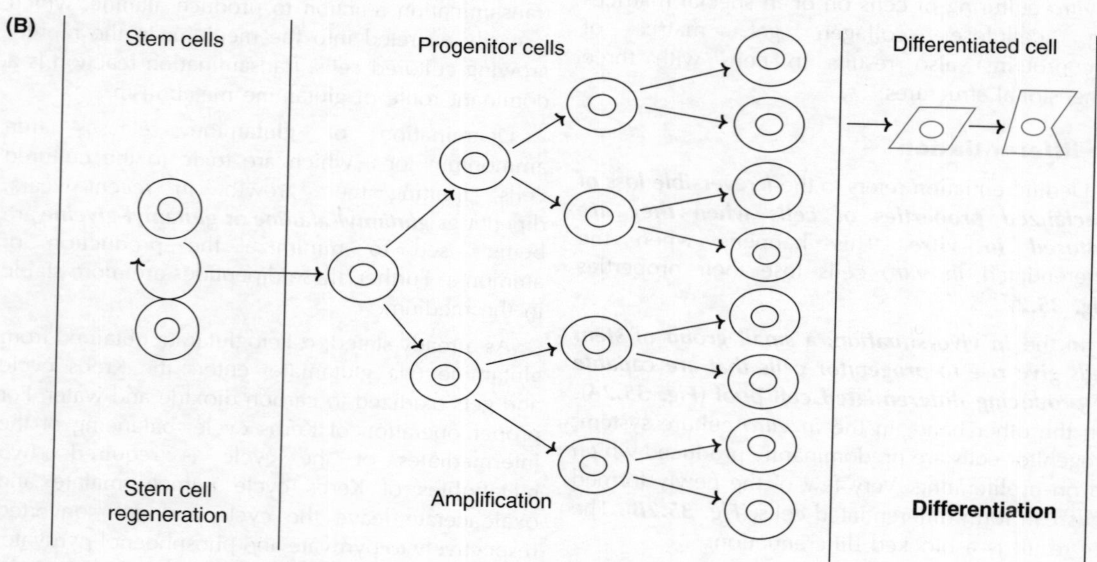

Fig. 35.2 : Differentiation of cells (A) In vivo *differentiation of stem cells (B) Blocked differentiation in cultured cells.*

monolayer cultures (by adhering to substrates) or as suspension cultures.

Among the cultured cells, some cells can grow and proliferate while some are unable to survive under the culture environment. The cells continue to grow in monolayer cultures, till the availability of the substrate is occupied.

The term ***confluence*** is used when ***the cultured cells make close contact with one another by fully utilizing the available growth area***. For certain cells, which are sensitive to growth limitation due to density, the cells stop growing once confluence is reached. However, the transformed cells are insensitive to confluence and continue to overgrow.

When the culture becomes confluent, the cells possess the following characters.

1. The closest morphological resemblance to the tissue of origin (i.e. parent tissue).

2. The expression of specialized functions of the cells comparable to that of the native cells.

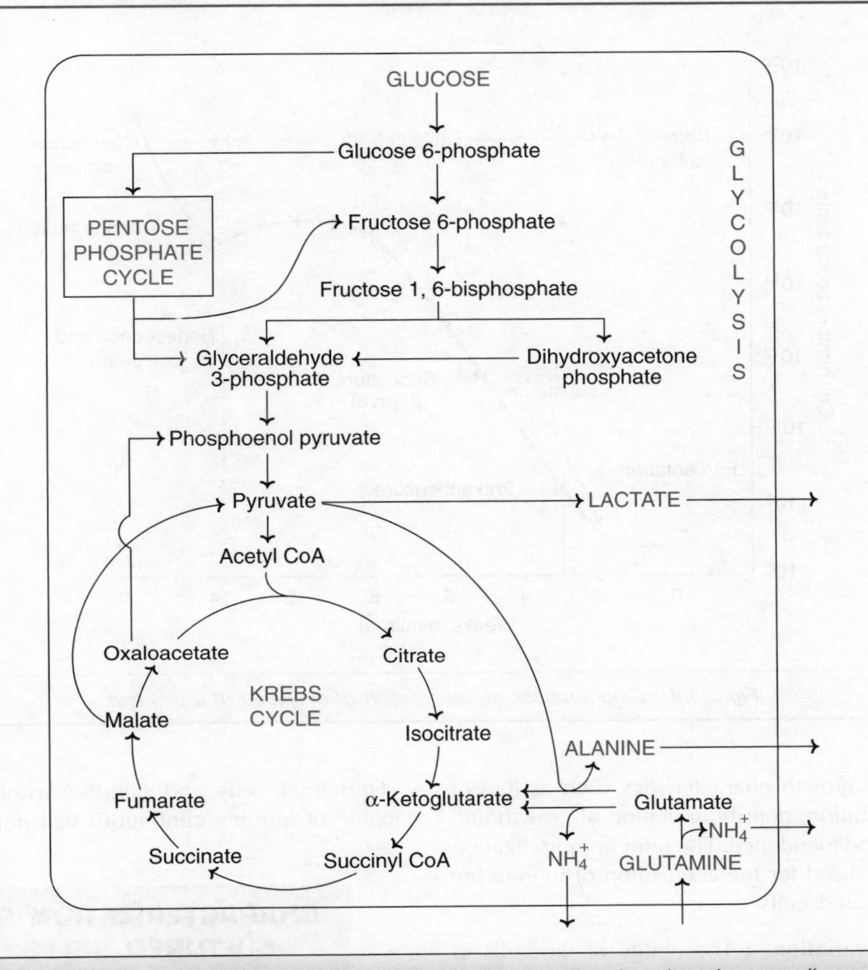

Fig. 35.3 : An outline of the glucose and glutamine metabolism in cultured mammalian cells.

EVOLUTION AND DEVELOPMENT OF CELL LINES

The primary culture grown after the first subculture is referred to as cell line. A given cell line may be propagated by further subculturing. As the subcultures are repeated, the most rapidly proliferating cells dominate while the non-proliferating or slowly proliferating cells will get diluted, and consequently disappear.

Senescence : The genetically determined event of cell divisions for a limited number of times (i.e. population doublings), followed by their ***death in a normal tissue is referred to as senescence***. However, germ cells and transformed cells are capable of continuously proliferating. In the *in vitro* culture, transformed cells can give rise to continuous cell lines.

The evolution of a continuous cell line is depicted in ***Fig. 35.4***. The cumulative cell number in a culture is represented on Y-axis on a log scale, while the X-axis represents the time in weeks. The time for development of a continuous cell line is variable. For instance, for human diploid fibroblasts, the continuous cell line arises at about 14 weeks while the senescence may occur between 10 to 20 weeks; usually after 30 and 60 cell doublings.

Development of continuous cell lines

Certain alterations in the culture, collectively referred to as ***transformation,*** can give rise to continuous cell lines. Transformation may be spontaneously occurring, chemically or virally-induced. Transformation basically involves an

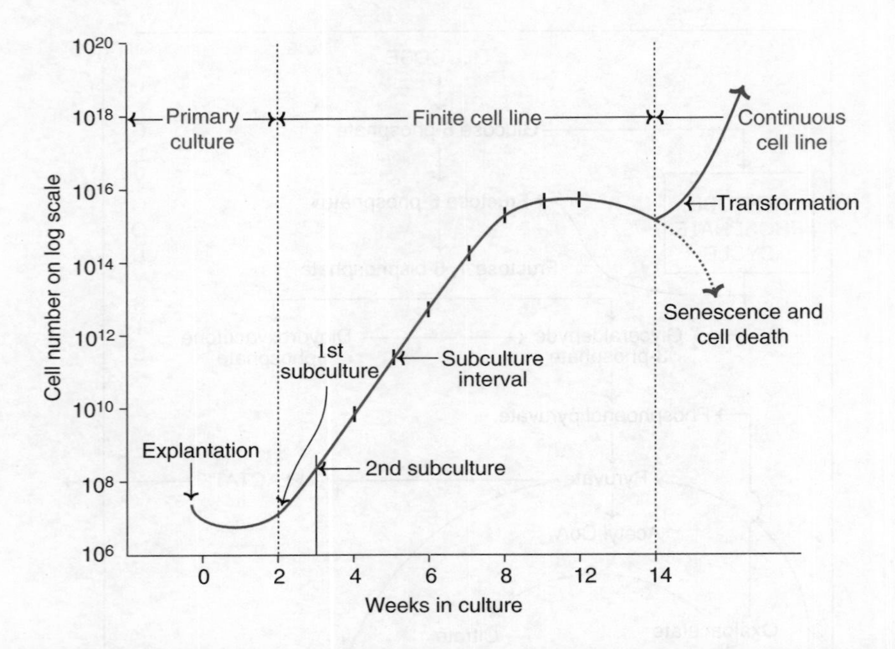

Fig. 35.4 : Diagrammatic representation of evolution of a cell line.

alteration in growth characteristics such as loss of contact inhibition, density limitation of growth and anchorage independence. The term immortalization is frequently used for the acquisition of infinite life span to cultured cells.

Genetic variations : The ability of the cells to grow continuously in cell lines represents genetic variation in the cells. Most often, the deletion or mutation of the p^{53} gene is responsible for continuous proliferation of cells. In the normal cells, the normal p^{53} gene is responsible for the arrest of cell cycle.

Most of the continuous cell lines are ***aneuploid***, possessing chromosome number between diploid and tetraploid value.

Normal cells and continuous cell lines

A great majority of normal cells are not capable of giving rise to continuous cell lines. For instance, normal human fibroblasts go on proliferating for about 50 generations, and then stop dividing. However, they remain viable for about 18 months. And throughout their life span, fibroblasts remain euploid. Chick fibroblasts also behave in a similar fashion.

Epidermal cells and lymphoblastoid cells are capable of forming continuous cell lines.

CHARACTERIZATION OF CULTURED CELLS

Characterization of cultured cells or cell lines is important for dissemination of cell lines through cell banks, and to establish contacts between research laboratories and commercial companies.

Characterization of cell lines with special reference to the following aspects is generally done.

1. Morphology of cells
2. Species of origin.
3. Tissue of origin.
4. Whether cell line is transformed or not.
5. Identification of specific cell lines.

MORPHOLOGY OF CELLS

A simple and direct identification of the cultured cells can be done by observing their morphological characteristics. However, the morphology has to be viewed with caution since it is largely dependent on the culture environment. For instance, the epithelial cells growing at the center (of the culture) are regular polygonal with clearly defined edges, while those growing at the periphery are irregular and distended (swollen). The composition of the culture medium, and the alterations in the substrate also influence the cellular morphology. In a tissue culture laboratory, the terms fibroblastic and epithelial are commonly used to describe the appearance of the cells rather than their origin.

Fibroblastic cells : For these cells, the length is usually more than twice of their width. Fibroblastic cells are bipolar or multipolar in nature.

Epithelial cells : These cells are polygonal in nature with regular dimensions and usually grow in monolayers.

The terms ***fibroblastoid*** (fibroblast-like) and ***epitheloid*** (epithelial-like) are in use for the cells that do not possess specific characters to identify as fibroblastic or epithelial cells.

SPECIES OF ORIGIN OF CELLS

The identification of the species of cell lines can be done by.

- Chromosomal analysis.
- Electrophoresis of isoenzymes.
- A combination of both these methods.

In recent years, chromosomal identification is being done by employing molecular probes.

IDENTIFICATION OF TISSUE OF ORIGIN

The identification of cell lines with regard to tissue of origin is carried out with reference to the following two characteristics.

1. The lineage to which the cells belong.

2. The status of the cells i.e. stem cells, precursor cells.

Tissue markers for cell line identification

Some of the important tissue or lineage markers for cell line identification are briefly described.

Differentiated products as cell markers : The cultured cells, on complete expression, are capable of producing differentiation markers, which serve as cell markers for identification. Some examples are given below.

- Albumin for hepatocytes.
- Melanin for melanocytes
- Hemoglobin for erythroid cells
- Myosin (or tropomyosin) for muscle cells.

Enzymes as tissue markers : The identification of enzymes in culture cells can be made with reference to the following characters.

- Constitutive enzymes.
- Inducible enzymes.
- Isoenzymes.

The commonly used enzyme markers for cell line identification are given in ***Table 35.1***.

Tyrosine aminotransferase is specific for hepatocytes, while tyrosinase is for melanocytes. Creatine kinase (MM) in serum serves as a marker for muscle cells, while creatine kinase (BB) is used for the detection of neurons and neuroendocrine cells.

Filament proteins as tissue markers : The intermediate filament proteins are very widely used as tissue or lineage markers. For example—

TABLE 35.1 Some common enzyme markers for cell line identification

Enzyme	*Cell type*
Tyrosine aminotransferase	Hepatocytes
Tysosinase	Melanocytes
Glutamyl synthase	Brain (astroglia)
Creatine kinase (isoenzyme MM)	Muscle cells
Creatine kinase (isoenzyme BB)	Neurons, neuroendocrine cells
Non-specific esterase	Macrophages
DOPA-decarboxylase	Neurons
Alkaline phosphatase	Enterocytes, type II pneumocytes
Angiotensin–converting enzyme	Endothelium
Sucrase	Enterocytes
Neuron-specific esterase	Neurons

DOPA–Dihydroxy phenylalanine; MM–Two polypeptide subunits of muscle; BB–Two polypeptide subunits of brain.

TABLE 35.2 A selected list of antibodies used for the detection of cell types

Antibody	*Cell type*
Cytokeratin	Epithelium
Epithelial membrane antigen	Epithelium
Albumin	Hepatocytes
α-Lactalbumin	Breast epithelium
Carcinoembryonic antigen (CEA)	Colorectal and lung adenocarcinoma
Prostate specific antigen (PSA)	Prostatic epithelium
Intracellular cell adhesion molecule (I-CAM)	T-cells and endothelium
α-Fetoprotein	Fetal hepatocytes
Human chorionic gonadotropin (hCG)	Placental epithelium
Human growth hormone (hGH)	Anterior pituitary
Vimentin	Mesodermal cells
Integrins	All cells
Actin	All cells

- Astrocytes can be detected by glial fibrillary acidic protein (GFAP).
- Muscle cells can be identified by desmin.
- Epithelial and mesothelial cells by cytokeratin.

Cell surface antigens as tissue markers : The antigens of the cultured cells are useful for the detection of tissue or cells of origin. In fact, many antibodies have been developed (commercial kits are available) for the identification cell lines (***Table. 35.2***). These antibodies are raised against cell surface antigens or other proteins.

The antibodies raised against secreted antigen α-fetoprotein serves as a marker for the identification of fetal hepatocytes. Antibodies of cell surface antigens namely integrins can be used for the general detection of cell lines.

TRANSFORMED CELLS

Transformation is the phenomenon of the ***change in phenotype due to the acquirement of new genetic material***. Transformation is associated with promotion of genetic instability. The transformed and cultured cells exhibit alterations in many characters with reference to

- Growth rate
- Mode of growth
- Longevity
- Tumorigenicity
- Specialized product formation.

While characterizing the cell lines, it is necessary to consider the above characters to determine whether the cell line has originated from tumor cells or has undergone transformation in culture.

For more details on transformation, Refer Chapter 6.

IDENTIFICATION OF SPECIFIC CELL LINES

There are many approaches in a culture laboratory to identify specific cell lines.

- Chromosome analysis
- DNA detection
- RNA and protein analysis
- Enzyme activities
- Antigenic markers.

Chromosome analysis

The species and sex from which the cell line is derived can be identified by chromosome analysis. Further, it is also ***possible to distinguish normal and malignant cells by the analysis of chromosomes***. It may be noted that the normal cells contain more stable chromosomes. The important techniques employed with regard to chromosome analysis are briefly described.

Chromosome banding : By this technique, it is possible to identify individual chromosome pairs when there is little morphological difference between them. Chromosome banding can be done by using Giemsa staining.

Chromosome count : A direct count of chromosomes can be done per spread between 50–100 spreads. A camera Lucida attachment or a closed circuit television may be useful.

Chromosome karyotyping : In this technique, the chromosomes are cut, sorted into sequence, and then pasted on to a sheet. The image can be recorded or scanned from the slide. Chromosome karyotyping is time consuming when compared to chromosome counting.

DNA detection

The ***total quantity of DNA per normal cell*** is quite constant, and ***is characteristic to the species of origin***. e.g. normal cell lines from human, chick and hamster fibroblasts. However, the DNA content varies in the normal cell lines of mouse, and also the cell lines obtained from cancerous tissues.

As already stated, most of the transformed cells are aneuploid and heteroploid. DNA analysis is particularly useful for characterization of such cells.

Analysis of DNA can be carried out by ***DNA hybridization and DNA fingerprinting.***

DNA hybridization : The popular ***Southern blotting technique*** (For details, Refer Chapter 7), can be used to detect unique DNA sequences. Specific molecular probes with radioisotope, fluorescent or luminescent labels can be used for this purpose.

The DNA from the desired cell lines is extracted, cut with restriction endonucleases, subjected to electrophoresis, blotted on to nitrocellulose, and then hybridized with a molecular (labeled) probe, or a set of probes. By this approach, specific sequences of DNA in the cell lines can be detected.

DNA fingerprinting : There are certain regions in the DNA of a cell that are not transcribed. These regions, referred to as satellite DNA, have no known functions, and it is believed that they may provide reservoir for genetic evolution. Satellite DNA regions are considered as regions of hypervariability. These regions may be cut with specific restriction endonucleases, and detected by using cDNA probes.

By using electrophoresis and autoradiography, the patterns of satellite DNA variations can be detected. Such patterns referred to as DNA fingerprints are cell line specific.

In recent years, the technique of DNA fingerprinting has become a very popular and a powerful tool to determine the origin of cell lines.

RNA and protein analysis

The phenotype characteristics of a cell line can be detected by gene expression i.e. identification of RNAs and/or proteins. ***mRNAs can be identified by Northern blot technique while proteins can be detected by Western blot technique.***

Enzyme activities

Some of the *in vivo* enzyme activities are lost when the cells are cultured *in vitro.* For instance, arginase activity of the liver cells is lost within a few days of culturing. However, ***certain cell lines express specific enzymes that can be employed for their detection*** e.g. tyrosine aminotransferase for hepatocytes, glutamyl synthase activity for astroglia in brain. For more examples of enzymes useful in cell line detection, refer ***Table 35.1***.

Isoenzymes : The multiple forms of an enzyme catalysing the same reaction are referred to as isoenzymes or isozymes. Isoenzymes differ in many physical and chemical properties—structure, electrophoretic and immunological properties, K_m and V_{max} values.

The isoenzymes can be separated by analytical techniques such as electrophoresis and chromatography. Most frequently, electrophoresis by employing agarose, cellulose acetate, starch and polyacrylamide is used. The crude enzyme is applied at one point on the electrophoretic medium. As the isoenzymes migrate, they distribute in different bands, which can be detected by staining with suitable chromogenic substrates.

Isoenzymes are characteristic to the species or tissues. Isoenzymes of the following enzymes are commonly ***used for cell line detection.***

- Lactate dehydrogenase
- Malate dehydrogenase
- Glucose 6-phosphate dehydrogenase
- Aspartate aminotransferase
- Peptidase B.

Isoenzyme analysis is also useful for the detection of interspecies cross-contamination of cell lines. For instance, contamination of mouse cell line with hamster cell line can be identified by using peptidase B isoenzymes.

Antigenic markers

Cell lines can be characterized by detection of antigenic markers through the use of antibodies. The antigenic markers may be located on the cell surface or secreted by the cells into the culture medium.

Some of the antibodies in common use for the detection of different cell types are given in ***Table 35.2*** (See p. 430).

MEASUREMENT OF GROWTH PARAMETERS OF CULTURED CELLS

Information on the growth state of a given culture is required to :

- Design culture experiments.
- Routine maintenance of culture.
- Measurement of cell proliferation.
- Know the time for subculture.
- Determine the culture response to a particular stimulus or toxin.

Some of the commonly used terms in relation to the measurement of growth of cultured cells are explained.

Population doubling time (PDT) : The time interval for the cell population to double at the middle of the logarithmic (log) phase.

Cell cycle time or generation time : The interval from one point in the cell division to the same point in the cycle, one division later. Thus cell cycle time is measured form one point in the cell cycle until the same point is reached again.

Confluence : It denotes the culture stage wherein all the available substrate (growth area) is utilized, and the cells are in close contact with each other.

Contact inhibition : Inhibition of cell motility and plasma membrane ruffling when the cells are in complete contact with other adjacent cells. This mostly occurs at confluence state, and results in the ceasation of the cell proliferation.

Cell density : The number of cells per ml of the medium.

Saturation density : The density of the cells (cells/ml^2 surface area) in the plateau phase.

GROWTH CYCLE OF CULTURED CELLS

The growth cycle of cultured cells is conventionally represented by three phases — the ***lag phase***, the ***log (exponential) phase*** and the ***plateau phase*** (*Fig. 35.5*). The properties of the cultured cells vary in the phases.

The lag phase

The lag phase represents a period of adaptation during which the cell forms the cell surface and extracellular matrix (lost during trypsinization),

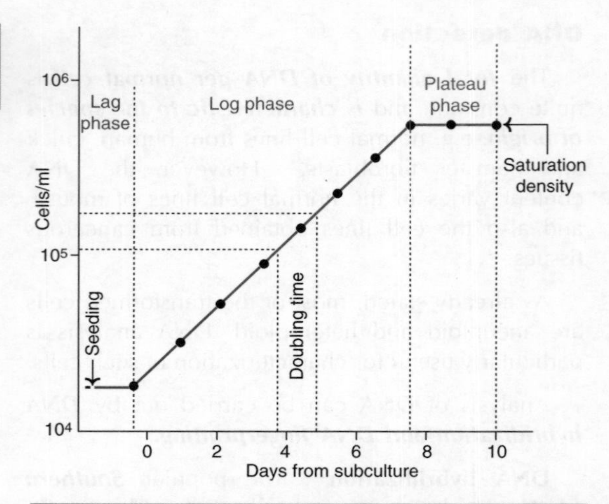

*Fig. 35.5 : Growth curve of cultured cells (**Note** : The cell concentration is expressed in semilog plot).*

attaches to the substrate and spreads out. There is an increased synthesis of certain enzymes (e.g. DNA polymerase) and structural proteins, preparing the cells for proliferation. The production of specialized products disappears which may not reappear until the cell proliferation ceases.

The lag phase represents preparative stage of the cells for proliferation following subculture and reseeding.

The log phase

The log phase is characterized by an exponential growth of cells, following the lag phase. The duration of log phase depends on the cells with reference to :

- Seeding density.
- Growth rate.
- Density after proliferation.

During the log phase, the cultured cells are in the most uniform and reproducible state with high viability. This is an ideal time for sampling.

The log phase terminates after confluence is reached with an addition of one or two population doublings.

The plateau phase

As the cells reach confluence, the growth rate is much reduced, and the proliferation of cultured

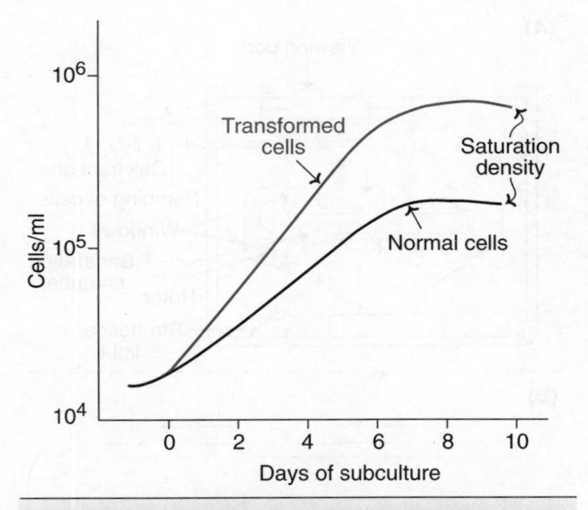

*Fig. 35.6 : Growth curves of transformed and normal cells (**Note :** The cell concentration is expressed in semilog plot).*

cells almost stops. This stage represents plateau or stationary phase, and is characterized by.

- Low motility of cells.
- Reduced ruffling of plasma membrane.
- Cells occupying minimum surface area.
- Contact inhibition.
- Saturation density.
- Depletion of nutrients and growth factors.
- Reduced synthesis of structural proteins.
- Increased formation of specialized products.

The majority of normal cultured cells that form monolayers stop growing as they reach confluence. Some of the cells however, with replenishment of medium continue to grow (at a reduced rate) after confluence, forming multilayers of cells.

The transformed cultured cells usually reach a higher cell density compared to the normal cells in the plateau phase (***Fig. 35.6***).

PLATING EFFICIENCY OF CULTURED CELLS

Plating efficiency, representing colony formation at low cell density, is a measure used for analyzing cell proliferation and survival.

When the cells, at low densities, are cultured in the form of single cell suspensions, they grow as discrete colonies. Plating efficiency is calculated as follows.

$$\text{Plating efficiency} = \frac{\text{No. of colonies formed}}{\text{No. of cells seeded}} \times 100$$

The term ***cloning efficiency*** is used (instead of plating efficiency) when each colony grows from a single cell.

Seeding efficiency representing the survival of cells at higher densities, is calculated as follows.

$$\text{Seeding efficiency} = \frac{\text{No. of cells recovered}}{\text{No. of cells seeded}} \times 100$$

CELL SYNCHRONIZATION

Synchronization literally means to make two or more things happen exactly simultaneously. For instance, two or more watches can be synchronized to show exactly the same time.

The ***cells at different stages of the cell cycle in a culture can be synchronized so that the cells will be at the same phase.*** Cell synchrony is required to study the progression of cells through cell cycle. Several laboratory techniques have been developed to achieve cell synchronization. They are broadly categorized into two groups.

1. Physical fractionation for cell separation.
2. Chemical blockade for cell separation.

CELL SEPARATION BY PHYSICAL MEANS

Physical fractionation or cell separation techniques, based on the following characteristics are in use.

- Cell density.
- Cell size.
- Affinity of antibodies on cell surface epitopes.
- Light scatter or fluorescent emission by labeled cells.

The two commonly used techniques namely centrifugal elutriation and fluorescence-activated cell separation are briefly described hereunder.

Centrifugal elutriation

The physical characteristics — ***cell size and sedimentation velocity are operative*** in the technique of centrifugal elutriation.

Centrifugal elutriator (from Beckman) is an advanced device for increasing the sedimentation rate so that the yield and resolution of cells is better. The cell separation is carried out in a specially designed centrifuge and rotor (***Fig. 35.7***). The cells in the medium are pumped into the separating chamber while the rotor is turning. Due to centrifugal force, the cell will be pushed to the edges. As the medium is then pumped through the chamber in such a way that the centripetal flow is equal to the sedimentation rate of cells. Due to differences in the cells (size, density, cell surface configuration), the cells tend to sediment at different rates, and reach equilibrium at different positions in the chamber. The entire operation in the elutriator can be viewed through the port, as the chamber is illuminated by stroboscopic light. At the equilibrium the flow rate can be increased and the cells can be pumped out, and separated in collecting vessels in different fractions. It is possible to carry out separation of cells in a complete medium, so that the cells can be directly cultured after separation.

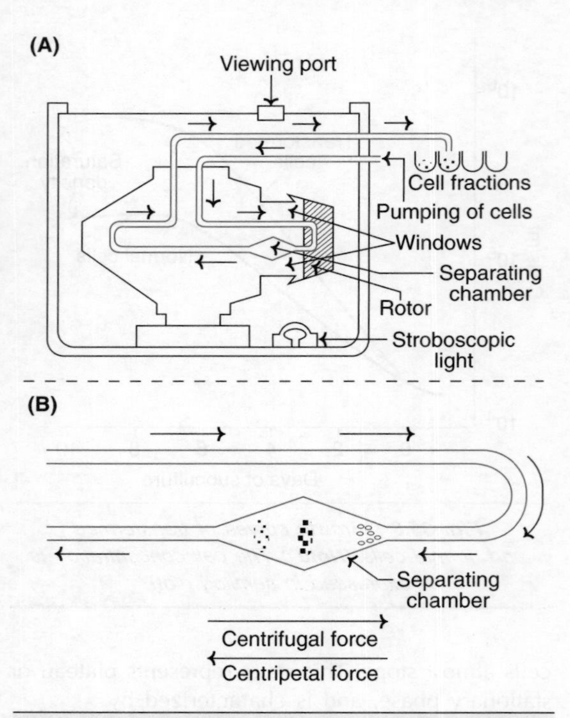

Fig. 35.7 : (A) Diagrammatic view of a centrifugal elutriator, (B) Separation chamber of elutriator.

Fluorescence-activated cell sorting

Fluorescence-activated cell sorting is a technique for sorting out the cells ***based on*** the differences that can be detected by light scatter (e.g. cell size) ***or fluorescence emission*** (by pretreated DNA, RNA, proteins, antigens).

The procedure involves passing of a single stream of cells through a laser beam so that the scattered light from the cells can be detected and recorded. When the cells are pretreated with a fluorescent stain (e.g. chromomycin A for DNA), the fluorescent emission excited by the laser can be detected.

There are two instruments in use based on the principle of fluorescent-activated cell sorting.

1. **Flow cytometer :** This instrument is capable of sorting out cells (from a population) in different phases of the cell cycle based on the measurements of a combination of cell size and DNA fluorescence.

2. **Fluorescent-activated cell sorter** (**FACS**) **:** In this instrument, the emission signals from the cells are measured, and the cells sorted out into collection tubes.

Comparison between physical methods

For separation of a large number of cells, centrifugal elutriator is preferred. On the other hand, fluorescent-activated cell sorting is mostly used to obtain high grade pure fractions of cells from small quantities of cells.

CELL SEPARATION BY CHEMICAL BLOCKADE

The cells can be separated by blocking metabolic reactions. Two types of metabolic blockades are in use — inhibition of DNA synthesis and nutritional deprivation.

Inhibition of DNA synthesis

During the S phase of cell cycle, DNA synthesis can be inhibited by using inhibitors such as thymidine, aminopterine, hydroxyurea and cytosine arabinoside. The effects of these inhibitors are variable. The cell cycle is predominantly blocked in S phase that results in viable cells.

Nutritional deprivation

Elimination of serum or isoleucine from the culture medium for about 24 hours results in the accumulation of cells at G_1 phase. This effect of nutritional deprivation can be restored by their addition by which time the cell synchrony occurs.

SOME HIGHLIGHTS OF CELL SYNCHRONIZATION

- Cell separation by physical methods is more effective than chemical procedures.
- Chemical blockade is often toxic to the cells.
- Transformed cells cannot be synchronized by nutritional deprivation.
- A high degree of cell synchrony (>80%) can be obtained in the first cycle, and in the second cycle it would be <60%. The cell distribution may occur randomly in the third cycle.

SENESCENCE AND APOPTOSIS

As the cells grow in culture, they become old due to aging, and they cannot proliferate any more. The ***end of the proliferative life span of cells is referred to as senescence***.

CELLULAR SENESCENCE

The ***growth of the cells*** is usually ***measured*** as ***population doublings (PDs)***. The PDs refer to the number of times the cell population doubles in number during the period of culture and is calculated by the following formula.

$$PD = \frac{\log_{10} \text{(No. of cells harvested)} - \log_{10} \text{(No. of cells seeded)}}{\log_{10} 2}$$

The phenomenon of senescence has been mostly studied with human fibroblast cultures. After 30-60 populations doublings, the culture is mainly composed of senescent fibroblasts. These senescent fibroblast are unable to divide in response to mitotic stimuli. It must be noted that the cells do not appear suddenly, but they gradually accumulate and increase in number during the life span of the culture.

The different parameters used for the measurement of cell growth in cultures are listed below.

- Direct measure of cell number.
- Determination of DNA/RNA content.
- Estimation of protein/ATP concentration.

MEASUREMENT OF SENESCENCE

The direct measurement of senescent cells is rather difficult. Some of the indirect measures are

- Loss of metabolic activity
- Lack of labeled precursor (^{3}H-thymidine) incorporation into DNA.
- Certain histochemical techniques.

Senescence-associated β-galactosidase activity assay

There occurs an overexpression of the lysosomal enzyme β-galactosidase at senescence. This enzyme elevation is also associated with an increase in the cell size as the cell enters a permanent non-dividing state.

The number of senescent cells in a culture can be measured by senescence-associated β-galactosidase (SA-β) assay. The assay consists of the following stages.

1. Wash the cells and fix them using a fixative (e.g. para formaldehyde), and wash again.
2. Add the staining solution (X-gal powder in dimethylformamide dissolved in buffer) to the fixed cells and incubate.
3. The senescent cells display a dense blue colour which can be counted.

APOPTOSIS

The process of ***programmed cell death (PCD)*** is referred to as apoptosis. The cell death may be initiated by a specific stimulus or as a result of several signals received from the external environment.

Apoptosis occurs as a result of inherent cellular mechanisms, which finally lead to self destruction. The cell activates a series of molecular events that cause an orderly degradation of the cellular constituents with minimal impact on the neighbouring tissues.

Reasons for *in situ* apoptosis

1. **For proper development :** The formation of fingers and toes of the fetus requires the removal of the tissues between them. This is usually carried out by apoptosis.

2. **Destruction of cells that pose threat to the integrity of the organism :** Programmed cell death is needed to destroy and remove the cells that may

otherwise damage the organisms. Some examples are listed

- Cells with damaged DNA during the course of embryonic development. If they are not destroyed, they may result in birth defects.
- Cells of the immune system, after their appropriate immune function, undergo apoptosis. This is needed to prevent autoimmune diseases e.g. rheumatoid arthritis.
- Cells infected with viruses are destroyed by apoptosis.

3. **Cell destruction due to negative signals :** There are several negative signals within the cells that promote apoptosis. These include accumulation of free radicals, exposure to UV rays, X-rays and chemotherapeutic drugs.

Mechanism of apoptosis

The programmed cell death may occur due to three different mechanisms.

1. Apoptisis due to internal signals.

2. Apoptosis triggered by external signals e.g. tumor necrosis factor-α (TNF-α), lymphotoxin.

3. Apoptosis triggered by reactive oxygen species.

Role of caspases in apoptosis

A group of enzymes namely ***activated proteases*** play a crucial role in the programmed cell death. These proteases are actually ***c***ysteinyl ***a***spartate ***s***pecific ***p***rotein***ases*** or in short, commonly referred to as ***caspases***. There are about ten different types of caspases acting on different substrates ultimately leading to cell death. For instance, capsase I cleaves interleukin 1β.

Inhibition of caspase activities

Since the caspases are closely involved in apoptosis, it is possible to prevent cell death by inhibiting their activities. Certain specific peptides that can inhibit caspases, and thus apoptosis have been identified.

MEASUREMENT OF APOPTOSIS

A simple and easy way of detecting dead or dying cells is the direct microscopic observation. The ***dying cells are rounded with dense bodies*** which can be identified under phase contrast microscope.

The ***cells that have undergone apoptosis contain fragmented chromatin*** which can be detected by conventional staining techniques.

In recent years, more sensitive and reliable techniques have been developed for measuring apoptosis. Some of them are briefly described.

Determination ADP/ATP ratio

Both the growth and apoptosis of cells require ATP. But when there is growth arrest, an elevation of ADP occurs. Thus measuring ADP/ATP ratio will throw light on the dead cells. In fact, some assay systems for measuring ADP/ATP ratios are commercially available.

TUNEL assay

A significant biochemical event for the apoptosis is the activation of endogenous nuclease activity. This enzyme cleaves DNA into fragments with free 3-hydroxyl groups. The newly formed small DNA fragments can be extended by employing the enzyme DNA polymerase. If labeled nucleotides are used for DNA fragment extension, they can be detected.

TUNEL is an abbreviation for **T**dT-mediated dUTP **n**ick **e**nd-**l**abeling assay. TUNEL is very fast and effective for the determination of DNA fragments formed by endogenous nuclease activity. The apoptotic nuclei can be identified by a fluorescent technique using fluorescein isothiocyanate (FITC) and 4,6-diaminophenylindole.

DNA laddering test

During the course of apoptosis, the genomic DNA is cleaved to mono — and oligonucleosomal DNA fragments. These fragments can be separated by agarose electrophoresis, and detected. The nucleosomal fragments of apoptotic cells give a characteristic ladder pattern on electrophoresis.

Limitations of the test : DNA laddering test is not very specific since several cells that have undergone apoptosis may not show DNA laddering. Further, some cells not subjected to apoptosis may also show DNA ladders, For these reasons, DNA laddering test is coupled with some other test for measurement of apoptosis.

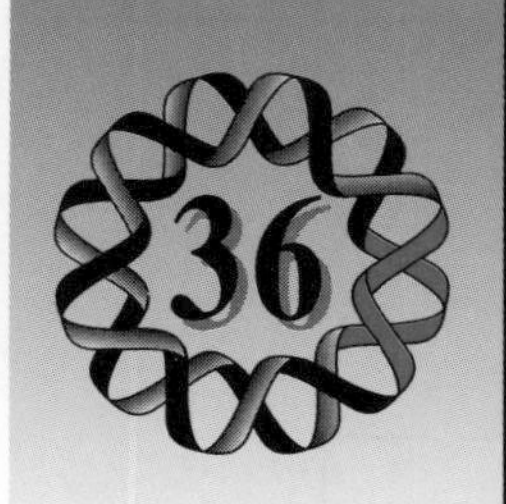

Primary Culture and Cell Lines

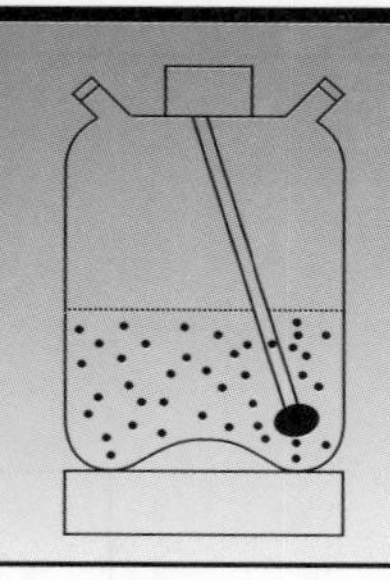

A primary culture refers to ***the starting culture of cells, tissues or organs, taken directly from an organism***. Thus, the primary culture is the initial culture before the first subculture. The term ***cell line is used for the propagation of cultures*** after the first subculture. Some basic and fundamental aspects of primary culture and cell lines are briefly described.

PRIMARY CELL CULTURE

As already stated, primary culture broadly involves ***the culturing techniques carried following the isolation of the cells, but before the first subculture***. Primary cultures are usually prepared from large tissue masses. Thus, these cultures may contain a variety of differentiated cells e.g. fibroblasts, lymphocytes, macrophages, epithelial cells.

With the experiences of the personnel working in tissue culture laboratories, the following criteria/ characteristics are considered for efficient development of primary cultures.

- Embryonic tissues rather than adult tissues are preferred for primary cultures. This is due to the fact that the embryonic cells can be disaggregated easily and yield more viable cells, besides rapidly proliferating *in vitro*.
- The quantity of cells used in the primary culture should be higher since their survival rate is substantially lower (when compared to subcultures).
- The tissues should be processed with minimum damage to cells for use in primary culture. Further, the dead cells should be removed.
- Selection of an appropriate medium (preferably a nutrient rich one) is advisable. For the addition of serum, fetal bovine source is preferred rather than calf or horse serum.
- It is necessary to remove the enzymes used for disaggregation of cells by centrifugation.

TECHNIQUES FOR PRIMARY CULTURE

Among the various techniques devised for the primary culture of isolated tissues, three techniques are most commonly used.

1. Mechanical disaggregation.
2. Enzymatic disaggregation.
3. Primary explant technique.

An outline of these techniques is depicted in ***Fig. 36.1***, and the procedures are briefly described.

MECHANICAL DISAGGREGATION

For the disaggregation of ***soft tissues*** (e.g. spleen, brain, embryonic liver, soft tumors), ***mechanical technique is usually employed***. This technique basically involves careful chopping or slicing of tissue into pieces and collection of spill out cells. The cells can be collected by two ways.

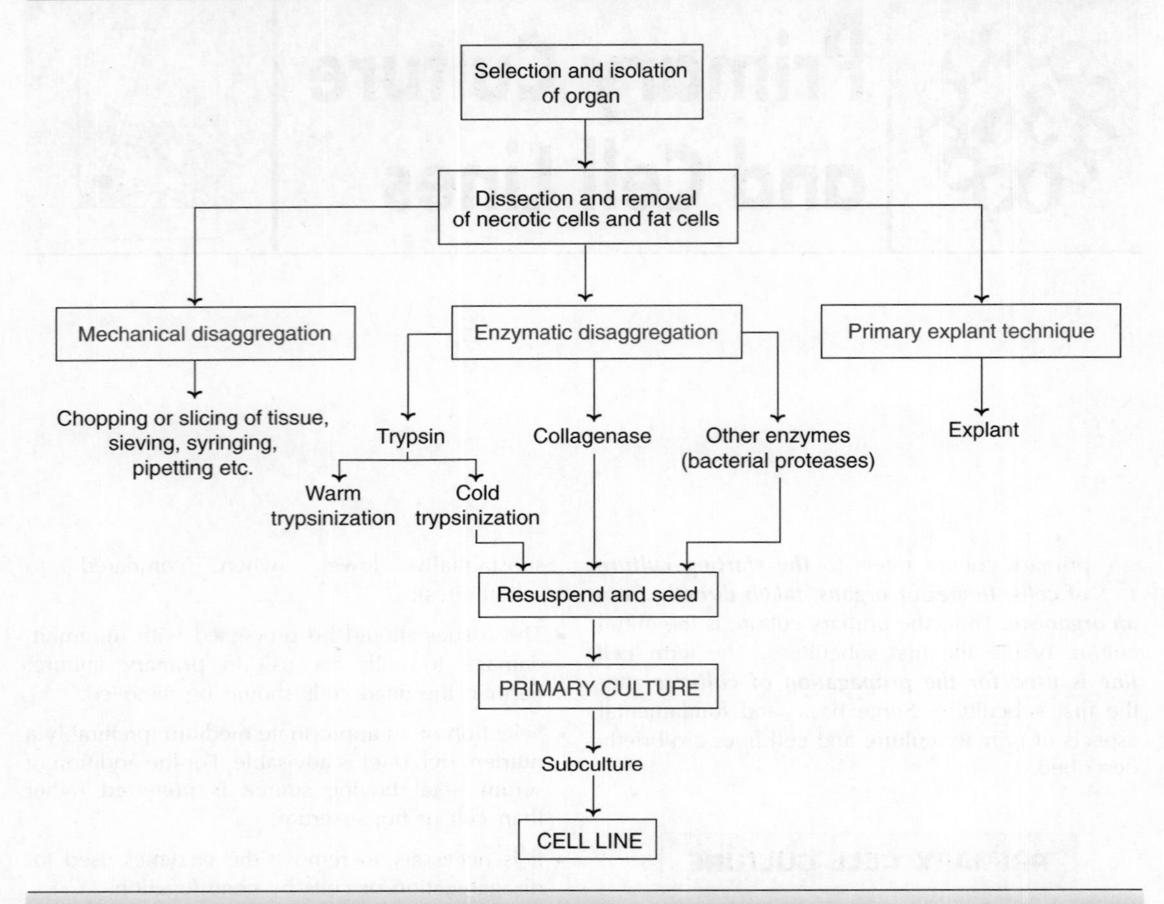

Fig. 36.1 : Different techniques used for primary culture.

- Pressing the tissue pieces through a series of sieves with a gradual reduction in the mesh size.
- Forcing the tissue fragments through a syringe and needle.

Although mechanical disaggregation involves the risk of cell damage, the procedure is less expensive, quick and simple. This technique is particularly useful when the availability of the tissue is in plenty, and the efficiency of the yield is not very crucial. It must however, be noted that the viability of cells obtained from mechanical techniques is much lower than the enzymatic technique.

ENZYMATIC DISAGGREGATION

Enzymatic disaggregation is mostly ***used when high recovery of cells is required from a tissue***. Disaggregation of embryonic tissues is more efficient with higher yield of cells by use of enzymes. This is due to the presence of less fibrous connective tissue and extracellular matrix. Enzymatic disaggregation can be carried out by using trypsin, collagenase or some other enzymes.

Disaggregation by trypsin

The term ***trypsinization*** is commonly used for disaggregation of tissues by the enzyme, trypsin. Many workers prefer to use crude trypsin rather than pure trypsin for the following reasons.

- The crude trypsin is more effective due to the presence of other proteases
- Cells can tolerate crude trypsin better.
- The residual activity of crude trypsin can be easily neutralized by the serum of the culture media (when serum-free media are used, a trypsin inhibitor can be used for neutralization).

Disaggregation of cells can also be carried out by using pure trypsin which is less toxic and more specific in its action.

The desired tissue is chopped to 2-3 mm pieces and then subjected to disaggregation by trypsin. There are two techniques of trypsinization-warm trypsinization and cold trypsinization (***Fig. 36.2***).

Warm trypsinization (*Fig. 36.2A*) : This method is widely used for disaggregation of cells. The chopped tissue is washed with dissection basal salt solution (DBSS), and then transferred to a flask containing warm trypsin (37° C). The contents are stirred, and at an interval of every thirty minutes, the supernatant containing the dissociated cells can be collected. After removal of trypsin, the cells are dispersed in a suitable medium and preserved (by keeping the vial on ice).

The process of addition of fresh trypsin (to the tissue pieces), incubation and collection of dissociated cells (at 30 minutes intervals) is carried out for about 4 hours. The disaggregated cells are pooled, counted, appropriately diluted and then incubated.

Cold trypsinization (*Fig. 36.2B*) : This technique is more appropriately referred to as ***trypsinization with cold preexposure***. The risk of damage to the cells by prolonged exposure to trypsin at 37°C (in warm trypsinization) can be minimized in this technique.

After chopping and washing, the tissue pieces are kept in a vial (on ice) and soaked with cold trypsin for about 6–24 hours. The trypsin is removed and discarded. However, the tissue pieces contain residual trypsin. These tissue pieces in a medium are incubated at 37°C for 20–30 minutes. The cells get dispersed by repeated pipettings. The dissociated cells can be counted, appropriately diluted and then used.

The ***cold trypsinization method usually results in a higher yield of viable cells with an improved survival of cells*** after 24 hours of incubation. This method does not involve stirring or centrifugation, and can be conveniently adopted in a laboratory. The major limitation of cold trypsinization is that it is not suitable for disaggregation of cells from large quantities of tissues.

Limitations of trypsin disaggregation

Disaggregation by trypsin may damage some cells (e.g. epithelial cells) or it may be almost ineffective for certain tissues (e.g. fibrous connective tissue). Hence other enzymes are also in use for dissociation of cells.

Disaggregation by collagenase

Collagen is the most abundant structural protein in higher animals. It is mainly present in the extra-cellular matrix of connective tissue and muscle. The enzyme collagenase (usually a crude one contaminated with non-specific proteases) can be effectively used for the disaggregation of several tissues (normal or malignant) that may be sensitive to trypsin. Highly purified grades of collagenase have been tried, but they are less effective when compared to crude collagenase.

The important stages in collagenase disaggregation, depicted in ***Fig. 36.3***, are briefly described hereunder.

The desired tissue suspended in basal salt solution, containing antibiotics is chopped into pieces. These pieces are washed by settling, and then suspended in a complete medium containing collagenase. After incubating for 1-5 days, the tissue pieces are dispersed by pipetting. The clusters of cells are separated by settling. The epithelial cells and fibroblastic cells can be separated.

Collagenase disaggregation has been successfully used for human brain, lung and several other epithelial tissues, besides various human tumors, and other animal tissues. Addition of another enzyme hyaluronidase (acts on carbohydrate residues on cell surfaces) promotes disaggregation. Collagenase in combination with hyaluronidase is found to be very effective for dissociating rat or rabbit liver. This can be done by perfusing the whole organ *in situ*.

Some workers use collagenase in conjunction with trypsin, a formulation developed in chick serum, for disaggregation of certain tissues.

Use of other enzymes in disaggregation

Trypsin and collagenase are the most widely used enzymes for disaggregation. Certain bacterial proteases (e.g. pronase, dispase) have been used with limited success. Besides hyaluronidase (described above), neuraminidase is also used in conjunction with collagenase for effective degradation of cell surface carbohydrates.

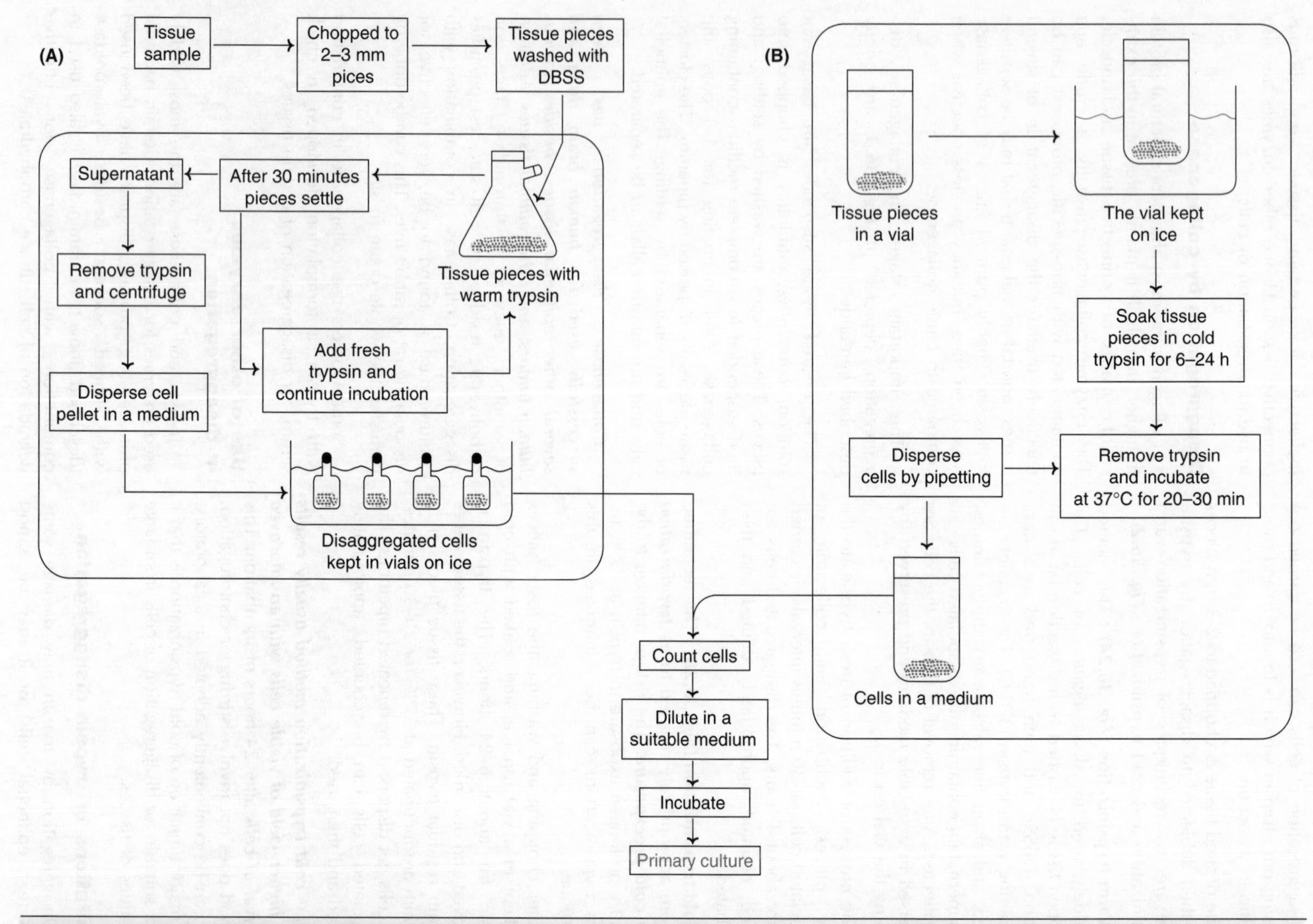

Fig. 36.2 : Preparation of primary culture by trypsin disaggregation (A) Warm trypsinization (B) Cold trypsinization (DBSS–Dissection basal salt solution).

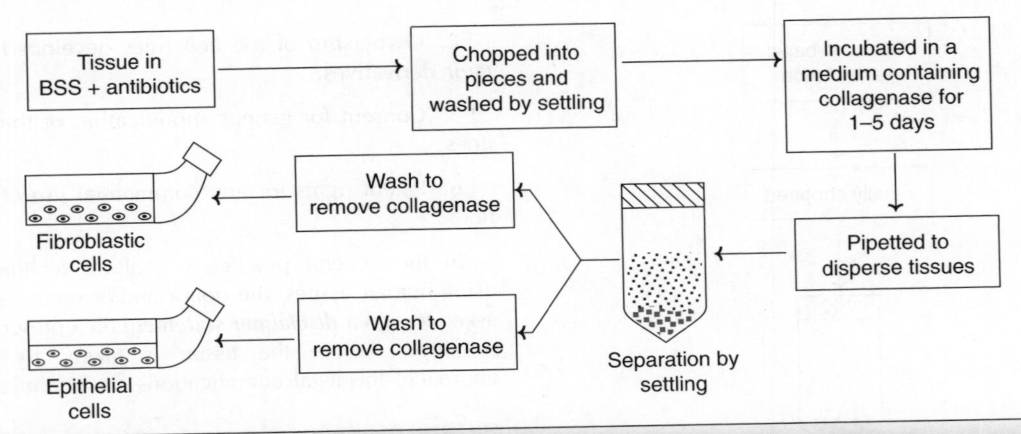

Fig. 36.3 : *Important stages in collagenase disaggregation of tissue for primary culture (BSS–Basal salt solution).*

PRIMARY EXPLANT TECHNIQUE

The primary explant technique was, in fact the original method, developed by Harrison in 1907. This technique has undergone several modifications, and is still in use. The simplified procedure adopted for primary explant culture is depicted in ***Fig. 36.4***, and briefly described below.

The tissue in basal salt solution is finely chopped, and washed by settlings. The basal salt solution is then removed. The tissue pieces are spread evenly over the growth surface. After addition of appropriate medium, incubation is carried out for 3-5 days. Then the medium is changed at weekly intervals until a substantial out-growth of cells is observed. Now, the explants are removed and transferred to a fresh culture vessel.

The ***primary explant technique is particularly useful for disaggregation of small quantities of tissues*** (e.g. skin biopsies). The other two techniques-mechanical or enzymatic disaggregation however, are not suitable for small amounts of tissues, as there is a risk of losing the cells. The limitation of explant technique is the poor adhesiveness of certain tissues to the growth surface, and the selection of cells in the outgrowth. It is however, observed that the primary explant technique can be used for a majority of embryonic cells e.g. fibroblasts, myoblasts, epithelial cells, glial cells.

SEPARATION OF VIABLE AND NON-VIABLE CELLS

It is a common practice to remove the non-viable cells while the primary culture is prepared from the disaggregated cells. This ***is usually done when the first change of the medium is carried out***. The very few left over non-viable cells get diluted and gradually disappear as the proliferation of viable cells commences.

Sometimes, the non-viable cells from the primary cultures may be removed by centrifugation. The cells are mixed with ficoll and sodium metrizoate, and centrifuged. The dead cells form a pellet at the bottom of the tube.

MEDICAL ETHICS AND SAFETY MEASURES IN CULTURE TECHNIQUES

Since the culture techniques involve the use of animal or human tissues, it is absolutely necessary to follow several safety measures and medical ethics. In fact, in some countries there are established legislation/norms for selection and use of tissues in cultures. For example, in United Kingdom, Animal Experiments (Scientific Procedures) Act of 1986 is followed.

The ***handling of human tissues poses several problems that are not usually encountered with animal tissues***. While dealing with fetal materials and human biopsies, the consent of the patient and/his or her relatives, besides the consent of local ethical committee is required. Further, taking any tissue (even in minute quantities) from human donors requires the full consent of the donor in a prescribed format. The following issues need to be fully considered while dealing with human tissues.

1. The consent of the patient and/or relatives for using tissues for research purposes.

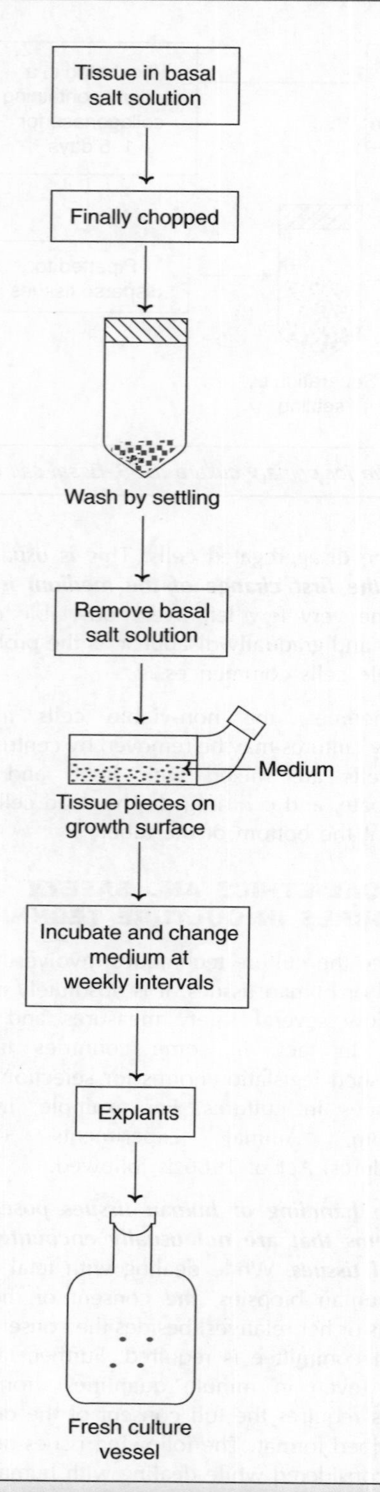

Fig. 36.4 : Primary explant technique for primary culture.

2. Ownership of the cell lines developed and their derivatives.

3. Consent for genetic modification of the cell lines.

6. Patent rights for any commercial use of cell lines.

In the general practice of culture techniques using human tissues, the donor and/or relatives are asked to sign a ***disclaimer statement*** (in a prescribed proforma) before the tissue is taken. By this approach, the legal complications are minimized.

Safety measures

Handling of ***human tissues*** is associated with a heavy ***risk of exposure for various infections.*** Therefore, it is absolutely necessary that the human materials are handled in a ***biohazard cabinet.*** The tissues should be screened for various infections such as hepatitis, tuberculosis, HIV, before their use. Further, the media and apparatus, after their use must be autoclaved or disinfected, so that the spread of infections is drastically reduced.

CELL LINES

The development and various other aspects of primary culture are described above. The term cell line refers to the ***propagation of culture after the first subculture.*** In other words, once the primary culture is subcultured, it becomes a cell line. A given cell line contains several cell lineages of either similar or distinct phenotypes.

It is possible to select a particular cell lineage by cloning or physical cell separation or some other selection method. Such a ***cell line derived by selection or cloning is referred to as cell strain.*** Cell strains do not have infinite life, as they die after some divisions.

FINITE CELL LINES

The cells in culture divide only a limited number of times, before their growth rate declines and they eventually die. The ***cell lines with limited culture life spans are referred to as finite cell lines.*** The cells normally divide 20 to 100 times (i.e. is 20-100 population doublings) before extinction. The actual number of doublings depends on the species, cell

TABLE 36.1 Comparison of properties of finite and continuous cell lines

Property	*Finite cell line*	*Continuous cell line*
Growth rate	Slow	Fast
Mode of growth	Monolayer	Suspension or monolayer
Yield	Low	High
Transformation	Normal	Immortal, tumorigenic
Ploidy	Euploid (multiple of haploid chromosomes)	Aneuploid (not an exact multiple of haploid chromosomes)
Anchorage dependence	Yes	No
Contact inhibition	Yes	No
Cloning efficiency	Low	High
Serum requirement	High	Low
Markers	Tissue specific	Chromosomal, antigenic or enzymatic

lineage differences, culture conditions etc. The human cells generally divide 50-100 times, while murine cells divide 30-50 times before dying.

CONTINUOUS CELL LINES

A few cells in culture may acquire a different morphology and get altered. Such cells are capable of growing faster resulting in an independent culture. The progeny derived from these altered cells has unlimited life (unlike the cell strains from which they originated). They are designated as continuous cell lines. The ***continuous cell lines are transformed, immortal and tumorigenic.*** The transformed cells for continuous cell lines may be obtained from normal primary cell cultures (or cells strains) by treating them with chemical carcinogens or by infecting with oncogenic viruses.

In the ***Table. 36.1***, the different properties of finite cell lines and continuous cell lines are compared.

The most commonly used terms while dealing with cell lines are explained below.

Split ratio : The divisor of the dilution ratio of a cell culture at subculture. For instance, when each subculture divided the culture to half, the split ratio is 1 : 2.

Passage number : It is the number of times that the culture has been subcultured.

Generation number : It refers to ***the number of doublings that a cell population has undergone.***

It must be noted that the passage number and generation number are not the same, and they are totally different.

NOMENCLATURE OF CELL LINES

It is a common practice to give codes or designations to cell lines for their identification. For instance, the code ***NHB 2-1*** represents the cell line from ***n***ormal ***h***uman ***b***rain, followed by cell strain (or cell line number) 2 and clone number **1**. The usual practice in a culture laboratory is to maintain a log book or computer database file for each of the cell lines.

While naming the cell lines, it is absolutely necessary to ensure that each cell line designation is unique so that there occurs no confusion when reports are given in literature. Further, at the time of publication, the cell line should be prefixed with a code designating the laboratory from which it was obtained e.g. NCI for National Cancer Institute, WI for Wistar Institute.

Commonly used cell lines

There are thousands of cell lines developed from different laboratories worldover. A selected list of some commonly used cell lines along with their origin, morphology and other characters are given in ***Table. 36.2***.

SELECTION OF CELL LINES

Several factors need to be considered while selecting a cell line. Some of them are briefly described.

Table 36.2 A selected list of commonly used cell lines

Cell line	*Species of origin*	*Tissue of origin*	*Morphology*	*Ploidy*	*Characteristics*
IMR-90	Human	Lung	Fibroblast	Diploid	Susceptible to human viral infections.
3T3-A31	Mouse	Connective tissue	Fibroblast	Aneuploid	Contact inhibited, readily transformed
BHK21-C13	Hamster (Syrian)	Kidney	Fibroblast	Aneuploid	Readily transformable
CHO-k1	Chinese hamster	Ovary	Fibroblast	Diploid	Simple karyotype
NRK49F	Rat	Kidney	Fibroblast	Aneuploid	Induction of suspension growth by TGF-α, β.
BRL 3A	Rat	Liver	Epithelial	Diploid	Produces IGF-2
Vero	Monkey	Kidney	Fibroblast	Aneuploid	Viral substrate and assay
HeLa-S_3	Human	Cervical carcinoma	Epithelial	Aneuploid	Rapid growth, high plating efficiency.
Sk/HEP-I	Human	Hepatoma	Endothelial	Aneuploid	Factor VIII
Caco-2	Human	Colo-rectal carcinoma	Epithelial	Aneuploid	Forms tight monolayer with polarised support.
MCF-7	Human	Breast tumor (effusion)	Epithelial	Aneuploid	Estrogen receptor positive.
Friend	Mouse	Spleen	Suspension	Aneuploid	Hemoglobin, growth hormone.

1. **Species :** In general, non-human cell lines have less risk of biohazards, hence preferred. However, species differences need to be taken into account while extrapolating the data to humans.

2. **Finite or continuous cell lines :** Cultures with continuous cell lines are preferred as they grow faster, easy to clone and maintain, and produce higher yield. But it is doubtful whether the continuous cell lines express the right and appropriate functions of the cells. Therefore, some workers suggest the use of finite cell lines, although it is difficult.

3. **Normal or transformed cells :** The transformed cells are preferred as they are immortalized and grow rapidly.

4. **Availability :** The ready availability of cell lines is also important. Sometimes, it may be necessary to develop a particular cell line in a laboratory.

5. **Growth characteristics :** The following growth parameters need to be considered.

- Population doubling time
- Ability to grow in suspension
- Saturation density (yield per flask)
- Cloning efficiency.

6. **Stability**: The stability of cell line with particular reference to cloning, generation of adequate stock and storage are important.

7. **Phenotypic expression**: It is important that the cell lines possess cells with the right phenotypic expression.

MAINTENANCE OF CELL CULTURES

For the routine and good maintenance of cell lines in culture (primary culture or subculture) the examination of cell morphology and the periodic change of medium are very important.

Cell morphology : The cells in the culture must be examined regularly to check the health status of the cells, the absence of contamination, and any other serious complications (toxins in medium, inadequate nutrients etc).

Replacement of medium : Periodic change of the medium is required for the maintenance of cell lines in culture, whether the cells are proliferating or non-proliferating. ***For the proliferating cells, the***

medium need to be changed more frequently when compared to non-proliferating cells. The time interval between medium changes depends on the rate of cell growth and metabolism. For instance, for rapidly growing transformed cells (e.g. HeLa), the medium needs to be changed twice a week, while for slowly growing non-transformed cells (e.g. IMR-90), the medium may be changed once a week. Further, for rapidly proliferating cells, the subculturing has to be done more frequently than for the slowly growing cells.

The following ***factors*** need to be considered ***for the replacement of the medium.***

1. **Cell concentration :** The cultures with high cell concentration utilize the nutrients in the medium faster than those with low concentration, hence the medium is required to be changed more frequently for the former.

2. **A decrease in pH :** A fall in the pH of the medium is an indication for change of medium. Most of the cells can grow optimally at pH 7.0, and they almost stop growing when the pH falls to 6.5. A further drop in pH (between 6.5 and 6.0), the cells may lose their viability. The rate of fall in pH is generally estimated for each cell line with a chosen medium. If the fall is less than 0.1 pH units per day, there is no harm even if the medium is not immediately changed. But when the fall is 0.4 pH units per day, medium should be changed immediately.

3. **Cell type :** Embryonic cells, transformed cells and continuous cell lines grow rapidly and require more frequent subculturing and change of medium. This is in contrast to normal cells, which grow slowly.

4. **Morphological changes:** Frequent examination of cell morphology is very important in culture techniques. Any deterioration in cell morphology may lead to an irreversible damage to cells. Change of the medium has to be done to completely avoid the risk of cell damage.

SUBCULTURE

Subculture (or passage) refers to the ***transfer of cells from one culture vessel to another culture vessel.*** Subculture usually (not always) involves the subdivision of proliferating cells that enables the propagation of a cell line. The term ***passage number*** is used to indicate the number of times a culture has been subcultured.

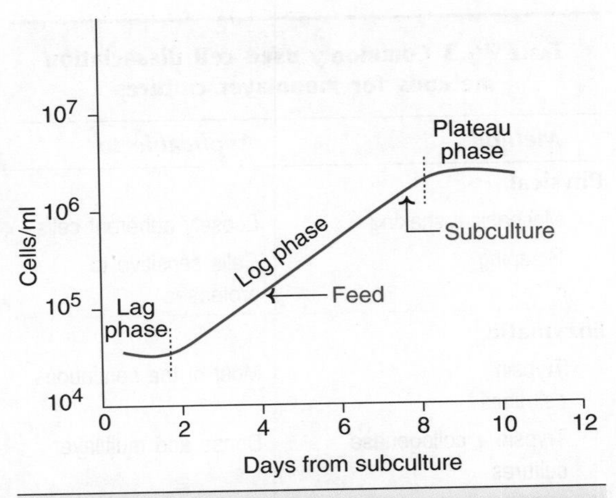

Fig. 36.5 : Depiction of a standard growth of cells in a culture (Note : the cell concentration is expressed in semilog plot).

The standard growth curve of cells in a culture is depicted in ***Fig. 36.5.*** The initial lag phase is followed by exponential or log phase and a plateau phase. During the active growth period in the log phase, the medium must be changed frequently, or else growth ceases. As the cell concentration exceeds the capacity of the medium, the culture has to be divided to subculture.

There are two types of subcultures-monolayer subculture and suspension subculture.

MONOLAYER CULTURES

When the ***bottom of the culture vessel is covered with a continuous layer of cells, usually one cell in thickness,*** they are referred to as monolayer cultures. The attachment of cells among themselves and to the substrate (i.e. culture vessel) is mediated through surface glycoproteins (cell adhesion molecules) and calcium ions (Ca^{2+}). For subculturing of monolayer cultures, it is usually necessary to remove the medium and dissociate the cells in the monolayer by degrading the cell adhesion molecules, besides removing Ca^{2+}.

Methods of cell dissociation

There are ***physical*** and ***enzymatic methods*** for dissociation of monolayer cultures (***Table. 36.3***).

TABLE 36.3 Commonly used cell dissociation methods for monolayer cultures

Method	*Applicable to*
Physical	
Mechanical shaking	Loosely adherent cells
Scraping	Cells sensitive to proteases
Enzymatic	
Trypsin	Most of the continuous cell lines
Trypsin + collagenase	Dense and multilayer cultures
Dispase	Removal of epithelium in sheets
Pronase	Single–cell suspensions

Mechanical shaking and cell scraping are employed for cultures which are loosely adhered, and the use of proteases has to be avoided. Among the enzymes, ***trypsin is the most frequently used***. For certain cell monolayers, which cannot be dissociated by trypsin, other enzymes such as pronase, dispase and collagenase are used. Prior to cell dissociation by enzymes, the monolayers are usually subjected to pretreatment of EDTA for the removal of Ca^{2+}.

Criteria for subculture of monolayers

The subculturing is ideally carried out between the middle of the log phase and the time before they enter plateau phase (***Fig. 36.6***). Subculture of cells should ***not be done when they are in lag phase***. The other important criteria for subculture of monolayers are briefly described.

Culture density : It is advisable to subculture the normal or transformed monolayer cultures, as soon as they reach confluence. Confluence denotes the culture stage wherein all the available growth area is utilized and the cells make close contact with each other.

Medium exhaustion : A drop in pH is usually accompanied by an increase in culture cell density. Thus, when the pH falls, the medium must be changed, followed by subculture.

Scheduled timings of subculture : It is now possible to have specified schedule timings for subculture of each cell line. For a majority of cell cultures, the medium change is usually done after 3-4 days, and subculturing after 7 days.

Purpose of subculture : The purpose for which the cells are required is another important criteria for consideration of subculturing. Generally, if the cells are to be used for any specialized purpose, they have to be subcultured more frequently.

Techniques of monolayer subculture

The subculture of monolayer cells basically consists of the following steps (***Fig. 36.6***)

1. Removal of the medium
2. Brief exposure of the cells to trypsin.
3. Removal of trypsin and dispersion in a medium.
4. Incubation of cells to round up.
5. Resuspension of the cells in a medium for counting and reseeding.
6. Cells reseeded and grown to monolayers.

Cell concentration at subculture : Most of the continuous cell lines are subcultured at a seeding concentration between 1×10^4 and 5×10^4 cells/ml. However for a new culture, subculture has to be started at a high concentration and gradually reduced.

SUSPENSION CULTURES

Majority of continuous cell lines grow as monolayers. Some of the cells which are ***non-adhesive*** e. g. cells of leukemia or certain cells ***which can be mechanically kept in suspension, can be propagated in suspension***. The transformed cells are subcultured by this method. Subculture by suspension is comparable to culturing of bacteria or yeast.

Advantages of cell propagation by suspension

- The process of propagation is faster.
- The lag period is usually shorter.
- Results in homogeneous suspension of cells.
- Treatment with trypsin is not required.
- Scale-up is convenient.
- No need for frequent replacement of the medium.

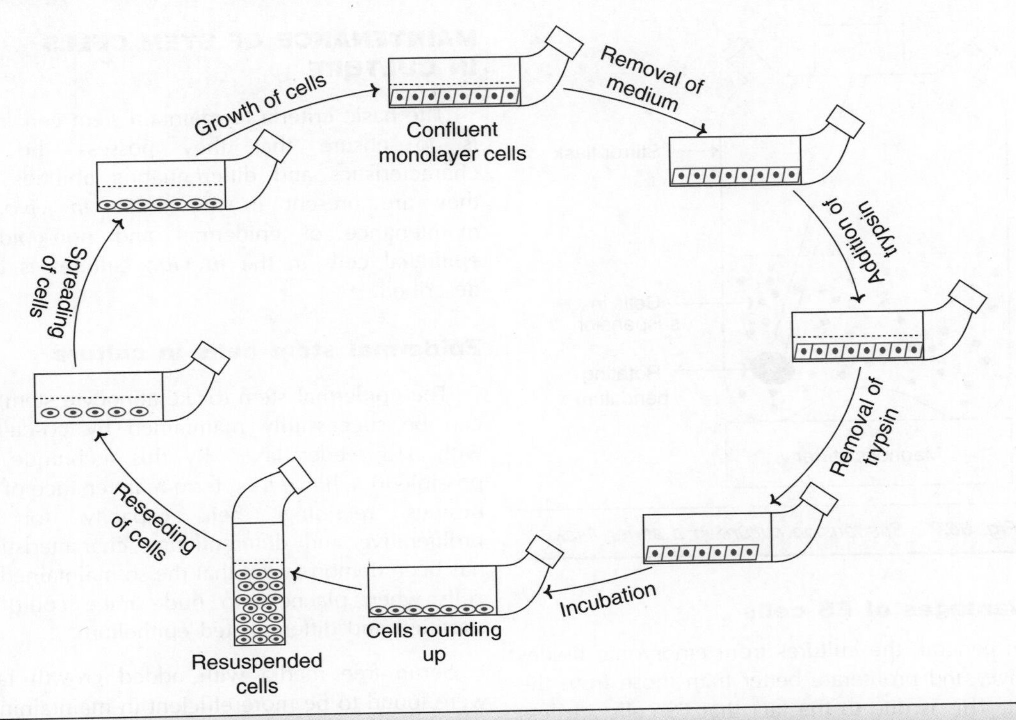

Fig. 36.6 : Technique of monolayer subculture.

- Maintenance is easy.
- Bulk production of cells can be conveniently achieved.

Criteria for suspension subculture

The criteria adopted for suspension subculture are the same as that already described for monolayer subcultures (See p. 446). The following aspects have to be considered.

- Culture density.
- pH change representing medium exhaustion.
- Schedule timings of subculture.
- Purpose of subculture.

Technique of suspension culture

The cells can be suspended in a culture flask (a stirrer flask) containing the desired medium (***Fig. 36.7***). The medium is continuously stirred with a magnetic pendulum rotating at the base of the flask. The cells have to periodically examined for contamination or signs of deterioration.

STEM CELL CULTURES

The ***cells that retain their proliferative capacity throughout life*** are regarded as ***stem cells***. When the stem cells divide, they can generate differentiated cells and/or some more stem cells. These stem cells are capable of regenerating tissue after injury. The lack of tissue-specific differentiation markers is a characteristic feature of stem cells.

EMBRYONIC STEM (ES) CELLS

As the embryonic development occurs, cells of the ***inner mass of embryo*** (i.e. those contributing to future fetus) represent embryonic stem (ES) cells. They continue to divide and remain in an un-differentiated to totipotent state. It has been possible to establish and maintain cell lines for ES cells. The ES cells isolated from mouse blastocyst are the most commonly used in the laboratory.

The most widely used embryonic stem lines are the various 3T3 lines, WI-38, MRC-5 and other human fetal lung fibroblasts.

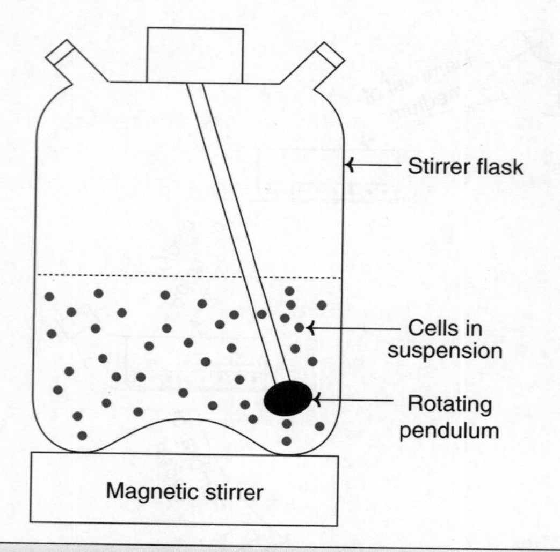

Fig. 36.7 : Suspension culture in a stirrer flask.

Advantages of ES cells

In general, the cultures from embryonic tissues survive, and proliferate better than those from the adult. This is due to the fact that ES cells are less specialized with higher proliferative potential.

Limitations of ES cells

In some cases, the ES cells will be different from the adult cells, and thus there is no guarentee that they will mature to adult-type cells. Therefore, it is necessary to characterize the cells by appropriate methods.

EPITHELIAL STEM CELLS

The epithelial cells (e.g. epidermis lining of gut) are constantly being shed from their outer surface. This cellular loss is compensated by a continuous replacement process. The replacement occurs in a highly organized and a regulated fashion.

It is estimated that in humans the entire outer layer of skin is shed daily. The entire epithelial lining of the mouse gut is replaced once in 3-4 days. This process of shedding and replacement continues throughout life.

The epidermis of the skin has a proliferative compartment containing stem cells and post-mitotic cells, besides some transit amplifying population of cells. The transit amplifying cells, produced from stem cells with limited life span are shed from the epidermis.

MAINTENANCE OF STEM CELLS IN CULTURE

The basic criteria to maintain stem cell *in vitro* is to ensure that they possess the same characteristics and differentiating abilities when they are present in the tissue *in vivo*. The maintenance of epidermal and non-epidermal epithelial cells in the *in vitro* cultures is briefly described.

Epidermal stem cells in culture

The epidermal stem (or keratinocyte stem) cells can be successfully maintained by co-culturing with 3T3 feeder layer. By this technique, it is possible to achieve long term maintenance of cells, besides retaining their capacity for both proliferative and differentiating characteristics. It has been demonstrated that the so maintained stem cells when placed into nude mice could form stratified and differentiated epithelium.

Serum-free media with added growth factors were found to be more efficient in maintaining the epidermal stem cells in culture.

Epithelial cells in culture

Several types of non-epidermal epithelial cells can be grown and maintained in cultures. As in the case with epidermal stem cells, use of feeder layer is advantageous for epithelial cell culture.

Epithelial cells of prostate gland have been successfully grown in suspension cultures in the presence of 3T3 feeder layer. The same method is also used for culturing human breast epithelial cells and colorectal carcinoma cells.

CHARACTERIZATION OF STEM CELLS

Immunological techniques are widely used for the characterization of different populations of stem cells. These techniques are mostly based on immunocytochemistry using fluorescent microscopy or staining technique involving colour reactions.

The cells of the tissues produce specific cell surface and cytoplasmic proteins. The cell surface proteins such as integrins and the members of CD (cluster of differentiation) antigens (e.g. CD_{10}, CD_{31}, CD_{44}) can be used as markers of epithelial cell types. Further, the cytoplasmic proteins of epithelial cells (of cytokeratin family) are also useful for their identification.

APPLICATIONS OF CULTURED STEM CELLS

Embroynic stem cells in tissue repair

The culture stem cells can be used for the repair of tissues with functional impairment that may occur due to damage or ageing. The cultured embryonic stem cells can be manipulated to produce cultures characteristic of a particular tissue. Thus, there exists a possibility of treating the following diseases.

- Diabetes with pancreatic insulin producing cells.
- Parkinson's disease with cultured dopamine-producing neurons.

Embryonic stem cells are useful for the production of defined transgenic animals. It is also possible to modify ES cell genome by gene targeting using *in vitro* transformation and selection.

Applications of tissue specific stem cells

Stem cells, isolated from different tissues of humans and animals, and cultured *in vitro* are less toitpotent than ES cells. They usually differentiate into a single cell type and are referred to as ***unipotent.*** However, stem cells from bone marrow and brain are capable of forming different cell types though to a lesser extent when compared to ES cells. In mouse lacking bone marrow, when the cultured neuronal cells are placed, they develop into blood cells.

Tissue specific culture stem cells are used for the following purposes.

- In surgical repair and tissue grafting.
- In gene therapy.

Some more details on ES cells, with particular reference to stem cell engineering, are given in Chapter 40.

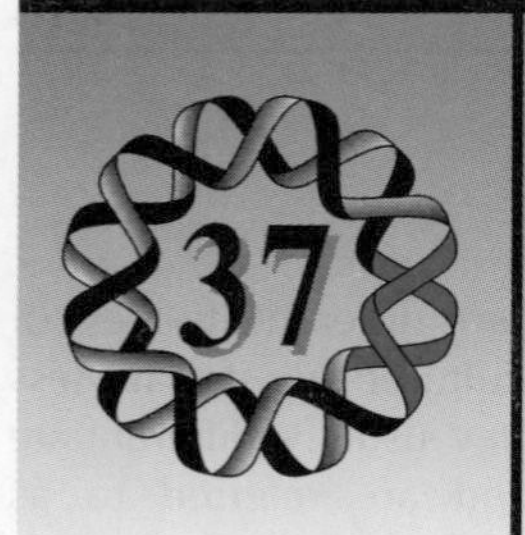

Animal Cell Culture — General Considerations and Scale-up

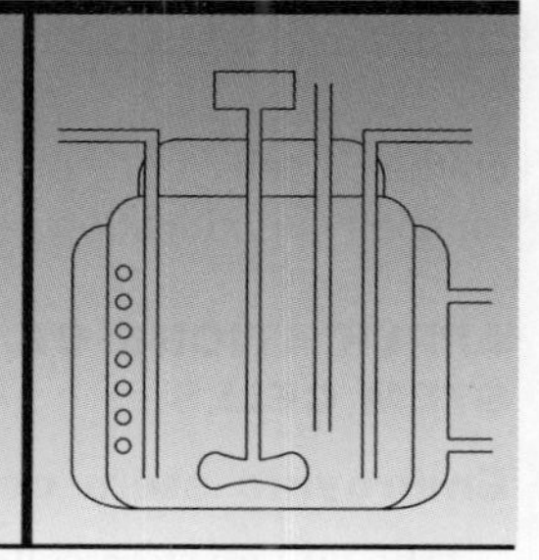

In the laboratories, small scale cultures of cells in flasks (usually 1-5 litre volume) are done for establishing the cell lines. Such cell cultures are useful for studying the morphology, growth, metabolism etc. Large-scale cultures are required for semi-industrial (100–1,000 l capacity) and ***large-scale industrial*** (5,000–20,000 l capacity) ***use of cells for production of wide range of biologically important compounds*** (e.g. enzymes, antibodies, hormones, interferons, plasminogen activator, interleukins).

The terms ***fermenter*** and ***bioreactor*** are in common use while dealing with the ***industrial use of cells***. A fermenter usually refers to the containment system for the cultivation of prokaryotic cells (bacteria, fungi), while a bioreactor grows the eukaryotic cells (mammalian, insect).

Scale-up refers to the process of developing the culture systems in stages from a laboratory to the industry. Scale-up although tedious, labour intensive and expensive, is required for the production of commercially important products.

For a better understanding of scale-up, certain basic and fundamental concepts of cell culture should be clear.

CELL CULTURE — GENERAL CONSIDERATIONS

There are several parameters that need to be considered for appropriate growth, proliferation and maintenance of cells in culture. A good understanding of these parameters, listed below is also necessary for scale-up.

- Cell quantitation.
- Equipment and medium.
- pH and buffer systems.
- Oxygen.
- Growth kinetics.
- Types of culture processes.
- Other practical considerations.

CELL QUANTITATION

The total number of cells in a culture can be measured by counting in a haemocytometer. It is however, not possible to identify the viable and non-viable cells by this method.

Cell viability : The viability of cells can be detected by use of dyes e.g. tryphan blue. The principle is based on the fact that the dye is permeable to dead cells while the viable cells do not take up dye.

Indirect measurements for cell viability : The viability of cells can be measured by their metabolic activity. Some of the most commonly used parameters are listed.

- Glucose utilization.
- Oxygen consumption.
- Pyruvate production.
- Carbon dioxide formation.

In recent years, many laboratories have started measuring the activity of lactate dehydrogenase (LDH) to detect cell viability. Dead cells release LDH and therefore, this enzyme can be used to quantitatively measure the loss of cell viability.

EQUIPMENT AND MEDIUM

The various aspects of equipment and medium used in culture laboratory are described in Chapters 33 and 34.

Culture vessels : The materials made up of ***glass or stainless steel*** are commonly used for cell cultures. Borosilicate glass (e.g. Pyrex) is preferred as it can better withstand autoclaving for suspension cultures, wherein cell attachment to the surface has to be discouraged; the culture vessels are usually treated with silicone (siliconization).

Medium and nutrients : Appropriate selection of the medium is done based on the nutritional requirements, and the purpose for which the cultured cells are required. ***Eagle's basal medium and minimal essential medium are the most commonly used***. The media may be supplemented with serum.

Additional feeding of certain nutrients is often required as they are quickly utilized and get exhausted. These include glucose, glutamine and cystine.

For ***suspension cultures, media lacking calcium and magnesium are used***, since their absence minimizes the surface attachment.

Non-nutrient medium supplements : Certain non-nutrient compounds are often added to the medium for improvement of cell cultures. Sodium carboxymethyl cellulose addition to medium helps to minimize mechanical damage that may occur due to forced aeration or the forces generated by stirred impeller. Polyglycol (trade name Pluronic F-68) in the medium reduces foaming in stirred and aerated cultures.

pH AND BUFFER SYSTEMS

The ***ideal pH*** for animal cell cultures is ***around 7.4***. A pH below 6.8 inhibits cell growth. The factors that can alter pH include the stability of the medium, type of buffer and its buffering capacity, concentration of glucose and headspace.

The commonly used buffer of the *in vitro* culture carbon dioxide-bicarbonate system (2-5% CO_2 with 10–25 mM $NaHCO_3$) is comparable to the blood buffer. The presence of phosphates in the medium improves the buffering capacity. Some laboratories use HEPES instead of bicarbonate for more efficient buffering.

As glucose is utilized by the cells, pyruvic acid and lactic acid are produced which can alter the pH. If fructose and galactose (instead of glucose) are used, the acid formation is less, but the cell growth is reduced.

OXYGEN

Oxygen ***has to be continuously supplied*** to the medium throughout the life of the culture. This has to be done without causing damage to the cells. Oxygen can be supplied to the cultures in one of the following ways.

Surface aeration : In closed system static cultures, the headspace is used for the supply of oxygen. For instance, in a 1 litre flask with 100 ml medium 900 ml of the space containing air has about 0.27 g of O_2. This O_2 is capable of supporting 10^8 cells for about 450 hours.

Sparging : The process of ***bubbling gas through the culture*** is referred to as sparging. This is an efficient means of O_2 supply, but may often damage the cells due to effects of the bubble on the cell membrane surfaces. Use of higher air bubbles minimizes the damaging effect.

Membrane diffusion : Adequate diffusion of oxygen into the culture can be obtained through silicone tubing which is highly permeable to gases. This approach however, is inconvenient, besides the high cost of silicone tubing.

Medium perfusion : The medium is perfused through an ***oxygenation*** chamber before it enters the culture system. This method ensures good O_2 saturation. Medium perfusion is in fact used in glass bead system and microcarrier systems.

GROWTH KINETICS

The standard pattern of growth of cultured cells follows a lag phase, an exponential (log) phase and a stationary phase. For more details, refer Chapter 35 and ***Fig. 35.5***.

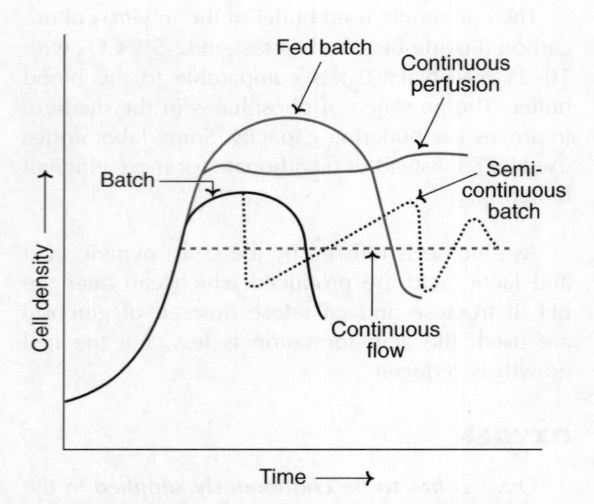

Fig. 37.1 : Comparison of different culture processes.

Growth of cells usually means an increase in cell numbers. However, increase in cell mass may occur without replication.

The following terms are in common use to represent growth of cultured cells.

Specific growth rate : The rate of cell growth per unit amount of biomass.

Doubling time : The time required for a population of cells to double in number or mass.

Degree of multiplication (number of doublings) : The number of times a given inoculum has replicated.

TYPES OF CULTURE PROCESSES

The different culture processes and the growth patterns of cells (represented by cell density) are depicted in ***Fig 37.1***. They are briefly described.

Batch culture

In this technique, when the cells are inoculated into a fixed volume of the medium, they utilize the nutrients and grow, and simultaneously accumulate metabolites. As the nutrients get exhausted, toxic waste products accumulate and the cell multiplication ceases. Further, the cell density drops due to death of the cells.

Batch culture is a standard technique. Several modifications have been made to increase proliferation of cells, besides prolonging their life. The other culture processes described below are the modified batch cultures.

Fed batch culture

There is a gradual addition of fresh medium so that the cell proliferation is much higher than the batch culture. Thus, in the fed batch culture there is an increase in the volume of culture.

Semi-continuous batch culture

A portion of the culture medium is intermittently replaced with an equal volume of fresh medium. The growth pattern of the cells is fluctuating, with a rapid increase in cell density after each replacement of the medium.

Continuous perfusion culture

There is a continuous addition of the medium to the culture and a withdrawal of an equal volume of used cell-free medium. The continuous perfusion process may close or open for circulation of the medium.

Continuous-flow culture

In the continuous-flow culture, a homeostatic condition with no change in the cell numbers, nutrients and metabolites is attained. This is made possible by a balance between the addition of the medium and withdrawal of medium along with cells. This is mostly suitable for suspension cultures.

OTHER PRACTICAL CONSIDERATIONS

Besides the parameters described above, there are several other practical considerations for *in vitro* culture and scale-up. Some important ones are given below.

Culture surface area : The available surface is important for the cells to grow. In general, the culture processes are planned in such a way that the surface area is not a limiting factor.

Inoculation density of cells : As such, there is no set rule for the density of inoculation. However, inoculation with high density is preferred for better growth.

Growth phase of cells : ***Cells in the late exponential (log) phase are most suitable for inoculation***. The cells at the stationary phase should be avoided since they have either prolonged lag phase or no growth at all.

Stirring rate of culture : The stirring rates of different culture lines are developed in the laboratories. It is usually in the range of 100-500 rpm for most of the cultures.

Temperature of the medium : It is advisable to warm the medium to 37°C before adding to the culture.

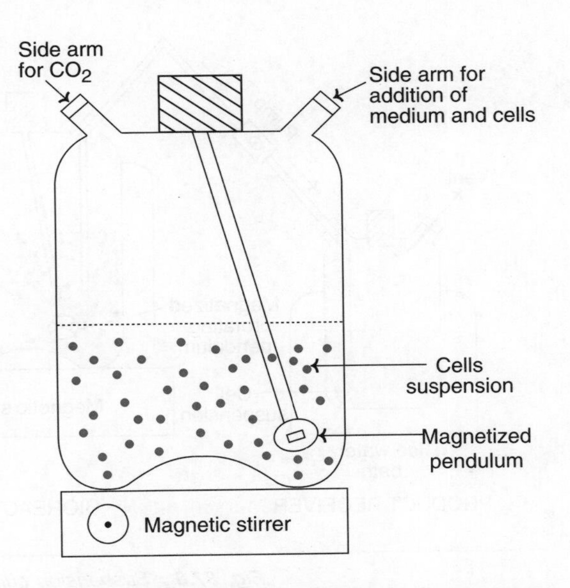

Fig. 37.2 : Diagrammatic representation of a stirrer flask.

SCALE-UP

Scale-up involves the ***development of culture systems in stages from (small scale) laboratory to (large scale) industry***. The methodology adopted to increase the scale of a culture depends on the proliferation of cells and is broadly divided into two categories.

1. Scale-up in suspension.
2. Scale-up in monolayer.

SCALE-UP IN SUSPENSION

Scale-up in suspension is the preferred method as it is simpler. Scale-up of suspension culture primarily involves an increase in the volume of the culture. Small scale generally means the culture capacity less than 2 litres volume (or sometimes 5 litres).

Stirred suspension cultures

It is usually necessary to maintain cell strains in ***stirred suspension cultures, by agitation*** (or stirring) ***of the medium***. The stirring of the culture medium is achieved by a magnet encased in a glass pendulum or by a large surface area paddle. The stirring is usually done at a speed of 30–100 rpm. This is sufficient to prevent sedimentation of cells without creating shear forces that would damage cells.

Static suspension cultures

Some cells can grow in suspension cultures, without stirring or agitation of the medium, and form monolayer cells. However, static suspension cultures are unsuitable for scale-up.

FACTORS IN SCALING-UP

For appropriate scale-up, the physical and chemical requirements of cells have to be satisfied.

Physical parameters

- Configuration of the bioreactor.
- Supply of power.
- Stirring of the medium.

Chemical parameters

- Medium and nutrients.
- Oxygen.
- pH and buffer systems.
- Removal of waste products.

Some of the relevant aspects of the factors in scale-up have already been described under cell culture-general considerations (See p. 450).

The most commonly used ***techniques for stirred suspension cultures*** are briefly described hereunder.

STIRRER CULTURE

A diagrammatic representation of a stirrer flask is shown in ***Fig 37.2.*** The size of the stirrer flask is in the range of 2–10 litres. It is fitted with a magnetized rotating pendulum, and two side arms — one for the addition of cells and medium, and the other for the supply of CO_2.

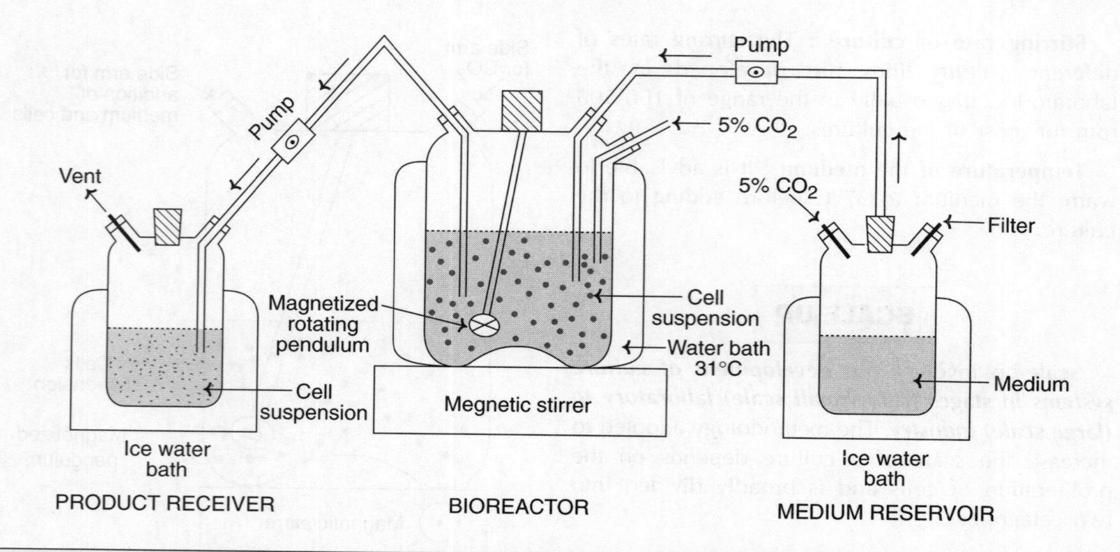

Fig. 37.3 : Suspension culture in a biostat (chemostat).

The stirrer culture vessel is autoclaved (at 15 lb/in^2 for 15 minutes), and is then set up as in ***Fig. 37.2***. The flask is seeded with the culture.

Then medium along with an antifoam agent is added. The flask is connected to CO_2 and stirred at a speed of 60 rpm. The flask is incubated for about 2 hours.

The contents of the small stirrer flask are transferred to a large flask and the entire set up is restarted. Incubation at 37°C is carried out for 4-7 days. The growth of the cells is monitored daily, and the cells are counted. There is a tendency of the cells to enter apoptosis, if the concentration exceeds 1×10^6 cells/ml.

CONTINUOUS FLOW CULTURE

In a continuous flow culture, it is possible to keep the cells at a desired and set concentration, and maintain. This is carried out by a ***biostat or chemostat*** (***Fig 37.3***).

Continuous flow culture consists of growing the cells at the mid-log phase, removal of a measured volume of cells, and replacement by an equal volume of medium. The equipment, specially designed for this purpose has the facility for removal of the cells and addition of medium. The flow rate of the medium addition can be determined from the growth rate of the culture. The medium flow can be regulated by a peristaltic pump. By this technique, it is possible to keep the culture conditions constant rather than to produce large number of cells.

The continuous flow cultures are useful for monitoring metabolic changes in relation to cell density. However, these cultures are more susceptible to contamination.

AIR-LIFT FERMENTER CULTURE

The major limitation of scale-up in suspension culture is inadequate mixing and gas exchange. For small cultures, stirring of the medium is easy, but the problem is with large cultures. The design of fermenter should be such that maximum movement of liquid is achieved with minimum shear to damage the cells.

A diagrammatic representation of an air-lift fermenter is depicted in ***Fig. 37.4***. A 5% CO_2 in air is pumped through the bottom of the fermenter. The bubbles formed move up to agitate and aerate the culture. These bubbles carry a flow of liquid along with them and release at the top which goes to the bottom for recycling.

It is possible to continuously supply O_2 to the culture in this technique. ***Air-lift fermenter culture technique is suitable for fragile animal as well as plant cells***. This fermenter is extensively used in the

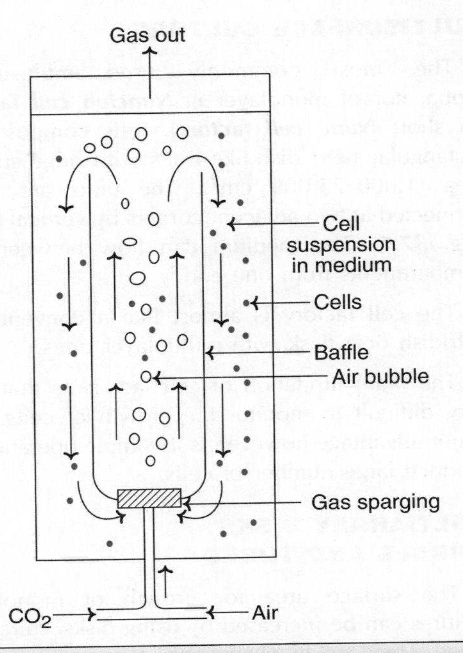

Fig. 37.4 : Diagrammatic representation of airlift fermenter.

biotechnology industry for culture capacities upto 20,000 litres.

NASA bioreactor

NASA (National Aeronautics Space Administration, USA) constructed a bioreactor to grow the cells at zero gravity by slowly rotating the chamber (*Fig. 37.5*). The cells remain stationary and form three-dimensional aggregates and this enhances the product formation. In the NASA bioreactor, there is almost no shear force; hence the cells are not damaged.

As the culture chamber stops its rotations, the cell aggregates sediment and the medium can be replaced.

OTHER SYSTEMS FOR SUSPENSION CULTURE

Rotating chambers : The mixing and aeration of the culture medium can be achieved by 2 or 3 rotating chambers. The chambers are so designed that the cell suspension and mixing are high in one chamber while the product and spent medium remain in the other chamber. These chambers are separated by semipermeable membrane.

Perfused suspension culture : This also has two compartments. The cells are kept in a low-volume compartment at high concentration, while the medium is perfused in adjacent compartment. The product can be collected in a third compartment.

SCALE-UP IN MONOLAYER

The monolayer culture are anchorage-dependent. Therefore, for the scale-up of monolayer cultures, it is necessary to increase the surface area of the substrate in proportion to the number of cells and volume of the medium.

As already stated, suspension cultures are preferred as they are simple. The advantages and disadvantages of monolayer cultures are listed.

Advantages

- Change of medium and washing of cells easy.
- It is easy to perfuse immobilized monolayer cells.

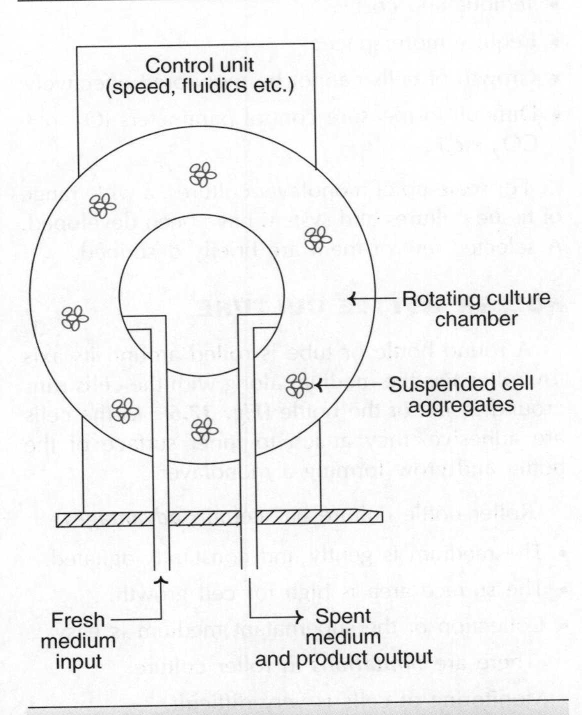

Fig. 37.5 : A bioreactor developed by NASA.

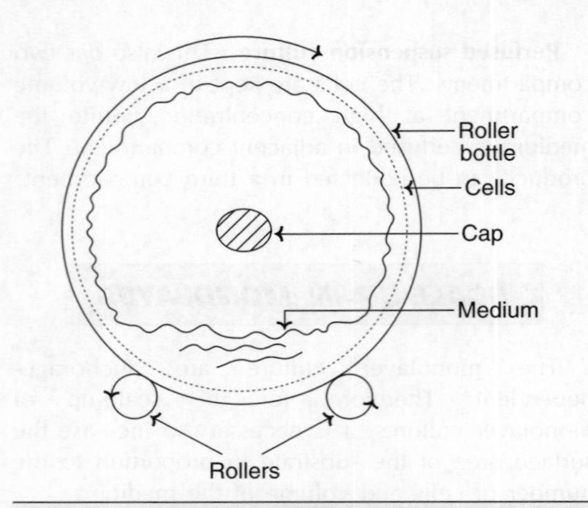

Fig. 37.6 : Roller bottle culture.

- The cell product formation (pharmaceutically important compounds e.g. interferon, antibodies) is much higher.
- The same set up and apparatus can be repeatedly used with different media and cells.

Disadvantages

- Tedious and costly.
- Require more space.
- Growth of cells cannot be monitored effectively.
- Difficult to measure control parameters (O_2, pH, CO_2 etc.)

For scale-up of monolayer cultures, a wide range of tissue cultures and system have been developed. A selected few of them are briefly described.

ROLLER BOTTLE CULTURE

A round bottle or tube is rolled around its axis (by rollers) as the medium along with the cells runs around inside of the bottle (***Fig. 37.6***). As the cells are adhesive, they attach to inner surface of the bottle and grow forming a monolayer.

Roller bottle culture has certain ***advantages***.

- The medium is gently and constantly agitated.
- The surface area is high for cell growth.
- Collection of the supernatant medium is easy.

There are ***limitations*** in roller culture.

- Monitoring of cells is very difficult.
- Investment is rather high.

MULTISURFACE CULTURE

The most commonly used multisurface propagator of monolayer is ***Nunclon cell factory*** (in short ***Nunc cell factory***). It is composed of rectangular petri dish-like units with huge surface area (1,000–25,000 cm^2). The units are inter-connected at two adjacent corners by vertical tubes (***Fig. 37.7***). The medium can flow between the compartments from one end.

The cell factory is almost like a conventional petridish or a flask with multiplayer units.

The main limitation of cell factory is that it is very difficult to monitor the growth of cells. The major advantage however, is its simple operation to produce large number of cells.

MULTIARRAY DISKS, SPIRALS AND TUBES

The surface area for growth of monolayer cultures can be increased by using disks, spirals or tubes. They are however, not in common use as their commercial importance is limited.

MICROCARRIER CULTURE

Monolayers can be ***grown on small spherical carriers or microbeads*** (80–300 μm diameter) referred to as microcarriers. The microcarriers are made up of any one the following materials (trade names given in brackets).

- Plastic (acrobeads, bioplas).
- Glass (bioglass, ventreglas).
- Gelatin (ventregel, cytodex-3).
- Collagen (biospex, biospheres)
- Cellulose (DE-52/53).
- DEAE Dextran (cytodex I, dormacell).

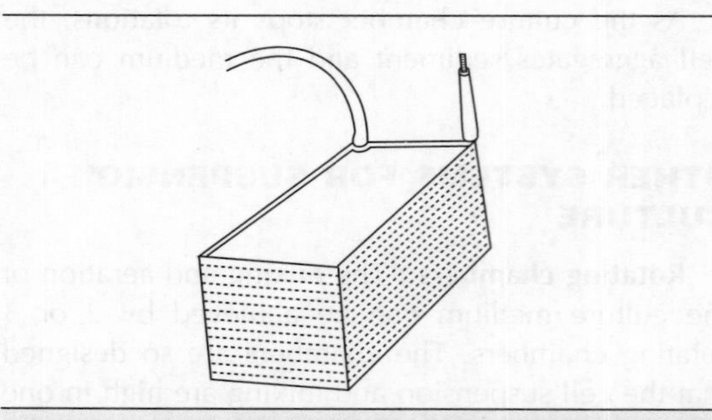

Fig. 37.7 : A diagrammatic representation of Nunc cell factory.

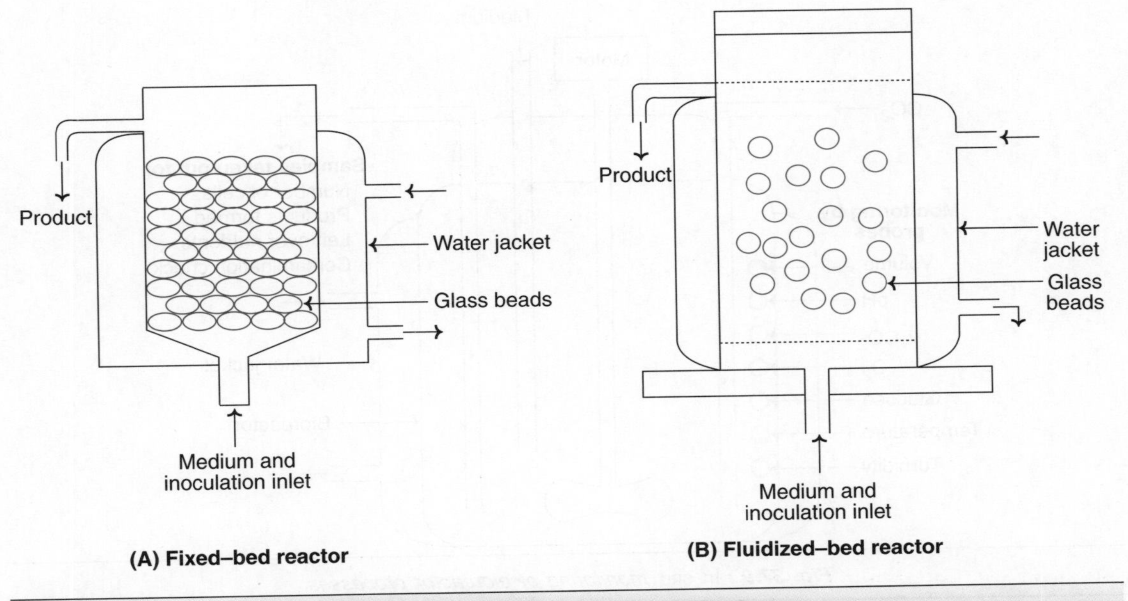

Fig. 37.8 : Fixed and fluidized–bed reactors.

The microbeads ***provide maximum surface area for monolayer cultures***. This actually depends on the size and density of the beads. The cells can grow well on the smooth surface at the solid-liquid interface. However, microcarriers need efficient stirring without grinding the beads. The main advantage with microcarrier culture is that it can be treated as a suspension culture for all practical purposes.

Microcarriers can be cultured in stirrer flask (See ***Fig. 37.2***) or in continuous suspension (See ***Fig. 37.3***). In fact, the suppliers of microcarriers provide the technical literature and other relevant information for setting up a microcarrier culture.

Factors affecting microcarrier culture

- Composition and coating of beads (gelatin and collagen beads are preferred as they can be solubilised by proteases).
- Higher stirring speed is usually required.
- Glass beads are used when the microcarriers need to be recycled.

Analysis of microcarrier culture

The cell counting techniques are difficult to be used for microcarrier cultures. The growth rate can be detected by analyzing DNA or protein.

PERFUSED MONOLAYER CULTURE

The growth surface areas of the monolayer cultures can be ***perfused to facilitate medium replacement and improved product formation and recovery***. The perfusion can be carried out with pumps, oxygenator and other controllers. Perfusion of fixed and fluid-bed reactor is briefly described.

Fixed-bed reactors

The fixed-bed reactor has a bed of glass beads (***Fig. 37.8A***). The medium is perfused upwards through the bed. The cells are grown on the surfaces of the beads. The products can be collected from the top along with the spent medium.

Instead of glass beads, porous ceramic matrix with microchannels can also be used in fixed-bed reactors.

Fluidized-bed reactors

In a fluidized-bed reactor, ***the beads are suspended in a stream of medium*** (***Fig. 37.8B***). These beads are porous in nature, and are made up of ceramics or a mixture of ceramics mixed with natural products such as collagen. They are of low density and float in the medium. The flow rate of the perfused medium is equal to the sedimentation

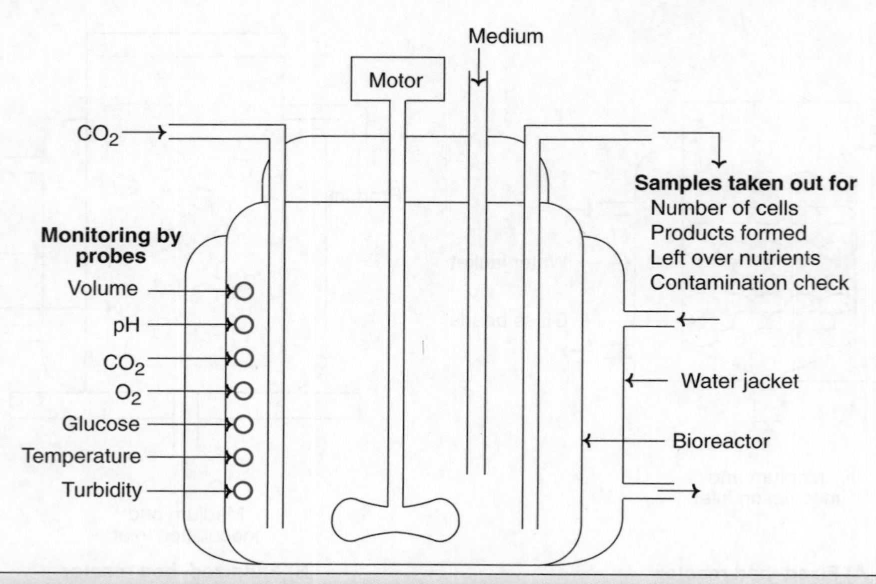

Fig. 37.9 : In situ *monitoring of bioreactor processes.*

rate of the beads. The cells can grow as monolayers on the outer surfaces and inside of the porous beads.

Other perfused monolayer cultures

Membrane perfusion, hollow-fiber perfusion, matrix perfusion and microencapsulation are among the other techniques for perfusion of monolayer cultures.

MONITORING OF CELL GROWTH IN SCALE-UP

Monitoring of the progress of cell growth and the culture systems are very important in scale-up.

MONITORING OF SUSPENSION CULTURES

The progress of suspension cultures can be monitored *in situ* ***by measuring glucose, O_2, CO_2, pH or metabolites produced*** (lactate, ammonia) or specialized products formed (e.g. immunoglobulins by hybridoma cells).

The cell proliferation and rate of biomass formation can also be determined by estimating DNA, protein and ATP.

The different parameters for monitoring of a bioreactor for suspension culture are depicted in ***Fig 37.9***.

MONITORING OF MONOLAYER CULTURES

It is rather difficult to monitor monolayer cell cultures for scale-up. This is due to the fact that in most of the techniques employed for monolayer cultures, the cells cannot be observed directly to monitor the progress of the culture.

In recent years, nuclear magnetic resonance (NMR) technique is used to assay the contents of culture. The characteristic NMR spectra generated by specific metabolites enables the identification and quantitation of metabolites, besides detecting the progress of cell growth.

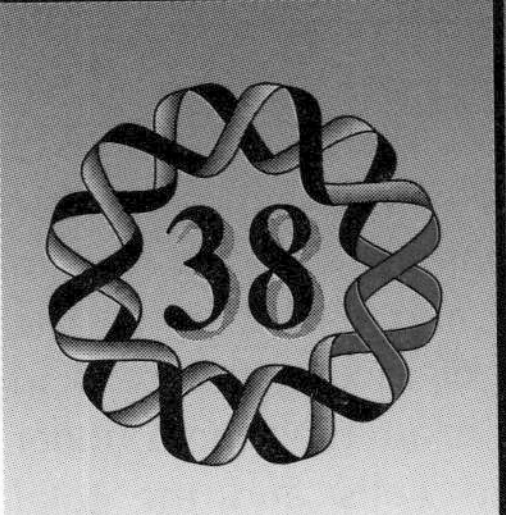

Cell Viability and Cytotoxicity

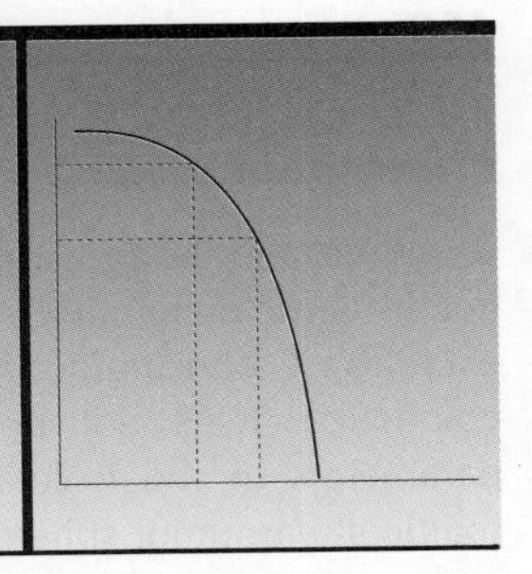

As the cells are removed from the living (*in vivo*) environment and subjected to experimental manipulations in the culture systems (*in vitro*), their viability assumes significance. ***Viability*** of the cells ***represents the capability of their existence, survival and development***.

Many experiments are carried out with cells in the culture rather than using the animal models. This is particularly so with regard to the determination of safety and cytotoxicity of several compounds (pharmaceuticals, cosmotics, anticancer drugs, food additives). *In vitro* testing for cytotoxicity and safety evaluation is in fact cost-effective, besides reducing the use of animals. Studies on ***cytotoxicity*** broadly involve the ***metabolic alterations of the cells, including the death of cells as a result of toxic effects of the compounds***. For instance, in case of anti-cancer drugs, one may look for death of cells, while for cosmetics the metabolic alterations and allergic responses may be more important.

LIMITATION OF *IN VITRO* CYTOTOXICITY STUDIES

Toxicity of a given compound is a complex process as it occurs *in vivo*. This may result in direct damage to cells, alterations in physiological and biochemical functions, inflammatory changes and other systemic effects, not only at the site of application but also at the other sites. Some of the important *in vitro* limitations are briefly described with special reference to systemic responses, metabolism and pharmacokinetics.

Tissue and systemic responses

The cultured cells represent the cells in isolation, and not an integral part of a tissue or an organ. As already stated, the nature of the *in vitro* effect is measured by cell survival or by an altered metabolic effect. On the other hand, the *in vivo* reactions are complicated that may lead to tissue responses (fibrosis, inflammatory reaction) or systemic responses (pyrexia, vascular dilation). Therefore, the *in vitro* cytotoxic responses have to be considered carefully.

In recent years, some attempts are made to create *in vitro* organotypic cultures by assembly of different cell types. Even with this approach, it is not possible to observe all the tissue, and systemic responses.

Metabolism

The whole body metabolism is complex and well integrated. Some of the compounds that are toxic *in vitro* are detoxified by the liver. On the other hand, certain non-toxic or less toxic compounds may be converted to more toxic ones in the liver. For these reasons, it is necessary that the *in vitro* cells are exposed to the same type of compound that is formed in liver after detoxification.

Pharmacokinetics

When the body is exposed to a drug, there occurs tissue penetration, metabolism, clearance and excretion, constituting an organized pharmacokinetics. It is not possible to stimulate these parameters in the isolated cells. However, use of multicellular tumor spheroids has certain advantages with regard to understanding of drug penetration.

ASSAYS FOR CELL VIABILITY AND CYTOTOXICITY

Despite the limitation stated above, there are several assays developed in the laboratory for measuring the cell viability and cytotoxicity. They are broadly categorized into the following types.

- Cytotoxicity and viability assays.
- Survival assays.
- Metabolic assays.
- Transformation assays.
- Inflammation assays.

CYTOTOXICITY AND VIABILITY ASSAYS

A majority of the cytotoxicity and viability assays are based on the measurement of membrane integrity, cellular respiration, radioisotope incorporation, colorimetric assays and luminescence-based tests.

Based on membrane integrity

The most common measurements of cell viability are based on membrane integrity. The damage to membrane may occur due to cell disaggregation, cell separation or freezing and thawing. Membrane integrity can be determined by uptake of dyes to which viable cells are impermeable (e.g. naphthalene black, trypan blue, erythrosin) or release of dyes normally taken up and retained by viable cells (e.g. neutral red, diacetyl fluorescein).

The other assays for membrane integrity are release of labeled chromium (^{51}Cr), enzymes and use of fluorescent probes. Cell viability measurements, based on membrane integrity are immediate that can be detected within a few hours. However, these measurements cannot predict the ultimate survival of cells.

Dye exclusion assay : The principle of this assay is based on the fact that viable cells are impermeable to several dyes such as naphthalene black, trypan blue, eosin Y, nigrosin green and erythrocin B. The technique basically consists of mixing the cells in suspension with the dye and examining them under the microscopy. The stained cells and the total number of cells are counted. The ***percentage of unstained cells represents the viable cells.***

Dye exclusion assay is convenient and suitable to suspension cultures than to monolayers. This is due to the fact that as the dead cells detatch from the monolayers they are lost from the assay.

The major limitation of this assay is that reproductively dead cells do not take up the dye, and will be counted as though they are viable.

Dye uptake assay : The viable cells can take up the dye diacetyl fluorescein and hydrolyse it to fluorescein. The latter is held up by the viable cells, as it is impermeable to membrane. The ***viable cells*** therefore ***emit fluorescin green*** while the dead cells do not. Thus, the viable cells can be identified.

Labeled chromium uptake assay : Labeled chromium (^{51}Cr) binds to the intracellular proteins through basic amino acids. When the cell membrane is damaged, the labeled proteins leak out of the cell, and the degree of leakage is proportional to the amount of damage. Labeled ^{51}Cr uptake method is used in the immunological studies to determine the cytotoxic activity of T-lymphocytes against target cells.

Enzyme release assays : The membrane integrity of cells can also be assessed by estimating the enzymes released. ***Lactate dehydrogenase (LDH)*** has been the most widely used enzyme for this purpose.

Based on cellular respiration

Respiration of the cells measured by oxygen utilization or carbon dioxide production can be used to assess cell viability. This is usually done by using Warburg manometer.

Based on radioisotope incorporation

By using radiolabeled substrates or metabolites, the radiolabel in the products formed can be detected. This method is particularly useful for the cytotoxicity assays of drugs. Some of the important radioisotope incorporation methods are briefly given.

Labeled nucleotides : Incorporation of (^{3}H) thymidine into DNA, and (^{3}H) uridine into RNA are widely used for the measurement of drug toxicity.

Labeled phosphate : The cells are prelabeled with ^{32}P. When the damage occurs to cells, they release labeled phosphate which can be measured. The efficacy of drugs can be evaluated by this approach.

Based on colorimetric assays

The recent developments in the colorimetric assays by using sophisticated microplate readers are fruitfully utilized for quantitation of cells. A good correlation between the cell number and colorimetric assay are observed. Some highlights of this approach are given below.

- ***Protein*** content can be estimated by methylene blue, amido black, sulforhodamine. In the Lowry method for protein estimation, Folin-Ciocalteau reagent is used.
- ***DNA*** can be quantitated by staining with fluorescence dyes e.g. 2-diaminodino-phenylindone.
- ***Lysosomal and Golgi body activity*** by using neutral red.
- ***Enzyme activity*** assays e.g. hexosaminidase, mitochondrial succinate dehydrogenase.

Based on luminescence test

The viability of cells can be measured with good sensitivity by estimating ATP levels by luminescence based test. The principle is based on the following reaction.

$$\text{ATP} + \text{D-Luciferin} + O_2 \xrightarrow{\text{Luciferase}} \text{AMP} + 2\text{Pi} + CO_2 + \textbf{\textit{Light}}$$

A good sensitivity of this test is reported for the cells in the range of 20 to 2×10^7 cells/ml.

Based on apoptosis

Most of the anticancer drugs kill cells by apoptosis which can be measured for the assessment of cytotoxicity. Apoptosis can be detected by the following ways.

- Changes in the morphology.
- Detection of phosphatidyl serine in the membrane by using annexin V conjugated to fluorescein isothiocyanate (FITC) or biotin.
- DNA laddering.

SURVIVAL ASSAYS

The tests described above for measurement of cell viability and cytotoxicity are short-term, and they identify the dead/live cells at the time of assay. Many times, when the cells are subjected to toxicity (i.e. exposed to drugs, irradiated), the effects are not immediate, but may be observed after several hours or sometimes even days. The assays based on the survival of cells (i.e. retention of regenerative capacity or reproductive integrity) are preferred.

Clonogenic assay

In clonogenic assay, the survival of the cells is ***measured by plating efficiency*** (i.e. the percentage of cells seeded at subculture that give rise to colonies). The plating efficiency measures the proliferative capacity for several cell generations. Clonogenic assay broadly consists of the following stages.

1. Treatment of the cells with varying concentrations of experimental agent for about 24 hours.
2. Trypsinization followed by seeding of cells at low density.
3. Incubation of the cells for 1-3 weeks.
4. Staining and counting of the colonies.

A survival curve (semilog plot) representing the survival fraction of the cells against drug concentration is depicted in ***Fig 38.1.*** The ***inhibitory concentration*** (***IC***) refers to the drug concentration required to inhibit the viability of cells. Thus, IC_{50} and IC_{90} represent the concentrations of a compound that respectively inhibit 50% and 90% of colony formation.

As is evident from the graph, the curve has a knee wherein IC_{50} lies, while IC_{90} falls in the linear range. Therefore, the differences will be more significant in the linear range.

The clonogenic assay is influenced by several factors, the important ones are listed.

- Concentration of the toxic agent.
- Duration of exposure.

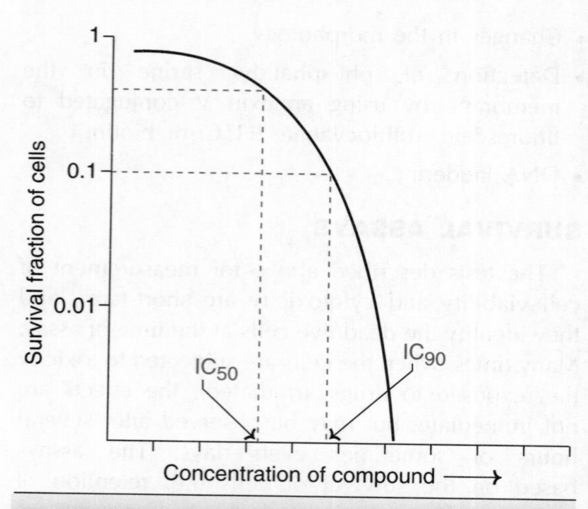

Fig. 38.1 : Survival curve in clonogenic assay.

- Cell density during exposure.
- Cell density during cloning.
- Size of colony.

MTT-based cytotoxicity assay

The tetrazolium salt 3, (4.5-dimethyl-thiazol-2-yl)-2, 5-diphenyl tetrazolium bromide) is commonly known as MTT. It is dye, and is widely used in cytotoxicity assays.

The growing cells in the log phase are exposed to cytotoxic drug. The drug is then removed and the cells are allowed to proliferate for 2-3 population doubling times (PDTs). The number of surviving cells can be detected by MTT dye reduction. The concentration of MTT-formazan formed can be determined spectrophotometrically.

MTT-based cytotoxicity assay is carried out in the following stages.

1. Incubation of monolayer cultures with varying drug concentrations in microtitration plates.

2. Removal of drug and feeding of plates to achieve 2-3 PDTs.

3. Treatment of plates with MTT, and removal of medium and MTT.

4. Measurement of MTT-formazan in an ELISA plate reader.

When the absorbance of test wells/control wells of the microplate is plotted against the concentration of the cytotoxic drug, a sigmoid curve is obtained.

METABOLIC ASSAYS

The metabolic assays are based on the measurements of metabolic responses of the cells. These test are carried out after exposure of the cells to cytotoxic drugs (either immediately or after 2-3 population doublings).

The most commonly used metabolic measurements are DNA, RNA or protein synthesis (by estimating their concentration), besides the assay of certain dehydrogenase enzymes. Some details on the estimation of DNA and protein are already given (See p. 493).

Limitations of metabolic assays : The estimation of the total content of DNA protein may or may not be indicative of increase in cell number. This is because these assays cannot discriminate between the proliferative and metabolic activity of cells. Some workers, therefore prefer to confirm the metabolic measurements by colonogenic survival assay.

TRANSFORMATION ASSAYS

The following are the commonly used assays for measurement of *in vitro* transformation.

- Evidence of mutagenesis.
- Anchorage independence.
- Reduced density limitation of cell proliferation.

Mutagenesis

Mutagenesis can be assayed by ***sister chromatid exchange*** (***SCE***). SCE basically involves the reciprocal exchange of DNA segments between sister chromatids at identical loci in the S-phase of cell cycle. Sister chromatid exchanges are more sensitive to mutagenesis than chromosomal breaks. For this reason, SCEs are preferred in mutagenesis research and transformation assay.

The SCE technique basically involves the incorporation of radioactive nucleotides into replicating DNA and detection of SCEs by fluorescence plus Giemsa (FPG) technique.

INFLAMMATION ASSAYS

Inflammation assays are required for testing the various forms of allergy induced by cosmotics, pharmaceuticals and other xenobiotics. These assays are at the early stages of development in the culture cells.

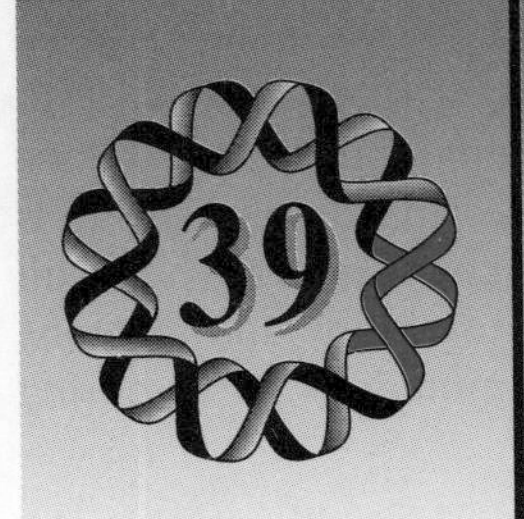

Cell Transformation and Cell Cloning

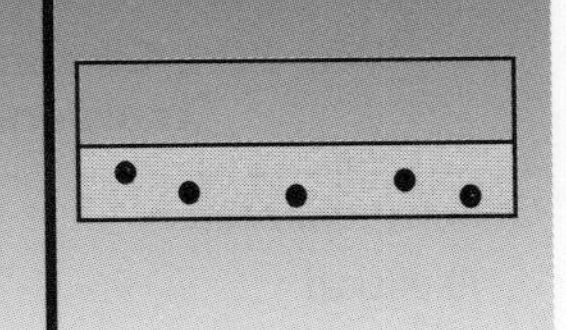

Cell transformation due to changes in the genetic material, and cell cloning involving the production of a population single cell are described in this chapter.

TRANSFORMATION OF CELLS

Transformation broadly refers to the ***change in phenotype of a cell due to a new genetic material***. As regards the cultured cells, transformation involves spontaneous or induced permanent phenotypic alterations as a result of heritable changes in DNA, and consequently gene expression.

Transformation of cells may occur due to any one of the following causes that ultimately result in a changed genetic material.

- Spontaneous
- Infection with transforming virus.
- From gene transfection.
- Exposure to chemical carcinogens.
- Exposure to ionizing radiations.

Characteristics of transformed cells

The general characters of transformed cells are given in ***Table 39.1***. They are grouped as ***genetic***, ***structural***, ***growth*** and ***neoplastic***, and listed.

Transformation is associated with ***genetic instability***, ***immortalization***, ***aberrant growth control*** and ***malignancy***. These aspects are briefly described.

GENETIC INSTABILITY

In general, the cell lines in culture are prone to genetic instability. A majority of normal finite cell lines are usually genetically stable while cell lines from other species (e.g. mouse) are genetically unstable, and can get easily transformed. The continuous cell lines derived from tumors of all species are unstable.

The normally occurring genetic variations in the cultured cells are due to the following causes.

1. High rate of spontaneous mutations in the *in vitro* conditions, possibly due to high rate of cell proliferation.

2. The continued presence of mutant cells in the culture, as they are not normally eliminated.

IMMORTALIZATION

The ***acquisition of an infinite life span by a cell*** is referred to as immortalization.

Most of the normal cells (from different species) have a finite life span of 20-100 generations. But some cells from mouse, most of the tumor cells have infinite life span, as they go on producing continuous cell lines.

Control of finite life span of cells

The finite life span of cultured cells is regulated by about 10 ***senescence genes***. These dominantly

Table 39.1 General characteristics of transformed cells

Genetic characters
Aneuploid
Heteroploid
High spontaneous mutation rate
Overexpressed oncogenes
Mutated or deleted suppressor genes
Structural characters
Altered cytoskeleton
Changed extracellular matrix
Modified expression of cell adhesion molecules
Disrupted cell polarity
Growth characters
Immortalized cells
Loss of contact inhibition
Anchorage independent
Density limitation of growth reduced
Growth factor independent
Low serum requirement
Shorter population doubling time
Neoplastic characters
Tumorigenic
Invasive
Increased protease secretion

acting genes synthesize products which inhibit the cell cycle progression.

It is strongly believed that immortalization occurs due to inactivation of some of the cell cycle regulatory genes e.g. Rb, p^{53} genes.

Immortalization of cells by viral genes

Several viral genes can be used to immortalize cells. Some of these genes are listed below.

SV40LT
HPV16E6/E7
hTRT
Ad5E1a
EBV.

Among the above viral genes, ***SV4OLT is most commonly used to induce immortalization***. The product of this gene (T antigen) binds to senescence genes such as Rb and p^{53}. This binding restricts surveillance activity of senescence genes. The result is an increased genomic instability and activity, leading to further mutations favouring immortalization.

For the process of immortalization, the cells are infected with retroviruses containing immortalizing gene before they enter senescence. By this way, the life span of the cells can be extended by 20-30 population doublings. Thereafter, the cells cease to proliferate, and enter a ***crisis phase*** that may last for several months. At the end of the crisis phase, a small portion of cells can grow, and eventually become immortalized.

Immortalization of human fibroblasts : The human fibroblasts are most successfully immortalized by the viral gene namely SV40LT. The process of fibroblast immortalization is complex and indirect with a very low probability i.e. about 1 in 10^7 cells.

Immortalization of cells by telomerase-induction

The most important cause of finite life span of cells (i.e. senescence) is due to telomeric shortening, followed by cell death (apoptosis).

If the cells are transfected with telomerase gene ***htrt***, the life span of the cells can be extended. And a small proportion of these cells become immortal.

ABERRANT GROWTH CONTROL

The transformed cells and the cells from tumors, grown in culture show many aberrations with respect to growth and its control. The growth characteristics of these cell are listed in ***Table 39.1***, and some of them briefly described hereunder.

Anchorage independence

There occur several changes on the cell surfaces of transformed cells. These include alterations in the cell surface glycoproteins and integrins, and loss of fibronectin. Some of the transformed cells ***may*** totally ***lack cell adhesion molecules (CAMs)***.

The modifications on the surface of transformed cells leads to a decrease in cell — cell, and cell-substrate adhesion. The net result is that there is a reduced requirement for attachment and spreading of the cells to proliferate. This phenomenon is referred to as anchorage independence.

Anchorage independent cells grow in a disorganized fashion. These cells may be comparable with the tumor cells detached from the native tissue which can grow in foreign tissues i.e. formation of metastases.

Contact inhibition

The ***transformed cells*** are characterized by ***loss of contact inhibition***. This can be observed by the morphological changes in the disoriented and disorganized monolayer cells. This results in a reduced density limitation of growth, consequently leading to higher saturation density compared to normal cells (Refer Chapter 35 and ***Fig. 35.6***).

Low serum requirement

In general, transformed cells or tumor cells have lower serum dependence than the normal cells. This is mostly due to the secrection of autocrine growth factors by the transformed cells (**Note :** The normal cells in culture are dependent on the serum for the supply of growth factors). Some of the growth factors produced by tumor cells are given.

- Colony stimulating factor (CSF).
- Transforming growth factor (TGFa).
- Interleukins 1,2 and 3.
- Vasoactive intestinal peptide (VIP).
- Gastrin releasing peptide.

It may be noted that many normal cells (fibroblasts, endothelial cells) also produce autocrine factors during active stage of cell proliferating. Hence, these factors will not be of much use to serve as markers of cell transformation.

TUMORIGENICITY

Cell transformation is a complex process that often results in the formation of neoplastic cells. The cell lines obtained from malignant tumors are already transformed. Such cells may undergo further transformation in the *in vitro* culture due to

- Increased growth rate.
- Immortalization.
- Reduced anchorage dependence.

For the malignant transformation of cells, several steps may be required. The following two approaches are in use to understand malignant-associated properties of cultured cells.

1. The cells can be cultured from malignant tumors and characterized.

2. Viral genes or chemical carcinogens can be used to transform the untransformed cells.

CELL CLONING

In the traditional culture techniques, the cells are heterogenous in nature. Isolation of pure cell strains is often required for various purposes. ***Cell cloning broadly involves*** the processes connected with the ***production of a population of cells derived from a single cell***. Cloning of continuous cell lines is much easier compared to that of the primary cultures, and finite cell lines.

There are certain limitations for cloning of culture cells derived from normal tissues. These cells survive for a limited number of generations, and therefore cloning may not result in any significant number of cells. On the other hand, cloning of continuous cell lines due to their transformed status is much easier. Thus, the transformed cells have higher cloning efficiency compared to normal cells.

Cloning may be carried out by two approaches-monolayer and suspension cultures.

1. **Monolayer culture :** Petri dishes, multiwell plates or flasks can be used for cloning by monolayer culture. It is relatively easy to remove the individual colonies of cells from the surfaces where they are attached.

2. **Suspension culture :** Cloning can be carried out in suspension by seeding cells into viscous solutions (Methocel) or gels (agar). As the daughter cells are formed in suspension, they remain intact and form colonies in suspension.

DILUTION CLONING

Dilution cloning is the most commonly used technique for cloning of monolayer cells, and involves the following stages (***Fig 39.1***).

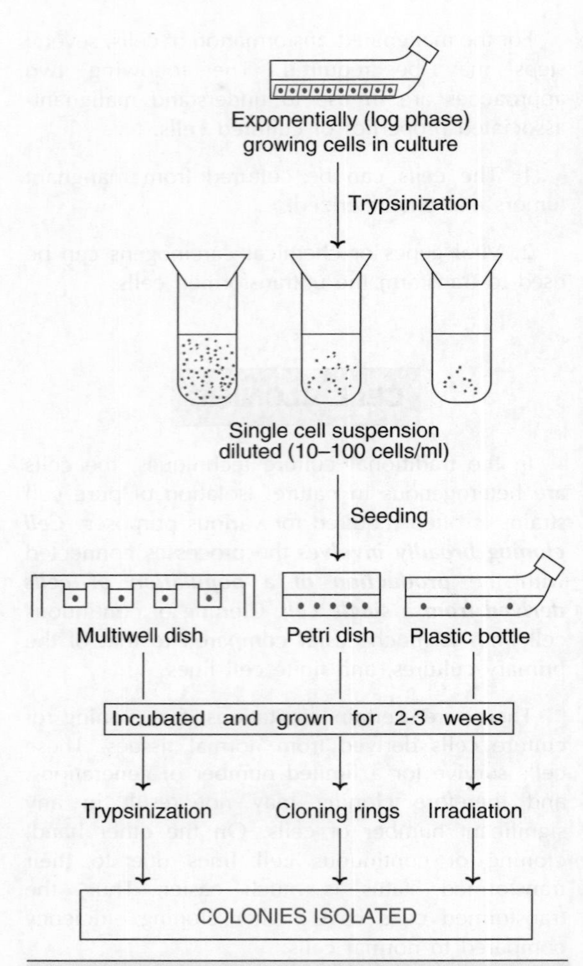

Fig. 39.1 : Dilution cell cloning technique for monolayer cultures.

1. Trypsinization of cells (at log phase) to produce single cell suspensions.

2. Dilution of the cells to about 10-100 cells/ ml.

3. Seed the cells in multiwell dishes, petri dishes or plastic bottles.

4. Incubate under appropriate conditions for 1-3 weeks.

5. Isolate individual colonies.

The clones can be isolated directly from the multiwell dishes (by trypsinization), by cloning ring technique from petridishes, and by irradiating the plastic bottle.

STIMULATION OF PLATING EFFICIENCY

Plating efficiency represents the ***percentage of cells seeded at subculture that gives rise to colonies.*** The plating efficiency and ***cloning efficiency*** are said to be identical, if each colony is derived from a single cell.

The plating efficiency is around 10% for continuous cell lines, while for primary cultures and finite cell lines, it is quite low — 0.5 to 5% or sometimes even zero. Several attempts are made to improve the plating efficiency in the culture laboratories. These approaches are based on the assumption that the cells at low densities require more nutrients and/or growth factors.

The stimulation of plating efficiency with regard to ***culture factors***, ***conditioned medium*** and feeder layers is briefly described

Culture factors

Medium : A medium rich in various nutrients is better suited for improving the plating efficiency.

Serum : Fetal bovine serum is better than horse or calf serum, if the addition of serum is required.

Addition of metabolites : Supplementing the medium with intermediary metabolites (e.g. pyruvate, α-ketoglutarate) and nucleosides stimulates plating efficiency.

Addition of hormones : Dexamethasone, a synthetic analogue of hydrocortisone, improves plating efficiency e.g. fibroblasts, melanoma cells, chick myoblasts. Insulin also stimulates plating efficiency of several cell types.

Carbon dioxide : CO_2 significantly influences plating efficiency. Most of the cells require 5% CO_2 while for some cells, a lower CO_2 concentration (around 2% CO_2) is better e.g. human fibroblasts. HEPES is used to protect the medium from pH fluctuations.

Pretreatment of substrate : The plates pretreated with fibronectin or polylysine show an improved plating efficiency.

Use of purified trypsin : Some workers prefer to use purified trypsin instead of crude trypsin for trypsinization so that the plating efficiency is better.

Conditioned medium

A medium that has already been used for the growth of other cells contains certain metabolites, growth factors and other products that stimulate growth. Such a medium, referred to as conditioned medium, when added to cell cloning medium ***improves plating efficiency***.

Feeder layers

A layer growth-arrested living cells, referred to as feeder layer, promotes plating efficiency. This is because the feeder cells provide nutrients, growth factors and matrix constituents that support survival, growth and proliferation of cells.

SUSPENSION CLONING

Certain cells, particularly the transformed fibroblasts and hematopoietic stem cells, can be more conveniently cloned in suspension rather than monolayers.

Suspension cloning can be carried out by using agar or Methocel, which can hold the cells of a given colony together, and prevent mixing of colonies.

The technique of cloning in agar suspension, is carried out in the following stages (***Fig 39.2***).

1. Cells from suspension culture or monolayers can be used. The monolayer cells have to trypsinized while the suspension cells can be directly used.

2. Count the cells and dilute serially so that 10-200 cells/ml are finally present.

3. Freshly prepared agar medium with appropriate dilution is used.

4. The agar medium is inoculated with the diluted cells.

5. Incubation for 1-3 weeks given clones in culture.

ISOLATION OF CLONES

After the cloning is complete, selection and isolation of specific cell strains is the next important step. This is essentially required for the propagation of cells.

If the monolayer cells are cloned directly in the multiwell plates, the colonies can be isolated by trypsinization of the individual wells. However, when the cloning is carried out in petri dishes, the colonies can be separated from the medium by placing stainless steel or ceramic rings around the colonies.

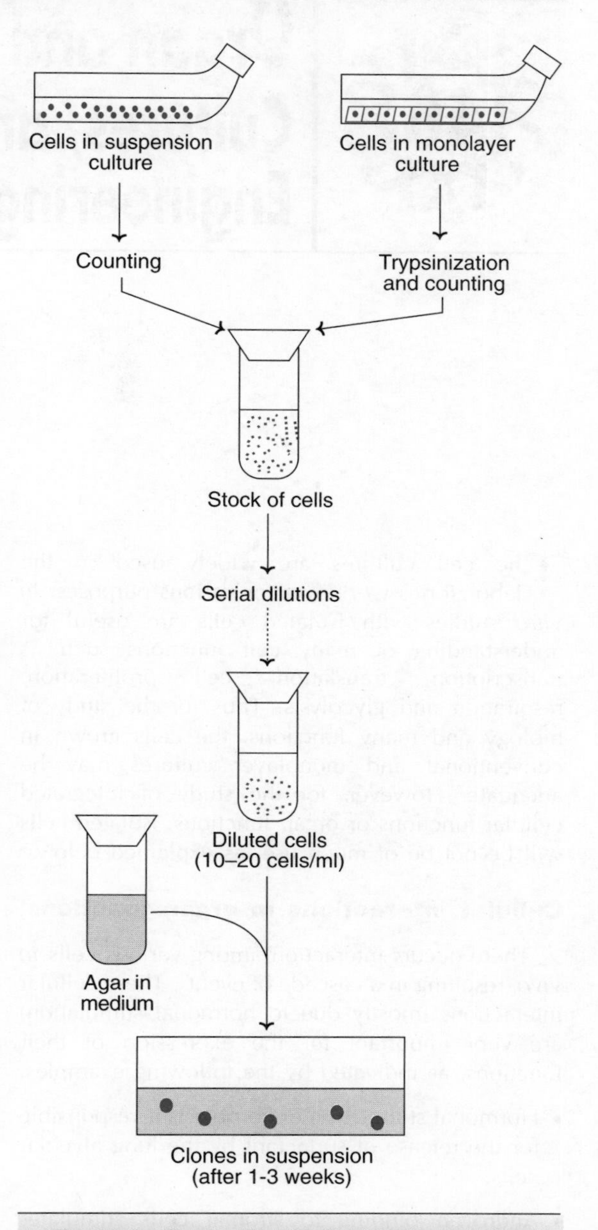

Fig. 39.2 : Suspension cloning technique in agar.

Micromanipulation

The genuineness of a colony, that is the colony is derived from a single cell can be done by micromanipulation. This can be achieved by ***monitoring the colony formation at the early stages of cell cloning***. Micromanipulation, if properly done, is believed to be the conclusive method for determining the genuine clonality of a clone.

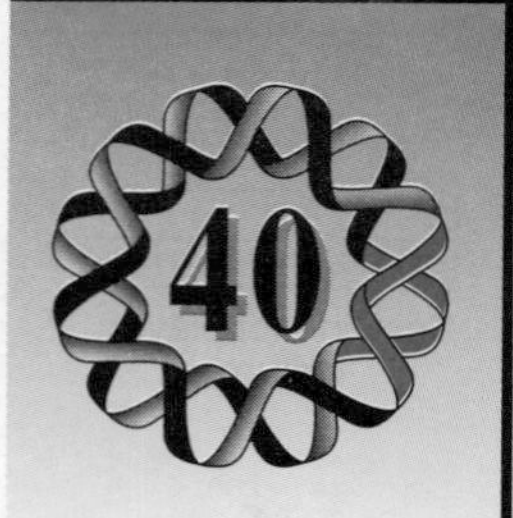

Organ and Histotypic Cultures, and Tissue Engineering

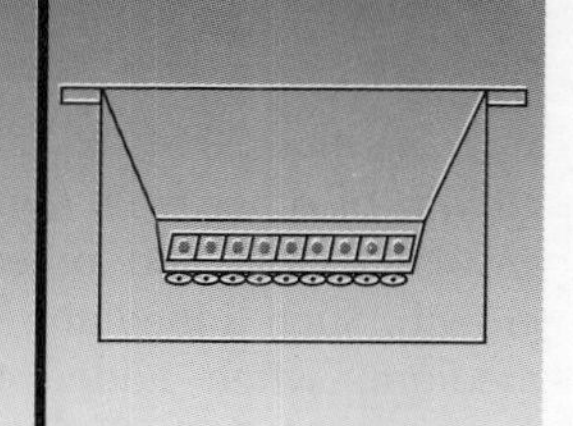

The cell cultures are widely used in the laboratories worldover for various purposes. *In vitro* studies with isolated cells are useful for understanding of many cell functions such as transcription, translation, cell proliferation, respiration and glycolysis. Thus for the study of biology and many functions, the cells grown in conventional and monolayer cultures may be adequate. However, for the study of integrated cellular functions or organ functions, isolated cells will be not be of much use, as explained below.

Cellular interactions in organ functions

There occurs interaction among various cells *in vivo*, resulting in a cascade of events. These cellular interactions (mostly due to hormonal stimulation) are very important for the expression of their functions, as indicated by the following examples.

- Hormonal stimulation of fibroblasts is responsible for the release of surfactant by the lung alveolar cells.
- Androgen binding to stromal cells stimulates prostate epithelium.

Besides hormones, nutritional factors and xenobiotics also exert stimulatory effects on the cells to function in a coordinated fashion.

ORGANOTYPIC MODELS

As explained above, the cellular interactions that occur in the *in vivo* system are not possible with isolated cells. The ***recent developments in the organ and histotypic cultures focus to create in vitro models comparable*** (as far as possible in biology and functions) ***to the in vivo systems***. The purpose of this organotypic models is to retain the original structural and functional interactive relationships of the organ. There are three broad approaches in this direction.

1. **Organ cultures :** The whole organs or small fragments of the organs that retain the special and intrinsic properties are used in culture.

2. **Histotypic cultures :** The cell lines grown in three dimensional matrix to high density represent histotypic cultures.

3. **Organotypic cultures :** In this case, the cells from different lineages are put together in the desired ratio and spatial relationships to create a component of an organ in the laboratory.

ORGAN CULTURES

The use of organ cultures (organs or their representative fragments) with reference to structural integrity, nutrient and gas exchange, growth and differentiation, along with the advantages and limitations is briefly described.

Structural integrity

As already stated, the isolated cells are individual, while in the organ culture, the cells are integrated as a single unit. The cell to cell association, and interactions found in the native tissues or organs are retained to a large extent.

As the structural integrity of the original tissue is preserved, the associated cells can exchange signals through cell adhesion or communications.

Nutrient and gas exchange

There is ***no vascular system*** in the organ culture. This ***limits the nutrient supply and gas exchanges*** of the cells. This happens despite the adequate care taken in the laboratory for the rapid diffusion of nutrients and gases by placing the organ cultures at the interface between the liquid and gaseous phases. As a consequence, some degree of necrosis at the central part of the organ may occur.

Some workers prefer to use high O_2 concentration (sometimes even pure O_2) in the organ cultures. Exposure of cells to high O_2 content is associated with the risk of O_2 induced toxicity e.g. nutrient metabolite exchange is severely affected.

Growth and differentiation

In general, the organ cultures do not grow except some amount of proliferation that may occur on the outer cell layers.

Advantages of organ cultures

- Provide a direct means of studying the behaviour of an integrated tissue in the laboratory.
- Understanding of biochemical and molecular functions of an organ/tissue becomes easy.

Limitations of organ cultures

- Organ cultures cannot be propagated, hence for each experiment there is a need for a fresh organ from a donor.
- Variations are high and reproducibility is low.
- Difficult to prepare, besides being expensive.

TECHNIQUES OF ORGAN CULTURE

The most important requirement of organ or tissue culture is to place them at such a location so that optimal nutrient and gas exchanges occur. This is mostly achieved by keeping the tissue at gas-limited interface of the following supports.

- Semisolid gel of agar.
- Clotted plasma.
- Microporous filter.
- Lens paper.
- Strip of Perspex or Plexiglas.

In recent years, ***filter-well inserts*** are in use to attain the natural geometry of tissues more easily.

Procedure for organ culture

The basic technique of organ culture consists of the following stages.

1. Dissection and collection of the organ tissue.
2. Reduce the size of the tissue as desired, preferably to less than I mm in thickness.
3. Place tissue on a support (listed above) at the gas medium interface.
4. Incubate in a humid CO_2 incubator.
5. Change the medium (M199 or CMRL 1066) as frequently as desired.
6. The organ culture can be analysed by histology, autoradiography and immunochemistry.

Organ culture on stainless steel support grid

Small fragments of tissue can be cultured on a filter laid on top of a stainless steel grid (***Fig. 40.1***).

Organ culture on filter-well inserts

Filter-well inserts have become very popular for organ cultures. This is mainly because the cellular interaction, stratification and polarization are better in these culture systems. Further, the recombination of cells to form tissue — like densities, and access to medium and gas exchange are better.

The four different types of filter wells for growing tissues in the form of cell layers are depicted in ***Fig. 40.2***.

- Growth of cell layer on top of filter (***Fig. 40.2A***).
- Growth of cell layers on matrix (collagen or matrigel) on top of filter (***Fig. 40.2B***).
- Cell layers grown on the interactive cell layers placed on the underside of filter (***Fig. 40.2C***).

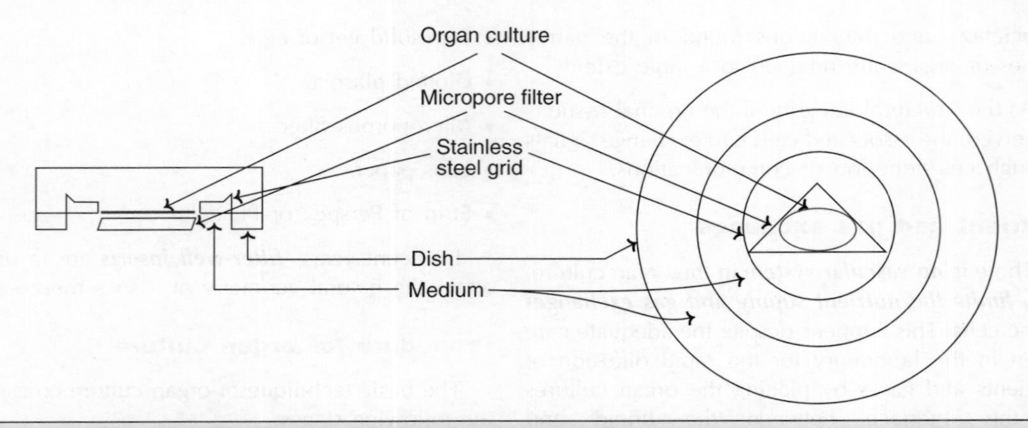

Fig. 40.1 : Organ culture on stainless steel support grid.

- Cell layer grown on the matrix with interactive cell layer on the underside of the filter (*Fig. 40.2D*).

Filter well-inserts with different materials (ceramic, collagen, nitrocellulose) are now commercially available for use in culture laboratories.

Filter-well inserts have been successfully used to develop functionally integrated thyroid epithelium, stratified epidermis, intestinal epithelium and renal (kidney) epithelium.

HISTOTYPIC CULTURES

Growth and propagation of cell lines in ***three-dimensional matrix to high cell density*** represent histotypic cultures. The advantage with this culture system is that dispersed monolayer cultures can be used to regenerate tissue-like structures.

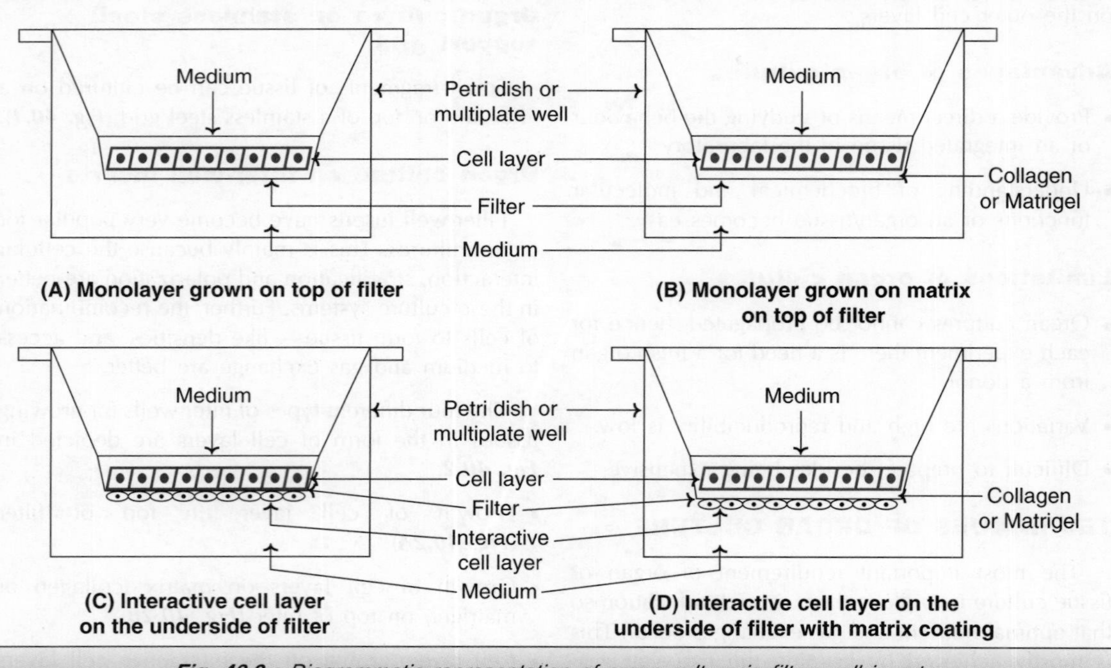

Fig. 40.2 : Diagrammatic representation of organ culture in filter–well inserts.

The commonly used techniques in histotypic cultures use gel and sponge hollow fibers and spheroids.

Gel and sponge technique

The cells (normal or tumor) in culture can penetrate gels (collagen) or sponges (gelatin) which provides a matrix for morphogenesis of primitive cells. This approach has been used for the development of mammary epithelium, and some tubular and glandular structures.

Hollow fibers technique

In recent years, perfusion chambers with a bed of plastic capillary fibers have been developed. The advantage of using hollow fibers in histotypic cultures is that nutrient and gas exchange is more efficient. As the cells attached to capillary fibers grow, there occurs an increase in cell density to form tissue-like structures. Many workers claim that the behaviour of high-density cells formed on hollow fibers is comparable to their *in vivo* behaviour. For instance, choriocarcinoma cells grown in hollow fiber cultures release more chorionic gonadotrophin than in a conventional monolayer.

Hollow fiber culture techniques are regarded as ideal systems for the industrial production of several biologically important compounds. Work is progressing in this direction.

THREE DIMENSIONAL CULTURES

Spheroids in histotypic culture

Spheroids represent the ***clusters of cells usually formed by the reassociation of dissociated cultured cells***. It is known for some years that the dissociated embryonic cells reassemble to form a specialized structure.

The basic principle of using spheroids in histotypic culture is that the cells in heterotypic or homotypic aggregates are capable of sorting out themselves into groups to form tissue-like architecture.

The major drawback of spheroids is the limitation in the diffusion and exchange of nutrients and gases.

Multicellular tumor spheroids (MCTS)

Multicellular tumor spheroids provide an *in vitro* proliferating model for studies on tumor cells. The three dimensional structure of MCTS allows the experimental studies related to drug therapy, penetration of drugs, resistance to radiation etc. Further, MCTS have also been used to study several biological processes.

- Regulation of cell proliferation and differentiation.
- Immune responses.
- Cell death.
- Cell invasion.
- Gene therapy.

The main advantage of three dimensional cell culture (in the form of MCTS) is that they ***provide a well-defined geometry of cells planar or spherical*** which is directly related to the structure and function. It is now well accepted that the MCTS behave like the initial avascular stages of solid tumors *in vivo*. However, beyond a critical size (≥ 500 mm), most of the MCTS develop necrosis (death of cells) at the centre surrounded by viable cells. A diagrammatic representation of MCTS in comparison with tumor is depicted in ***Fig. 40.3***.

Technique of MCTS production

Single-cell suspension obtained from trypsinized monolayer cells or disaggregated tumor is inoculated into the medium in magnetic stirrer flasks or roller tubes. As the incubation is carried out for about 3-5 days, aggregates of cells representing spheroids are formed. It is observed that spheroid formation is more efficient under static conditions on stationary and non-adhesive surfaces. For this reason, agar/agarose-coated culture dishes to which cells do not adhere are frequently used to initiate spheroid formation.

Once the spheroids are formed, they are transferred to 24 well plates for analysis. Spheroid growth is quantified by measuring their diameters regularly. This can be done by using a microscope eyepiece micrometer or an image analysis scanner. Good growth of spheroids is observed when grown in wells.

Transfectant mosaic spheroids : It is now possible to produce spheroids from cells that have been transfected with different genes. Mosaic spheroids are formed by mixing transfected and non-transfected spheroids in the desired proportion.

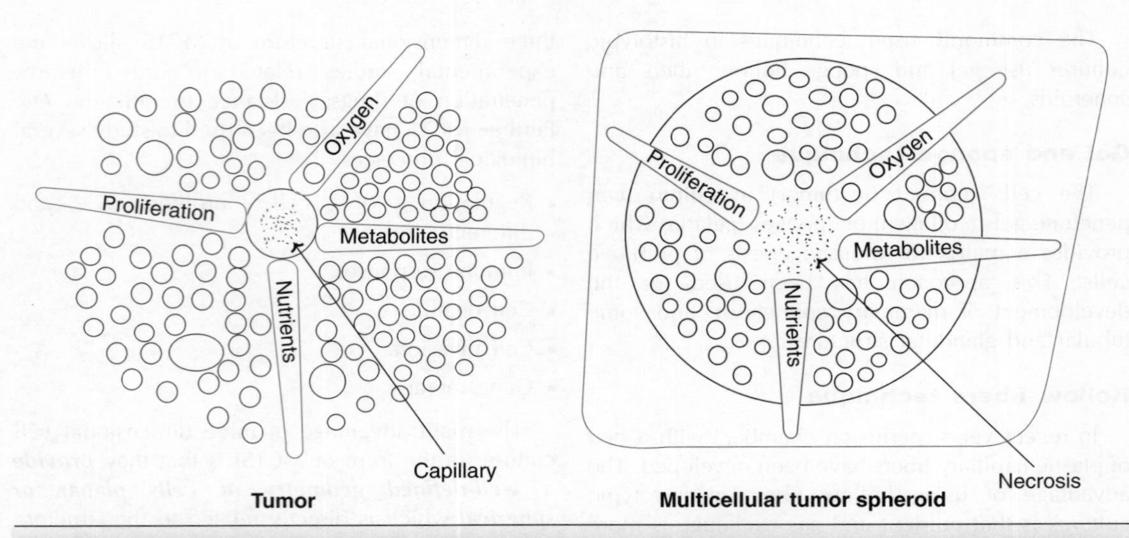

Fig. 40.3 : A diagrammatic representation of a tumor in comparison with a multicellular tumor spheroid.

MCTS co-cultures : MCTS can be produced from heterogenous cells also, forming MCTS co-cultures. This is comparable to heterologous spheroids (in short heterospheroids) consisting of tumor cells in combination with host cells. Some of the MCTS co-cultures are listed.

- MCTS and immune cells.
- MCTS and fibroblasts.
- MCTS and endothelial cells.

Heterospheroids with heterotypic cell interaction serve as good models for studying several *in vivo* processes e.g. inflammation. MCTS co-cultures are very useful in tissue modelling and tissue engineering, the details of which are given later.

Applications of spheroids or MCTS

Spheroids have a wide range of applications. Some of the important ones are listed.

- Serve ***as models for a vascular tumor growth***.
- For the ***study of gene expression*** in a three dimensional configuration of cells.
- To determine the effect cytotoxic drugs, antibodies, radionucleotides used for therapeutic purposes.
- ***To study certain disease processes*** e.g. rheumatoid arthritis.
- For the development of ***gene therapies*** for several diseases e.g. cancer.
- To evaluate radiation effects on target tissues.
- For the development of tissues and tissue models.

ORGANOTYPIC CULTURES

Organotypic culture basically involves the combination of cells from different lineages in a determined ratio to create a component of an organ. With the advances in the organotypic culture techniques, it is now possible to develop certain tissues or tissue models.

- Skin equivalents have been created by co-culturing dermis with epidermis with interviewing layers of collagen.
- Models for prostate and breast.
- Models for control of growth and differentiation of lung.

TISSUE ENGINEERING

Tissue engineering (TE) refers to the ***application of the principles of engineering to cell culture for the construction of functional anatomical units*** (tissues/organs**)**. The ultimate purpose of TE is to supply various body parts for the repair or replacement of damaged tissues or organs. Tissue engineering may be regarded as the ***backbone of reconstructive surgery***. It is possible to supply almost all surgical implants (skin, blood vessels, ligaments, heart valves, joint surfaces, nerves) through the developments in tissue engineering.

There are two schools of thought while dealing with tissue engineering techniques.

1. Some workers believe that the ***living cells possess an innate potential of biological regeneration***. This implies that when suitable cells are allowed to grow on an appropriate support matrix, the cells proliferate, and ultimately result in an organized and functional tissue. This tissue resembles the original tissue in structure and function. This approach is very simple, and economical, although the success is limited.

2. According the second school of thought, there are several control processes to produce a new and functional tissue. Thus, tissue regeneration *in vivo* or tissue production *in vitro* are very complex. Therefore, tissue engineering is not a simple regeneration of cells, and it requires a comprehensive approach with a thorough understanding of cellular configuration, spacial arrangement and control process.

Tissue engineering is a complicated process. Some fundamental and basic aspects of TE with special reference to the following aspects are briefly described.

- Cell sources and culture
- Cell orientation
- Cell support materials
- Design and engineering of tissues.

CELL SOURCES AND CULTURE

Adequate quantities of cells are required for tissue engineering. There are three types of cell sources-autologous, allogeneic and xenogeneic.

Autologous cell sources

The cell source is said to be autologous when the ***patient's own cells are used in TE***. This is a straight forward approach. A piece of desired tissue is taken by biopsy. It may be enzymatically digested or explant cultured, and the cells are grown to the required number.

The main ***advantages*** of autologous cells in TE are :

- Avoidance of immune complications
- Reduction in the possible transfer of inherent infections.

There are certain ***disadvantages*** associated with autologous cells.

- It is not always possible to obtain sufficient biopsy material from the patient.
- Disease state and age of the patient will be limiting factors.

Allogeneic cell sources

If the ***cells*** are ***taken from a person other than the patient***, the source is said to be allogeneic. The ***advantages*** of allogeneic cell source are listed.

- Obtained in good quantity from a healthy donor.
- Cells can be cultured in a large scale.
- Cost-effective with consistent quality.
- Available as and when required by a patient.

The major ***problem*** of allogeneic cell source is the ***immunological complications*** that may ultimately lead to graft rejection. The immune responses however, are variable depending on the type of cells used. For instance, endothelial cells are more immunogenic while fibroblasts and smooth muscle cells are less immunogenic. The age of the donor is another important factor that contributes to immunological complications. Thus, cells from adult donors are highly immunogenic while fetal or neonatal cells elicit little or no immune response.

Xenogeneic cell sources

When the ***cells are taken from different species*** (e.g. pig source for humans) the source is said to be xenogeneic. This approach is not in common use due to immulogical complications.

CULTURE OF CELLS

The methods adapted for culturing of cells required for tissue engineering depend on the type and functions of cells. For most of the cells, the conventional monolayer cultures serve the purpose. The major drawback of monolayer cultures is that cells may lose their morphology, functions and proliferative capacity after several generations.

Some workers prefer three dimensional cultures for the cells to be used in tissue engineering. For details on these techniques, See p. 471. The nutrient and gaseous exchanges are the limiting factors in three dimensional cultures.

Genetic alterations of cultured cells for use in TE

Gene therapy can be successfully employed in tissue engineering. This can be achieved by transferring the desired genes to cells in culture. The new genes may increase the production of an existing protein or may synthesize a new protein. Some success has been achieved in this direction.

- Genetically altered fibroblasts can produce transferrin, clotting factor VIII and clotting factor IX.
- Modified endothelial cells can synthesize tissue plasminogen activator.
- Genetically engineered keratinocytes can produce transglutaminase-I (This enzyme is lacking in patients suffering from a dermal disorder, lamellar icthyosis). The altered keratinocytes proved successful when transplanted in animal (rat) models of this disease.

CELL ORIENTATION

The orientation of cells with regard to specific shape and spatial arrangement is influenced by the following environmental factors.

1. Substrate or contact guidance.
2. Chemical gradients.
3. Mechanical cues.

Substrate guidance

The topographical features of the substrate determine the contact guidance. These features may be in the form of ridges, aligned fibers etc. It is possible to use differential attachment to substrates as a means of producing different alignment of cells. In recent years, synthetic polymer substrate collagen fibrils and fibronectin are used as bioresorbable templates for tissue engineering.

Chemical gradients

Development of chemical gradients is required for cellular orientation and ***for the stimulation of cellular functions***. Certain growth factors and extracellular macromolecules are capable of creating chemical gradients e.g. vascular endothelial growth factor (VEGF), oligosaccharide fragments of hyaluronan, fibronectin, collagen.

There are certain practical difficulties in maintaining effective chemical gradients for the cells in three dimensional cultures. This is particularly the limiting factor when the cells become dense.

Mechanical cues

The response of the cells to mechanical signals is complex and this may result in any one or more of the following.

- Changes in the cell alignment.
- Deformation of cytoskeleton.
- Altered matrix formation.
- Synthesis of regulatory molecules (e.g growth factors, hormones).

There are mainly three mechanical cues governing cell populations.

1. Tensional forces.
2. Compressional forces.
3. Shear forces.

CELL SUPPORT MATERIALS

The support materials of cells largely determine the nature of adherent cells or cell types, and consequently tissue engineering. There are a large number of support materials which may be broadly categorized as follows.

- Traditional abiotic materials.
- Bioprosthesis materials.
- Synthetic material.
- Natural polymers.
- Semi-natural materials.

Traditional abiotic materials

The traditional abiotic support materials include plastics, ceramics and metals. These materials cannot be resorbed or become biologically integrated into the tissues. Therefore, it is preferable to avoid the traditional materials in tissue engineering.

Bioprosthesis materials

The ***natural materials modified to become biologically inert represent bioprosthesis materials***. They are formed by extensive chemical cross linking of natural tissues. For instance, the natural collagen-based connective tissue (e.g. porcine heart values) can be stabilized by treatment with glutaraldehyde. The product formed is non-immunogenic that remains unchanged at the site of transplantation for several years. However, growth of some cells or even connective tissue can occur on bioprosthesis materials. The design and fabrication of these materials is done in such a way that their functions are not affected by the surrounding host tissues.

Synthetic materials

A wide range of synthetic bioresorbable polymers are available as support materials. The most commonly used ***polymers in tissue engineering*** are poly (glycolic acid) (PGA), poly (lactic acid) (PLA), and copolymer PLGA (poly (lactic-co-glycolic acid). The composition and dimensions of these polymers can be so adjusted to make them stable *in vivo*, besides supporting *in vivo* cell growth.

There are certain ***advantages*** in using synthetic polymers.

- Production is easy and relatively cheap.
- Composition of polymers is reproducible even in large scale production.

There are however, some ***disadvantages*** also.

- Compatibility with cells is not as good as natural polymers.
- On degradation, they may form some products which cause undesirable cellular effects.

Natural polymers

The most widely used natural polymer materials are collagen-chondroitin sulfate aggregates. These materials are commercially available with varying composition under the trade name ***Integra***. The other natural polymers for cell support are usually obtained by their aggregation in culture as it occurs *in vivo* e.g. collagen gels, fibrin glue, Matrigel and some polysaccharides. Among the polysaccharides, chitosan and hyaluronan are used as hydrated gels.

The natural polymers mainly act on the principle of intermolecular interaction within the polymers to promote intimate molecular packing. The so formed molecules can effectively serve as support materials.

Semi-natural materials

Semi-natural materials are derived from the natural macromolecular polymers or whole tissues. They are the modified materials to achieve aggregation or stabilization. Some examples of semi-natural materials are listed below.

- Chemically cross-linked hyaluronan, stabilized by benzyl esterification.
- Collagen cross-linked with agents such as tannic acid or carbodiimide.

DESIGN AND ENGINEERING OF TISSUES

The following surgical criteria are taken into consideration while dealing with tissue engineering.

- Rapid restoration of the desired function.
- Ease of fixing the tissue.
- Minimal patient discomfort.

For designing tissue engineering, the ***source of donor cells is very critical*** (See cell sources p. 473). Use of patients own cells (autologous cells) is favoured to avoid immunological complications. Allogeneic cells are also used, particularly when the TE construct is designed for temporary repair. It is observed that when the cells are cultured and/or preserved (i.e. cryopreservation), the antigenicity of allogeneic cells is reduced.

Another important criteria in TE is the ***support material***, its degradation products, cell adhesion characteristics and mechanical cues.

The design and tissue engineering with respect to skin, urothelium and peripheral nerve are briefly described hereunder.

Tissue engineered skin

It was first demonstrated in 1975 that ***human keratinocytes could be grown in the laboratory in a form suitable for grafting***. Many improvements have been made since then. It is now possible to grow epithelial cells to produce a continuous sheet which progresses to form cornified layers. The major difficulty with TE skin is the dermal layer

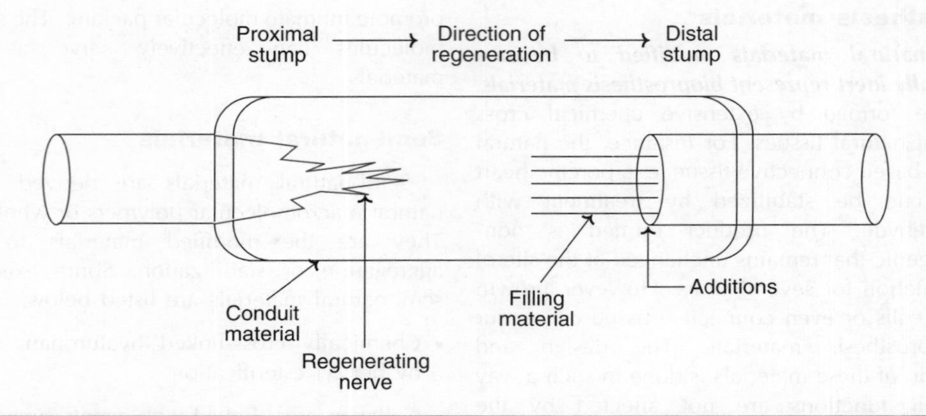

Fig. 40.4 : A diagrammatic representation of the basic design for peripheral nerve implant.

possessing blood capillaries, nerves, sweat glands and other accessory organs.

Some developments have occurred in recent years to produce implantable skin substitutes which may be regarded as tissue engineering skin constructs.

Integra™ : This is a bioartificial material composed of collagen-glycosaminoglycan. Integra™ is not a true TE construct. It is mainly used to carry the seeded cells.

Dermagraft™ : This is composed of poly (glycolic acid) polymer mesh seeded with human dermal fibroblasts from neonatal foreskins.

Apligraf™ : This has human dermal fibroblasts seeded into collagen gel. A layer of human keratinocytes is then placed on the upper surface.

The tissue constructs described above have limited shelf-life (about 5 days). However, they can integrate into the surrounding normal tissue and form a good skin cover. Further, there is no evidence of immunological complications with TE constructs.

Tissue engineered urothelium

It is now possible to culture urothelial cells and bladder smooth muscle cells. This raises the hope that the construction of TE urothelium is possible. In fact, some success has been reported in the development of a functional bladder in dogs. For this purpose, poly (glycolic acid) polymer base was shaped into a bladder and muscle cells were coated on the outer surface. The lumenal surface (i.e. inner surface) coated with pre-cultured urothelial cells. The bladder constructed in this way functioned almost like a normal one, and was maintained for about one year.

Tissue engineered peripheral nerve implants

Peripheral nerve injury is a common occurrence of trauma and tumor resection surgery, often leading to irreversible muscle atrophy. Therefore, the repair of injured peripheral nerves assumes significance.

A diagrammatic representation of the basic design of a peripheral nerve implant is depicted in *Fig 40.4*.

The regeneration of the injured nerve occurs from the proximal stump to rejoin at distal stump. The regeneration is guided by three types of substances.

Conduct material : This is the outer layer and is the primary source of guidance. Conduct material is composed of collagen-glycosaminoglycans, PLGA (poly lactic-co-glycolic acid), hyaluronan and fibronectin. All these are bioresorbable materials.

Filling material : This supports the neural cells for regeneration, besides guiding the process of regeneration. Filling material contains collagen, fibrin, fibronectin and agarose.

Additives : Additives include a large number of growth factors; neurotrophic factors (in different forms, combinations, ratios) e.g. fibroblast growth factor (FGF), nerve growth factor (NGF). Additions of Schwann cells or transfected fibroblasts promote nerve generation process.

TISSUE MODELLING

Research is in progress to create tissue models in the form of artificial organs. Some of the recent development on experimental tissue modelling are briefly outlined.

Artificial liver

Hepatocytes, cultured as spheroids or hepatocytes and fibroblasts cultured as hetero-spheroids can be used. They are held in the artificial support systems such as porous gelatin sponges, agarose or collagen. Addition of exogenous molecules is useful for the long - term culture of liver cells. Some progress has been reported in creating artificial liver as is evident from the hepatocytes three-dimensional structure and metabolic functions.

Artificial pancreas

Spheroids of insulin secreting cells have been developed from mouse insulinoma beta cells. Some workers could implant fetal islet-like cell clusters under the kidneys of mice, although the functions were not encouraging due to limitation of oxygen supply.

Other tissue models

Pituitary gland : Multicellular spheroids could be created to study certain hormonal release e.g. luteinizing hormone (LH), following stimulation by luteinizing hormone releasing hormone (LHRH). Some success has also been achieved to create spheroids for the production of melatonin.

Thyroid gland : Thyroid cell spheroids can be used for the study of cell adhesion, motility, and thyroid follicle biogenesis.

Brain cell cultures : Three dimensional brain cell cultures have been used for the study of neural myelination and demyelination, neuronal regeneration, and neurotoxicity of lead. Aggregated brain cells are also used for the study of Alzheimer's disease and Parkinson's disease.

Heart cell cultures : Aggregated heart cells have been used for the study of cardiac development and physiology.

EMBRYONIC STEM CELL ENGINEERING

The cells of the body, when grown in culture generally maintain their original character. Thus, liver cells behave like liver cells, and keratinocytes as keratinocytes. This is possible since each type of specialized cell has a memory of its developmental history.

Stem cells are ***undifferentiated cells*** that can divide continuously (indefinitely) to produce daughter cells. The daughter cells undergo differentiation into particular cell types.

Embryonic stem (ES) cells are an extraordinary class of stem cells that can ***proliferate indefinitely*** in culture, as they possess very high developmental potential. The cultured ES cells when put back into the animal can develop into different cell types and tissues. This depends on the site at which they are introduced. For instance, ES cells in liver adopt the character and behaviour of normal liver cells.

ES CELL CULTURES TO PRODUCE DIFFERENTIATED CELLS

The ES cells obtained from an early mouse embryo can be cultured indefinitely. The cultures may be continued as monolayers or allowed to form aggregates called embryoid bodies. The cells of the embryoid bodies can specialize and differentiate under suitable conditions (by using various combinations of signal proteins) into different cells (***Fig. 40.5***). For instance, when treated with certain growth factors, ES cells can form astrocytes and oligodendrocytes. These are the main types of glial cells of the central nervous system.

Cultured ES cells, appropriately treated with growth factors, when injected into the brain can serve as progenitors of glial cells. Thus, it is possible to correct a mouse dificient in myelin-forming oligodendrocytes. The grafted cells are capable of forming myelin sheaths around axons lacking them.

HUMAN EMBRYONIC STEM CELL RESEARCH

It was in 1998, researchers for the first time reported the establishment of human embryonic stem cell lines. These cells, existing indefinitely in culture, are capable of giving rise to any human cell type.

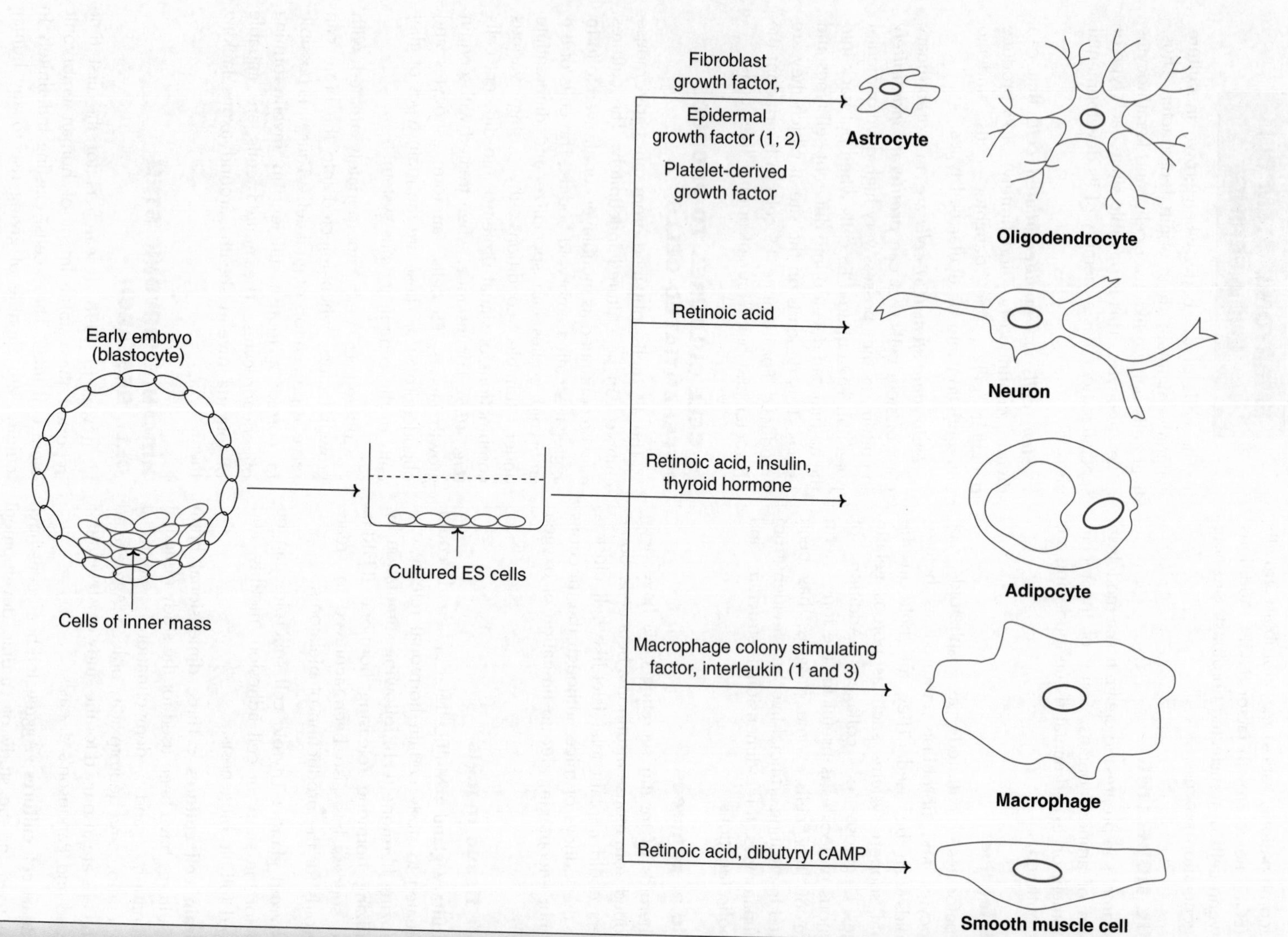

Fig. 40.5 : Culturing of embryonic stem (ES) cells and their differentiation into various cells.

Applications of human ES cells

The applications of human embryonic stem cell research are extraordinary. Some of them are listed below

- Corrections of disorders with loss of normal cells-diabetes, Alzheimer's disease, Parkinson's disease. This can be achieved by appropriate cell therapy.
- Engineering and replacement of various tissues.
- For the discovery of new drugs, and testing safety of drugs.
- To study the development of humans.

Limitations of human ES cells

There are several practical and technical difficulties associated with ES cell cultures and their utility. It is recently (2004) found that contamination with medium (the most commonly used being animal-derived media) created immunological complications when such cells are utilized for therapeutic purposes in humans. This contamination is identified to be due to a non-human molecule namely N-glycolylneuraminic acid. It is suggested that for human ES cell cultures, products of animal origin of any kind should not be used. An ideal alternative is to use human embryo-derived connective tissue cells as the feeder layer in ES cell cultures.

Ethical issues of ES cell research

Many people object to growing of human embryos in the laboratories, even if it is limited to the early stages of development. Some countries have, in fact, banned the use of Government funds for human embryo research. However, some private companies are conducting/financing research on human embryonic cells.

There are many serious ethical, legal and political issues surrounding human ES cell research. This is in addition to the enormous technical difficulties. If may take some more years before the appropriate applications of ES cell research to human welfare becomes a reality.

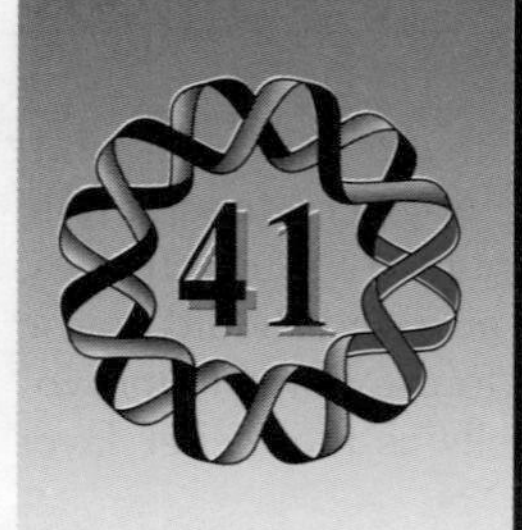

Transgenic Animals

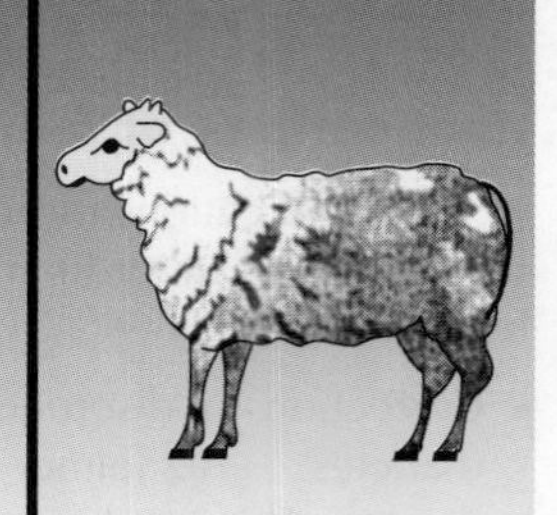

The dependence of man on animals such as cattle, sheep, poultry, pig and fish for various purposes (milk, meat, eggs, wool etc.) is well known. Improvement in the genetic characteristics of livestock and other domestic animals (e.g., high milk yield, weight gain, etc.), in the early days, was carried out by ***selective breeding methods***. This technique primarily involves a combination of mating and selection of animals with improved genetic triats. Although selective breeding is very time consuming and costly, it was the only method available, till some years ago, to enhance the genetic characteristics of animals. For larger animals with long gestation period, it might take several decades to create a desired character by conventional breeding. With the advent of modern biotechnology, it is now possible to carry out manipulations at the genetic level to get the desired characteristics in animals. ***Transgenesis refers to the phenomenon of introduction of exogeneous DNA into the genome to create and maintain a stable heritable character***. The foreign DNA that is introduced is called ***transgene***. And the animal whose genome is altered by adding one or more transgenes is said to be transgenic. The transgenes behave like other genes present in the animals' genome and are passed on to the offsprings. Thus, transgenic animals are ***genetically engineered*** or ***genetically modified organisms (GMOs)*** with a new heritable character. It was in 1980s, the genetic manipulation of animals by introducing genes into fertilized eggs became a reality.

IMPORTANCE OF TRANSGENIC ANIMALS-GENERAL

Transgenesis has now become a powerful tool for studying the gene expression and developmental processes in higher organisms, besides the improvement in their genetic characteristics. Transgenic animals serve as good models for understanding the human diseases. Further, several proteins produced by transgenic animals are important for medical and pharmaceutical applications. Thus, the transgenic farm animals are a part of the lucrative world-wide biotechnology industry, with geat benefits to mankind.

Transgenesis is important ***for improving the quality and quantity of milk, meat, eggs and wool production***, besides creating drug resistant animals.

Milk as the medium of protein production

Milk is the secretion of mammary glands that can be collected frequently without causing any harm to the animal. Thus, milk from the transgenic animals can serve as a good and authenticated source of human proteins for a wide range of applications. Another advantage with milk is that it contains only a few proteins (casein, lactalbumin, immunoglobuline etc.) in the native state, therefore isolation and purification of a new protein from milk is easy.

Commonly used animals for transgenesis

The first animals used for transgenesis was a mouse. The '***Super Mouse***', was created by inserting a rat gene for growth hormone into the mouse genome. The offspring was much larger than the parents. Super Mouse attracted a lot of public attention, since it was a product of genetic manipulation rather than the normal route of sexual reproduction.

Mouse continues to be an ***animal of choice for*** most ***transgenic experiments***. The other animals used for transgenesis include rat, rabbit, pig, cow, goat, sheep and fish.

TRANSGENIC MICE

As already stated, mouse is the animal of choice for transgenic experiments. Being a small animal, it can be easily handled, and mouse is regarded as researcher-friendly by biotechnologists. Another improtant reason of choosing mice for transgenic experiments is it produces more eggs (normal mouse 5–10 eggs, superovulated mouse can yield up to 40 eggs) unlike the large domestic animals. In the last two decades, hundreds of different genes have been introduced into the various mouse strains. And as such, the methodology of transgenesis is well developed with laboratory mouse.

Transgenic mice have significantly contributed to the understanding of molecular biology, genetics, immunology and cancer, besides creating animal models for several human genetic diseases.

There are three ***methods for introducing a foreign gene*** (transgene) into mice, and in fact the same methods are applicable to other animals as well.

1. ***Retroviral vector method.***
2. ***Microinjection method.***
3. ***Embryonic stem cell method.***

It may be noted here that the term ***transfection*** is used for introducing a foreign gene into animals. This is quite comparable to transformation that is carried out in lower organisms (Refer Chapter 6).

RETROVIRAL VECTOR METHOD

The transfer of small pieces (8 kb) of DNA can be effectively carried out by retroviruses. This method, however, is unsuitable for transfer of larger genes. Further, even for small genes, there is a risk of losing some regulatory sequences. Above all, the biggest drawback is the ***risk of retroviral contamination*** in the products (particularly in foods for human consumption), obtained from transgenic animals. Because of these limitations, the retroviral vector method is not in regular use for transgenesis.

MICROINJECTION METHOD

The introduction of DNA by microinjection method involves the following steps (***Fig. 41.1***).

1. The young virgin female mice (4–5 weeks age) are subjected to superovulation. This is achieved by administration of follicle-stimulating hormone (pregnant mare's serum), followed by (2 days later) human chorionic gonadotropin. The superovulated mouse produces 30–35 eggs (instead of normal 5–10 eggs).

2. The above female mice are mated with males and sacrificed on the following day. The fertilized eggs are removed from the fallopian tubes.

3. By micromanipulation using a micro-injection needle and a holding pipette, the ***DNA is injected into the male pronucleus of the fertilized egg***. Adequate care must be taken to ensure that while the elastic nuclear membrane is punctured, the needle does not touch the nucleoli. A dissection microscope can be used for identifying the male pronucleus (larger in size) and for microinjection.

4. The eggs with the transgenes are kept overnight in an incubator to develop to a 2-cell stage. These eggs are then implanted microsurgically into a foster mother i.e., pseudo-mouse pregnant female mouse which has been mated the previous might with vasectimized (or infertile) male. The foster mother can deliver pups after 3 weeks of implantation.

The presence of transgene in the pups can be identified by polymerase chain reaction or Southern blot hybridization.

The mouse carrying the foreign gene is the transgenic founder from which pure transgenic lines can be established.

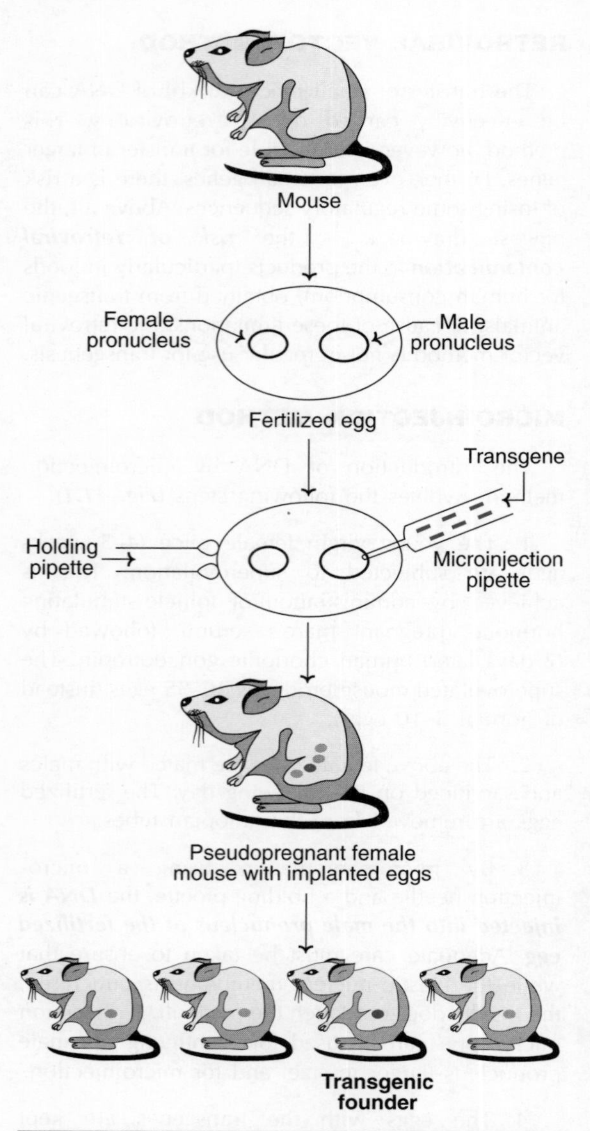

Fig. 41.1 : DNA microinjection method to produce transgenic mice.

The microinjection method involves several steps and none of them is 100% efficient for any animal to develop into transgenic animal. In case of mouse, it was found that about 65% of the fertilized eggs survive microinjection procedure, about 25% of the implanted eggs develop into pups, and only 25% of them are transgenic. Thus, if one starts with 1000 fertilized eggs, only 30 to 50 transgenic pups may be produced i.e., 3–5% of the inoculated eggs develop into transgenic animals.

Limitations of microinjection method

Besides the ***low efficiency*** (discussed above), there are some other disadvantages in this technique. The foreign DNA randomly integrates into the host genome. Sometimes, even many pieces of DNA get incorporated at a single site. Further, ***transgenes may not be expressed*** at all or sometimes underexpressed, or even overexpressed. All these processes will disturb the normal physiology of the transgenic animal. In addition, microinjection procedures are time consuming, costly and labour intensive. Despite all these limitations, this technique is routinely used for producing transgenic animals.

EMBRYONIC STEM CELL METHOD

Cells from the inner cell mass of the blastocyst stage of a developing mouse embryo can proliferate in cell culture. These cells, referred to as pluripotent ***embryonic stem*** (ES) cells, are capable of differentiating into other types of cells (including germ line cells) when transferred to another blastocyst embryo.

The embryonic stem cell technology basically involves the ***introduction of a foreign DNA into ES cell*** (***Fig. 41.2***). Embryonic stem cells in culture can be subjected to genetic manipulations without changing their plutipotency. ***Foreign DNA can be introduced into ES cells by electroporation or microinjection***. The desired genetically engineered cells with transgene can be identified by a selection procedure using a marker gene or PCR analysis (described below). The transfected cells can be cultured, introduced (by microinjection) into blastocyst and then implanted into foster mother (i.e., pseudopregnant female mouse). By this way, transgenic founder mice are produced. Transgenic lines can be established by suitable breeding strategies of the founder mice.

Selection of transgene containing cells

Several strategies have been developed for the selection of transgene containing cells. The important ones are briefly described.

Selection by use of marker gene coding for thymidine kinase : It is worthwhile to know the role of thymidine kinase to understand its utility as a marker gene. There are two pathways for the synthesis of deoxyribonucleotides (dATP, dGTP, dCTP and dTTP), the basic units of DNA structure.

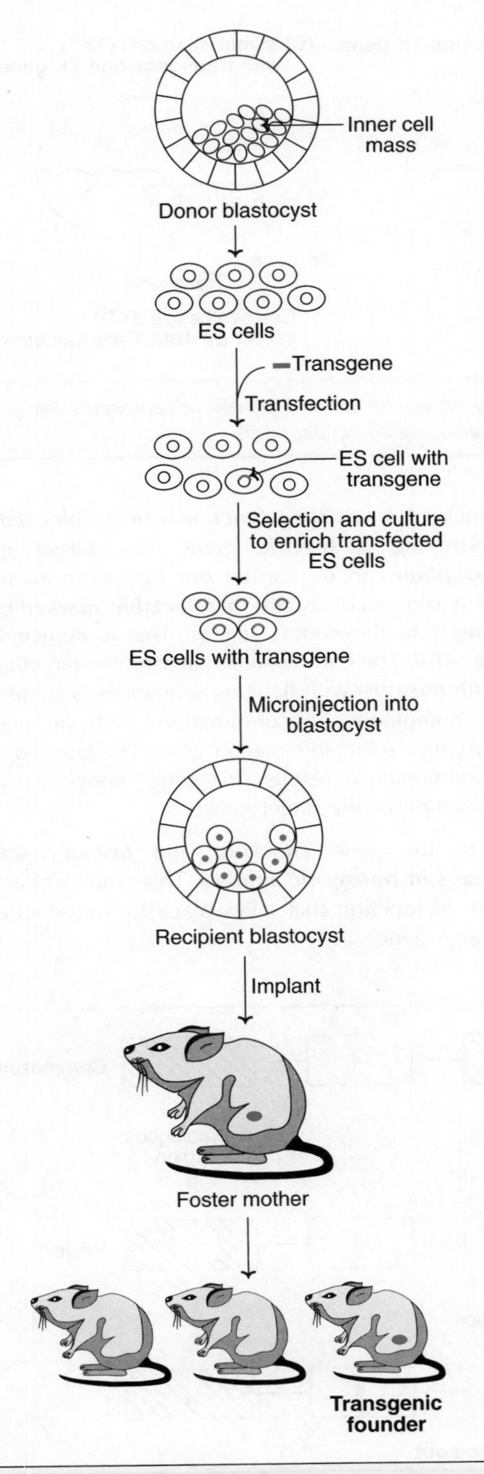

Fig. 41.2 : Embryonic stem cell (ES) method to produce transgenic mice.

One is the ***salvage pathway*** that recycles the degraded nitrogenous bases formed from DNA. The other alternate pathway is an ***endogenous synthetic pathway*** from different precursors (glycine, aspartate, glutamine, methyl tetrahydrofolate etc.).

The enzyme thymidine kinase (TK) is involved in the salvage pathway. TK phosphorylates thymidine to produce thymidine monophosphate (dTMP) which is finally converted to thymidine triphosphate (dTTP).

The gene that encodes the enzyme thymidine kinase can be used as a marker to determine whether the transgene has been inserted. This is illustrated in ***Fig. 41.3***. The mammalian cells are capable of synthesizing dTTP by salvage pathway and endogenous synthetic pathway. The cells lacking TK gene cannot produce dTTP. If such cells are cultured in a ***HAT*** medium containing ***h***ypoxanthine (H), ***a***minopterine (A) and ***t***hymidine (T), they cannot grow and therefore die. This is because thymidine cannot be utilized in the salvage pathway due to lack the enzyme thymidine kinase. Further, aminopterine blocks the endogenous pathway (by inhibiting the enzyme dihydrofolate reductase, required for one carbon metabolism).

If a transgene is joined to a TK gene, inserted into a mammalian cell (TK^-) and then the cells can grow in HAT medium. This is possible only if the TK gene is incorporated into the mammalian cells. And logically, the cells that survive in HAT medium carry the transgene. In this fashion, thymidine kinase can be effectively used as a marker gene.

There are other enzymes that serve as markers for identifying transgene insertion. These include dihydrofolate reductase (resistant to methotrexate) and neomycin phosphotransferase (resistant to antibiotic G418) and ***PCR analysis for selecting transgene containing cells***. The last one is a more direct and recent method, and is successfully used for detecting transgene containing cells.

Promoter sequence to facilitate transgenesis

In the early experiments on transgenesis, the ***mouse metallothionein (MMT)*** gene promoter was used. MMT gene encodes for a metal binding protein that is involved in metal homeostasis. The foreign gene (i.e., a rat growth hormone gene) can be linked to a promoter sequence of MMT. By

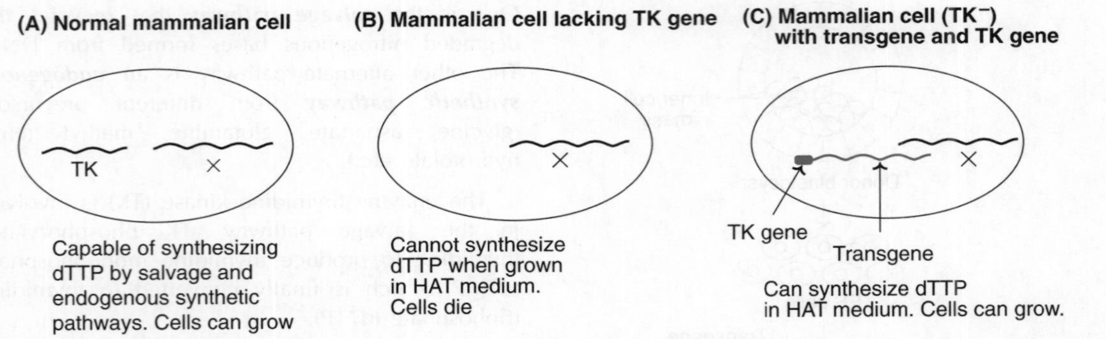

(A) Normal mammalian cell

TK ×

Capable of synthesizing dTTP by salvage and endogenous synthetic pathways. Cells can grow

(B) Mammalian cell lacking TK gene

×

Cannot synthesize dTTP when grown in HAT medium. Cells die

(C) Mammalian cell (TK^-) with transgene and TK gene

×

TK gene

Transgene

Can synthesize dTTP in HAT medium. Cells can grow.

Fig. 41.3 : Thymidine kinase (TK) marker gene for selecting transgene containing cells (X-represents the genes for synthesizing dTTP by endogenous synthetic pathway).

doing so, the promoter switches on the growth hormone gene when the MMT is activated by a metal in the environment (e.g., cadmium). Thus, the metal inducer (Cd) can stimulate the promoter (MMT promoter) to facilitate the transgene (growth hormone gene) to express. Therefore, addition of cadmium triggers the growth hormone production.

GENE KNOCKOUT

By inserting a transgene (foreign gene) into a chromosome, a new function is introduced while producing transgenic animals (described above). On the other hand, in a process referred to as gene knockout an ***existing function can be blocked by destroying a specific gene***. The ***target gene disruption*** can be carried out ***by*** incorporating a DNA sequence, usually ***a selectable marker gene*** (***smg***) into the coding region. This is depicted in ***Fig. 41.4***. The chromosome carrying the target gene (with 4 exons) with flanking sequences is subjected to homologous recombination with a vector carrying a selectable marker gene. The homologous recombination results in gene knockout i.e., disruption of the target gene.

In the gene knockout, the ***loss-of-function occurs in transgenic animals***. This is in contrast to gain of function that takes place by introducing a foreign gene.

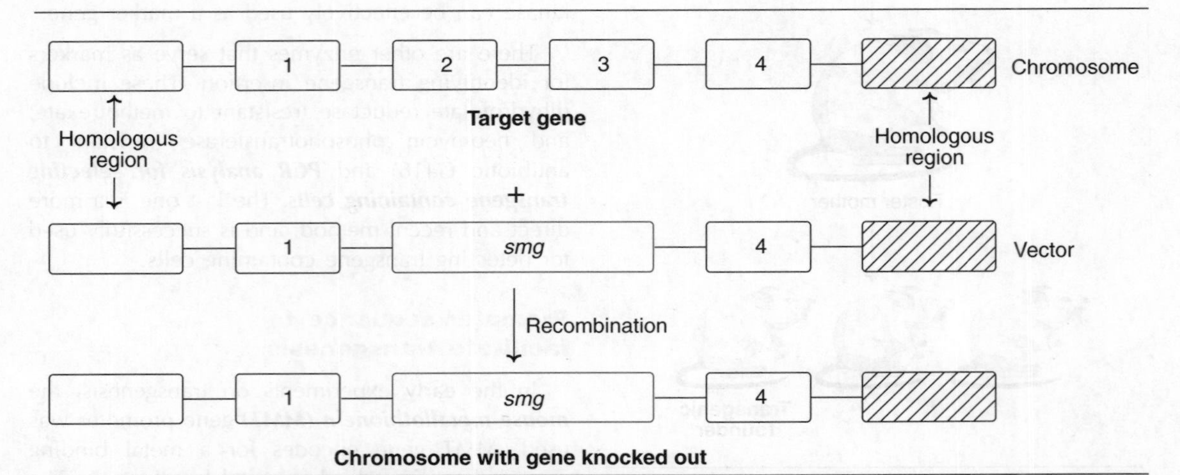

Fig. 41.4 : Gene knockout by homologous recombination (1-4 represent exons of target gene; smg-Selectable marker gene).

Applications of gene knockout

Disruption of the target genes (gene knockout) is important for understanding the development and physiological consequences in an organism. Further, the biochemical and pathological basis of several human diseases can be appropriately understood by inactivating specific genes. About 200 knockout mice have been so far created to serve as animal models for the study of a large number of human abnormalities and disorders. In fact, knockout mouse which lack genes for a single organ or organ system can be produced (For more details, See p. 486).

YEAST ARTIFICIAL CHROMOSOME IN TRANSGENESIS

In the conventional transgenesis, small sized transgenes (≤ 20 kb) are transferred through vectors. This involves a risk of losing some important sequences including the regulatory ones. Further, several genes exist as complexes and are too large to be handled by conventional vectors. Yeast artificial chromosomes (***YACs***) can carry large-sized genes (size range 100–1,000 kb), and are effectively used in transgenesis.

By using microinjection technique or transfection of ES cells with YACs, transgenic mice have been produced. Selected examples are cited below.

1. YACs are used to carry human β-globin gene complex (5 genes with 250 kb size) and produce transgenic mice.

2. YACs are employed for producing human antibodies in transgenic mice. Synthesis of antibodies is very complex process. YACs carrying varying sizes of DNA sequences (800–1,000 kb YACs) have been employed to generate different antibodies.

TRANSGENIC MICE AND THEIR APPLICATIONS

Mouse, although not close to humans in its biology, has been and continues to be the most exploited animal model in transgenesis experiments. The common feature between man and mouse is that both are mammals. Transgenic mice are extensively used as animal models for understanding human diseases and for the production of therapeutic agents. Adequate care, however, must be exercised before extrapolating data of transgenic mice to humans.

Mouse models for several human diseases (cancers, muscular dystrophy, arthritis, Alzheimer's disease, hypertension, allergy, coronary heart disease, endocrine diseases, neurodegenerative disorders etc.) have been developed. A selected few of them are briefly discussed.

THE HUMAN MOUSE

The transgenic mice with ***human immune system*** were produced, and they are commonly referred to as human mice (***Fig. 41.5***). For this purpose, mice with severe combined immuno-deficiency (SCID-a condition characterized by total lack of immune system cells) were chosen. Human thymus tissue from an aborted fetus was transplanted under the capsule membrane of the kidney of the mouse. Human lymph node was placed under the opposite kidney. After about a week, immature immune cells (T-lymphocytes) from a human fetus were injected into the mouse tail vein. These lymphocytes enter the thymus tissue under the kidney and mature to T-lymphocytes. The so produced T-lymphocytes enter the circulation and in the lymph node (present under the second kidney), they multiply to form a full-pledged functional immune system. It takes about two weeks after the transplant for the ***mice*** to ***display*** the ***human immune system*** (characteristics of both T-lymphocytes and B-lymphocytes).

The human mouse, being a close ***animal model for human immune system*** is a boon for immunologists, particularly working on ***AIDS***. This is because the various immunological aspects of AIDS including the possible development of an AIDS vaccine can be explored by using human mouse (**Note :** There is no good animal model for AIDS research except chimpanzee).

THE ALZHEIMER'S MOUSE

Alzheimer's disease affects about 1% of the population between 60–65 years old, and about 30% of the population over 80 years old. This disease is characterized by ***progressive loss of memory and personality changes*** (decline in thinking, judgement etc.). The postmortem analysis of brains of Alzheimer's patients revealed plaques of ***dead nerve cells entangled in a protein called amyloid***. This protein was purified and its amino

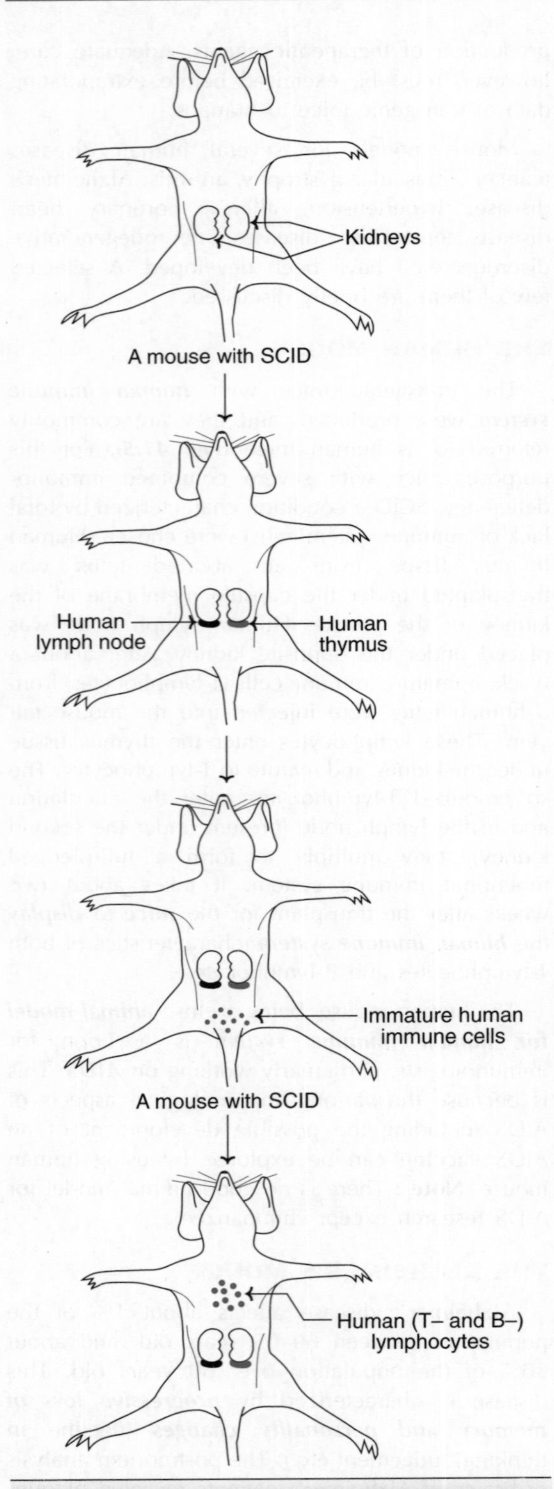

Fig. 2.5 : The human mouse (SCID-Severe combined immunodeficiency).

acid sequence determined. Later, ***amyloid precursor protein*** (***APP***) and its gene sequence were also identified. Alzheimer's disease is more prevalent in some families, clearly indicating a genetic basis for this disease.

Transgenic mice were developed by introducing amyloid precursor gene into fertilized egg cells of mice. The synthesis of human amyloid protein and its accumulation as typical plaques in the mice brain were observed. The Alzheimer's mouse is very useful in understanding the pathological basis of the disease. Certain mutations in APP gene, and the involvement of some other genes are believed to be responsible for Alzheimer's disease.

THE ONCOMOUSE

The ***animal model for cancer*** is the oncomouse (onco refers to cancer). First developed for breast cancer, the oncomouse is useful for understanding of cancer and evolving modalities for cancer therapy.

The ***oncogene c-myc*** in association with mouse mammary tumor (MMT) virus was found to be responsible for breast cancer in animals. Transgenic mice were produced by introducing chimeric DNA consisting of *c-myc* gene and sections MMT virus into fertilized mouse egg cells. Breast cancer developed in adult female mice and the trait was passed on to the offspring.

Oncomouse (the mouse that is genetically altered and is susceptible for cancer) was patented by U.S. Patent office ***in 1988***. In fact, it was the ***very first animal to be patented***.

THE PROSTATE MOUSE

The prostate gland, surrounding the urethra of males is responsible for secreting semen fluid. In the older men, particularly above 60 years of age, prostate gland gets elarged and may become cancerous. The oncogene for prostate cancer was identified (***int-2***). A chimeric DNA by joining ***int-2*** with viral promoter was prepared and introduced into fertilized mouse eggs. In the transgenic mice so developed, enlargement of prostate gland was observed. There prostate mice were also patented in 1991.

THE KNOCKOUT MOUSE

The basic principles underlying gene knockout have been described (See p. 484). Several knockout mice have been developed. It is not an exaggeration that the knockout mice have become as common as a test tube in the laboratory for a biotechnologist. It must be noted that not all the knockout mice are immediately useful for human health and welfare. A selected few of the knockout mice are described.

SCID mouse

Severe combined immunodeficiency (SCID) is a condition with a total lack of immune system. SCID mice were developed ***by eliminating a single gene and the resultant mice lost the ability to produce B-lymphocytes and T-lymphocytes***. The human mouse was later developed from the SCID mouse (See p. 485).

Knockout mouse for allergy

The receptor sites on certain body cells for ***IgE antibodies*** are believed to be responsible for triggering allergy reactions. Knockout mice were developed for allergy by ***removing the gene encoding for receptor protein***. The result is that antibodies cannot bind to cells due to lack of receptors and the mice are unaffected by allergic reactions. It is expected that some breakthrough may occur in the near future to benefit the millions of sufferers of allergic reactions, spread throughout the world.

Knockout mouse for transplantation

By using a ***suicide gene***, the liver cells were destroyed in a mouse that already lacks immune system. Sample human liver cells were transplanted in this mouse. Encouraged by lack of immune system, the human liver cells can develop. In this fashion, organ replacement in animals is possible.

Knockout mouse with memory loss

The memory processes in brain are believed to be carried out by a specialized area called hippocampus. By a gene knockout technique, researchers have developed ***mice that lack hippocampus***. These knockout mice lacked the ability to remember.

Knockout mouse with retinitis pigmentosa

By inactivating the mouse rhodopsin gene, rods cells of the retinal deteriorate in the transgenic mice. This retinal degeneration is comparable to human retinitis pigmentosa. The ***rhodopsin knockout mouse*** is useful for understanding the retinal degeneration, besides evolving therapeutic strategies.

TRANSGENIC MICE FOR HUMAN DISEASES

Transgenic mice are important for the development of therapeutic drugs and possible gene therapies, besides the understanding of the human disease. Many transgenic mice with human disease equivalents have been developed and a selected few of them are given in ***Table 41.1***.

TRANSGENESIS IN LARGE ANIMALS

In general, transgenesis in large animals is more difficult than with mice. There are several factors for the lower efficiency of transgenesis in large animals. These include less number of eggs they

TABLE 41.1 Transgenic mice with human disease equivalents (selected examples)

Human disease equivalent	*Genetic change in mice*
Sickle-cell anemia	Insertion of β-globin of sickle-cell hemoglobin.
Lesch-Nyhan syndrome	Inactivation of mouse gene encoding hypoxanthine-guanine phosphoribosyltransferase
Kaposis sarcoma	Introduction of HIV *tat* gene
Development of malignancy	Insertion of human *ras* and *c-myc* oncogenes
X-Linked muscular dystrophy	Mutation at a locus on X-chromosome
Hypertension*	Introduction of mouse renin gene

**This was done in transgenic rats.*

produce and technical difficulties in handling, besides long gestational periods to get the offspring (It takes about 2 years to produce a calf from a fertilized egg).

Some of the early experiments to produce transgenic large animals were far from satisfactory. For instance, transgenic sheep overproducing growth hormone grow leaner with increased feed efficiency. But they are more susceptible to infection, become infertile and tend to die at young age. All this might be due to ineffective control of gene regulation. Several improvements have been made to produce transgenic animals with desirable characters.

Biotechnologists are particularly interested to improve the quality of animals, with improved resistance to diseases, besides enhancing their ability produce foods. '***Building a better animal***', ***being the motto***. Further, production of commercial and pharmaceutical compounds by transgenic animals is also gaining importance in recent years.

The protocol adopted for producing other transgenic animals is comparable with that already described for transgenic mice, with certain modifications.

TRANSGENIC CATTLE

The ***mammary gland*** of the dairy cattle is an ***ideal bioreactor*** for producing several new proteins (of pharmaceutical importance), besides improving the quality and quantity of the existing ones. For instance, a transgenic cow, with an over-expressed casein transgene, can give milk with higher content of casein. If lactase transgene is introduced and expressed in the mammary gland, milk free from lactose will be secreted. Such a milk will be a boon for lactose intolerant people who experience indigestion and other complications, after consuming normal milk and milk products.

Some success has been achieved in creating transgenic cattle with improved resistance to viral, bacterial and parasitic diseases. However, this is not an easy job due to the complexicity of genetic control to combat the disease-producing organisms.

Attempts have been made in recent years to produce cattle with inherited immunological protection by transgenesis. Introduction of genes that code for heavy and light chains of monoclonal antibodies has met with some success in this direction.

In vivo immunization of an animal although not yet fully successful, is ideal for disease protection. *In vivo* immunization primarily involves the insertion of a transgene for an antibody that specifically binds to an antigen.

TRANSGENIC SHEEP AND GOATS

Transgenesis experiments in sheep and goats mostly involve the development of mammary glands as bioreactors for the production of proteins for pharmaceutical use. This is possible despite the fact that quantity of milk produced by sheep and goats is less than that of dairy cattle (cow, buffalo). Some proteins produced by sheep and goats have good pharmaceutical use (***Table 41.2***).

Transgenic sheep with increased wool production

Keratin is the wool protein with highly cross-linked disulfide bridges. For good production of quality wool, the amino acid cysteine (or its precursor methionine) is required in large quantities. However, cysteine supply to sheep is always inadequate, since the microbes harboring the rumen utilize it and release in the form of sulfide. This problem can be overcome by producing transgenic sheep containing bacterial genes for the synthesis of cysteine. The two enzymes, synthesized by the transgenes, are capable of trapping the hydrogen sulfide liberated in the intestine to produce cysteine. Thus, ***good supply of cysteine to the sheep improves the quality and quantity of wool***.

TRANSGENIC PIGS

Transgenic pigs that can ***produce human hemoglobin*** have been successfully developed. This human hemoglobin can be separated from pig hemoglobin by simple analytical techniques. Hemoglobin, the oxygen carrying protein of RBC, can be used as a substitute in blood transfusion experiments. In fact, hemoglobin can be stored for longer period (a few months) than whole blood (weeks only). Further, there is no problem of contamination (like HIV) as is the case with whole blood. However, the free hemoglobin (naked hemoglobin) cannot transport oxygen as effectively as the hemoglobin of RBC. In addition, naked hemoglobin is easily degraded and the breakdown products cause damage to kidney. There also exists a risk of contamination by pig viruses and other

TABLE 41.2 Transgenic animals as bioreactors for the production of therapeutically important proteins

Transgenic animal	*Protein product*	*Biological importance*
Cow	Lactoferrin	Promotes intestinal iron absorption and hence can be used to overcome iron-deficiency anemias. Possesses antibacterial activity
Cow	Interferon	Provides resistance against viral infections
Sheep	α_1-Antitrypsin	Used in the treatment of emphysema (promotes the exchange of gases in lungs)
Goat	Cystic fibrosis transmembrane regulator (CFTR)	For the treatment of patients suffering from cystic fibrosis (promotes transport of ions)
Goat	Tissue plasminogen activator (tPA)	Used in treating the patients of myocardial infarction (dissolves blood clots)
Goat	Antithrombin III	Regulates blood clotting
Rabbits	α-Glucosidase	Treatment of Pompe's disease (a genetic disorder characterized by block in glycogen degradation)
Mouse	Urokinase	For dissolving blood clots
Mouse	Immunoglobulins (antibodies)	Administration enhances immunity
Pig	Hemoglobin	Blood transfusion
Goat and other animals	Vaccines (?)	To immunize against various diseases

compounds to cause allergic reactions. With these limitations, the initial enthusiasm for substituting blood transfusion with free hemoglobin has remained short-lived.

It is now advised not to use naked hemoglobin for transfusion, when there is a heavy blood loss. However, it can be used during major surgeries for supplementing the whole blood transfusion.

Pig in organ farms

The human organs such as heart, liver, pancreas, kidney and lungs are in great demand for transplantation surgery. The shortage of these transplantable organs can be overcome by developing them in animals. ***Pig is a favourite animal for harvesting human organs***. This is because the physiology of pigs is close to that of humans. Further, pigs do not carry any major infectious diseases transmissible to humans. The use of pigs in organ farming is still at the experimental stages.

In the preliminary experiments, organ transplantation from transgenic pigs into primates showed some promising results. The day may not be very far for utilizing transgenic pigs as donors of human organs (For more details, See p. 492).

TRANSGENIC CHICKENS

The production of transgenic chickens (or other birds) is rather complicated. This is mainly because during fertilization in chickens, several sperms enter the ovum instead of one. This is in contrast to mammals where usually only one sperm enters the egg. The identification of male pronuclei that will fuse with female pronuclei is quite difficult. Further, embryonic stem (ES) cells have not been identified in chicken. Despite all these limitations, transgenic chickens have been developed.

The blastoderm cells (from an egg) can be removed from a donor chicken. They are transfected with transgenes (usually by lipofection with liposomes). The so modified blastoderm cells are reintroduced into the subgerminal space of irradiated blastoderm of freshly laid eggs. Some of the resulting chickens may carry the transgene. Transgenic lines of chickens can be established.

Transgenesis in chicken can be used to develop low fat and cholesterol, and high protein containing eggs. Transgenic chickens that are ***resistant to viral and bacterial diseases have also been developed***. Some attempts have also been made to develop pharmaceutical proteins in the eggs of transgenic chickens.

TRANSGENIC FISH

Several transgenic fish (catfish, salmon, trout etc.) have been developed ***with increase in their growth and size***. This was carried out by introducing ***growth hormone transgene*** (by microinjection or electroporation). The fertilized eggs with inserted transgene are incubated in temperature-regulated holding tanks. (**Note :** The fish egg development is external in contrast to the mammalian embryogenesis). The efficiency of fish transgenesis is as high as 70%.

It was found that the transgenic salmon fish (with growth hormone transgene) were 10 times heavier than the normal ones, at the end of one year.

POSITION EFFECTS

Position effect is the phenomenon of ***different levels of gene expression that is observed after insertion of a new gene at different position in the eukaryotic genome***. This is commonly observed in transgenic animals as well as plants. These transgenic organisms show variable levels and patterns of transgene expression. In a majority of cases, position effects are dependent on the site of transgene integration.

In general, the defective expression is due to the insertion of transgene into a region of highly packed chromatin. The transgene will be more active if inserted into an area of open chromatin.

The positional effects are overcome by a group of DNA sequences called ***insulators***. The sequences referred to as ***specialized chromatin structure (SCS)*** are known to perform the functions of insulators. It has been demonstrated that the expression of the gene is appropriate if the transgene is flanked by insulators.

ANIMAL BIOREACTORS

Transgenesis is wonderfully utilized for production proteins of pharmaceutical and medical use. In fact, any protein synthesized in the human body can be made in the transgenic animals, provided that the genes are correctly programmed. The advantage with transgenic animals is to produce scarce human proteins in huge quantities. Thus, the ***animals serving as factories for production of biologically important products*** are referred to as ***animal bioreactors or*** sometimes ***pharm animals***. Frankly speaking, transgenic animals as bioreactors can be commercially exploited for the benefit of mankind.

Once developed, animal bioreactors are cost-effective for the production of large quantities of human proteins. Routine breeding and healthful living conditions are enough to maintain transgenic animals.

The importance of transgenic animals has already been discussed under the respective individual animals. A selected list of the therapeutically important proteins produced by animal bioreactors is given ***Table 41.2***.

DOLLY-THE TRANSGENIC CLONE

Dolly, the first ever mammal clone was developed by Wilmut and Campbell in 1997. It is a ***sheep*** (female lamb) ***with a mother and no father.***

The ***technique primarily involves nuclear transfer and the phenomenon of totipotency***. The character of a cell to develop to different cells, tissues, organs, and finally an organism is referred to as ***totipotency*** or ***pluropotency***. Totipotency is the basic character of embryonic cells. As the embryo develops, the cells specialize to finally give the whole organism. As such, the cells of an adult lack totipotency. Totipotency was induced into the adult cells for developing Dolly.

The cloning of sheep for producing Dolly, illustrated in ***Fig. 41.6***, is briefly described here. The mammary gland cells from a donor ewe were isolated. They were subjected to total nutrient deprivation (starvation) for five days. By this process, the mammary cells abandon their normal growth cycle, enter a dormant stage and regain totipotency character. An ovum (egg cell) was taken from another ewe, and its nucleus was removed to form an enucleated ovum. The dormant mammary gland cell and the enucleated ovum were fused by pulse electricity. The mammary cell outer

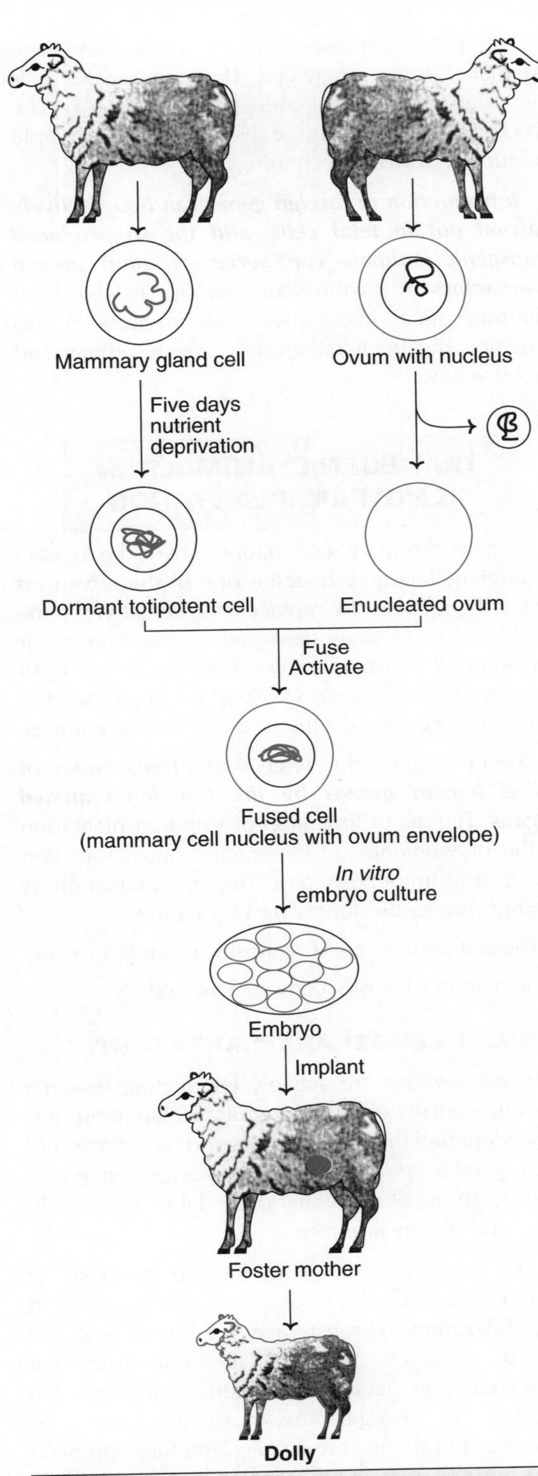

Fig. 41.6 : The cloning of sheep for developing Dolly.

membrane was broken, allowing the ovum to envelope the nucleus. The fused cell, as it had gained totipotency, can multiply and develop into an embryo. This embryo was then implanted into another ewe which serves as a surrogate/foster mother. Five months later, Dolly was born.

As reported by Wilmut and Campbell, they fused 277 ovum cells, achieved 13 pregnancies, and of these only one pregnancy resulted in live birth of the offspring-Dolly.

CLONING OF PET ANIMALS

Some of the companies involved in transgenic experiments have started cloning pet animals like cats and dogs. Little Nicky was the first pet cat that was cloned at a cost of $50,00 by an American company (in Dec. 2004). More cloned cats and dogs will be made available to interested parties (who can afford) in due course.

Some people who own pet animals are interested to continue the same pets which is possible through cloning. There is some opposition to this approach as the cloned animals are less healthy, and have shorter life span, besides the high cost factor.

TRANSGENIC ANIMALS PRODUCED BY CLONING FETAL CELLS

Fetal cells such as fibroblasts are totipotent. Fetal cell cloning was successfully carried out by some workers to produce ***transgenic sheep (Polly), transgenic bull calf (Gene)*** and other animals. Transgenes (foreign genes) can be inserted into the fetal cell genomes to produce desired products by transgenic animals.

As an example, the development of transgenic calves produced by cloning with fetal cells is shown in ***Fig. 41.7***. Fibroblasts were collected from a fifty five day old bovine fetus. These fibroblasts with totipotent character are cultivated in a nutritious medium. The desired foreign genes (transgenes) can be introduced into fibroblasts. The nucleus with the genetically altered DNA (fibroblast nucleus) is removed from the cell. It is then inserted into a bovine enucleated ovum. This ovum cell multiplies to form embryos. They are implanted in a surrogate (foster) mother cow to give birth to transgenic calves.

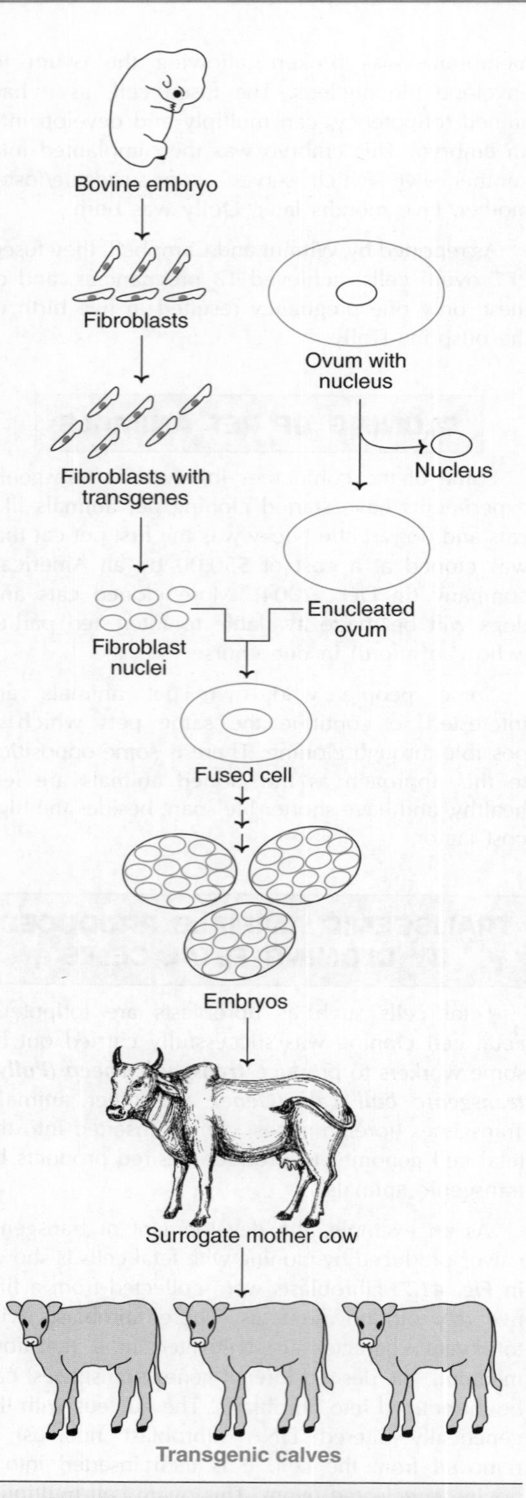

Fig. 41.7 : Transgenic calves produced by cloning fetal fibroblasts.

The calves represent clones, since they have originated from a single cell. They are transgenic as they carry the transgenes (foreign genes). The production of transgenic calves is a good example of ***nuclear transfer*** technology.

Introduction of foreign genes can be effectively carried out in fetal cells, and the so produced transgenic animals can serve as good animal bioreactors to synthesize several products of pharmaceutical importance. The progress in this direction has been rather slow due to ethical and moral issues.

TRANSGENIC ANIMALS IN XENOTRANSPLANTATION

Organ transplantation (kidney, liver, heart etc.) in humans has now become one of the advanced surgical practices to replace the defective, non–functional or severaly damaged organs. The major limitation of transplantation is the shortage of organ donors. This often results in long waiting times and many unnecessary deaths of organ failure patients.

Xenotransplantation refers to the ***replacement of failed human organs by the functional animal organs***. The major limitation of xenotransplantation is the phenomenon of hyperacute organ rejection due to host immune system. The organ rejections is mainly due to the following two causes

- The antibodies raised against the foreign organ.
- Activation of host's complement system.

PIGS IN XENOTRANSPLANTATION?

Some workers are actively conducting research to utilize organs of pigs in xenotransplantation. It is now identified that the major reason for rejection of pig organs by primates is due to the presence of a special group of disaccharides (Gal-α 1,3-Gal) in pigs, and not in primates.

The enzyme responsible for the synthesis of specific disaccharides in pigs has been identified. It is ***α 1,3-galactosyltransferase***, present in pigs and not in primates. Scientists are optimistic that ***knockout pigs*** lacking the gene encoding the enzyme α 1,3-galactosyltransferase can be developed in the next few years. Another approach is to introduce genes in primates that can degrade or modify Gal-α 1,3-Gal disaccharide groups (of pigs). This will reduce immunogenecity.

Besides the above, there are other strategies to avoid hyperactive organ rejection by the hosts in xenotransplantation.

- Expression of antibodies against the pig disaccharides.
- Expression of complement — inactivating protein on the cell surfaces.

By the above approaches, it may be possible to overcome immediate hyperactive rejection of organs. The next problem is the delayed rejection which involves the macrophages and natural killer cells of the host.

Another concern of xenotransplantation is that the endogenous pig retroviruses could get activated after organ transplantation. This may lead to new genetic changes with unknown consequences.

The use of transgenic animals in xenotransplantation is only at the laboratory experimental stages, involving animals. It is doubtful whether this will become a reality in the near future.

There is a vigorous debate concerning the ***ethics of xenotransplantation and the majority of general public are against it***.

TRANSGENIC ORGANISMS TO INTERRUPT DISEASE CYCLES

Several human diseases have a second host in the life cycle of the parasite. Transgenesis will be useful for disease control by interrupting the life cycle. Attempts are being made in the recent years in this direction, although the sucess has been limited. ***Transgenic organisms may soon serve as environmental replacements to control several diseases***.

TRANSGENIC SNAILS

Schistosomiasis is a parasitic diseases caused by *Schistosoma* which develops in the snails. The parasite infects humans by penetrating through skin when contacted in water. It is estimated that about 100 million people worldwide are the victims of schistosomiasis. This disease is characterized by chills, fever, intestinal ulcerations and diarrhea.

By developing transgenic snails, it is possible to interrupt the life cycle of *Schistosoma*. Some workers have attempted to ***create transgenic snails that will resist the invasion of the parasite***. If such snails are released into the environment, they will break the life cycle of schistosoma.

TRANSGENIC MOSQUITOES

Mosquitoes are responsible for the transmission of malaria. Some workers have identified certain critical ***genes in mosquitoes*** (*Anopheles* genus that transmits *Plasmodium* species malarial parasite) that are ***responsible for harbor and transmission of the parasite***. Theoretically, it is possible to alter these genes and produce transgenic mosquito. If such mosquitoes are released into the environment in large numbers, they will dilute the population of native mosquitoes, and halt the transmission of malarial parasite.

Another approach to control malaria is to understand ***vector incompetence*** i.e., the genetic basis of the vector to sustain a parasite and how to alter it so as to make the vector inhospitable for the parasite. Some success has been achieved in developing transgenic mosquitoes with vector incompetence. If such mosquitoes are released into the environment, the life cycle of the malarial parasite will be interrupted.

TRANSGENIC TSETSE FLIES

A protozoal disease African sleeping sickness is transmitted by tsetse fly. This disease affects the nervous system and is often accompanied by coma. Transgenic tsetse flies were developed with a novel approach. Researchers found a ***protein that can kill disease-producing protozoa***. They identified the protein encoding gene and inserted it into the bacteria of tsetse fly gut. These bacteria produce antiprotozoal protein that kills tsetse flies. In this manner the disease transmission can be prevented.

TRANSGENIC BOLLWORMS

Bollworms are the caterpillars that damage the cotton crop. Researches have developed ***transgenic bollworms with a suicide gene***. When released into the environment, the transgenic bollworms will mate with wild bollworms and produce caterpillars that die. The cotton crop can be saved from the damage.

TRANSGENIC MEDFLIES

Medflies (Mediterranean fruit flies) destroy fruit and coffee crops throughout the world. Attempts are being made to develop transgenic medflies to replace wild medflies and save the crops.

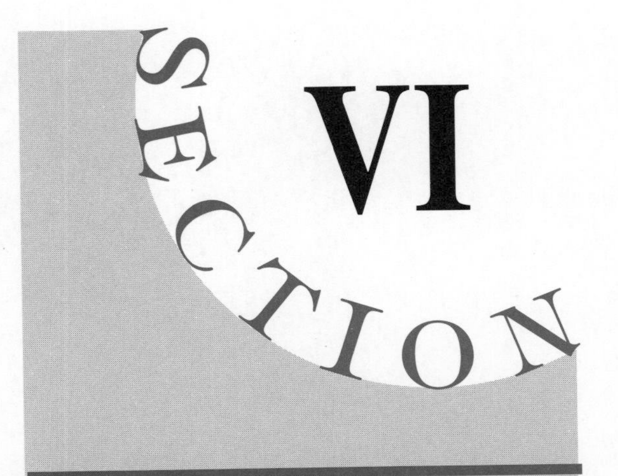

PLANT/ AGRICULTURAL BIOTECHNOLOGY

CONTENTS

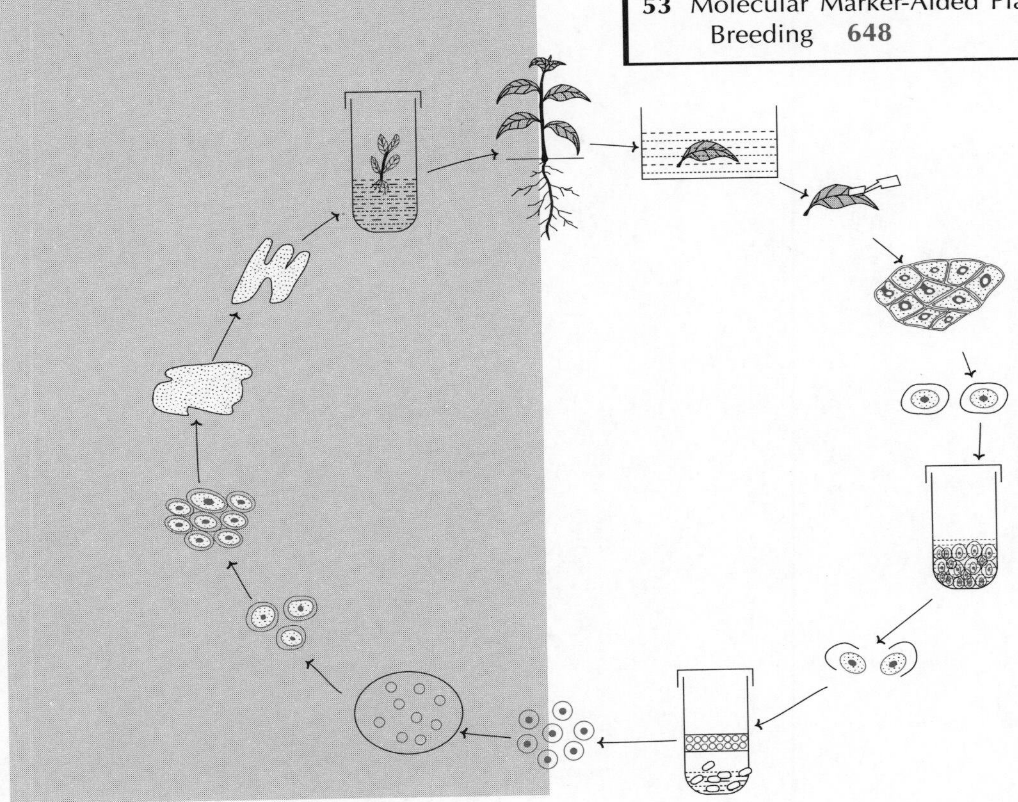

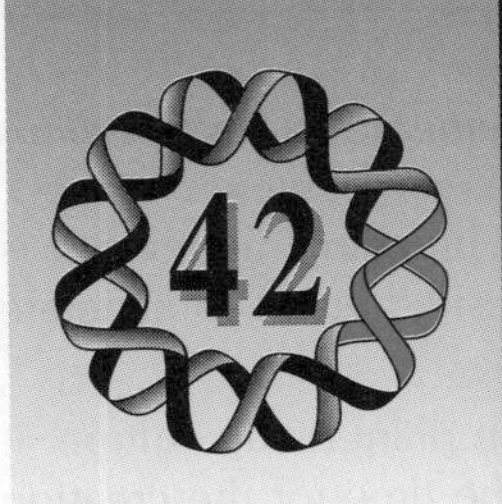

Plant Tissue Culture — General

PLANT TISSUE CULTURE
- Callus culture
- Organ culture (embryo, seed, anther, ovary, meristem, nucellus)
- Cell culture
- Protoplast culture

Plant tissue culture broadly refers to the ***in vitro* cultivation of plants, seeds and various parts of the plants** (organs, embryos, tissues, single cells, protoplasts). The cultivation process is invariably carried out in a nutrient culture medium under aseptic conditions.

Plant cells have certain advantages over animal cells in culture systems. Unlike animal cells, highly ***mature*** and differentiated ***plant cells retain the ability of totipotency*** i.e. the ability of change to meristematic state and differentiate into a whole plant.

BENEFITS OF PLANT TISSUE CULTURE

Plant tissue culture is one of the most rapidly growing areas of biotechnology because of its high potential to develop improved crops and ornamental plants. With the advances made in the tissue culture technology, it is now possible to regenerate species of any plant in the laboratory. To achieve the target of creating a new plant or a plant with desired characteristics, tissue culture is often coupled with recombinant DNA technology. The techniques of plant tissue culture have largely helped in the ***green revolution by improving the crop yield and quality***.

The knowledge obtained from plant tissue cultures has contributed to our understanding of metabolism, growth, differentiation and morphogenesis of plant cells. Further, developments in tissue culture have helped to produce several ***pathogen-free plants***, besides the ***synthesis of many biologically important compounds***, including pharmaceuticals. Because of the wide range of applications, plant tissue culture attracts the attention of molecular biologists, plant breeders and industrialists.

BASIC STRUCTURE AND GROWTH OF A PLANT

An adult plant basically consists of a stem and a root, each with many branches (***Fig. 42.1***). Both the stem and root are characterized by the presence of ***apical growth regions*** which are composed of ***meristematic cells***. These cells are the primary source for all the cell types of a plant.

The plant growth and development occur in two different ways.

1. **Determinate growth :** This is characterized by ceasation of growth as the plant parts attain certain size and shape. e.g., leaves, flowers, fruits.

2. **Indeterminate growth :** This refers to the continuous growth of roots and stems under suitable conditions. It is possible due to the presence of meristems (in stems and roots) which can proliferate continuously.

As the seed germinates and seedling emerges, the meristematic cells of the root apex multiply. Above the root apex, the cells grow in length without multiplication. Some of the elongated cells of the outer layer develop into root hairs to absorb

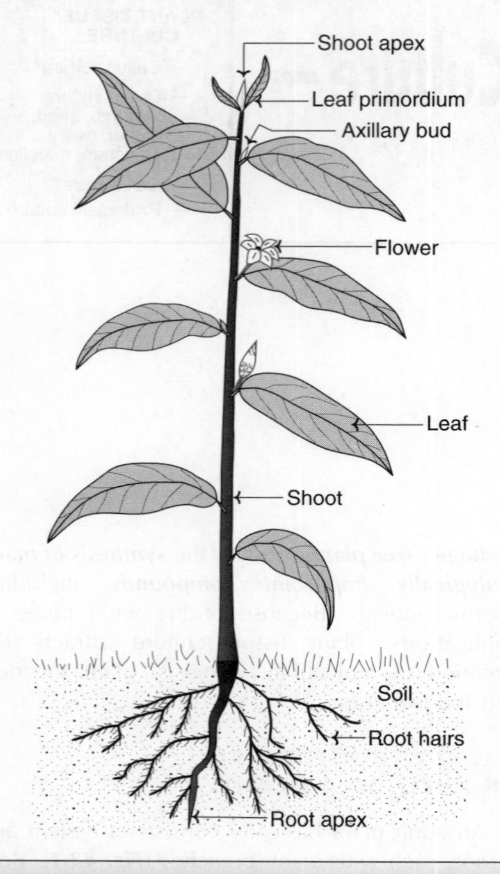

Fig. 42.1 : A diagrammatic view of a plant structure.

water and nutrients from the soil. As the plant grows, root cells differentiate into ***phloem*** and ***xylem***. Phloem is responsible for the absorption of nutrients while xylem absorbs water.

The meristematic cells of the shoot apex divide leading to the growth of stem. Some of the stem cells differentiate and develop into ***leaf primordia***, and then leaves. Axillary buds present between the leaf primordia and elongated stem also possess meristems which can multiply and give rise to branches and flowers.

A diagrammatic view of a plant and a flower are respectively depicted in ***Fig. 42.1*** and ***Fig. 42.2***.

CONVENTIONAL PLANT BREEDING AND PLANT TISSUE CULTURE

Since the time immemorial, man has been closely involved in the improvement of plants to meet his basic needs. The ***conventional*** methods employed for ***crop improvement are very tedious and long time processes*** (sometimes decades). Further, in the conventional breeding methods, it is not possible to introduce desired genes to generate new characters or products.

With the developments in plant tissue culture, it is now possible to reduce the time for the creation of new plants with desired characteristics, transfer of new genes into plant cells and large scale production of commercially important products.

TERMS USED IN TISSUE CULTURE

A selected list of the most commonly used terms in tissue culture are briefly explained

Explant : An excised piece of differentiated tissue or organ is regarded as an explant. The explant may be taken from any part of the plant body e.g., leaf, stem, root.

Callus : The unorganized and undifferentiated mass of plant cells is referred to as callus. Generally, when plant cells are cultured in a suitable medium, they divide to form callus i.e., a mass of parenchymatous cells.

Dedifferentiation : The phenomenon of mature cells reverting to meristematic state to produce callus is dedifferentiation.

Dedifferentiation is possible since the non-dividing quiescent cells of the explant, when grown

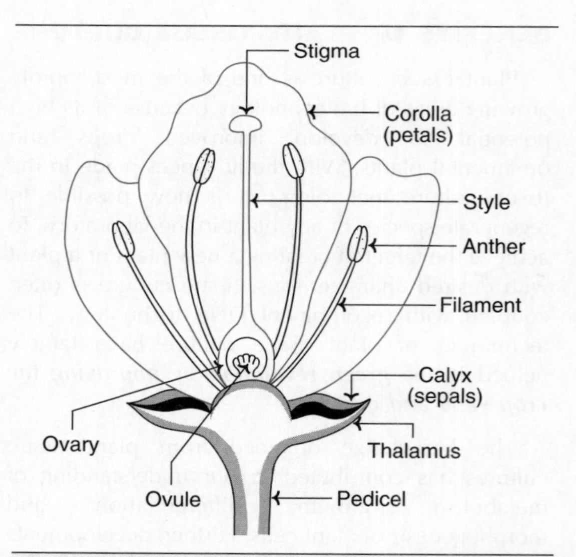

Fig. 42.2 : A diagrammatic representation of important parts in a flower.

in a suitable culture medium revert to meristematic state.

Redifferentiation : The ability of the callus cells to differentiate into a plant organ or a whole plant is regarded as redifferentiation.

Totipotency : The ability of an individual cell to develop into a whole plant is referred to as cellular totipotency. The inherent characteristic features of plant cells namely dedifferentiation and redifferentiation are responsible for the phenomenon of totipotency.

The other terms used in plant tissue culture are explained at appropriate places.

BRIEF HISTORY OF PLANT TISSUE CULTURE

About 250 years ago (1756), Henri-Louis Duhamel du Monceau' demonstrated callus formation on the decorticated regions of elm plants. Many botanists regard this work as the forward for the discovery of plant tissue culture. In 1853, Trecul published pictures of callus formation in plants.

German botanist ***Gottlieb Haberlandt*** (1902), regarded as ***the father of plant tissue culture***, first developed the concept of *in vitro* cell culture. He was the first to culture isolated and fully differentiated plant cells in a nutrient medium.

During 1934–1940, three scientists namely Gautheret, White and Nobecourt largely contributed to the developments made in plant tissue culture.

Good progress and rapid developments occurred after 1940 in plant tissue culture techniques. Steward and Reinert (1959) first discovered somatic embryo production *in vitro*. Maheswari and Guha (1964) from India were the first to develop anther culture and poller culture for the production of haploid plants.

TYPES OF CULTURE

There are different types of plant tissue culture techniques, mainly based on the explant used (***Fig. 42.3***).

Callus culture

This involves the culture of differentiated tissue from explant which dedifferentiates *in vitro* to form callus.

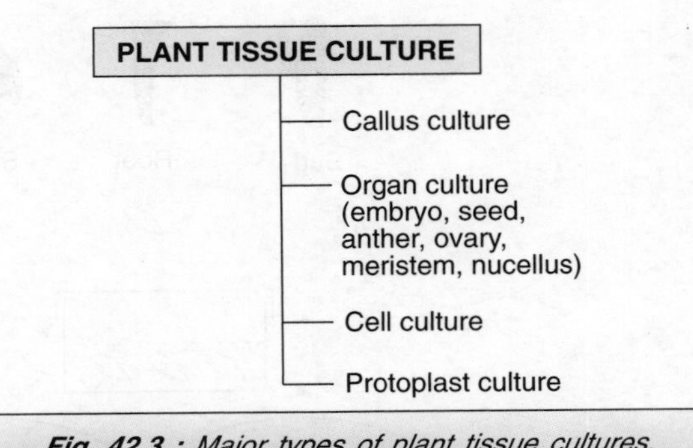

Fig. 42.3 : *Major types of plant tissue cultures.*

Organ culture

Culture of isolated plant organs is referred to as organ culture. The organ used may be embryo, seed, root, endosperm, anther, ovary, ovule, meristem (shoot tip) or nucellus.

The organ culture may be organized or unorganized.

Organized organ culture : When a well organized structure of a plant (seed, embryo) is used in culture, it is referred to as organized culture. In this type of culture, the characteristic individual organ structure is maintained and the progeny formed is similar in structure as that of the original organ.

Unorganized organ culture : This involves the isolation of cells or tissues of a part of the organ, and their culture *in vitro*. Unorganized culture results in the formation of callus. The callus can be dispersed into aggregates of cells and/or single cells to give a suspension culture.

Cell culture

The culture of isolated individual cells, obtained from an explant tissue or callus is regarded as cell culture. These cultures are carried out in dispension medium and are referred to as ***cell suspension cultures***.

Protoplast culture

Plant protoplasts (i.e., cells devoid of cell walls) are also used in the laboratory for culture.

BASIC TECHNIQUE OF PLANT TISSUE CULTURE

The general procedure adopted for isolation and culture of plant tissues is depicted in ***Fig. 42.4*** and briefly described in the next page.

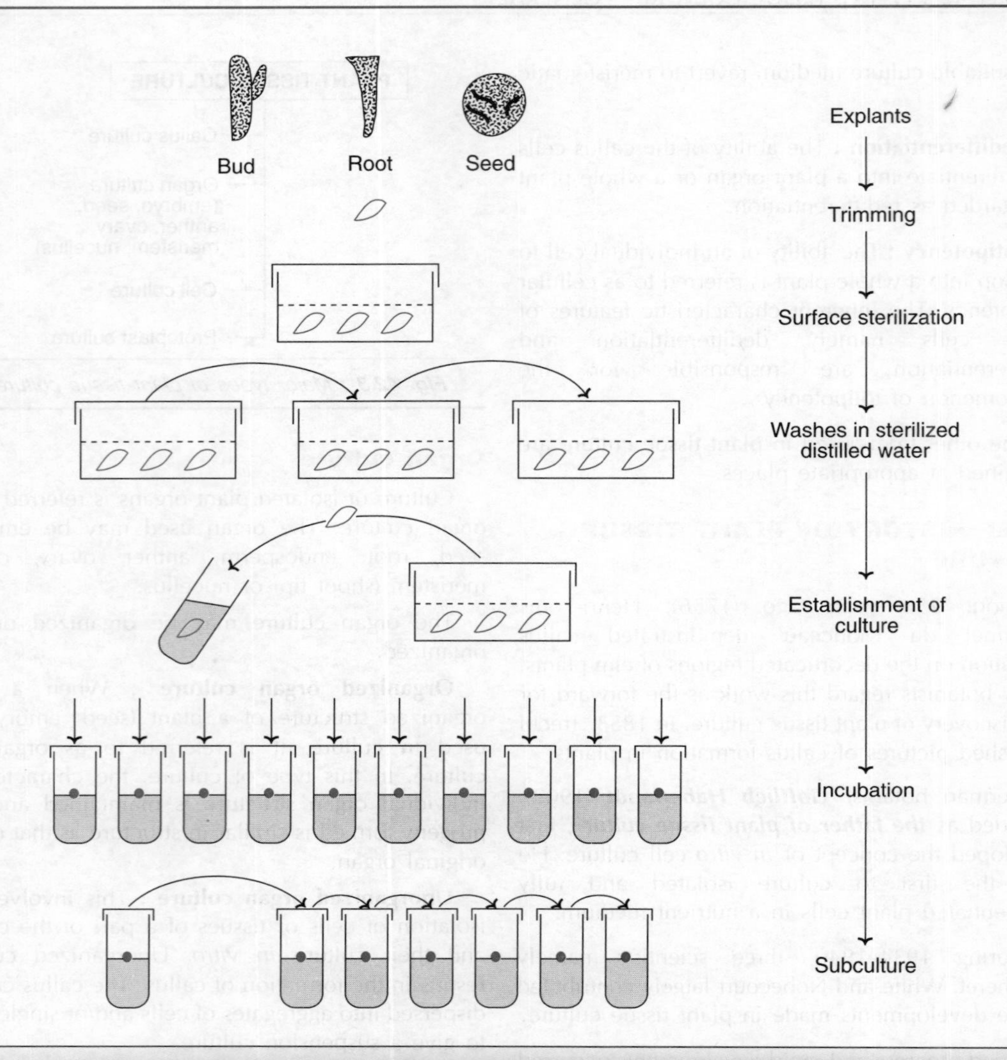

Fig. 42.4 : A diagrammatic outline of the basic procedure in plant tissue culture.

The requisite explants (buds, stem, seeds) are trimmed and then subjected to sterilization in a detergent solution. After washing in sterile distilled water, the explants are placed in a suitable culture medium (liquid or semisolid form) and incubated. This results in the establishment of culture. The mother cultures can be subdivided, as frequently as needed, to give daughter cultures.

The most important aspect of *in vitro* culture technique is to carry out all the operations under aseptic conditions. Bacteria and fungi are the most common contaminants in plant tissue culture. They grow much faster in culture and often kill the plant tissue. Further, the contaminants also produce certain compounds which are toxic to the plant tissue. Therefore, it is absolutely essential that ***aseptic conditions*** are maintained ***throughout the tissue culture operations***.

Some of the culture techniques are described here while a few others are discussed at appropriate places.

CALLUS CULTURE

Callus is the undifferentiated and unorganized mass of plant cells. It is basically a tumor tissue which usually forms on wounds of differentiated tissues or organs. Callus cells are parenchymatous in nature although not truely homogenous. On careful examination, callus is found to contain some quantity of differentiated tissue, besides the bulk of non-differentiated tissue.

Callus formation *in vivo* is frequently observed as a result of wounds at the cut edges of stems or roots. Invasion of microorganisms or damage by insect feeding usually occurs through callus.

An outline of technique used for callus culture, and initiation of suspension culture is depicted in *Fig. 42.5*.

Explants for callus culture

The starting materials (explants) for callus culture may be the differentiated tissue from any part of the plant (root, stem, leaf, anther, flower etc.). The selected explant tissues may be at different stages of cell division, cell proliferation and organization into different distinct specialized structures. If the explant used possesses meristematic cells, then the cell division and multiplication will be rapid.

Factors affecting callus culture

Many factors are known to influence callus formation in *in vitro* culture. These include the source of the explant and its genotype, composition of the medium (MS medium most commonly used), physical factors (temperature, light etc.) and growth factors. Other important factors affecting callus culture are — age of the plant, location of explant, physiology and growth conditions of the plant.

Physical factors : A temperature in the range of 22–28°C is suitable for adequate callus formation. As regards the effect of light on callus, it is largely dependent on the plant species-light may be essential for some plants while darkness is required by others.

Growth regulators : The growth regulators to the medium strongly influence callus formation. Based on the nature of the explant and its genotype, and the endogenous content of the hormone, the requirements of growth regulators may be categorized into 3 groups

1. Auxin alone
2. Cytokinin alone
3. Both auxin and cytokinin.

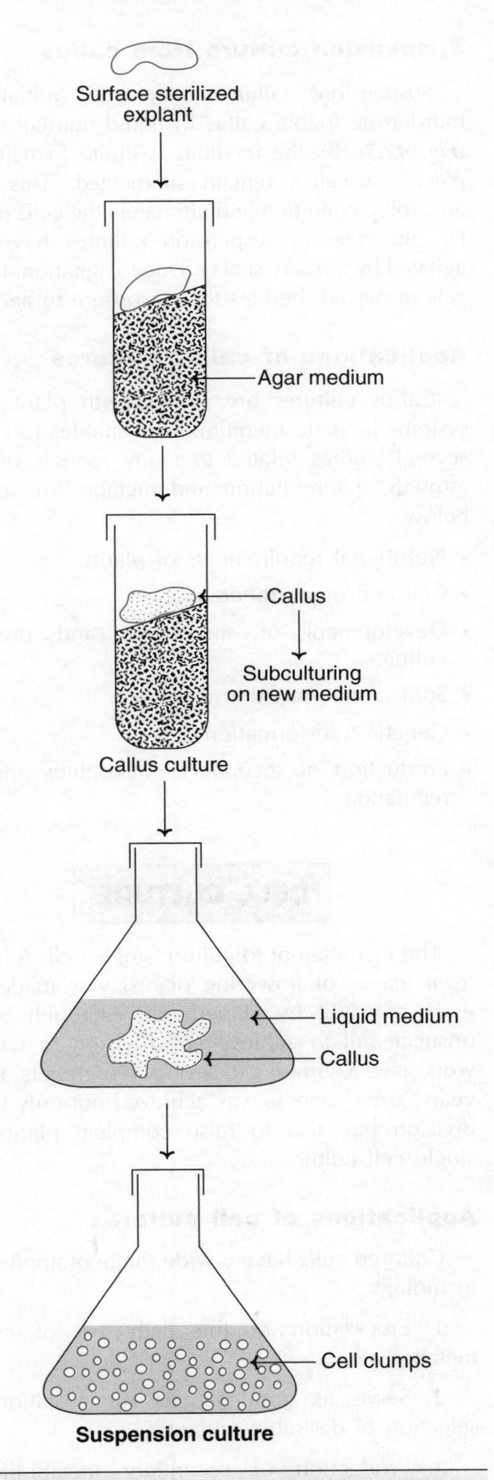

Fig. 42.5 : A diagrammatic representation of callus culture and initiation of suspension culture.

Suspension culture from callus

Suspension cultures can be initiated by transferring friable callus to liquid nutrient medium (*Fig. 42.5*). As the medium is liquid in nature, the pieces of callus remain submerged. This creates anaerobic condition and ultimately the cells may die. For this reason, suspension cultures have to be agitated by a rotary shaker. Due to agitation, the cells gets dispersed, besides their exposure to aeration.

Applications of callus cultures

Callus cultures are slow-growth plant culture systems in static medium. This enables to conduct several studies related to many aspects of plants (growth, differentiation and metabolism) as listed below.

- Nutritional requirements of plants.
- Cell and organ differentiation.
- Development of suspension and protoplast cultures.
- Somaclonal variations.
- Genetic transformations.
- Production of secondary metabolites and their regulation.

CELL CULTURE

The first attempt to culture single cells (obtained from leaves of flowering plants) was made in as early as 1902 by Haberlandt. Although he was unsuccessful to achieve cell division *in vitro*, his work gave a stimulus to several researchers. In later years, good success was achieved not only for cell division but also to raise complete plants from single cell cultures.

Applications of cell cultures

Cultured cells have a wide range of applications in biology.

1. Elucidation of the pathways of cellular metabolism.

2. Serve as good targets for mutation and selection of desirable mutants.

3. Production of secondary metabolites of commercial interest.

4. Good potential for crop improvement.

For more detailed information on the application of cell cultures, See p. 506.

Cell culture technique

The *in vitro* cell culture technique broadly involves the following aspects :

1. Isolation of single cells.
2. Suspension cultures growth and subculturing.
3. Types of suspension cultures.
4. Synchronization of suspension cultures.
5. Measurement of growth of cultures.
6. Measurement of viability of cultured cells.

The salient features of the above steps are briefly described.

ISOLATION OF SINGLE CELLS

The cells employed for *in vitro* culture may be obtained from plant organs, and from cultured tissues.

From plant organs : Plant leaves with homogenous population of cells are the ideal sources for cell culture. Single cells can be isolated from leaves by mechanical or enzymatic methods.

Mechanical method : Surface sterilized leaves are cut into small pieces (< 1 cm^2), suspended in a medium and subjected to grinding in a glass homogeniser tube. The homogenate is filtered through filters and then centrifuged at a low speed to remove the cellular debris. The supernatant is removed and diluted to achieve the required cell density.

Enzymatic method : The enzyme ***macerozyme*** (under suitable osmotic pressure) can release the individual cells from the leaf tissues. Macerozyme degrades middle lamella and cell walls of parenchymatous tissues.

From cultured tissues : Single cells can be isolated from callus cultures (grown from cut pieces of surface sterilized plant parts). Repeated subculturing of callus on agar medium improves the friability of callus so that fine cell suspensions are obtained.

SUSPENSION CULTURES — GROWTH AND SUBCULTURE

The isolated cells are grown in suspension cultures. Cell suspensions are maintained by routine subculturing in a fresh medium. For this purpose, the cells are picked up in the early stationary phase and transferred.

As the cells are incubated in suspension cultures, the cells divide and enlarge. The incubation period is dependent on :

- Initial cell density
- Duration of lag phase
- Growth rate of cells.

Among these, cell density is very crucial. The initial cell density used in the subcultures is very critical, and largely depends on the type of suspension culture being maintained. With low initial cell densities, the lag phase and log phases of growth get prolonged. Whenever a new suspension culture is started, it is necessary to determine the optical cell density in relation the volume of culture medium, so that maximum cell growth can be achieved. With low cell densities, the culture will not grow well, and requires additional supplementation of metabolites to the medium.

The normal incubation time for the suspension cultures is in the range of 21–28 days.

TYPES OF SUSPENSION CULTURES

There are mainly two types of suspension cultures — batch cultures and continuous cultures.

Batch cultures

A batch culture is a cell suspension culture ***grown in a fixed volume of nutrient culture medium***. In batch culture, cell division and cell growth coupled with increase in biomass occur until one of the factors in the culture environment (nutrient, O_2 supply) becomes limiting. The cells exhibit the following five phases of growth when the cell number in suspension cultures is plotted against the time of incubation (***Fig. 42.6***).

1. ***Lag phase*** characterized by preparation of cells to divide.

2. ***Log phase*** (exponential phase) where the rate of cell multiplication is highest.

3. ***Linear phase*** represented by slowness in cell division and increase in cell size expansion.

4. ***Deceleration phase*** characterized by decrease in cell division and cell expansion.

5. ***Stationary phase*** represented by a constant number of cells and their size.

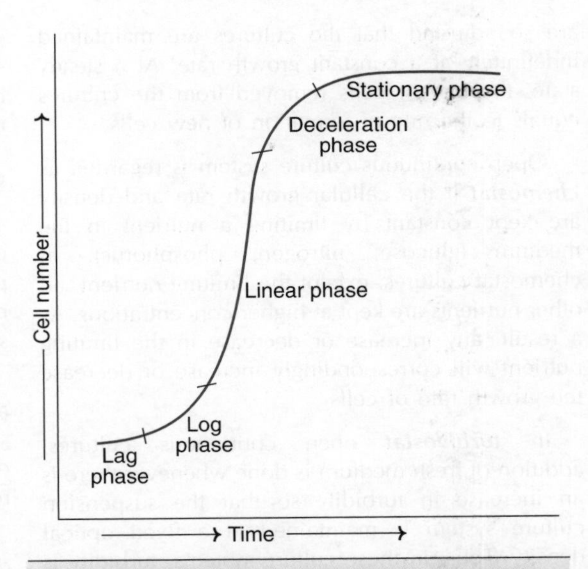

Fig. 42.6 : A graphic representation of different phases of batch suspension culture.

The batch cultures can be maintained continuously by transferring small amounts of the suspension medium (with inoculum) to fresh medium at regular intervals (2-3 days).

Batch cultures are characterized by a constant change in the pattern of cell growth and metabolism. For this reason, these cultures are not ideally suited for the studies related to cellular behaviour.

Continuous cultures

In continuous cultures, there is a regular ***addition of fresh nutrient medium and draining out the used medium*** so that the culture volume is normally constant. These cultures are carried out in specially designed culture vessels (bioreactors).

Continuous cultures are carried out under defined and controlled conditions—cell density, nutrients, O_2, pH etc. The cells in these cultures are mostly at an exponential phase (log phase) of growth.

Continuous cultures are of two types—open and closed.

Open continuous cultures : In these cultures, the inflow of fresh medium is balanced with the outflow of the volume of spent medium along with the cells. The addition of fresh medium and culture harvest are so adjusted that the cultures are maintained indefinitely at a constant growth rate. At a steady state, the rate of cells removed from the cultures equals to the rate of formation of new cells.

Open continuous culture system is regarded as ***chemostat*** if the cellular growth rate and density are kept constant by limiting a nutrient in the medium (glucose, nitrogen, phosphorus). In chemostat cultures, except the limiting nutrient, all other nutrients are kept at higher concentrations. As a result, any increase or decrease in the limiting nutrient will correspondingly increase or decrease the growth rate of cells.

In ***turbidostat*** open continuous cultures, addition of fresh medium is done whenever there is an increase in turbidity so that the suspension culture system is maintained at a fixed optical density. Thus, in these culture systems, turbidity is preselected on the basis of biomass density in cultures, and they are maintained by intermittent addition of medium and washout of cells.

Closed continuous cultures : In these cultures, the cells are retained while the inflow of fresh medium is balanced with the outflow of corresponding spent medium. The cells present in the outflowing medium are separated (mechanically) and added back to the culture system. As a result, there is a continuous increase in the biomass in closed continuous cultures. These cultures are useful for studies related to cytodifferentiation, and for the production of certain secondary metabolites e.g., polysaccharides, coumarins.

SYNCHRONIZATION OF SUSPENSION CULTURES

In the normal circumstances, the cultured plant cells vary greatly in size, shape, cell cycle etc., and are said to be ***asynchronous***. Due to variations in the cells, they are not suitable for genetic, biochemical and physiological studies. For these reasons, synchronization of cells assumes significance.

Synchronization of cultured cells broadly refers to the ***organized existence of majority of cells in the same cell cycle phase simultaneously***.

A synchronous culture may be regarded as a culture in which the cell cycles or specific phase of cycles for majority of cultured cells occur simultaneously.

Several methods are in use to bring out synchronization of suspension cultures. They may be broadly divided into physical and chemical methods.

Physical methods

The environmental culture growth influencing physical parameters (light, temperature) and the physical properties of the cell (size) can be carefully monitored to achieve reasonably good degree of synchronization. A couple of them are described

Cold treatment : When the suspension cultures are subjected to low temperature (around 4°C) shock synchronization occurs. Cold treatment in combination with nutrient starvation gives better results.

Selection by volume : The cells in suspension culture can be selected based on the size of the aggregates, and by this approach, cell synchronization can be achieved.

Chemical methods

The chemical methods for synchronization of suspension cultures include the use of chemical inhibitors, and deprivation of an essential growth factor (nutrient starvation). By this approach, the ***cell cycle can be arrested at a particular stage***, and then allowed to occur simultaneously so that synchronization is achieved.

Chemical inhibition : Inhibitors of DNA synthesis (5-aminouracil, hydroxyurea, 5-fluorodeoxypurine), when added to the cultures results in the accumulation of cells at G_1 phase. And on removal of the inhibitor, synchronization of cell division occurs.

Colchicine is a strong inhibitor to arrest the growth of cells at metaphase. It inhibits spindle formation during the metaphase stage of cell division. Exposure to colchicine must be done for a short period (during the exponential growth phase), as long duration exposure may lead to mitoses.

Starvation : When an essential nutrient or growth promoting compound is deprived in suspension cultures, this results in stationary growth phase. On supplementation of the missing nutrient compound, cell growth resumption occurs synchronously. Some workers have reported that deprivation and subsequent addition of growth hormone also induces synchronization of cell cultures.

MEASUREMENT OF GROWTH OF CULTURES

It is necessary to assess the growth of cells in cultures. The parameters selected for the measuring growth of suspension cultures include cell counting, packed cell volume and weight increase.

Cell counting

Although cell counting to assess culture growth is reasonably accurate, it is tedious and time consuming. This is because cells in suspension culture mostly exist as colonies in varying sizes. These cells have to be first disrupted (by treating with pectinase or chromic acid), separated, and then ***counted using a haemocytometer***.

Packed cell volume

Packed cell volume (PCV) is expressed as ***ml of pellet per ml of culture***. To determine PCV, a measured volume of suspension culture is centrifuged (usually at 2000 xg for 5 minutes) and the volume of the pellet or packed cell volume is recorded.

After centrifugation the supernatant can be discarded, the pellet washed, dried overnight and weighed. This gives ***cell dry weight***.

Cell fresh weight

The wet cells are collected on a preweighed nylon fabric filter (supported in funnel). They are washed to remove the medium, drained under vacuum and weighed. This gives the fresh weight of cells. However, ***large samples have to be used*** for accurate weights.

MEASUREMENT OF VIABILITY OF CULTURED CELLS

The viability of cells is the most important factor for the growth of cells. Viability of cultured cells can be measured by microscopic examination of cells directly or after staining them.

Phase contrast microscopy

The viable cells can be detected by the presence of healthy nuclei. Phase contrast microscope is used for this purpose.

Evan's blue staining

A dilute solution of Evan's blue (0.025% w/v) dye ***stains the dead or damaged cells*** while the living (viable) cells remain unstained.

Fluorescein diacetate method

When the cell suspension is incubated with fluorescein diacetate (***FDA***) at a final concentration of 0.01%, it is cleaved by esterase enzyme of living cells. As a result, the polar portion of fluorescein which emits green fluoroscence under ultraviolet (UV) light is released. The ***viable cells can be detected by their fluoroscence***, since fluorescein accumulates in the living cells only.

CULTURE OF ISOLATED SINGLE CELLS (SINGLE CELL CLONES)

A ***clone is a mass of cells***, all of them ***derived*** through mitosis ***from a single cell***. The cells of the clone are expected to be identical with regard to genotype and karyotype. However, changes in these cells may occur after cloning. Single cells separated from plant tissues under suitable conditions can form clones.

The various methods for the isolation of single cells have already been described (See p. 502). Single cells can be cultured by the following methods :

1. Filter paper raft-nurse tissue technique
2. Microchamber technique
3. Microdrop method
4. Bergman's plating technique.

Filter paper raft-nurse tissue technique

Small pieces of sterile filter papers are placed on established callus cultures several days before the start of single cell culture. Single cell is now placed on the filter paper (***Fig. 42.7A***). This filter paper, wetted by the exudates from callus tissue (by diffusion) supplies the nutrients to the single cell. The ***cell divides and forms clonies on the filter paper***. These colonies can be isolated and cultured.

Microchamber technique

A microscopic ***slide or a coverslip can be used to create a microchamber***. Sometimes, a cavity

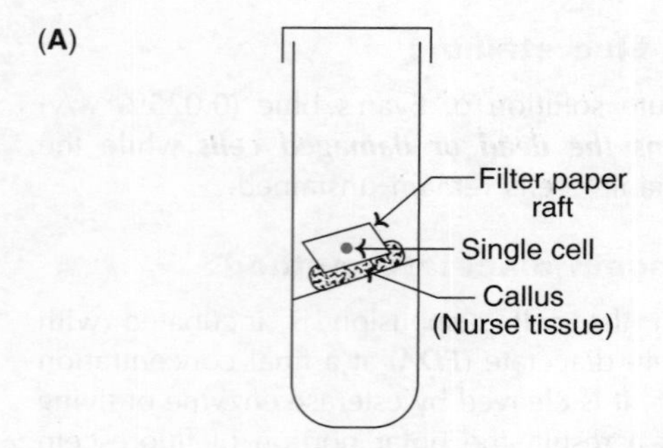

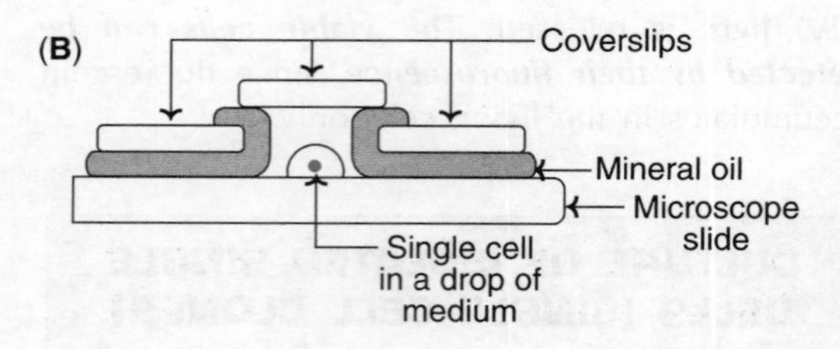

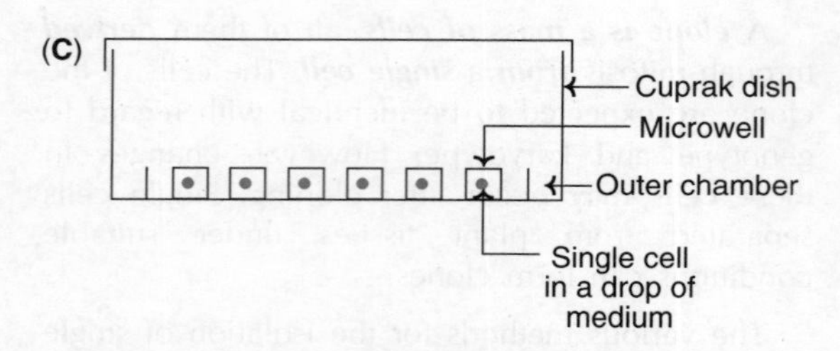

Fig. 42.7 : Techniques for the culture of single cells (A) Filter paper raft-nurse tissue technique (B) Microchamber technique (side view), (C) Microdrop method (Refer Fig. 42.8 for Bergmann's plating technique).

slide can be directly used. A drop of the medium containing a single cell is placed in the microchamber. A drop of mineral oil is placed on either side of the culture drop which is covered with a coverslip (***Fig. 42.7B***). On incubation, single cell colonies are formed.

Microdrop method

For the culture of single cells by microdrop method, a specially designed dish (cuprak dish) is used. It has a small outer chamber (to be filled with sterile distilled water) and a large inner chamber with a number of microwells (***Fig. 42.7C***). The cell density of the medium is adjusted in such a way that it contains one cell per droplet.

Bergmann's plating technique

Bergmann (1960) developed a technique for cloning of single cells. Now a days, Bergmann's plating technique is the ***most widely used method*** for culture of isolated single cells. This method is depicted in ***Fig. 42.8*** and briefly described hereunder.

The cell suspension is filtered through a sieve to obtain single cells in the filtrate. The free cells are suspended in a liquid medium, at a density twice than the required density for cell plating. Now, equal volumes of melted agar (30–35°C) and medium containing cells are mixed. The agar medium with single cells is poured and spread out in a petridish so that the cells are evenly distributed on a thin layer (of agar after it solidifies). The petridishes (culture dishes) are sealed with a parafilm and incubated at 25°C in dark or diffused light. The single cells divide and develop into clones.

The viability of cells in single clones can be measured by the same techniques that have been described for suspension cultures.

APPLICATIONS OF PLANT TISSUE CULTURES

Plant tissue cultures are associated with a wide range of applications—the most important being the ***production of pharmaceutical, medicinal and other industrially important compounds***. In addition, tissue cultures are useful for several other purposes listed below.

1. To study the respiration and metabolism of plants.
2. For the evaluation of organ functions in plants.
3. To study the various plant diseases and work out methods for their elimination.
4. Single cell clones are useful for genetic, morphological and pathological studies.
5. Embryonic cell suspensions can be used for ***large scale clonal propagation***.
6. Somatic embryos from cell suspensions can be stored for long term in germplasm banks.
7. In the production of variant clones with new characteristics, a phenomenon referred to as ***somaclonal variations***.

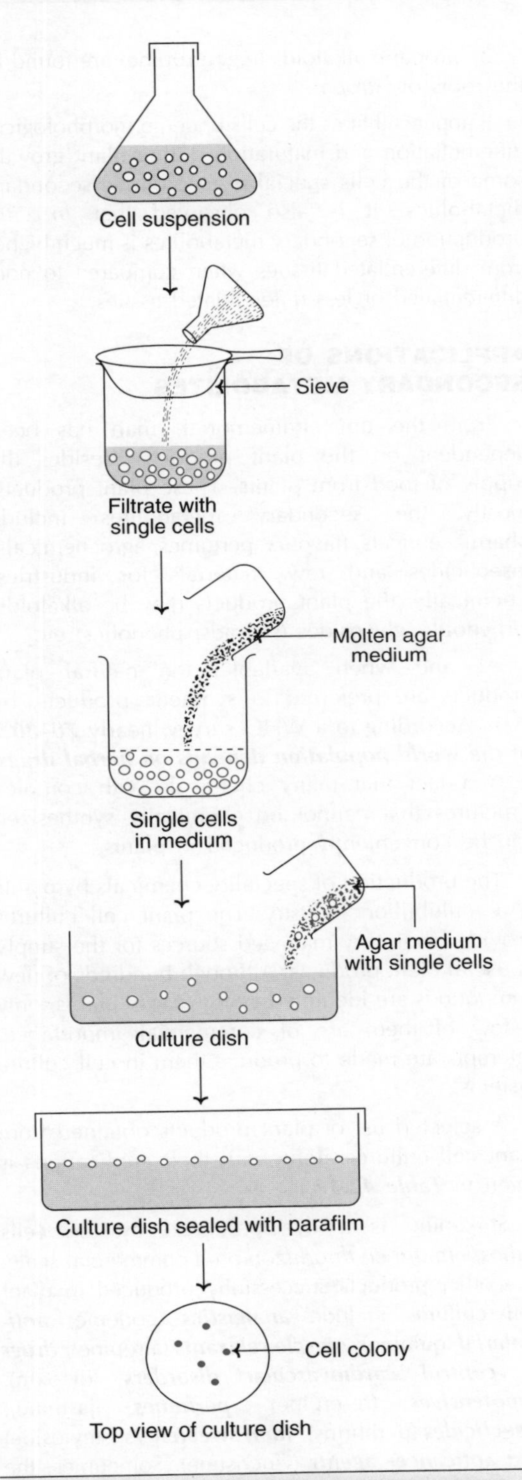

Fig. 42.8 : A diagrammatic representation of Bergmann's cell plating technique.

8. ***Production of haploids*** (with a single set of chromosomes) for improving crops.

9. Mutant cells can be selected from cultures and used for crop improvement.

10. Immature embryos can be cultured *in vitro* to produce hybrids, a process referred to ***as embryo rescue***.

SECONDARY METABOLITES IN PLANT CULTURES

The chemical compounds produced by plants are collectively referred to as ***phytochemicals***. Biotechnologists have special interest in plant tissue culture for the large scale production of commercially important compounds. These include pharmaceuticals, flavours, fragrances, cosmetics, food additives, feedstocks and antimicrobials. Most of these products are ***secondary metabolites—chemical compounds that do not participate in metabolism of plants***. Thus, secondary metabolites are not directly needed by plants as they do not perform any physiological function (as is the case with primary metabolites such as amino acids, nucleic acids etc.).

Although the native plants are capable of producing the secondary metabolites of commercial interest, tissue culture systems are preferred. The advantages and limitations are listed.

Major advantages

1. Compounds can be produced under controlled conditions as per market demands.

2. Culture systems are ***independent of environmental factors***, seasonal variations, pest and microbial diseases and geographical constraints.

3. Cell growth can be controlled to facilitate improved product formation.

4. The quality of the product will be consistent as it is produced by a specific cell line.

5. Recovery of the product will be easy.

6. Plant cultures are particularly useful in case of plants which are difficult or expensive to be grown in the fields.

7. Mutant cell lines can be developed for the ***production of novel compounds*** of commercial importance, which are not normally found in plants.

8. Biotransformation reactions (converting specific substrates to valuable products) can be carried out with certain cultured cells.

9. The production control is not at the mercy of political interference.

10. The production time is less and labour costs are minimal.

Considering the advantages listed above, ***about 25–30% of medicines for human use***, and the various chemical materials for industrial purposes are ***obtained from plant tissue cultures***. In general, tissue culture production of natural materials is cheaper compared to synthetic production. However, there are certain limitations associated with tissue cultures.

Limitations/disadvantages

1. In general, ***in vitro production of secondary metabolites is lower*** when compared to intact plants.

2. Many a times, secondary metabolites are formed in differentiated tissues/organs. In such a case, culture cells which are non-differentiated can produce little.

3. ***Cultured cells are genetically unstable and may undergo mutation***. The production of secondary metabolite may be drastically reduced, as the culture ages.

4. Vigorous stirring is necessary to prevent aggregation of cultured cells. This may often damage the cells.

5. Strict aseptic conditions have to be maintained during culture technique. Any infection to the culture adversely affects product formation.

Why do plants produce secondary metabolites?

Based on the existing evidence, it is believed that the production of some secondary metabolites is linked to the induction of morphological differentiation.

Consider the following examples

1. Cardiac glycosides are found in the leaves of *Digitalis*.

2. Quinine and quinidine are present in the bark of *Cinchona*.

3. Tropane alkaloids (e.g. atropine) are found in the roots of *Atropa*.

It appears that as the cells undergo morphological differentiation and maturation during plant growth, some of the cells specialise to produce secondary metabolites. It is also observed that *in vitro* production of secondary metabolites is much higher from differentiated tissues when compared to non-differentiated or less differentiated tissues.

APPLICATIONS OF SECONDARY METABOLITES

From the time immemorial, man has been dependent on the plant products, besides the supply of food from plants. These plant products, mostly the secondary metabolites include pharmaceuticals, flavours, perfumes, agrochemicals, insecticides and raw materials for industries. Chemically, the plant products may be alkaloids, terpenoids, glycosides (steroids, phenolics) etc.

As and when available, the natural plant products are preferred to synthetic products, by man. According to a WHO survey, nearly ***70–80% of the world population depends on herbal drugs***. It is a fact that many chemicals with complex structures that cannot be chemically synthesized can be conveniently produced in plants.

The production of speciality chemicals by plants is a multibillion industry. The plant cell cultures provide laboratory managed sources for the supply of useful plant products. Although hundreds of new compounds are identified every year in plants, only a few of them are of commercial importance. Attempts are made to produce them in cell culture systems.

A selected list of plant products obtained from plant cell cultures along with their applications is given in ***Table 42.1***.

Shikonine is a dye produced by the cells *Lithospermum erythrorhizon* on a commercial scale. The other products successfully produced in plant cell cultures include ***analgistics*** (codeine) ***anti-malarial*** (quinine), ***muscle relaxants*** (atropine), ***drugs to control cardiovascular disorders*** (digoxin), ***hypotensives*** (reserpine), ***perfumes*** (jasmine), ***insecticides*** (pyrithrins), ***food sweeteners*** (stevioside) and ***anticancer agents*** (vincristine). Sometimes, the cost of the plant products is unimaginably high. For instance, one kg of vincristine and vinblastine respectively cost \$ 3,500,00 and \$ 1,000,000!

TABLE 42.1 A selected list of secondary metabolites obtained from plant cell cultures along with their application(s)

Product	*Plant species*	*Uses*
Shikonine	*Lithospermum erythrorhizon*	Dye, pharmaceutical
Codeine, morphine	*Papaver somniferum*	Analgistic
Quinine	*Cinchona officinalis*	Antimalarial
Atropine	*Atropa belladonna*	Muscle relaxant
Digoxin	*Digitalis lanata*	Cardiovascular disorders
Reserpine	*Rauwolfia serpentina*	Hypotensive
Diosgenin	*Dioscorea deltoidea*	Antifertility
Vanillin	*Vanilla* sp	Vanilla
Jasmine	*Jasmium* sp	Perfume
Vinblastine, ajmalicine, vincristine	*Catharanthus roseus*	Anticancer
Taxol	*Taxus brevifolia*	Anticancer
Baccharine	*Baccharis megapotanica*	Anticancer
Cesaline	*Caesalpinia gillisesii*	Anticancer
Fagaronine	*Fagara zanthoxyloides*	Anticaner
Maytansine	*Maytenus bucchananii*	Anticancer
Harring tonine	*Cephalotaxus harringtonia*	Anticancer
Thalicarpine	*Thalictrum dasycarpum*	Anticancer
Ellipticine, 3-deoxycolchine	*Ochrosia moorei*	Anticancer
Pyrithrins	*Tagetus erecta* *Chrysanthemum cincerariefolium*	Insecticide
Rotenoids	*Derris elliptica* *Tephrosia* sp	Insecticide
Nicotine	*Nicotiana tabacum* *Nicotiana rustica*	Insecticide
Saffron	*Crocus sativus*	Food colour and flavouring agent
Stevioside	*Stevia rabaudiana*	Sweetener
Thaumatin	*Thaumatococcus damielli*	Sweetener
Capsaicin	*Capsicum frutesus*	Chilli
Rosamarinic acid	*Coleus blunei*	Spice, antioxidant
Anthraquinones	*Morinda citrifolia*	Laxative, dye
Berberine	*Coptis japonica*	Antibacterial
Sarcoplasmine (hyoscine)	*Datura stramonium*	Treatment of nausea

PRODUCTION OF SECONDARY METABOLITES

The process of *in vitro* culture of cells for the large scale production of secondary metabolites is complex, and involves the following aspects

1. Selection of cell lines for high yield of secondary metabolites.
2. Large scale cultivation of plant cells.
3. Medium composition and effect of nutrients.
4. Elicitor-induced production of secondary metabolites.
5. Effect of environmental factors.
6. Biotransformation using plant cell cultures.
7. Secondary metabolite release and analysis.

SELECTION OF CELL LINES FOR HIGH YIELD OF SECONDARY METABOLITES

The very purpose of tissue culture is to produce high amounts of secondary metabolites. However, in general, majority of callus and suspension cultures produce less quantities of secondary metabolites. This is mainly due to the lack of fully differentiated cells in the cultures. Some special techniques have been devised to select cell lines that can produce higher amounts of desired metabolites. These methods are ultimately useful for the ***separation of producer cells from the non-producer cells***. The techniques commonly employed for cell line selection are cell cloning, visual or chemical analysis and selection for resistance.

Cell cloning

This is a simple procedure and involves the growth of single cells (taken from a suspension cultures) in a suitable medium. Each cell population is then screened for the secondary metabolite formation. And only those cells with high-yielding ability are selected and maintained by subcloning.

Single cell cloning : There are certain practical difficulties in the isolation and culture of single cells.

Cell aggregate cloning : Compared to single cell cloning, cell aggregate cloning is much easier, hence preferred by many workers.

A schematic representation of cell aggregate cloning for the selection of cells yielding high quantities of secondary metabolites is given in *Fig. 42.9*. A high yielding plant of the desired metabolite is selected and its explants are first cultured on a solid medium. After establishing the callus cultures, high metabolite producing calluses are identified, and they are grown in suspension cultures. Cell aggregates from these cultures are grown on solid medium. The freshly developed cell aggregates (calluses) are divided into two parts. One half is grown further, while the other half is used for the quantitative analysis of the desired metabolite produced. The cell lines with high yield of secondary metabolites are selected and used for scale-up in suspension cultures. This is followed by large scale tissue culture in a bioreactor.

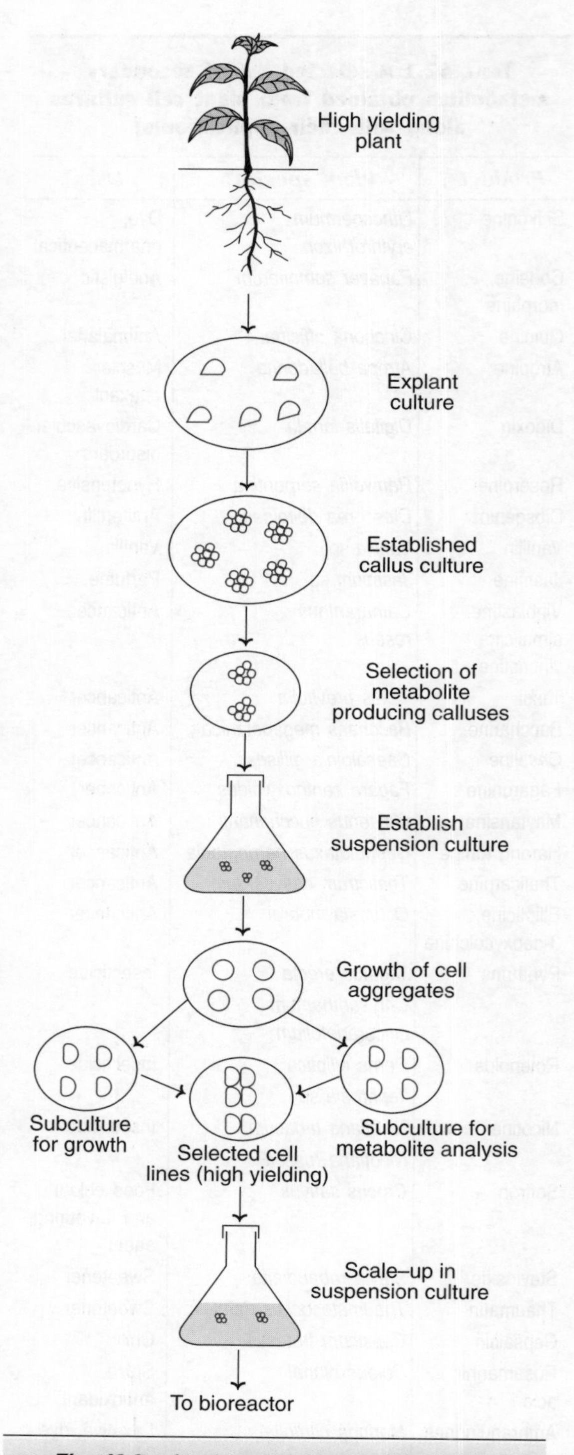

Fig. 42.9 : A schematic representation of cell aggregate cloning for the selection of high yielding cell lines.

Visual or chemical analysis

A direct measurement of some of the secondary metabolites produced by cell lines can be done either by visual or chemical analysis.

Visual identification of cell lines producing ***coloured secondary metabolites*** (pigments e.g., β-carotene, shikonin) will help ***in the selection*** of high-yielding cells. This method is quite simple and non-destructive. The major limitation is that the desired metabolite should be coloured.

Certain secondary metabolites emit fluorescence under UV light, and the corresponding clones can be identified.

Some workers use simple, sensitive and inexpensive chemical analytical methods for quantitative estimation of desired metabolites. Analysis is carried out in some colonies derived from single cell cultures. Radioimmunoassay is the most commonly used analytical method. Microspectrophotometry and fluorescent antibody techniques are also in use.

Selection for resistance

Certain cells resistant to toxic compounds may lead to the ***formation of mutant cells*** which can overproduce a primary metabolite, and then a secondary metabolite. Such mutants can be selected and used to produce the desired metabolite in large quantities. One example is described.

Cell lines selected for resistance of 5-methyl-tryptophan (analogue of tryptophan) produce strains which can overproduce tryptophan. These tryptophan overproducing strains can synthesize 10–50 times higher levels of the natural auxin namely indole acetic acid (**Note :** The secondary metabolite indole acetic acid is derived from the primary metabolite tryptophan).

LARGE SCALE (MASS) CULTIVATION OF PLANT CELLS

In order to achieve industrial production of the desired metabolite, large scale cultivation of plant cells is required. Plant cells (20–150 μm in diameter) are generally 10–100 times larger than bacterial or fungal cell. When cultured, plant cells exhibit changes in volumes and thus variable shapes and sizes. Further, cultured cells have low growth rate and genetic instability. All these aspects have to be considered for mass cultivation of cells. The following four different culture systems are widely used

1. Free-cell suspension culture
2. Immobilized cell culture
3. Two-phase system culture
4. Hairy root culture.

Free-cell suspension culture

Mass cultivation of plant cells is most frequently carried out by cell suspension cultures. Care should be taken to achieve good growth rate of cells and efficient formation of the desired secondary metabolite. Many specially designed bioreactors are in use for free-cell suspension cultures. Some of these are listed below :

- Batch bioreactors
- Continuous bioreactors
- Multistage bioreactors
- Airlift bioreactors
- Stirred tank bioreactors.

Two important aspects have to be considered for good success of suspension cultures.

1. Adequate and continuous oxygen supply.

2. Minimal generation of hydrodynamic stresses due to aeration agitation.

Immobilized cell cultures

Plant cells can be made immobile or immovable and used in culture systems. The cells are physically immobilized by entrapment. Besides individual cells, it is also possible to immobilize aggregate cells or even calluses. Homogenous suspensions of cells are most suitable for immobilization.

Surface immobilized plant cell (SIPC) technique efficiently retains the cells and allows them to ***grow at a higher rate***. Further, through immobilization, there is better cell-to-cell contact, and the cells are protected from high liquid shear stresses. All this helps in the maximal production the secondary metabolite.

The common methods adopted for entrapment of cells are briefly described.

1. **Entrapment of cells in gels :** The cells or the protoplasts can be entrapped in several gels e.g., alginate, agar, agarose, carrageenin. The gels may be used either individually or in combination. The techniques employed for the immobilization of plant cells are comparable to those used for immobilization of microorganisms or other cells (Refer Chapter 21).

2. **Entrapment of cells in nets or foams :** Polyurethane foams or nets with various pore sizes are used. The actively growing plant cells in suspension can be immobilized on these foams. The cells divide within the compartments of foam and form aggregates.

3. **Entrapment of cells in hollow-fibre membranes :** Tubular hollow fibres composed of cellulose acetate silicone polycarbonate and organized into parallel bundles are used for immobilization of cells. It is possible to entrap cells within and between the fibres.

Membrane entrapment is mechanically stable. However, it is more expensive than gel or foam immobilization.

Bioreactors for use of immobilized cells

Fluidized bed or fixed bed bioreactors are employed to use immobilized cells for large scale cultivation.

In the fluidized-bed reactors, the immobilized cells are agitated by a flow of air or by pumping the medium. In contrast, in the fixed-bed bioreactor, the immobilized cells are held stationary (not agitated) and perfused at a slow rate with an aerated culture medium.

Table 42.2 A selected list of plant species with immobilized cells employed for the production secondary metabolite(s)

Plant culture species	*Immobilization method*	*Substrate*	*Product*
Catharanthus roseus	Entrapment in agarose	Cathenamine	Ajmalicine
Digitalis lanata	Entrapment in alginate	Digitoxin	Digoxin
Capsicum frutescens	Entrapment in polyurethane foam	Sucrose	Capsaicin
Catheranthus roseus	Entrapment in alginate, agarose, carrageenin	Sucrose	Ajmalicine
Petunia hybrida	Entrapment in hollow fibres	Sucrose	Phenolics
Morinda citrifolia	Entrapment in alginate	Sucrose	Anthraquinone
Solanum aviculare	Attachment polyphenylene beads	Sucrose	Steroid glycosides
Glycine max	Entrapment in hollow fibre	Sucrose	Phenolics

Biochemicals produced by using immobilized cells

A selected list of the immobilized cells from selected plants and their utility to produce important biochemicals is given in ***Table 42.2***.

Two-phase system culture

Plant cells can be cultivated in an aqueous two phase system for the production of secondary metabolites. In this technique, the cells are kept apart from the product by separation in the bioreactor. This is advantageous since the product can be removed continuously. Certain polymers (e.g., dextran and polyethylene glycol for the separation of phenolic compounds) are used for the separation of phases.

Hairy root culture

Hairy root cultures are used ***for the production of root-associated metabolites***. In general, these cultures have high growth rate and genetic stability.

For the production of hairy root cultures, the explant material (plant tissue) is inoculated with the cells of the pathogenic bacterium, *Agrobacterium rhizogenes*. This organism contains root-inducing (Ri) plasmid that causes genetic transformation of plant tissues, which finally results in hairy root cultures. Hairy roots produced by plant tissues have metabolite features similar to that of normal roots.

Hairy root cultures are most recent organ culture systems and are successfully used for the commercial production of secondary metabolites. A selected list of the plants employed in hairy root cultures and the secondary metabolites produced is given in ***Table 42.3***.

MEDIUM COMPOSITION AND EFFECT OF NUTRIENTS

The *in vitro* growth of the plant cells occurs in a suitable medium containing all the requisite elements. The ingradients of the medium effect the growth and metabolism of cells.

For optimal production of secondary metabolites, a two-medium approach is desirable. The first medium is required for good growth of cells (biomass growth) while the second medium, referred to as ***production medium promotes secondary metabolite*** formation. The effect of

Table 42.3 A selected list of plant species used in hairy root cultures for the production of secondary metabolite(s)

Plant species	*Secondary metabolite(s)*
Nicotiana tabacum	Nicotine, anatabine
Atropa belladonna	Atropine
Datura stramonium	Hyoscyamine
Lithospermum erythrorhizon	Shikonin
Catharanthus roseus	Ajmalicine, serpentine
Cinchona ledgeriana	Quinine alkaloids
Mentha vulgaris	Monoterpenes
Solanum laciniatum	Steroid alkaloids

nutrients (carbon and nitrogen sources, phosphate, growth regulators, precursors, vitamins, metal ions) on different species in relation to metabolite formation are variable, some of them are briefly described.

Effect of carbon source

Carbohydrates influence the production of phytochemicals. Some examples are given below.

1. Increase in sucrose concentration (in the range 4–10%) increases allkaloid production in *Catharanthus roseus* cultures.

2. ***Sucrose is a better carbon source*** than fructose or galactose for diosgenin production by *Dioscorea deltoidea* or *Dalanites aegyptiaca* cultures.

3. Low concentration of sucrose increases the production of ubiquinone-10 in tobacco cell cultures.

Effect of nitrogen source

The standard culture media usually contain a mixture of nitrate and ammonia as nitrogen source. Majority of plant cells can tolerate high levels of ammonia. The cultured cells utilize nitrogen for the biosynthesis of amino acids, proteins (including enzymes) and nucleic acids. The ***nitrogen containing primary metabolites directly influence the secondary metabolites.***

In general, high ammonium ion concentrations inhibit secondary metabolite formation while lowering of ammonium nitrogen increases. It is reported that addition of KNO_3 and NH_4NO_3 inhibited anthocyanin (by 90%) and alkaloid (by 80%) production.

Effect of phosphate

Inorganic phosphate is essential for photosynthesis and respiration (glycolysis). In addition, many secondary metabolites are produced through phosphorylated intermediates, which subsequently release the phosphate e.g., phenylpropanoids, terpenes, terpenoids. In general, high phosphate levels promote cell growth and primary metabolism while low phosphate concentrations are beneficial for secondary product formation. However, this is not always correct.

Increase in phosphate concentration in the medium may increase, decrease or may not affect product formation e.g.

1. Increased phosphate concentration increases alkaloid (in *Catharanthus roseus*), anthraquinone (in *Morinda citrifolia*) and diosgenin (in *Dioscorea deltoidea*) production.

2. Decreased phosphate level in the medium increases the formation of anthocyanins and phenolics (in *Catharanthus roseus*), alkaloids (in *Peganum harmala*) and solasodine (in *Solanum lanciatum*).

3. Phosphate concentration (increase or decrease) has no effect on protoberberine (an alkaloid) production by *Berberis* sp.

Effect of plant growth regulators

Plant growth regulators (auxins, cytokinins) ***influence growth, metabolism and differentiation of cultured cells***. (For more details on the nature and different types of auxins and cytokinins, Refer Chapter 43). There are a large number of reports on the influence of growth regulators for the production of secondary metabolites in cultured cells. A few examples are given.

1. Addition of ***auxins*** (indole acetic acid, indole pyruvic acid, naphthalene acetic acid) enhanced the production of diosgenin in the cultures of *Balanites aegyptiaca*.

2. Auxins may inhibit the production of certain secondary metabolites e.g., naphthalene acetic acid and indole acetic acid inhibited the synthesis of anthocyanin in carrot cultures.

3. Another auxin, 2, 4-dichlorophenoxy acetate (2, 4-D) inhibits the production of alkaloids in the cultures of tobacco, and shikonin formation in the cultures of *Lithospermum erythrorhizon*.

4. ***Cytokinins*** promote the production of secondary metabolites in many tissue cultures e.g., ajmalicine in *Catharanthus roseus*; scopolin and scopoletin in tobacco; carotene in *Ricinus* sp.

5. In some tissue cultures, cytokinins inhibit product formation e.g., anthroquinones in *Morinda citrifolia*; shikonin in *Lithospermum erythroshizon*; nicotine in tobacco.

In the above examples, auxins and cytokinins are separately discussed. In actual practice, a combination of auxins and cytokinins is used to achieve maximum production of secondary metabolites in culture systems.

Effect of precursors

The substrate molecules that are incorporated into the secondary metabolites are referred to as precursors. ***In general, addition of precursors to the medium enhances product formation***, although they usually inhibit the growth of the culture e.g., alkaloid synthesis in *Datura* cultures in increased while growth is inhibited by the addition of ornithine, phenylalanine, tyrosine and sodium phenylpyruvate; precursors tryptamine and secologanin increase ajmalicine production in *C. roseus* cultures.

ELICITOR-INDUCED PRODUCTION OF SECONDARY METABOLITES

The production of secondary metabolites in plant cultures is generally low and does not meet the commercial demands. There are continuous efforts to understand the mechanism of product formation at the molecular level, and exploit for increased production. The synthesis of majority of secondary metabolites involves multistep reactions and many enzymes. It is possible to stimulate any step to increase product formation.

Elicitors are the compounds of biological origin which stimulate the production of secondary metabolites, and the phenomenon of such stimulation is referred to as ***elicitation***.

Elicitors produced within the plant cells are ***endogenous elicitors*** e.g., pectin, pectic acid, cellulose, other polysaccharides. When the elicitors are produced by the microorganisms, they are referred to as ***exogenous elicitors*** e.g., chitin, chitosan, glucans. All the elicitors of biological origin are ***biotic elicitors***. The term ***abiotic elicitors*** is used to represent the physical (cold, heat, UV light, osmotic pressure) and chemical agents (ethylene, fungicides, antibiotics, salts of heavy metals) that can also increase the product formation. However, the term abiotic stress is used for abiotic elicitors, while elicitors exclusively represent biological compounds.

Phytoalexins

Plants are capable of defending themselves when attacked by microorganisms, by producing ***antimicrobial compounds*** collectively referred to as phytoalexins. Phytoalexins are the chemical weapons of defense against pathogenic microorganisms. Some of the phytoalexins that induce the production of secondary metabolites are regarded as elicitors. Some chemicals can also act as elicitors e.g., actinomycin-D, sodium salt of arachidonic acid, ribonuclease-A, chitosan, poly-L-lysine, nigeran. These compounds are ***regarded as chemically defined elicitors.***

Interactions for elicitor formation

Elicitors are compounds involved in plant-microbe interaction. Three different types of interactions between plants and microorganisms are known that lead to the formation of elicitors.

1. Direct release of elicitor by the microorganisms.

2. Microbial enzymes that can act as elicitors. e.g. endopolygalacturonic acid lyase from *Erwinia carotovara.*

3. Release of phytoalexins by the action of plant enzymes on cell walls of microorganisms which in turn stimulate formation elicitors from plant cell walls e.g., chitosan from *Fusarium* cell walls; α-1, 3-endoglucanase from *Phytophthora* cell walls.

Methodology of elicitation

Selection of microorganisms : A wide range of microorganisms (viruses, bacteria, algae and fungi) that need not be pathogens have been tried in cultures for elicitor induced production of secondary metabolites. Based on the favourable elicitor response, an ideal microorganism is selected. The quantity of the microbial inoculum is important for the formation elicitor.

Co-culture : Plant cultures (frequently suspension cultures) are inoculated with the selected microorganism to form co-cultures. The cultures are transferred to a fresh medium prior to the inoculation with microorganism. This helps to stimulate the secondary metabolism.

Co-cultures of plant cells with microorganisms may sometimes have inhibitory effect on the plant cells. In such a case, elicitor preparations can be obtained by culturing the selected microorganism on a tissue culture medium, followed by homogenisation and autoclaving of the entire culture. This process releases elicitors. In case of heat labile elicitors, the culture homogenate has to be filter sterilized (instead of autoclaving).

In some co-culture systems, direct contact of plant cells and microorganisms can be prevented by immobilization (entrapment) of one of them. In these cultures, plant microbial interaction occurs by diffusion of the elicitor compounds through the medium.

Mechanism of action of elicitors

Elicitors are found to activate genes and increase the synthesis of mRNAs encoding enzymes responsible for the ultimate biosynthesis secondary metabolites.

There are some recent reports suggesting the involvement of elicitor mediated calcium-based signal transduction systems that promotes the product formation. When the cells are pretreated with a calcium chelate (EDTA) prior to the addition of elicitor, there occurs a decrease in the production of secondary metabolite.

Elicitor-induced products in cultures

In ***Table 42.4***, a selected list of elicitor-induced secondary metabolites produced in culture systems are given.

TABLE 42.4 A selected list of elicitor-induced secondary metabolite production in plant cell cultures

Elicitor microorganism	*Plant cell culture(s)*	*Secondary metabolite(s)*
Aspergillus niger	*Cinchona ledgeriana, Rubia tinctoria*	Anthraquinones
Pythium aphanidermatum	*Catharanthus roseus*	Ajmalicine, Strictosidine Catharanthine
Botrytis sp	*Papaver somniferum*	Sanguinarine
Phytophthora megasperma	*Glycine max*	Isoflavonoids Gluceollin
Dendryphion sp	*Papaver somniferum*	Sanguinarine
Alternaria sp	*Phaseolus vulgaris*	Phaseollin
Fusarium sp	*Apium graveolens*	Furanocoumarins
Phythium aphanidermatum	*Daucus carota*	Anthocynins
Penicillium expansum	*Sanguinaria canadensis*	Benzophenan-thridine Alkaloids

EFFECT OF ENVIRONMENTAL FACTORS

The physical factors namely light, incubation temperature, pH of the medium and aeration of cultures influence the production of secondary metabolites in cultures.

Effect of light

Light is absolutely essential for the carbon fixation (photosynthesis) of field-grown plants. Since the carbon fixation is almost absent or very low in plant tissue cultures, light has no effect on the primary metabolism. However, the ***light-mediated enzymatic reactions indirectly influence the secondary metabolite formation***. The quality of light is also important. Some examples of light-stimulated product formations are given

1. Blue light enhances anthocyanin production in *Haplopappus gracilis* cell suspensions.

2. White light increases the formation of anthocyanin in the cultures of *Catharanthus roseus, Daucus carota* and *Helianthus tuberosus.*

3. White or blue light inhibits naphthoquinone biosynthesis in callus cultures of *Lithospermum erythrorhizon.*

Effect of incubation temperature

The growth of cultured cells is increased with increase in temperature up to an optimal temperature (25–30°C). However, at least for the production some secondary metabolites lower temperature is advantageous. For instance, in *C. roseus* cultures, indole alkaloid production is increased by two fold when incubated at 16°C instead of 27°C. Increased temperature was also found to reduce the production of caffeine (by *C. sineneis*) and nicotine (by *N. tabacum*).

Effect of pH of the medium

For good growth of cultures, the pH of the medium is in the range of 5 to 6. There are reports indicating that pH of the medium influences the formation of secondary metabolites. e.g., production of anthocyanin by cultures of *Daucus carota* was much less when incubated at pH 5.5 than at pH 4.5. This is attributed to the increased degradation of anthocyanin at higher pH.

Aeration of cultures

Continuous aeration is needed for good growth of cultures, and also for the efficient production of secondary metabolites.

BIOTRANSFORMATION USING PLANT CELL CULTURES

The ***conversion of one chemical into another*** (i.e., a substrate into a final product) ***by using biological systems*** (i.e. cell suspensions) as biocatalysts is regarded as biotransformation or bioconversion. The biocatalyst may be free or immobilized, and the process of biotransformation may involve one or more enzymes. Biotransformation involving microorganisms and animal cells are described elsewhere (Chapter 22).

The biotechnological application of plant cell cultures in biotransformation reactions involves the conversion of some less important substances to valuable medicinal or commercially important products. In biotransformation, it is necessary to select such cell lines that possess the enzymes for catalysing the desired reactions. Bioconversions may involve many types of reactions e.g., hydroxylation, reduction, glycosylation.

A good example of biotransformation by plant cell cultures is the large scale ***production of cardiovascular drug digoxin*** from digitoxin by *Digitali lanata*. Digoxin production is carried out by immobilized cells of *D. lanata* in airlift bioreactors. Cell cultures of *Digitalis purpurea* or *Stevia rebaudiana* can convert steviol into steviobiocide and steviocide which are 100 times sweeter than cane sugar.

A selected list of biotransformations carried out in plant cell cultures is given in ***Table 42.5***.

TABLE 42.5 Selected examples of biotransformations by plant cell cultures

Plant cell culture	*Substrate*	*Product*
Digitalis lanata	Digitoxin	Digoxin
Papaver somniferum	Codeinone	Codeine
Nicotiana tobacum	Carvoxine	Cavaxone
Daucus carota	Digitoxigenin	Periplogenin
Mucuna pruriens	L-Tyrosine	L-Dihydroxy-phenylalanine (L-DOPA)
Mentha sp	(–)-Menthone	(+)-Neomenthol
Coffea arabica	Vanillin	Vanillin-D-glucoside
Solanum tuberosum	Solavetivone	Hydroxylated derivatives
Galium mollugo	2-Succinyl benzoate	Anthra quinones
Datura sp	Hydroquinone	Arbutin
Citrus sp	Valencene	Nootkatone
Choisya ternata	Ellipticine	5-Formyl-ellipticine
Digitalis purpurea / *Stvia rebandiana*	Steviol	Steviocide, Steviobiocide

SECONDARY METABOLITE RELEASE AND ANALYSIS

The methods employed for the separation and purification of secondary metabolites from cell cultures are the same as that used for plants.

Sometimes, the products formed within the cells are released into the medium, making the isolation and analysis easy. For the secondary metabolites stored within the vacuoles of cells, two membranes (plasma membrane and tonoplast) have to be disrupted. Permeabilizing agents such as dimethyl sulfoxide (DMSO) can be used for the release of products.

In general, separation and purification of products from plant cell cultures are expensive, therefore every effort is made to make them cost-effective. Two approaches are made in this direction :

1. Production of secondary metabolite should be as high as possible.

2. Formation of side product(s) which interfere with separation must be made minimal.

Once a good quantity of the product is released into the medium, separation and purification techniques (e.g. extraction) can be used for its recovery. These techniques largely depend on the nature of the secondary metabolite.

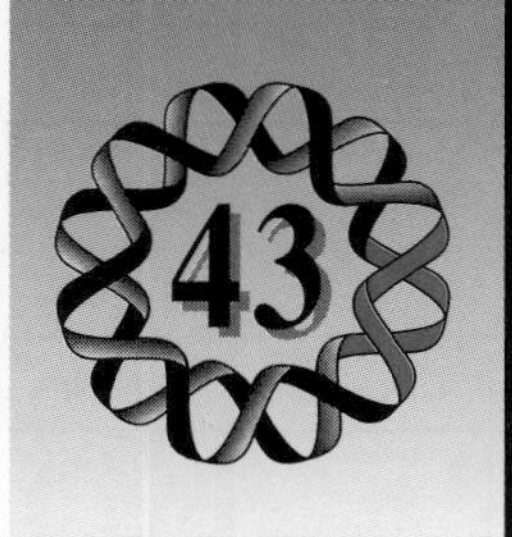

Plant Tissue Culture Media

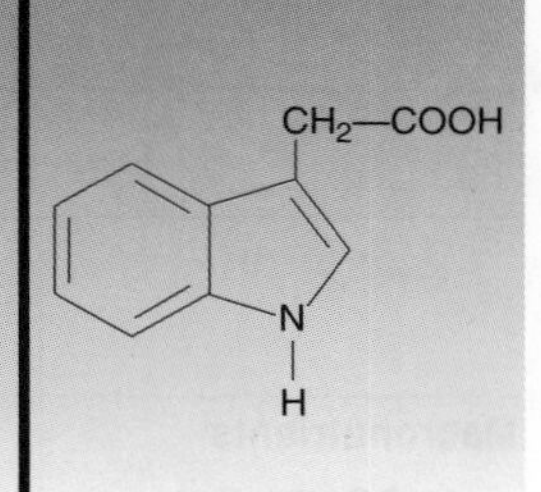

Culture media are largely responsible for the *in vitro* growth and morphogenesis of plant tissues. The success of the plant tissue culture depends on the choice of the nutrient medium. In fact, the cells of most plant cells can be grown in culture media.

Basically, the plant tissue culture media should contain the same nutrients as required by the whole plant. It may be noted that plants in nature can synthesize their own food material. However, ***plants growing in vitro are mainly heterotrophic i.e. they cannot synthesize their own food***.

Composition of media

The composition of the culture media is primarily dependent on two parameters.

1. The particular species of the plant.

2. The type of material used for culture i.e. cells, tissues, organs, protoplasts.

Thus, the composition of a medium is formulated considering the specific requirements of a given culture system. The media used may be solid (***solid medium***) or liquid (***liquid medium***) in nature. The selection of solid or liquid medium is dependent on the better response of a culture.

MAJOR TYPES OF MEDIA

The composition of the most commonly used tissue culutre media is given in ***Table 43.1***, and briefly discribed below.

White's medium : This is one of the earliest plant tissue culture media developed for root culture.

MS medium : Murashige and Skoog (MS) originally formulated a medium to induce organogenesis, and regeneration of plants in cultured tissues. These days, MS medium is widely used for many types of culture systems.

B5 medium : Developed by Gamborg, B5 medium was originally designed for cell suspension and callus cultures. At present with certain modifications, this medium is used for protoplast culture.

N6 medium : Chu formulated this medium and it is used for cereal anther culture, besides other tissue cultures.

Nitsch's medium : This medium was developed by Nitsch and Nitsch and frequently used for anther cultures.

Among the media referred above, MS medium is most frequently used in plant tissue culture work due to its success with several plant species and culture systems.

Synthetic and natural media : When a medium is composed of chemically defined components, it is referred to as a synthetic medium. On the other hand, if a medium contains chemically undefined compounds (e.g., vegetable extract, fruit juice, plant extract), it is regarded as a natural medium.

TABLE 43.1 Composition of commonly used plant tissue culture media

Components	*Amount (mg l^{-1})*				
	White's	*Murashige and Skoog (MS)*	*Gamborg (B5)*	*Chu(N6)*	*Nitsch's*
Macronutrients					
$MgSO_4.7H_2O$	750	370	250	185	185
KH_2PO_4	—	170	—	400	68
$NaH_2PO_4.H_2O$	19	—	150	—	—
KNO_3	80	1900	2500	2830	950
NH_4NO_3	—	1650	—	—	720
$CaCl_2.2H_2O$	—	440	150	166	—
$(NH_4)_2.SO_4$	—	—	134	463	—
Micronutrients					
H_3BO_3	1.5	6.2	3	1.6	—
$MnSO_4.4H_2O$	5	22.3	—	4.4	25
$MnSO_4.H_2O$	—	—	10	3.3	—
$ZnSO_4.7H_2O$	3	8.6	2	1.5	10
$Na_2MoO_4.2H_2O$		0.25	0.25	—	0.25
$CuSO_4.5H_2O$	0.01	0.025	0.025	—	0.025
$CoCl_2.6H_2O$	—	0.025	0.025	—	0.025
KI	0.75	0.83	0.75	0.8	—
$FeSO_4.7H_2O$	—	27.8		27.8	27.8
$Na_2EDTA.2H_2O$	—	37.3	—	37.3	37.3
Sucrose (g)	20	30	20	50	20
Organic supplements					
Vitamins					
Thlamine HCl	0.01	0.5	10	1	0.5
Pyridoxine (HCl)	0.01	0.5	1	0.5	0.5
Nicotinic acid	0.05	0.5	1	0.5	5
Myoinositol	—	100	100	—	100
Others					
Glycine	3	2	—	—	2
Folic acid	—	—	—	—	0.5
Biotin	—		—	—	0.05
pH	5.8	5.8	5.5	5.8	5.8

Synthetic media have almost replaced the natural media for tissue culture.

Expression of concentrations in media : The concentrations of inorganic and organic constituents in culture media are usually expressed as mass values (mg/l or ppm or mg l^{-1}). However, as per the recommendations of the International Association of Plant Physiology, the concentrations of macronutrients should be expressed as mmol/l⁻ and micronutrients as μmol/l⁻.

CONSTITUENTS OF MEDIA

Many elements are needed for plant nutrition and their physiological functions. Thus, these elements have to be supplied in the culture medium to support adequate growth of cultures *in vitro*. A selected list of the elements and their functions in plants is given in ***Table 43.2***.

The culture media usually contain the following constituents

1. Inorganic nutrients
2. Carbon and energy sources
3. Organic supplements
4. Growth regulators
5. Solidifying agents
6. pH of medium

Inorganic nutrients

The inorganic nutrients consist of ***macronutrients*** (concentration >0.5 mmol/l⁻) and ***micronutrients*** (concentration <0.5 mmol/l⁻). A wide range of mineral salts (elements) supply the macro- and micronutrients. The inorganic salts in water undergo dissociation and ionization. Consequently, one type of ion may be contributed by more than one salt. For instance, in MS medium, K^+ ions are contributed by KNO_3 and KH_2PO_4 while NO_3^- ions come from KNO_3 and NH_4NO_3.

Macronutrient elements : The six elements namely ***nitrogen, phosphorus, potassium, calcium, magnesium and sulfur*** are the essential macronutrients for tissue culture. The ideal concentration of nitrogen, and potassium is around 25 mmol l^{-1} while for calcium, phosphorus, sulfur and magnesium, it is in the range of 1-3 mmol l^-. For the supply of nitrogen in the medium, nitrates and ammonium salts are together used.

Micronutrients : Although their requirement is in minute quantities, micronutrients are essential for plant cells and tissues. These include iron, manganese, zinc, boron, copper and molybdenum. Among the microelements, ***iron requirement is very critical***. Chelated forms of iron and copper are commonly used in culture media.

Carbon and energy sources

Plant cells and tissues in the culture medium are heterotrophic and therefore, are dependent on the external carbon for energy. Among the energy sources, ***sucrose is the most preferred***. During the course of sterilization (by autoclaving) of the medium, sucrose gets hydrolysed to glucose and fructose. The plant cells in culture first utilize glucose and then fructose. In fact, glucose or fructose can be directly used in the culture media. It may be noted that for energy supply, glucose is as efficient as sucrose while fructose is less efficient.

TABLE 43.2 A selected list of elements and their functions in plants

Element	*Function(s)*
Nitrogen	Essential component of proteins, nucleic acids and some coenzymes. (Required in most abundant quantity)
Calcium	Synthesis of cell wall, membrane function, cell signalling.
Magnesium	Component of chlorophyll, cofactor for some enzymes.
Potassium	Major inorganic cation, regulates osmotic potential.
Phosphorus	Component of nucleic acids and various intermediates in respiration and photosynthesis, involved in energy transfer.
Sulfur	Component of certain amino acids (methionine, cysteine and cystine, and some cofactors).
Manganese	Cofactor for certain enzymes.
Iron	Component of cytochromes, involved in electron transfer.
Chlorine	Participates in photosynthesis.
Copper	Involved in electron transfer reactions, Cofactor for some enzymes.
Cobalt	Component of vitamin B_{12}.
Molybdenum	Component of certain enzymes (e.g., nitrate reductase), cofactor for some enzymes.
Zinc	Required for chlorophyll biosynthesis, cofactor for certain enzymes.

It is a common observation that ***cultures grow better on*** a medium with ***autoclaved sucrose*** than on a medium with filter-sterilized sucrose. This clearly indicates that the hydrolysed products of sucrose (particularly glucose) are efficient sources of energy. Direct use of fructose in the medium subjected to autoclaving, is found to be detrimental to the growth of plant cells.

Besides sucrose and glucose, other carbohydrates such as lactose, maltose, galactose, raffinose, trehalose and cellobiose have been used in culture media but with a very limited success.

Organic supplements

The organic supplements include vitamins, amino acids, organic acids, organic extracts, activated charcoal and antibiotics.

Vitamins : Plant cells and tissues in culture (like the natural plants) are capable of synthesizing vitamins but in suboptimal quantities, inadequate to support growth. Therefore the medium should be supplemented with ***vitamins to achieve good growth of cells***. The vitamins added to the media include thiamine, riboflavin, niacin, pyridoxine, folic acid, pantothenic acid, biotin, ascorbic acid, myo-inositol, para-amino benzoic acid and vitamin E.

Amino acids : Although the cultured plant cells can synthesize amino acids to a certain extent, media supplemented with ***amino acids stimulate cell growth and help in establishment of cells lines***. Further, organic nitrogen (in the form of amino acids such as L-glutamine, L-asparagine, L-arginine, L-cysteine) is more readily taken up than inorganic nitrogen by the plant cells.

Organic acids : Addition of Krebs cycle intermediates such as citrate, malate, succinate or fumarate allow the growth of plant cells. Pyruvate also enhances the growth of cultured cells.

Organic extracts : It has been a practice to supplement culture media with organic extracts such as ***yeast***, ***casein hydrolysate***, coconut milk, orange juice, tomato juice and potato extract.

It is however, preferable to avoid the use of natural extracts due to high variations in the quality and quantity of growth promoting factors in them. In recent years, natural extracts have been replaced by specific organic compounds e.g., replacement of yeast extract by L-asparagine; replacement of fruit extracts by L-glutamine.

Activated charcoal : Supplementation of the medium with activated charcoal stimulates the growth and differentiation of certain plant cells (carrot, tomato, orchids). Some ***toxic/inhibitory compounds*** (e.g. phenols) produced by cultured plants are ***removed*** (by adsorption) ***by activated charcoal***, and this facilitatis efficient cell growth in cultures.

Addition of activated charcoal to certain cultures (tobacco, soybean) is found to be inhibitory, probably due to adsorption of growth stimulants such as phytohormones.

Antibiotics : It is sometimes necessary to add antibiotics to the medium ***to prevent the growth of microorganisms***. For this purpose, low concentrations of streptomycin or kanamycin are used. As far as possible, addition of antibiotics to the medium is avoided as they have an inhibitory influence on the cell growth.

Growth regulators

Plant hormones or ***phytohormones*** are a group of natural organic compounds that promote growth, development and differentiation of plants. Four broad classes of growth regulators or hormones are used for culture of plant cells-***auxins, cytokinins, gibberellins*** (***Fig. 43.1***) and ***abscisic acid***. They promote growth, differentiation and organogenesis of plant tissues in cultures.

Auxins : Auxins ***induce cell division***, cell elongation, and formation of callus in cultures. At a low concentration, auxins promote root formation while at a high concentration callus formation occurs. A selected list of auxins used in tissue cultures is given in ***Table 43.3***.

Among the auxins, 2, 4-dichlorophenoxy acetic acid is most effective and is widely used in culture media.

Cytokinins : Chemically, cytokinins are derivatives of a purine namely adenine. These adenine derivatives are involved in cell division, ***shoot differentiation and somatic embryo formation***. Cytokinins promote RNA synthesis and thus stimulate protein and enzyme activities in tissues. The most commonly used cytokinins are given in ***Table 43.3***.

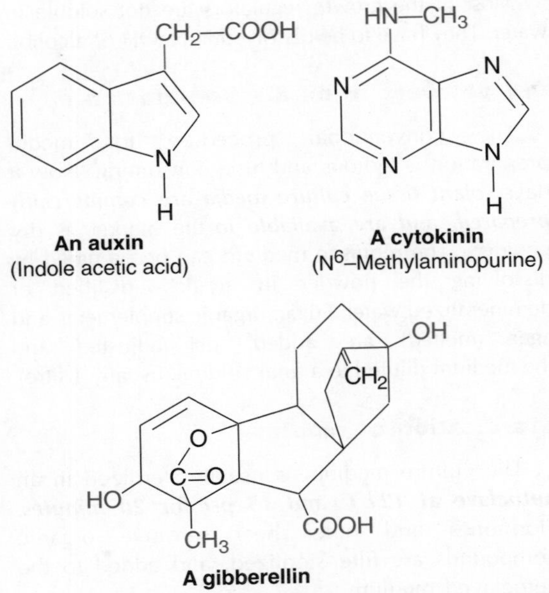

An auxin
(Indole acetic acid)

A cytokinin
(N^6–Methylaminopurine)

A gibberellin

Fig. 43.1 : Structures of selected plant growth regulators.

Among the cytokinins, kinetin and benzylaminopurine are frequently used in culture media.

Ratio of auxins and cytokinins : The relative concentrations of the growth factors namely auxins and cytokinins are crucial for the morphogenesis of culture systems. When the ***ratio of auxins to cytokinins is high, embryogenesis, callus initiation and root initiation occur. On the other hand, for axillary and shoot proliferation, the ratio of auxins to cytokinins is low***. For all practical purposes, it is considered that the formation and maintenance of callus cultures require both auxin and cytokinin, while auxin is needed for root culture and cytokinin for shoot culture.

The actual concentrations of the growth regulators in culture media are variable depending on the type of tissue explant and the plant species.

Gibberellins : About 20 different gibberellins have been identified as growth regulators. Of these, gibberellin A_3 (GA_3) is the most commonly used for tisue culture. GA_3 promotes growth of cultured cells, ***enhances callus growth*** and induces dwarf plantlets to elongate.

Gibberellins are capable of promoting or inhibiting tissue cultures, depending on the plant species. They usually inhibit adventitious root and shoot formation.

Abscisic acid (ABA) : The callus growth of cultures may be stimulated or inhibited by ABA. This largely depends on the nature of the plant species. Abscisic acid is an important growth regulation for induction of embryogenesis.

Solidifying agents

For the preparation of semisolid or solid tissue culture media, solidifying or ***gelling agents*** are required. In fact, solidifying agents extend support to tissues growing in the static conditions.

Agar : Agar, a polysaccharide obtained from seaweeds, is most commonly used as a gelling agent for the following reasons (next page).

TABLE 43.3 A selected list of plant growth regulators used in culture media

Growth regulator (abbreviation/name)	*Chemical name*
Auxins	
IAA	Indole 3-acetic acid
IBA	Indole 3-butyric acid
NAA	1-Naphthyl acetic acid
2, 4-D	2, 4-Dichlorophenoxy acetic acid
2, 4, 5-T	2, 4, 5-Trichlorophenoxy acetic acid
4—CPA	4-Chlorophenoxy acetic acid
NOA	2-Naphthyloxy acetic acid
MCPA	2-Methyl 4-chlorophenoxy acetic acid
Dicamba	2-Methoxy 3, 6-dichlorobenzoic acid
Picloram	4-Amino 2, 5, 6-trichloropicolinic acid
Cytokinins	
BAP	6-Benzyl aminopurine
BA	Benzyl adenine
2 iP (IPA)	N^6-(2-isopentyl) adenine
DPU	Diphenyl urea
Kinetin	6-Furfuryl aminopurine
Zeatin	4-Hydroxy 3-methyltrans 2-butenyl aminopurine
Thidiazuron	1-Phenyl 3-(1, 2, 3-thiadiazol-5 yl) urea

1. It does not react with media constituents.

2. It is not digested by plant enzymes and is stable at culture temperature.

Agar at a concentration of 0.5 to 1% in the medium can form a gel.

Gelatin : It is used at a high concentration (10%) with a limited success. This is mainly because gelatin melts at low temperature (25°C), and consequently the gelling property is lost.

Other gelling agents : Biogel (polyacrylamide pellets), phytagel, gelrite and purified agarose are other solidifying agents, although less frequently used. It is in fact advantageous to use synthetic gelling compounds, since they can form gels at a relatively low concentration (1.0 to 2.5 g l^{-1}).

pH of medium

The optimal pH for most tissue cultures is ***in the range of 5.0-6.0***. The pH generally falls by 0.3-0.5 units after autoclaving. Before sterilization, pH can be adjusted to the required optimal level while preparing the medium. It is usually not necessary to use buffers for the pH maintenance of culture media.

At a pH higher than 7.0 and lower than 4.5, the plant cells stop growing in cultures. If the pH falls during the plant tissue culture, then fresh medium should be prepared. In general, pH above 6.0 gives the medium hard appearance, while pH below 5.0 does not allow gelling of the medium.

PREPARATION OF MEDIA

The general methodology for a medium preparation involves preparation of stock solutions (in the range of 10x to 100x concentrations) using high purity chemicals and demineralized water. The stock solutions can be stored (in glass or plastic containers) frozen and used as and when required.

Most of the growth regulators are not soluble in water. They have to be dissolved in NaOH or alcohol.

Dry powders in media preparation

The conventional procedure for media preparation is tedious and time consuming. Now a days, ***plant tissue culture media are commercially prepared, and are available in*** the market as dry powders. The requisite medium can be prepared by dissolving the powder in a glass distilled or demineralized water. Sugar, organic supplements and agar (melted) are added, pH adjusted and the medium diluted to a final volume (usually 1 litre).

Sterilization of media

The culture medium is usually sterilized in an ***autoclave at 121°C and 15 psi for 20 minutes***. Hormones and other heat sensitive organic compounds are filter-sterilized, and added to the autoclaved medium.

SELECTION OF A SUITABLE MEDIUM

In order to select a suitable medium for a particular plant culture system, it is customary to start with a known medium (e.g. MS medium, B5 medium) and then develop a new medium with the desired characteristics. Among the constituents of a medium, growth regulators (auxins, cytokinins) are highly variable depending on the culture system. In practice, 3-5 different concentrations of growth regulators in different combinations are used and the best among them are selected.

For the selection of appropriate concentrations of minerals and organic constituents in the medium, similar approach referred above, can be employed.

Medium-utmost important for culture

For tissue culture techniques, it is absolutely essential that the medium preparation and composition are carefully followed. Any mistake in the preparation of the medium is likely to do a great harm to the culture system as a whole.

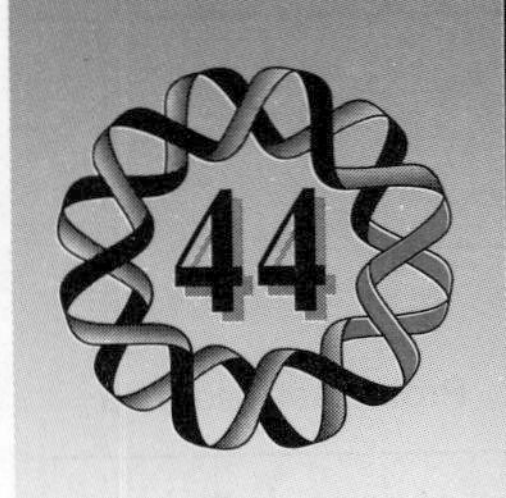

Protoplast Culture and Somatic Hybridization

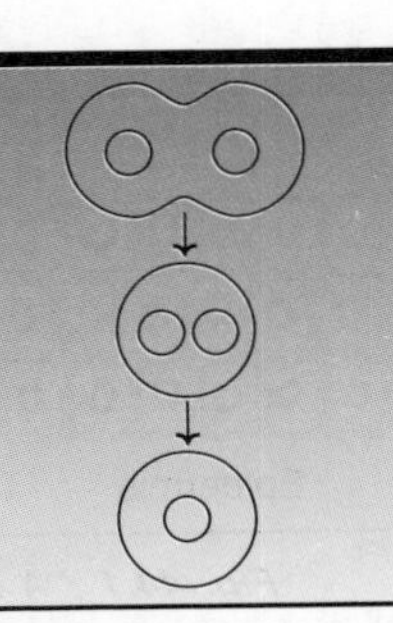

Protoplasts are ***naked plant cells without the cell wall***, but they possess plasma membrane and all other cellular components. They represent the functional plant cells but for the lack of the barrier, cell wall. ***Protoplasts of different species can be fused*** to generate a hybrid and this process is referred to as ***somatic hybridization*** (or protoplast fusion). Cybridization is the phenomenon of fusion of a normal protoplast with an enucleated (without nucleus) protoplast that results in the formation of a ***cybrid*** or ***cytoplast*** (cytoplasmic hybrids).

Historical developments

The term protoplast was introduced in 1880 by Hanstein. The first isolation of protoplasts was achieved by Klercker (1892) employing a mechanical method. A real beginning in protoplast research was made in 1960 by Cocking who used an enzymatic method for the removal of cell wall. Rakabe and his associates (1971) were successful to achieve the regeneration of whole tobacco plant from protoplasts. Rapid progress occurred after 1980 in protoplast fusion to improve plant genetic material, and the development of transgenic plants.

IMPORTANCE OF PROTOPLASTS AND THEIR CULTURES

The isolation, culture and fusion of protoplasts is a fascinating field in plant research. Protoplast isolation and their cultures provide ***millions of single cells*** (comparable to microbial cells) ***for a viriety of studies***. Protoplasts have a wide range of applications, some of them are listed below.

1. The protoplast in culture can be regenerated into a whole plant.

2. Hybrids can be developed from protoplast fusion.

3. It is easy to perform single cell cloning with protoplasts.

4. Genetic transformations can be achieved through genetic engineering of protoplast DNA.

5. Protoplasts are excellent materials for ultrastructural studies.

6. Isolation of cell organelles and chromosomes is easy from protoplasts.

7. Protoplasts are useful for membrane studies (transport and uptake processes).

8. Isolation of mutants from protoplast cultures is easy.

ISOLATION OF PROTOPLASTS

Protoplasts are isolated by two techniques

1. Mechanical method

2. Enzymatic method

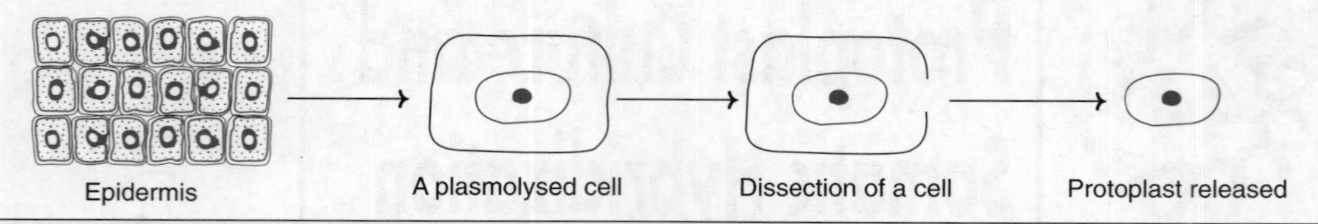

Fig. 44.1 : A diagrammatic representation of mechanical method for the isolation of protoplasts.

MECHANICAL METHOD

Protoplas isolation by mechanical method is a crude and tedious procedure. This results in the isolation of a very small number of protoplasts. The technique involves the following stages (***Fig. 44.1***).

1. A small piece of epidermis from a plant is selected.

2. The cells are subjected to plasmolysis. This causes protoplasts to shrink away from the cell walls.

3. The tissue is dissected to release the protoplasts.

Mechanical method for protoplast isolation is no more in use because of the following limitations

- Yield of protoplasts and their viability is low.
- It is restricted to certain tissues with vacuolated cells.
- The method is laborious and tedious.

However, some workers ***prefer mechanical methods if the cell wall degrading enzymes*** (of enzymatic method) ***cause deleterious effects to protoplasts***.

ENZYMATIC METHOD

Enzymatic method is ***a very widely used technique*** for the isolation of protoplasts. The advantages of enzymatic method include good yield of viable cells, and minimal or no damage to the protoplasts.

Sources of protoplasts

Protoplasts can be isolated from a wide variety of tissues and organs that include leaves, roots, shoot apices, fruits, embryos and microspores. Among these, the mesophyll tissue of fully expanded leaves of young plants or new shoots are most frequently used. In addition, callus and suspension cultures also serve as good sources for protoplast isolation.

Enzymes for protoplast isolation

The enzymes that can digest the cell walls are required for protoplast isolation. Chemically, the plant cell wall is mainly composed of cellulose, hemicellulose and pectin which can be respectively degraded by the enzymes cellulase, hemicellulase and pectinase. The different enzymes for protoplast isolation and the corresponding sources are given in ***Table 44.1***.

In fact, the various enzymes for protoplast isolation are commercially available. The enzymes are usually used at a pH 4.5 to 6.0, temperature 25–30°C with a wide variation in incubation period that may range from half an hour to 20 hours. The enzymatic isolation of protoplasts can be carried out by two approaches.

TABLE 44.1 A selected list of commercially available enzymes for protoplast isolation, and their sources

Enzyme	*Source*
Cellulases	
Cellulase onozuka R-10	*Trichoderma viride*
Cellulase YC	*Trichoderma viride*
Cellulysin	*Trichoderma viride*
Driselase	*Irpex lactus*
Hemocellulases	
Hemicellulase	*Aspergillus niger*
Helicase	*Helix pomatia*
Rhozyme HP-150	*Aspergillus niger*
Hemicellulase H-2125	*Rhizopus* sp
Pectinases	
Macerase	*Rhizopus arrhizus*
Pectolyase	*Aspergillus japonicus*
Macerozyme R-10	*Rhizopus arrhizus*
Zymolyase	*Arthrobacter luteus*

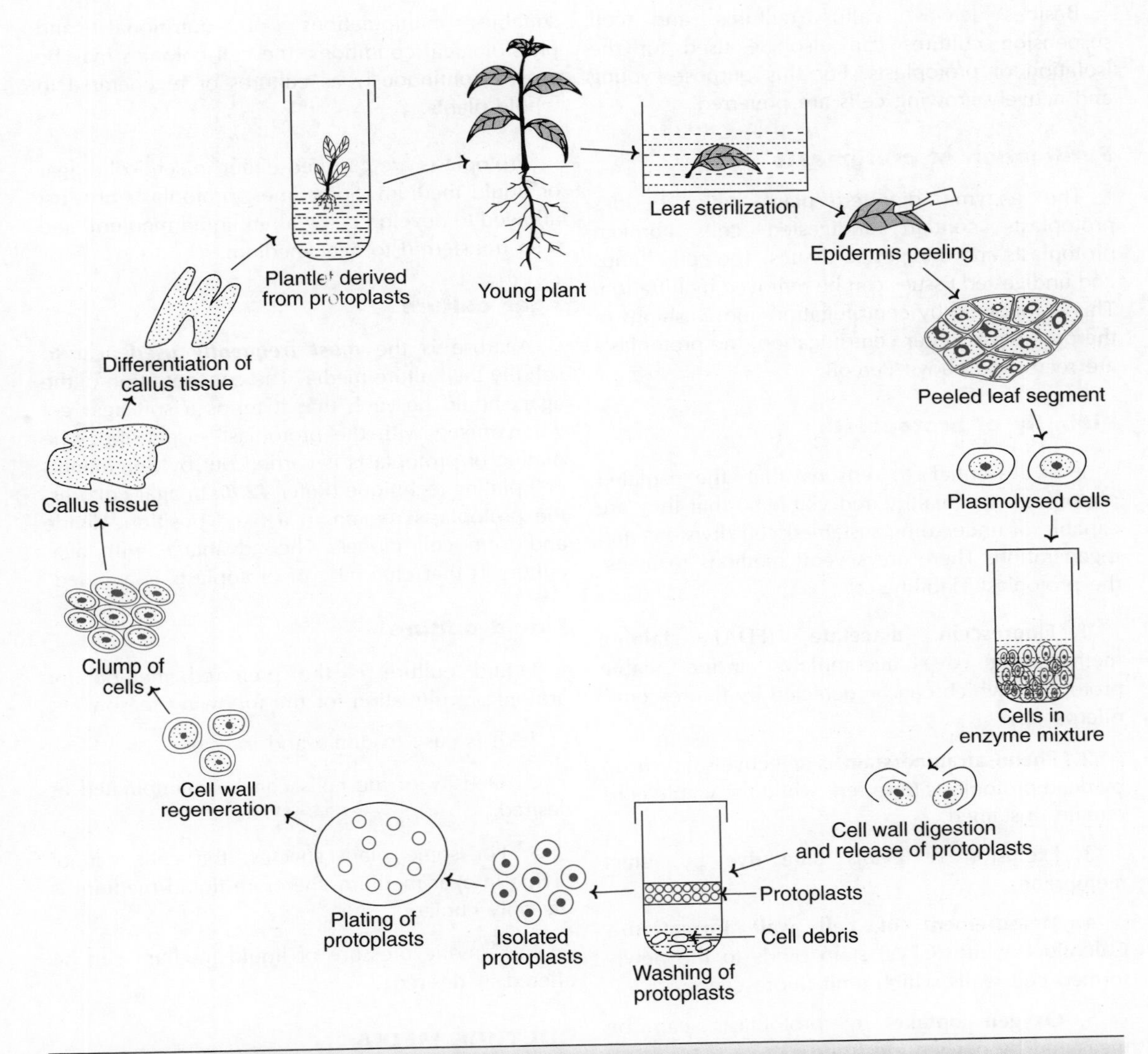

Fig. 44.2 : Major steps involved in protoplast isolation, culture and regeneration of plants.

1. **Two step or sequential method :** The tissue is first treated with pectinase (macerozyme) to separate cells by degrading middle lamella. These free cells are then exposed to cellulase to release protoplasts. Pectinase breaks up the cell aggregates into individual cells while cellulase removes the cell wall proper.

2. **One step or simultaneous method :** This is the preferred method for protoplast isolation. It involves the simultaneous use of both the enzymes — macerozyme and cellulase.

Isolation of protoplasts from leaves

Leaves are ***most commonly used***, for protoplast isolation, since it is possible to isolate uniform cells in large numbers. The procedure broadly involves the following steps (***Fig. 44.2***).

1. Sterilization of leaves.
2. Removal of epidermal cell layer.
3. Treatment with enzymes.
4. Isolation of protoplasts.

Besides leaves, callus cultures and cell suspension cultures can also be used for the isolation of protoplasts. For this purpose, young and actively growing cells are preferred.

Purification of protoplasts

The enzyme digested plant cells, besides protoplasts contain undigested cells, broken protoplasts and undigested tissues. The cell clumps and undigested tissues can be removed by filtration. This is followed by centrifugation and washings of the protoplasts. After centrifugation, the protoplasts are recovered above Percoll.

Viability of protoplasts

It is essential to ensure that the isolated protoplasts are healthy and viable so that they are capable of undergoing sustained cell divisions and regeneration. There are several methods to assess the protoplast viability.

1. **Fluorescein diacetate (FDA) staining** method—The dye accumulates inside viable protoplasts which can be detected by fluorescence microscopy.

2. **Phenosafranine stain** is selectively taken up by dead protoplasts (turn red) while the viable cells remain unstained.

3. Exclusion of **Evans blue dye** by intact membranes.

4. **Measurement of cell wall formation**—Calcofluor white (CFW) stain binds to the newly formed cell walls which emit fluorescence.

5. **Oxygen uptake** by protoplasts can be measured by oxygen electrode.

6. **Photosynthetic activity** of protoplasts.

7. The ability of protoplasts to undergo continuous **mitotic divisions** (this is a direct measure).

CULTURE OF PROTOPLASTS

The very ***first step*** in protoplast culture is the ***development of a cell wall*** around the membrane of the protoplast. This is followed by the cell divisions that give rise to a small colony. With suitable manipulations of nutritional and physiological conditions, the cell colonies may be grown continuously as cultures or regenerated to whole plants.

Protoplasts are cultured either in semisolid agar or liquid medium. Sometimes, protoplasts are first allowed to develop cell wall in liquid medium, and then transferred to agar medium.

Agar culture

Agarose is the ***most frequently used*** agar to solidify the culture media. The concentration of the agar should be such that it forms a soft agar gel when mixed with the protoplast suspension. The plating of protoplasts is carried out by Bergmann's cell plating technique (Refer ***42.8***). In agar cultures, the protoplasts remain in a fixed position, divide and form cell clones. The advantage with agar culture is that clumping of protoplasts is avoided.

Liquid culture

Liquid culture is the preferred method for protoplast cultivation for the following reasons.

1. It is easy to dilute and transfer.

2. Density of the cells can be manipulated as desired.

3. For some plant species, the cells cannot divide in agar medium, therefore liquid medium is the only choice.

4. Osmotic pressure of liquid medium can be altered as desired.

CULTURE MEDIA

The culture media with regard to nutritional components and osmoticum are briefly described.

Nutritional components

In general, the nutritional requirements of protoplasts are ***similar to those of cultured plant cells*** (callus and suspension cultures). Mostly, MS and B5 media (Refer Chapter 43) with suitable modifications are used. Some of the special features of protoplast culture media are listed below.

1. The medium should be devoid of ammonium, and the quantities of iron and zinc should be less.

2. The concentration of calcium should be 2-4-times higher than used for cell cultures. This is needed for membrane stability.

3. High auxin/kinetin ratio is suitable to induce cell divisions while high kinetin/auxin ratio is required for regeneration.

4. Glucose is the preferred carbon source by protoplasts although a combination of sugars (glucose and sucrose) can be used.

5. The vitamins used for protoplast cultures are the same as used in standard tissue culture media.

Osmoticum and osmotic pressure

Osmoticum broadly refers to the ***reagents/chemicals that are added to increase the osmotic pressure of a liquid.***

The isolation and culture of protoplasts require osmotic protection until they develop a strong cell wall. In fact, if the freshly isolated protoplasts are directly added to the normal culture medium, they will burst. Thus, addition of an osmoticum is essential for both isolation and culture media of protoplast to prevent their rupture. The osmotica are of two types — non-ionic and ionic.

Non-ionic osmotica : The non-ionic substances most commonly used are soluble carbohydrates such as mannitol, sorbitol, glucose, fructose, galactose and sucrose. Mannitol, being metabolically inert, is most frequently used.

Ionic osmotica : Potassium chloride, calcium chloride and magnesium phosphate are the ionic substances in use to maintain osmotic pressure.

When the protoplasts are transferred to a culture medium, the use of metabolically active osmotic stabilizers (e.g., glucose, sucrose) along with metabolically inert osmotic stabilizers (mannitol) is advantageous. As the growth of protoplasts and cell wall regeneration occurs, the metabolically active compounds are utilized, and this results in the reduced osmotic pressure so that proper osmolarity is maintained.

CULTURE METHODS

The culture techniques of protoplasts are almost the same that are used for cell culture with suitable modifications. Some important aspects are briefly given.

Feeder layer technique

For culture of protoplasts at low density feeder layer technique is preferred. This method is also important for selection of specific mutant or hybrid cells on plates. The technique consists of exposing protoplast cell suspensions to X-rays (to inhibit cell division with good metabolic activity) and then plating them on agar plates.

Co-culture of protoplasts

Protoplasts of ***two different plant species*** (one slow growing and another fast growing) ***can be co-cultured.*** This type of culture is advantageous since the growing species provide the growth factors and other chemicals which helps in the generation of cell wall and cell division. The co-culture method is generally used if the two types of protoplasts are morphologically distinct.

Microdrop culture

Specially designed dishes namely cuprak dishes with outer and inner chambers are used for microdrop culture. The inner chamber carries several wells wherein the individual protoplasts in droplets of nutrient medium can be added. The outer chamber is filled with water to maintain humidity. This method allows the culture of fewer protoplasts for droplet of the medium.

REGENERATION OF PROTOPLASTS

Protoplast regeneration which may also be regarded as ***protoplast development*** occurs in two stages.

1. Formation of cell wall.
2. Development of callus/whole plant.

Formation of cell wall

The process of cell wall formation in cultured protoplasts starts within a few hours after isolation that ***may take two to several days*** under suitable conditions. As the cell wall development occurs, the protoplasts lose their characteristic spherical shape. The newly developed cell wall by protoplasts can be identified by using calcofluor white fluorescent stain.

The freshly formed cell wall is composed of loosely bound microfibrils which get organized to form a typical cell wall. This process of cell wall development ***requires continuous supply of nutrients***, particularly a readily metabolised carbon source (e.g. sucrose). Cell wall development is found to be improper in the presence of ionic osmotic stabilizers in the medium.

The protoplasts with proper cell wall development undergo normal cell division. On the other hand, protoplasts with poorly regenerated cell wall show budding and fail to undergo normal mitosis.

Development of callus/whole plant

As the cell wall formation around protoplasts is complete, the cells increase in size, and the first division generally occurs within 2-7 days. Subsequent divisions result in small colonies, and by the end of third week, visible colonies (macroscopic colonies) are formed. These colonies are then transferred to an osmotic-free (mannitol or sorbitol-free) medium for further development to form callus. With induction and appropriate manipulations, the callus can undergo organogenic or embryogenic differentiation to finally form the whole plant. A general view of the protoplast isolation, culture and regeneration is represented in ***Fig. 44.2*** (See p. 525).

Plant regeneration can be done from the callus obtained either from protoplasts or from the culture of plant organs. There are however, certain differences in these two calluses. The callus derived from plant organs carries preformed buds or organized structures, while the callus from protoplast culture does not have such structures.

The first success of regeneration of plants from protoplast cultures of *Nicotiana tabacum* was achieved by Takebe *et al* (in 1971). Since then, several species of plants have been regenerated by using protoplasts (***Table 44.2***).

TABLE 44.2 Selected examples of plant species regenerated from protoplasts

Category	*Plant species*
Cereals	*Oryza sativa*
	Zea mays
	Hordeum vulgare
Vegetables	*Cucumis sativus*
	Brassica oleracea
	Capsicum annuum
Woody trees	*Larix eurolepsis*
	Coffea canephora
	Prunus avium
Ornamentals	*Rosa sp*
	Chrysanthemum sp
	Pelargonium sp
Tubers and roots	*Beta vulgaris*
	Ipomoca batatas
Oil crops	*Helianthus annuces*
	Brassica napus
Legumes	*Glycine max*

SUB-PROTOPLASTS

The ***fragments derived from protoplasts*** that do not contain all the contents of plant cells are referred to as sub-protoplasts. It is possible to experimentally induce fragmentation of protoplasts to form sub-protoplasts. This can be done by application of different centrifugal forces created by discontinuous gradients during centrifugation. Exposure of protoplasts to cytochalasin B in association with centrifugation is a better approach for fragmentation of protoplasts. There are three types of sub-protoplasts (***Fig. 44.3***).

1. **Miniprotoplasts :** These are also called as ***karyoplasts*** and contain the nucleus. Miniprotoplasts can divide and are capable of regeneration into plants.

2. **Cytoplasts :** These are sub-protoplasts containing the original cytoplasmic material (in part or full) but lack nucleus. Thus, cytoplasts are ***nuclear-free sub-protoplasts*** which cannot divide, but they can be used for ***cybridization***.

3. **Microprotoplasts :** This term was suggested for sub-protoplasts that contain not all but a few chromosomes.

SOMATIC HYBRIDIZATION

The conventional method to improve the characteristics of cultivated plants, for years, has been ***sexual hybridization***. The major limitation of sexual hybridization is that it can be performed

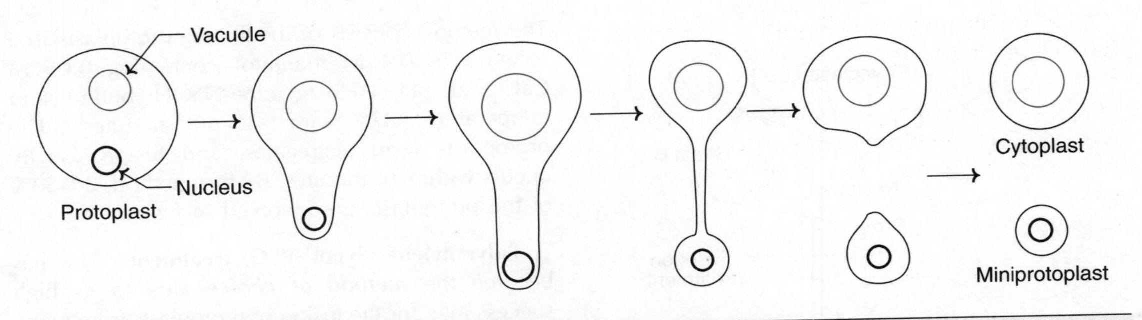

Fig. 44.3 : A diagrammatic representation of fragmentation of protoplast to form sub–protoplasts (cytoplasts and miniprotoplasts)

within a plant species or very closely related species. This restricts the improvements that can be done in plants.

The species barriers for plant improvement encountered in sexual hybridization can be overcome by somatic cell fusion that can form a viable hybrids. Somatic hybridization broadly involves ***in vitro fusion of isolated protoplasts to form a hybrid cell and its subsequent development to form a hybrid plant***. Plant protoplasts are of immense utility in somatic plant cell genetic manipulations and imporovement of crops. Thus, protoplasts provide a novel opportunity to create cells with new genetic constitution. And protoplast fusion is a wonderful approach to overcome sexual incompatibility between different species of plants. More details on the applications of somatic hybridization are given later.

Somatic hubridization involves the following aspects :

1. Fusion of protoplasts
2. Selection of hybrid cells
3. Identification of hybrid plants.

FUSION OF PROTOPLASTS

As the isolated protoplasts are devoid of cell walls, their *in vitro* fusion becomes relatively easy. There are no barriers of incompatibility (at interspecific, intergeneric or even at interkingdom levels) for the protoplast fusion.

Protoplast fusion that involves mixing of protoplasts of two different genomes can be achieved by spontaneous, mechanical, or induced fusion methods.

Spontaneous fusion

Cell fusion is a natural process as is observed in case of egg fertilization. During the course of enzymatic degradation of cell walls, some of the adjoining protoplasts may fuse to form ***homokaryocytes*** (homokaryons). These fused cells may sometimes contain high number of nuclei (2-40). This is mainly bacause of expansion and subsequent coalescence of plasmodermal connections between cells. The frequency of homokaryon formation was found to be high in protoplasts isolated from dividing cultured cells.

Spontaneously fused protoplasts, however, cannot regenerate into whole plants, except undergoing a few cell divisions.

Mechanical fusion

The protoplasts can be pushed together mechanically to fuse. Protoplasts of *Lilium* and *Trillium* in enzyme solutions can be fused by gentle trapping in a depression slide. Mechanical fusion may damage protoplasts by causing injuries.

Induced fusion

Freshly isolated protoplasts can be fused by induction. There are several ***fusion-inducing agents*** which are collectively referred to as ***fusogens*** e.g. $NaNO_3$, high pH/Ca^{2+}, polyethylene glycol, polyvinyl alcohol, lysozyme, concavalin A, dextran, dextran sulfate, fatty acids and esters, electrofusion. Some of the fusogens and their use in induced fusion are described. A diagrammatic representation of protoplast fusion is depicted in ***Fig. 44.4***.

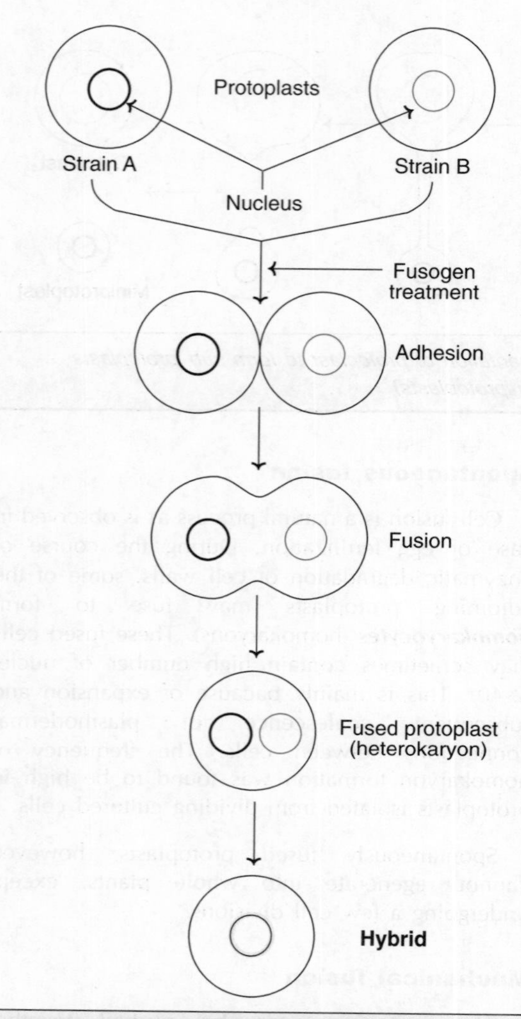

Fig. 44.4 : A diagrammatic representation of protoplast fusion.

Treatment with sodium nitrate : The isolated protoplasts are exposed to a mixture of 5.5% $NaNO_3$ in 10% sucrose solution. Incubation is carried out for 5 minutes at 35°C, followed by centrifugation (200 xg for 5 min). The protoplast pellet is kept in a water bath at 30°C for about 30 minutes, during which period protoplast fusion occurs. $NaNO_3$ treatment results in a low frequency of heterokaryon formation, particularly when mesophyll protoplasts are fused.

High pH and high Ca^{2+} ion treatment : This method was first used for the fusion of tobacco protoplasts, and is now in use for other plants also. The method consists of incubating protoplasts in a solution of 0.4 M mannitol containing 0.05 M $CaCl_2$ at pH 10.5 (glycine-NaOH buffer) and temperature 37°C for 30–40 minutes. The protoplasts form aggregates, and fusion usually occurs within 10 minutes. By this method, 20–50% of the protoplasts are involved in fusion.

Polyethylene glycol (PEG) treatment : This has become the ***method of choice***, due to its high success rate, for the fusion of protoplasts from many plant species. The isolated protoplasts in culture medium (1 ml) are mixed with equal volume (1 ml) of 28–56% PEG (mol. wt. 1500–6000 daltons) in a tube. PEG enhances fusion of protoplasts in several species. This tube is shaken and then allowed to settle. The settled protoplasts are washed several times with culture medium.

PEG treatment method is widely used for protoplast fusion as it has several ***advantages***

- It results in a reproducible high-frequency of heterokaryon formation.
- Low toxicity to cells.
- Reduced formation of binucleate heterokaryons.
- PEG-induced fusion is non-specific and therefore can be used for a wide range of plants.

Electrofusion : In this method, electrical field is used for protoplast fusion. When the protoplasts are placed in a culture vessel fitted with micro-electrodes and an electrical shock is applied, protoplasts are induced to fuse. Electrofusion technique is simple, quick and efficient and hence preferred by many workers. Further, the cells formed due to electrofusion do not show cytotoxic responses as is the case with the use of fusogens (including PEG). The major ***limitation*** of this method is the ***requirement of specialized and costly equipment***.

Mechanism of fusion

The fusion of protoplasts involves three phases agglutination, plasma membrane fusion and formation of heterokaryons.

1. **Agglutination (adhesion) :** When two protoplasts are in close contact with each other, adhesion occurs. Agglutination can be induced by fusogens e.g. PEG, high pH and high Ca^{2+}.

2. **Plasma membrane fusion :** Protoplast membranes get fused at localized sites at the points of adhension. This leads to the formation of cytoplasmic bridges between protoplasts. The plasma membrane fusion can be ***increased by high pH and high Ca^{2+}, high temperature and PEG***, as explained below.

(a) High pH and high Ca^{2+} ions neutralise the surface charges on the protoplasts. This allows closer contact and membrane fusion between agglutinated protoplasts.

(b) High temperature helps in the intermingling of lipid molecules of agglutinated protoplast membranes so that membrane fusion occurs.

(c) PEG causes rapid agglutination and formation of clumps of protoplasts. This results in the formation of tight adhesions of membranes and consequently their fusion.

3. **Formation of heterokaryons :** The fused protoplasts get rounded as a result of cytoplasmic bridges leading to the formation of spherical homokaryon or heterokaryon.

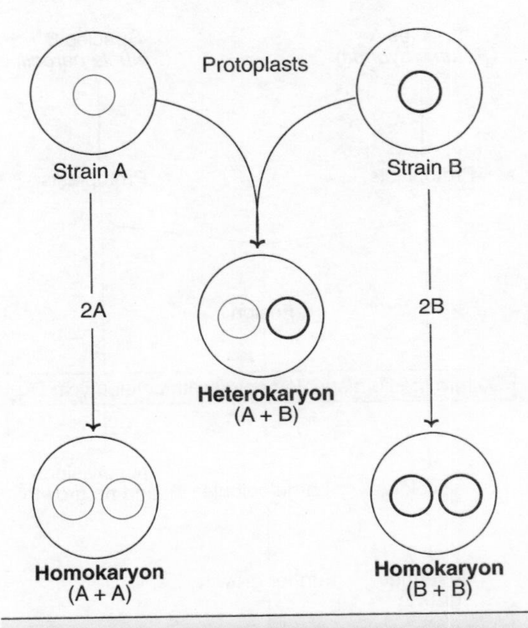

Fig. 44.5 : Fusion products of protoplasts.

SELECTION OF HYBRID CELLS

About 20–25% of the protoplasts are actually involved in the fusion. After the fusion process, the protoplast population consists of a heterogenous mixture of unfused chloroplasts, ***homokaryons*** and ***heterokaryons*** (***Fig. 44.5***). It is therefore necessary to select the hybrid cells (heterokaryons). The commonly used methods employed for the selection of hybrid cells are ***biochemical***, ***visual*** and ***cytometric methods***.

Biochemical methods

The biochemical methods for selection of hybrid cells are based on the use of biochemical compounds in the medium (selection medium). These compounds help to sort out the hybrid and parental cells based on their differences in the expression of characters. Drug sensitivity and auxotrophic mutant selection methods are described below.

1. **Drug sensitivity :** This method is useful for the selection hybrids of two plant species, if one of them is sensitive to a drug. Protoplasts of *Petunia hybride* (species A) can form macroscopic callus on MS medium, but are sensitive to (inhibited by) actinomycin D. *Petunia parodii* protoplasts (species B) form small colonies, but are resistant to actinomycin D. When these two species are fused, the fused protoplasts derive both the characters — formation of macroscopic colonies and resistance to actinomycin D on MS medium. This helps in the selection of hybrids (***Fig. 44.6***). The parental protoplasts of both the species fail to grow. Protoplasts of *P. parodii* form very small colonies while that of *P. hybrida* are inhibited by actinomycin D.

Drug sensitivity technique was originally developed by Power *et al* (1976) for the selection of hybrids of *Petunia* sp (described above). A similar procedure is in use for the selection of other somatic hybrids e.g., hybrids between *Nicotiana sylvestris* and *Nicotiana knightiana*.

2. **Auxotrophic mutants :** Auxotrophs are mutants that cannot grow on a minimal medium and therefore require specific compounds to be added to the medium. Nitrate reductase deficient mutants of tobacco (*N. tabacum*) are known. The parental protoplasts of such species cannot grow with nitrate as the sole source of nitrogen while the hybrids can grow. Two species of nitrate reductase deficiency— one due to lack of apoenzyme (nia-type mutant) and the other due to lack of molybdenum cofactor (cnx-

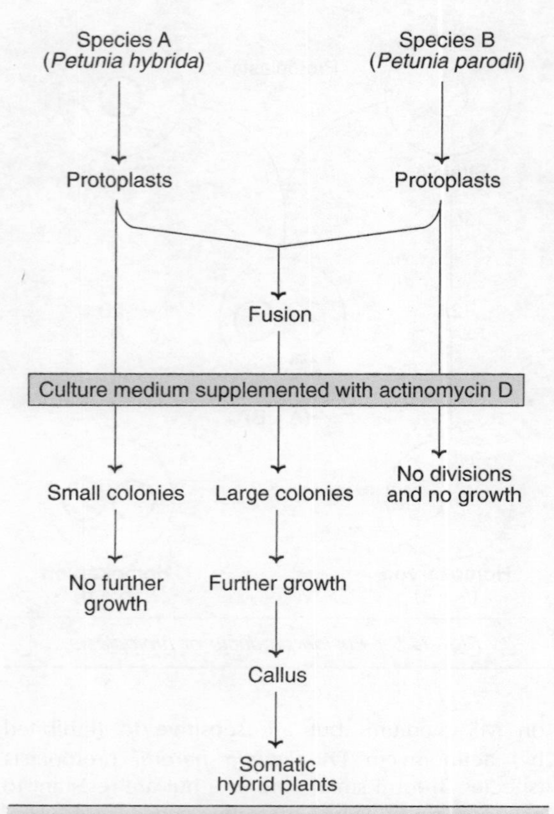

Fig. 44.6 : A diagrammatic representation of drug sensitivity method for the isolation of hybrid cells.

type mutant) are known. The parental protoplasts cannot grow on nitrate medium while the hybrid protoplasts can grow (***Fig. 44.7***).

The selection of auxotrophic mutants is possible only if the hybrid cells can grow on a minimal medium. Another limitation of the technique is the paucity of higher plant auxotrophs.

Visual methods

Visual selection of hybrid cells, although tedious is very efficient. In some of the somatic hybridization experiments, chloroplast deficient (albino or non-green) protoplasts of one parent are fused with green protoplasts of another parent. This facilitates the visual identification of haterokaryons under light microscope. The ***heterokaryons are bigger and green in colour while the parental protoplasts are either small or colourless.*** Further identification of these heterokaryons has to be carried out to develop the specific hybrid plant.

There are two approaches in this direction — growth on selection medium, and mechanical isolation.

1. **Visual selection coupled with differential media growth :** There exist certain natural differences in the sensitivity of protoplasts to the nutrients of a given medium. Thus, some media can selectively support the development of hybrids but not the parental protoplasts.

A diagrammatic representation of visual selection coupled with the growth of heterokaryons on a selection medium is given in ***Fig. 44.8.***

2. **Mechanical isolation :** The visually identified heterokaryons under the microscope can be isolated by mechanical means. This involves the use of a special pipette namely Drummond pipette. The so isolated heterokaryons can be cloned to finally produce somatic hybrid plants. The major limitation of this method is that each type of hybrid

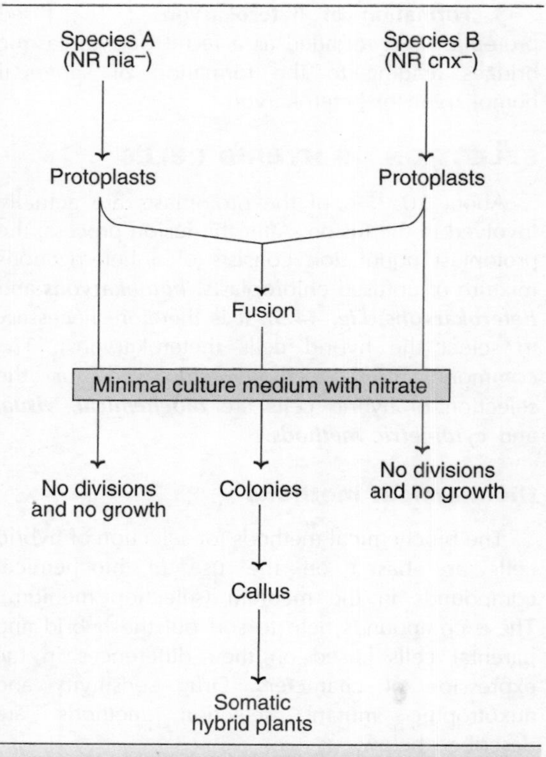

Fig. 44.7 : A diagrammatic representation of hybrid selection based on auxotrophic mutant (NR nia⁻— Nitrate reductase apoenzyme deficient; NR cnx⁻— Nitrate reductase lacking molybdenum cofactor).

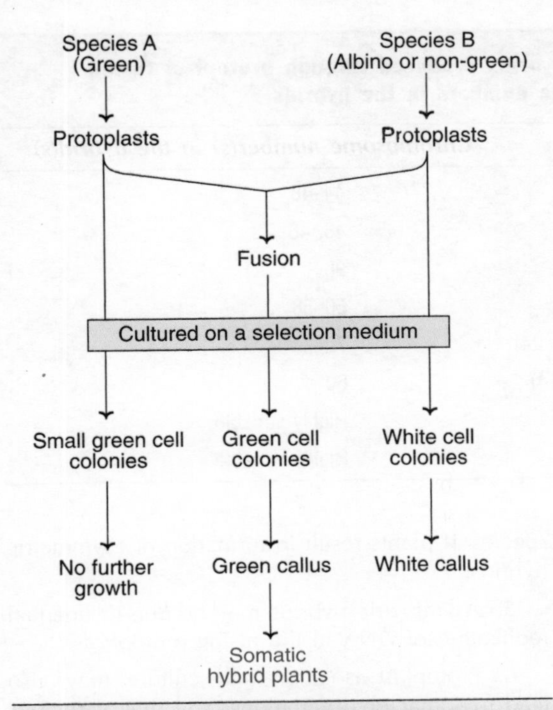

Fig. 44.8 : A diagrammatic representation of visual selection of hybrids coupled with growth on selection medium.

cell requires a special culture medium for its growth. This can be overcome by employing microdrop culture of single cells using feeder layers (Refer p. 506).

Cytometric methods

Some workers use flow cytometry and fluorescent-activated cell sorting techniques for the analysis of plant protoplasts while their viability is maintained. The same techniques can also be applied for sorting and selection of heterokaryons. The hybrid cells derived from such selections have proved useful for the development of certain somatic hybrid plants.

IDENTIFICATION OF HYBRID (CELLS) PLANTS

The development of hybrid cells followed by the generation of hybrid plants requires a clear proof of genetic countribution from both the parental protoplasts. The hybridity must be established only from euploid and not from aneuploid hybrids. Some of the commonly used approaches for the identification of hybrid plants are briefly described.

Morphology of hybrid plants

Morphological features of hybrid plants which ***usually are intermediate between two parents*** can be identified. For this purpose, the vegetative and floral characters are considered. These include leaf shape, leaf area, root morphology, flower shape, its structure, size and colour, and seed capsule morphology.

The somatic hybrids such as ***pomatoes*** and ***topatoes*** which are the fused products of potato and tomato show abnormal morphology, and thus can be identified.

Although the genetic basis of the morphological characters has not been clearly known, intermediate morphological features suggest that the traits are under the control of multiple genes. It is preferrable to support hybrid morphological characters with evidence of genetic data.

Isoenzyme analysis of hybrid plants

The multiple forms of an enzyme catalysing the same reaction are referred to as isoenzymes. Electrophoretic patterns of isoenzymes have been widely used to verify hybridity. ***Somatic hybrids posses specific isoenzymes*** (of certain enzymes) of one or the other parent or both the parents simultaneously.

There are many enzymes possessing unique isoenzymes that can be used for the identification of somatic hybrids e.g. amylase, esterase, aspartate aminotransferase, phosphodiesterase, isoperoxidase, and hydrogenases (of alcohol, lactate, malate). If the enzyme is dimeric (having two subunits), somatic hybrids usually contain an isoenzyme with an intermediate mobility properties.

The isoenzymes are often variable within the same plant. Therefore, it is necessary to use the same enzyme from each plant (parents and somatic hybrids), from a specific tissue with the same age.

Chromosomal constitution

The number of chromosomes present in the hybrid cells can be directly counted. This provides information on the ploidy state of the cells. The somatic hybrids are expected to possess chromosomes that are equal to the total number of

TABLE 44.3 A selected list of interspecific hybrids produced through protoplast fusion along with the chromosome numbers in the hybrids

Plant species with their chromosome number	*Chromosome number(s) in the hybrid(s)*
Petunia parodii (2n = 48) + *P. hybrida* (2n = 14)	44–48
Datura innoxia (2n = 24) + *D. stramonium* (2n = 24)	46, 48, 72
Nicotiana tabacum (2n = 48) + *N. nesophila* (2n = 48)	96
Nicotiana tabacum (2n = 48) + *N. glutinosa* (2n = 24)	50–58
Lycopersicon esculentum (2n = 24) + *L. peruvianum* (2n = 24)	72
Solanum tuberosum (2n = 24, 48) + *S. chacoense* (2n = 14)	60
Brassica oleracea (2n = 18) + *B. campestris* (2n = 18)	Highly variable
Brassica napus (2n = 38) + *B. juncea* (2n = 36)	Highly variable

chromosomes originally present in the parental protoplasts. Sometimes, the hybrids are found to contain more chromosomes than the total of both the parents. The presence of chromosomal markers is greatly useful for the genetic analysis of hybrid cells.

Molecular techniques

Many recent developments in molecular biology have improved the understanding of genetic constitution of somatic plant hybrids. Some of them are listed below.

1. Differences in the restriction patterns of chloroplast and mitochondrial DNAs.

2. Molecular markers such as RFLP, AFLP, RAPD and microsatellites.

3. PCR technology.

CHROMOSOME NUMBER IN SOMATIC HYRBIDS

The chromosome number in the somatic hybrids is ***generally more than the total number of both of the parental protoplasts***. However, wide variations are reported which may be due to the following reasons

1. Fusion of more than two protoplasts.

2. Irregularities in mitotic cell divisions.

3. In fusogen or electro-induced fusions, about one third of the fusions occur between more than two protoplasts.

4. Differences in the status of protoplasts (actively dividing or quiescent) from the two species of plants result in formation of asymmetric hybrids.

5. Asymmetric hybrids may be due to unequal replication of DNA in the fusing protoplasts.

6. Protoplast isolation and culture may also lead to somaclonal variations, and thus variations in chromosome number.

A selected list of interspecific hybrids produced through protoplast fusion along with the number of chromosomes in the hybrids is given in ***Table 44.3***.

Symmetric and asymmetric hybrids

If the ***chromosome number in the hybrid is the sum of the chromosomes*** of the two parental protoplasts, the hybrid is said to be ***symmetric***. Symmetric hybrids between incompatible species are usually sterile. This may be due to production of 3n hybrids by fusing 2n of one species with n of another species.

Asymmetric hybrids have abnormal or wide variations in the chromosome number than the exact total of two species. These hybrids are usually formated with full somatic complement of one parental species while all or nearly all of the chromosomes of other parental species are lost during mitotic divisions. Asymmetric hybrids may be regarded as cybrids but for the introgressed genes.

As given in ***Table 44.3***, protoplast fusion between *N. tabacum* (2n = 48) and *N. nesophila* (2n = 24) results in a symmetric hybrids, while asymmetric hybrids are formed when *B. napus* and *B. junea* are fused.

CYBRIDS

The ***cytoplasmic hybrids where the nucleus is derived from only one parent and the cytoplasm is derived from both the parents*** are referred to as cybrids. The phenomenon of formation of cybrids is regarded as ***cybridization***. Normally, cybrids are prduced when protoplasts from two phytogenetically distinct species are fused. Genetically, ***cybrids are hybrids only for cytoplasmic traits.***

Hybrids and somatic incompatibility

Many a times, production of full-pledged hybrids through fusion of ***protoplasts of distantly related higher plant species*** is rather difficult due to instability of the two dissimilar genomes in a common cytoplasm. This phenomenon is referred to as ***somatic incompatibility***. Hybrids formed despite somatic incompatibility may exhibit structural and developmental abnormalities. Several generations may be required to eliminate the undesirable genes. Due to this limitation in somatic hybridization, cybridization involving protoplast fusion for partial genome transfer is gaining importance in recent years.

Methodology of cybridization

A diagrammatic representation of the formation of hybrids and cybrids is given in ***Fig. 44.9***.

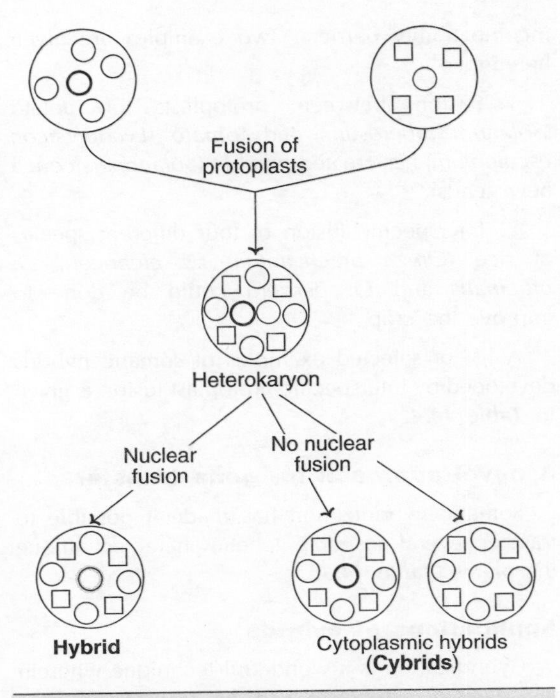

*Fig. 44.9 : A diagrammatic representation of hybridization and cybridization (**Note** : The plastids are shown as □ and ○)*

As the formation of heterokaryon occurs during hybridization, the nuclei can be stimulated to segregate so that one protoplast contributes to the cytoplasm while the other contributes nucleus alone (or both nucleus and cytoplasm). In this way cybridization can be achieved. Some of the approaches of cybridization are given hereunder.

1. The protoplasts of cytoplasm donor species are ***irradiated with X-rays*** or ***γ-rays***. This treatment renders the protoplasts inactive and non-dividing, but they are efficient donors of cytoplasmic constituents when fused with recipient protoplasts.

2. Normal ***protoplasts can be*** directly ***fused with enucleated protoplasts.*** Enucleated protoplasts can be isolated by high-speed centrifugation.

3. Protoplasts are ***inactivated by metabolic inhibitors*** such as iodoacetate. In practice, iodoacetate treated protoplasts are fused with X-rays irradiated protoplasts for more efficient formation of cybrids.

4. It is possible to suppress nuclear division in some protoplasts and fuse them with normal protoplasts.

Genetic recombination in asexual or sterile plants

There are many plants that cannot reproduce sexually. Somatic hybridization is a novel approach through which two parental genomes of a sexual or sterile plants can be brought together. Thus, by fusing parental protoplasts, fertile diploids and polyploids can be produced.

Overcoming barriers of sexual incompatibility

Sexual crossing between two different species (interspecific) and two different genus (intergeneric) is impossible by conventional breeding methods. Somatic hybridization overcomes the sexual incompatibility barriers. Two examples are given hereunder.

1. Fusion between protoplasts of ***po***tato (*Solanum tuberosum*) and to***mato*** (*Lycopersicon esculentum*) has created ***pomato*** (*Solanopersicon*, a new genus).

2. Interspecific fusion of four different species of rice (*Oryza brachyantha, O. eichngeri, O. officinalis* and *O. perrieri*) could be done to improve the crop.

A list of selected examples of somatic hybrids developed by interspecific protoplast fusion is given in ***Table 44.4***.

TABLE 44.4 Selected examples of somatic hybrids developed by interspecific protoplast fusion

Common name (botanical name)	*Common name (botanical name)*
Tomato (*Lycopersicon esculentum*)	Potato (*Solanum tuberosum*)
Petunia (*Petunia parodii*)	Petunia (*Petunia parviflora*)
Thorn apple (*Datura innoxia*)	Deadly nightshade (*Atropa belladonna*)
Turnip (*Brassica campestis*)	Thale cress (*Arabidopsis thaliana*)

A novel approach for gene transfer

Somatic hybridization has made it possible to transfer several desirable genetic characters among the plants (***Table 44.5***).

Applications of cybrids

Cybridization is a wonderful technique wherein the ***desired cytoplasm can be transferred in a single step***. Cybrids are important for the transfer of cytoplasmic male sterility (CMS), antibiotic and herbicide resistance in agriculturally useful plants.

Some of the genetic triats in certain plants are cytoplasmically controlled. This includes some types of ***male sterility, resistance to certain antibiotics and herbicides***. A selected list of agronomic characters transferred through cybrids is given in ***Table 44.5*** (along with somatic hybrids).

Cybridization has been successfully used to transfer CMS in rice. Cybrids of *Brassica raphanus* that contain nucleus of *B. napus,* chloroplasts of atrazinc resistant *B. campestris* and male sterility from *Raphanus sativas* have been developed.

APPLICATIONS OF SOMATIC HYBRIDIZATION

Somatic hybridization has opened new possibilites for the *in vitro* ***genetic manipulation of plants to improve the crops***. Some of the practical application are briefly given

1. **Disease resistance :** Several interspecific and intergeneric hybrids with disease resistance have been created. Many disease resistance genes (e.g., tobacco mosaic virus, potato virus X, club rot disease) could be successfully transferred from one species to another. For example, resistance has been introduced in tomato against diseases such as TMV, spotted wilt virus and insect pests.

2. **Environmental tolerance :** The genes responsible for the tolerance of cold, frost and salt could be successfully introduced through somatic hybridization. e.g., introduction of cold tolerance gene in tomato.

3. **Quality characters :** Somatic hybrids for the production of high nicotine content, and low erucic acid have been developed (***Table 44.5***).

4. **Cytoplasmic male sterility :** A modification of hybridization in the form of cybridization has made it possible to transfer cytoplasmic male sterility. Details given in the preceeding section.

Other application of somatic hybridization

1. Somatic hybridization has helped to study the cytoplasmic genes and their functions. In fact, the information is successfully used in plant breeding programmes.

2. Protoplast fusion will help in the combination of mitochondria and chloroplasts to result in a unique nuclear-cytoplasmic genetic combination.

3. Somatic hybridization can be done in plants that are still in juvenile phase.

4. Protoplast transformation (with traits like nitrogen fixation by incorporating exogenous DNA) followed by somatic hybridization will yield innovative plants.

TABLE 44.5 A selected list of genetic traits transferred through protoplast fusion in crop plant species

Somatic hybrids	*Genetic trait in new plant/ resistance (or tolerance) trait*
Nicotiana tobaccum + N. nesophila	Tobacco mosaic virus
	Tobacco horn worm
Solanum tuberosum + S. chacoense	Potato virus X
Solanum tuberosum + S. commersounii	Frost tolerance
Solanum tuberosum + S. brevidens	Potato leaf roll virus
Solanum ochranthum + Lycopersicon esculentum	Cold tolerance
Brassica oleracea + B. napus	Black rot
Citrullus lanatus + Cucumis melo	Club rot
Raphanus sativus + Brassica napus	Beet cyst nematode
Hordeum vulgare + Daucus carota	Frost and salt tolerance
Somatic hybrids	***Quality character***
Nicotiana tabacum + N. rustica	High nicotine content
Brassica napus + Eruca sativa	Low erucic acid
Cytoplasmic hybrids (cybrids)	***Agronomic character***
Nicotiana tabacum + N. sylvestris	Streptomycin resistance
Nicotiana nigrum + Solanum tuberosum	Triazine resistance
Brassica nigra + B. napus	Hygromycin resistance
Solanum nigrum + S. tuberosum	Triazine resistance
Nicotiana tabacum + N. sylvestris	Cytoplasmic male sterility
Brassica napus + B. tournefortii	Cytoplasmic male sterility
Brassica campestris + B. napus	Cytoplasmic male sterility
Lycopersicon esculentum + Solanum acaule	Cytoplasmic male sterility
Brasica napus + B. campestris + Raphanus sativa	Cytoplasmic male sterility and triazine resistance

LIMITATIONS OF SOMATIC HYBRIDIZATION

Although somatic hybridization is a novel approach in plant biotechnology, there are several problems and limitations. The success of the technique largely depends on overcoming these limitations, some of which are listed below.

1. Somatic hybridization does ***not always produce plants that give fertile and visible seeds***.

2. Regenerated plants obtained from somatic hybridization are often ***variable due to somaclonal variations***, chromosomal elimination, organelle segregation etc.

3. Protoplast culture is frequently associated with genetic instability.

4. Protoplast fusion between different species/ genus is easy, but the production of viable somatic hybrids is not possible in all instances.

5. Some of the somatic hybrids, particularly when produced by the fusion of taxonomically different partners, are unbalanced and not viable.

6. There are limitations in the selection methods of hybrids, as many of them are not efficient.

7. There is no certainity as regards the expression of any specific character in somatic hybridization.

8. Somatic hybridization between two diploids results in the formation of an amphidiploid which is not favourable. For this reason, haploid protoplasts are recommended in somatic hybridization.

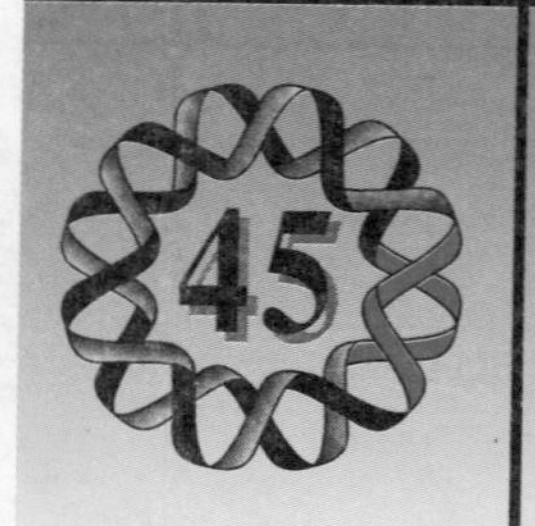

Production of Haploid Plants

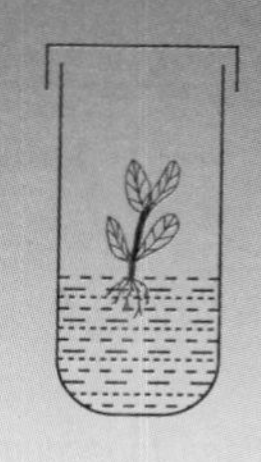

Haploid plants are characterized by ***possessing only a single set of chromosomes*** (gametophytic number of chromosomes i.e. n) in the sporophyte. This is in contrast to diploids which contain two sets (2n) of chromosomes. Haploid plants are of great significance for the production of ***homozygous lines*** (homozygous plants) and for the improvement of plants in plant breeding programmes.

Brief history

The existence of haploids was discovered (as early as 1921) by Bergner in *Datura stramonium*. Plant breeders have been conducting extensive research to develop haploids. The Indian scientists ***Guha and Maheswari (1964) reported the direct development of haploid embryos and plantlets from microspores of Datura innoxia*** by the cultures of excised anthers. Subsequently, Bourgin and Hitsch (1967) obtained the first full-pledged haploid plants from *Nicotiana tabacum*. Thereafter, much progress has been made in the anther cultures of wheat, rice, maize, pepper and a wide range of economically important species.

Grouping of haploids

Haploids may be divided into two broad categories.

1. **Monoploids (monohaploids) :** These are the haploids that possess half the number of chromosomes from a diploid species e.g. maize, barley.

2. **Polyhaploids :** The haploids possessing half the number of chromosomes from a polyploid species are regarded as polyhaploids e.g. wheat, potato.

It may be noted that when the term haploid is generally used it applies to any plant originating from a sporophyte (2n) and containing half the number (n) of chromosomes.

IN VIVO AND *IN VITRO* APPROACHES

The importance of haploids in the field of plant breeding and genetics was realised long ago. Their practical application, however, has been restricted due to very a low frequency (< 0.001%) of their formation in nature. The process of apomixis or ***parthenogenesis*** (***development of embryo from an unfertilized egg***) is responsible for the spontaneous ***natural production of haploids***. Many attempts were made, both by *in vivo* and *in vitro* methods to develop haploids. The success was much higher by *in vitro* techniques.

In vivo techniques for haploid production

There are several methods to induce haploid production *in vivo*. Some of them are listed below.

1. **Androgenesis :** Development of an egg cell containing ***male nucleus*** to a haploid is referred to as androgenesis. For a successful *in vivo* androgenesis, the egg nucleus has to be inactivated or eliminated before fertilization.

2. **Gynogenesis :** An ***unfertilized egg*** can be manipulated (by delayed pollination) to develop into a haploid plant.

3. **Distant hybridization :** Hybrids can be produced by elimination of one of the parental genomes as a result of distant (interspecific or intergeneric crosses) hybridization.

4. **Irradiation effects :** Ultra violet rays or X-rays may be used to induce chromosomal breakage and their subsequent elimination to produce haploids.

5. **Chemical treatment :** Certain chemicals (e.g., chloramphenicol, colchicine, nitrous oxide, maleic hydrazide) can induce chromosomal elimination in somatic cells which may result in haploids.

In vitro techniques for haploid production

In the plant biotechnology programmes, haploid production is achieved by two methods.

1. **Androgenesis :** Haploid production occurs through anther or pollen culture, and they are referred to as ***androgenic haploids***.

2. **Gynogenesis :** Ovary or ovule culture that results in the production of haploids, known as ***gynogenic haploids***.

ANDROGENESIS

In androgenesis, the male gametophyte (microspore or immature pollen) produces haploid plant. The basic principle is to ***stop the development of pollen cell into a gamete*** (sex cell) ***and force it to develop into a haploid plant***.

There are two approaches in androgenesis—anther culture and pollen (microspore) culture. Young plants, grown under optimal conditions of light, temperature and humidity, are suitable for androgenesis.

ANTHER CULTURE

The selected flower buds of young plants are surface-sterilized and anthers removed along with their filaments. The anthers are excised under aseptic conditions, and crushed in 1% acetocarmine to test the stage of pollen development. If they are at the correct stage, each anther is gently separated (from the filament) and the intact anthers are inoculated on a nutrient medium. Injured anthers should not be used in cultures as they result in callusing of anther wall tissue.

The anther cultures are maintained in alternating periods of light (12–18 hr) and darkness (6–12 hrs) at 28°C. As the anthers proliferate, they produce callus which later forms an embryo and then a haploid plant (***Fig. 45.1***).

POLLEN (MICROSPORE) CULTURE

Haploid plants can be produced from immature pollen or microspores (male gametophytic cells). The pollen can be extracted by pressing and squeezing the anthers with a glass rod against the sides of a beaker. The pollen suspension is filtered to remove anther tissue debris. Viable and large pollen (smaller pollen do not regenerate) are concentrated by filtration, washed and collected. These pollen are cultured on a solid or liquid medium. The callus/embryo formed is transferred to a suitable medium to finally produce a haploid plant (***Fig. 45.1***), and then a diploid plant (on colchicine treatment).

Comparison between anther and pollen cultures

Anther culture is easy, quick and practicable. Anther walls act as conditioning factors and promote culture growth. Thus, anther cultures are reasonably efficient for haploid production. The major limitation is that the plants not only originate from pollen but also from other parts of anther. This results in the population of plants at different ploidy levels (diploids, aneuploids). The disadvantages associated with anther culture can be overcome by pollen culture.

Many workers prefer pollen culture, even though the degree of success is low, as it offers the following ***advantages***

- Undesirable effects of anther wall and associated tissues can be avoided.
- Androgenesis, starting from a single cell, can be better regulated.
- Isolated microspores (pollen) are ideal for various genetic manipulations (transformation, mutagenesis).
- The yield of haploid plants is relatively higher.

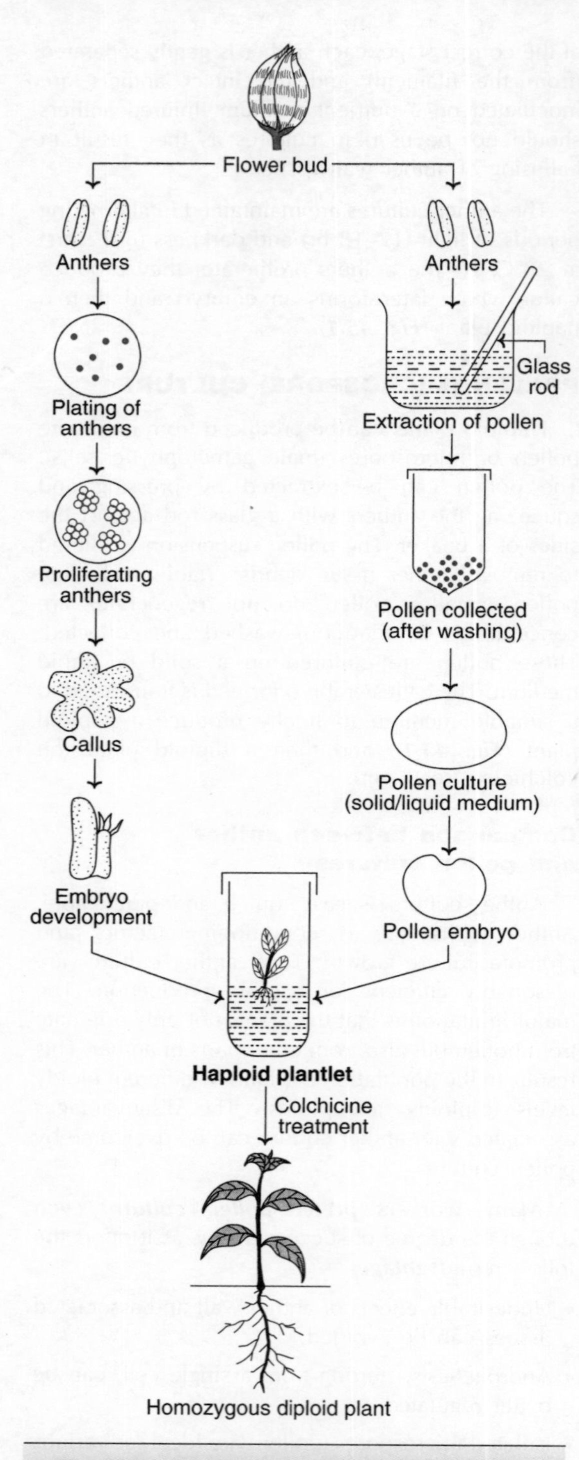

Fig. 45.1 : Diagrammatic representation of anther and pollen cultures for the production of haploid and diploid plants.

DEVELOPMENT OF ANDROGENIC HAPLOIDS

The process of *in vitro* androgenesis for the ultimate production of haploid plants is depicted in *Fig. 45.2*.

The cultured microspores mainly follow four distinct pathways during he initial stages of *in vitro* androgenesis.

Pathway I : The uninucleate microspore undergoes equal division to form ***two daughter cells*** of equal size e.g. *Datura innoxia*.

Pathway II : In certain plants, the microspore divides unequally to give bigger vegetative cell and a smaller generative cell. It is the ***vegetative cell*** that undergoes further divisions to ***form callus*** or embryo. The generative cell, on the other hand, degenerates after one or two divisions—e.g., *Nicotiana tabacum, Capsicum annuum.*

Pathway III : In this case, the microspore undergoes unequal division. The ***embryos are formed from the generative cell*** while the vegetative cell does not divide at all or undergoes limited number of divisions e.g. *Hyoscyamus niger.*

Pathway IV : The microspore divides unequally as in pathways I and II. However, in this case, both ***vegetative and generative cells*** can further divide and ***contribute to the development of haploid*** plant e.g. *Datura metel, Atropa belladonna.*

At the initial stages, the microspore may follow any one of the four pathways described above. As the cells divide, the pollen grain becomes multicellular and burst open. This multicelluar mass may form a callus which later differentiates into a plant (through ***callus phase***). Alternately, the multicellular mass may produce the plant through ***direct embryogenesis*** (***Fig. 45.1***).

FACTORS AFFECTING ANDROGENESIS

A good knowledge of the various factors that influence androgenesis will help to improve the production of androgenic haploids. Some of these factors are briefly described.

Genotype of donar plants

The success of anther or pollen culture largely depends on the genotype of the donor plant. It is therefore important to ***select*** only ***highly responsive genotypes***. Some workers choose a breeding approach for improvement of genotype before they are used in androgenesis.

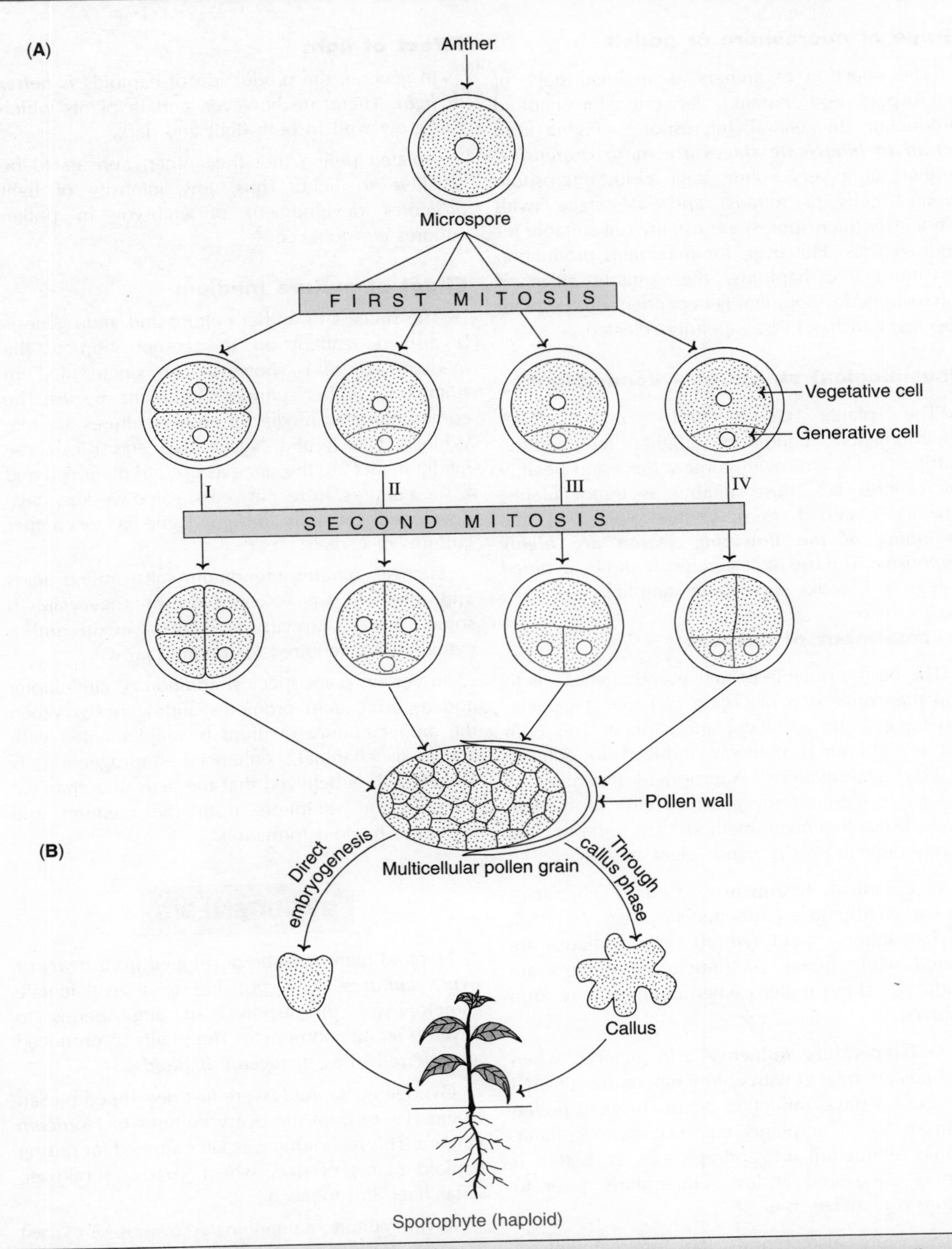

***Fig. 45.2 :** Diagrammatic representation of microscope divisions leading to the formation of a multicelluar pollen grain (**A**), followed by the formation of haploid sporophyte (**B**) (**Note :** I, II, III and IV indicate respective pathways).*

Stage of microspore or pollen

The selection of anthers at an ideal stage of microspore development is very critical for haploid production. In general, microspores ranging from ***tetrad to binucleate stages are more responsive***. Anthers at a very young stage (with microspore mother cells or tetrads) and late stage (with binucleate microspores) are usually not suitable for androgenesis. However, for maximum production of androgenic haploids, the suitable stage of microspore development is dependent on the plant species, and has to be carefully selected.

Physiological status of a donar plant

The plants grown under best natural environmental conditions (light, temperature, nutrition, CO_2 etc.) with good anthers and healthy microspores are most suitable as donor plants. Flowers obtained from young plants, at the ***beginning of the flowering season are highly responsive***. The use of pesticides should be avoided at least 3-4 weeks preceeding sampling.

Pretreatment of anthers

The basic principle of native androgenesis is to stop the conversion of pollen cell into a gamete, and force its development into a plant. This is in fact an abnormal pathway induced to achieve *in vitro* androgenesis. Appropriate treatment of anthers is required for good success of haploid production. Treatment methods are variable and largely depend on the donor plant species.

1. **Chemical treatment :** Certain chemicals are known to induce parthenogenesis e.g. 2-chloro-ethylphosphonic acid (ethrel). When plants are treated with ethreal, multinucleated pollens are produced. These pollens when cultured may form embryos.

2. **Temperature influence :** In general, when the buds are treated with cold temperatures (3-6°C) for about 3 days, induction occurs to yield pollen embryos in some plants e.g. *Datura, Nicotiana*. Further, induction of androgenesis is better if anthers are stored at low temperature, prior to culture e.g. maize, rye.

There are also reports that pretreatment of anthers of certain plants at higher temperatures (35°C) stimulates androgenesis e.g. some species of *Brassica* and *Capsicum*.

Effect of light

In general, the production of haploids ***is better in light***. There are however, certain plants which can grow well in both light and dark.

Isolated pollen (not the anther) appears to be sensitive to light. Thus, low intensity of light promotes development of embryos in pollen cultures e.g. tobacco.

Effect of culture medium

The success of anther culture and androgenesis is also dependent on the composition of the medium. There is, however, no single medium suitable for anther cultures of all plant species. The commonly used media for anther cultures are MS, White's, Nitsch and Nitsch, N6 and B5. These media in fact are the same as used in plant cell and tissue cultures. In recent years, some workers have developed specially designed media for anther cultures of cereals.

Sucrose, nitrate, ammonium salts, amino acids and minerals are essential for androgenesis. In some species, growth regulators — auxin and/or cytokinin are required for optimal growth.

In certain plant species, addition of glutathione and ascorbic acid promotes androgenesis. When the anther culture medium is supplemented with activated charcoal, enhanced androgenesis is observed. It is believed that the activated charcoal removes the inhibitors from the medium and facilitates haploid formation.

GYNOGENESIS

Haploid plants can be developed from ***ovary*** or ***ovule cultures***. It is possible to trigger female gametophytes (megaspores) of angiosperms to develop into a sporophyte. The plants so produced are referred to as ***gynogenic haploids***.

Gynogenic haploids were first developed by San Noem (1976) from the ovary cultures of *Hordeum vulgare*. This technique was later applied for raising haploid plants of rice, wheat, maize, sunflower, sugar beet and tobacco.

In vitro culture of unpollinated ovaries (or ovules) is usually employed when the anther cultures give unsatisfactory results for the production of haploid plants. The procedure for gynogenic haploid production is briefly described.

The flower buds are excised 24–48 hr prior to anthesis from unpollinated ovaries. After removal of calyx, corolla and stamens, the ovaries (see *Fig. 45.3)* are subjected to surface sterilization. The ovary, with a cut end at the distal part of pedicel, is inserted in the solid culture medium. Whenever a liquid medium is used, the ovarier are placed on a filter paper or allowed to float over the medium with pedicel inserted through filter paper. The commonly used media are MS, White's, N6 and Nitsch, supplemented growth factors.

Production of ***gynogenic haploids is particularly useful in plants with male sterile genotype***. For such plant species, this technique is superior to anther culture technique.

Limitations of gynogenesis

In practice, production of haploid plants by ovary/ ovule cultures is not used as frequently as anther/ pollen cultures in crop improvement programmes. The major limitations of gynogenesis are listed.

1. The dissection of unfertilized ovaries and ovules is rather difficult.
2. The presence of only one ovary per flower is another disadvantage. In contrast, there are a large number of microspores in one anther.

However, the future of gynogenesis may be more promising with improved and refined methods.

IDENTIFICATION OF HAPLOIDS

Two approaches based on morphology and genetics are commonly used to detect or identify haploids.

MORPHOLOGICAL APPROACH

The vegetative and floral parts, and the cell sizes of haploid plants are relatively reduced when compared to diploid plants. By this way haploids can be detected in a population of diploids. Morphological approach, however, is not as effective as genetic approach.

GENETIC APPROACH

Genetic markers are widely used for the specific identification of haploids. Several markers are in use.

- 'a_1' marker for brown coloured aleurone.
- 'A' marker for purple colour.
- 'Lg' marker for liguleless character.

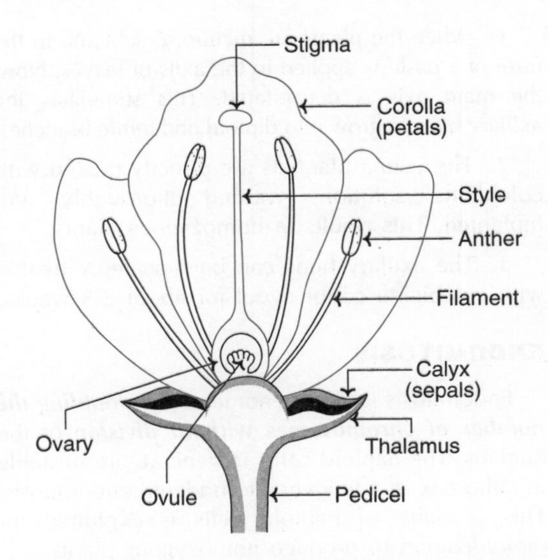

Fig. 45.3 : A diagrammatic representation of important parts in a flower.

The above markers have been used for the development of haploids of maize.

It may be noted that for the detection of androgenic haploids, the dominant gene marker should be present in the female plant.

DIPLOIDIZATION OF HAPLOID PLANTS (PRODUCTION OF HOMOZYGOUS PLANTS)

As described in the preceeding pages, haploid plants are obtained either by androgenesis or gynogenesis. These plants may grow up to a flowering stage, but viable gametes cannot be formed due to lack of one set of homologous chromosomes. Consequently, there is no seed formation.

Haploids can be diploidized (by duplication of chromosomes) to produce homozygous plants. There are mainly two approaches for diploidization—colchicine treatment and endomitosis.

COLCHICINE TREATMENT

Colchicine is very widely used for diploidization of homologous chromosomes. It acts as an inhibitor of spindle formation during mitosis and ***induces chromosome duplication***. There are many ways of colchicine treatment to achieve diploidization for production of homozygous plants.

1. When the plants are mature, colchicine in the form of a paste is applied to the axils of leaves. Now, the main axis is decapitated. This stimulates the axillary buds to grow into diploid and fertile branches.

2. The young plantlets are directly treated with colchicine solution, washed thoroughly and replanted. This results in homozygous plants.

3. The axillary buds can be repeatedly treated with colchicine cotton wool for about 2-3 weeks.

ENDOMITOSIS

Endomitosis is the phenomenon of ***doubling the number of chromosomes without division*** of the nucleus. The haploid cells, in general, are unstable in culture with a tendency to undergo endomitosis. This property of haploid cells is exploited for diploidization to produce homozygous plants.

The procedure involves growing a small segment of haploid plant stem in a suitable medium supplemented with growth regulators (auxin and cytokinin). This induces callus formation followed by differentiation. During the growth of callus, chromosomal doubling occurs by endomitosis. This results in the production of diploid homozygous cells and ultimately plants.

APPLICATIONS OF HAPLOIDS

In vitro production of haploids is of great ***significance in plant breeding programmes***. Some of them are listed.

Development of homozygous lines

It is now possible to develop ***homozygous lines within a span of few months or a year*** by employing anther/pollen culture. This is in contrast to the conventional plant breeding programme that might take several years (6–10 yrs). In this way, production of haploids is highly useful for research related to plant genetics and breeding.

Generation of exclusive male plants

By the process of androgenesis to produce haploids, followed by chromosome doubling, it is possible to develop exclusive male plants. The male plants are particularly useful when their productivity and applications are much more than female plants.

Induction of mutations

In general, majority of induced mutations are recessive and therefore are not expressed in diploid cells (due to the presence of dominant allele). Haploids provide a convenient system for the induction of mutations and selection of mutants with desired traits. In fact, the haploid cells can be cultured and handled in a fashion similar to microorganisms.

Mutants from several plant species that are ***resistant to antibiotics, toxins, herbicides*** etc. have ***been developed***. When the haploid cells of tobacco plant (*Nicotiana tabacum*) were exposed to methionine sulfoximine (a mutagen), mutants which showed lower level of infection to *Pseudomonas tabaci* were produced.

Production of disease resistance plants

Disease resistance genes can be introduced while producing haploids. The so developed haploids are screened for the desired resistance, and then diploidized. Some examples of disease resistance plants are listed.

1. Hwansambye, a rice variety resistant to leaf blast, bacterial leaf blight and rice stripe tenui virus.

2. Barley accession Q21681 resistant to stem rust, leaf rust and powdery mildew.

More examples of disease resistance crops are given in ***Table 45.1***.

Production of insect resistance plants

Some varieties of rice resistant to insects have been developed e.g. Hwacheongbyeo resistant to brown plant hopper. Other varieties of rice that are resistant to pests have also been produced.

Production of salt tolerance plants

The plant species with salt tolerance are needed for their cultivation in some areas. Anther cultures have resulted in some varieties of rice and wheat with good salt tolerance e.g. wheat Hua Bain 124–4.

Cytogenetic research

Haploids are useful in several areas of cytogenetic research. These include

- Production of aneuploids

TABLE 45.1 A selected list of improved varieties of crops developed by using anther culture

Crop	*Varieties*	*Improvements made*
Wheat (*Triticum aestivum*)	Lunghua 1, Zing Hua 1, Zing Hua 2 Huapei 1, Florin, Ambitus, Jingdan 2288	High yield, rust resistance, cold resistance, large spikes, more tillers.
Rice (*Oryza sativa*)	Tangfong 1, Xin Xiu, Zhog Hua 8 Zhong Hua 9, Hua yu 1, Hua Yu 2, Huapei Shanyou 63, Zhe keng 66, Ta Be 78, Nonhua 5, Hirohikari, Hirohonami.	High yield, good quality, disease resistance
Tobacco (*Nicotiana tabacum*)	Tanyu 1, Tanyu 2, Tanyu 3, F 211 Hai Hua 19, Hai Hua 30	Mild smoking, disease resistance
Brassica napus	Jai kisan	Low erucic acid

- Determination of the nature of ploidy
- Determination of basic chromosome number
- Evaluation of origin of chromosomes.

Induction of genetic variability

Besides the development of haploid mutants, it is also possible to produce plants with various ploidy levels through androgenesis.

Doubled haploids in genome mapping

Genome mapping, a recent development in molecular biology, can be more conveniently achieved by using doubled haploid plant species.

Evolutionary studies

A comparison of dihaploids (doubled haploids) with diploid wild plant species will be useful to trace the evolutionary origin of various plants. The close evolutionary relationship between tomato and potato has been evaluated by this approach.

CROPS DEVELOPED THROUGH ANTHER CULTURES

Anther culture has made it possible to develop many new varieties of plants, a selected list is given in ***Table 45.1***.

In general, the new crops are high-yielding varieties with disease resistance. Some of them are resistance to cold, salt etc. Many plant breeders these days use anther cultures in their regular breeding programmes.

LIMITATIONS OF HAPLOIDS

It has been possible to raise several haploid plants through anther cultures. However, haploid breeding programmes have not yielded the expected and desired results, despite heavy investments made during the past 3 decades. There are many problems encountered with haploid production. Some of them are listed below.

1. The ***frequency of haploid production is very low***, hence selection is often difficult.

2. The operation of tissue culture to develop haploids requires high level expertise and management.

3. Besides haploids, ***different ploidy levels are also produced***.

4. Haploids with deleterious traits frequently develop in cultures.

5. The callus derived from anther culture is usually detrimental to haploid production.

6. Isolation of haploids from cultures is often difficult since ***polyploids outgrow haploids***.

7. The embryos derived from haploids often get aborted.

8. Haploid production is associated with high incidence of albino (colourless) plants.

9. The doubling of haploids (***diploidization***) may ***not always lead to the formation of homozygous plant***.

10. *In vitro* haploid production is not economically viable due to very low success rate.

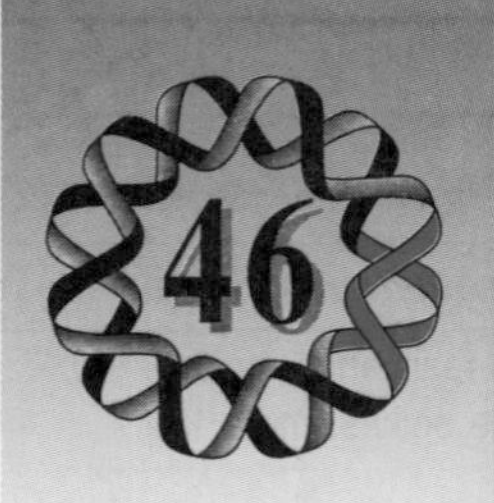

Somaclonal Variations

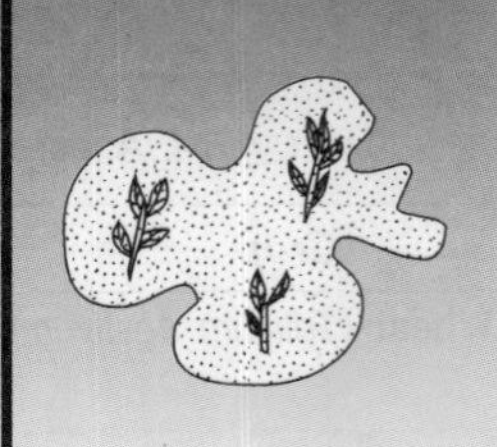

The ***genetic variations found in the in vitro cultured cells*** are collectively referred to as somaclonal variations. The plants derived from such cells are referred to ***somaclones.***

Some authors use the terms ***calliclones*** and ***protoclones*** to represent cultures obtained from callus and protoplasts respectively.

The growth of plant cells *in vitro* is an asexual process involving only mitotic division of cells. Thus, culturing of cells is the method to clone a particular genotype. It is therefore expected that plants arising from a given tissue culture should be the exact copies of the parental plant. The occurrence of phenotypic variants among the regenerated plants (from tissue cultures) has been known for several years. These variations were earlier dismissed as tissue culture artefacts.

The term somaclonal variations was first used by Larkin and Scowcraft (1981) for variations arising due to culture of cells. i.e., ***variability generated by a tissue culture***. This term is now universally accepted.

As described elsewhere (Chapter 42), the explant used in tissue culture may come from any part of the plant organs or cells. These include leaves, roots, protoplasts, microspores and embryos. Somaclonal variations are reported in all types of plant tissue cultures.

In recent years, the term ***gametoclonal variations*** is used for the variations observed in the regenerated plants from gametic cells (e.g., anther cultures). For the plants obtained from protoplast cultures, ***protoclonal variations*** is used.

BASIS OF SOMACLONAL VARIATIONS

Somaclonal variations occur as a result of ***genetic heterogeneity*** (change in chromosome number and/or structure) in plant tissue cultures. This may be due to

- Expression of chromosomal mosaicism or genetic disorders.
- Spontaneous mutations due to culture conditions.

The genetic changes associated with somaclonal variations include polyploidy, aneuploidy, chromosomal breakage, deletion, translocation, and gene amplifications, besides several mutations. In fact, the presence of several chromosomal aberrations—reciprocal translocation, deletions, inversions, chromosomal breakage, multicentric, acentric fragments have been found among the somaclones of barley, garlic and oat.

The occurrence of mutations in cultures is relatively low. Mutations may be due varied nutrients, culture conditions and mutagenic effects of metabolic products that accumulate in the medium.

Somaclonal variations due to transposable elements, mitotic crossing over and changes in the cytoplasmic genome have also been reported.

Nomenclature of somaclones

The somaclones that are regenerated from tissue cultures directly are regarded as R_0 or R plants. The self-fertilized progeny of R_0 plants represent R_1 plants. R_2, R_3, R_4 etc. plants are the subsequent generations. Some workers use other nomenclature — somaclones ($SC_1 = R_0$), SC_2, SC_3, SC_4 etc. for subsequent generations.

ISOLATION OF SOMACLONAL VARIANTS

There are two procedures commonly used for obtaining the crop plants with somaclonal variations

1. Without *in vitro* selection
2. With *in vitro* selection.

WITHOUT *IN VITRO* SELECTION

An explant (leaf, stem, root etc.) is cultured on a suitable medium, supplemented with growth regulators. The unorganized callus and cells do not contain any selective agent (toxic or inhibitory substance). These cultures are normally subcultured, and transferred to shoot induction medium for regeneration of plants. The so produced plants are grown in pots, transferred to field, and analyzed for somaclonal variants (***Fig. 46.1***).

Somaclonal variants of several crops have been successfully obtained by this approach e.g., sugarcane, potato, tomato, cereals etc. A selected list of disease resistant crop plants obtained from somaclonal variations without *in vitro* selection along with the pathogenic organisms is given in ***Table 46.1***.

Limitations of without *in vitro* selection approach

There is no directed and specific approach for the isolation of somaclones without *in vitro* selection. Consequently, the appearance of a desired trait is purely by chance. Further, this procedure is time consuming and requires screening of many plants.

WITH *IN VITRO* SELECTION

Isolation of somaclones with *in vitro* selection method basically involves handling of plant cells in cultures (protoplast, callus) like microorganisms and selection of biochemical mutants. The cell lines are screened from plant cultures for their ability to survive in the presence of a toxic/inhibitory substance in the medium or under conditions of environmental stress.

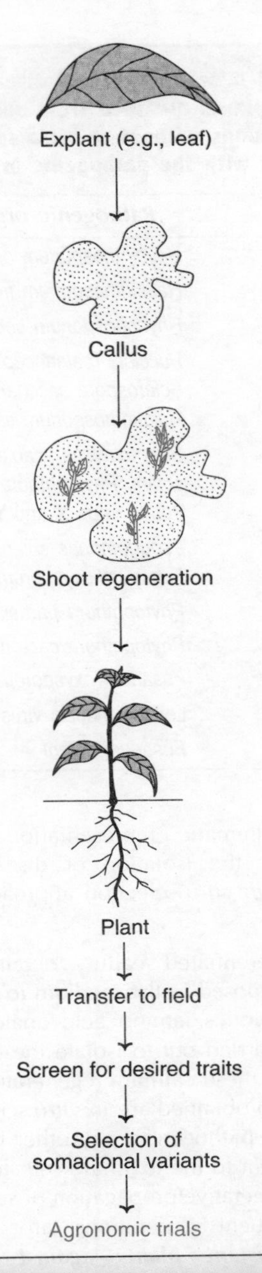

***Fig. 46.1 :** A diagrammatic representation of isolation of somaclones without* in vitro *selection.*

Table 46.1 A selected list of disease resistant crop plants obtained from somaclonal variations without *in vitro* selection, along with the pathogenic organisms

Crop	Pathogenic organism(s)
Rice	*Helminthosporium oryzae*
Maize	*Helminthosporium maydis*
Barley	*Rhynchosporium secalis*
Sugarcane	*Puccinia melanocephala, Sclerospora sacchari Helminthosporium sacchari*, Fiji virus
Potato	*Streptomyces scabie, Alternaria solani, Phytophthora infestans,* Potato virus X and Y.
Tomato	*Pseudomonas solanacearum, Fusarium oxysporum*
Tobacco	*Phytophthora parasitica*
Apple	*Phytophthora cactorum*
Banana	*Fusarium oxysporum*
Lettuce	Lettuce mosaic virus
Alfalfa	*Fusarium solani*

A diagrammatic representation of *in vitro* protocol for the isolation of disease resistance plants with *in vitro* selection approach is given in ***Fig. 46.2***.

The differentiated callus, obtained from an explant is exposed in the medium to inhibitors like toxins, antibiotics, amino acid analogs. Selection cycles are carried out to isolate the tolerant callus cultures and these calli are regenerated into plants. The plants so obtained are *in vitro* screened against the toxin (or pathogen or any other inhibitor). The plants resistant to the toxin are selected and grown further by vegetative propagation or self pollination. The subsequent generations are analysed for ***disease resistant plants against the specific pathogenic organism.***

A selected list of disease resistant crop plants obtained from somaclonal variations by *in vitro* selection along with pathogenic organisms and selection agents is given in ***Table 46.2***.

Besides the disease resistant plants (described above), plants with herbicide resistance and antibiotic resistance have also been developed with *in vitro* selection approach.

Environmental stress tolerance

High salt concentration in the soil is the major constraint limiting the crop development and yield. Many plants with salt tolerance (salinity) have been developed e.g. rice, tobacco.

Several attempts are being made by plant biotechnologists to develop cold tolerant crops, although the success rate has been very limited.

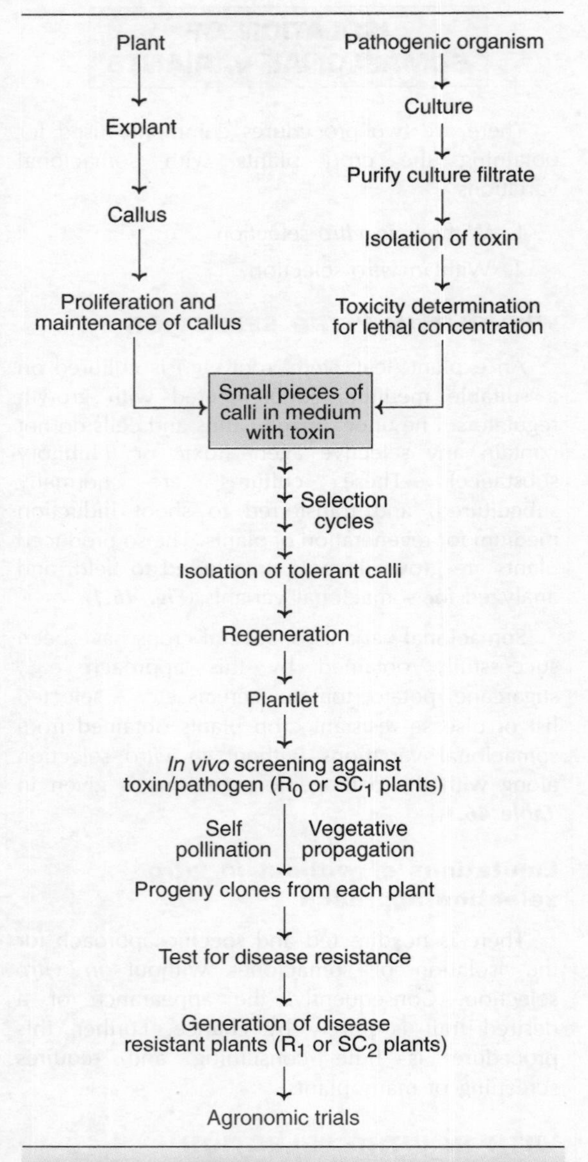

***Fig. 46.2 :** A diagrammatic representation of isolation of disease resistant plants with* in vitro *selection.*

TABLE 46.2 A selected list of disease resistant crop plants obtained from somaclonal variations with *in vitro* selection along with pathogenic organisms and selection agents

Crop	*Pathogenic organism(s)*	*Selection agent*
Rice	*Xanthomonas oryzae*	Bacterial cells
Wheat	*Helminthosporium sativum*	Crude toxin
	Pseudomonas syringae	Syringomycin
Barley	*Fusarium* sp	Fusaric acid
	Helminthosporium sativum	Crude toxin
Maize	*Helminthosporium maydis*	Hm T toxin
Sugarcane	*Helminthosporium sacchari*	Toxin
Potato	*Fusarium oxysporum*	Culture filtrate
	Ercoinia carotovora	Pathogen
Tomato	*Pseudomonas solanacearum*	Crude filtrate
	Tobacco mosaic virus	Virus
Alfalfa	*Foxysporum* sp	Crude filtrate
Tobacco	Tobacco mosaic virus	Virus
	Pseudomonas syringae	Methionine sulfoximine

Advantages of with *in vitro* selection appraoch

The major advantage of with *in vitro* selection method is the specific selection of the desired trait rather than a general variation found at the plant level. This procedure is less time consuming when compared to without *in vitro* selection approach.

FACTORS AFFECTING PRODUCTION OF SOMACLONAL VARIANTS

Some of the important factors that influence development of somaclonal variants by without *in vitro* selection and with *in vitro* selection are briefly described.

Genotype and explant source

The nature of genotype of the plants ***influences the frequency of regeneration and frequency of production of somaclones***.

Explants can be taken from any part of plant— leaves, roots, internodes, ovaries etc. The source of explant is very critical for somaclonal variations. For instance, potato plants regenerated from callus of rachis and petiole are much higher (~50%) compared to those regenerated from callus of leaves (~12%).

Duration of cell culture

In general, for many plant cultures, somaclonal variations are higher with increased duration of cultures. For example, it was reported that genetic variability increased in tobacco protoplasts from 1.5 to 6% by doubling the duration of cultures.

Growth hormone effects

The plant growth regulators in the medium will influence the karyotypic alterations in cultured cells, and therefore development of somaclones. Growth hormones such as 2, 4-dichlorophenoxy acetic acid (2, 4-D) and naphthalene acetic acid (NAA) are frequently used to achieve chromosomal variability.

Besides the factors discussed above, selection of somaclones with *in vitro* selection are dependent on the following parameters.

- Selection propagule (cells, protoplasts, calli).
- Selection agent (toxin, herbicide, amino acid analogue).
- Technique used for selection.
- Stability of resistant substance.
- *In vivo* testing procedure.
- Ability for regeneration of plants.

APPLICATIONS OF SOMACLONAL VARIATIONS

Somaclonal variations (and also gametoclonal variations, described later) are highly useful in plant breeding programmes. The genetic variations with desirable (or improved characters), besides the existing favourable characters can be introduced into the plants. In general, the ***methodology*** adopted for induction of somaclonal variations are ***simpler and easier compared to recombinant DNA technology***. Hence, they are ***preferred by some workers***. The important applications of somaclonal variations are briefly described.

TABLE 46.3 A selected list of somaclonal variants obtained from different crop species with their morphological characters

Crop	*Character(s)*
Rice	Flowering period, panicle size; tiller number; plant height; leaf length, shape and colour; frequency of fertile seed; sterility mutants.
Wheat	Plant height; tiller number; grain colour; seed storage protein.
Maize	Reduced pollen fertility and male sterility; twin stalks from a single node.
Sugarcane	High sugar yield; increased stalk length, diameter, weight and density.
Barley	Increased grain yield; leaf shape; heading date; ash content.
Oats	Plant height; heading date; morphology and fertility.
Soybean	Variable height; maturity; seed protein and oil content.
Potato	Higher yield; growth habit, maturity and morphology.
Tomato	Dwarf habit; early flowering; orange fruit colour.
Carrot	Higher carotene content.
Pineapple	Foliage density; leaf colour, width and spine formation.
Brassica	Multiple branching stem; altered leaf; slow growth; failure to flower or delay in flowering; large pollen grains.
Tobacco	Increased yield; plant height; leaf number, shape, width and yield; type of inflorescence and yield.

Production of agronomically useful plants

As a result of somaclonal variations, several novel variants of existing crops have been developed. e.g., pure thornless blackberries.

In ***Table 46.3***, somaclonal variations in a selected list of crops with useful and improved morphological characters are given. The crops include rice, wheat, maize, sugarcane, potato, carrot etc.

Resistance to diseases

Somaclonal variations have largely contributed towards the development of disease resistance in many crops e.g. rice, wheat, maize, sugarcane, tobacco, apple, tomato.

Selected crops somaclonal variants, with increased disease resistance developed, without *in vitro* selection and with *in vitro* selection are respectively given in ***Tables 46.1 and 46.2***.

Resistance to abiotic stresses

It has been possible to develop biochemical mutants with abiotic stress resistance.

- Freezing tolerance e.g. wheat.
- Salt tolerance e.g., rice, maize, tobacco.
- Aluminium tolerance e.g., carrot, sorghum, tomato.

Resistance to herbicides

Certain somaclonal variants with herbicide resistance have been developed. Selected examples are given

- Tobacco resistant to glyphosate, sulfonylurea and picloram.
- Carrot resistant to glyphosate.
- Lotus resistant to 2, 4-dichlorophenoxy acetic acid (2, 2-D).

Improved seed quality

A new variety of *Lathyrus sativa* seeds (Lathyrus Bio L 212) with a ***low content of neurotoxin*** has been developed through somaclonal variations. (**Note :** Lathyrism is a crippling disease caused by consumption of Lathyrus seeds i.e. kesari dal, in many parts of central India).

LIMITATIONS OF SOMACLONAL VARIATIONS

Despite several applications of somaclonal variations, there are certain limitations/ disadvantages also.

- Most of the somaclonal variations ***may not be useful***.
- The variations occur in an unpredictable and uncontrolled manner.

- Many a times the genetic traits obtained by somaclonal variations are ***not stable and heritable***.
- Somaclonal variations are cultivar-dependent which is frequently a time consuming process.
- Somaclones can be produced in only those species which regenerate to complete plants.
- Many cell lines (calli) may not exhibit regeneration potential.

GAMETOCLONAL VARIATIONS

The ***variations*** observed while ***culturing*** the ***gametic cells*** are regarded as gametoclonal variations. This is in contrast to the somaclonal variations detected in the cultures of somatic tissues.

The term ***gametoclones*** (in place of somaclones) is used for the products of gametoclonal variations.

As the somatic cells divide by mitosis, the genetic material is equally distributed to the daughter cells. In contrast, the gametes, being the products of meiosis, possess only half of the parent cell genetic material.

The gametoclonal variations differ from somaclonal variations by three distinct features.

1. Mutants obtained from gametoclonal variations give rise to haploid plants since a single set of chromosomes are present.

2. Meiotic crossing over is the recombination process observed in gametoclonal variations.

3. The gametoclones can be stabilized by doubling the chromosome number.

TABLE 46.4 A selected list of plants regenerated from gametoclonal variations

Crop	*Characteristics*
Oryza sativa	Plant height; time of flowering; seed size and protein content; level of tillering; waxy mutant; chloroplast content.
Nicotiana tabacum	Plant size; leaf shape; number of leaves; alkaloid content; virus resistance; time of flowering.
Brassica napus	Leaf shape and colour; time to flower; type of flower; glucinolate content; pod size and shape.
Hordeum vulgare	Plant height; days to maturity; grain yield; fertility.

Production of gametoclones

Gametoclones can be developed by culturing male or female gametic cells. The cultures of anthers or isolated microspores are widely used. (For details, Refer Chapter 43).

A selected list of plants regenerated from gametoclonal variations is given in ***Table 46.4***. Improvements have been made in several plant species through development of gametoclones e.g., rice, wheat, tobacco.

Source of gametoclonal variations

There are three sources of genetic variations in the gametoclones.

1. Cell culture technique may induce genetic variations.

2. Variations may be induced while doubling the haploid chromosomes.

3. Genetic variations may occur due to heterozygosity of the diploids.

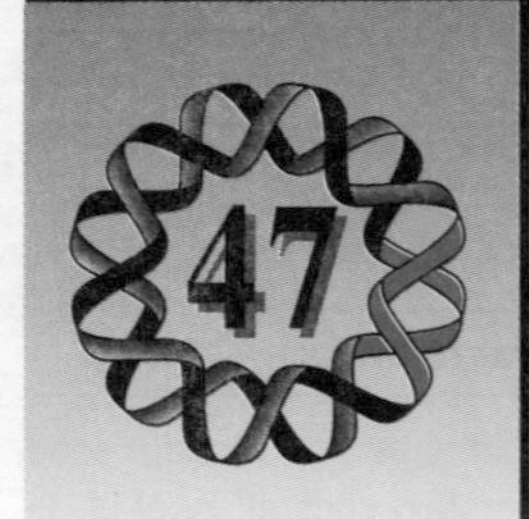

Clonal Propagation (Micropropagation)

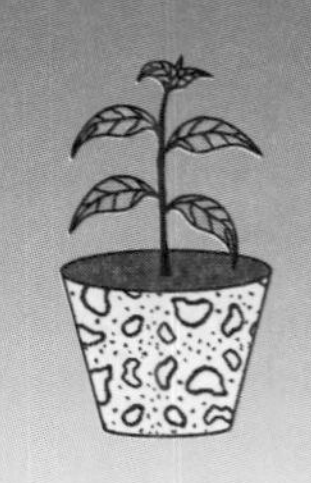

Plants can be propagated by sexual (through generation of seeds) or asexual (through multiplication of vegetative parts) means. Clonal propagation refers to the process of ***asexual reproduction by multiplication of genetically identical copies of individual plants***. The term ***clone*** is used to represent a plant population derived from a single individual by asexual reproduction.

Asexual reproduction through ***multiplication of vegetative parts*** is the only method for the *in vivo* propagation of certain plants, as they do not produce viable seeds e.g. banana, grape, fig, chrysanthemum. Clonal propagation has been successfully applied for the propagation of apple, potato, tuberous and several ornamental plants.

Advantages of vegetative propagation

Asexual (vegetative) propagation of plants has certain advantages over sexual propagation.

- Faster multiplication — large number of plants can be produced from a single individual in a short period.
- Possible to produce genetically identical plants.
- Sexually — derived sterile hybrids can be propagated.
- Seed — raised plants pass through an undesirable juvenile phase which is avoided in asexual propagation.
- Gene banks can be more easily established by clonally propagated plants.

In vitro clonal propagation

The *in vivo* clonal propagation of plants is tedious, expensive and frequently unsuccessful. ***In vitro clonal propagation through tissue culture is referred to as micropropagation***. Use of tissue culture technique for micropropagation was first started by Morel (1960) for propagation of orchids, and is now applied to several plants. Micropropagation is a handy technique for rapid multiplication of plants.

TECHNIQUE OF MICROPROPAGATION

Micropropagation is a complicated process and mainly involves 3 stages (I, II and III). Some authors add two more stages (stage 0 and IV) for more comprehensive representation of micro-propagation. All these stages are represented in ***Fig. 47.1***, and briefly described hereunder.

Stage 0 : This is the initial step in micro-propagation, and involves the selection and growth of stock plants for about 3 months under controlled conditions.

Stage I : In this stage, the initiation and establishment of culture in a suitable medium is achieved. Selection of appropriate explants is important. The most commonly used explants are organs, shoot tips and axillary buds. The chosen explant is surface sterilized and washed before use.

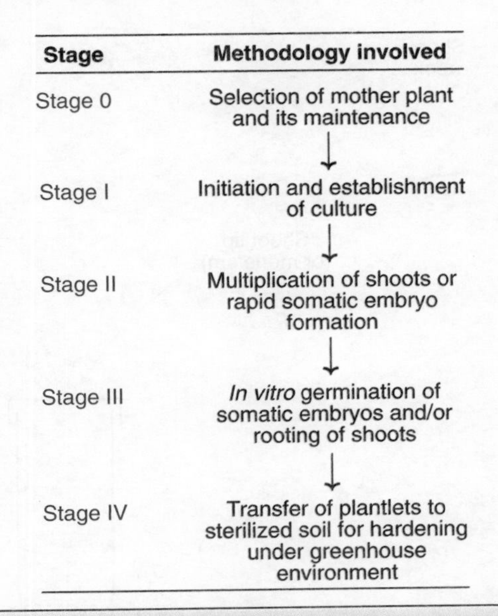

Stage
Methodology involved
Stage 0
Selection of mother plant and its maintenance
Stage I
Initiation and establishment of culture
Stage II
Multiplication of shoots or rapid somatic embryo formation
Stage III
In vitro germination of somatic embryos and/or rooting of shoots
Stage IV
Transfer of plantlets to sterilized soil for hardening under greenhouse environment

Fig. 47.1 : Major stages involved in micropropagation.

Stage II : It is in this stage, the major activity of micropropagation occurs in a defined culture medium. Stage II mainly involves multiplication of shoots or rapid embryo formation from the explant.

Stage III : This stage involves the transfer of shoots to a medium for rapid development into shoots. Sometimes, the shoots are directly planted in soil to develop roots. *In vitro* rooting of shoots is preferred while simultaneously handling a large number of species.

Stage IV : This stage involves the establishment of plantlets in soil. This is done by transferring the plantlets of stage III from the laboratory to the environment of greenhouse. For some plant species, stage III is skipped, and unrooted stage II shoots are planted in pots or in suitable compost mixture.

The different stages described above for micropropagation are particularly useful for comparison between two or more plant systems, besides better understanding. It may however, be noted that not all plant species need to be propagated *in vitro* through all the five stages referred above.

Micropropagation mostly involves *in vitro* clonal propagation by two approaches.

1. Multiplication by axillary buds/apical shoots.
2. Multiplication by adventitious shoots.

Besides the above two approaches, the ***plant regeneration*** processes namely ***organogenesis*** and ***somatic embryogenesis*** may also be treated as micropropagation, hence they are also described in this chapter.

3. **Organogenesis** : The formation of individual organs such as shoots, roots, directly from an explant (lacking preformed meristem) or from the callus and cell culture induced from the explant.

4. **Somatic embryogenesis** : The regeneration of embryos from somatic cells, tissues or organs.

MULTIPLICATION BY AXILLARY BUDS AND APICAL SHOOTS

Quiescent or actively dividing meristems are present at the axillary and apical shoots (shoot tips). The axillary buds located in the axils of leaves are ***capable of developing into shoots***. In the *in vivo* state, however only a limited number of axillary meristems can form shoots. By means of induced *in vitro* multiplication in micropropagation, it is possible to develop plants from meristem and shoot tip cultures and from bud cultures.

Meristem and shoot tip cultures

Apical meristem is a dome of tissue located at the extreme tip of a shoot. The apical meristem along with the young leaf primordia constitutes the shoot apex. For the development of disease-free plants, meristem tips should be cultured.

Meristem or shoot tip is isolated from a stem by a V-shaped cut. The size (frequently 0.2 to 0.5 mm) of the tip is critical for culture. In general, the larger the explant (shoot tip), the better are the chances for culture survival. For good results of micropropagation, explants should be taken from the actively growing shoot tips, and the ideal timing is at the end of the plants dormancy period.

The most widely used media for meristem culture are MS medium and White's medium. A diagrammatic representation of shoot tip (or meristem) culture in micropropagation is given in ***Fig 47.2***, and briefly described hereunder.

In stage I, the culture of meristem is established. Addition of growth regulators namely cytokinins (kinetin, BA) and auxins (NAA or IBA) will support the growth and development.

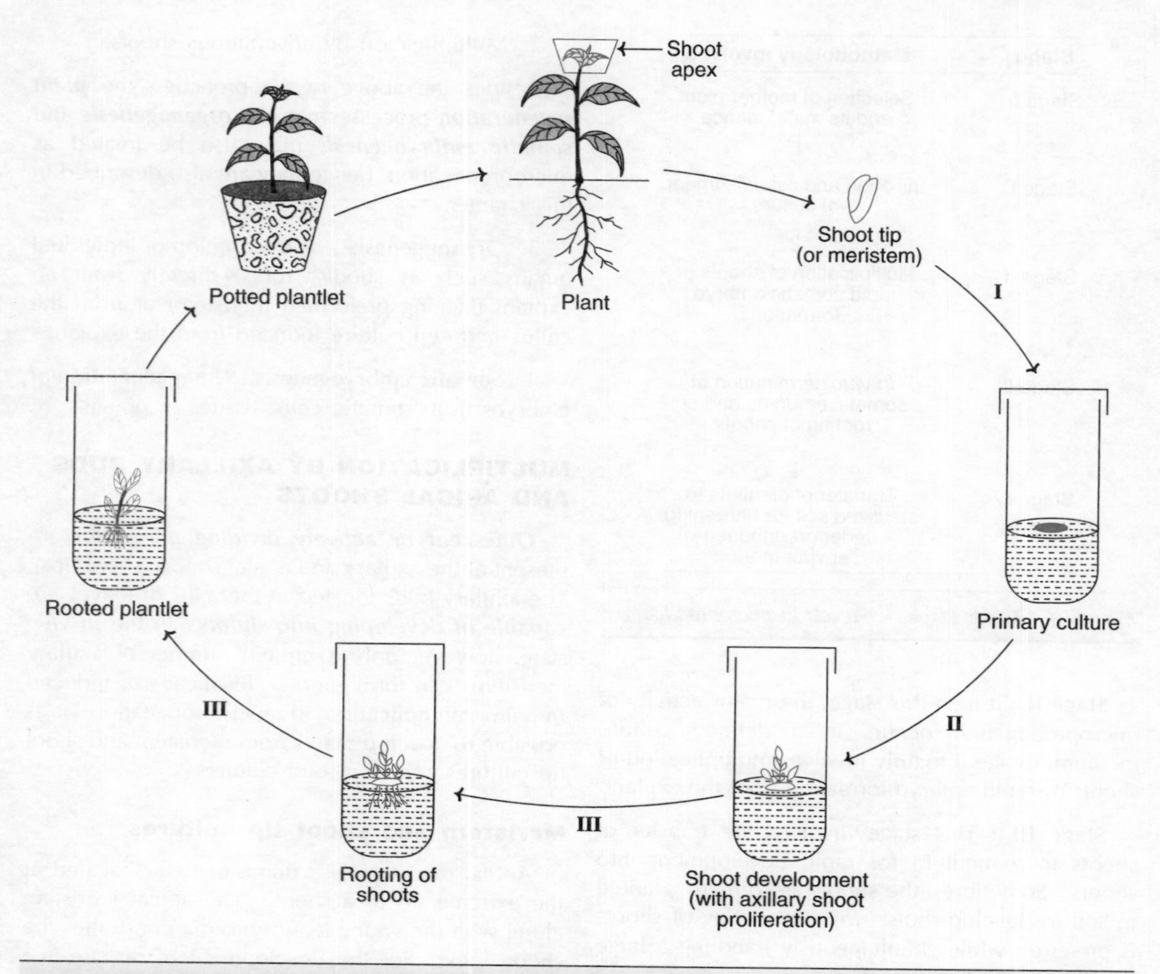

Fig. 47.2 : A diagrammatic representation of shoot tip (or meristem) culture in micropropagation (Note : I, II and III represent stages in micropropagation)

In stage II, shoot development along with axillary shoot proliferation occurs. High levels of cytokinins are required for this purpose.

Stage III is associated with rooting of shoots and further growth of plantlet. The root formation is facilitated by low cytokinin and high auxin concentration. This is opposite to shoot formation since high level of cytokinins is required (in stage II). Consequently, ***stage II medium and stage III medium should be different in composition***.

The optimal temperature for culture is in the range of 20–28°C (for majority 24-26°C). Lower light intensity is more appropriate for good micropropagation.

Bud cultures

The plant buds possess quiescent or active meristems depending on the physiological state of the plant. Two types of bud cultures are used—single node culture and axillary bud culture.

Single node culture : This is a natural method for vegetative propagation of plants both in *in vivo* and *in vitro* conditions. The bud found in the axil of leaf is comparable to the stem tip, for its ability in micropropagation. A bud along with a piece of stem is isolated and cultured to develop into a plantlet. Closed buds are used to reduce the chances of infections.

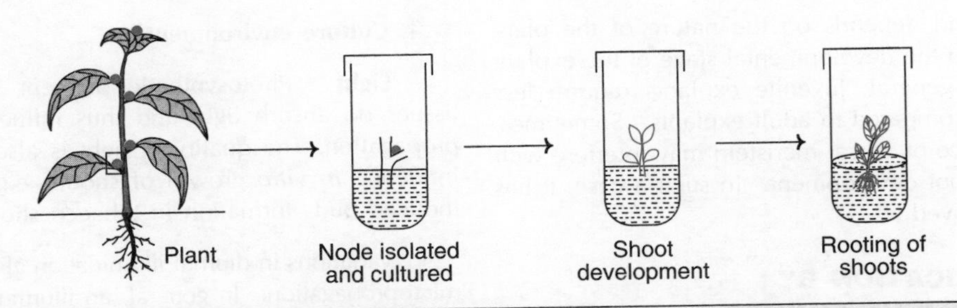

Fig. 47.3 : A diagrammatic representation of micropropagation by single node technique.

A diagrammatic representation of single node culture is depicted in ***Fig 47.3***. In single node culture, no cytokinin is added.

Axillary bud culture : In this method, a shoot tip along with axillary bud is isolated. The cultures are carried out with high cytokinin concentration. As a result of this, apical dominance stops and axillary buds develop. A schematic representation of axillary bud culture for a rosette plant and an elongate plant is given in ***Fig 47.4***.

For a ***good axillary bud culture, the cytokinin/auxin ratio is around 10 : 1***. This is however,

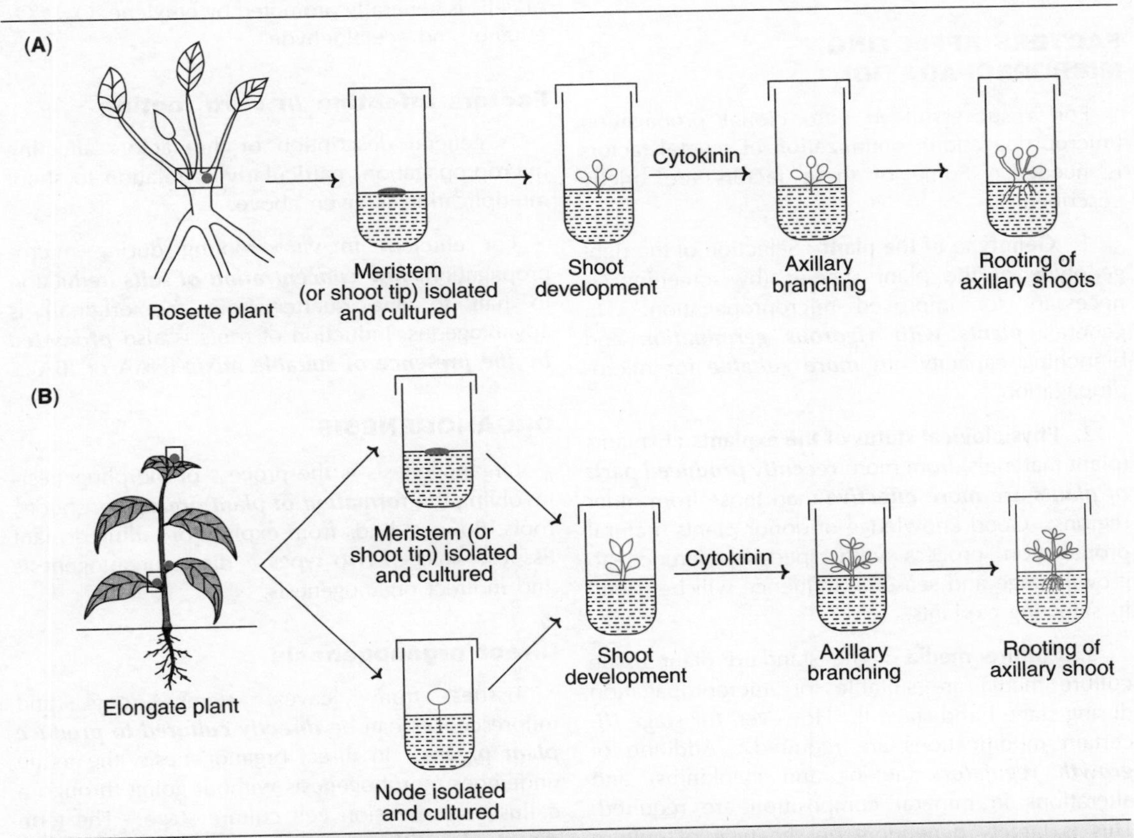

Fig. 47.4 : A diagrammatic representation of micropropagation of plants by axillary bud (or shoot tip) method (A) Rosette plant (B) Elongate plant.

variable and depends on the nature of the plant species and the developmental stage of the explant used. In general, juvenile explants require less cytokinin compared to adult explants. Sometimes, the presence of apical meristem may interfere with axillary shoot development. In such a case, it has to be removed.

MULTIPLICATION BY ADVENTITIOUS SHOOTS

The stem and leaf structures that are naturally formed on plant tissues located in sites other than the normal leaf axil regions are regarded as adventitious shoots. There are many adventitious shoots which include stems, bulbs, tubers and rhizomes. The adventitious shoots are useful for *in vivo* and *in vitro* clonal propagation.

The meristematic regions of adventitious shoots can be induced in a suitable medium to regenerate to plants.

FACTORS AFFECTING MICROPROPAGATION

For a successful *in vitro* clonal propagation (micropropagation), optimization of several factors is needed. Some of these factors are briefly described.

1. **Genotype of the plant :** Selection of the right genotype of the plant species (by screening) is necessary for improved micropropagation. In general, ***plants with vigorous germination*** and branching capacity are ***more suitable*** for micropropagation.

2. **Physiological status of the explants :** Explants (plant materials) from more ***recently produced parts of plants are more effective*** than those from older regions. Good knowledge of donor plants' natural propagation process with special reference to growth stage and seasonal influence will be useful in selecting explants.

3. **Culture media :** The standard plant tissue culture media are suitable for micropropagation during stage I and stage II. However, ***for stage III***, certain modifications are required. Addition of ***growth regulators*** (auxins and cytokinins) and alterations in mineral composition are required. This is largely dependent on the type of culture (meristem, bud etc).

4. **Culture environment**

Light : Photosynthetic pigment in cultured tissues do absorb light and thus influence micropropagation. The quality of light is also known to influence *in vitro* growth of shoots. e.g blue light induced bud formation in tobacco shoots.

Variations in diurnal illumination also influence micropropagation. In general, an illumination of 16 hours day and 8 hours night is satisfactory for shoot proliferation.

Temperature : Majority of the culture for micropropagation requires an ***optimal*** temperature ***around 25°C***. There are however, some exceptions e.g. *Begonia* X *Cheimantha* hybrid tissue grow at a low temperature (around 18°C).

Composition of gas phase : The constitution of the gas phase in the culture vessels also influences micropropagation. Unorganized growth of cells is generally promoted by ethylene, O_2, CO_2 ethanol and acetaldehyde.

Factors affecting *in vitro* rooting

A general description of the factors affecting micropropagation, particularly in relation to shoot multiplication is given above.

For efficient *in vitro* rooting during micropropagation, ***low concentration of salts*** (reduction to half to one quarter from the original) is advantageous. Induction of roots is also ***promoted by the presence of suitable auxin*** (NAA or IBA).

ORGANOGENESIS

Organogenesis is the process of morphogenesis involving the ***formation of plant organs*** i.e. shoots, roots, flowers, buds from explant or cultured plant tissues. It is of two types — direct organogenesis and indirect organogenesis.

Direct organogenesis

Tissues from leaves, stems, roots and inflorescences can be ***directly cultured to produce plant organs.*** In direct organogenesis, the tissue undergoes morphogenesis without going through a callus or suspension cell culture stage. The term ***direct adventitious organ formation*** is also used for direct organogenesis.

Induction of adventitious shoot formation directly on roots, leaves and various other organs of intact plants is a widely used method for plant propagation. This approach is particularly useful for herbaceous species.

For appropriate organogenesis in culture system, exogenous addition of growth regulators—auxin and cytokinin is required. The concentration of the growth promoting substance depends on the age and nature of the explant, besides the growth conditions.

Indirect organogenesis

When the organogenesis occurs ***through callus or suspension cell culture formation***, it is regarded as indirect organogenesis (***Fig 47.5 B and C***). Callus growth can be established from many explants (leaves, roots, cotyledons, stems, flower petals etc.) for subsequent organogenesis.

The explants for good organogenesis should be mitotically active immature tissues. In general, the bigger the explant the better the chances for obtaining viable callus/cell suspension cultures. It is advantageous to select meristematic tissues (shoot tip, leaf, petiole) for efficient indirect organogenesis. This is because their growth rate and survival rate are much better.

For indirect organogenesis, the cultures may be grown in liquid medium or solid medium. Many culture media (MS, B5, White's etc.) can be used in organogenesis. The concentration of growth regulators in the medium is critical for organogenesis. By varying the concentrations of auxins and cytokinins, *in vitro* organogenesis can be manipulated.

- Low auxin and low cytokinin concentration will induce callus formation.
- Low auxin and high cytokinin concentration will promote shoot organogenesis from callus.
- High auxin and low cytokinin concentration will induce root formation.

SOMATIC EMBRYOGENESIS

The process of ***regeneration of embryos from somatic cells***, tissues or organs is regarded as somatic (or asexual) embryogenesis. Somatic embryogenesis may result in non-zygotic embryos or somatic embryos (directly formed from somatic

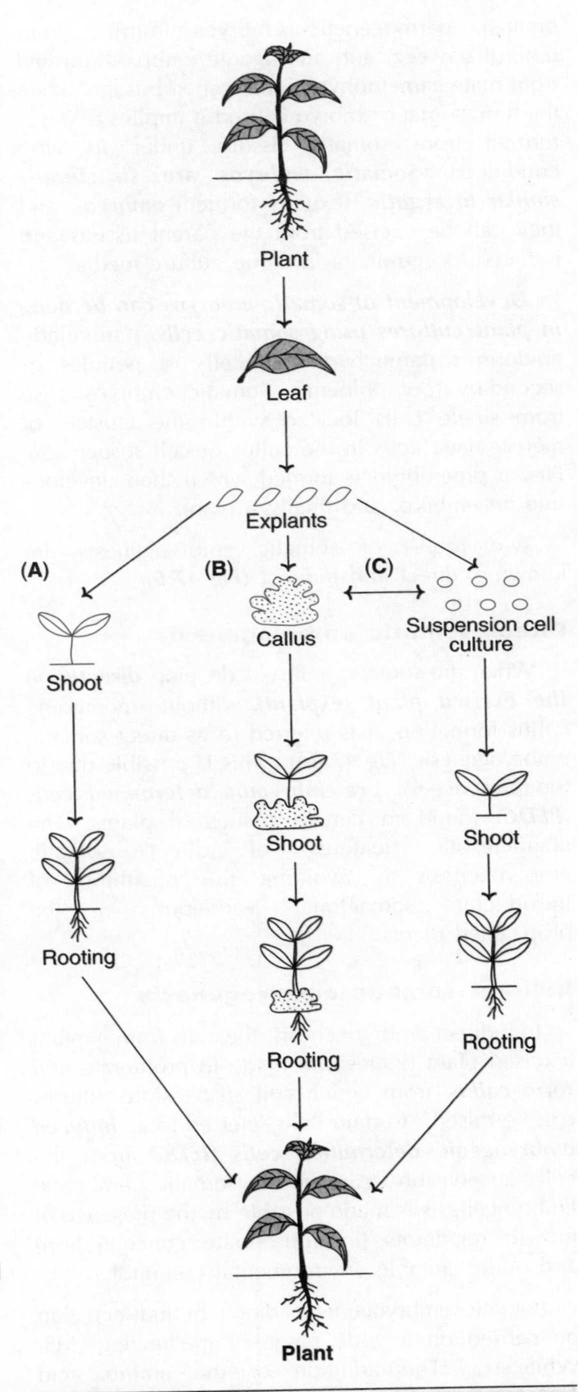

Fig. 47.5 : Micropropagation of plants by organogenesis (A) Direct organogenesis (B) Indirect organogenesis through callus (C) Indirect organogenesis through suspension cell culture.

organs), parthogenetic embryos (formed from unfertilized egg) and androgenic embryos (formed from male gametophyte). In a general usage, when the term somatic embryo is used it implies that it is formed from somatic tissues under *in vitro* conditions. ***Somatic embryos are structurally similar to zygotic*** (sexually formed) ***embryos***, and they can be excised from the parent tissues and induced to germinate in tissue culture media.

Development of somatic embryos can be done in plant cultures using somatic cells, particularly epidermis, parenchymatous cells of petioles or secondary root phloem. Somatic embryos arise from single cells located within the clusters of meristematic cells in the callus or cell suspension. First a proembryo is formed which then develops into an embryo, and finally a plant.

Two routes of somatic embryogenesis are known — direct and indirect (***Fig 47.6***).

Direct somatic embryogenesis

When the somatic embryos develop ***directly on the excised plant (explant)*** without undergoing callus formation, it is referred to as direct somatic embryogenesis (***Fig 47.6A***). This is possible due to the presence of ***pre-embryonic determined cells*** (***PEDC***) found in certain tissues of plants. The characteristic features of direct somatic embryogenesis is avoiding the possibility of introducing somaclonal variations in the propagated plants.

Indirect somatic embryogenesis

In indirect embryogenesis, the cells from explant (excised plant tissues) are made to proliferate and ***form callus***, from which cell suspension cultures can be raised. Certain cells referred to as ***induced embryogenic determined cells*** (***IEDC***) from the cell suspension can form somatic embryos. Embryogenesis is made possible by the presence of growth regulators (in appropriate concentration) and under suitable environmental conditions.

Somatic embryogenesis (direct or indirect) can be carried on a wide range of media (e.g. MS, White's). The addition of the amino acid ***L-glutamine promotes embryogenesis***. The presence of auxin such as 2, 4-dichloro-phenoxy acetic acid is essential for embryo initiation. On a low auxin or no auxin medium, the embryogenic clumps develop into mature embryos.

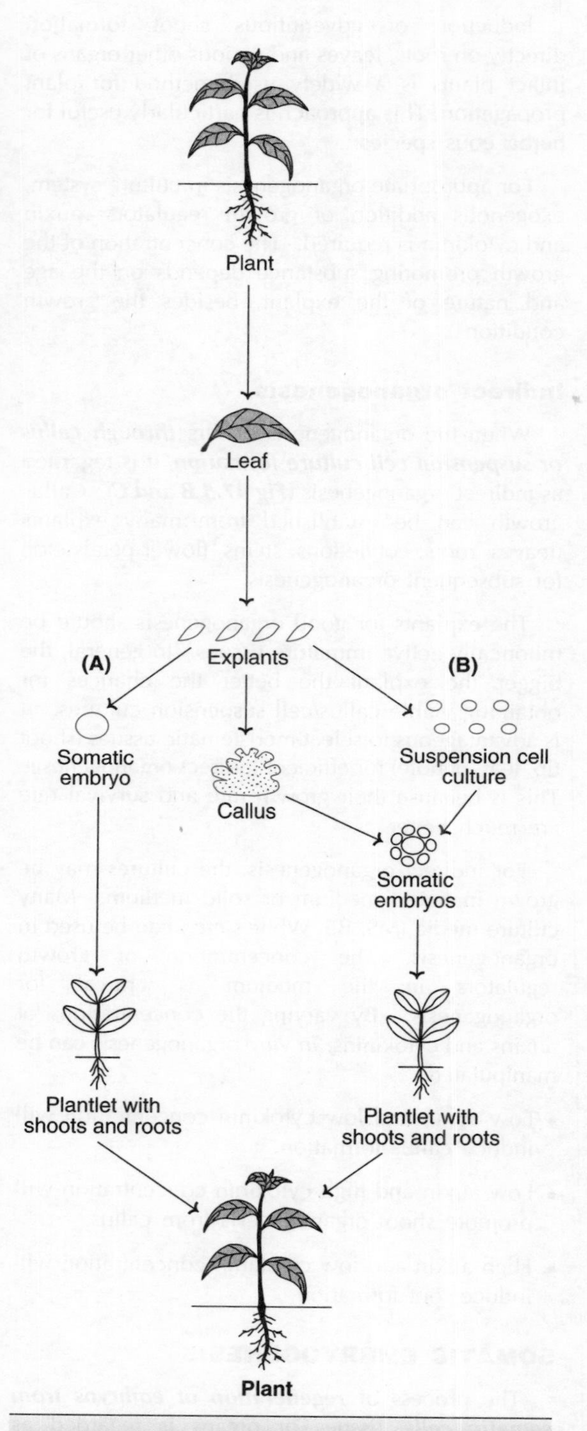

Fig. 47.6 : *Micropropagation of plants by embryogenesis* ***(A)*** *Direct embryogenesis* ***(B)*** *Indirect embryogenesis*

Indirect somatic embryogenesis is commercially very attractive since a large number of embryos can be generated in a small volume of culture medium. The somatic embryos so formed are synchronous and with good regeneration capability.

Artificial seeds from somatic embryos

Artificial seeds can be made by ***encapsulation of somatic embryos***. The embryos, coated with sodium alginate and nutrient solution, are dipped in calcium chloride solution. The calcium ions induce rapid cross-linking of sodium alginate to produce small gel beads, each containing an encapsulated embryo. These artificial seeds (encapsulated embryos) can be maintained in a viable state till they are planted.

APPLICATIONS OF MICROPROPAGATION

Micropropagation has become a suitable alternative to conventional methods of vegetative propagation of plants. There are ***several advantages*** of micropropagation.

High rate of plant propagation

Through micropropagation, a ***large number of plants can be grown from a piece of plant tissue within a short period.*** Another advantage is that micropropagation can be carried out throughout the year, irrespective of the seasonal variations. Further, for many plants that are highly resistant to conventional propagation, micropropagation is the suitable alternative.

The small sized propagules obtained in micropropagation can be easily stored for many years (germplasm storage), and transported across international boundaries.

Production of disease-free plants

It is possible to produce disease-free plants through micropropagation. ***Meristem tip cultures*** are generally employed to ***develop pathogen-free plants*** (details given later in this chapter). In fact, micropropagation is successfully used for the production of virus-free plants of sweet potato (*Ipomea batatus*), cassava (*Manihot esculenta*) and yam (*Discorea rotundata*).

Production of seeds in some crops

Micropropagation, through axillary bud proliferation method, is suitable for seed production in some plants. This is required in certain plants where the limitation for seed production is high degree of genetic conservation e.g. cauliflower, onion.

Cost-effective process

Micropropagation requires minimum growing space. Thus, millions of plant species can be maintained inside culture vials in a small room in a nursery.

The production cost is relatively low particularly in developing countries (like India) where the manpower and labour charges are low.

Automated micropropagation

It has now become possible to automate micropropagation at various stages. In fact, bio-reactors have been set up for large scale multi-plication of shoots and bulbs. Some workers employ robots (in place of labourers) for micro-propagation, and this further reduces production cost of plants.

DISADVANTAGES OF MICROPROPAGATION

Contamination of cultures

During the course of micropropagation, several slow-growing microorganisms (e.g. *Eswinia* sp, *Bacillus* sp) contaminate and grow in cultures. The microbial infection, can be controlled by addition of antibiotics or fungicides. However, this will ***adversely influence propagation of plants.***

Brewing of medium

Micropropagation of certain plants (e.g. woody perennials) is often associated with accumulation of growth inhibitory substances in the medium. Chemically, these substances are phenolic compounds, which can turn the medium into dark colour. ***Phenolic compounds are toxic and can inhibit the growth of tissues.***

Brewing of the medium can be prevented by the addition of ascorbic acid or citric acid or polyvinyl pyrrolidone to the medium.

Genetic variability

When micropropagation is carried out through shoot tip cultures, genetic variability is very low. However, use of adventitious shoots is often associated with pronounced genetic variability.

Vitrification

During the course of repeated *in vitro* shoot multiplication, the cultures exhibit water soaked or almost translucent leaves. Such ***shoots cannot grow and even may die***. This phenomenon is referred to as vitrification. Vitrification may be prevented by increasing the agar concentration (from 0.6 to1%) in the medium. However, increased agar concentration reduces the growth rate of tissues.

Cost factor

For some micropropagation techniques, expensive equipment, sophisticated facilities and trained manpower are needed. This limits its use.

PRODUCTION OF DISEASE-FREE PLANTS

Many plant species are infected with pathogens — viruses, bacteria, fungi, mycoplasma and nematodes that cause systemic diseases. Although these diseases do not always result in the death of plants, they reduce the quality and yield of plants. The plants infected with bacteria and fungi frequently respond to chemical treatment by bactericides and fungicides. However, it is very difficult to cure the virus-infected plants. Further, viral disease are easily transferred in seed-propagated as well as vegetatively propagated plant species. Plant breeders are always interested to develop disease-free plants, particularly viral disease-free plants. This have become ***a reality through tissue cultures.***

Apical meristems with low concentration of viruses

In general, the apical meristems of the pathogen infected and disease harbouring plants are either free or carry a low concentration of viruses, for the following reasons.

- Absence of vascular tissue in the meristems through which viruses readily move in the plant body.
- Rapidly dividing meristematic cells with high metabolic activity do not allow viruses to multiply.
- Virus replication is inhibited by a high concentration of endogenous auxin in shoot apices. Tissue culture techniques employing ***meristem-tips*** are successfully ***used for the production of disease-free plants,*** caused by several pathogens — viruses, bacteria, fungi, mycoplasmas.

METHODS TO ELIMINATE VIRUSES IN PLANTS

In general, plants are infected with many viruses; the nature of some of them may be unknown. The usage virus-free plant implies that the given plant is free from all the viruses, although this may not be always true. The commonly used methods for virus elimination in plants are listed below, and briefly described next.

- Heat treatment of plant
- Meristem-tip culture
- Chemical treatment of media
- Other *in vitro* methods

Heat treatment (thermotherapy) of plants

In the early days, before the advent of meristem cultures, *in vivo* eradication of viruses from plants was achieved by heat treatment of whole plants. The underlying principle is that many viruses in plant tissues are either partially or completely inactivated at higher temperatures with minimal injury to the host plant. Thermotherapy (at temperatures 35–40°C) was carried out by using hot water or hot air for elimination viruses from growing shoots and buds.

There are two ***limitations*** of viral elimination by heat treatment.

1. Most of the viruses are not sensitive to heat treatment.

2. Many plant species do not survive after thermotherapy.

With the above disadvantages, heat treatment has not become popular for virus elimination.

Meristem-tip culture

A general description of the methodology adopted for meristem and shoot tip cultures has been described (see ***Fig 47.2***).

TABLE 47.1 A selected list of the plants with virus elimitation by meristem cultures

Plant species	Virus eliminated
Solanum tuberosum (potato)	Leaf roll, potato viruses — A, X, Y, S
Nicotiana tabacum (tobacco)	Tobacco mosaic virus
Saccharum officinarum (sugar cane)	Mosaic virus
Allium sativum (garlic)	Mosaic virus
Anenas sativus (pineapple)	Mosaic virus
Brassica oleracea (cauliflower)	Cauliflower/mosaic virus turnip mosaic virus
Ipomoea batata (sweet potato)	Fealthery mottle virus
Ribes grassularia	Vein banding virus
Humulus lupulus	Hop latent virus
Armoracia rusticena	Turnip mosaic virus
Musa sp (Banana)	Cucumber mosaic virus
Hycinthus sp	Hycinth mosaic virus
Dahlia sp	Dahlia mosaic virus
Chrysanthemum sp	Virus B
Petunia sp	Tobacco mosaic virus
Iris sp	Iris mosaic virus
Cymbidium sp	Cymbidium mosaic virus
Fragaria sp	Pallidosis virus, yellow virus complex
Freesia sp	Freesia mosaic virus

For viral elimination, the size of the meristem used in cultures is very critical. This is due to the fact that most of the viruses exist by establishing a gradient in plant tissues. ***In general, the regeneration of virus-free plants through cultures is inversely proportional to the size of the meristem*** used. The meristem-tip explant used for viral elimination cultures are too small. A stereoscopic microscope is usually employed for this purpose.

Meristem-tip cultures are influenced by the following factors.

- Physiological condition of the explant — actively growing buds are more effective.
- Thermotherapy prior to meristem-tip culture — for certain plants (possessing viruses in the meristematic regions), heat treatment is first given and then the meristem-tips are isolated and cultured.
- Culture medium — MS medium with low concentrations of auxins and cytokinins is ideal.

A selected list of the plants from which viruses have been eliminated by meristem cultures is given in ***Table 47.1.***

Chemical treatment of media

Some workers have attempted to eradicate viruses from infected plants by chemical treatment of the tissue culture media. The commonly used chemicals are growth substances (e.g. cytokinins) and antimetabolites (e.g thiouracil, acetyl salicylic acid). There are however, conflicting reports on the elimination viruses by chemical treatment of the media. For instance, addition of cytokinin suppressed the multiplication of certain viruses while for some other viruses, it actually stimulated.

Other *in vitro* methods

Besides meristem-tip culture, other *in vitro* methods are also used for raising virus-free plants. In this regard ***callus cultures*** have been successful to some extent. The callus derived from the infected tissue does not carry the pathogens throughout the cells. In fact, the uneven distribution of tobacco mosaic virus in tobacco leaves was exploited to develop virus-free plants of tobacco.

Somatic cell hybridization, gene transformation and ***somaclonal variations*** also useful to raise disease-free plants.

ELIMINATION OF PATHOGENS OTHER THAN VIRUSES

Besides the elimination of viruses, meristem-tip cultures and callus cultures are also useful for eradication bacteria, fungi and mycoplasmas. Some examples are given

- The fungus *Fusarium roseum* has been successfully eliminated through meristem cultures from carnation plants.
- Certain bacteria (*Pseudomonas carophylli, Pectobacterium parthenii*) are eradicated from carnation plants by using meristem cultures.

MERITS AND DEMERITS OF DISEASE-FREE PLANT PRODUCTION

Among the culture techniques, ***meristem-tip culture is the most reliable method*** for virus and other pathogen elimination. This, however, requires good knowledge of plant pathology and tissue culture.

Virus-free plants exhibit increased growth and vigour of plants, higher yield (e.g. potato), increased flower size (e.g. *Chrysanthemum*), improved rooting of stem cuttings (e.g. *Pelargonium*)

Virus-free plants are more susceptible to the same virus when exposed again. This is the major limitation. Reinfection of disease-free plants can be minimized with good knowledge of greenhouse maintenance.

EMBRYO CULTURE

Embryo culture deals with the sterile isolation and *in vitro* growth of a mature or an immature embryo with an ultimate objective of obtaining a viable plant. Conventionally, the term embryo culture refers to the sexually produced zygotic embryo culture. This is different from the somatic embryogenesis, already described in this chapter.

There are two types of embryo culture — mature embryo culture and immature embryo culture (embryo rescue).

MATURE EMBRYO CULTURE

Mature embryos are isolated from ripe seeds and cultured *in vitro*. Mature embryo cultures are carried out in the following conditions.

- When the embryos remain dormant for long periods.
- Low survival of embryos *in vivo*.
- To avoid inhibition in the seed for germination.
- For converting sterile seeds to viable seedlings.

Seed dormancy in plant species is a common occurrence. This may be due to chemical inhibitors or mechanical resistance exerted by the structures covering the embryo. Seed dormancy can be successfully bypassed by culturing the embryos *in vitro*.

Embryo culture is relatively easy as they can be grown on a simple inorganic medium supplemented with energy source (usually sucrose). This is possible since the mature embryos excised from the developing seeds are autotrophic in nature.

EMBRYO RESCUE

Embryo rescue involves the ***culture of immature embryos*** to rescue them from unripe or hybrid seeds ***which fail to germinate***. This approach is very useful to avoid embryo abortion and produce a viable plant.

Wild hybridization involving crossing of two different species of plants from the same genus or different genera often results in failure. This is mainly because the normal development of zygote and seed is hindered due to genetic barriers. Consequently, hybrid endosperm fails to develop leading the abortion of hybrid embryo. The endosperm may also produce toxins that ultimately kill the embryo.

In the normal circumstances, endosperm first develops and supports embryo development nutritionally. Thus, majority of embryo abortions are due to failure in endosperm development. Embryo abortion can be avoided by isolating and culturing the hybrid embryos prior to abortion.

The most important ***application*** of embryo rescue is the ***production of interspecific and intergeneric hybrids from wild plant species.***

Culture technique for embryo rescue

The isolation of immature embryos often poses some difficulty. The aseptically isolated embryos can be grown in a suitable medium under optimal conditions. In general, a complex nutrient medium is required for culture methods involving embryo rescue.

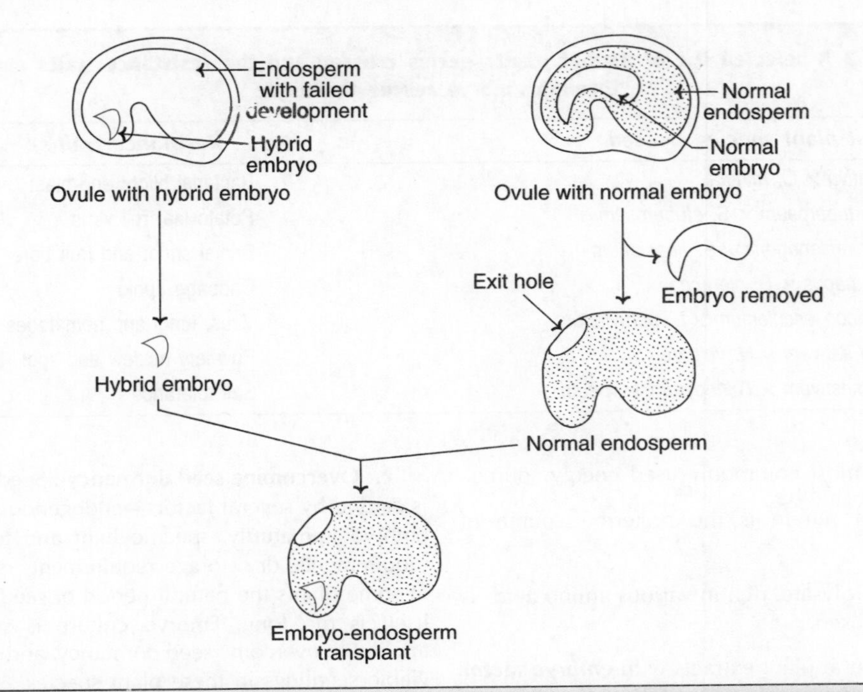

Fig. 47.7 : Embryo–endosperm transplant technique used in embryo rescue (or immature embryo culture).

For adequate nutritional support of immature embryos, embryo-endosperm transplant is used.

Embryo-endosperm transplant : The endosperm transplant technique used for culturing immature embryos is given in ***Fig. 47.7***, and briefly described below.

The hybrid embryo from the ovule in which endosperm development has failed is taken out by excision. Another normally developed ovule with endosperm enclosing an embryo is chosen. This ovule is dissected and the normal embryo is pressed out. This leaves a normal endosperm with an exit hole. Now, the hybrid embryo can be inserted into the normal endosperm through exit hole. This results in embryo-endosperm transplant which can be cultured in a suitable medium.

By using embryo-endosperm transplant, many interspecific and intergeneric plants have been raised e.g., hybrid plants of legumes.

NUTRITIONAL REQUIREMENTS OF EMBRYO CULTURES

There are two phases in the embryo development and the nutritional requirement varies accordingly

1. **Heterotrophic phase :** This is an early phase and the embryo is mostly dependent on the endosperm and maternal tissues for nutrient supply.

2. **Autotrophic phase :** This phase is characterized by the metabolic capability of the embryo to synthesize substances required for its growth which slowly makes it independent.

The critical stage is the intervening phase between the heterotrophic and autotrophic phases. The nutrient supply is highly variable at this phase which mostly depends on the plant species.

In general, the composition of the medium for culturing immature embryos is more complex than that required by mature embryos which can grow on a simple inorganic medium. Further, the transfer of embryos from one medium to another is frequently needed in order to achieve full development of embryos.

Composition of the medium : Some salient features of medium and culture conditions are listed below

- Inorganic constituents of MS, B5 or White's media are adequate.

TABLE 47.2 A selected list of distant plant species crossed and the resistance traits developed through embryo rescue technique

Distant plant species crossed	*Resistance trait(s)*
Oryza sativa × *O. minuta*	Bacterial blight and blast
Solanum tuberosum × *S. etuberosum*	Potato leaf roll virus
Solanum melanogena × *S. khasianum*	Brinjal shoot and fruit borer
Brassica napus × *B. oleracea*	Cabbage aphid
Lycopersicon esculentum × *L. peruvianum*	Virus, fungi and nematodes
Hordeum sativum × *H. vulgare*	Powdery mildew and spot blotch
Triticum aestivum × *Thinopyrum scirpeum*	Salt tolerance

- Sucrose is most commonly used energy source.
- Ammonium nitrate is the preferred source of nitrogen.
- Casein hydrolysate, rich in various amino acids is frequently used.
- Certain natural plant extracts with ***embryo factor*** promote embryo cultures e.g. liquid endosperm of coconut milk. The embryo factor is believed to supply certain amino acids, sugars, growth regulators etc.
- In general, growth regulators are not required, as they induce callus formation.
- Embryos grow well in the pH range of 5-7.5.
- An incubation temperature of 24–26°C is ideal.
- Better growth of embryos is observed in darkness which are then transferred to light for germination.

During the culture conditions, the embryos are grown into plantlets, and then transferred to sterile soil for full-pledged growth to maturity.

APPLICATIONS OF EMBRYO CULTURE

1. **Prevention of embryo abortion :** Incompatibility barriers in interspecific and intergeneric hybridization programmes leading to embryo abortion can be successfully overcome by embryo rescue. In fact, many distant hybrids have been obtained through embryo rescue techniques. A selected list of distant plant species crossed and the resistance traits developed by employing embryo rescue technique is given in ***Table 47.2***.

2. **Overcoming seed dormancy :** Seed dormancy is caused by several factors—endogenous inhibitors, embryo immaturity, specific light and temperature requirements, dry storage requirements etc. Further, in some plants the natural period of seed dormancy itself is too long. Embryo culture is successfully applied to overcome seed dormancy, and to produce viable seedlings in these plant species.

3. **Shortening of breeding cycle :** Some of the plants in their natural state have long breeding cycles. This is mostly due to seed dormancy attributed to seed coat and/or endosperm. The embryos can be excised and cultured *in vitro* to develop into plants within a short period. For instance, Hollies, a Christmas decoration plant can be ***grown in 2-3 weeks*** time through embryo cultures ***in contrast to 3 years*** period required through seed germination.

4. **Production of haploids :** Embryo culture has been successfully used for the production of haploid (or monoploid) plants e.g. barley.

5. **Overcoming seed sterility :** Certain plant species produce sterile seeds that do not germinate e.g. early ripening varieties of cherry, apricot, plum. Seed sterility is mostly associated with incomplete embryo development which leads to the death of the germinating embryo. Using embryo cultures, it is possible to raise seedlings from sterile seeds of early ripening fruits e.g. apricot, plum.

6. **Clonal propagation :** Embryos are ideally suited for *in vitro* clonal propagation. This is due to the fact that embryos are juvenile in nature with high regenerative potential. Further, it is possible to induce organogenesis and somatic embryogenesis from embryonic tissues.

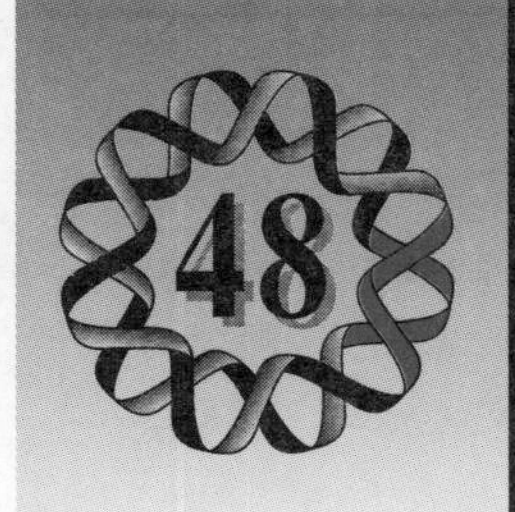

Germplasm Conservation and Cryopreservation

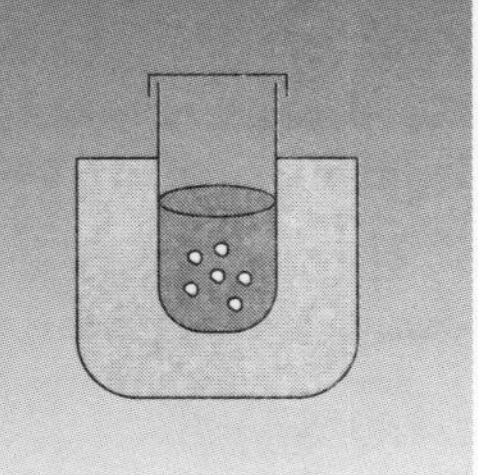

Germplasm broadly refers to the ***hereditary material*** (total content of genes) transmitted to the offspring through germ cells. Germplasm provides the raw material for the breeder to develop various crops. Thus, conservation of germplasm assumes significance in all breeding programmes.

As the primitive man learnt about the utility of plants for food and shelter, he cultivated the habit of saving selected seeds or vegetative propagules from one season to the next one. In other words, this may be regarded as ***primitive*** but ***conventional germplasm preservation*** and management, which is highly valuable in breeding programmes.

The very ***objective*** of germplasm conservation (or storage) ***is to preserve the genetic diversity of a particular plant or genetic stock for its use at any time in future***. In recent years, many new plant species with desired and improved characteristics have started replacing the primitive and conventionally used agricultural plants. It is important to conserve the endangered plants or else some of the valuable genetic traits present in the primitive plants may be lost.

A global body namely ***International Board of Plant Genetic Resources (IBPGR)*** has been established for germplasm conservation. Its main objective is to provide necessary support for collection, conservation and utilization of plant genetic resources throughout the world.

There are two approaches for germplasm conservation of plant genetic materials.

1. *In-situ* conservation
2. *Ex-situ* conservation

IN-SITU CONSERVATION

The ***conservation*** of germplasm ***in their natural environment*** by establishing biosphere reserves (or national parks/gene sanctuaries) is regarded as *in-situ* conservation. This approach is particularly useful for preservation of land plants in a near natural habitat along with several wild relatives with genetic diversity. The *in-situ* conservation is considered as a high priority germplasm preservation programme.

The major ***limitations*** of *in-situ* conservation are listed below.

- The risk of losing germplasm due to environmental hazards
- The cost of maintenance of a large number of genotypes is very high.

EX-SITU CONSERVATION

Ex-situ conservation is the ***chief method*** for the preservation of germplasm obtained from cultivated and wild plant materials. The ***genetic materials*** in the form of seeds or from *in vitro* cultures (plant cells, tissues or organs) can be ***preserved as gene banks for long term storage*** under suitable conditions. For successful establishment of gene banks, adequate knowledge of genetic structure of plant populations, and the techniques involved in sampling, regeneration, maintenance of gene pools etc. are essential.

Germplasm conservation in the form of seeds

Usually, seeds are the most ***common and convenient materials*** to conserve plant germplasm. This is because many plants are propagated through seeds, and seeds occupy relatively ***small space***. Further, seeds can be ***easily transported*** to various places.

There are however, certain ***limitations*** in the conservation of seeds

- Viability of seeds is reduced or lost with passage of time.
- Seeds are susceptible to insect or pathogen attack, often leading to their destruction.
- This approach is exclusively confined to seed propagating plants, and therefore it is of no use for vegetatively propagated plants e.g. potato, *Ipomoea, Dioscorea*.
- It is difficult to maintain clones through seed conservation.

Certain seeds are heterogeneous and therefore, are not suitable for true genotype maintenance.

In vitro methods for germplasm conservation

In vitro methods employing shoots, meristems and embryos are ideally suited for the conservation of germplasm of vegetatively propagated plants. The plants with recalcitrant seeds and genetically engineered materials can also be preserved by this *in vitro* approach.

There are several advantages associated with *in vitro* germplasm conservation

- Large quantities of materials can be preserved in small space.
- The germplasm preserved can be maintained in an environment, free from pathogens.
- It can be protected against the nature's hazards.
- From the germplasm stock, large number of plants can be obtained whenever needed.
- Obstacles for their transport through national and international borders are minimal (since the germplasm is maintained under aspectic conditions).

There are mainly three approaches for the *in vitro* conservation of germplasm

1. Cryopreservation (freeze-preservation)
2. Cold storage
3. Low-pressure and low-oxygen storage

CRYOPRESERVATION

Cryopreservation (Greek, krayos-frost) literally means ***preservation in the frozen state***. The principle involved in cryopreservation is to bring the ***plant cell and tissue cultures to a zero metabolism or non-dividing state*** by reducing the temperature in the presence of cryoprotectants.

Cryopreservation broadly means the storage of germplasm at very low temperatures.

- Over solid carbon dioxide (at –79°C)
- Low temperature deep freezers (at –80°C)
- In vapour phase nitrogen (at –150°C)
- In liquid nitrogen (at –196°C)

Among these, the most commonly used cryopreservation is by employing ***liquid nitrogen***. At the temperature of liquid nitrogen (–196°C), the cells stay in a completely inactive state and thus can be conserved for long periods. In fact, cryopreservation has been successfully applied for germplasm conservation of a wide range of plant species e.g. rice, wheat, peanut, cassava, sugarcane, straberry, coconut. Several plants can be regenerated from cells, meristems and embryos stored in cryopreservation.

Mechanism of cryopreservation

The technique of freeze preservation is based on the transfer of water present in the cells from a liquid to a solid state. Due to the presence of salts and organic molecules in the cells, the cell water requires much more lower temperature to freeze (even up to –68°C) compared to the freezing point of pure water (around 0°C). When stored at low temperature, the metabolic processes and biological deteriorations in the cells/tissues almost come to a standstill.

Precautions/limitations for successful cryopreservation

Good technical and theoretical knowledge of living plant cells and as well as cryopreservation

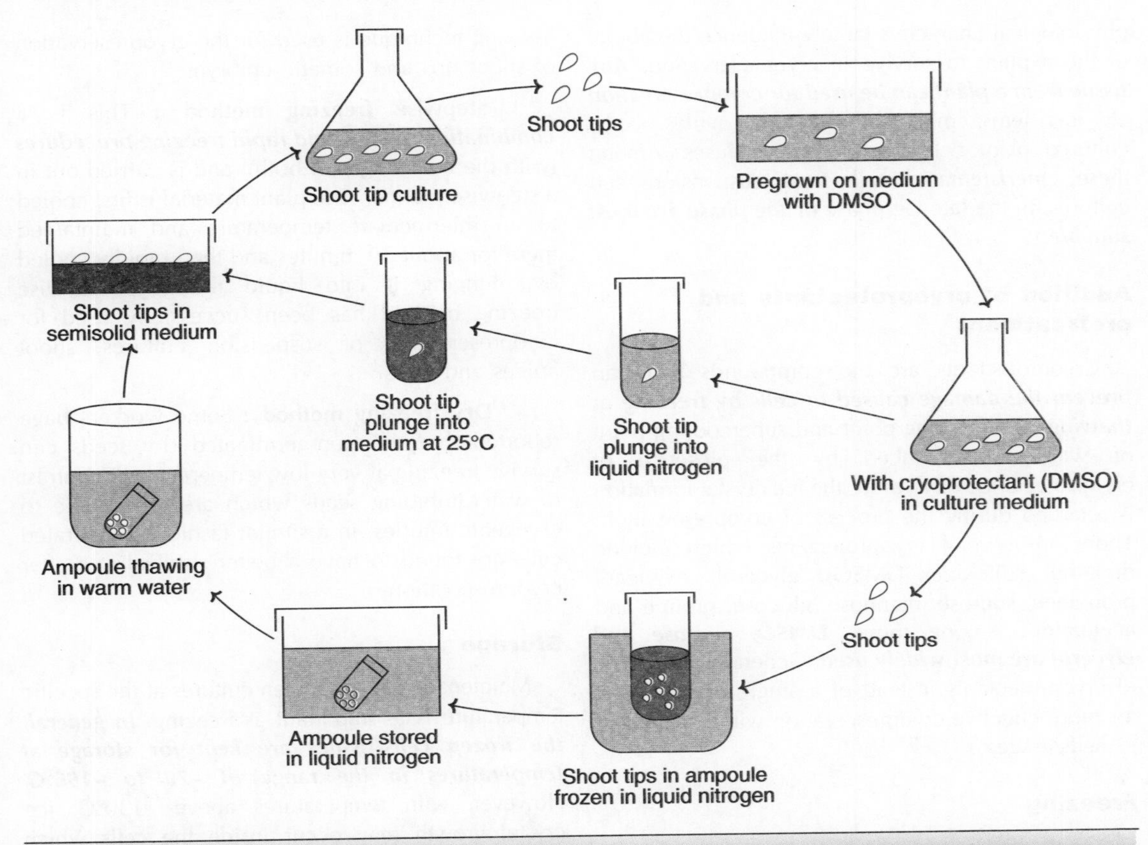

Fig. 48.1 : An outline of the protocol for cryopreservation of shoot tip (DMSO–Dimethyl sulfoxide).

technique are essential. Other ***precautions*** (the limitations that should be overcome) for successful cryopreservation are listed below

- Formation ice crystals inside the cells should be prevented as they cause injury to the organelles and the cell.
- High intracellular concentration of solutes may also damage cells.
- Sometimes, certain solutes from the cell may leak out during freezing.
- Cryoprotectants also affect the viability of cells.
- The physiological status of the plant material is also important.

TECHNIQUE OF CRYOPRESERVATION

An outline of the protocol for cryopreservation of shoot tip is depicted in ***Fig. 48.1***. The cryopreservation of plant cell culture followed by the regeneration of plants broadly involves the following stages

1. Development of sterile tissue cultures
2. Addition of cryoprotectants and pretreatment
3. Freezing
4. Storage
5. Thawing
6. Reculture
7. Measurement of survival/viability
8. Plant regeneration.

The salient features of the above stages are briefly described.

Development of sterile tissue culture

The selection of plant species and the tissues with particular reference to the morphological and physiological characters largely influence the ability of the explant to survive in cryopreservation. ***Any tissue from a plant can be used for cryopreservation*** e.g. meristems, embryos, endosperms, ovules, seeds, cultured plant cells, protoplasts, calluses. Among these, ***meristematic cells*** and suspension cell cultures, in the late lag phase or ***log phase are most suitable***.

Addition of cryoprotectants and pretreatment

Cryoprotectants are the compounds that can ***prevent the damage caused to cells by freezing*** or ***thawing***. The freezing point and supercooling point of water are reduced by the presence of cryoprotectants. As a result, the ice crystal formation is retarded during the process of cryopreservation. There are several cryoprotectants which include dimethyl sulfoxide (DMSO), glycerol, ethylene, propylene, sucrose, mannose, glucose, proline and acetamide. Among these, ***DMSO, sucrose and glycerol are most widely used***. Generally, a mixture of cryoprotectants instead of a single one, is used for more effective cryopreservation without damage to cells/tissues.

Freezing

The sensitivity of the cells to low temperature is variable and largely depends on the plant species. Four different types of freezing methods are used.

1. **Slow-freezing method :** The tissue or the requisite plant material is slowly frozen at a slow ***cooling rates of 0.5-5°C/min*** from 0°C to –100°C, and then transferred to liquid nitrogen. The advantage of slow-freezing method is that some amount of water flows from the cells to the outside. This promotes extracellular ice fromation rather than intracellular freezing. As a result of this, the plant cells are partially dehydrated and survive better. The slow-freezing procedure is successfully used for the ***cryopreservation of suspension cultures***.

2. **Rapid freezing method :** This technique is quite simple and involves plunging of the vial containing plant material into liquid nitrogen. During rapid freezing, a ***decrease in temperature –300° to –1000°C/min occurs***. The freezing process is carried out so quickly that small ice crystals are formed within the cells. Further, the growth of intracellular ice crystals is also minimal. Rapid freezing technique is used for the cryopreservation of shoot tips and somatic embryos.

3. **Stepwise freezing method :** This is a ***combination of slow and rapid freezing procedures*** (with the advantages of both), and is carried out in a stepwise manner. The plant material is first cooled to an intermediate temperature and maintained there for about 30 minutes and then rapidly cooled by plunging it into liquid nitrogen. Stepwise freezing method has been successfully used for cryopreservation of suspension cultures, shoot apices and buds.

4. **Dry freezing method :** Some workers have reported that the non-germinated dry seeds can survive freezing at very low temperature in contrast to water-imbibing seeds which are susceptible to cryogenic injuries. In a similar fashion, dehydrated cells are found to have a better survival rate after cryopreservation.

Storage

Maintenance of the frozen cultures at the specific temperature is as important as freezing. ***In general, the frozen cells/tissues are kept for storage at temperatures in the range of –70 to –196°C***. However, with temperatures above –130°C, ice crystal growth may occur inside the cells which reduces viability of cells. Storage is ideally done in liquid nitrogen refrigerator — at 150°C in the vapour phase, or at –196°C in the liquid phase.

The ultimate objective of storage is to stop all the cellular metabolic activities and maintain their viability. ***For long term storge***, temperature at ***–196°C in liquid nitrogen is ideal***. A regular and constant supply of liquid nitrogen to the liquid nitrogen refrigerator is essential. It is necessary to check the viability of the germplasm periodically in some samples.

Proper documentation of the germplasm storage has to be done. The documented information must be comprehensive with the following particulars.

- Taxonomic classification of the material
- History of culture
- Morphogenic potential
- Genetic manipulations done
- Somaclonal variations
- Culture medium
- Growth kinetics

Thawing

Thawing is usually carried out by ***plunging*** the frozen samples in ***ampoules into a warm water*** (temperature 37–45°C) bath with vigorous swirling. By this approach, rapid thawing (at the rate of 500–750°C min^{-1}) occurs, and this protects the cells from the damaging effects ice crystal formation.

As the thawing occurs (ice completely melts) the ampoules are quickly transferred to a water bath at temperature 20–25°C. This transfer is necessary since the cells get damaged if left for long in warm (37–45°C) water bath.

For the cryopreserved material (cells/tissues) where the water content has been reduced to an optimal level before freezing, the process of thowing becomes less critical.

Reculture

In general, thawed germplasm is washed several times to remove cryoprotectants. This material is then recultured in a fresh medium following standard procedures.

Some workers prefer to directly culture the thawed material without washing. This is because certain vital substances, released from the cells during freezing, are believed to promote *in vitro* cultures.

Measurement of survival/viability

The viability/survival of the frozen cells can be measured at any stage of cryopreservation or after thawing or reculture.

The techniques employed to determine viability of cryopreserved cells are the same as used for cell cultures (Refer Chapter 42). ***Staining techniques*** using triphenyl tetrazolium chloride (TTC), Evan's blue and fluorescein diacetate (FDA) are ***commonly used.***

The best indicator to measure the viability of cryopreserved cells is their entry into cell division and regrowth in culture. This can be evaluated by the following expression.

$$\frac{\text{No. of cells/organs growing}}{\text{No. of cells/organs thawed}} \times 100$$

Plant regeneration

The ultimate purpose of cryopreservation of germplasm is to regenerate the desired plant. For appropriate plant growth and regeneration, the cryopreserved cells/tissues have to be carefully nursed, and grown. Addition of certain growth promoting substances, besides maintenance of appropriate environmental conditions is often necessary for successful plant regeneration.

A selected list of plants (in various forms) that have been successfully used for cryopreservation is given in ***Table 48.1***.

TABLE 48.1 A selected list of plants in various forms that are successfully cryopreserved

Plant material	*Plant species*
Cell suspensions	*Oryza sativa*
	Glycine max
	Zea mays
	Nicotiana tabacum
	Capsicum annum
Callus	*Oryza sativa*
	Capsicum annum
	Saccharum sp
Protoplast	*Zea mays*
	Nicotiana tabacum
Meristems	*Solanum tuberosum*
	Cicer arietinum
Zygotic embryos	*Zea mays*
	Hordeum vulgare
	Manihot esculenta
Somatic embryos	*Citrus sinensis*
	Daucus carota
	Coffea arabica
Pollen embryos	*Nicotiana tabacum*
	Citrus sp
	Atropa belladona

COLD STORAGE

Cold storage basically involves germplasm conservation at a ***low and non-freezing temperatures (1-9°C)***. The growth of the plant material is slowed down in cold storage in contrast to complete stoppage in cryopreservation. Hence,

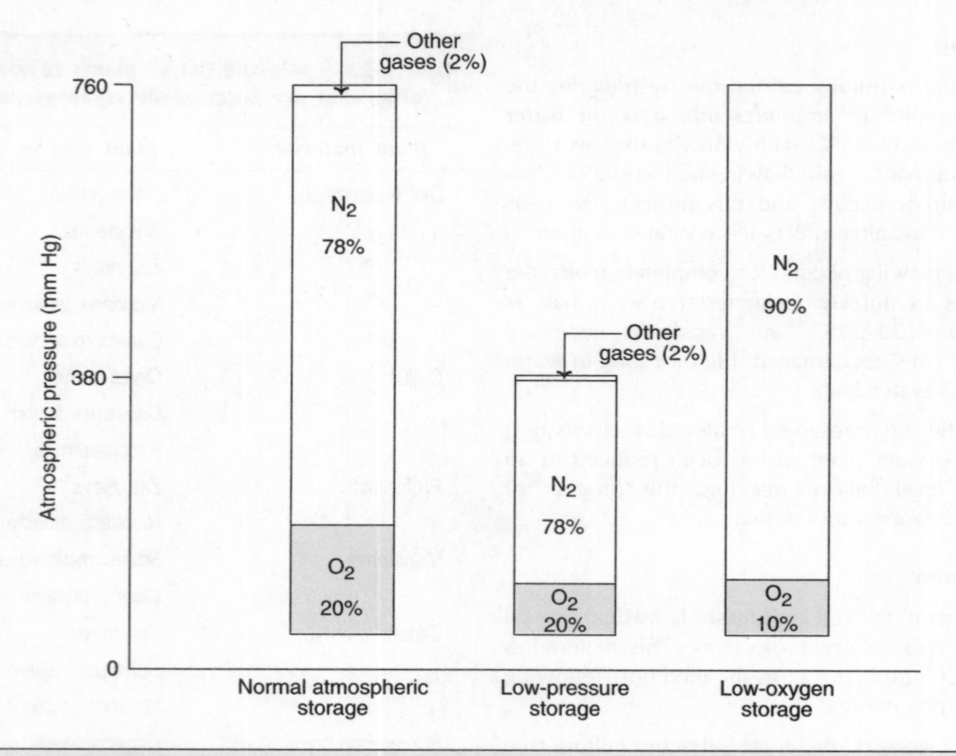

Fig. 48.2 : A graphic representation of tissue culture storage under normal atmospheric pressure, low-pressure, and low-oxygen.

cold storage is regarded as a ***slow growth germplasm conservation*** method. The major advantage of this approach is that the plant material (cells/tissues) is not subjected to cryogenic injuries.

Long-term cold storage is simple, cost-effective and yields germplasm with good survival rate. Many *in vitro* developed shoots/plants of fruit tree species have been successfully stored by this approach e.g. grape plants, strawberry plants. Virus-free strawberry plants could be preserved at 10°C for about 6 years, with the addition of a few drops of medium periodically (once in 2-3 months). Several grape plants have been stored for over 15 years by cold storage (at around 9°C) by transferring them yearly to a fresh medium.

LOW-PRESSURE AND LOW-OXYGEN STORAGE

As alternatives to cryopreservation and cold storage, low-pressure storage (LPS) and low-oxygen storage (LOS) have been developed for germplasm conservation. A graphic representation of tissue culture storage under normal atmospheric pressure, low-pressure and low-oxygen is depicted in ***Fig. 48.2***.

Low-pressure storage (LPS)

In low-pressure storage, the atmospheric pressure surrounding the plant material is reduced. This results in a partial decrease of the pressure exerted by the gases around the germplasm. The ***lowered partial pressure reduces the in vitro growth of plants*** (of organized or unorganized tissues).

Low-pressure storage systems are useful for short-term and long-term storage of plant materials. The short-term storage is particularly useful to increase the shelf life of many plant materials e.g. fruits, vegetables, cut flowers, plant cuttings. The germplasm grown in cultures can be stored for long term under low pressure.

Besides germplasm preservation, LPS reduces the activity of pathogenic organisms and inhibits spore germination in the plant culture systems.

Low-oxygen storage (LOS)

In the low-oxygen storage, the oxygen concentration is reduced, but the atmospheric pressure (260 mm Hg) is maintained by the addition of inert gases (particularly nitrogen).

The partial pressure of oxygen below 50 mm Hg reduces plant tissue growth (organized or unorganized tissue). This is due to the fact that with reduced availability of O_2, the production of CO_2 is low. As a consequence, the ***photosynthetic activity is reduced, thereby inhibiting the plant tissue growth and dimension***.

Limitations of LOS : The long-term conservation of plant materials by low-oxygen storage is likely to inhibit the plant growth after certain dimensions.

APPLICATIONS OF GERMPLASM STORAGE

The germplasm storage has become a boon to plant breeders and biotechnologists. Some of the applications are briefly described.

1. **Maintenance of stock cultures :** Plant materials (cell/tissue cultures) of several species can be cryopreserved and maintained for several years, and used as and when needed. This is in contrast to an *in vitro* cell line maintenance which has to be subcultured and transferred periodically to extend viability. Thus, germplasm storage is an ideal method to avoid subculturing, and maintain cells/ tissues in a viable state for many years.

2. Cryopreservation is an ideal method ***for long term conservation of cell cultures*** which produce secondary metabolites (e.g. medicines).

3. Disease (pathogen)-free plant materials can be frozen, and propagated whenever required.

4. Recalcitrant seeds can be maintained for long.

5. Conservation of somaclonal and gametoclonal variations in cultures.

6. Plant materials from ***endangered species can be conserved.***

7. Conservation of pollen for enhancing longevity.

8. Rare germplasms developed through somatic hybridization and other genetic manipulations can be stored.

9. Cryopreservation is a good method for the selection of cold resistant mutant cell lines which could develop into frost resistant plants.

10. Establishment of ***germplasm banks for exchange of information at the international level.***

LIMITATIONS OF GERMPLASM STORAGE

The major limitations of germplasm storage are the ***expensive equipment and the trained personnel***. It may, however, be possible in the near future to develop low cost technology for cryopreservation of plant materials.

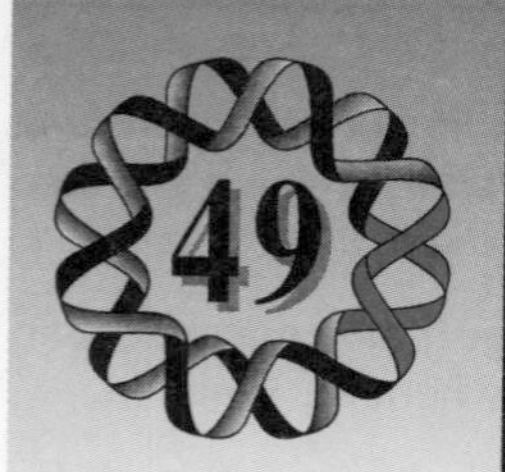

Genetic Engineering of Plants — Methodology

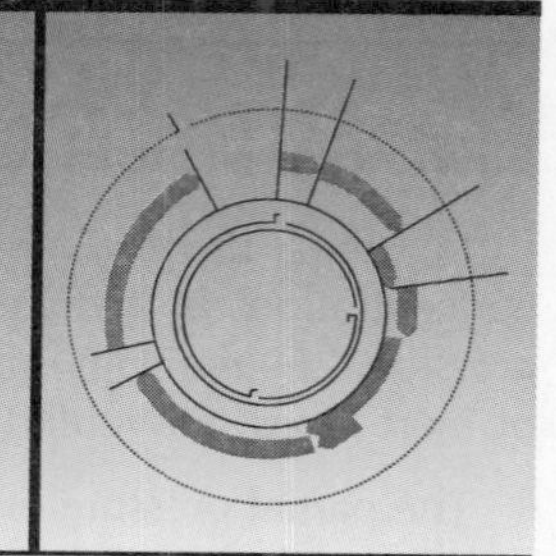

By the ***conventional plant breeding techniques***, significant achievements have been made in the improvement of several food crops. These age-old classical methods, involving gene transfer through sexual and vegetative propagation, ***take very long time***. For instance, about 6-8 years may be required to develop a new rice or a wheat by sexual propagation. Rapid advances in gene structure and function, coupled with the recent developments made in the genetic engineering techniques have dramatically improved the plant breeding methods to yield the desired results in a short period.

Plant genetic transformation technology basically deals with ***the transfer of desirable gene(s) from one plant species to another*** (or insertion of totally new genes) with subsequent integration and expression of the foreign gene(s) in the host genome. The term ***transgene*** is used to ***represent the transferred gene***, and the genetic transformation in plants is broadly referred to as ***plant transgenesis***. The ***genetically transformed*** new plants are regarded as ***transgenic plants***.

The development of transgenic plants is the outcome of an integrated application of recombinant DNA (rDNA) technology, gene transfer-methods and tissue culture techniques. (**Note :** The reader must ***refer Chapters 6 and 7*** for basic information on genetic engineering, and for common techniques employed in rDNA technology).

Why transgenic plants?

It is only through the recombinant approach (genetic engineering) of biotechnology, new genes with desired characters (that may or may not be present in other plants) can be introduced into the plants. Further, it is possible to manipulate the existing genes to make the proteins with suitable alterations e.g. increase in the content of an essential amino acid. The most important ***reasons for developing transgenic plants*** are listed

- To improve agricultural, horticultural or ornamental value of plants.
- To develop ***plant bioreactors*** for inexpensive manufacture of commercially important products e.g. proteins, medicines, pharmaceutical compounds.
- To study the action of genes in plants during development and various biological processes.

Genetic traits introduced into transgenic plants

Since plant cells are ***totipotent*** (i.e. a single plant cell can regenerate into a whole plant), the genetically engineered cells with new gene(s) can produce a transgenic plant. This plant carrying the desired trait will give raise to successive generations. ***Many genetic traits have been introduced*** into plants through genetic engineering

- Resistance to herbicides

TABLE 49.1 Gene transfer (DNA delivery) methods in plants

Method	*Salient features*
I. Vector–mediated gene transfer	
Agrobacterium (Ti plasmid)-mediated gene transfer	Very efficient, but limited to a selected group of plants
Plant viral vectors	Ineffective method, hence not widely used
II. Direct or vectorless DNA transfer	
(A) Physical methods	
Electroporation	Mostly confined to protoplasts that can be regenerated to viable plants. Many cereal crops developed.
Microprojectile (particle bombardment)	Very successful method used for a wide range of plants/tissues. Risk of gene rearrangement high.
Microinjection	Limited use since only one cell can be microinjected at a time. Technical personnel should be highly skilled.
Liposome fusion	Confined to protoplasts that can be regenerated into viable whole plants.
Silicon carbide fibres	Requires regenerable cell suspensions. The fibres, however, require careful handling.
(B) Chemical methods	
Polyethylene glycol (PEG)-mediated	Confined to protoplasts. Regeneration of fertile plants is frequently problematical.
Diethylaminoethyl (DEAE) dextran-mediated	Does not result in stable transformants.

- Protection against viral infections
- Insecticidal activity
- Improved nutritional quality
- Altered flower pigmentation
- Tolerance to environmental stresses
- Self incompatibility

Criteria for commercial use of genetically transformed plants

For large-scale commercial application of genetically engineered plants, the following requirements have to be satisfied

- Introduction of desirable gene(s) to all plant cells.
- Expression of cloned genes in the appropriate cells at the right time.
- Stable maintenance of new gene(s) inserted.
- Transmission of new genetic information to subsequent generations.

GENE TRANSFER METHODS

The gene transfer techniques in plant genetic transformation are broadly grouped into two categories

I. Vector-mediated gene transfer

II. Direct or vectorless DNA transfer

The salient features of the commonly used gene (DNA) transfer methods are given in ***Table 49.1***.

VECTOR-MEDIATED GENE TRANSFER

Vector-mediated gene transfer is carried out either by *Agrobacterium*-mediated transformation or by use of plant viruses as vectors.

AGROBACTERIUM-MEDIATED GENE TRANSFER

Agrobacterium tumefaciens is a soil-borne, Gram-negative bacterium. It is rod shaped and motile, and belongs to the bacterial family of

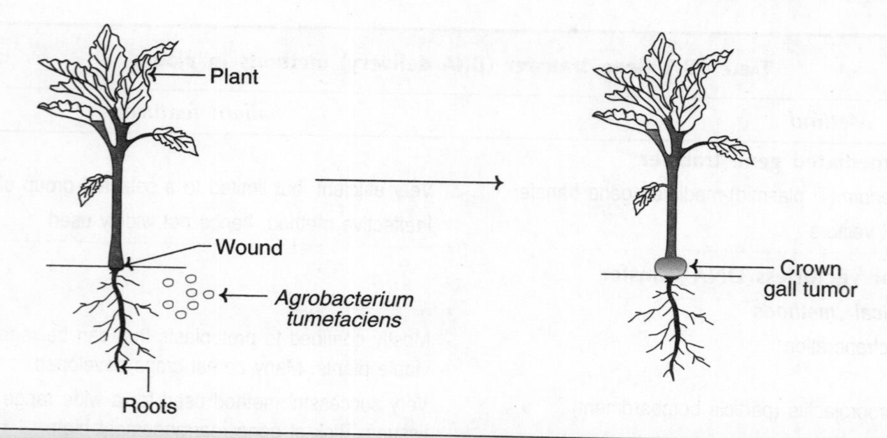

Fig. 49.1 : Formation of a crown gall tumor in a plant infected with Agrobacterium tumefaciens.

Rhizobiaceae. ***A. tumefaciens*** is a phytopathogen, and is treated as the ***nature's most effective plant genetic engineer***. Some workers consider this bacterium as the ***natural expert of interkingdom gene transfer***. In fact, the major credit for the development of plant transformation techniques goes to the natural unique capability of *A. tumefaciens*. Thus, this bacterium is the most beloved by plant biotechnologists.

There are mainly two species of *Agrobacterium* :

- *A. tumefaciens* that induces crown gall disease.
- *A. rhizogenes* that induces hairy root disease.

CROWN GALL DISEASE AND Ti PLASMID

Almost 100 years ago (1907), Smith and Townsend postulated that a bacterium was the causative agent of crown gall tumors, although its importance was recognized much later.

As ***A. tumefaciens*** infects wounded or damaged plant tissues, in induces the formation of a ***plant tumor called crown gall*** (***Fig. 49.1***). The entry of the bacterium into the plant tissues is facilitated by the release of certain phenolic compounds (acetosyringone, hydroxyacetosyringone) by the wounded sites. Crown gall formation occurs when the bacterium releases its ***Ti plasmid*** (**t**umor-**i**nducing plasmid) into the plant cell cytoplasm. A ***fragment*** (segment) ***of Ti plasmid***, referred to as ***T-DNA***, is actually transferred from the bacterium into the host where it gets integrated into the plant cell chromosome (i.e. host genome). Thus, ***crown gall disease is a naturally evolved genetic engineering process***.

The T-DNA carries genes that code for proteins involved in the biosynthesis of growth hormones (auxin and cytokinin) and novel plant metabolites namely ***opines*** — amino acid derivatives and ***agropines*** — sugar derivatives (***Fig. 49.2***). The growth hormones cause plant cells to proliferate and form the gall while opines and agropines are utilized by *A. tumefaciens* as sources of carbon and energy. As such, opines and agropines are not normally part of the plant metabolism (neither produced nor metabolised). Thus, *A. tumefaciens* genetically transforms plant cells and creates a biosynthetic machinery to produce nutrients for its own use.

As the bacteria multiply and continue infection, grown gall develops which is a visible mass of the accumulated bacteria and plant material. Crown gall formation is the consequence of the transfer, integration and expression of genes of T-DNA (or Ti plasmid) of *A. tumefaciens* in the infected plant. The genetic transformation leads to the formation of crown gall tumors, which interfere with the normal growth of the plant. Several ***dicotyledonous plants (dicots)*** are affected by crown gall disease e.g. grapes, roses, stone-fruit trees.

Organization of Ti plasmid

The Ti plasmids (approximate size 200 kb each) exist as independent replicating circular DNA molecules within the *Agrobacterium* cells. The T-DNA (transferred DNA) is variable in length in

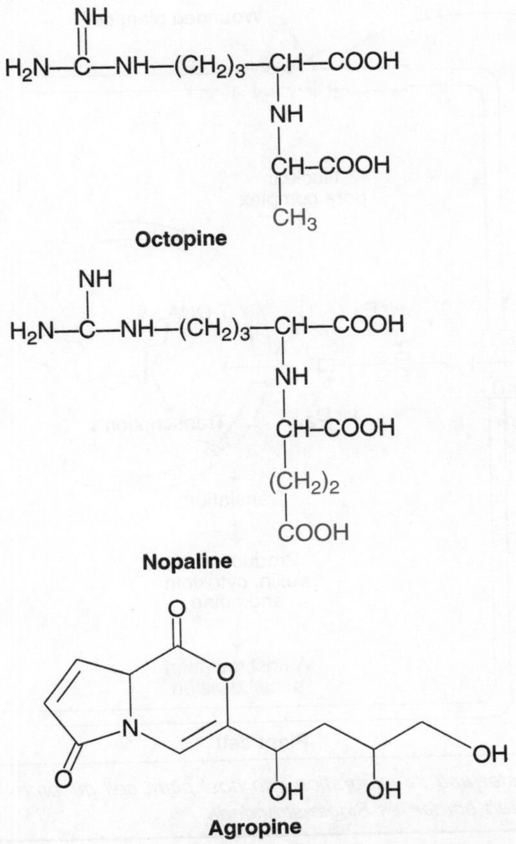

Fig. 49.2 : Structures of three opines–octopine, nopaline, and agropine.

the range of 12 to 24 kb, which depends on the bacterial strain from which Ti plasmids come. Nopaline strains of Ti plasmid have one T-DNA with length of 20 kb while octopine strains have two T-DNA regions referred to as T_L and T_R that are respectively 14 kb and 7 kb in length.

A diagrammatic representation of a Ti plasmid is depicted in ***Fig. 49.3***. The Ti plasmid has three important regions.

1. **T-DNA region :** This region has the genes for the biosynthesis of ***auxin (aux)***, ***cytokinin (cyt)*** and ***opine (ocs)***, and is flanked by left and right borders. These three genes-*aux*, *cyto* and *ocs* are referred to as ***oncogenes***, as they are the determinants of the tumor phenotype.

T-DNA borders — A set of 24 kb sequences present on either side (right and left) of T-DNA are also transferred to the plant cells. It is now clearly established that the right border is more critical for T-DNA transfer and tumorigenesis.

2. **Virulence region :** The genes responsible for the transfer of T-DNA into the host plant are located outside T-DNA and the rigion is referred to as *vir* or virulence region. *Vir* region codes for proteins involved in T-DNA transfer. At least nine *vir*-gene operons have been identified. These include *vir A*, *vir G*, *vir* B_1, *vir* C_1, *vir* D_1, D_2 and D_4, and *vir* E_1 and E_2.

3. **Opine catabolism region :** This region codes for proteins involved in the uptake and metabolisms of opines.

Besides the above three, there is ***ori region*** that is responsible for the origin of DNA replication which permits the Ti plasmid to be stably maintained in *A. tumefaciens*.

T-DNA transfer and integration

The process of T-DNA transfer and it integration into the host plant genome is depicted in ***Fig. 49.4***, and is briefly described.

1. **Signal induction to *Agrobacterium* :** The wounded plant cells release certain chemicals-phenolic compounds and sugars which are recognized as signals by *Agrobacterium*. The signals induced result in a sequence of biochemical events in *Agrobacterium* that ultimately helps in the transfer of T-DNA of T-plasmid.

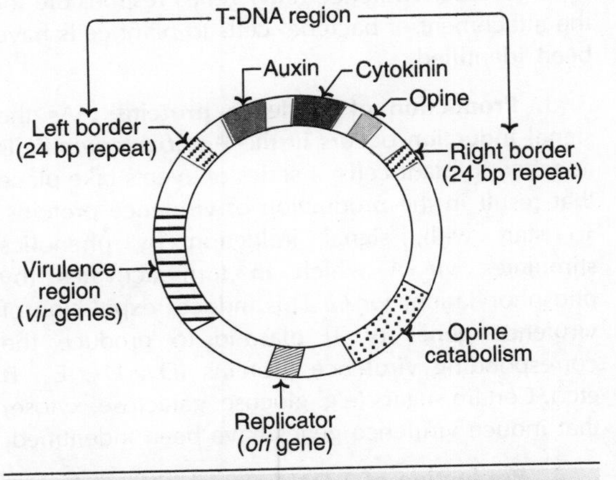

Fig. 49.3 : A dagrammatic representation of a Ti plasmid.

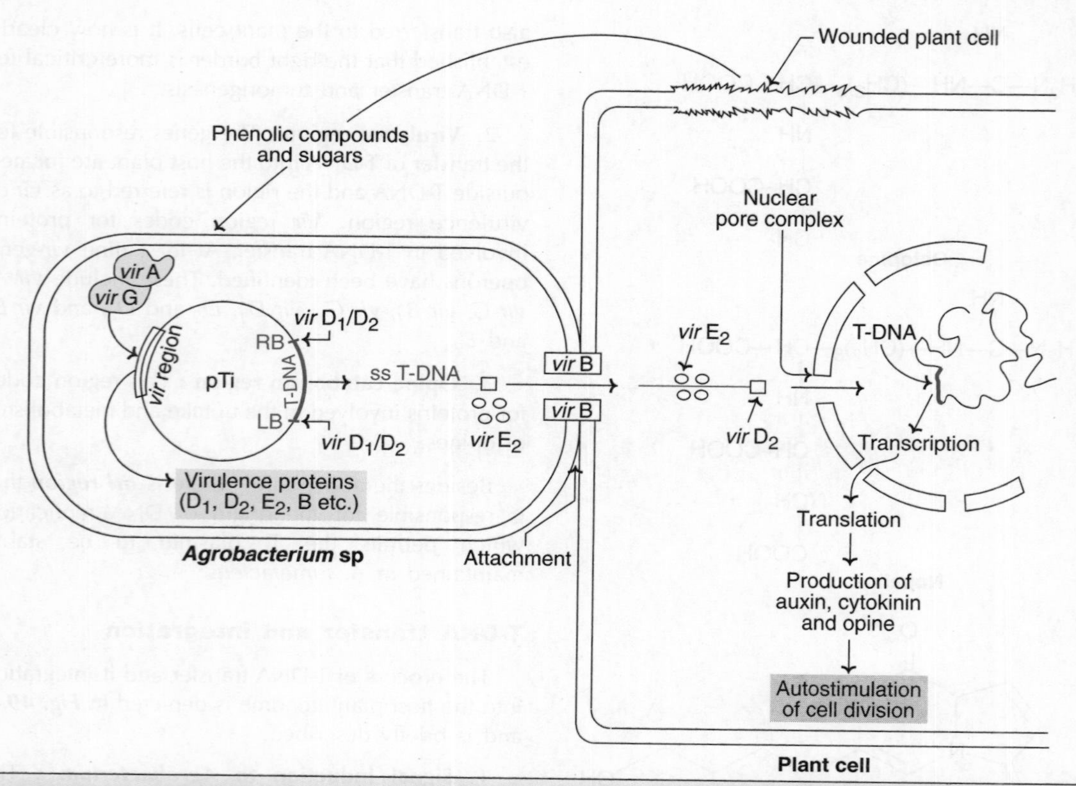

Fig. 49.4 : A diagrammatic representation of T-DNA transfer and its integration into host plant cell genome (pTi-Ti plasmid; RB-Right border; LB-Left border; ss-Single-stranded).

2. **Attachment of *Agrobacterium* to plant cells :** The *Agrobacterium* attaches to plant cells through polysaccharides, particularly cellulose fibres produced by the bacterium. Several chromosomal virulence (*chv*) genes responsible for the attachment of bacterial cells to plant cells have been identified.

3. **Production of virulence proteins :** As the signal induction occurs in the *Agrobacterium* cells attached to plant cells, a series of events take place that result in the production of virulence proteins. To start with, signal induction by phenolics stimulates *vir A* which in turn activates (by phosphorylation) *vir G*. This induces expression of virulence genes of Ti plasmid to produce the corresponding virulence proteins (D_1, D_2, E_2, B etc.). Certain sugars (e.g. glucose, galactose, xylose) that induce virulence genes have been indentified.

4. **Production of T-DNA strand :** The right and left borders of T-DNA are recognized by vir D_1/vir D_2 proteins. These proteins are involved in the production single-stranded T-DNA (ss DNA), its protection and export to plant cells. The ss T-DNA gets attached to vir D_2.

5. **Transfer of T-DNA out of *Agrobacterium* :** The ss T-DNA — vir D_2 complex in association with vir G is exported from the bacterial cell. *Vir B* products form the transport apparatus.

6. **Transfer of T-DNA into plant cells and integration :** The T-DNA-vir D_2 complex crosses the plant plasma membrane. In the plant cells, T-DNA gets covered with vir E_2. This covering protects the T-DNA from degradation by nucleases. vir D_2 and vir E_2 interact with a variety of plant proteins which influences T-DNA transport and integration. The T-DNA-vir D_2-vir E_2 — plant protein complex enters the nucleus through nuclear pore complex. Within the nucleus, the T-DNA gets integrated into the plant chromosome through a process referred to ***illegitimate recombination***. This is different from the homologous recombination, as it does not depend on the sequence similarity.

HAIRY ROOT DISEASE OF A. RHIZOGENES — R_i PLASMIDS

Agrobacterium rhizogenes can also infect plants. But this results in hairy roots and not crown galls as is the case with *A. tumefaciens*. The plasmids, of *A. rhizogenes* have been isolated and characterized. These plasmids, referred to as ***Ri plasmids***, (Ri stands for ***R***oot ***i***nducing) are of different types. Some of the Ri plasmid strains possess genes that are homologous to Ti plasmid e.g. auxin biosynthetic genes.

Instead of virulence genes, Ri plasmids contain a series of open reading frames on the T-DNA. The products of these genes are involved in the metabolism of plant growth regulators which gets sensetized to auxin and leads to root formation.

Vectors of A. *rhizogenes*

As it is done with *A tumefaciens*, vectors can be constructed by using *A. rhizogenes*. These vectors are alternate strategies for gene transfer. However, employment of *A. rhizogene*-based vectors for plant transformation is not common since more efficient systems of *A. tumefaciens* have been developed.

Importance of hairy roots

Hairy roots can be cultured *in vitro*, and thus are important in plant biotechnology. Hairy root systems are useful for the production of secondary metabolites, particularly pharmaceutical proteins.

Ti PLASMID-DERIVED VECTOR SYSTEMS

The ability of Ti plasmid of *Agrobacterium* to genetically transform plants has been described. It is possible to insert a desired DNA sequence (gene) into the T-DNA region (of Ti plasmid), and then use *A. tumefaciens* to deliver this gene(s) into the genome of plant cell. In this process, Ti plasmids serve as natural vectors. However, there are several ***limitations to use Ti plasmids directly as cloning vectors***.

- Ti plasmids are large in size (200–800 kb). Smaller vectors are preferred for recombinant experiments. For this reason, large segments of DNA of Ti plasmid, not essential for cloning, must be removed.
- Absence of unique restriction enzyme sites on Ti plasmids.
- The phytohormones (auxin, cytokinin) produced prevent the plant cells being regenerated into plants. Therefore auxin and cytokinin genes must be removed.
- Opine production in transformed plant cells lowers the plant yield. Therefore opine synthesizing genes which are of no use to plants should be removed.
- Ti plasmids cannot replicate in *E. coli*. This limits their utility as *E. coli* is widely used in recombinant experiments. An alternate arrangement is to add an origin of replication to Ti plasmid that allows the plasmid to replicate in *E. coli*.

Considering the above limitations, ***Ti plasmid-based vectors with suitable modifications have been constructed***. These vectors are mainly composed of the following components.

1. The right border sequence of T-DNA which is absolutely required for T-DNA integration into plant cell DNA.

2. A multiple cloning site (polylinker DNA) that promotes the insertion of cloned gene into the region between T-DNA borders.

3. An origin of DNA replication that allows the plasmids to multiply in *E. coli*.

4. A selectable marker gene (e.g. neomycin phosphotransferase) for appropriate selection of the transformed cells.

Two types of Ti plasmid-derived vectors are used for genetic transformation of plants— ***cointegrate vectors*** and ***binary vectors***.

Cointegrate vector

In the cointegrate vector system, the disarmed and modified Ti plasmid combines with an intermediate cloning vector to produce a recombinant Ti plasmid (***Fig. 49.5***).

Production of disarmed Ti plasmid : The T-DNA genes for hormone biosynthesis are removed (disarmed). In place of the deleted DNA, a bacterial plasmid (pBR322) DNA sequence is incorporated. This disarmed plasmid, also referred to as ***receptor plasmid***, has the basic structure of T-DNA (right and left borders, virulence genes etc.) necessary to transfer the plant cells.

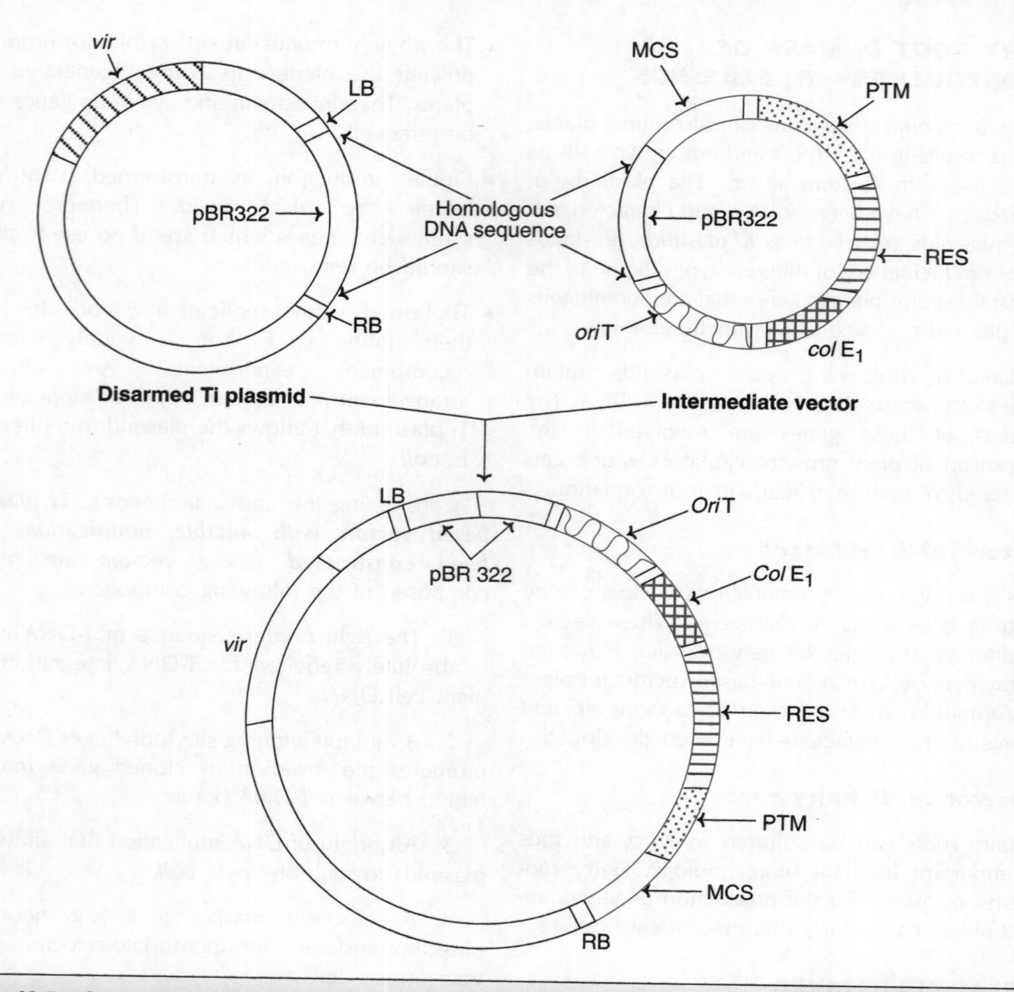

*Fig. 49.5 : Cointegrate vector system (*vir*-Ti plasmid virulence region; pBR322-Bacterial plasmid 322; LB-Left border; RB-Right border; MCS-Multiple cloning site; PTM-Plant transformation marker; RES-Bacterial resistance marker;* col *E_1-Origin of a replication from col E_1 plasmid;* ori *T-Origin of transfer site for conjugative plasmid mobilization).*

Construction of intermediate vector : The intermediate vector is constructed with the following components.

- A pBR322 sequence ***DNA homologous*** to that found in the receptor Ti plasmid.
- A ***plant transformation marker*** (***PTM***) e.g. a gene coding for neomycin phosphotransferase II (*npt* II). This gene confers resistance to kanamycin in the plant cells and thus permits their isolation.
- A ***bacterial resistance marker*** e.g. a gene coding for spectinomycin resistance. This gene confers spectinomycin resistance to recipient bacterial cells and thus permits their selective isolation.
- A ***multiple cloning site*** (***MCS***) where ***foreign genes*** can be ***inserted***.
- A *Col*E_1 origin of replication which allows the replication of plasmid in *E. coli* but not in *Agrobacterium*.
- An *ori*T sequence with basis of mobilization (*bom*) site for the transfer of intermediate vector from *E. coli* to *Agrobacterium*.

Production and use of cointegrate vectors : The desired foreign gene (target-gene) is first cloned in the multiple cloning site of the intermediate vector.

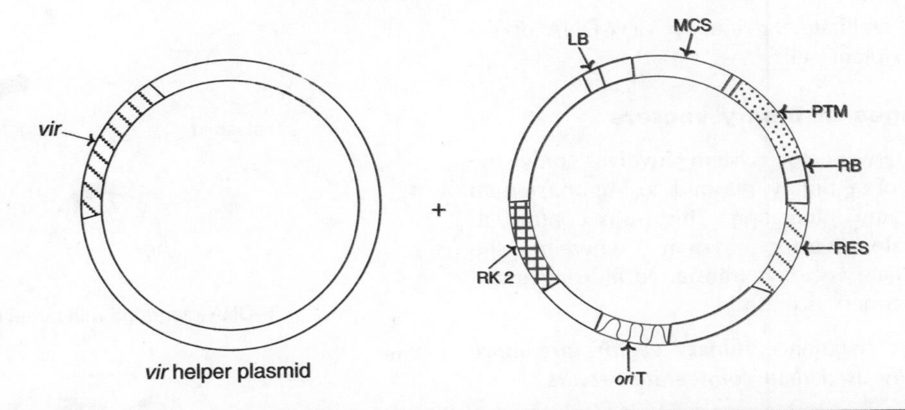

Fig. 49.6 : Binary vector system (vir- Ti plasmid virulence region; LB-Left border; RB-Right border; MCS-Multiple cloning site; PTM-Plant transformation marker; RES-Bacterial resistance marker; oriT-Origin of transfer site for conjugative plasmid mobilization; RK_2-Origin of replication from plasmid).

The cloning process is carried out in *E. coli*, the bacterium where the cloning is most efficient. The intermediate vector is mated with *Agrobacterium* so that the foreign gene is mobilised into the latter. The transformed *Agrobacterium* cells with receptor Ti plasmid and intermediate vector are selectively isolated when grown on a minimal medium containing spectinomycin. The selection process becomes easy since *E. coli* does not grow on a minimal medium in which *Agrobacterium* grows. Within the *Agrobacterium* cells, intermediate plasmid gets integrated into the receptor Ti plasmid to produce cointegrate plasmid. This plasmid containing plant transformation marker (e.g. *npt II*) gene and cloned target gene between T-DNA borders is transferred to plant cells. The transformed plant cells can be selected on a medium containing kanamycin when the plant and *Agrobacterium* cells are incubated together.

Advantages of cointegrate vector

- Target genes can be easily cloned
- The plasmid is relatively small with a number of restriction sites.
- Intermediate plasmid is conveniently cloned in *E. coli* and transferred to *Agrobacterium*.

Binary vector

The binary vector system ***consists of an Agrobacterium strain along with a disarmed Ti plasmid called vir helper*** plasmid (the entire T-DNA region including borders deleted while *vir* gene is retained). It may be noted that both of them are not physically linked (or integrated). A binary vector with T-DNA can replicate in *E. coli* and *Agrobacterium*.

A diagrammatic representation of a typical binary vector system is depicted in ***Fig. 49.6***. The binary vector has the following components.

1. Left and right borders that delimit the T-DNA region.

2. A plant transformation marker (PTM) e.g. *npt II* that confers kanamycin resistance in plant transformed cells.

3. A multiple cloning site (MCS) for introducing target/foreign genes.

4. A bacterial resistance marker e.g. tetracycline resistance gene for selecting binary vector colonies in *E. coli* and *Agrobacterium*.

5. *oriT* sequence for conjugal mobilization of the binary vector from *E. coli* to *Agrobacterium*.

6. A broad host-range origin of replication such as RK_2 that allows the replication of binary vector in *Agrobacterium*.

Production and use of binary vector : The target (foreign) gene of interest is inserted into the multiple cloning site of the binary vector. In this way, the target gene is placed between the right and left border repeats and cloned in *E. coli*. By a mating process, the binary vector is mobilised from *E. coli* to *Agrobacterium*. Now, the virulence gene proteins of T-DNA facilitate the transfer of T-DNA of the vector into plant cells.

Advantages of binary vectors

- The binary vector system involves only the transfer of a binary plasmid to *Agrobacterium* without any integration. This is in contrast to cointegrate vector system wherein the intermediate vector is transferred and integrated with disarmed Ti plasmid.
- Due to convenience, ***binary vectors are more frequently used than cointegrate vectors.***

PLANT TRANSFORMATION TECHNIQUE USING *AGROBACTERIUM*

Agrobacterium-mediated technique is the ***most widely used*** for the transformation of plants and generation of transgenic plants. The important requirements for gene transfer in higher plants through *Agrobacterium* mediation are listed.

- The explants of the plant must produce phenolic compounds (e.g. autosyringone) for activation of virulence genes.
- Transformed cells/tissues should be capable to regenerate into whole plants.

In general, most of the *Agrobacterium*-mediated plant transformations have the following basic protocol (***Fig. 49.7***)

1. Development of *Agrobacterium* carrying the cointegrate or binary vector with the desired gene.
2. Identification of a suitable explant e.g. cells, protoplasts, tissues, calluses, organs.
3. Co-culture of explants with *Agrobacterium.*
4. Killing of *Agrobacterium* with a suitable antibiotic without harming the plant tissue.
5. Selection of transformed plant cells.
6. Regeneration of whole plants.

Advantages of *Agrobacterium*-mediated transformation

- This is a natural method of gene transfer.
- *Agrobacterium* can conveniently infect any explant (cells/tissues/organs).
- Even large fragments of DNA can be efficiently transferred.

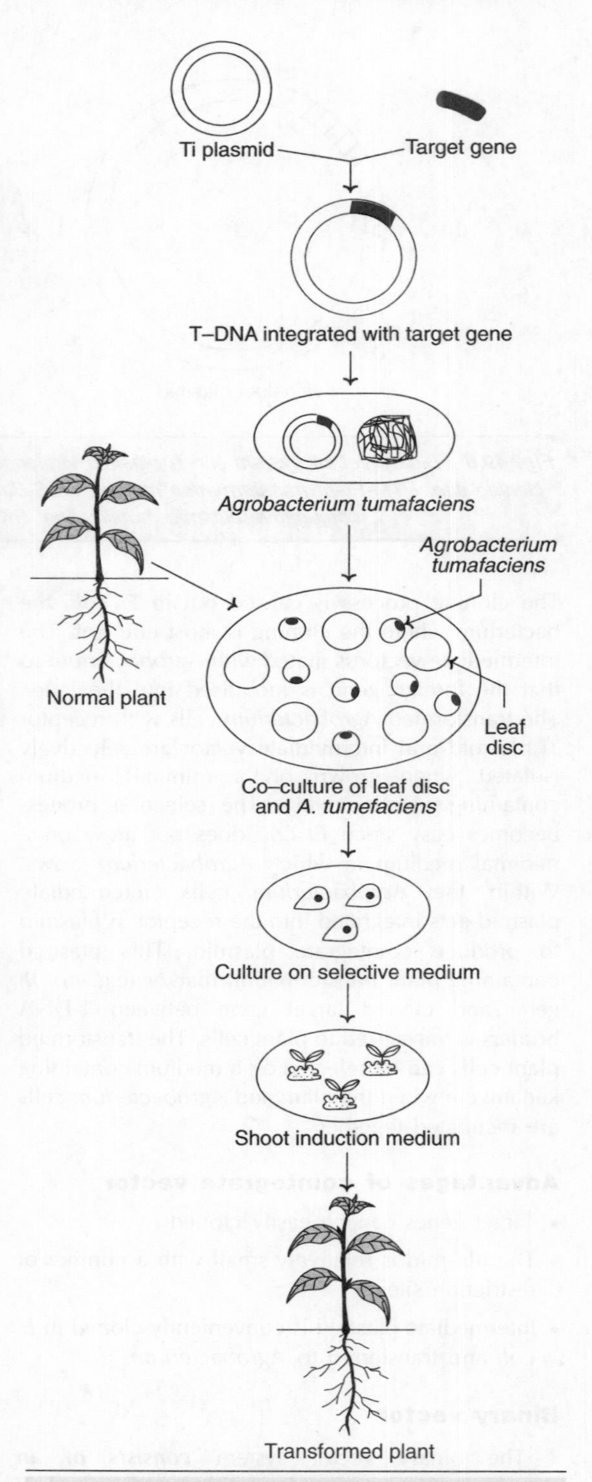

***Fig. 49.7 :** Transformation technique using* Agrobacterium*-mediated gene transfer.*

- Stability of transferred DNA is reasonably good.
- Transformed plants can be regenerated effectively.

Limitations of *Agrobacterium*-mediated transformation

- There is a limitation of host plants for *Agrobacterium*, since many crop plants (***monocotyledons*** e.g. cereals) are ***not infected*** by it. In recent years, virulent strains of *Agrobacterium* that can infect a wide range of plants have been developed.
- The cells that regenerate more efficiently are often difficult to transform. e.g. embryonic cells lie in deep layers which are not easy targets for *Agrobacterium*.

VIRUS-MEDIATED GENE TRANSFER (PLANT VIRUSES AS VECTORS)

Plant viruses are considered as ***efficient gene transfer agents*** as they can infect the intact plants and amplify the transferred genes through viral genome replication. Viruses are natural vectors for genetic engineering. They can introduce the desirable gene(s) into almost all the plant cells since the viral infections are mostly systemic.

Plant viruses are nonintegrative vectors

The plant viruses do not integrate into the host genome in contrast to the vectors based on T-DNA of *A. tumefaciens* which are integrative. The viral genomes are suitably modified by introducing desired foreign genes.

These recombinant viruses are transferred, multiplied and expressed in plant cells. They spread systemically within the host plant where the new genetic material is expressed.

Criteria for a plant virus vector

An ideal plant virus for its effective use in gene transfer is expected to posses the following characteristics.

- The virus must be capable of spreading from cell to cell through plasmodesmata.
- The viral genome shoule be able to replicate in the absence of viral coat protein and spread from cell to cell. This is desirable since the insertion of foreign DNA will make the viral genome too big to be packed.
- The recombinant viral genome must elicit little or no disease symptoms in the infected plants.
- The virus should have a broad host range.
- The virus with DNA genome is preferred since the genetic manipulations involve plant DNA.

The three groups of viruses — ***caulimoviruses***, ***geminiviruses*** and ***RNA viruses*** that are used as vectors for gene transfer in plants are briefly described.

CAULIMOVIRUSES AS VECTORS

The caulimoviruses contain circular double-stranded DNA, and are spherical in shape. Caulimoviruses are widely distributed and are responsible for a number of economically important diseases in various crops. The caulimovirus group has around 15 viruses and among these ***cauliflower mosaic virus*** (CaMV) is the most ***important for gene transfer***. The other caulimoviruses include carnation etched virus, dahlia mosaic virus, mirabilis mosaic virus and strawberry vein banding virus.

Cauliflower mosaic virus (CaMV)

CaMV infects many plants (e.g. members of Cruciferae, Datura) and can be easily transmitted, even mechanically. Another attractive feature of CaMV is that the ***infection is systemic***, and large quantities of viruses are found in infected cells.

A diagrammatic view of the CaMV genetic map is depicted in ***Fig. 49.8***. The genome of CaMV consists of a 8 kb (8024 bp) relaxed but tightly packed circular DNA with six major and two minor coding regions. The genes II and VII are not essential for viral infection.

Use of CaMV in gene transfer

For appropriate transmission of CaMV, the foreign DNA must be encapsulated in viral protein. Further, the newly inserted foreign DNA must not interfere with the native assembly of the virus. CaMV genome does not contain any non-coding regions wherein foreign DNA can be inserted. It is fortunate that two genes namely ***gene II and gene VII have no essential functions*** for the virus. It is therefore possible to ***replace one of them and insert the desired foreign gene***.

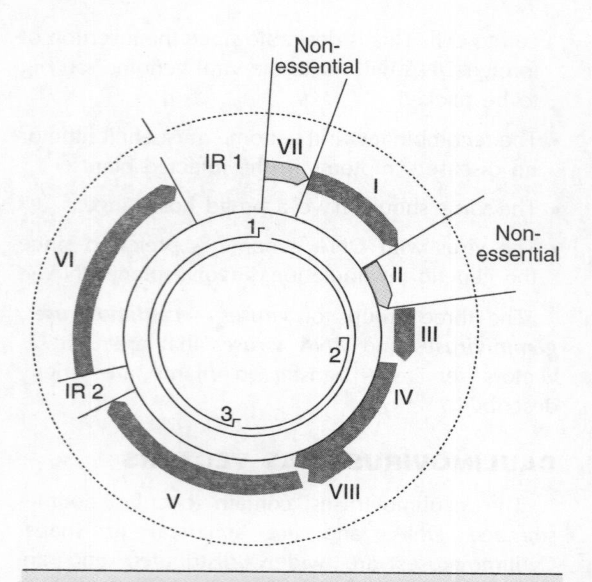

Fig. 49.8 : A diagrammatic representation of the genetic map of cauliflower mosaic virus genome (I...VIII represent coding regions; IR 1and IR 2 are intergeneric regions; The outside dotted circle represents 30S transcript; The two circular lines at the centre indicate viral DNA strands).

Gene II of CaMV has been successfully replaced with a bacterial gene encoding dihydrofolate reductase that provides resistance to methotrexate. When the chimeric CaMV was transmitted to turnip plants, they were systemically infected and the plants developed resistance to methotrexate.

Limitations of CaMV as a vector

- CaMV vector has a limited capacity for insertion of foreign genes.
- Infective capacity of CaMV is lost if more than a few hundred nucleotides are introduced.
- Helper viruses cannot be used since the foreign DNA gets expelled and wild-type viruses are produced.

GEMINIVIRUSES AS VECTORS

The geminiviruses are so named because they have geminate (Gemini literally means heavenly twins) morphological particles i.e. twin and paired capsid structures. These viruses are characterized by possessing one or two single-stranded circular DNAs (ss DNA). On replications, ss DNA forms an intermediate double-stranded DNA.

The geminiviruses can infect a wide range of crop plants (monocotyledons and dicotyledons) which attract plant biotechnologists to employ these viruses for gene transfer. Curly top virus (CTV) and maize streak virus (MSV) and bean golden mosaic virus (BGMV) are among the important geminiviruses.

It has been observed that a large number of replicative forms of a geminivirus genome accumulate inside the nuclei of infected cells. The single-stranded genomic DNA replicates in the nucleus to form a double-stranded intermediate.

Geminivirus vectors can be used to deliver, amplify and express foreign genes in several plants/ explants (protoplasts, cultured cells). However, the serious drawback in employing geminiviruses as vectors is that it is very difficult to introduce purified viral DNA into the plants. An alternate arrangement is to take the help of *Agrobacterium* and carry out gene transfer.

RNA PLANT VIRUSES AS VECTORS

There are mainly two types single-stranded RNA viruses.

1. **Monopartite viruses :** These viruses are usually large and contain undivided genomes for all the genetic information e.g. tobacco mosaic virus (TMV).

2. **Multipartite viruses :** The genome in these viruses is divided into small RNAs which may be in the same particle or different particles. e.g. brome mosaic virus (BMV). HMV contains four RNAs divided between three particles.

Plant RNA viruses, in general, are characterized by high level of gene expression, good efficiency to infect cells and spread to different tissues. But the major limitation to use them as vectors is the difficulty of joining RNA molecules *in vitro*.

Use of cDNA for gene transfer

Complementary DNA (cDNA) copies of RNA viruses are prepared *in vitro*. The cDNA so generated can be used as a vector for gene transfer in plants. This approach is tedious and cumbersome. However, some success has been reported. A gene sequence encoding chloramphenicol resistance (enzyme-chloramphenicol acetyltransferase) has been inserted into brome mosaic virus genome. This gene expression, however, has been confined to protoplasts.

LIMITATIONS OF VIRAL VECTORS IN GENE TRANSFER

The ultimate objective of gene transfer is to ***transmit the desired genes to subsequent generations***. With virus vectors, this is ***not possible*** unless the virus is seed-transmitted. However, in case of vegetatively propagated plants, transmission of desired traits can be done e.g. potatoes. Even in these plants, there is always a risk for the transferred gene to be lost anytime.

For the reasons referred above, plant biotechnologists prefer to insert the desired genes of interest into a plant chromosome.

DIRECT OR VECTORLESS DNA TRANSFER

The term direct or vectorless transfer of DNA is used when the ***foreign DNA is directly introduced into the plant genome***. Direct DNA transfer methods rely on the delivery of naked DNA into the plant cells. This is in contrast to the *Agrobacterium* or vector-mediated DNA transfer which may be regarded as indirect methods.

Majority of the direct DNA transfer methods are simple and effective. And in fact, several transgenic plants have been developed by this approach.

Limitations of direct DNA transfer

The major disadvantage of direct gene transfer is that the frequency of ***transgene rearrangements is high***. This results in higher transgene copy number, and ***high frequencies of gene silencing*** (described on p. 593).

Types of direct DNA transfer

The direct DNA transfer can be broadly divided into three categories.

1. ***Physical gene transfer methods***—electroporation, particle bombardment, microinjection, liposome fusion, silicon carbide fibres.

2. ***Chemical gene transfer methods***—Polyethylene glycol (PEG)-mediated, diethyl aminoethyl (DEAE) dextran-mediated, calcium phosphate precipitation.

3. DNA imbibition by cells/tissues/organs.

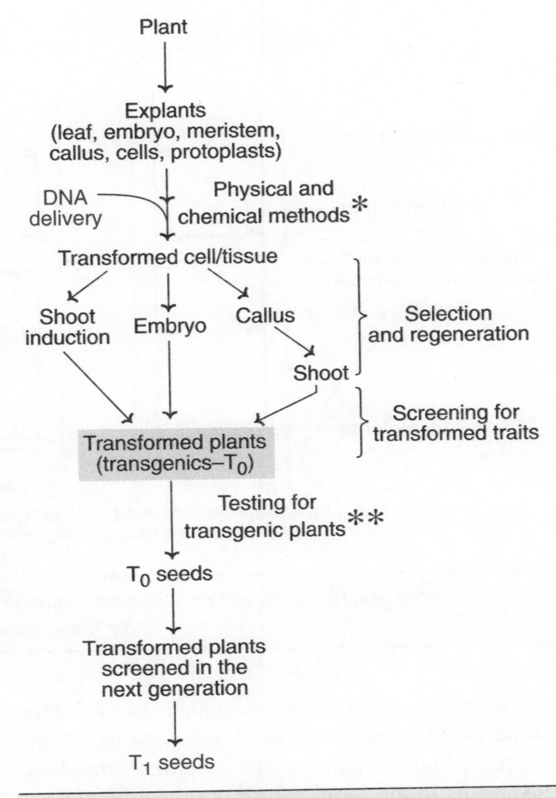

***Fig. 49.9 :** An overview of the protocol for the production of transgenic plants using direct DNA delivery methods (*Electroporation, microinjection, macroinjection, bombardment, etc.; **Polymerase chain reaction, Southern hybridization)*

The salient features of the different methods for direct DNA transfer are given in ***Table 49.1*** (See p. 573). The commonly used methods are briefly described in the following pages.

PHYSICAL GENE TRANSFER METHODS

An overview of the general scheme for the production of transgenic plants by employing physical transfer methods is depicted in ***Fig. 49.9***. Some details of the different techniques are described.

ELECTROPORATION

Electroporation basically involves the use of high field strength ***electrical impulses to reversibly permeabilize the cell membranes for the uptake of DNA***. This technique can be used for the delivery of DNA into intact plant cells and protoplasts.

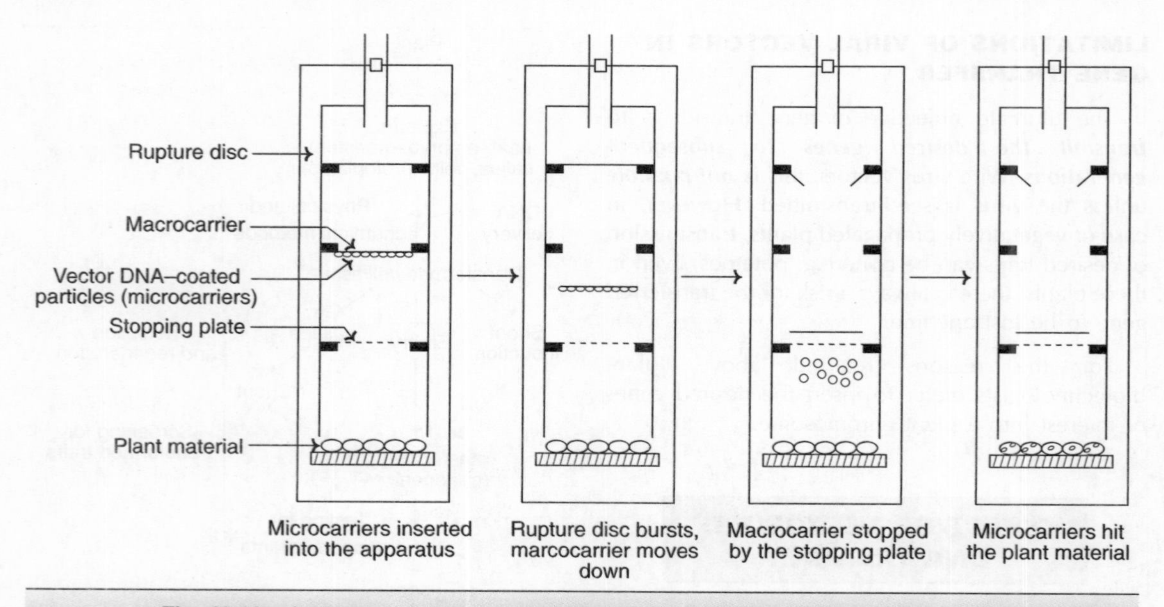

Fig. 49.10 : A diagrammatic representation of particle bombardment (biolistics) system for gene transfer in plants.

The plant material is incubated in a buffer solution containing the desired foreign/target DNA, and subjected to high voltage electrical impulses. This results in the formation of pores in the plasma membrane through which DNA enters and gets integrated into the host cell genome. In the early years, only protoplasts were used for gene transfer by electroporation. Now a days, intact cells, callus cultures and immature embryos can be used with suitable pre- and post-electroporation treatments. Electroporation has been successfully used for the production of transgenic plants of many cereals e.g. rice, wheat, maize.

Advantages of electroporation

- This technique is simple, convenient and rapid, besides being cost-effective.
- The transformed cells are at the same physiological state after electroporation.
- Efficiency of transformation can be improved by optimising the electrical field strength, and addition of spermidine.

Limitations of electroporation

- Under normal conditions, the amount of DNA delivered into plant cells is very low.
- Efficiency of electroporation is highly variable depending on the plant material and the treatment conditions.
- Regeneration of plants is not very easy, particularly when protoplasts are used.

PARTICLE BOMBARDMENT (BIOLISTICS)

Particle (or ***microprojectile***) ***bombardment*** is the most effective method for gene transfer, and creation of transgenic plants. This method is versatile due to the fact that it can be successfully used for the DNA transfer in mammalian cells and microorganisms.

The microprojectile bombardment method was initially named as biolistics by its inventor Sanford (1988). ***Biolistics*** is a combination of ***bio***logical and bal***listics***. There are other names for this technique-***particle gun, gene gun, bioblaster***.

A diagrammatic representation of micro-projectile bombardment system for the transfer of genes in plants is depicted in ***Fig. 49.10***, and briefly described below.

Microcarriers (microprojectiles), the tungsten or gold particles coated with DNA, are carried by macrocarriers (macroprojectiles). These macrocarriers are inserted into the apparatus and pushed downward by rupturing the disc. The stopping plate does not permit the movement of macrocarrier while the microcarriers (with DNA) are propelled at a high speed into the plant material. Here the DNA segments are released which enter the plant cells and integrate with the genome.

Plant material used in bombardment

Two types of plant tissue are commonly used for particle bombardment.

1. ***Primary explants*** which can be subjected to bombardment that are subsequently induced to become embryogenic and regenerate.

2. ***Proliferating embryonic tissues*** that can be bombarded in cultures and then allowed to proliferate and regenerate.

In order to protect plant tissues from being damaged by bombardment, cultures are maintained on high osmoticum media or subjected to limited plasmolysis.

Transgene integration in bombardment

It is believed (based on the gene transfer in rice by biolistics) that the gene transfer in particle bombardment is a two stage process.

1. In the ***preintegration phase***, the vector DNA molecules are spliced together. This results in fragments carrying multiple gene copies.

2. ***Integrative phase*** is characterized by the insertion of gene copies into the host plant genome.

The integrative phase facilitates further transgene integration which may occur at the same point or a point close to it. The net result is that particle bombardment is frequently associated with high copy number at a single locus. This type of single locus may be beneficial for regeneration of plants.

The success of bombardment

The particle bombardment technique was first introduced in 1987. It has been successfully used for the transformation of many cereals. e.g. rice, wheat, maize. In fact, the ***first commercial genetically modified (GM) crops such as maize*** containing ***Bt-toxin gene were developed*** by this approach.

TABLE 49.2 A selected list of transgenic plants (along with cell sources) developed by microprojectile bombardment

Plant	*Cell source(s)*
Rice	Embryonic callus, immature zygotic embryos
Wheat	Immature zygotic embryos
Sorghum	Immature zygotic embryos
Corn	Embryonic cell suspension, immature zygotic embryos
Barley	Cell suspension, immature zygotic embryos
Banana	Embryonic cell suspension
Sweet potato	Callus cells
Cotton	Zygotic embryos
Grape	Embryonic callus
Peas	Zygotic embryos
Peanut	Embryonic callus
Tobacco	Pollen
Alfalfa	Embryonic callus

A selected list of the ***transgenic plants*** (developed by biolistics) along with the sources of the plant materials used is given in ***Table 49.2***.

Factors affecting bombardment

Several attempts are made to study the various factors, and optimize the system of particle bombardment for its most efficient use. Some of the important parameters are described.

Nature of microparticles : Inert metals such as tungsten, gold and platinum are used as microparticles to carry DNA. These ***particles with relatively higher mass will have a better chance*** to move fast when bombarded and ***penetrate the tissues***.

Nature of tissues/cells : The target cells that are capable of undergoing division are suitable for transformation. Some more details on the choice of plant material used in bombardment are already given.

Amount of DNA : The transformation may be low when too little DNA is used. On the other hand, too much DNA may result is high copy number and rearrangement of transgenes.

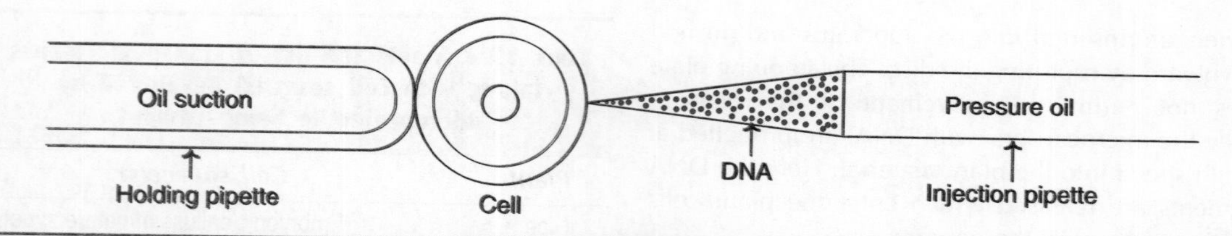

Fig. 49.11 : Microinjection of DNA by holding pipette method.

Therefore, the quantity of ***DNA used should be balanced***. Recently, some workers have started using the chemical aminosiloxane to coat the microparticles with low quantities of DNA adequate enough to achieve high efficiency of transformation.

Environmental parameters : Many environmental variables are known to influence particle bombardment. These factors (temperature, humidity, photoperiod etc.) influence the physiology of the plant material, and consequently the gene transfer. It is also observed that some explants, after bombardment may require special regimes of light, humidity, temperature etc.

The technology of particle bombardment has been improved in recent years, particularly with regard to the use of equipment. A ***commercially produced particle bombardment apparatus*** namely ***PDS-1000/HC*** is widely used these days.

Advantages of particle bombardment

- Gene transfer can be efficiently done in organized tissues.
- Different species of plants can be used to develop transgenic plants.

Limitations of particle bombardment

- The major complication is the production of high transgene copy number. This may result in instability of transgene expression due to ***gene silencing***.
- The target tissue may often get damaged due to lack of control of bombardment velocity.
- Sometimes, undesirable chimeric plants may be regenerated.

MICROINJECTION

Microinjection is a ***direct physical method involving the mechanical insertion of the desirable DNA into a target cell***. The target cell may be the one identified from intact cells, protoplasts, callus, embryos, meristems etc. Microinjection is used for the transfer of cellular organelles and for the manipulation of chromosomes.

The technique of microinjection involves the transfer of the gene through a micropipette (0.5–10.0 μm tip) into the cytoplasm/nucleus of a plant cell or protoplast. While the gene transfer is done, the recipient cells are kept immobilized in agarose embedding, and held by a suction holding pipette (***Fig. 49.11***).

As the process of microinjection is complete, the transformed cell is cultured and grown to develop into a transgenic plant. In fact, transgenic tobacco and *Brassica napus* have been developed by this approach.

The major limitations of microinjection are that it is slow, expensive, and has to be performed by trained and skilled personnel.

LIPOSOME-MEDIATED TRANSFORMATION

Liposomes are artificially created lipid vesicles containing a phospholipid membrane. They are successfully used in mammalian cells for the delivery of proteins, drugs etc. Liposomes carrying genes can be employed to fuse with protoplasts and transfer the genes. The efficiency of transformation increases when the process is carried out in conjunction with polyethylene glycol (PEG).

Liposome-mediated transformation involves ***adhesion of liposomes to the protoplast surface, its fusion at the site of attachment and release of plasmids inside the cell*** (***Fig. 49.12***).

Advantages of liposome fusion

- Being present in an encapsulated form of liposomes, DNA is protected from environmental insults and damage.

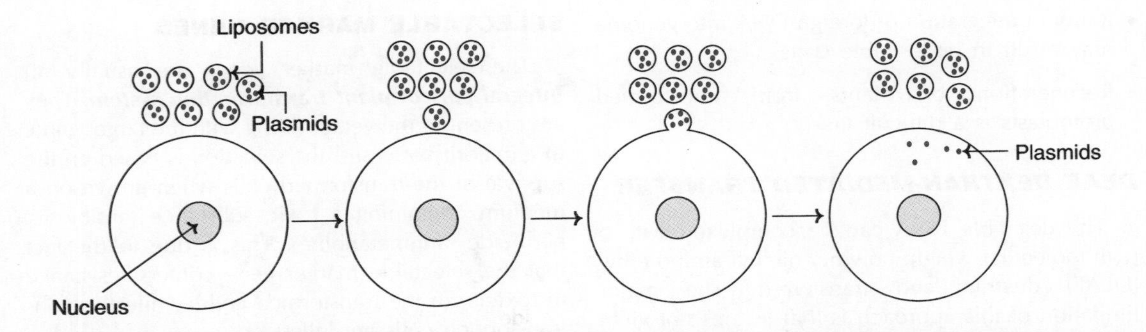

Fig. 49.12 : A diagrammatic representation of fusion of plasmid–filled liposomes with protoplasts.

- DNA is stable and can be stored for sometime in liposomes prior to transfer.
- Applicable to a wide range of plant cells.
- There is good reproducibility in the technique.

Limitations of liposome fusion

The major problem with liposome-mediated transformation is the difficulty associated with the regeneration of plants from transformed protoplasts.

SILICON CARBIDE FIBRE-MEDIATED TRANSFORMATION

The silicon carbide fibres (***SCF***) are about 0.3-0.6 μm in diameter and 10–100 μm in length. These fibres are capable of penetrating the cell wall and plasma membrane, and thus can deliver DNA into the cells.

The DNA coated silicon carbide fibres are vortexed with plant material (suspension culture, calluses). During the mixing, DNA adhering to the fibres enters the cells and gets stably integrated with the host genome. The silicon carbide fibres with the trade name ***Whiskers*** are available in the market.

Advantages of SCF-mediated transformation

- Direct delivery of DNA into intact walled cells. This avoids the protoplast isolation.
- Procedure is simple and does not involve costly equipment.

Disadvantages of SCF-mediated transformation

- Silicon carbide fibres are cancinogenic and therefore have to be carefully handled.
- The embryonic plant cells are hard and compact and are resistant to SCF penetration.

In recent years, some improvements have been made in SCF-mediated transformation. This has helped in the transformation of rice, wheat, maize and barley by using this technique.

CHEMICAL GENE TRANSFER METHODS

POLYETHYLENE GLYCOL-MEDIATED TRANSFORMATION

Polyethylene glycol (PEG), in the presence of divalent cations (using Ca^{2+}), ***destabilizes the plasma membrane of protoplasts and renders it permeable to naked DNA***. In this way, the DNA enters nucleus of the protoplasts and gets integrated with the genome.

The procedure involves the isolation of protoplasts and their suspension, addition of plasmid DNA, followed by a slow addition of 40% PEG-4000 (w/v) dissolved in mannitol and calcium nitrate solution. As this mixture is incubated, protoplasts get transformed.

Advantages of PEG-mediated transformation

- A large number of protoplasts can be simultaneously transformed.
- This technique can be successfully used for a wide range of plant species.

Limitations of PEG-mediated transformation

- The DNA is susceptible for degradation and rearrangement.

- Random integration of foreign DNA into genome may result in undesirable traits.
- Regeneration of plants from transformed protoplasts is a difficult task.

DEAE DEXTRAN-MEDIATED TRANSFER

The desirable DNA can be complexed with a high molecular weight polymer diethyl amino ethyl (DEAE) dextran and transferred. The major limitation of this approach is that it does not yield stable transformants.

CALCIUM PHOSPHATE CO-PRECIPITATION-MEDIATED TRANSFER

The DNA is allowed to mix with calcium chloride solution and isotonic phosphate buffer to form DNA-calcium phosphate precipitate. When the actively dividing cells in culture are exposed to this precipitate for several hours, the cells get transformed. The success of this method is dependent on the high concentration of DNA and the protection of the complex precipitate. Addition of ***dimethyl sulfoxide*** (DMSO) ***increases the efficiency of transformation.***

DNA IMBIBITION BY CELLS/TISSUES

Some workers have seriously tried to transform cells by incubating cell suspensions, tissues, embryos and even seeds with DNA. The belief is that the DNA gets imbibed, and the cells get transformed. DNA imbibition approach has met with little or no success.

MARKER GENES FOR PLANT TRANSFORMATION

In general, genetic transformation of plants is a low-frequency event. Some ***methods for selecting the transformed plant materials*** (cells/tissues) have been devised ***by using a set of genes*** referred to as marker genes. These marker genes are introduced into the plant material along with the target gene. The marker genes are of two types.

I. Selectable marker genes

II. Reporter genes

SELECTABLE MARKER GENES

The selectable marker genes are usually an ***integral part of plant transformation system***. They are present in the vector along with the target gene. In a majority of cases, the selection is based on the survival of the transformed cells when grown on a medium containing a toxic substance (antibiotic, herbicide, antimetabolite). This is due to the fact that the selectable marker gene confers resistance to toxicity in the transformed cells, while the non-transformed cells get killed.

A large number of selectable marker genes are available and they are grouped into three categories—antibiotic resistance genes, antimetabolite marker genes, and herbicide resistance genes (***Table 49.3***).

ANTIBIOTIC RESISTANCE GENES

In many plant transformation systems, antibiotic resistance genes (particularly of *E. coli*) are used as selectable markers. Despite the plants being eukaryotic in nature, antibiotics can effectively inhibit the protein biosynthesis in the cellular organelles, particularly in chloroplasts. Some of the antibiotic resistance selectable marker genes are briefly described.

Neomycin phosphotransferase II (*npt II* gene)

The ***most widely used selectable marker*** is *npt II* gene encoding the enzyme neomycin phosphotransferase II (NPT II). This marker gene confers resistance to the antibiotic kanamycin. The transformants and the plants derived from them can be checked by applying kanamycin solution and the resistant progeny can be selected.

Hygromycin phosphotransferase (*hpt* gene)

The antibiotic hygromycin is more toxic than neomycin and therefore can kill non-transformed plant cells much faster. Hygromycin phosphotransferase (*hpt*) gene thus provides resistance to transformed cells.

Aminoglycoside adenyltransferase (*aadA* gene)

Aminoglycoside 3′-adenyltransferase (*aadA*) gene confers resistance to transformed plant cells against the antibiotics streptomycin and spectionomycin.

TABLE 49.3 A selected list of selectable marker genes used for gene transfer in plants, their source and substrates used for their selection

Selectable marker gene (encoded enzyme)	Abbreviation	Source of gene	Substrate(s) used for selection
Antibiotic resistance			
Neomycin phosphotransferase II	*nptII*	*E. coli*	Kanamycin, geneticin (G418)
Neomycin phosphotransferase III	*nptIII*	*Streptococcus faecalis*	Kanamycin, geneticin (G418)
Hygromycin phosphotransferase	*hpt/hyg*	*E. coli*	Hygromycin
Bleomycin resistance	*ble*	*E. coli*	Bleomycin
Aminoglycoside adenyltransferase	*aadA*	*Shigella flexneri*	Streptomycin, spectinomycin
Antimetabolite markers			
Dihydrofolate reductase	*dhfr*	Mouse	Methotrexate
Dihydropteroate synthase	*dhps/sul*	*E. coli*	Sulfonamides
Herbicide resistance			
Phosphinothricin acetyltransferase	*bar/pat*	*Streptomyces hygroscopicus/ S. viridochromogenes*	Glufosinate, L-phosphinothricin, Bialophos
Enolpyruvyl shikimate phosphate synthase	*epsps/aroA*	*Agrobacterium* sp/ *Petunia hybrida*	Glyphosate
Acetolactase synthase	*als*	*Arabidopsis* sp/maize/tobacco	Sulfonylureas
Glyphosate oxidoreductase	*gox*	*Achromobacter LBAA*	Glyphosate
Bromoxynil nitrilase	*bxn*	*Klebsiella pneumoniae*	Bromoxynil
Others			
β-Glucuronidase	*gus/uidA*	*E. coli*	Cytokinin glucuronide
Xylose isomerase	*xylA*	*Thermoanaerobcterium thermosulfurogenes*	Xylose
Mannose 6-phosphate isomerase	*pmi/manA*	*E. coli*	Mannose
Betaine aldehyde dehydrogenase	*badh*	Spinach	Betaine aldehyde

ANTIMETABOLITE MARKER GENES

Dihydrofolate reductase (*dhfr* gene)

The enzyme dihydrofolate reductase, produced by *dhfr* gene is inhibited by the antimetabolite methotrexate. A mutant *dhfr* gene in mouse that codes for this enzyme which has a low affinity to methotrexate has been identified. This *dhfr* gene fused with CaMV promoter results in a methotrexate resistant marker which can be used for the selection of transformed plants.

HERBICIDE RESISTANCE MARKERS

Genes that confer resistance to herbicides are in use as markers for the selection of transgenic plants.

Phosphinothricin acetyltransferase (*pat/bar* gene)

Bialophos, phosphinothricin and glufosinate are commonly used herbicides. The *pat/bar* genes code for phosphinothricin acetyltransferase which converts these herbicides into acetylated forms that are non-herbicidal. Thus, *pat/bar* genes confer resistance to the transformed plants.

Enolpyruvylshikimate phosphate synthase (*epsps/aroA* genes)

The herbicide glyphosate inhibits photosynthesis. It blocks the activity of enolpyruvylshikimate phosphate (EPSP) synthase, a key enzyme involved in the biosynthesis of phenylalanine, tyrosine and tryptophan. Mutant strains of *Agrobacterium* and *Petunia hybrida* that are resistant to glyphosate have been identified. The genes *epsps/aroA* confer resistance to transgenic plants which can be selected.

Bromoxynil nitrilase (*bxn* gene)

The herbicide bromoxynil inhibits photosynthesis (photosystem II). Bromoxynil nitrilase enzyme coded by the gene *bxn* inactivates this herbicide. The gene *bxn* can be successfully used as a selectable marker for the selection of transformed plants.

PRODUCTION OF MARKER-FREE TRANSGENIC PLANTS

There is a growing ***concern among the public*** regarding the use of ***antibiotic or herbicide resistance genes as selectable markers*** of plant transformation

- The products of some marker genes may be toxic or allergic.
- The antibiotic resistance might be transferred to pathogenic microorganisms in the soil.
- There is a possibility of creation of superweeds that are resistant to normally used herbicides.
- A transgenic plant with selectable marker genes cannot be transformed again by using the same selectable markers.

In light of the apprehensions listed above, the public is concerned about the safety of transgenic technology, particularly related to the selectable marker genes (antibiotic/herbicide resistance genes). There are fears about the safety of consumption of foodstuffs derived from genetically engineered plants. This is despite the fact that ***so far none of the marker genes have been shown to adversely affect human, animal or environmental safety***.

CLEAN GENE TECHNOLOGY

The process of ***developing transgenic plants without the presence of selectable marker genes*** or by use of more acceptable marker genes is regarded as clean gene technology. And this will result in the production of many marker-free transgenic plants that will be readily acceptable by the public. Some of the approaches for clean gene technology are given.

Avoiding selectable marker genes

Theoretically, it is possible to totally avoid marker genes and introduce only the transgene of interest. The transformed palnts can then be screened by an advanced technique like polymerase chain reaction and the desirable plants selected. This approach is not practicable due to cost factor.

Cotransformation with two DNAs

The transgenic plants can be produced by employing two separate DNAs — one carrying the desired target gene and the other the marker gene. The transformed plants contain both the genes, but at different sites on the chromosomal DNA. Traditional breeding techniques (a few rounds) can be used to get rid of the transgenic plants with selectable markers.

Removal of selectable markers

It is possible to selectively remove the selectable marker genes from the plant genome. For this purpose, ***site-specific recombinase systems*** are utilized. Several recombinase systems are in fact available which can be used to selectively excise the marker genes from the plant genome.

Cloning of selectable markers between transposable elements

A selectable marker gene can be cloned between plant transposable elements (Ds elements) and then inserted. The selectable marker is planked by the sequences that increase the intrachromosomal recombination. This results in the excision of the marker gene.

REPORTER GENES

A reporter gene may be regarded as the ***test gene whose expression can be quantified***. The plant transformation can be assessed by the expression of reporter genes (also called as screenable or scoreable genes). In general, an assay for the reporter gene is carried out by estimating the quantity of the protein it produces or the final products formed.

A selected list of the reporter genes along with the detection assays is given in ***Table 49.4***, some of the important ones are discussed below.

TABLE 49.4 A selected list of reporter genes used for gene transfer in plants, their sources, and detection assays

Reporter gene (enzyme/protein encoded)	*Abbreviation*	*Source of gene*	*Detection assay*
Octopine synthase	*ocs*	*Agrobacterium tumefaciens*	Electrophoresis, chromatography
Nopaline synthase	*nos*	*Agrobacterium tumefaciens*	Electrophoresis, chromatography
β-Glucuronidase	*gus/uidA*	*E. coli*	Fluorometric or histochemical or colorimetric
Green fluorescent protein	*gfp*	*Aequorea victoria* (jelly fish)	Fluorescence
Luciferase (bacterial)	*luxA/luxB*	*Vibrio harveyi*	Bioluminescence
Luciferase (firefly)	*luc*	*Photonus pyralis*	Bioluminescence
Chloramphenicol acetyltransferase	*cat*	*E. coli*	Autoradiography

Opine synthase (*ocs, nos* genes)

The common opines present in T-DNA of Ti or Ri plasmids of *Agrobacterium* are octopine and nopaline, respectively produced by the synthase genes *ocs* and *nos*. The transformed status of the plant cells can be easily detected by the presence of these opines. ***Opines*** can be ***separated*** by electrophoresis ***and identified***. Alternately, the enzyme activities responsible for the production of opines can also be assayed.

β-Glucuronidase (*gus/uidA* gene)

β-Glucuronidase producing gene (*gus/uidA*) is the ***most commonly used reporter gene*** in assessing plant transformation for the following reasons.

- β-Glucuronidase assays are very sensitive.
- Quantitative estimation of the enzyme can be done by fluorometric method (using substrate 4-methylumbelliferryl β-D-glucuronide which is hydrolysed to 4-methylumbelliferone).
- Qualitative data on the enzyme can be obtained by histochemical means (enzyme localization can be detected by chromogenic substance such as substrate X-gluc).
- No need to extract and identify DNA.

Green fluorescent protein (*gfp* gene)

Green fluorescent protein (GFP), coded by *gfp* gene, is being widely used in recent years. In fact, in many instances, GFP has replaced GUS since ***assays of GFP are easier and non-destructive***. Thus, screening of even the primary transplants can be done by GFP which is not possible with other reporter genes.

Gene for GFP has been isolated from jelly fish *Aequorea victoria* which is a luminescent organism. The original *gfp* gene has been significantly modified to make it more useful as a reporter gene. GFP emits fluorescence which can be detected under a fluorescent microscope.

Bacterial luciferase (*luxA/luxB* genes)

The bacterial luciferase genes (*luxA* and *luxB*) have originated from *Vibrio harveyi*. They can be detected in some plant transformation vectors. The ***detection assay*** of the enzyme is based on the principle of ***bioluminescence***. Bacterial luciferase catalyses the oxidation of long-chain fatty aldehydes that results in the emission of light which can be measured.

Firefly luciferase (*luc gene*)

The enzyme firefly luciferase, encoded by the gene *luc*, catalyses the oxidation of D-luciferin (ATP dependent) which results in the ***emission of light*** that can be detected by sensitive luminometers.

The firefly luciferase gene, however, is not widely used as a marker gene since the assay of the enzyme is rather cumbersome.

Chloramphenicol acetyl transferase (*cat* gene)

The *cat* gene producing chloramphenicol acetyl transferase (CAT) is a widely used reporter gene in mammalian cells. Due to the availability of GUS and GFP reporter systems for plant transformants, CAT is not commonly used. However, some workers continue to use CAT by a sensitive radioactive assay, for the detection of the reporter gene *cat*.

PROMOTERS AND TERMINATORS

The ultimate objective of gene transfer is its correct expression to provide the desired character/ trait. The ***appropriate expression of genes is made possible by the presence of promoters and terminators***. The DNA sequence upstream the coding region is the promoter while the terminator is the sequence at the 3′ terminus. The promoters are responsible for the commencement of transcription whereas the terminators ensure the ceasation of transcription at the correct position.

Promoters possess certain inherent characters such as promoter strength, tissue specificity and developmental regulation which determine the efficiency of promoter function in gene expression.

Agrobacterium-derived promoters and terminators

The genes coding for ***napaline synthase*** (*nos*) in Ti plasmid of *Agrobacterium* are frequently used as promoters and terminators in plant transformation vectors. Originally derived from bacteria, the genes coding for opine synthesis are well adapted to function in plants. In fact, *nos* promoter is regarded as constitutive by many plant biotechnologists.

The 30S promoter of CaMV

The cauliflower mosaic virus (CaMV) 30S promoter is the ***most widely used as a promoter in plants***. This promoter, (a 30S RNA gene) is expressed in almost all the tissues of the transgenic plants. The driving strength of 30S promoter is much higher in dicots compared to monocots.

The 30S promoter is preferred for the appropriate expression of sclectable marker genes and reporter genes. In recent years, the efficiency of 30S promoter has been further increased by suitable modifications in the enhancer region.

Promoters for monocots : Since 30S promoter is not very efficient for monocots, alternates are used. ***Ubiquitin I promoter*** or the ***rice actin promoter*** are frequently used for high expression of transgenes in monocots.

Inducible promoters

In recent years, certain inducible promoter systems for transgene expression have been developed. These promoters differ from 30S promoter which is constitutive in nature. There are mainly three inducible expression systems :

1. **Non-plant-derived systems :** These inducible promoters are independent of the normal plant processes. A specific exogenous chemical will induce their expression. e.g. tetracycline, ethanol, steroid, copper. Non-plant-derived inducible promoters are useful, but not economically viable.

2. **Plant-derived systems based on response to environmental signals :** These systems are not independent, since they are plant-derived and actually form a part of normal plant processes. Plant-derived systems respond to a variety of environmental signals e.g. wound, heat shock.

3. **Plant-derived systems based on developmental control of gene expression :** Certain genes that express at a particular stage of plant development have been identified. The promoters of some of these developmental genes are useful for transgene expression. e.g.

- Senescence-specific gene expression
- Abscisic acid inducible gene expression
- Auxin inducible gene expression

Although plant-derived systems (2 and 3) are not independent as non-plant derived one (1), they are still useful in plant biotechnology since no exogenous inducer is required.

Tissue-specific promoters

Efforts are on in recent years to isolate promoters that can drive gene expression in a tissue specific manner. The advantage with tissue-specific promoters is that the expression (which may produce a harmful compound) is confined to selected tissues that are not consumed by humans or animals. In fact, some tissue-specific promoters have been isolated, and are in use.

TRANSGENE STABILITY, EXPRESSION AND GENE SILENCING

The genetically transformed plant cells are grown *in vitro* to finally regenerate to plants. At the initial stages of plant cell growth, some evidence for the success of plant transformation can be obtained e.g. resistance to antibiotics, herbicides etc.

The ***integration of transgenes with the host plant genome can be confirmed by some molecular techniques***— Southern hybridization, polymerase chain reaction. This is usually carried out by analysing the seeds at T_1 generation.

What is actually required for the success of plant transformation is the efficient and stable expression of transgene, and not just its presence in plant genome. It is just useless to have a desired gene without appropriate expression.

SCAFFOLD ATTACHMENT REGIONS AND GENE STABILITY

Scaffold attachment regions (***SARs***; also known as ***matrix attachment/associated regions, MARs***) are the regions of DNA isolated based on their ability to bind to the nuclear scaffold (protein depleted chromosome forms a central scaffold surrounded by DNA). SARs are known to stabilize gene expression in transgenic plants. During the course of transformation, SARs are ligated to the flanking regions of foreign gene. It is observed that the transformation efficiency by particle bombardment is increased by use of SARs.

The ***presence of SARs along with transgene stabilizes or normalizes gene expression***. e.g. SARs from yeast and tobacco have helped to stabilize gene expression in plants. The degree of stabilization of genes by SARs is dependent on the affinity of SARs towards the nuclear matrix of the target plant cells. SARs are particularly useful for stabilizing the gene expression when the copy number of DNA introduced is high. In the absence of SARs, high DNA copy number would result in an instable and highly variable gene expression.

INTRONS AND GENE EXPRESSION

The presence of introns between the promoter and coding regions of a gene will significantly influence the gene expression. The gene expression is enhanced when introns are used in monocotyledonous plant species. For instance, introduction of introns between cauliflower mosaic virus 35S promoter and β-glucuronidase significantly improved gene expression in maize. It is believed that introns may stabilize mRNAs and increase the protein biosynthesis.

There are conflicting reports on the affect of introns on the gene expression in dicotyledonous plants. Some workers have reported stimulation while others contradict this claim.

It is now accepted that the ***intron-containing constructs will enhance gene expression*** in ***transgenic monocots***, although the picture is less clear as regards dicots.

GENE SILENCING

There are in fact many instances of gene transfer that are not properly expressed. The ***instability of gene expression*** (or inadequate gene expression) in ***transgenic plants is*** referred to as ***gene silencing***. The mechanism of gene silencing is not well understood although it is predominantly due to the phenomenon of ***homology dependent gene silencing*** (***HDGS***).

Two types of gene silencing are known in plant biotechnology—transcriptional gene silencing and post-transcriptional gene silencing. The two differ at the level of gene expression where silencing occurs.

Transcriptional gene silencing (TGS)

When the transgenes share homology in their promoter regions, TGS occurs. It is due to altered methylation patterns and altered chromatin conformation. Gene silencing occurs by repression of transcription.

Post-transcriptional gene silencing (PTGS)

Sometimes, the expression of a homologous transgene may inhibit the expression of the transgene and endogenous gene. This primarily occurs by decreasing the stability of RNA, and thus a reduced expression. This is often observed when strong promoters are used to drive the transgene expression which may result in co-suppresion or PTGS, and thus a lower level of gene expression. For this reason, some workers prefer to use weak promoters rather than strong promoters.

Post-transcriptional gene silencing is due to the production of double-stranded RNA either in the nucleus or cytoplasm. The double-stranded RNA is formed when antisense RNA is produced due to the activity of RNA dependent RNA polymerase.

Strategies to avoid gene silencing

The control of gene silencing is not an easy job, since it occurs in an unpredictable fashion. Some general recommendations, are, however, made to minimize the impact of gene silencing in transgenic plants

- Reduction in the number of transgenes inserted (i.e. reduced copy number).
- Avoiding the use of promoters and transgenes with high degree of homology.
- Minimizing/avoiding the use of multiple copies of the same promoter or terminator.

Gene silencing is not observed in chloroplast (plastid) transformation, hence it is preferred in recent years.

CHLOROPLAST TRANSFORMATION

The chloroplasts (plastids) and mitochondria are believed to have evolved from prokaryotes during the course of evolution. Both these organelles have their own genome, although it is much simpler when compared to nuclear genome. Further, many of the proteins that function in chloroplasts and mitochondria are encoded by nuclear genes and then transported to the organelle.

Chloroplast genome

Most of the higher plants have about 100 chloroplasts per leaf cell. Each chloroplast contains approximately 100 copies of chloroplast DNA genome. The chloroplast genome (the ***plastome***) is a ***circular double-stranded DNA*** molecule (or chromosome) located in the stroma. Majority of chloroplast genomes are in the size of 120–160 kbp and contain about 120–140 genes. About 100 chloroplast genes are known to code for proteins. The protein synthesis in chloroplasts resembles that of prokaryotes.

CHLOROPLAST ENGINEERING

Genetic engineering of chloroplast that leads to chloroplast (plastid) transformation is an important and exciting field in modern biotechnology as it offers the following advantages.

1. ***Chloroplasts are maternally inherited,*** hence there is no danger of gene transfer through pollen to related weeds. This is because pollen does not contain transgenes.

2. Multigene transfer can be conveniently carried out in chloroplasts which is rather difficult with nuclear genome.

3. Chloroplasts genome is functionally comparable to prokaryotic genome. A single promoter can control the expression of group of genes (transgenes). It is therefore possible to introduce desirable multiple genes which can be expressed under the control of a single promoter.

4. High level of transgene expression is possible with chloroplasts. There are about 100 chloroplasts per cell, each containing about 100 copies of genome. Thus, there is possibility of 10,000 copies of transgenes per cell! This is a tremendous number of transgenes carried by transformed chloroplasts. There is a tremendous ***potential for a very high level of gene expression*** and large scale production of active proteins.

5. Chloroplast transformation is ***not associated with gene silencing*** which is a major problem with nuclear genome transformation.

6. Antibiotic resistance genes need not be used as selectable markers, Even if used, they can be easily excised.

7. Toxicity associated with foreign protein production in chloroplasts is much less when compared to nuclear-controlled foreign proteins.

Design of vectors for chloroplast transformation

A diagrammatic representation of two vector constructs for chloroplast transformation is depicted in ***Fig. 49.13***.

1. **A construct for expression of a single gene :** The vector for chloroplast transformation is based on the selectable marker gene *aadA* that provides resistance to antibiotic spectinomycin. The single foreign (desirable) gene is fused to regulatory sequences (promoter and terminator) which in turn is flanked on either side by chloroplast DNA (Cp DNA) (***Fig. 49.13A***).

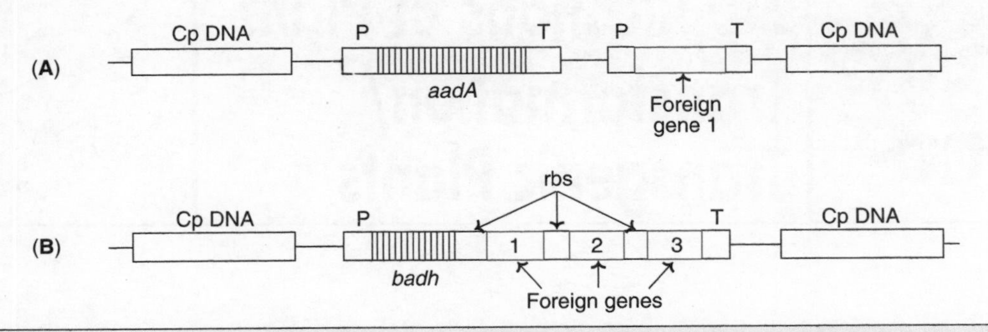

Fig. 49.13 : A diagrammatic representation of vectors for chloroplast transformation (A) A construct designed for a single foreign gene (B) A construct designed for multiple foreign genes (Cp DNA-Chloroplast DNA; P-Promoter; aadA *-A selectable marker gene that confers resistance to antibiotic spectinomycin; T-Terminator;* badh *-A selectable marker gene encoding betaine aldehyde dehydrogenase; rbs-Ribosome binding site).*

2. **A construct for expression of multiple genes :** In this case, the selectable marker is the betaine-aldehyde dehydrogenase (*badh*) gene.

It is flanked by a promoter and the multiple transgenes are flanked by a terminator. At both ends chloroplast DNA sequences are present. In between the transgenes, these are ribosome-binding sites (one between two transgenes) to ensure efficient translation (***Fig. 49.13B***).

Introduction of foreign genes into chloroplast genome

Most of the methods used for introducing the foreign genes into nuclear genome are not useful for chloroplast transformation. The most successful method for inserting foreign genes into chloroplasts is ***particle gun bombardment***.

After the bombardment, homologous recombination occurs between the chloroplast DNA sequences on the vector and those of on the genome. This is a site-specific integration and thus avoids the frequent problems associated with randon insertion of foreign genes into nuclear genome.

The regenerated plants derived from the modified plastome (chloroplast genome) are regarded as ***transplastomic plants***.

The future of chloroplast transformation

The technology of chloroplast transformation is ***in the developing stages***. In fact, it has not become as routine as transformation of nuclear genomes of plants.

Chloroplast engineering, however, ***holds a great promise in plant biotechnology*** being an efficient, clean and environmental-friendly approach for the production of transgenic plants.

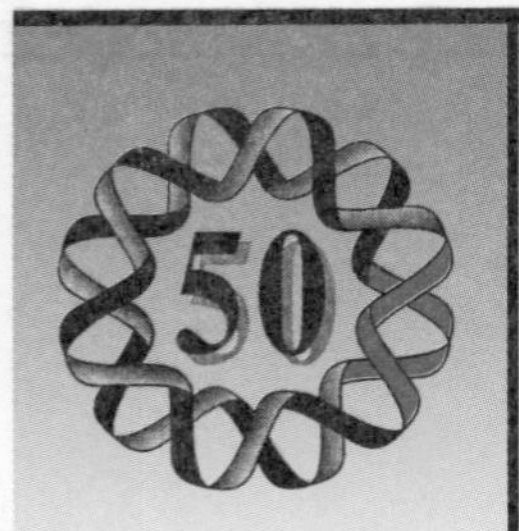

Applications of Plant Transformation/ Transgenic Plants

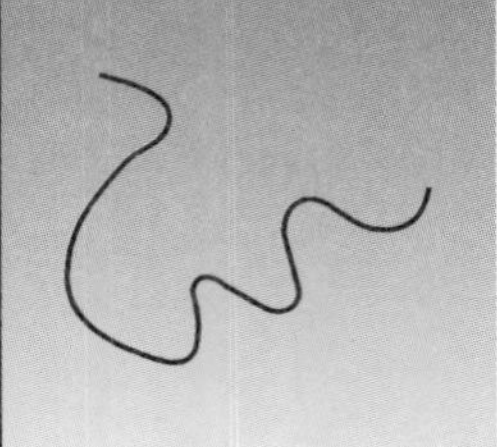

The genetic manipulations carried out in plants for the production of transgenic plants have been described (Chapter 49). The ultimate goal of transgenics (involving introduction, integration, and expression of foreign genes) is ***to improve the crops, with the desired traits***. Some of the important ones are listed.

- Resistance to biotic stresses i.e. resistance to diseases caused by insects, viruses, fungi and bacteria.
- Resistance to abiotic stresses-herbicides, temperature (heat, chilling, freezing), drought, salinity, ozone, intense light.
- Improvement of crop yield, and quality e.g. storage, longer shelf life of fruits and flowers.
- Transgenic plants with improved nutrition.
- Transgenic plants as bioreactors for the manufacture of commercial products e.g. proteins, vaccines, and biodegradable plastics.

Environmental stresses to plants

The different types of external stresses that influence the plant growth and development are depicted in ***Fig. 50.1***, These stresses are grouped based on their characters—***biotic and abiotic stresses.*** The biotic stresses are caused by insects, pathogens (viruses, fungi, bacteria), and wounds. The abiotic stresses are due to herbicides, water deficiency (caused by drought, temperature, salinity), ozone and intense light.

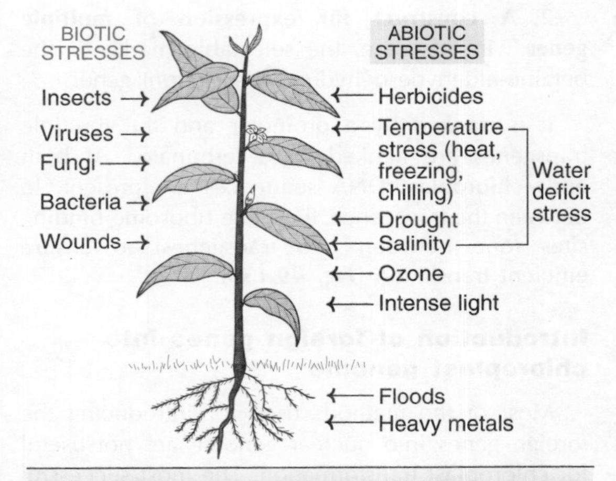

Fig. 50.1 : Biotic and abiotic stresses that affect plant growth, development and yield.

Almost all the stresses, either directly or indirectly, lead to the production of reactive oxygen species (ROS) that create oxidative stress to plants. This damages the cellular constitutents of plants which is associated with a reduction in plant yield.

The major ***objective of plant biotechnology is to develop plants that are resistant to biotic and abiotic stresses.***

RESISTANCE TO BIOTIC STRESSES

Genetic engineering of plants has led to the development of crops with increased resistance to

TABLE 50.1 A selected list of common insect pests along with the major crops damaged by them

Common name of pest	*Botanical name*	*Crop(s) damaged*
Cotton bollworm	*Helicoverpa zea*	Cotton
Cotton leafworm	*Spodoptera littiralis*	Rice, maize, cotton, tobacco
Tobacco hornworm	*Manduca sexta*	Tobacco, tomato, potato
European corn borer	*Ostrinia nubilalis*	Maize
Locust	*Locusta migratoria*	Grasses
Tobacco budworm	*Heliothis virescens*	Tobacco, cotton
Tomato fruitworm	*Heliothis armigera*	Tomato, cotton
Cowpea seed beetle	*Callosobruchus maculatus*	Cowpea, soybean
Colorado beetle	*Leptinotarsa decemlineata*	Potato
Brown plant hopper	*Nilaparvata lugens*	Rice

biotic stresses which is described in three major categories

1. Insect resistance.
2. Virus resistance.
3. Fungal and bacterial disease resistance.

INSECT (PEST) RESISTANCE

It is estimated that about 15% of the world's crop yield is lost to insects or pests. A selected list of the common insects and the crops damaged is given in ***Table 50.1.***

The damage to crops is mainly caused by insect larvae and to some extent adult insects. The majority of the insects that damage crops belong to the following orders (with examples).

- Lipidoptera (bollworms).
- Coleoptera (beetles).
- Orthoptera (grasshoppers).
- Homoptera (aphids).

Till sometime ago, chemical pesticides are the only means of pest control. Scientists have been looking for alternate methods of pest control for the following reasons (i.e. limitations of pesticide use).

- About 95% of the pesticide sprayed is washed away from the plant surface and accumulates in the soil.
- It is difficult to deliver pesticides to vulnerable parts of plants such as roots, stems and fruits.
- Chemical pesticides are not efficiently degraded in the soil, causing environmental pollution.
- Pesticides, in general, are toxic to non-target organisms, particularly humans and animals.

It is fortunate that scientists have been able to discover new biotechnological alternatives to chemical pesticides thereby providing insect resistance to crop plants. Transgenic plants with insect resistance transgenes have been developed. About 40 genes obtained from microorganisms of higher plants and animals have been used to provide insect resistance in crop plants. Some of the approaches for the ***biocontrol of insects*** are briefly described.

RESISTANCE GENES FROM MICROORGANISMS

Bacillus thuringiensis (Bt) toxin

Bacillus thuringiensis was first discovered by Ishiwaki in 1901, although its commercial importance was ignored until 1951. *B. thuringiensis* is a Gram negative, soil bacterium. This bacterium produces a parasporal crystalline proteinous toxin with insecticidal activity. The protein produced by *B.thuringiensis* is referred to as ***insecticidal crystalline protein (ICP).*** ICPs are among the endotoxins produced by sporulating bacteria, and were originally classified as ***δ-endotoxins*** (to distinguish them from other classes of α-, β- and γ-endotoxins).

Bt toxin genes

Several strains of *B. thuringiensis* producing a wide range of ***crystal (cry) proteins*** have been identified. Further, the structure of *cry* genes and their corresponding toxin (δ-endotoxin) products have been characterized. The *cry* genes are classified (latest in 1998) into a large number of distinct families (about 40) designated as *cry 1......cry 40,* based on their size and sequence similarities. And within each family, there may be sub-families. Thus, the total number of genes producing *Bt* toxins (Cry proteins) is more than 100.

There are differences in the structure of different Cry proteins, besides certain sequence similarities. The molecular weights of Cry proteins may be either large (~130 KDa) or small (~70KDa). Despite the differences in the Cry proteins, they share a common active core of three domains.

Mode of action of Cry proteins

Most of the *Bt* toxins (Cry proteins) are active against Lepidopteran larvae, while some of them are specific against Dipteran and Coleopteran insects. The protoxin of Cry I toxin group has a molecular mass of 130 kilodaltons (130 KDa). When this parasporal crystal is ingested by the target insect, the protoxin gets activated within its gut by a combination of alkaline pH (7.5 to 8.5) and proteolytic enzymes. This results in the conversion of protoxin into an active toxin with a molecular weight of 68 KDa (***Fig. 50.2***).

The active form of toxin protein gets itself inserted into the membrane of the gut epithelial cells of the insect. This result in the formation of ion channels through which there occurs an excessive loss of cellular ATP. As a consequence, cellular metabolism ceases, insect stops feeding, and becomes dehydrated and finally dies. Some workers in the recent years suggest that the *Bt* toxin opens cation-selective pores in the membranes, leading to the inflow of cations into the cells that causes osmotic lysis and destruction of epithelial cells (and finally the death of insect larvae).

The *Bt* toxin is not toxic to humans and animals since the conversion of protoxin to toxin requires alkaline pH and specific proteases (These are absent humans and animals).

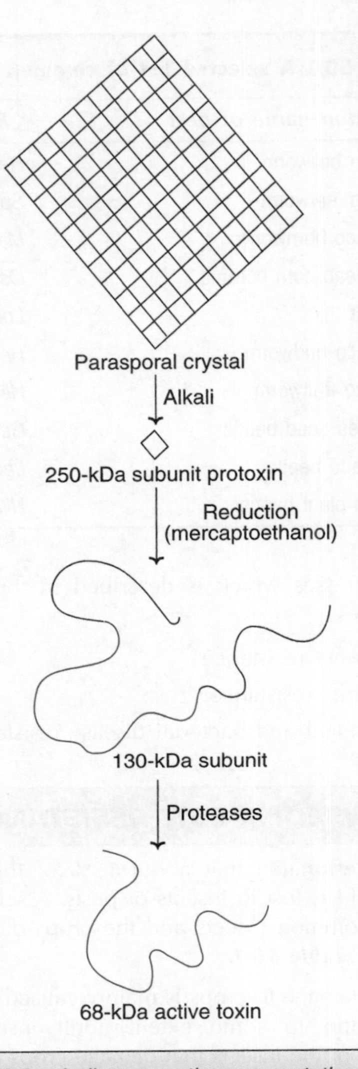

Fig. 50.2 : *A diagrammatic representation of the formation of active toxin from the parasporal crystal of* Bacillus thuringiensis.

Bt toxin as biopesticide

Preparations of *Bt* spores or isolated crystals have been used as organic biopesticide for about 50 years. This approach has not met with much success for the following reasons.

- Low persistence and stability (sunlight degrades toxin) of the toxin on the surface of plants.
- The *Bt* toxin cannot effectively penetrate into various parts of plants, particularly roots.
- Cost of production is high.

TABLE 50.2 *Bt*–based genetically modified crop plants developed for commercial use

Crop	*Trade name*	*Bt protein*	*Resistance to insect(s)*
Cotton	Bollgard	Cry 1Ac	Cotton bollworm, tobacco budworm
Maize	YieldGard knockout	Cry 1Ab	European corn borer
Maize	Starlink	Cry 9C	European corn borer
Maize	Herculex I	Cry 1F	European corn borer
Maize	Bt-Xtra	Cry 1Ac	European corn borer
Potato	New-leaf	Cry 3A	Colarado beetle

Bt-based genetic transformation of plants

It has been possible to genetically modify (***GM***) ***plants*** by inserting *Bt* genes and provide pest resistance to these transformed plants. For an effective pest resistance, the bacterial gene in transgenic plants must possess high level expression. This obviously means that the transgene transcription should be under the effective control of promoter and terminator sequences.

The early attempts to express cry 1A and cry 3A proteins under the control of CaMV 35S or *Agrobacterium* T-DNA promoters resulted in a very low expression in tobacco, tomato and potato plants.

Modification of *Bt* cry 1A gene : The wild type transgene *Bt* cry 1A(b) was found to express at a very low levels in transgenic plants. The nucleotide sequence of this gene was modified (G + C content altered, several polyadenylation signals removed, ATTTA sequence deleted etc). With appropriate sequence changes, an enormous increase (about 100 fold) in the *Bt* toxin product formation was observed.

The transgenic *Bt* crops that were found to provide effective protection against insect damage were given approval for commercial planting by USA in the mid-1990s (***Table 50.2***). Some biotechnological companies with their own trade names introduced several transgenic crops into the fields. Among these, only maize and cotton *Bt* crops are currently in use in USA. The other genetically modified plants met with failure for various reasons.

Advantages of transgenic plants with *Bt* genes

- *Bt* genes could be expressed in all parts of the plants, including the roots and internal regions of stems and fruits. This is not possible by any chemical pesticide.
- Toxic proteins are produced within the plants; hence they are environmental-friendly.
- *Bt* toxins are rapidly degraded in the environment.

The problem of insect resistance to *Bt* crops

The major limitation of *Bt*-gene possessing transgenic plants is the ***development of Bt-resistant insects.*** The *Bt* toxin is a protein, and the membrane receptor (of the gut) through which the toxin mediates its action is also a protein. It is possible that the appropriate mutations in the insect gene coding for receptor protein may reduce the toxin binding and render it ineffective. This may happen within a few generations by repeated growing of *Bt* crops.

Several approaches are made to avoid the development of resistance in insects.

- Introduction of two different *Bt* toxin genes for the same target insect.
- Development of transgenic plants with two types of insect resistance genes e.g. *Bt* gene and proteinase inhibitor gene.
- Rotating *Bt* crops with non-*Bt* crops may also prevent the build-up of resistance in insect population.

The environmental impact of *Bt* crops

The most serious impact of *Bt* crops on environment is the ***build-up of resistance in the pest population***.

In 1999, another issue was brought to light about *Bt* crops. It was reported that the pollen from

Table 50.3 A selected list of plant insecticidal (non-*Bt*) genes used for developing transgenic plants with insect resistance

Plant gene	Transgenic plant(s)	Encoded protein	Resistance to insect(s)
Protease inhibitors			
CpTi	Potato, apple, rice, sunflower, wheat, tomato	Trypsin	Coleoptera, Lepidoptera
CII	Tobacco, potato	Serine protease	Coleoptera, Lepidoptera
PI-IV	Potato, tobacco	Serine protease	Lebidoptera
OC-1	Tobacco, oilseed rape	Cysteine protease	Coleoptera, Homoptera
CMe	Tobacco	Trypsin	Lebidoptera
α-Amylase inhibitors			
α-A1-Pv	Pea, tobacco	α-Amylase	Coleoptera
WMAI-1	Tobacco	α-Amylase	Lepidoptera
Lectins			
GNA	Potato, rice, sugarcane sweet potato, tobacco	Lectin	Homoptera, Lepidoptera
WGA	Maize	Agglutin	Lepidoptera, Coleoptera
Others			
BCH	Potato	Chitinase	Homoptera, Lepidoptera
TDC	Tobacco	Tryptophan decarboxylase	Homoptera

Bt maize might be toxic to the larvae of Monarch butterfly. This generated considerable opposition to *Bt* crops by the public, since Monarch butterfly is one of the most colorful natives in USA. It was later proved that the fears about the impact of *Bt* crops on the monarch butterfly were without the required scientific evidence.

The lesson learnt from the monarch butterfly episode is that the risks of GM crops should be thoroughly assessed before they are reported.

Usage of *Bt* : The usage *Bt* is commonly used for a transgenic crop with a *cry* gene e.g. *Bt* cotton. In the same way, Cry proteins are also referred to as *Bt* proteins. It may also be stated here that the authors use four different names for the same group of proteins-δ-endotoxin, insecticidal crystal protein (ICP), Cry and now *Bt*.

Resistance genes from other microorganisms

The *Bt* toxin genes from *B.thuringiensis* have been described in the preceeding pages. There are certain other insect resistant genes from other microorganisms. Some of the important ones are listed.

1. ***Cholesterol oxidase*** of *Strepotmyces* culture filtrate was found to be toxic to boll weevil larvae. Cholesterol oxidase gene has been introduced into tobacco to develop a transgenic plant.

2. ***Isopentenyl transferase gene*** from *Agrobacterium tumefaciens* has been introduced into tobacco and tomato. This gene codes for an important enzyme in the synthesis of cytokinin. The transgenic plants with this transgene were found to reduce the leaf consumption by tobacco hornworm and decrease the survival of peach potato aphid.

RESISTANCE GENES FROM HIGHER PLANTS

Certain genes from higher plants were also found to result in the synthesis of products possessing insecticidal activity. Some authors regard them as ***non-Bt insecticidal proteins***. A selected list of plant insecticidal (non-*Bt*) genes used for developing transgenic plants with insect resistance is given ***Table 50.3***. Some of them are briefly described.

PROTEINASE (PROTEASE) INHIBITORS

Proteinase inhibitors are the proteins that inhibit the activity of proteinase enzymes. Certain plants naturally produce proteinase inhibitors to provide defence against herbivorous insects. This is possible since the inhibitors when ingested by insects interfere with the digestive enzymes of the insect. This results in the nutrient deprivation causing death of the insects.

It is possible to control insects by introducing proteinase inhibitor genes into crop plants that normally do not produce these proteins.

Cowpea trypsin inhibitor gene

It was observed that the wild species of cowpea plants growing in Africa were resistant to attack by a wide range of insects. Research findings revealed that insecticidal protein was a trypsin inhibitor that was capable of ***destroying insects*** belonging to the orders Lepidoptera (*e.g Heliothis virescans*), Orthaptera (e.g.*Locusta migratoria*) and Coleoptera (e.g.*Anthonous grandis*). Cowpea trypsin inhibitor (*CpTi*) has no affect on mammalian trypsins; hence it is ***non-toxic to mammals***.

CpTi gene was introduced into tobacco, potato and oilseed rape for developing transgenic plants. Survival of insects and damage to plants were much lower in plants possessing *CpTi* gene.

Advantages of proteinase inhibitors

- Many insects, not controlled by *Bt*, can be effectively controlled.
- Use of proteinase gene along with *Bt* gene will help to overcome *Bt* resistance development in plants.

Limitations of proteinase inhibitors

- Unlike *Bt* toxin, high levels of proteinase inhibitors are required to kill insects.
- It is necessary that the expression of proteinase inhibitors should be very low in the plant parts consumed by humans, while the expression should be high in the parts of plants utilized by insects.

α-Amylase inhibitors

The insect larvae secrete a gut enzyme α- amylase to digest starch. By blocking the activity of this enzyme by α-amylase inhibitor, the larvae can be starved and killed. α-Amylase inhibitor gene (α-AI-Pv) isolated from bean has been successfully transferred and expressed in tobacco. It provides ***resistance against Coleoptera*** (e.g. *Zabrotes subfasciatus*).

LECTINS

Lectins are plant glycoproteins and they provide resistance to insects by acting as toxins. The lectin gene (*GNA*) from snowdrop (*Galanthus nivalis*) has been transferred and expressed in potato and tomato. The major limitations of lectin are that it acts only against piercing and sucking insect, and high doses are required.

RESISTANCE GENES FROM ANIMALS

Proteinase inhibitor genes from mammals have also been transferred and expressed in plants to provide resistance against insects, although the success in this direction is very limited. Bovine pancreatic trypsin inhibitor (BPTI) and α_1-antitrypsin genes appear to be promising to offer insect resistance to transgenic plants.

INSECT RESISTANCE THROUGH COPY NATURE STRATEGY

Some of the limitations experienced by transferring the insecticidal genes (particularly *Bt*) and developing transgenic plants have prompted scientists to look for better alternatives. The copy nature strategy was introduced in 1993 (by Boulter) with the objective of ***insect pest control which is relatively sustainable and environmentally friendly.*** The copy nature strategy for the development of insect -resistant transgenic plants has the following stages.

1. **Identification of leads**: The first step in copy nature strategy is to identify the plants (from worldover) that are naturally resistant to insect damage.

2. **Isolation and purification of protein**: The protein with insecticidal properties (from the resistant plants) is isolated and purified. The sequence of the protein is determined, and the gene responsible for its production identified.

3. **Bioassay of isolated protein**: The activity of the protein against the target insects is determined by performing a bioassay in the laboratory.

4. **Testing for toxicity in mammals**: It is absolutely necessary to test the toxicity of the protein against mammals, particularly humans. If the protein is found to have any adverse affect, the copy nature strategy should be discontinued.

5. **Gene transfer :** By the conventional techniques of genetic engineering, the isolated gene corresponding to the protein toxin is introduced into the crop plants.

6. **Selection of transgenic plants** : After the gene transfer, the transgenic plants developed should be tested for the inheritance and appropriate expression of transgene. The efficiency of insecticidal protein to destroy insects is also evaluated.

7. **Evaluation for biosafety** : Field trails have to be conducted to evaluate the crop yield, damage to insects, influence on the environment with respect to the transgenic plant.

The copy nature strategy, though time consuming and many a times unsuccessful, takes into account the complex interplay in biological communities (between plants animals, microorganisms) and physical environment.

VIRUS RESISTANCE

Virus infections of crops may result in retarded cell division (***hypoplasia***), excessive cell division (***hyperplasia***), and cell death (***necrosis***). The overall effects of virus infections are growth retardation, lowered product yield and sometimes complete crop failure.

The ***chemical methods*** used to control various plant pathogens ***will be ineffective*** with respect to plant viruses since the viruses are intracellular obligate parasites.

There are however, certain ***safe agricultural practices*** to control/reduce viral infections to plants.

- Use of seeds that are virus - free.
- Control insects that spread plant viruses.
- Control weeds that serve as alternate hosts for viruses.
- Use cultivars that possess virus resistance.

It is possible to immunize plants against viral damages by expressing viral proteins in the plant cells. With the advances made in genetic engineering, it has become a reality to develop ***transgenic plants with virus resistance***. This is mostly done by employing ***virus-encoded genes -*** virus coat proteins, movement proteins, transmission proteins, satellite RNA, antisense RNAs and ribozymes. In recent years, some attempts are also made to provide virus resistance to plants by using ***animal genes***. Some of the developments are briefly described.

Virus coat proteins

The virus coat protein-mediated approach is the most successful one to provide virus resistance to plants. It was in 1986, transgenic tobacco plants expressing tobacco mosaic virus (TMV) coat protein gene were first developed. These plants exhibited high levels of resistance to TMV. Excited by this remarkable success, scientists have worked with many more viruses (around 30 or so) and developed crops with virus coat protein-mediated protection.

A selected list of the virus resistant transgenic plants with sources of virus coat protein genes is given in ***Table 50.4***. The transgenic plant providing coat protein-mediated resistance to virus are rice, potato, wheat, tobacco, peanut, sugar beet, alfalfa etc. The viruses that have been used include alfalfa mosaic virus (AIMV), cucumber mosaic virus (CMV), potato virus X (PVX), potato virus Y (PVY), citrus tristeza virus (CTV) and R rice stripe virus (RSV).

Advantages of virus coat proteins : The coat protein gene from one virus sometimes provides resistance (cross protection) to some other viruses, which may be unrelated e.g. TMV of tobacco plant provides resistance to potato virus X, alfalfa mosaic virus and cucumber mosaic virus.

Limitation of virus coat proteins

The virus coat protein-mediated protection is successful for viruses with single-stranded RNA genomes. However, this approach is of not much use for viruses with genomes containing double-stranded RNA and single-stranded DNA.

Mechanism of action of virus coat proteins : As the transgenic plant expresses the gene for coat protein of a given virus, the ability of the same virus to infect the plants again is drastically reduced. Despite a remarkable success in the virus coat protein-mediated protection, the molecular mechanism of the protection is not clearly known.

Movement proteins

As the virus infects the plant cells, its rapid spread through intercellular junctions (plasmadesmata) of vascular tissue occurs through the participation of movement proteins produced by the viruses. Good examples of movement proteins are 30KDa protein of tobacco mosaic virus (TMV) and 32KDa protein of brome mosaic virus (BMV).

Transgenic tobacco plants that express a mutated 30KDa movement protein have been developed. The TMV infection to these plants is much less. It is believed that the mutated movement protein competes with the wild-type TMV-coded protein thereby reducing the spread of the virus (TMV). In recent years, a recombinant movement protein having the components of golden mosaic virus and African cassava mosaic virus have been developed.

TABLE 50.4 A selected list of the virus-resistant transgenic plants with sources of virus protein coat genes

Plant	*Source(s) of virus coat protein gene*
Tobacco	*TMV, CMV, AIMV*
Rice	*RTSV, RSV, RYMV*
Wheat	*SBWMV, BYDV*
Potato	*PVX, PVY, PLRV*
Squash	*CMV, ZYMV*
Sugar beet	*BNYVV*
Peanut	*TSWV*
Papaya	*PRSV*
Citrus	*CTV*
Alfalfa	*AIMV*

TMV-Tobacco mosaic virus; CMV-Cucumber mosaic virus; AIMV-Alfalfa mosaic virus; RTSV-Rice tungro spherical virus; RSV-Rice stripe virus; RYMV-Rice yellow mottle virus; SBWMV-Soil-borne wheat mosaic virus; BYDV-Barley yellow dwarf virus; PVX-Potato virus X; PVY-Potato virus Y; PLRV-Potato leaf froll virus; ZYMV-Zucchini yellow mosaic virus; BNYVV-Beet necrotic yellow vein virus; TSWV-Tomato spotted wilt virus; PRSV-Papaya ringspot virus; CTV-Citrus tristeza virus.

This protein effectively interferes with the spread of both the viruses.

The ***advantage*** with movement protein strategy is that it is ***applicable to single-stranded DNA viruses*** (Geminiviruses) also.

Transmission proteins

There is a good coordination and interaction between plant viruses and insect vectors for the spread of viruses from one plant to another. Certain viral-encoded transmission proteins do this job effectively. It is possible to produce mutated transmission proteins and block the spread of viruses. Thus, the ***spread of insect-transmitted viruses*** can be ***prevented by*** engineering crops to express a ***defective virus-transmission protein***.

Satellite RNAs

Plant viral satellite RNAs are small RNA molecules that multiply in the host cells with the help of specific helper viruses. These satellite RNAs are encapsulated together with the respective helper viruses. In general, the presence of satellite RNAs reduces the severity of the viral disease and the symptoms, and thus reduces the effect of the virus. Transgenic plants containing satellite sequences have been developed to provide resistance to virus diseases. One example is given here. When cucumber mosaic virus (CMV) infects pepper plants, severe symptoms appear. These symptoms can be minimized with higher plant yield when CMV is coinoculated with a satellite RNA.

Satellite RNA approach is ***not widely used*** due to several ***limitations***.

- Some of the satellite RNA may increase the severity of disease symptoms in some plants.
- Satellite RNAs mutate very rapidly which may sometimes result in a highly virulent agent.
- Recombinations between satellite RNAs have been detected. This may lead to serious consequences.

Antisense RNAs

The antisense RNA approach is designed to specifically interfere with virus replication.

By use of genetic engineering, a complementary DNA strand of a gene (DNA sequence) can be inserted in reverse orientation ($3' \rightarrow 5'$ as opposed

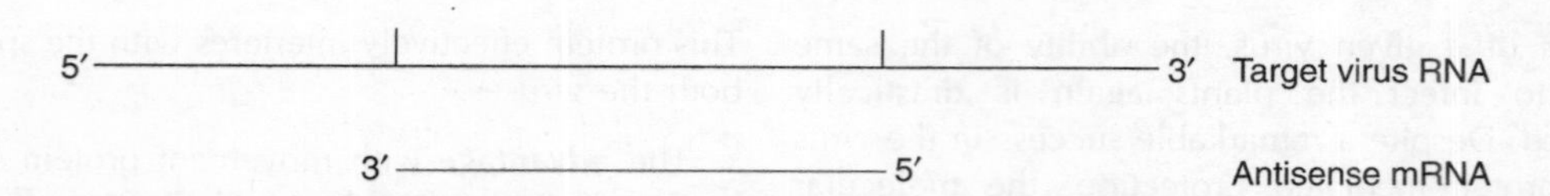

Fig. 50.3 : Hybridization of antisense mRNA with virus RNA to block replication.

to 5′ → 3′) and this is referred to as antisense gene. The mRNA produced by antisense gene is complementary to the mRNA synthesized by normal gene. As a result, both these mRNAs hybridize and thus the normal translation of mRNA is blocked. The net effect of employing an ***antisense gene*** into a cell is that it ***blocks a specific gene expression***.

It is possible to introduce viral antisense genes into plants and produce mRNAs complementary to viral sequences involved in virus replication. The antisense mRNAs can block the replication of viruses (***Fig 50.3***). Initially, antisense RNA approach was carried out in single-stranded RNA viruses. The success of this approach however, was limited probably due to the following reasons.

- High concentration of antisense mRNA may be required.
- Protein association with mRNA interferes with hybridization (between sense mRNA and antisense mRNA).

Antisense RNA approach may be more useful for DNA viruses. In fact, tomato golden mosaic virus (TGMV) replicase coding sequence was cloned in antisense orientation and introduced into tobacco plants. The transgenic tobacco plants expressed antisense RNA of TGMV replicase. These plants were resistant to TGMV infection.

Ribozymes

Ribozymes are small RNA molecules which promote the catalytic cleavage of RNA. For providing virus resistance, ribozymes in the form of antisense RNAs capable of cleaving the target viral (sense) RNAs have been developed. The ribozyme (antisense RNA) binds to a small sequence of viral RNA and splits (***Fig. 50.4***).

In this way, it is possible to block the replication of viral RNA. However, the ribozymes approach has not been very successful in plants.

FUNGAL AND BACTERIAL DISEASES

The plants do posses general defence systems against invading pathogens. This is however, not truely comparable with the immune system of the animals.

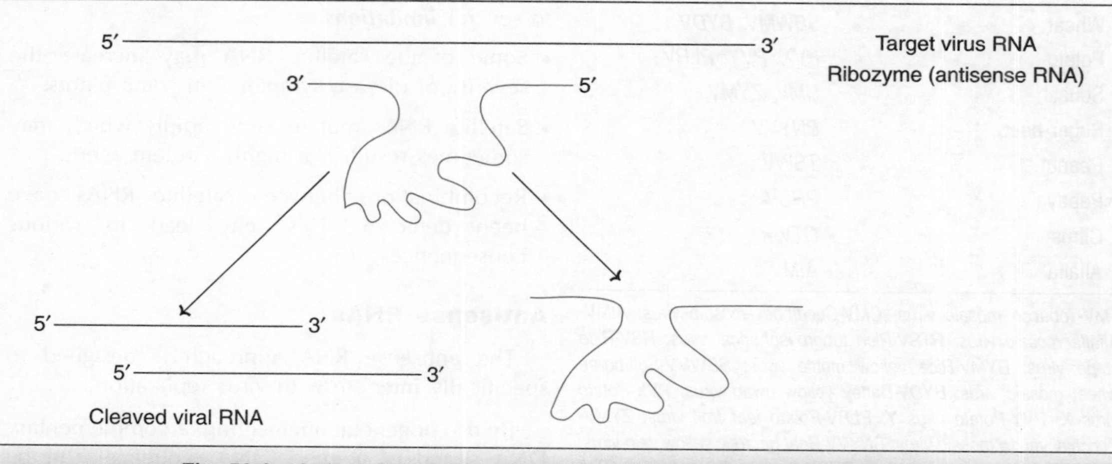

Fig. 50.4 : Action of ribozymes as antisense RNAs to block virus replication.

Whenever there is a cellular damage caused by pathogens (fungi, bacteria) and plant pests, the general defence system of plants get geared up to provide some amount of protection to the plant. This natural disease resistance of plants is inadequate. However, knowledge on the natural systems of plant resistance is useful for the biotechnological approaches to develop disease resistance.

Some of the defenses of plants and the biotechnological approaches are briefly described.

PATHOGENESIS-RELATED (PR) PROTEINS

To defend themselves against the invading pathogens (fungi and bacteria), plants accumulate ***low molecular weight proteins*** which are collectively regarded as pathogenesis-related (PR) proteins. The different types of PR proteins and their properties are given in ***Table 50.5***. Some of the most important ones are described.

Chitinase

Chitin is a constituent of fungal cell walls which can be hydrolysed by the enzyme chitinase. Certain chitinase genes from plants have been isolated and characterized. A bacterial chitinase gene obtained from a soil bacterium (*Serratia marcescens*) was introduced and expressed in tobacco leaves. Some other workers isolated a chitinase gene from bean (*Phaseolus vulgaris*) and developed transgenic plants of tobacco and *Brassica napus* with this gene.

The transformed tobacco plants were found to be resistant to infection of the pathogen *Rhizoctonia solani*. In case of *B.napus*, the protection however, was comparatively less.

Glucanase

Glucanase is another enzyme that degrades the cell wall of many fungi. The most widely used glucanase is β-1, 4-glucanase. The gene encoding for β-1, 4-glucanase has been isolated from barley, introduced, and expressed in transgenic tobacco plants. This gene provided good protection against soil-borne fungal pathogen *Rhizoctonia solani*.

The resistance to fungal pathogens is much higher if both chitinase and glucanase producing genes are present in transgenic plants. By this approach, fungal resistant tobacco, tomato and carrot have been developed.

TABLE 50.5 Different types of pathogenesis-related (PR) proteins produced in plants

Type	*Properties*
PR-1	Antifungal
PR-2	Endo β-1, 3-glucanases
PR-3	Endochitinases
PR-4	Antifungal, endochitinase
PR-5	Antifungal, thaumatin-like proteins, osmotins
PR-6	Protease inhibitors
PR-7	Endoprotease
PR-8	Chitinase/lysozyme
PR-9	Peroxidases
PR-10	Ribonucleases
PR-11	Endochitinase acitivty
PR-12	Defensins
PR-13	Thionins
PR-14	Lipid transfer proteins (non-specific)

RIBOSOME-INACTIVATING PROTEINS (RIPs)

Ribosome-inactivating proteins offer protection against fungal infections. They act on the large rRNA of eukaryote and prokaryote ribosomes (remove an adenine residue from a specific site), and thus inhibit protein biosynthesis. Certain RIPs that do not inhibit plant ribosomes were identified and the corresponding genes have been used to develop transgenic plants e.g. Type-I barley RIP is used to provide resistance to fungal infections.

Some authors use the term ***antimicrobial proteins*** to RIPs. The other examples of antimicrobial proteins are lectins, defensins, lysozyme, thionins etc.

Lysozyme

Lysozyme degrades chitin and peptidoglycan of cell wall, and in this way fungal infection can be reduced. Transgenic potato plants with lysozyme gene providing resistance to *Eswinia carotovora* have been developed.

Table 50.6 A selected list of transgenic plants developed along with the genes transferred and the resistance provided against the pathogens (fungus/bacterium)

Crop	*Gene(s) transferred*	*Resistance against pathogen*
Pathogenesis-related (PR) proteins		
Tobacco	Chitinase from bacterium (*Serratia marcescens*)	*Alternaria longipes*
	Bean chitinase	*Rhizoctonia solani, Phytophthora parasitica*
	Chitinase and 1, 3-β glucanase	*Cercospora nicotinae*
Rice	Chitinase	*Rhizoctonia solani*
Carrot	Chitinase and 1, 3-β glucanase	*Alternaria dauci, A. radicina*
Tomato	Chitinase and 1, 3-β glucanase	*Fusarium oxysporum*
Brassica napus	Chitinase	*Rhizoctonia solani*
Antimicrobial proteins		
Tobacco	Barley ribosome inactivating protein	*Rhizoctonia solani*
Tobacco	Defensin from radish	*Alternaria longipes*
Tobacco	α-Thionin gene from barley	*Pseudomonas syringae*
Potato	Bacteriophage T-4 lysozyme	*Erwinia carotovora*
Phytoalexins		
Rice	Stilbene synthase	*Pyricularia oryzae*
Tobacco	Stilbene synthase	*Botrytis cinerea*

Defensins

Defensins are antimicrobial peptides (26–50 amino acid residues) found in all the plant cells. They attack the microbial plasma membrane, however this is not adequate to provide resistance to pathogens.

In recent years, an artificial defensin gene has been developed and introduced into potatoes. These potatoes developed resistance to the bacterium *Eswinia carotovora*.

Thionins

Thionin proteins also offer protection against bacteria. Thionin coding genes have been introduced into tobacco and the transgenic plant so developed showed resistance to *Pseudomonas syringae*.

PHYTOALEXINS

Phytoalexins are secondary metabolites produced in plants in response to infection. They are low-molecular weight and antimicrobial in nature. The phytoalexins usually present in specialized cells or organelles are mobilized when infection occurs. Further, during infection there occurs induction of genes for increased production of phytoalexins. Stilbene synthase is a key enzyme for the synthesis of a common phytoalexin. The gene coding stilbene synthase has been isolated from peanut and introduced into tobacco, rice and *Brassica napus*. The transgenic plants carrying stilbene synthase gene were resistant against some fungi.

A selected list of transgenic plants developed, along with the genes transferred and the controlled pathogens is given in ***Table 50.6.***

NEMATODE RESISTANCE

Nematodes are simple worms found in the soil. They possess a complete digestive tract. The annual crop loss of the world due to nematode (roundworm) infestation is very high.

Some workers have identified and cloned a nematode resistance gene from wild beet plants. It is proposed that this gene encodes a protein that detects the pests (nematodes) and triggers a defensive reactions in the plant. It is believed that some chemical compounds that destroy the gut of the nematode are produced.

Attempts were also made to transfer the nematode resistance gene to sugar beet. Not much success was reported, the major limitation being the difficulty in cultivating the gene-altered cells of sugar beet.

RESISTANCE TO ABIOTIC STRESSES

Plants are constantly being subjected to environmental stresses (See ***Fig 50.1***) that may result in deterioration of crop plants, and a very low or even no yield. Plants are dependent on the subtle internal mechanisms for tolerance of various stresses. The *in situ* tolerance of crop plants, whenever present, is inadequate and therefore cannot give protection against the stresses. A wide range of strategies are required to engineer plants against a particular type of stress tolerance.

Some of the abiotic stresses and the recombinant strategies developed to overcome them are described.

HERBICIDE RESISTANCE

Weeds (***wild herbs)*** are unwanted and useless plants that grow along with the crop plants. Weeds compete with crops for light and nutrients, besides harbouring various pathogens. It is estimated that the world's crop yield is reduced by 10-15% due to the presence of weeds. To tackle the problem of weeds, modern agriculture has developed a wide range of ***weedkillers*** which are collectively referred to as ***herbicides***. In general, majority of the herbicides are broad-spectrum as they can kill a wide range of weeds. A good or an ***ideal herbicide*** is expected to possess the ***following characteristics***.

- Capable of killing weeds without affecting crop plants.
- Not toxic to animals and microorganisms.
- Rapidly translocated within the target plant.
- Rapidly degraded in the soil.

None of the commercially available herbicides fulfils all the above criteria. The major limitation of the herbicides is that they cannot descriminate weeds from crop plants. For this reason, the ***crops are*** also ***affected by herbicides, hence the need to develop herbicide-resistant plants.*** Thus, these plants provide an opportunity to effectively kill the weeds (by herbicides) without damaging the crop plants.

Strategies for engineering herbicide resistance

A number of biological manipulations particularly involving genetic engineering are in use to develop herbicide-resistant plants.

1. **Overexpression of the target protein** : The target protein, being acted by the herbicide can be produced in large quantities so that the affect of the herbicide becomes insignificant. Overexpression can be achieved by integrating multiple copies of the genes and/or by using a strong promoter.

2. **Improved plant detoxification** : The plants do possess natural defense systems against toxic compounds (herbicides). Detoxification involves the conversion of toxic herbicide to non-toxic or less toxic compound. By enhancing the plant detoxification system, the impact of the herbicide can be reduced.

3. **Detoxification of herbicide by using a foreign gene** : By introducing a foreign gene into the crop plant, the herbicide can be effectively detoxified.

4. **Mutation of the target protein**: The target protein which is being affected by the herbicide can be suitably modified. The changed protein should be capable of discharging the functions of the native protein but is resistant to inhibition by the herbicide. Once the resistant target protein gene is identified, it can be introduced into the plant genomes, and thus herbicide-resistant plants can be developed.

For success in the development of herbicide resistant plants, good knowledge of the target protein and the action of herbicides is required. Some of the developments made in the herbicide resistance of plant are briefly described.

GLYPHOSATE RESISTANCE

Glyphosate, is a glycine derivative. It acts as a broad-spectrum herbicide and is effective against 76 of the world's worst 78 weeds. Glyphosate is less toxic to animals and is rapidly degraded by microorganisms. In addition, it has a short half-life.

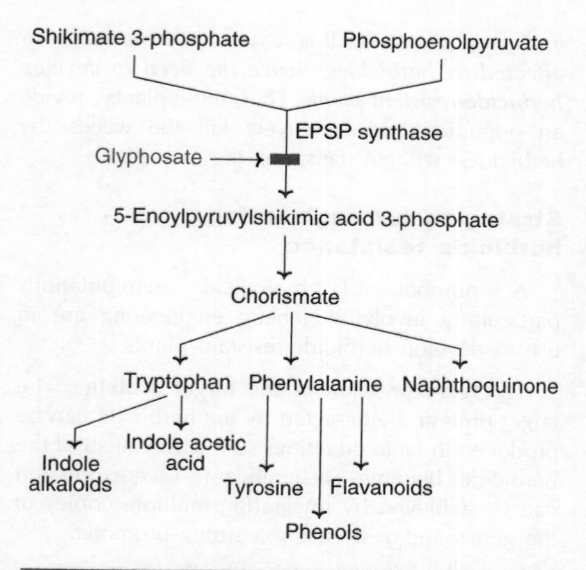

Fig. 50.5 : Shikimate pathway indicating the action of the herbicide glyphosate (EPSP synthase-5-Enolylpyruvylshikimate 3-phosphate synthase)

The American chemical company Monsanto markets glyphosate as ***Round up***.

Mechanism of action of glyphosate

Glyphosate is rapidly transported to the growing points of plants. It is capable of killing the plants even at a low concentration. Glyphosate acts as a ***competitive inhibitor*** of the enzyme ***5-enoylpyruvylshikimate 3-phosphate synthase (EPSPS).*** This is a key enzyme in ***shikimic acid pathway*** that results in the formation of aromatic amino acids (tryptophan, phenylalanine and tyrosine), phenols and certain secondary metabolites (***Fig. 50.5***).

The enzyme EPSPS catalyses the synthesis of 5-enoylpyruvylshikimate 3-phosphate from shikimate 3-phosphate and phosphoenoylpyruvate. Glyphosate has some structural similarily with the substrate phosphoenol pyruvate (***Fig 50.6***). Consequently, glyphosate binds more tightly with EPSPS and blocks the normal shikimic acid pathway. Thus, the herbicide glyphosate inhibits the biosynthesis of aromatic amino acids and other important products. This results in inhibition of protein biosynthesis (due to lack of aromatic amino acids). As a consequence, cell division and plant growth are blocked. Further, the plant growth regulator indole acetic acid (an auxin) is also produced from tryptophan. The net result of glyphosate is the death of the plants. Glyphosate is toxic to microorganisms as they also possess shikimate pathway.

Glyphosate is non-toxic to animals (including humans), since they do not possess shikimate pathway. Of the three aromatic amino acids (synthesized in this pathway), tryptophan and phenylalanine are essential and they have to be supplied in the diet, while tyrosine can be formed from phenylalanine.

Strategies for glyphosate resistance

There are three distinct strategies to provide glyphosphate resistance to plants.

1. **Overexpression of crop plant EPSPS gene** : An overexpressing gene of EPSPS was detected in *Petunia*. This expression was found to be due to gene amplification rather than an increased expression of the gene. EPSPS gene from *Petunia* was isolated and introduced into other plants. The increased synthesis of EPSPS (by about 40 fold) in transgenic plants provides resistance to glyphosate. These plants can tolerate glyphosate at a dose of 2-4 times higher than that required to kill wild-type plants.

2. **Use of mutant EPSPS genes** : An EPSPS mutant gene that conferred resistance to glyphosate was first detected in the bacterium *Salmonella typhimurium*. It was found that ***a single base substitution*** (***C*** to ***T***) resulted in the change of an amino acid from proline to serine in EPSPS. This ***modified enzyme cannot bind to glyphosate***, and thus provides resistance.

The mutant EPSPS gene was introduced into tobacco plants using *Agrobacterium* Ti plasmid vectors. The transgene produced high quantities of the enzyme EPSPS. However, the transformed tobacco plants provided only marginal resistance to

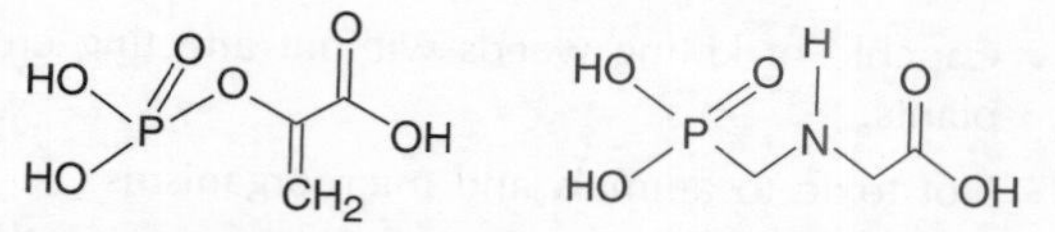

Phosphoenolpyruvate **Glyphosate**

Fig. 50.6 : Structures of phosphoenolpyruvate (the substrate) and the herbicide glyphosate (the competitive inhibitor).

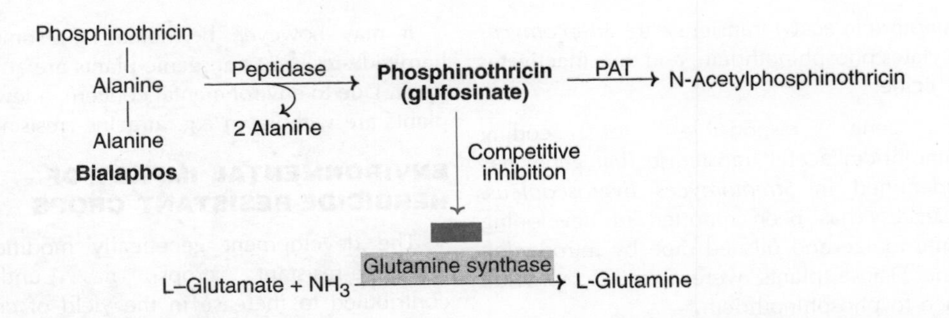

Fig. 50.7 : The formation, mode of action and detoxification of phosphinothricin (PAT-Phosphinothricin acetyl transferase).

glyphosate. The reason for this was not immediately identified. It was later known that the shikimate pathway occurs in the chloroplasts while the glyphosate resistant EPSPS was produced only in the cytoplasm. This enzyme was not transported to the chloroplasts, hence the problem to provide resistance. This episode made scientists to realize the importance of chloroplasts in genetic engineering.

In later years, the mutant EPSPS gene was tagged with a chloroplast-specific transit peptide sequence. By this approach, the glyphosate-resistant EPSPS enzyme was directed to freely ***enter chloroplast and confer resistance against the herbicide.***

3. **Detoxification of glyphosate** : The soil microorganisms possess the enzyme glyphosate oxidase that converts glyphosate to glyoxylate and aminomethylphosponic acid. The gene encoding glyphosate oxidase has been isolated from a soil organism *Ochrobactrum anthropi*. With suitable modifications, this gene was introduced into crop plants e.g. oilseed rape. The transgenic plants were found to exhibit very good glyphosate resistance in the field.

Use of a combined strategy : More efficient resistance of plants against glyphosate can be provided by employing a combined strategy. Thus, resistant (i.e. mutant) EPSPS gene in combination with glyphosate oxidase gene are used. By this approach, there occurs glyphosate resistance (due to mutant EPSPS gene) as well as its detoxification (due to glyphosate oxidase gene).

PHOSPHINOTHRICIN RESISTANCE

Phosphinothricin (or ***glufosinate***) is also a broad spectrum herbicide like glyphosate. Phosphinothricin is more effective against broad-leafed weeds but least effective against perennials. (**Note** : Phosphinothricin and glufosinate are two names for the same herbicide. However, to avoid confusion between glyphosate and glufosinate, phosphinothricin is more commonly used. ***Basta Aventis*** and ***Liberty*** are the ***trade names*** for phosphinothricin).

Phosphinothricin-a natural herbicide

Phosphinothricin is an unusual herbicide, being a derivative of a natural product namely ***bialaphos***. Certain species of *Streptomyces* produce bialaphos which is a combination of phosphinothricin bound to two alanine residues, forming a tripeptide. By the action of a peptidase, bialaphos is converted to active phosphinothricin (***Fig 50.7***).

Mechanism of action of phosphinothricin

Phosphinothricin acts as a competitive inhibitor of the enzyme glutamine synthase (***Fig 50.7***). This is possible since phosphinothricin has some structural similarity with the substrate glutamate. As a consequence of the inhibition of glutamine synthase, ammonia accumulates and kills the plant cells. Further, disturbance in glutamine synthesis also inhibits photosynthesis. Thus, the herbicidal activity of phosphinothricin is due to the combined effects of ammonia toxicity and inhibition of photosynthesis.

Strategy for phosphinothricin resistance

The natural detoxifying mechanism of phosphinothricin observed in *Streptomyces* sp has prompted scientists to develop resistant plants against this herbicide. The enzyme phosphinothricin acetyl transferase (of *Streptomyces* sp) acetylates phosphinothricin, and thus inactivates the herbicide.

The gene responsible for coding phosphinothricin acetyl transferase (*bar* gene) has been identified in *Streptomyces hygroscopicus*. Some success has been reported in developing transgenic maize and oilseed rape by introducing *bar* gene. These plants were found to provide resistance to phosphinothricin.

SULFONYLUREAS AND IMIDAZOLINONES RESISTANCE

The herbicides namely sulfonylureas and imidazolinones inhibit the enzyme acetolactate synthase (ALS), a key enzyme in the synthesis of branched chain amino acids namely isoleucine, leucine and valine. Mutant forms of this enzyme and the corresponding genes have been isolated, identified and characterized. Transgenic plants with the mutant genes of ALS were found to be resistant to sulfonylureas and imidazolinones e.g. maize, tomato, sugarbeet.

Resistance to other herbicides

Besides the above, some other herbicide resistant plants have also been developed e.g. bromoxynil, atrazine, phenocarboxylic acids, cyanamide. A list of selected examples of gene transferred herbicide resistant plants is given in **Table 50.7**.

It may however, be noted that some of the herbicide-resistant transgenic plants are at field-trial stage. Due to environmental concern, a few of these plants are withdrawn e.g. atrazine- resistant crops.

ENVIRONMENTAL IMPACT OF HERBICIDE-RESISTANT CROPS

The development genetically modified (GM) herbicide-resistant crops has undoubtedly contributed to increase in the yield of crops. For this reason, farmers particularly in the developed countries (e.g. USA) have started using these GM crops. Thus, the proportion of herbicide resistant soybean plants grown in USA increased from 17% in 1997 to 68% in 2001. The farmer is immensely benefited as there is a reduction in the cost of herbicide usage.

It is believed that the impact of herbicide-resistant plants on the environment is much lower than the direct use of the herbicides in huge quantities. There are however, other environmental concerns.

- Disturbance in biodiversity due to elimination of weeds.
- Rapid development of herbicide–resistance weeds that may finally lead to the production of ***super weeds***.

TOLERANCE TO WATER DEFICIT STRESSES

The environmental conditions such as ***temperature*** (heat, freezing, chilling), ***water***

TABLE 50.7 Selected examples of gene transferred herbicide resistant plants

Herbicide	*Gene transfer/mechanism of resistance*	*Transgenic crop(s)*
Glyphosate	Inhibition of EPSPS	Soybean, tomato
Glyphosate	Detoxification by glyphosate oxidase	Maize, soybean
Phosphinothricin	*bar* gene coding phosphinothricin acetyltransferase	Maize, rice, wheat, cotton, potato, tomato, sugarbeet
Sulfonylureas/imidazolinones	Mutant plant with acetolactate synthase	Rice, tomato, maize, sugarbeet
Bromoxynil	Nitrilase detoxification	Cotton, potato, tomato
Atrazine	Mutant plant with chloroplast *psb A* gene	Soybean
Phenocarboxylic acids	Monooxygenase detoxification (e.g. 2,4-D and 2,4,5-T)	Maize cotton
Cyanamide	Cyanamide hydratase gene	Tobacco

(EPSPS-5-Enoylpyruvylshikimate 3-phosphate synthase; 2,4-D-2,4-Dichlorophenoxy acetic acid; 2,4,5-T-2,4,5-Trichlorophenoxy acetic acid)

availability (shortage due to drought), and ***salinity*** influence the plant growth, development and yield. The abiotic stresses due to temperature, drought and salinity are collectively regarded as water deficit stresses (See ***Fig 50.1***).

Causes of water deficit

Water deficit may occur due to the following causes.

- Reduced soil water potential.
- Increased water evaporation (in dry, hot and windy conditions).
- High salt concentration in the soil (decrease soil water potential).
- Low temperature resulting in the formation of ice crystals.

Effects of water deficit

- Results in osmotic stress.
- Inhibits photosynthesis.
- Increases the concentration of toxic ions (reactive oxygen species) within the cells.
- Loss of water from the cell causing plasmolysis and finally cell death.

Tolerance to osmotic stress

The plant cells are subjected to severe osmotic stress due to water deficit. They however, produce certain compounds, collectively referred to as ***osmoprotectants*** or ***osmolytes***, to overcome the osmotic stress. Osmoprotectants are non-toxic compatable solutes and are divided into two groups.

1. **Sugar and sugar alcohols** e.g. mannitol, sorbitol, pinitol, ononitol, trehalose, fructans.

2. **Zwitterionic compounds** : These osmoprotectants carry positive and negative charges e.g. proline, glycine betaine.

The production of a given osmoprotectant is species dependent. The formation of mannitol, proline and glycine betaine are more closely linked to osmotic tolerance.

Strategies to develop water deficit tolerance plants

As explained above osmoprotectants offer good protection to plants against osmotic stress and therefore water deficit. It is therefore, logical to think of genetic engineering strategies for the increased production of osmoprotectants.

Some progress has been made in this direction. The biosynthetic pathways for the production of many osmoprotectants have been established and genes coding key enzymes isolated. In fact, some progress has been made in the development of transgenic plants with high production of osmoprotectants.

Transgenic plants with glycine betaine production

Glycine betaine is a quaternary ammonium compound and is electrically neutral. Besides functioning as a cellular osmolytes, glycine betaine stabilizes proteins and membrane structures.

Some of the key enzymes for the production of glycine betaine have been identified e.g. choline monooxygenase, choline dehydrogenase, betaine aldehyde dehydrogenase. The genes coding these enzymes were transferred to develop transgenic plants.

By using choline oxidase gene from *Arthrobacter* sp, transgenic rice that produces higher glycine betaine (which offers tolerance against water deficit stress) has been developed.

RESISTANCE AGAINST ICE-NUCLEATING BACTERIA

Formation of ice on the plant cells (outer membrane) is a complex chemical process. The importance of ice-nucleating bacteria is recognized in recent years. The occurrence of these bacteria has been reported in most of the plants — cereals, fruits and vegetable crops. The ice-nucleating bacteria synthesize proteins, which coalesce with water molecules to form ice crystals at temperature around 32°F. As the ice crystals grow, they can pierce the plant cells and severely damage the plants.

Chemical treatment of plants to protect from ice formation

Plants can be treated with copper containing compounds to kill the bacteria. Another approach is to use urea solution so that the ice formation is minimized.

Ice-minus bacteria to resist plants from cold temperatures

The bacterium *Pseudomonas syringae* is one of the highly prevalent ice-forming organisms in nature. With genetic manipulations, the gene that directs the synthesis of ice-related bacterial proteins in *P. syringae* was removed. These newly developed bacteria are referred to as ice-minus bacteria.

The researchers proposed to spray the transgenic ice-minus bacteria on to young plants. The intention was that these bacteria would ***give frost tolerance to the plants***; and thus increase the crop yield. The opponents of DNA technology were against this approach—the main fear being that the bacterial mutants may create some health complication in humans. The researchers argued and justified that no new genetic information is introduced into *P. syringae* and it is closely related in all aspect to the parent one which is already in the environment. After prolonged court proceedings in USA, clearance was given for spraying the ice-minus bacteria in the fields.

It was in 1987, ice-minus bacteria were sprayed on to the field of potato plants and strawberry plants. Another strain of *P. syringae* commercially labeled, as ***Frostban*** was later developed and used in crop fieds.

It may be noted here that ***ice-minus bacteria of P. syringae were the first transgenic bacteria*** that were ***used outside the laboratory***. Fortunately, the experiments yielded encouraging results, since crop damage due to frost formation was found to be reduced.

Arabidopsis with cold-tolerant genes

Scientists were successful in developing cold-tolerant genes (around 20) in *Arabidopsis* when this plant was gradually exposed to slowly declining temperatures. They also identified a ***coordinating gene*** that encodes a protein, which acts as a transcription factor for regulating the expression of cold-tolerant genes. By introducing the coordinating gene, expression of cold-tolerant genes was triggered, and this protected the plants against cold temperatures. More work is in progress in this direction.

IMPROVEMENT OF CROP YIELD AND QUALITY

With the advances made in plant genetic engineering, improvement in crop yield and quality have become a reality. The crop yield is primarily dependent on the photosynthetic efficiency and the harvest index (the fraction of the dry matter allocated to the harvested part of the crop). The quality of the crop is dependent on a wide range of desirable characters-nutritional composition of edible parts, flavour, processing quality, shelf-life etc.

GREEN REVOLUTION

The 'Green Revolution' led by Borlaug, Swaminathan and Khus enabled the ***world's food supply to be tripled during the last three decades of 20th century***. This was made possible by adopting genetically improved varieties of crops, coupled with advances in crop management.

The development of high-yielding varieties of wheat and rice has enabled several developing countries (a good example being India) to move from a position of food scarcity to become net exporter of these cereals. The Green Revolution became a reality as the farmers adopted to new cereal seeds, besides employing high-input methods of agriculture — use of nitrogen fertilizers, herbicides, pesticides, modern equipment of agriculture etc.

Selected examples of crops for quality and yield

There are a wide range of crops that have been manipulated by scientists for improved yield and quality. Only selected examples are briefly described.

GENETIC ENGINEERING FOR EXTENDED SHELF-LIFE OF FRUITS

The genetic manipulation of fruit ripening has become an important commercial aspect in plant genetic engineering. Delay in fruit ripening has many advantages.

- It extends the shelf-life, keeping the quality of the fruit intact.
- Long distance transport becomes easy without damage to fruit.
- Slow ripening improves the flavour.

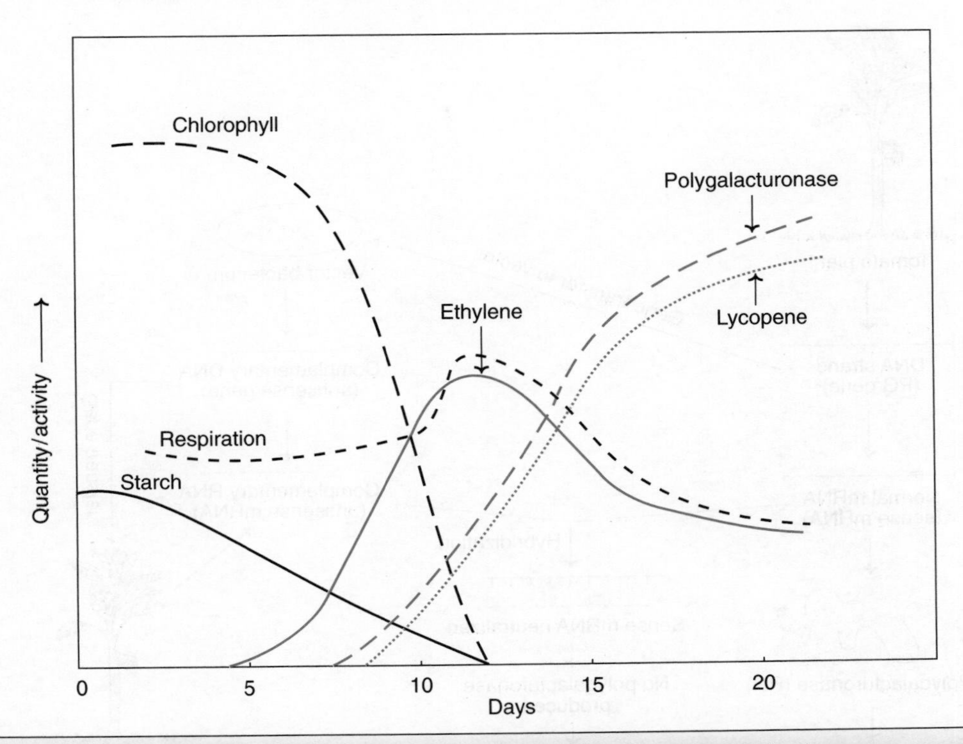

Fig. 50.8 : Biochemical changes during the process of tomato ripening.

Genetic engineering work has been extensively carried out in tomatoes, and some of the development are described.

BIOCHEMICAL CHANGES DURING TOMATO RIPENING

Fruit ripening is an active process. It is characterized by increased respiration accompanied by a rapid increase in ethylene synthesis. As the chlorophyll gets degraded, the green colour of the fruit disappears, and a red pigment, lycopene is synthesized (***Fig. 50.8***). The fruit gets softened as a result of the activity of cell wall degrading enzymes namely ***polygalacturonase*** (PG) and ***pectin methyl esterase***. The phytohormone ethylene production is intimately linked to fruit ripening as it triggers the ripening process of fruit. Addition of exogenous ethylene promotes fruit ripening, while inhibition of ethylene biosynthesis drastically reduces ripening.

The breakdown of starch to sugars, and accumulation of a large number of secondary products improves the flavour, taste and smell of the fruit.

Three distinct genes involved in tomato ripening have been isolated and cloned. The enzymes encoded by these genes and their respective role in fruit ripening are given in ***Table 50.8***.

TABLE 50.8 Clones of tomato ripening genes and their functions

Gene clone	*Enzyme synthesized*	*Function in ripening*
pTOM 5	Phytoene synthase	Lycopene synthesis that gives red colouration
pTOM 6	Polygalacturonase	Degradation of cell wall, resulting in fruit softening
pTOM 13	ACC oxidase	Ethylene formation that triggers fruit ripening

(ACC-1-Amino-cyclopropane-1-carboxylic acid)

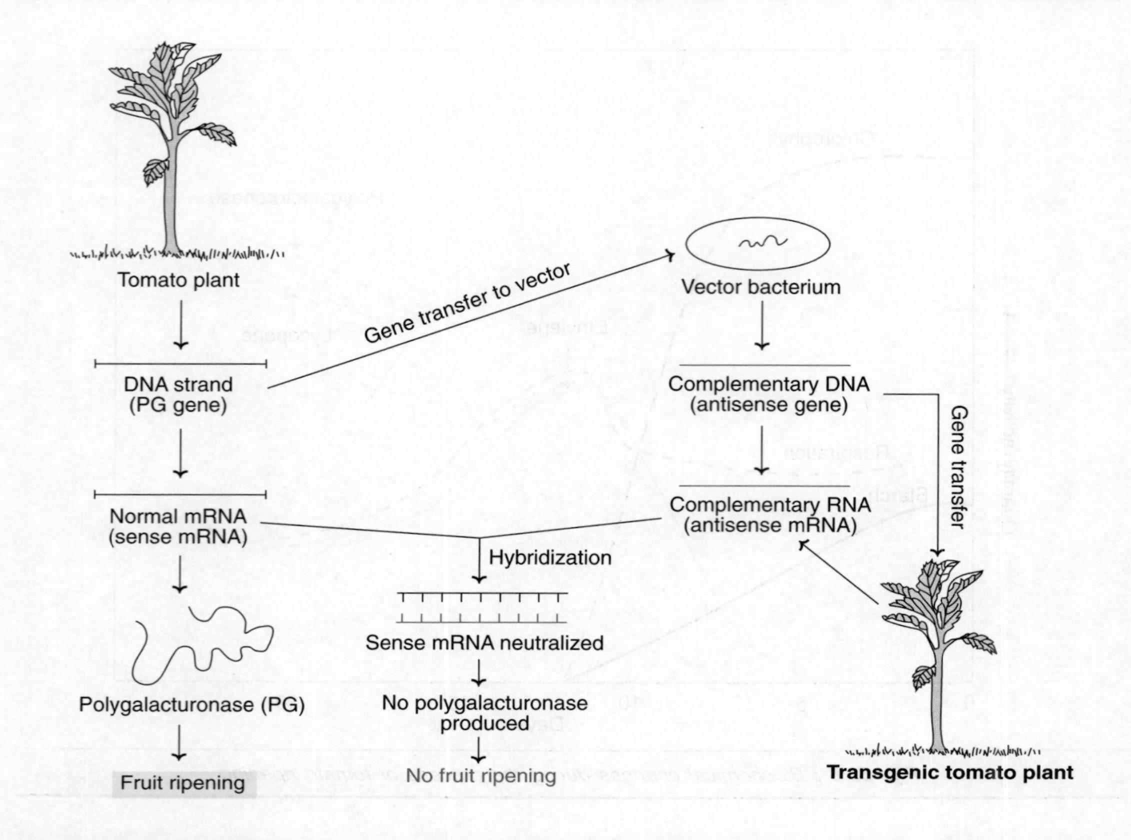

*Fig. 50.9 : Genetic manipulation of the enzyme polygalacturonase (PG) by antisense RNA approach (Production of **Flavr Savr** tomato plant)*

GENETIC MANIPULATIONS OF FRUIT RIPENING

Scientists have been trying to genetically manipulate and delay the fruit ripening process. Almost all the attempts involve ***antisense RNA approach***.

Manipulation of the enzyme polygalacturonase (development of Flavr Savr tomato)

As already stated, softening of the fruit is largely due to degradation of the cell wall (pectin) by the enzyme polygalacturonase (PG). The gene responsible for PG, the rotting enzyme, has been cloned (pTOM 6). The genetic manipulation of polygalacturonase by antisense RNA approach for the development of ***Flavr Savr tomato*** (by Calgene company in USA) is depicted in ***Fig. 50.9***, and mainly involves the following stages.

1. Isolation of the DNA from tomato plant that encodes the enzyme polygalacturonase (PG).

2. Transfer of PG gene to a vector bacteria and production of complementary DNA molecules.

3. Introduction of complementary DNA into a fresh tomato plant to produce a transgenic plant.

Mechanism of PG antisense RNA approach : In the normal tomato plant, PG gene encodes a normal (sense) mRNA that produces the enzyme polygalacturonase that is actively involved in fruit ripening. The complementary DNA of PG encodes for antisense mRNA, which is complementary to normal (sense) mRNA. The hybridization between the sense and antisense mRNAs renders the sense mRNA ineffective. Consequently, no polygalacturonase is produced, hence fruit ripening is delayed.

The rise and fall of Flavr Savr tomato

The genetically engineered tomato, known as Flavr Savr (pronounced flavour saver) by employing PG antisense RNA was approved by U.S. Food and Drug Administration on 18th May 1994. The FDA ruled that Flavr Savr tomatoes are as safe as tomatoes that are bred by conventional means, and therefore no special labeling is required. The new tomato could be shipped without refrigeration to far off places, as it was capable of resisting rot for more than three weeks (double the time of a conventional tomato).

Although Flavr Savr was launched with a great fanfare in 1995, it did not fulfill the expectation for the following reasons.

- Transgenic tomatoes could not be grown properly in different parts of U.S.A.
- The yield of tomatoes was low.
- The cost of Flavr Savr was high.

It is argued that the company that developed Flavr Savr, in its overenthusiasm to become the first Biotech Company to market a bioengineered food, had not taken adequate care in developing the transgenic plant. And unfortunately, within a year after its entry, Flavr Savr was withdrawn, and it is now almost forgotten!

Manipulation of ethylene biosynthesis

It has been clearly established that ethylene plays a key role in the ripening of fruits. The biosynthetic pathway of ethylene is depicted in ***Fig 50.10***. Ethylene is synthesized from S-adenosyl methonine via the formation of an intermediate, namely 1-***aminocyclopropane-1 carboxylic acid (ACC)***, catalysed by the enzyme ACC synthase. The next step is the conversion of ACC to ethylene by ACC oxidase.

Three different strategies have been developed to block ethylene biosynthesis, and thereby reduce fruit ripening.

1. **Antisense gene of ACC oxidase :** Transgenic plants with antisense gene of ACC oxidase have been developed. In these plants, production of ethylene was reduced by about 97% with a significant delay in fruit ripening.

2. **Antisense gene of ACC synthase :** Ethylene biosynthesis was inhibited to an extent of 99.5% by inserting antisense gene of ACC synthase, and the tomato ripening was markedly delayed.

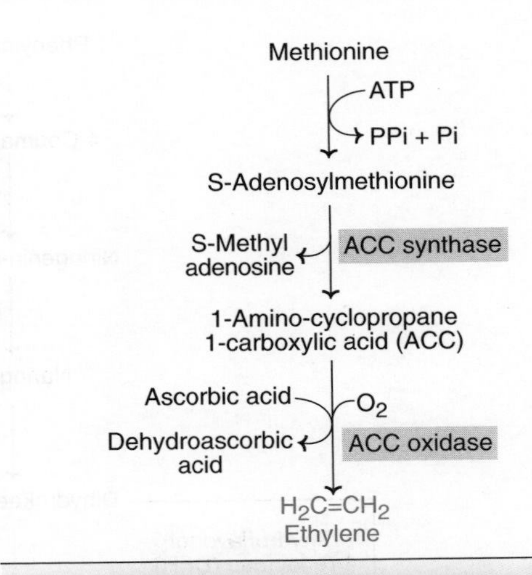

Fig. 50.10 : Biosynthesis of ethylene.

3. **Insertion of ACC deaminase gene :** ACC deaminase is a bacterial enzyme. It acts on ACC (removes amino group), and consequently the substrate availability for ethylene biosynthesis is reduced. The bacterial gene encoding ACC deaminase has been transferred and expressed in tomato plants. These transgenic plants inhibited about 90% of ethylene biosynthesis. The fruit ripening was delayed by about six weeks.

The strategies ***1 and 2*** may be referred to as ***antisense ethylene technology***.

LONGER SHELF-LIFE OF FRUITS AND VEGETABLES

The spoilage of fruits, vegetables and senescence of picked flowers, collectively referred to as ***post-harvest spoilage*** is major concern in agriculture. This hampers the distribution system particularly when the transport is done to far off places.

The successful manipulations to delay ripening, senescence and spoilage of various foods will significantly contribute to the appropriate food distribution and thus good economic practices in agriculture.

Suppressing the biosynthesis of ethylene appears to be a promising area to reduce the spoilage of fruits, vegetables and senescence of flowers. The three different strategies to block ethylene synthesis

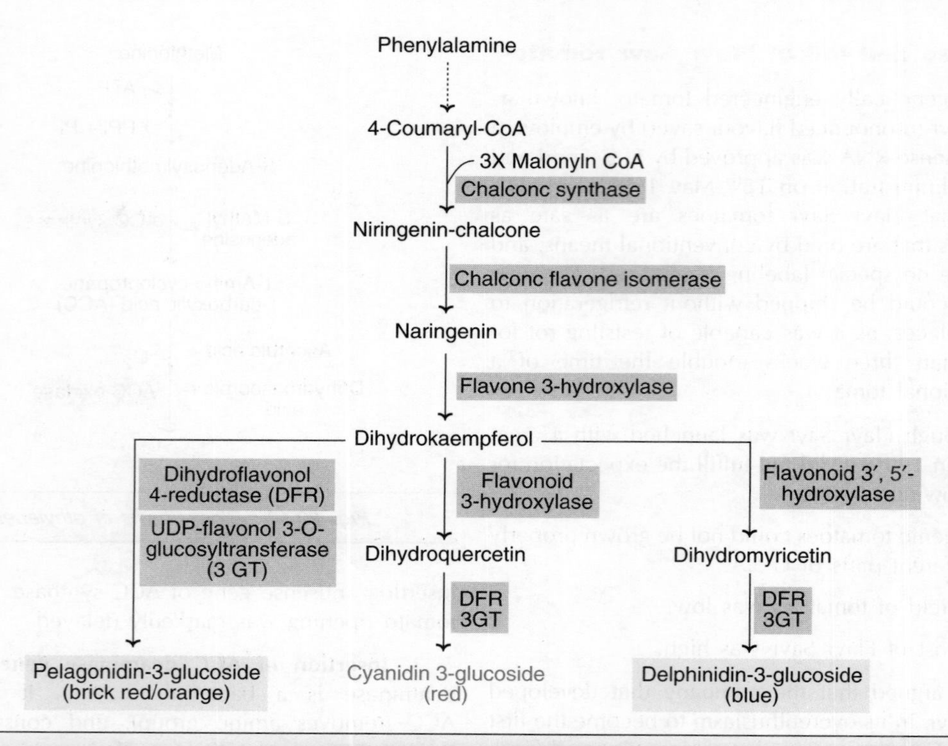

Fig. 50.11 : Biosynthesis of anthocyanins.

in tomato have been described. The same approaches in fact can be successfully used for other fruits, vegetables etc., to ***achieve longer shelf-life***

GENETIC ENGINEERING FOR PREVENTING DISCOLORATION

Discoloration of fruits and vegetables is a major postharvest problem encountered in food industry. Certain food additives are added to prevent discoloration. However, these additives may cause health complications in humans.

Biochemically, discoloration of fruits and vegetables is mainly due to the oxidation of phenols (mono- and diphenols) to quinones, catalysed by a group of enzymes namely ***polyphenol oxidases.*** These enzymes are localized in the membranes of mitochondria and chloroplasts.

Genetic manipulations using antisense approach to inhibit the synthesis of polyphenol oxidase has been carried. Some success has been reported in preventing the discoloration of potatoes by this strategy.

GENETIC ENGINEERING FOR FLOWER PIGMENTATION

There are continuous attempts in flower industry to make the ornamental flowers more attractive (by improving or creating new colours), besides prolonging post-harvest lifetime. The cut flower industry is mostly (about 70%) dominated by four plants—roses, tulips, chrysanthemums and carnations.

The most common type of flower pigments are anthocyanins, a group of flavonoids. They are synthesized by a series of reactions, starting from the amino acid phenylalanine (***Fig. 50.11***). The colour of the flower is dependent on the chemical nature of the anthocyanin produced.

- Pelagonidin 3-glucoside — brick red/orange.
- Cyanidin 3-glucoside — red.
- Delphinidin 3-glucoside — blue to purple.

Manipulation of anthocyanin pathway enzymes

The enzymes responsible for different reactions, in the anthocyanin pathway have been identified.

By genetic manipulations and mutations, it is possible to develop flowers with the desired colours.

Most of the flowers (roses, carnations chrysanthemums) lack blue colour due to the absense of the key enzyme flavonoids 3′, 5′-hydroxylase (F 3′5′ H) that produces delphinidine 3 glucoside. One company, by the name Florigene, has genetically manipulated and introduced the gene encoding the enzyme F 3′ 5′ H (from *Petunia hybrida*) into the following plants.

The ***world's first genetically modified (GM) flower*** was introduced in 1996. It was a mauve (bluish) coloured carnation with a trade name ***Moondust***™. Subsequently, many other flowers have been produced and marketed.

Can GM-flowers be eaten?

In majority of countries, flowers are used for ornamental purposes and not usually eaten. However, in some countries like Japan, flower petals are used for decoration of foods, and frequently eaten also. This raises an important question about the safety of GM flowers, since they are not thoroughly screened for human consumption. But the present belief is that the anthocyanins (the colouring chemical molecules) are natural plant materials, and their consumption may be in fact beneficial to health.

GENETIC ENGINEERING FOR MALE STERILITY

The plants may inherit male sterility either from the nucleus or cytoplasm. ***cytoplasmic male sterility (cms)*** is due to the defects in the mitochondiral genome. It is possible to introduce male sterility through genetic manipulations while the female plants maintain fertility.

In tobacco plants, male sterility was introduced by using a mitochondrial mutated gene encoding the enzyme ribonuclease. The gene encoding ribonuclease namely *barnase* gene from *Bacillus amyloliquefaciens* was transferred to tobacco plants. The ribonuclease is toxic to tapetal cells, and thus prevents the development of pollen, ultimately leading to male sterility. By this approach, transgenic plants of tobacco, cauliflower, cotton, tomato, corn, lettuce etc., with male sterility have been developed.

It is possible to restore male sterility in the above plants by crossing them with a second set of transgenic plants containing ribonuclease inhibitor gene.

TRANSGENIC PLANTS WITH IMPROVED NUTRITION

Genetic manipulations for improving the nutritional quality of plant products are of great importance in plant biotechnology. Some success has been achieved in this direction through conventional cross-breeding of plants. However, this approach is very slow and difficult, and many a times will not give the traits with the desired improvements in the nutritional quality. Selected examples of genetic engineering with improved nutritional contents are described.

AMINO ACIDS OF SEED STORAGE PROTEINS

Of the 20 amino acids present in the humans, 10 are essential while the other 10 can be synthesized by the body. The 10 essential amino acids (EAAs) have to be supplied through the diet. Cereals (rice, wheat, maize, corn) are the predominant suppliers of EAAs. However, cereals do not contain adequate quantity of the essential amino acid lysine. On the other hand, pulses (Bengal gram, red gram, soybean) are rich in lysine and limited in sulfur-containing amino acids (the essential one being methionine).

Transgenic routes have been developed to improve the essential amino acid contents in the seed storage proteins of various crop plants.

Overproduction of lysine by deregulation

The four essential amino acids namely lysine, methionine, threonine and isoleucine are produced from a non-essential amino acid aspartic acid (***Fig. 50.12***). The formation of lysine is regulated by feedback inhibition of the enzymes aspartokinase (AK) and dihydrodipicolinate synthase (DHDPS). Theoretically, it is possible to overproduce lysine by abolishing the feedback regulation. This is what has been accomplished.

The lysine feedback-insensitive genes encoding the enzymes AK and DHPDS have been respectively isolated from *E.coli* and *Cornynebacterium* with appropriate genetic

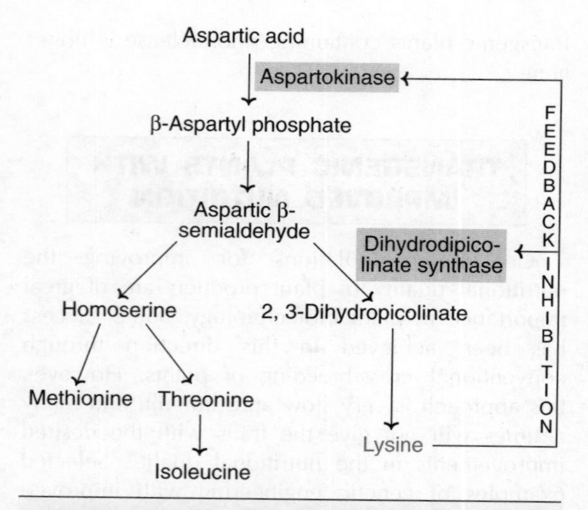

*Fig. 50.12 : An overview of the biosynthetic pathway of some essential amino acids derived from aspartic acid (**Note :** Lysine regulates its own synthesis by feedback inhibition).*

manipulations, these genes were introduced into soybean and canola plants. The transgenic plants so developed produced high quantities of lysine.

Transfer of genes encoding methionine-rich proteins

Several genes encoding methonine-rich proteins have been identified.

- In maize, 21 KDa zein with 28% methionine.
- In rice, 10 KDa prolamin with 20% methionine.
- In sunflower, seed albumin with 16% methionine.

These genes have been introduced into some crops such as soybean, maize and canola.

The transgenic plants produced proteins with high contents of sulfur-containing amino acids.

Production of lysine-rich glycinin in rice

Glycinin is a lysine-rich protein of soybean. The gene encoding glycinin has been introduced into rice and successfully expressed. The transgenic rice plants produced glycinin with high contents of lysine. Another added advantage of ***glycinin*** is that its consumption in humans is associated with a ***reduction in serum cholesterol*** (hypocholesterolaemic effect).

Construction of artificial genes to produce proteins rich in EAAs

Attempts are being made to construct artificial genes that code for proteins containing the essential amino acids in the desired proportion. Some success has been reported in the production of one synthetic protein containing 13% methionine residues.

GENETIC ENGINEERING FOR IMPROVING PALATABILITY OF FOODS

More than the nutritive value, taste of the food is important for attracting humans. It is customary to make food palatable by adding salt, sugar, flavors and many other ingradients. It would be nice if a food has an intrinsically appetizing character.

A protein ***monellin*** isolated from an African plant (*Dioscorephyllum cumminsii*) is about ***100,000 sweeter than sucrose*** on molar basis. Monellin gene has been introduced into tomato and lettuce plants. Some success has been reported in the production of monellin in these plants, improving the palatability.

GOLDEN RICE — THE PROVITAMIN A ENRICHED RICE

About one-third of the world's population is dependent on rice as staple food. The milled rice that is usually consumed is almost deficit in β-carotene, the provitamin A. As such, vitamin A deficiency (causing night blindness) is major nutritional disorder worldover, particularly in people subsisting on rice.

To overcome vitamin A deficiency, it was proposed to genetically manipulate rice to produce β-carotene, in the rice endosperm. The presence of ***β-carotene in the rice gives*** a characteristic ***yellow/orange colour***, hence the provitamin A-enriched rice are appropriately considered as Golden Rice.

In ***Fig. 50.13*** an outline of the biosynthetic pathway for the formation of β-carotene is given. The genetic manipulation to produce Golden Rice required the introduction of three genes encoding the enzymes phytoene synthase, carotene desaturase and lycopene β-cyclase. It took about 7 years to insert three genes for developing Golden Rice.

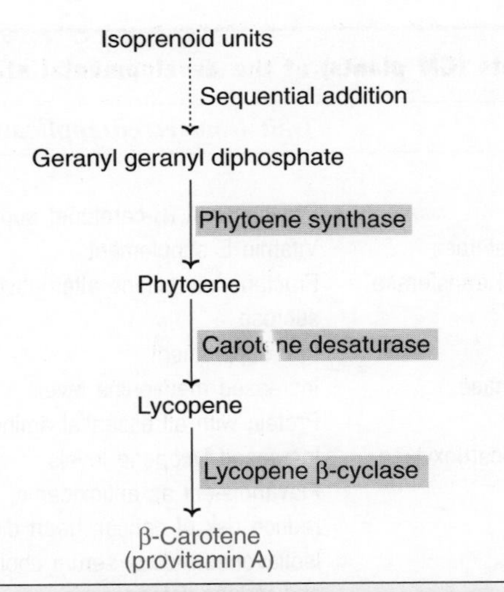

Fig. 50.13 : An outline of pathway for the biosynthesis of provitamin A (β-carotene).

Golden Rice has met almost all the objections raised by the opponents of GM foods. However, many people are still against the large scale production of Golden Rice, as this will open door to the entry of many other GM foods. Another argument put forth against the consumption of Golden Rice is that it can supply only about 20% of daily requirement of vitamin A. But the proponents justify that since rice is a part of a mixed diet consumed (along with many other foods), the contribution of provitamin A through Golden Rice is quite substantial.

Recently (in 2004), a group of British scientists have developed an improved version of Golden Rice. The new strain, Golden Rice 2 contains more than 20 times the amount of provitamin A than its predecessor. It is claimed that a daily consumption of 70 g rice can meet the recommended dietary allowance for vitamin A.

TABLE 50.9 A selected list of transgenic crop plants (GM crops approved in USA) for commercial use

Crop plant	*Genetically altered trait*	*Product name*
Cotton	Insect resistance	Bollguard
	Glyphosate resistance	Roundup ready
	Bromoxynil resistance	BXN
	Sulfonylurea resistance	—
Maize	Insect resistance	Yield Guard
	Insect resistance	Maximizer
	Glyphosate resistance	Roundup Ready
	Glufosinate resistance	Liberty Link
Rice	Vitamin A enrichment	Golden Rice
Tomato	Delayed ripening	Flavr Savr
	Delayed ripening	Endless Summer
	Virus resistance	—
Soybean	Glyphosate resistance	Roundup Ready
Potato	Insect resistance	Newleaf
	Modified starch	—
Oilseed rape (canola)	Glufosinate resistance	Innovator
	Glyphosate resistance	Roundup Ready
	High lauric acid	Laurical
	Male sterility hybrid	—
Squash	Virus resistance	Freedom II
Tobacco	Virus resistance	—
Capsicum	Virus resistance	—
Carnation	Modified flower colour	—

Table 50.10 Some examples of transgenic crop plants (GM plants) at the developmental stages

Plant	Gene transfer	Trait transferred/application(s)
For improving human health		
Tomato	Phytoene desaturase	Provitamin A (β-carotene) supplement
Canola	γ-Tocopherol methyl transferase	Vitamin E supplement
Sugar beet	Sucrose-sucrose fructosyl transferase	Fructans-low calorie alternatives to sucrose
Rice	Ferritin	Iron supplement
Potato	Antisense threonine synthase	Increased methionine levels
Potato	Seed albumin	Protein with all essential amino acids
Tomato	S-Adenosylmethionine decarboxylase	Increased lycopene levels
Tomato	Chalcone isomerase	Flavanols-act as antioxidants, reduce risk of cancer, heart diseases
Arabidopsis	Isoflavone synthase	Isoflavones-reduce serum cholesterol, and reduce osteoporosis
Canola	Modified acyl-acyl carrier protein thioesterase	*cis*-Stearates-lower the risk of heart diseases
For increased crop yield		
Rice	Phosphoenol pyruvate carboxylase	Increased efficiency of photosynthesis
Tobacco	Phytochrome A	Avoids shades
Lettuce	Gibberellic acid (GA) oxidase	Inhibits GA accumulation and stem growth (dwarfing)
Potato	Phytochrome B	Increased photosynthesis and longer life span
Others		
Tobacco and soybean	Cytochrome P_{450}	Synthesis of epoxy fatty acids for manufacture of adhesives and paints
Rice	Nicotianamine aminotransferase	Tolerance to low iron availability
Tobacco	Nitroreductase	Reduces land contamination by trinitrotoluene

GENETIC ENGINEERING TO INCREASE VITAMINS AND MINERALS

The transgenic rice (Golden Rice) developed with high provitamin A content is described above. Transgenic crop plants are also being developed for increased production of other vitamins and minerals.

A transgenic *Arabidopsis thaliana* that can produce ten-fold higher ***vitamin E*** (α-tocopherol) than the native plant has been developed. This was done by a novel approach. *A. thaliana* possesses the biochemical machinery to produce a compound close in structure to α-tocopherol. A gene that can finally produce α-tocopherol is also present, but is not expressed. This dormant gene was activated by inserting a regulatory gene from a bacterium. This resulted in an efficient production of vitamin E.

Some workers are trying to increase the mineral contents of edible plants by enhancing their ability to absorb from the soil. Some success has been reported with regard to increased concentration of iron.

COMMERCIAL TRANSGENIC CROP PLANTS

The very purpose of production of transgenic plants is for their commercial importance with high productivity. It was in 1995-96, transgenic plants (potato and cotton) were, for the first time, made available to farmers in USA. By the year 1998-99, five major transgenic crops (cotton, maize, soybean, canola and potato) were in widespread use. They accounted for about 75% of the total area planted by crops in USA.

A selected list of transgenic crop plants (approved in USA) for the commercial use is given in ***Table 50.9.*** Some examples of transgenic crop plants, which are at the developmental stages are given in ***Table 50.10***. These plants are carefully designed to give rise to products, which will improve human health and increase of crop yield.

Goals of biotechnological improvements in crops

There are about 30–40 crops that have been genetically modified, and many more are being added. However, very few of them have got the clearance for commercial use. A selected list is already given in ***Table 50.9.***

The ultimate goals of genetically modified (GM) crop plants are listed below.

- Resistance to diseases (insect, microorganisms).
- Improved nitrogen fixing ability.
- Higher yielding capacity.
- Resistance to drought and soil salinity.
- Better nutritional properties.
- Improved storage qualities.
- Production of pharmaceutically important compounds.
- Absence of allergens.
- Modified sensory attributes e.g. increased sweetness as in thaumatin.

Concerns about transgenic plants

The fears about the harmful environmental and hazardous health affects of transgenic plants still exists, despite the fact that there have been no reports so far in this regard.

The transfer of almost all the transgenic plants from the laboratory to the crop fields is invariably associated with legal and regulatory hurdles, besides the social and economic concerns.

The major concern expressed by public (also acknowledged by biotechnologists) is the development of resistance genes in insects, generation of super weeds etc. Several remedial measures are advocated to overcome these problems.

The farmers in developing countries are much worried about the ***seed terminator technology*** which forces them to buy seeds for every new crop. These farmers are traditionally habituated to use the seeds from the previous crop which is now not possible due to seed termintor technology.

TRANSGENIC PLANTS AS BIOREACTORS

Another important application of genetically transformed plants is their utility as bioreactors to produce a wide range of metabolic and industrial products. These aspects are described in the next chapter.

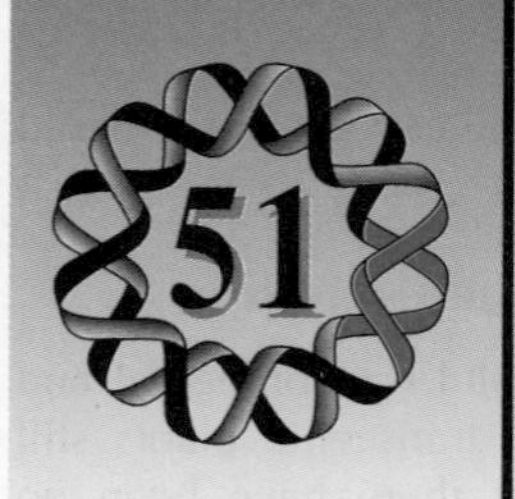

Transgenic Plants as Bioreactors

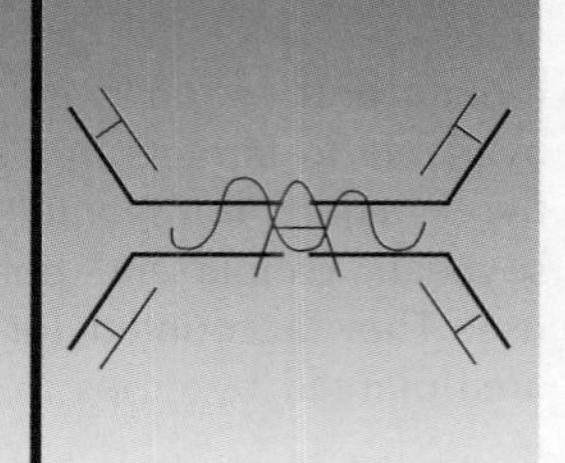

Genetically modified plants can be manipulated to act as bioreactors to produce a wide range of biologically important compounds. These include carbohydrates, lipids and proteins, besides the secondary products. The commercial products of plants are useful for industries or for improving the human or animal health.

The terms ***molecular farming/pharming or metabolic engineering of plants*** are also used to collectively represent the molecular biological techniques for the synthesis of commercial products in plants. Metabolic engineering of transgenic plants is gaining importance in recent years as an attractive alternative to animals and micro-organisms for the manufacture of biologically important products.

METABOLIC ENGINEERING OF CARBOHYDRATES

An outline of the biosynthetic pathways for the production of different carbohydrates is given in ***Fig 51.1***. As is evident, the important carbohydrates are synthesized and stored in different cellular compartments.

- Starch and its derivatives are synthesized in the plastids.
- Sugars and sugar derivatives are produced in the cytosol and accumulate throughout the cell.
- Fructans synthesized and stored in the vacuoles.

STARCH

Starch is a polymer of glucose, and is composed of amylose and amylopectin. Starch is used as a food, feed and for industrial purposes. Genetic engineering techniques can be used to manipulate the quantity and quality of starch.

Increasing the production of starch

Biosynthesis of starch in plants is a highly regulated process involving the key enzyme ***ADP-glucose pyrophosphorylase***. This enzyme is allosterically controlled (feedback inhibition) by metabolites such as phosphate.

ADP-glucose pyrophosphorylase in *E.coli* was mutated to alter its allosteric properties. This mutant gene was transferred and expressed in potato plants. The ***transgenic potato plants produced high quantities of starch***.

Synthesis of amylopectin starch

Starch normally contains 20–30% amylose and 70–80% amylopectin. The relative proportion of amylose and amylopectin determine the physico-chemical properties of starch. Amylopectin gels are more stable and therefore are preferred in food processing industries.

The enzyme namely ***granule-bound starch synthase (GBSS)*** is responsible for the synthesis of amylose while ***starch branching enzyme (SBE)*** produces amylopectin (***Fig 51.1***). By using an

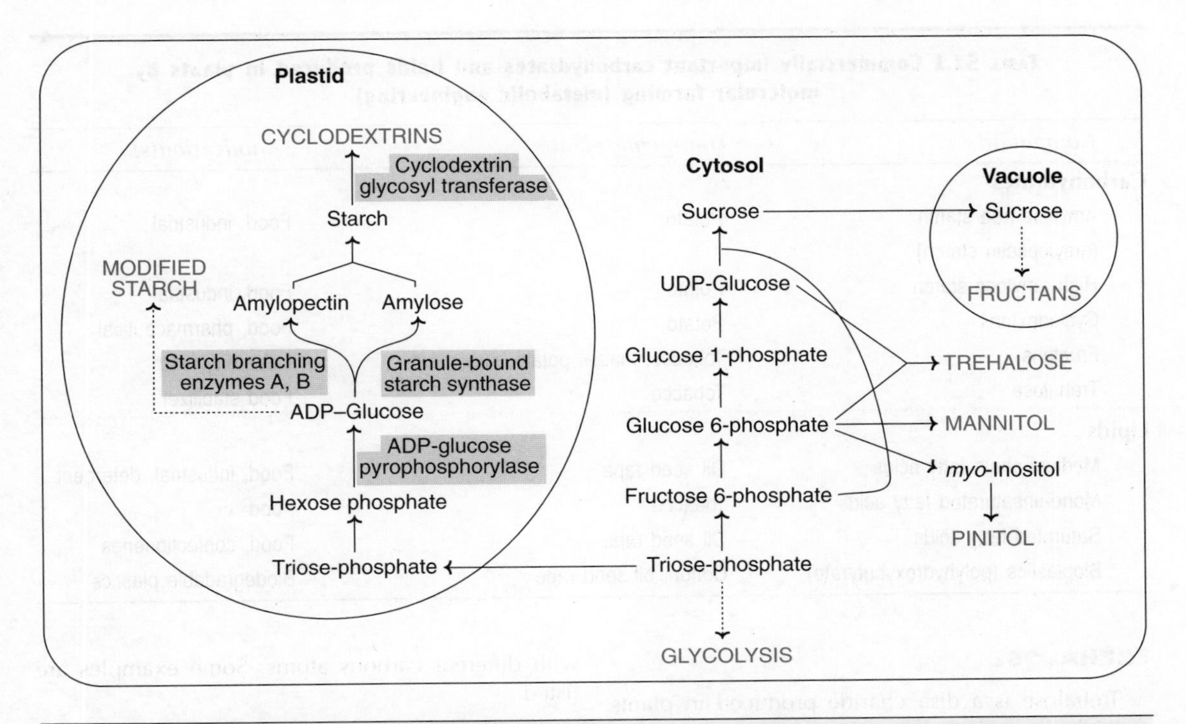

Fig. 51.1 : An outline of the metabolic pathway for the biosynthesis of carbohydrates and their important derivatives in a plant cell.

antisense approach, the enzyme GBSS was inhibited in potato plants. Consequently, amylose-free starch i.e. starch containing only amylopectin was produced.

Synthesis of high-amylose starch

High-amylose starch with limited branching is useful as a food, feed and for certain industrial purposes. It is possible to produce high-amylose starch in potatoes by antisense inhibition of starch branching enzyme A and B (SBE A and SBE B).

CYCLODEXTRINS

Cyclodextrins are cone-shaped rings formed by 6-8 glucopyranose subunits. They are hydrophilic in nature and can pocket hydrophobic compounds. Due to this property, cyclodextrins are used as therapeutic agents to solubilise hydrophobic pharmaceuticals such as steroids.

A key enzyme responsible for the synthesis of cyclodextrins from starch namely ***cyclodextrin glycosyl transferase*** has been identified. A bacterial gene coding for this enzyme was transferred to potato plants. However, the transgenic potato plants did not show any enhancement in the synthesis of cyclodextrins due to various reasons.

FRUCTANS

Fructans, also referred to as polyfructans, are soluble polymers of fructose. They are synthesized and stored in cellular vacuoles. Short-chain fructans (oligofructans) are almost as sweet as sucrose. Thus, they can be used as sugar substitutes in food and soft drink industries. Another advantage is that fructans are not digested in the gut and therefore, they serve as low-calorie sweeteners.

Transgenic potato plant with ***fructosyl transferase gene*** (from *Streptomyces*) has been developed. Fructosyl transferase, being a key enzyme enhanced the synthesis of fructans.

In recent years, oligofructans of sugarbeet (fructan beet) with suitable genetic manipulation have been produced. They serve as low calorie sweeteners.

TABLE 51.1 Commercially important carbohydrates and lipids produced in plants by molecular farming (metabolic engineering)

Compound	Transgenic plant(s)	Application(s)
Carbohydrates		
Amylose-free starch (amylopectin starch)	Potato	Food, industrial
High amylose starch	Potato	Food, industrial
Cyclodextrins	Potato	Food, pharmaceutical
Fructans	Tobacco, maize, potato, sugarbeet	Industrial, food
Trehalose	Tobacco	Food stabilizer
Lipids		
Medium chain fatty acids	Oil seed rape	Food, industrial, detergent
Mono-unsaturated fatty acids	Tobacco	Food
Saturated fatty acids	Oil seed rape	Food, confectioneries
Bioplastics (polyhydroxybutyrate)	Cotton, oil seed rape	Biodegradable plastics

TREHALOSE

Trehalose is a disaccharide produced in plants and microorganisms in response to osmotic stress. Genetic manipulations have been successfully carried out for enhanced synthesis of trehalose to withstand abiotic stress (that cause water deficit).

Trehalose is useful as a food preservative. Some workers are attempting to produce trehalose in bulk quantities for its utility in food industries.

METABOLIC ENGINEERING OF LIPIDS

Plant oils are useful as foods (about two thirds), and for industrial purposes (about one third). The industrial applications of plant oils include their use in the manufacture of soaps, detergents, lubricants and biofuels.

An outline of the synthesis of oils (chemically triacylglycerols) is depicted in ***Fig 51.2***. There is an involvement of plastids, cytoplasm and endoplasmic reticulum for the production of oils. After their synthesis, oils are stored in lipid bodies.

Acetate from the cytoplasm is taken up by the plastids and converted to acetyl CoA and malonyl CoA. These two molecules undergo a series of reactions, catalysed by the enzyme fatty acid synthase (FAS), to produce fatty acyl carrier proteins with different carbons atoms. Some examples are listed.

- Laurate — C_{12}
- Myristate — C_{14}
- Palmitate — C_{16}
- Stearate — C_{18}
- Oleate — $C_{18:1}$

By the action of acyl-ACP thioesterases, the fatty acids are released and exported to the cytoplasm. Here, they may undergo certain modifications — elongation, desaturation (insertion of double bonds), hydroxylation etc. These modified fatty acids react with glycerol 3-phosphate (in the endoplasmic reticulum) to finally form triacylglycerols (TG). TG are transported to lipid oil bodies and stored. The oil bodies of seeds also contain proteins called ***oleosins***, in the lipid monolayers (for discussion on oleosins, See p. 631).

Some of the approaches of genetic engineering for the manipulation of plant oil biosynthesis are briefly described.

PRODUCTION OF SHORTER CHAIN FATTY ACIDS

Majority of the plant oils contain more than 16-carbons e.g. palmitic, stearic, oleic acids. Oils with shorter chains (C_8—C_{14}) are more useful in

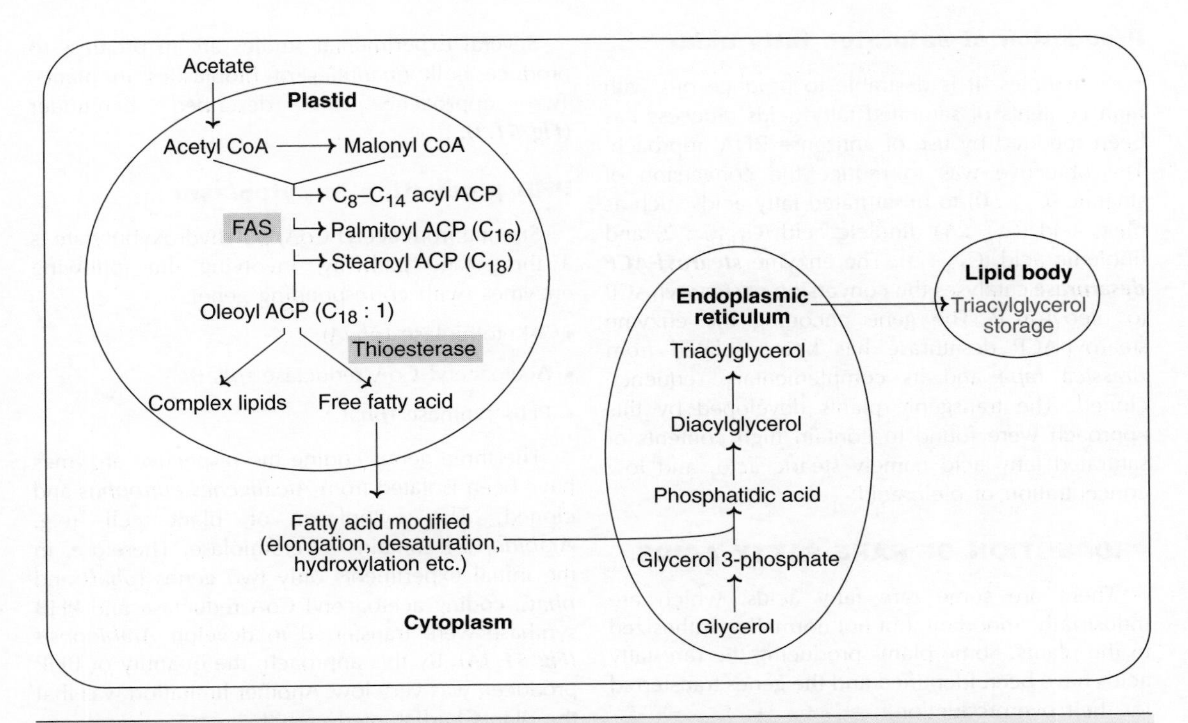

Fig. 51.2 : An outline of the biosynthesis of triacylglycerols in plants (FAS-Fatty acid synthase; ACP-Acyl carrier protein).

many industries — for the production of soaps, detergents, cosmetics etc.

It is possible to terminate the hydrolysis of acyl-ACP by specific thioesterases and produce high proportion of selected fatty acids. One acyl-ACP thioesterase that specifically hydrolyses lauroyl-ACP has been isolated from California bay tree (*Umbellularia californica*). The gene encoding this enzyme has been cloned and transferred to oilseed rape. The transgenic plants were found to produce oils with high proportion of lauric acid (12-carbon fatty acid).

PRODUCTION OF LONGER CHAIN FATTY ACIDS

For the application as industrial oils, triacylglycerols with longer chain fatty acids ($> C_{18}$) are preferred. Thus, erucic acid (22C) containing oils are useful in industries. However, erucic acid is unsuitable for human consumption.

By conventional plant breeding two distinct crops of oilseed rape have been developed — ***high-erucic acid rape (HEAR)*** and ***low-erucic acid rape (LEAR)***.

Some attempts are being made to genetically manipulate crops to yield oils with high contents of erucic acid. The approaches include to overexpress genes encoding the enzymes elongases and transfer of genes to produce enzymes that can preferentially incorporate erucic acid into triacylglycerols.

PRODUCTION OF FATTY ACIDS WITH MODIFIED DEGREE OF SATURATION

A fatty acid is said to be saturated if it has no double bonds. Saturated and unsaturated (with on or more double bonds) fatty acids occur in nature. It is possible to genetically manipulate the degree of saturation in fatty acids.

Production of unsaturated fatty acids

Oleic acid (C_{18} : 1) rich oils are useful as food, feed and in some industries. There has been some success in the transfer of antisense gene encoding the enzyme ***desaturase*** in oilseed rape and soybean plants. These transgenic plants were found to produce oils with very high proportion of oleic acid.

Production of saturated fatty acids

Sometimes, it is desirable to produce oils with high contents of saturated fatty acids. Success has been reported by use of antisense RNA approach. The objective was to reduce the conversion of stearate (C_{18} : 0) to unsaturated fatty acids such as oleic acid (C_{18} : 1), linoleic acid (C_{1818} : 2) and linolenic acid (C_{18} : 3). The enzyme ***stearoyl-ACP desaturase*** catalyses the conversion of stearoyl-ACP to oleoyl-ACP. The gene encoding the enzyme stearoyl-ACP desaturase has been isolated from *Brassica rapa* and its complementary sequence cloned. The transgenic plants developed by this approach were found to contain high contents of saturated fatty acid namely stearic acid, and low concentration of oleic acid.

PRODUCTION OF RARE FATTY ACIDS

There are some rare fatty acids, which are industrially important, but not normally synthesized in the plants. Some plants producing the rare fatty acids have been identified and the genes transferred for their overproduction.

One good example is the production of ***petroselenic acid*** that is found in coriander. Tobacco plants were transformed with coriander ***acyl-ACP desaturase*** that led to a high production of petroselenic acid in tobacco plants. Petroselenic acid is commercially important. On oxidation by ozone, it forms lauric acid (for use in soap and detergent production) and adipic acid (for the manufacture of nylon).

Some success has also been reported in the increased production of several unsaturated fatty acids through genetic manipulation by incorporating genes coding special enzymes namely ***front-end desaturases*** e.g. γ-linolenic acid, arachidonic acid, ricolenic acid.

BIODEGRADABLE PLASTICS (BIOPLASTICS)

Biodegradable plastics (or bioplastics) are chemically ***polyhydroxy alkanoates (PHAs)***. They are currently being produced in large quantities by microbial fermentation. The structures and the biosynthetic pathways for the production of PHAs are given in Chapter 30. Among the PHAs, ***polyhydroxy butyrate*** (PHB) is the most important one.

Several experimental studies are in progress to produce bulk quantities of bioplastics in plants. Two approaches are described hereunder (***Fig 51.3***).

PHB production in cytoplasm

Starting from acetyl CoA, polyhydroxybutyrate is a three-stage pathway, involving the following enzymes (with corresponding gene).

- 3-Ketothiolase (*phaA*).
- Acetoacetyl CoA reductase (*phaB*).
- PHB synthase (*phaC*).

The three genes coding the respective enzymes have been isolated from *Alcaligenes eutrophus* and cloned. The cytoplasm of plant cell (e.g. *Arabidopsis*) contains 3-ketothiolase. Therefore, in the initial experiments only two genes (*phaB* and *phaC*) coding acetoacetyl CoA reductase and PHB synthase were transferred to develop *Arabidopsis* (***Fig 51.3A***). By this approach, the quantity of BHP produced was very low. Another limitation was that the plants had stunted growth.

PHB production in plastids

The problems encountered in the above approach were overcome by transferring all three genes (*phaA, phaB, phaC*) of PHB synthesis and targeting them to chloroplast (***Fig 51.3B***). To achieve this, each gene was separately fused with a coding sequence of transit peptid bound to N-terminal fragment of ***Rubisco*** (ribulose 1,5-bisphosphate carboxylase) subunit protein. The genes expression was carried out by CaMV 35S promoter. Transgenic *Arabidopsis* plants with each gene construct were first developed. Then a series of sexual crossings were carried out between the individual transformants. The transgenic plants developed by this approach yielded good quantity of bioplastics (about 14% dry weight of the plant), and in addition there was no observable adverse affect on the growth or fertility of these plants.

Production of bioplastics in cotton fibres

Cotton fibres contains the enzyme β-ketothiolase. Therefore, the genes for the other two enzymes of PHB pathway (*phaB* and *phaC*) from *Alcaligenes eutrophus* were transferred into meristems of cotton

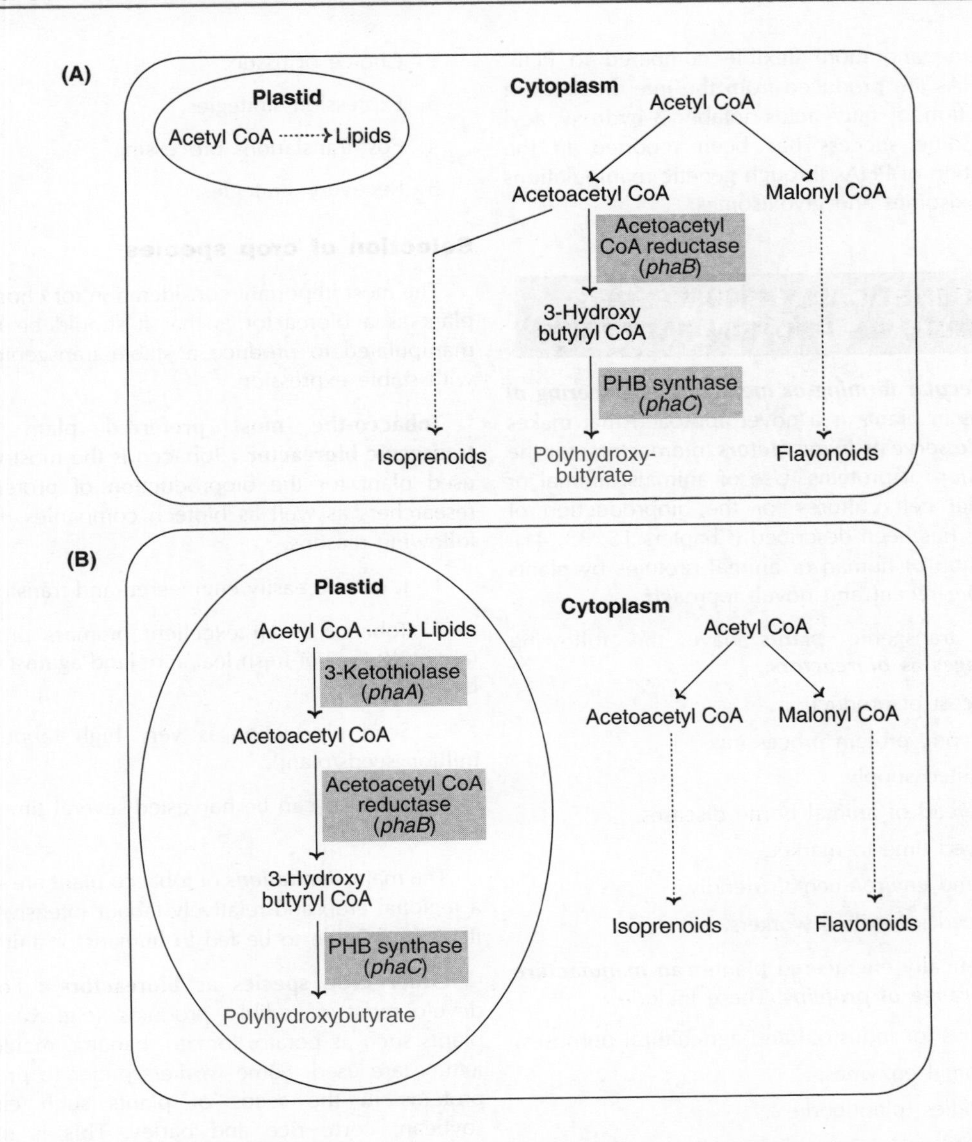

Fig. 51.3 :** Development of transgenic* Arabidopsis *for the biosynthesis of polyhydroxybutyrate (PHB) (A) Cytoplasmic synthesis of PHB (B) Chloroplast (plastid) synthesis of PHB (**Note : phaA, phaB *and* phaC *represent genes for the corresponding enzymes).*

plant by particle bombardment. Adequate synthesis of PHB was reported in the fibres of transgenic cotton plants.

Production of polyhydroxyalkanoate co-polymers

The most important bioplastic of commercial importance is polyhydroxybutyrate. The genetic engineering approaches for its manufacture in plants are described above. But the disadvantage with PHB production is that it is found as stiff and bristle plastics, since it forms highly crystalline polymers.

The other bioplastic, composed of polylydroxyalkanoate (PHA) co-polymer is a polymer made up of longer monomers. It is less crystalline and more flexible compared to PHB. The PHAs are produced from the intermediates of β-oxidation of fatty acids-notably 3-hydroxy acyl CoA. Some success has been reported in the production of PHAs through genetic manipulations of peroxisomes and glyoxisomes.

GENETICALLY ENGINEERED PLANTS AS PROTEIN FACTORIES

Molecular farming or metabolic engineering of proteins in plants is a novel approach that makes ***plants to serve as living factors*** (bioreactors) for the production of proteins. Use of animals, animal or microbial cell cultures for the bioproduction of proteins has been described (Chapters 15, 33, 41). Production of human or animal proteins by plants is a more recent and novel approach.

The transgenic ***plants*** have the following ***advantages as bioreactors.***

- Low cost of production.
- Eukaryotic protein processing.
- Unlimited supply.
- No spread of animal borne diseases.
- Reduced time to market.
- Safe and environmental friendly.
- No need for skilled workers.

Genetically engineered plants ***can manufacture a wide range of proteins***. These include :

- Enzymes for industrial and agricultural purposes.
- Lysosomal enzymes.
- Antibodies (plantibodies).
- Subunit vaccines.
- Other biopharmaceuticals or medically related proteins.

The general approaches for the production of desired proteins in plants are first described, followed by the different products of commercial importance.

APPROACHES FOR PROTEIN PRODUCTION IN PLANTS

The general methodology for the production of proteins in plants involves the following aspects

1. Selection of crop species.
2. Choice of tissue.
3. Expression strategies.
4. Post-translations processing.
5. Recovery strategies.

Selection of crop species

The most important consideration for choosing a plant as a bioreactor is that it should be readily manipulated to produce a stable transgenic line, with stable expression.

Tobacco-the most preferred plant as a transgenic bioreactor : Tobacco is the most widely used plant for the bioproduction of proteins by researchers as well as biotech companies, for the following reasons.

1. It can be easily engineered and transformed.

2. Tobacco is an excellent biomass producer (about 40 tons of fresh leaf/acre land against 4 tons by rice).

3. Seed production is very high (about one million seeds/plant).

4. Tobacco can be harvested several times in a year.

The major ***limitations*** of tobacco plant are — it is a regional crop and relatively labour intensive, and it is not suitable to be fed to humans or animals.

Other crop species as bioreactors : For the development of edible products (e.g. vaccines) plants such as potato, tomato, banana, maize and lettuce are used. Some workers prefer to produce proteins in the seeds of plants such canola, soybean, corn, rice and barley. This is mainly because seeds can accumulate and store good quantities of proteins.

Choice of tissue

The preferred tissues for protein production by plants include leaves, storage organs (e.g. tubers) and seeds. This choice of tissue mainly depends on the following factors.

- Compatibility with the desired protein.
- Correct processing.
- Stable accumulation.
- Efficiency of recovery.

Many proteins have been produced in leaves (particularly using tobacco plant) e.g. lysosomal enzymes, mammalian antibodies, human serum albumin.

In recent years, seeds have become an attractive high protein production (e.g. hirudin) vehicles due to good storage capacity and stability. It is no surprise that some of the seed proteins retain their biological activity for several years. One limitation of seeds is that it is sometimes difficult to recover the protein.

Expression strategies

There are two major approaches for the transgene expression in plants to produce proteins-stable integration approach and use of plant viruses as transient vectors.

1. **Stable integration approach** : This strategy is most suitable for the bulk production of proteins particularly in leaves. In this approach, the transgene is regulated by a strong constitutive promoter such as 35S promoter. Another alternative is to use tissue-specific promoter. By restricting the transgene expression to a particular tissue (e.g. seed), the yield of the protein can be substantially increased. In addition, the protein is stable for a long time from weeks to years.

A diagrammatic representation of stable gene expression approach for protein production is depicted in ***Fig 51.4.***

2. **Transient expression by using plant viruses :** Bioproduction strategies involving viruses are useful for the protein production at the desired period (discrete period). By genetic manipulations, it is possible to insert the desired gene (for protein) into the coat protein gene of the virus genome. The so developed infectious RNA viruses are introduced into the plants for the production of proteins.

Transient expression system by viruses has been successfully used in tobacco plants by employing tobacco mosaic virus (TMV). Tobacco plants at an appropriate age were inoculated with genetically modified TMV. Recombinant protein could be extracted within 2-3 weeks of harvesting.

Post-translational processing

The ultimate purpose of the use of plants as bioreactors is to produce proteins with native conformation, good biological activity and biocompatibility. The specific folding of the protein with disulfide bonds and suitably modified amino acids is important for this purpose.

The changes that occur after (or sometimes even during) the protein is synthesized are collectively referred to as post-translational modifications e.g. phosphorylation, hydroxylation, carboxylation, glycosylation, proteolytic processing etc. Variations in post-translational changes are often limiting the successful production and use of recombinant proteins either in plants or even in other systems (transgenic animals or cell cultures).

The major ***limitations of plants*** with regard to post-translational modifications of proteins are listed.

- Glycosylation (incorporation of carbohydrate moiety) is different in plants.
- Plant glycosylation results in the production of complex glycans containing fucose or xylose, which do not occur in humans.
- Plants cannot perform specialized carboxylation necessary for certain clotting factors (II, VII, IX, and X) and enzymes (protein C).

Due to above limitations, many a times proteins of transgenic plants are inefficient or less efficient in their function, besides exhibiting immunogenecity.

In recent years, cloning of genes responsible for post-translational modifications of proteins (e.g. glycation, carboxylation) have met with success to produce more biologically active proteins.

Recovery strategies (purification strategies)

A rational approach for a cost-effective purification strategy is desirable for the recovery of the proteins (downstream processing) produced in transgenic plants. The degree of purity is dependent on the purpose for which the protein is produced. For instance, industrial enzymes in general, do not require high degree of purity. Sometimes, purification may not be necessary at all. A good example is the production of the enzyme phytase in seeds. Phytase acts on phytate and increases the availability of phosphate to animals. For this purpose, milled transgenic seeds containing phytase can be directly added to the feed. This totally avoids the purification/downstream processing costs.

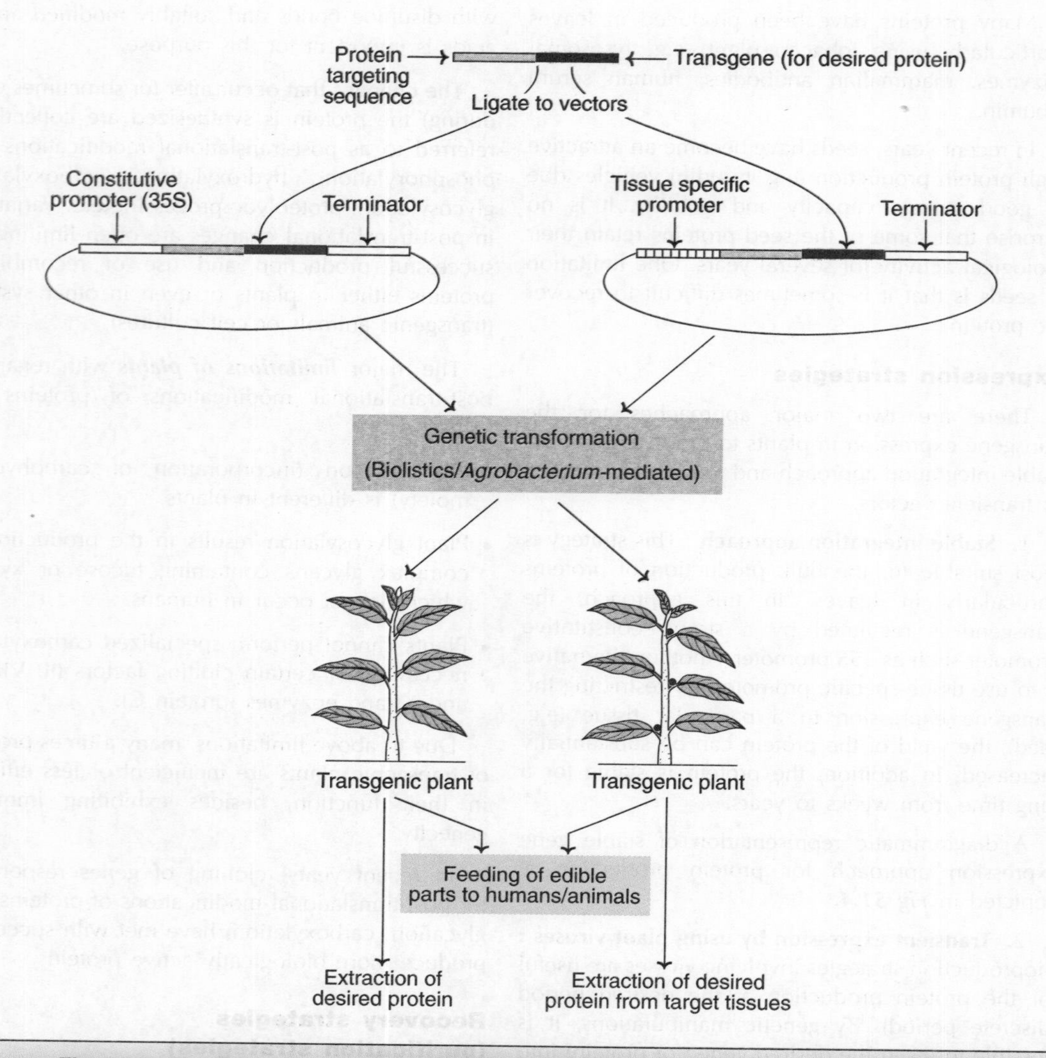

Fig. 51.4 : Stable gene expression strategy for the production of desired proteins in plants.

For a great majority of proteins, particularly pharmaceutical proteins, purification strategy is absolutely required. It is therefore necessary to develop efficient methods for downstream processing. Some of the recovery strategies are briefly described.

Affinity tag-based purification : The use of affinity tags for the purification of recombinant proteins has been described elsewhere (Chapter 11), and a similar strategy works in plant systems as well. The technique involves the fusion of desired protein with another protein or peptide (tag), which can bind to ligand, and thus the protein can be isolated. Following purification of the desired protein, the affinity tag can be removed. Some workers have been successful in purifying the enzyme ***glucocerebrosidase*** by this approach.

Purification through compartmentalization : It is possible to direct the accumulation of proteins in a specific sub-cellular organelle. This is achieved by using signal peptides or fusion peptides. Once the protein is localized, the technique of sub-cellular fractionation can be used for preliminary isolation of protein followed by its purification.

The human neuropeptide leu-eukephalin has been compartmentalized in the endoplasmic reticulum and vacuoles by this strategy. Then by appropriate purification techniques, it is isolated.

Protein purification by production in oil bodies : Oil bodies are natural sub-cellular organelles that store triacylglycerols (TG). Oil bodies are composed of triacylglycerols enveloped by a phospholipid monolayer. A group of proteins, referred to as ***oleosins*** are associated with the surface of the oil bodies.

Oil bodies are found in the oil/seeds that represent the storage form of energy (as TG). Oil seeds contain oleosin at a concentration in the range of 2–10% of the total seed proteins.

Oil bodies can be used for the production of foreign proteins in plants. The development of transgenic plants and the purification of the desired protein by employing oil bodies are shown in ***Fig. 51.5***.

A transgene with oleosin and desired protein can be constructed. By introducing this gene, transgenic plants are developed. Oleosins tolerate foreign proteins; hence it is possible to produce oleosin-fusion proteins that accumulate in the oil bodies.

The plant materials (mainly seeds oil bodies) are crushed and centrifuged to separate into three fractions.

- A pellet of insoluble plant material at the bottom of the tube.
- An aqueous phase containing soluble components of the seeds at the middle.
- A floating layer at the top with oil bodies and their associated oleosin fusion proteins.

The top layer of oil bodies is isolated, resuspended in a buffer and re-centrifuged. The concentrated oil bodies are treated with the proteolytic enzyme protease that cleaves the desired protein from oleosin. On further centrifugation, the pharmaceutically important protein (aqueous phase) can be separated from the oil bodies.

OLEOSIN PARTITION TECHNOLOGY

The ***purification of foreign proteins through their production in oil bodies*** (described above) is referred to as oleosin partition technology (***Fig 51.5***). The oil bodies along with the oleosin-fusion proteins are quite stable within the seed and during the course of processing. The pharmaceutical protein of interest remains stable retaining its biological activity within the seeds for years. Further, the purification oleosin-fusion proteins is relatively easier. Hence oleosin partition technology is preferred for the purification of many pharmaceutically important proteins. Two functional proteins namely ***hirudin*** and ***β-glucuronidase*** have been recovered by oleosin partition technology.

Production of hirudin in *Brassica napus*

Hirudin is a natural anticoagulant protein produced in the salivary glands of leeches (*Hirudo medicinalis*). It is an effective therapeutic agent as it specifically inhibits thrombin and blocks blood coagulation.

Till sometime ago, hirudin was produced by employing bacteria and yeasts. The annual requirement of hirudin is very high, and it is a good candidate for producing in transgenic plants.

A synthetic gene encoding hirudin was fused with *Arabidopsis* oleosin gene. An endopeptidase factor Xa gene was inserted between hirudin and oleosin genes. (The endopeptidase gene serves as a recognition site for the protease action). The transgene construct was introduced into *Brassica napus.* The so developed transgenic plants produce oil bodies containing ***oleosin-hirudin fusion protein***. Hirudin can be purified by the procedure described already and depicted in ***Fig 51.5.***

Oleosin partition technology holds a great promise for the successful commercial production of several pharmaceutically important proteins.

PRODUCTION OF INDUSTRIAL ENZYMES IN PLANTS

There is an ever-growing demand for industrial enzymes. Existing sources may not be able to meet the requirements. Large-scale production of plant-derived transgenic enzymes for commercial and industrial purposes are preferred. Besides several advantages of plants as bioreactors (See p. 628), there is no fear of spread of animal pathogens (like BSE) as is the case with animal production.

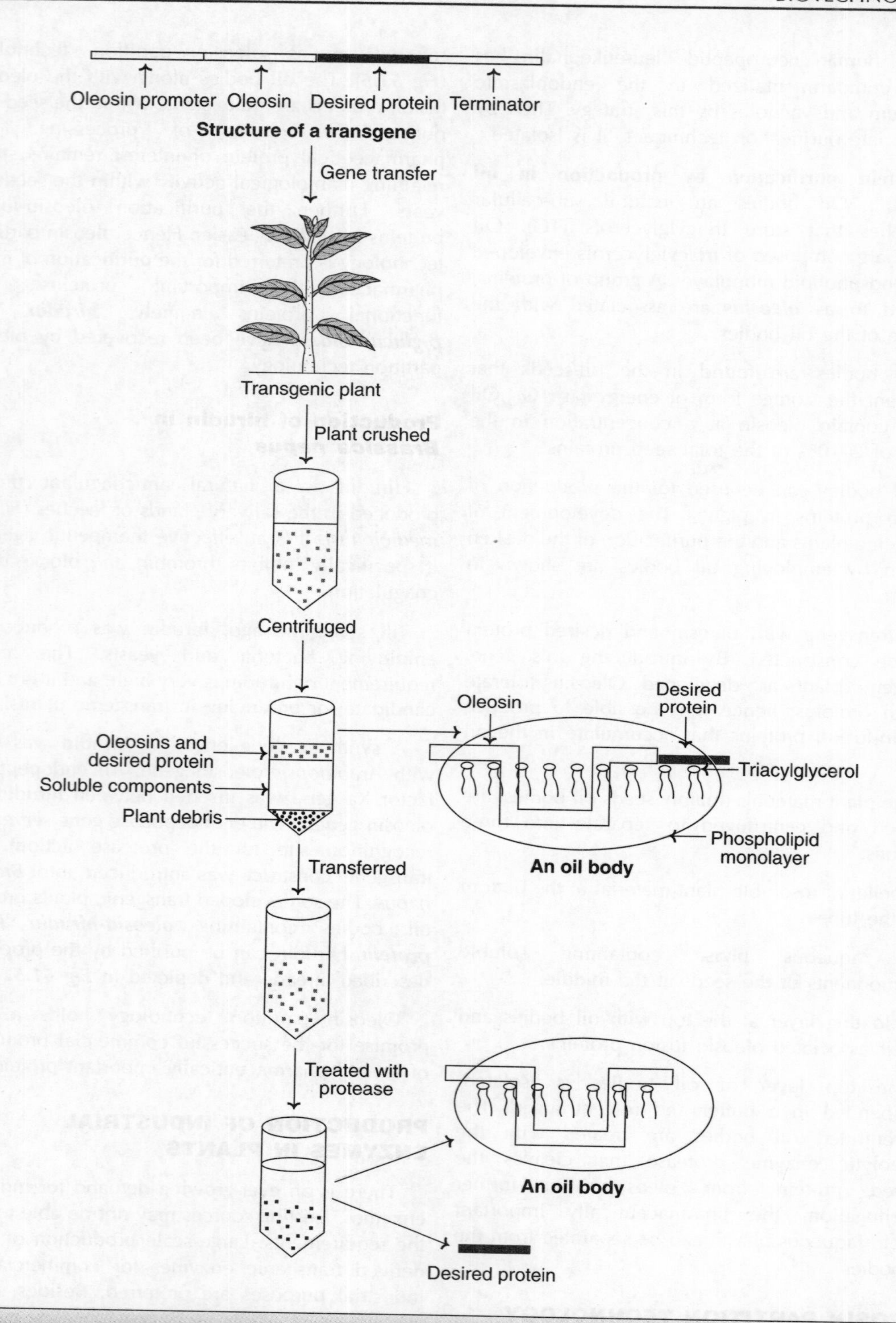

*Fig. 51.5 : The purification strategy of a desired (pharmaceutical) protein by production in oil bodies (**oleosin partition technology**).*

TABLE 51.2 Selected examples of industrial enzymes produced in plants and their application(s)

Enzyme	*Application(s)*
α-Amylase	Food processing
Avidin	In diagnostic kits
Cellulase	Production of alcohol from wastes (cellulose)
β-Glucanase	In brewing industry
β-Glucuronidase	In diagnostic kits
Lignin peroxidase	In paper manufacture
Phytase	Improved phosphate utilization (by phytate breakdown)
Trypsin	Pharmaceutical
Xylanase	Biomass processing, paper and textile industries

A selected list of industrial enzymes produced in transgenic plants and their important applications is given in ***Table 51.2.*** Some of the important enzymes are described.

Avidin and β-glucuronidase

The first proteins/enzymes that were produced in transgenic plants (maize) are avidin and β-glucuronidase. They are used in diagnostic kits.

Trypsin

Trypsin is an important proteolytic enzyme and its production by conventional recombinant approaches is rather difficult. Trypsin is now produced in plants. It has a wide range of applications-for the production of insulin, vaccines, wound care etc.

Phytase

Phytase is a hydrolytic enzyme that catalyses the hydrolysis of phytate (inositol hexaphosphate) to inositol and inorganic phosphate.

Phytate is present in high quantities in many plant seeds used as a feed to pigs and poultry (monogastric animals). These animals do not possess the enzyme phytase; hence they cannot derive the nutrient phosphate from phytate. The undigested phytate gets excreted and accumulates in the soil and water, leading to eutrophication.

Transgenic plants capable of synthesizing phytase in their seeds have been developed. These seeds (no need to isolate the enzyme) can be mixed with the feed of animals, and fed. The phytase enzyme has successfully solved nutritional (phosphate) and environmental (eutrophication) problems.

Cellulase and xylanase

The two enzymes namely cellulase and xylanase are used in several industries- bioethanol, textile, paper and pulp. In all these processes, they are basically involved in the degradation of plant materials (predominantly cellulose).

By a novel approach, it is possible to produce cellulase and xylanase in the plants for which the target itself is the digestion of plant cell. The risk of autodigestion of the plant cells (by these enzymes) is overcome by genetic manipulation to produce thermostable enzymes. Thus, cellulase and xylanase, produced by transgenic plants, are inactive at the temperatures at which plants normally grow. The activity of these enzymes is restored on heating the plant extracts. And these extracts are very successfully used in many industries.

While the recovery of enzymes from transgenic plants is often required, there are some instances where the crude extracts can be directly used. The industrial applications of cellulase, xylanase and phytase (described above) are some good examples.

PRODUCTION OF LYSOSOMAL ENZYMES IN PLANTS

Lysosomes are the cellular organelles responsible for the degradation of macromolecules. The degradative enzymes present in lysosomes include proteases, nucleases, lipases, glycosidases, phosphatases, phospolipases and sulfatases. Deficiency of a specific lysosomal enzyme results in the accumulation of undegraded substrate causing clinical manifestations. Some examples of lysosomal disorders and the corresponding enzyme deficiencies are listed below.

- Tay-Sachs disease — α-hexosaminidase.
- Gaucher's disease — glucocerebrosidase.
- Hurler syndrome — iduronidase.

- Mucopolysaccharidoses (a group of diseases) — Several enzyme of glycosaminoglycan degradation.

A couple of lysosomal enzymes produced in transgenic tobacco plants are described below.

Glucocerebrosidase

Glucocerebrosidase is a lysosomal enzyme that degrades glucocerebroside (predominantly produced when erythrocytes are destroyed due to aging or damage) to glucose and ceramide. The deficiency of this enzyme causes Gaucher's disease, characterized by swelling of spleen, liver, and bone damage causing extreme pain.

Gaucher's disease can be effectively ***treated by*** administering ***the enzyme glucocerebrosidase***. At present, this enzyme is obtained from human placenta or from mammalian cell cultures, both being very costly. It is estimated that a single patient requires 10–12 tons of human placenta annually costing $100,000 to 400,000!

Glucocerebroside was the first lysosomal enzyme ***produced*** in plants (***Nicotiana tobacum***). The production process of this enzyme has been patented, and FDA approved it for use in humans. It is hoped that through the plant-based production of glucocerebrosidase (marketed as ***Cerezyme***), the patients of Gaucher's disease can be treated in a cost-effective manner.

α-L-Iduronidase

The deficiency of the enzyme iduronidase causes Hurler's syndrome, the most common disorder of defective mucopolysaccharide degradation.

Tobacco plants have been genetically engineered to produce α-L-iduronidase.

Limitations for the production of lysosomal enzymes in plants

Both the enzymes referred above are glycoproteins (glucocerebrosidase and iduronidase). As described elsewhere (See p. 629), appropriate glycation of animal proteins is not feasible in plants. This poses a major problem for the production of lysosomal enzymes in plants. Through a series of genetic manipulations, biotechnologists were successful in achieving the desired glycation for the production glucocerebrosidase and iduronidase.

PRODUCTION OF ANTIBODIES (PLANTIBODIES) IN PLANTS

Antibodies or immunoglobulins are the defense proteins produced in mammals. For details on the structure and functions of different immunoglobulins, refer Chapter 68.

The use of plants for commercial production of antibodies, referred to as plantibodies, is a novel approach in biotechnology. The first successful production of a functional antibody, namely a mouse immunoglobulin IgGI in plants, was reported in 1989. This was achieved by developing two transgenic tobacco plants-one synthesizing heavy γ-chain and the other light κ-chain, and crossing them to generate progeny that can produce an assembled functional antibody.

Production of secretory IgA (sIgA)

Secretory IgA is an immunoglobulin that protects against dental caries produced by *Streptococcus mutans*. For the production of sIgA, transgenic plants were developed to synthesize different subunits and then crossed to produce the functional antibody (***Fig 51.6***).

Four separate transgenic plants synthesizing four distinct pieces of antibody (H-, L-, J-chains and secretory component) were developed. The plants expressing H- and L-chains were crossed (cross 1) giving plants that produce IgA. When these plants were crossed (cross 2) with plants expressing J-chain, the progeny produced dimeric IgA. The dimeric IgA synthesizing plants were then crossed (cross 3) with the plants expressing secretory component, the functional sIgA could be produced.

Secretory antibodies have many advantages. They are resistant to proteolytic degradation; hence their yield in plants is substantially higher. sIgA are the predominant antibodies that protect against mucosal infections of microorganisms. They bind to antigens more effectively and offer good protection.

The secretory antibodies produced in transgenic plants have been tested on humans. When sIgA was topically applied to teeth, it could prevent the colonization by *Streptococcus mutans* up to 4 months. This is comparable to the protection offered by immunoglobulins produced through hybridoma technology. This was possible despite some structural differences between plantibodies and monoclonal antibodies. It appears that there is no difference in the binding properties between the two types of antibodies.

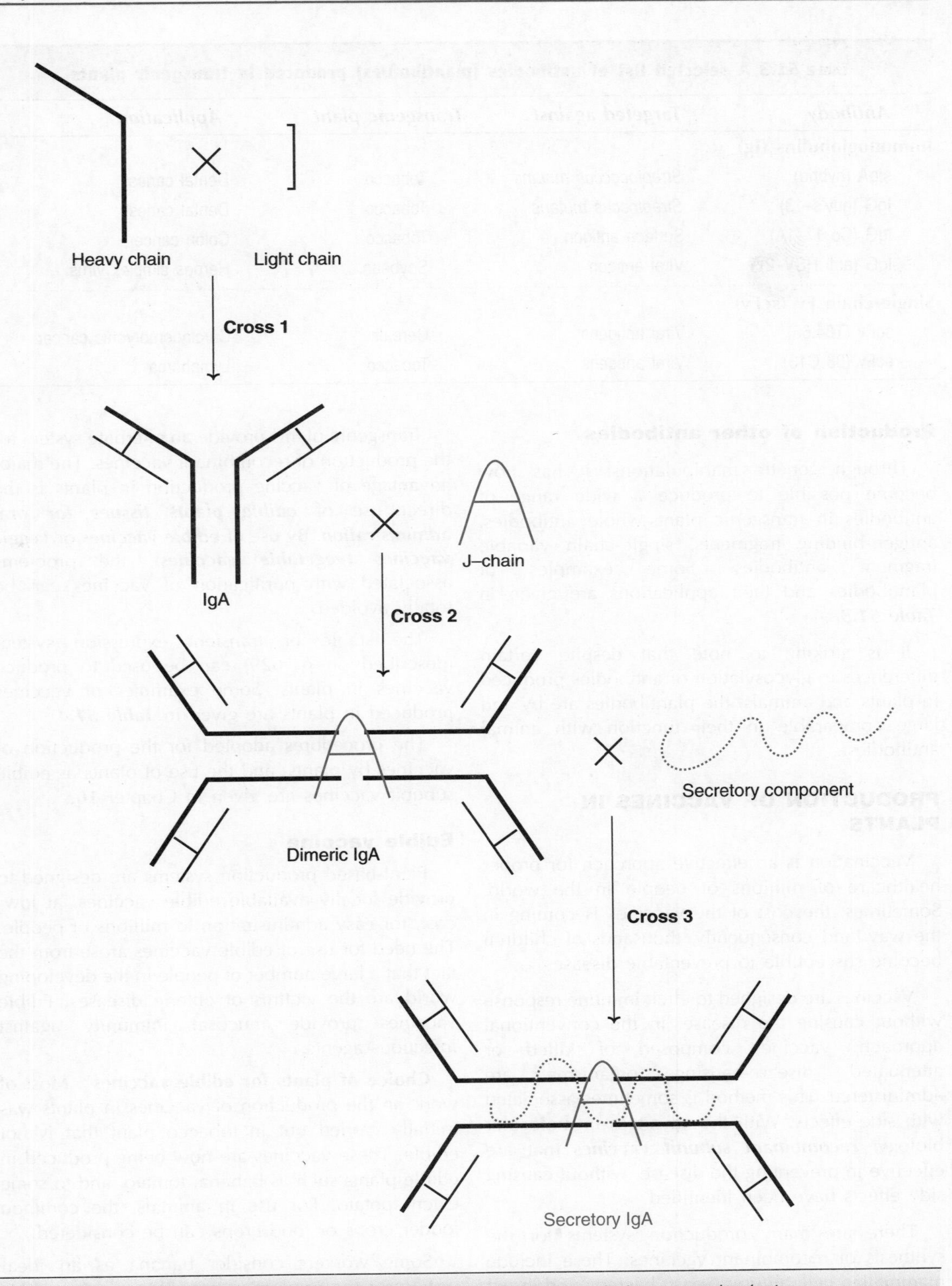

Fig. 51.6 : Production of secretory IgA (sIgA) molecule in transgenic plants.

Table 51.3 A selected list of antibodies (plantibodies) produced in transgenic plants

Antibody	*Targeted against*	*Transgenic plant*	*Application*
Immunoglobulins (Ig)			
sIgA (hybrid)	*Streptococcus mutans*	Tobacco	Dental caries
IgG (guy's–13)	*Streptoccus mutans*	Tobacco	Dental caries
IgG (Co 17–1A)	Surface antigen	Tobacco	Colon cancer
IgG (anti HSV–2)	Viral antigen	Soybean	Herpes simplex virus
Single-chain Fv (scFv)			
scFv (T84.66)	Viral antigens	Cereals	Carcinoembryonic cancer
scFv (38 C13)	Viral antigens	Tobacco	Lymphoma

Production of other antibodies

Through genetic manipulations, it has now become possible to produce a wide range of antibodies in transgenic plants-whole antibodies, antigen-binding fragments, single-chain variable fragment antibodies. Some examples of plantibodies and their applications are given in ***Table 51.3.***

It is striking to note that despite certain differences in glycosylation of antibodies produced in plants and animals, the plantibodies are by and large comparable in their function with animal antibodies.

PRODUCTION OF VACCINES IN PLANTS

Vaccination is an effective approach for proper healthcare of millions of people in the world. Sometimes, the cost of the vaccines is coming in the way, and consequently, thousands of children become susceptible to preventable diseases.

Vaccines are designed to elicit immune response without causing the disease. In the conventional approach, vaccines composed of killed or attenuated disease-causing organisms are administered. This method is sometimes associated with side effects. With the advances in molecular biology, ***recombinant subunit vaccines*** that are effective in preventing the disease, without causing side effects have been identified.

There are many production systems for the synthesis of recombinant vaccines. These include mammalian cell cultures, yeast, bacteria and insect cell cultures, and transgenic animals.

Transgenic plants provide an alternate system for the production of recombinant vaccines. The major advantage of vaccine production in plants is the direct use of ***edible plants tissues for oral administration***. By use of ***edible vaccines*** or ***veggie vaccines*** (***vegetable vaccines***), the problems associated with purification of vaccines can be totally avoided.

The stable or transient expression system (described on p. 629) can be used to produce vaccines in plants. Some examples of vaccines produced in plants are given in ***Table 51.4***.

The procedures adopted for the production of vaccines by plants, and the use of plants as edible subunit vaccines are given in Chapter 16.

Edible vaccine

Plant-based production systems are designed to provide locally available edible vaccines, at low-cost, for easy administration to millions of people. The need for use of edible vaccines arose from the fact that a large number of people in the developing world are the victims of enteric diseases. Edible vaccines provide mucosal immunity against infectious agents.

Choice of plants for edible vaccines : Most of work on the production of vaccines in plants was initially carried out in tobacco plant that is not edible. These vaccines are now being produced in edible plants such as banana, tomato, and to some extent potato. For use in animals, the common fodder crops or food crops can be considered.

Some workers consider banana as an ideal system for the production of edible vaccines. This is mainly because it is grown in most parts of the

Table 51.4 Some examples of vaccines produced in transgenic plants

Recombinant protein (vaccine)	*Transgenic plant*	*Application (protection against)*
Human		
Heat-labile enterotoxin B	Tobacco	*E. coli*
Cholera Ctox A and Ctox B subunits	Potato	*Vibrio cholerae*
Envelope surface protein	Tobacco/potato	Hepatitis B
Capsid protein	Tobacco/potato	Morwalk virus
Rabies virus glycoprotein	Tomato	Rabies virus
Animal		
Virus epitope VP_1	Alfalfa/*Arabidopsis*	Foot and mouth virus
Viral epitope VP_2	Blackeyed bean	Milk enteritis virus
Viral glycoprotein	Maize/tobacco	Porcine coronavirus
Peptide from VP_2 capsid protein	*Arabidopsis*	Canine parvovirus

world, and eaten raw. Another advantage is that children (to whom vaccines are most needed) like eating banana.

The procedures adopted for the production of vaccines by plants, and the use of plants as edible subunit vaccines are given in Chapter 16.

Delivery of vaccine to the gut : Vaccines, being proteins, are likely to be degraded in the stomach. This is true to some extent. However, it is now known that the orally administered plant materials (edible vaccine) can induce immune response. The particulate materials of plants are more effective in this regard.

Food-based tablets to replace edible vaccines : It is true that the edible vaccines may work well in the laboratory or under controlled conditions. There is a difficulty of dose adjustment when edible vaccines are consumed as a part of foodstuff. Some workers prefer to discontinue the direct use of plant materials, and prefer to opt for food-based tablets containing a known dose of vaccine. This approach is being applied to vaccines produced in tomatoes.

Limitations of edible vaccines : Direct consumption of transgenic fruit or vegetable or food-based tablets may create some problems.

- The risk of loss of vaccines by the action of enzymes in stomach and intestine.
- The possibility of allergic reactions as they enter circulation.

The future of edible vaccines : Despite several limitations, biotechnologists see a great hope for the new wave of ***transgenic veggie vaccines.*** But it may take several years before the banana or tomato replaces the needle as a vehicle for vaccine delivery!

PRODUCTION OF THERAPEUTIC PROTEINS IN PLANTS

The general approaches, and the production of industrial enzymes, lysosomal enzymes, antibodies and vaccines in transgenic plants have been described in the proceeding pages. Many of these products actually represent therapeutic proteins or biopharmaceuticals e.g. lysosomal antibodies, vaccines. Therefore, they must also be referred again.

In ***Table 51.5,*** a selected list of therapeutic proteins, and the plants producing them, along with the applications is given.

The major ***limitations*** of protein production by transgenic plants are the ***low product yield and*** the difficulties associated with ***recovery.*** With improvements in genetic engineering and recovery processes, it is hoped that the production of therapeutic proteins will substantially increase in the coming years.

Chloroplasts in the production of therapeutic proteins

Chloroplasts are capable of folding the foreign proteins, besides bringing out most of the post-

TABLE 51.5 Selected examples of therapeutic proteins produced in transgenic plants

Therapeutic protein	*Transgenic plant*	*Application(s)*
Hemoglobin	Tobacco	Blood substitute
Serum albumin	Tobacco	Burns/fluid replacement, blood extender
Protein C	Tobacco	Anticoagulant
Hirudin	Canola	Anticoagulant
α_1-Interferon	Rice	Viral protection, anticancer
β-Interferon	Rice/tobacco/turnip	Treatment for hepatitis B + C
γ-Interferon	Tobacco	Phagocyte activator
Collagen	Tobacco	As collagen
Somatotrophin	Tobacco	As growth hormone
Trypsin inhibitor	Maize	Transplant surgery
α_1-Antitrypsin	Rice	Cystic fibrosis
Erythropoietin	Tobacco	As mitogen
Lactoferrin	Potato	Antimicrobial
Tissue growth factor	Tobacco	As mitogen
Enkephalin	Canola/*Arabidopsis*	Opiate
Angiotension converting enzyme	Tobacco/tomato	Hypertension
Glucocerebrosidase	Tobacco	Gaucher's disease
α-Galactosidase	Tobacco	Fabry disease
Trichosanthin-α	Tobacco	HIV therapy, cancer

translational modification. As the chloroplasts are inherited maternally, they will not spread via pollen to non-transgenic systems. This type of biotechnological approach will help to get clearance from the regulatory bodies of biotechnology. Some of the therapeutic proteins produced in chloroplasts are listed.

- Interferons
- Serum albumin
- Hemoglobin
- Proinsulin
- Monoclonal antibodies
- Protective antigen of *Bacillus anthracis.*

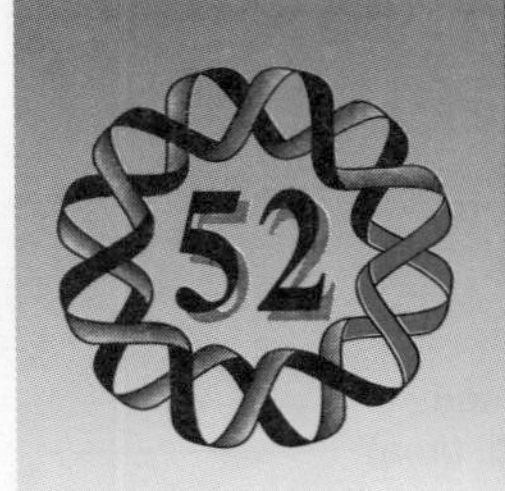

Growth-Promoting Bacteria in Plants

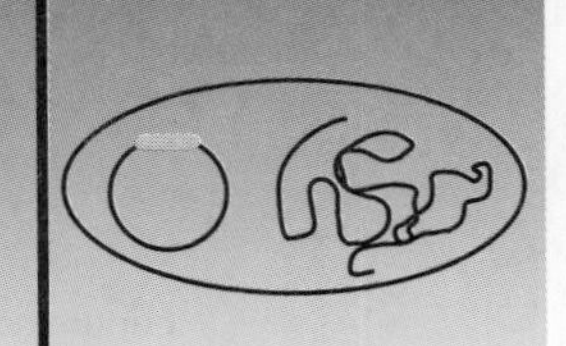

Certain beneficial microorganisms, present in the soil, are known to influence the plant growth, development and yield. These ***bacteria and fungi*** may ***provide growth-promoting products to plants or inhibit the growth of soil pathogenic microorganisms*** (phytopathogens), which hinder the plant growth. The former is the direct effect while the latter is the indirect effect of growth-promoting bacteria in plants.

The growth-promoting activity of micro-organisms and the biotechnological approaches are described briefly with respect to the following aspects.

1. Biological nitrogen fixation.
2. Biocontrol of phytopathogens.
3. Biofertilizers.

BIOLOGICAL NITROGEN FIXATION

Nitrogen is an essential element of many biomolecules, the most important being nucleic acids and amino acids. Although nitrogen is the most abundant gas (about 80%) in the atmosphere, neither animals nor plants can use this nitrogen to synthesize biological compounds. However, there are certain microorganisms on which the living plants (and animals) are dependent to bring nitrogen into their biological systems.

The phenomenon of ***fixation of atmospheric nitrogen by microorganisms*** is known as ***diazotrophy*** and these organisms are collectively referred to as ***diazotrophs***. Diazotrophs are biological nitrogen fixers, and are prokaryotic in nature.

NITROGEN CYCLE

An outline of the nitrogen cycle is depicted in ***Fig. 52.I.*** Nitrogen enters the soil with the deposits of dead animals and plants, and urea of urine. These waste materials (proteins, urea) are decomposed by soil bacteria into ammonia and other products. The ammonia is converted to nitrite (NO_2) and then nitrate (NO_3) by certain bacteria belonging to the genera *Nitrosomonas* and *Nitrobacter*. The nitrate is degraded by various microorganisms to release nitrogen that enters atmosphere. This atmospheric nitrogen is taken up by the nitrogen fixing bacteria (present on the roots of leguminous plants) and used for the synthesis of biomolecules (e.g. amino acids). As the animals consume the leguminous plants as food, the nitrogen cycle is complete.

NITROGEN FIXING BACTERIA

It is estimated that about 50% of the nitrogen needed by the plant comes from nitrogen fixing bacteria. These are two types of nitrogen fixing microorganisms-asymbiotic and symbiotic.

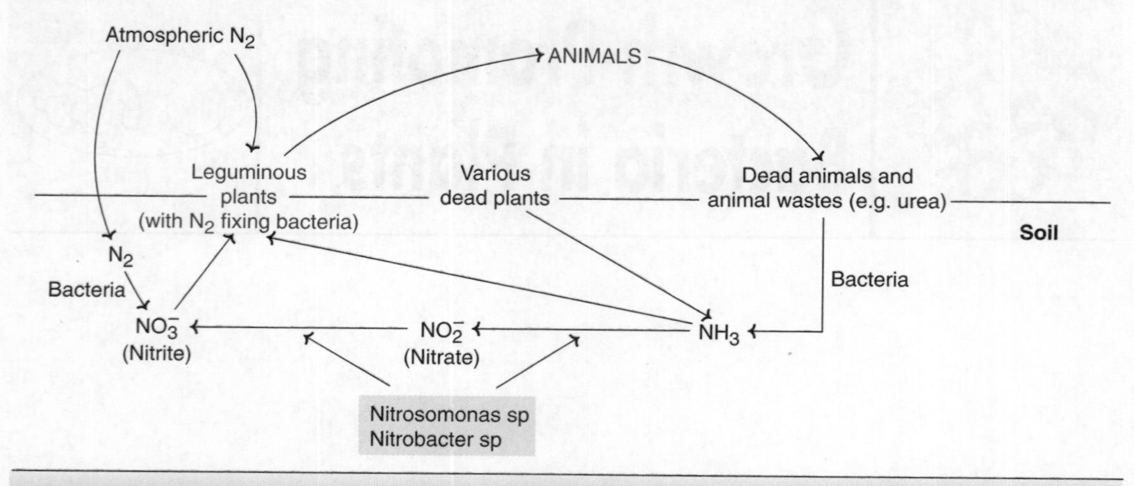

Fig. 52.1 : An outline of the nitrogen cycle.

Asymbiotic nitrogen fixing microorganisms

The gaseous nitrogen of the atmosphere is directly and independently utilized to produce nitrogen-rich compounds. When these non-symbiotic organisms die, they enrich the soil with nitrogenous compounds. Several species of bacteria and fungi can do this job e.g. *Clostridium pasturianum, Azatobacter chrooccum.*

The mechanism of nitrogen fixation by asymbiotic bacteria is not clearly understood. It is believed that nitrogen is first converted to hydroxylamine or ammonium nitrate, and then incorporated into biomolecules.

Symbiotic nitrogen fixing microorganisms

These microorganisms live together with the plants in a mutually beneficial relationship, phenomenon referred to as ***symbiosis***. The most important microorganisms involved in symbiosis belong to two related genera namely *Rhizobium* and *Bradyrhizobium*. These symbiotic bacteria also referred to as nodule bacteria are Gram negative, flagellated and rod-shaped. The host plants harbouring these bacteria are known as ***legumes*** e.g. soybean, peas, beans, alfalfa, peanuts, and clover.

Each one of the species of *Rhizobium* and *Bradyrizobium* are specific for a limited number of plants, which survive as the natural hosts (***Table 52.1***). It is now clearly known that these bacteria do not interact with plants other than the natural hosts.

The relationship between the symbiotic bacteria and the legumes is well recognized. On the roots of legumes, there are a number of nodules (swellings) in which *Rhizobium* sp thrive. These bacteria trap atmospheric nitrogen and synthesize nitrogen-rich compounds (amino acids, proteins etc) used by the legumes. At the same time, the legumes supply important nitrogen compounds for the metabolism of Rhizobia.

The growth of legumes has been known to enrich the soil fertility. This is due to the fact that the concentration of nitrogen compounds in the soil increases as a result of the presence of symbiotic bacteria. For this reason normally,

TABLE 52.1 Symbiotic nitrogen fixing bacteria along with the host plant(s)

Bacterial species	*Host plant(s)*
Rhizobium leguminosarum	Pea, broad bean
Rhizobium meliloti	Alfalfa
Rhizobium fredii	Soybean
Rhizobium loti	Lotus
Rhizobium elti	Mung bean, kidney bean
Rhizobium ciceri	Chickpea
Bradyrhizobium japonicum	Soybean
Bradyrhizobium elkanii	Soybean

nitrogen fertilizers are not needed in the fields cultivated legumes.

MECHANISM OF NITROGEN FIXATION

Inside the root nodules of leguminous plants, the bacteria proliferate. These bacteria exist in a form that has no cell wall.

The bacteria of the nodules are capable of fixing nitrogen by means of the specific enzyme namely ***nitrogenase.***

Nitrogenase

Nitrogenase is a complex enzyme containing two oxygen sensitive components. Component I has two α-protein subunits and two β-protein subunits, 24 molecules of iron, two molecules of molybdenum and an ***iron molybdenum cofactor (FeMoCo).*** Component II possesses two α-protein subunits (different from that of component I) and a large number of iron molecules.

Component I of nitrogenase catalyses the actual conversion of N_2 to ammonia while component II donates electrons to component I (***Fig. 52.2***).

Leghemoglobin

A protein comparable of hemoglobin in animals has been identified ***in the nodules of leguminous plants***. Leghemoglobin (***LHb***) contains iron and is red in colour. It is an oxygen binding protein. The heme part of leghemoglobin is synthesized by the bacterium while the protein (globin) portion is produced by the host plant. Leghemoglobin is absolutely necessary for nitrogen fixation. The nodules that lack LHb are not capable of fixing nitrogen.

It is LHb that facilitates the appropriate transfer of oxygen (by forming oxyLHb) to the bacteria for respiration to produce ATP. And energy in the form of ATP is absolutely required for nitrogen fixation.

Another important function of LHb is that it prevents the damaging effects of direct exposure of O_2 on nitrogenase.

In ***Fig. 52.2***, the fixation of nitrogen by symbiotic bacteria is depicted. As the oxyLHb supplies O_2, bacterial respiration occurs. The ATP generated is used for fixing nitrogen to produce ammonia. The complex reaction is summarized below.

$$N_2 + 8H^+ + 8e^- + 16\ ATP \downarrow 2NH_3 + H_2\uparrow + 16\ ADP + 16\ Pi$$

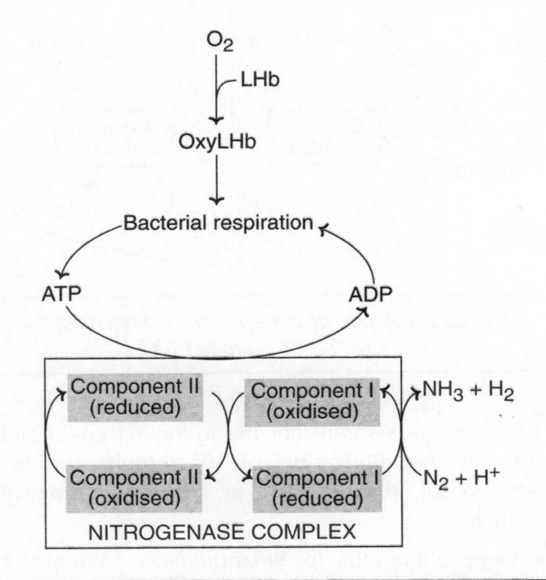

Fig. 52.2 : Nitrogen fixation in symbiotic bacteria.

Hydrogenase

During the course of nitrogen fixation by nitrogenase, an undesirable reaction also occurs. That is reduction of H^+ to H_2 (hydrogen gas). For the production of hydrogen, ATP is utilized, rather wasted. Consequently the efficiency of nitrogen fixation is drastically lowered. It is possible theoretically to reduce the energy wastage by recycling H_2 to form H^+.

In fact, some strains of ***Bradyrhizobium japonicum*** in soybean plants were found to use hydrogen as the energy source. These strains were found to ***possess*** an enzyme namely ***hydrogenase.*** Recycling of the hydrogen gas that is formed as a byproduct in nitrogen fixation is shown in ***Fig. 52.3.***

It is advantageous for nitrogen fixation if the symbiotic bacteria possess the enzyme hydrogenase. However, the naturally occurring strains of *Rhizobium* and *Bradhyrhizobium* do not normally possess the gene encoding hydrogenase.

GENETIC MANIPULATIONS FOR NITROGEN FIXATION

The nitrogen-fixing bacteria that are closely associated with the world's food supply are among the favoured organisms for genetic manipulations.

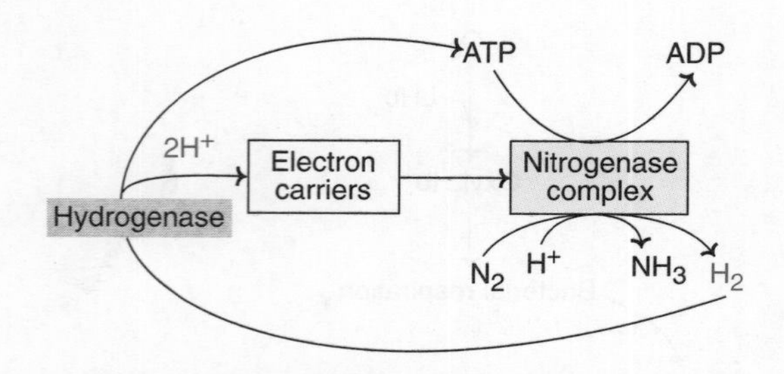

Fig. 52.3 : Action of the enzyme hydrogenase for recycling of hydrogen gas.

Biotechnologists consider the following possibities for effective utilization of diazotrophs (or the process of diazotrophy) as natural biological fertilizers.

- Gene alterations in *Rhizobium* sp to improve nitrogen fixing efficiency, and bacteria-host plant interactions
- Genetic engineering of *Rhizobium* sp so that it can form a symbiotic relationship with non-leguminous plants such as wheat, rice and corn.
- Transfer of genes for nitrogen fixation from *Rhizobium* sp to other bacteria such as *Agrobacterium tumefaciens.* The so developed *A. tumefaciens* can infect several important crops (e.g. tomato, tobacco, petunia) and fix nitrogen.

Some other considerations include the insertion of nitrogen-fixing genes into plants or even animals including humans. This approach, which enables the plants, animals and humans to directly trap and utilize nitrogen from the atmosphere is rather theoretical. Life would be certainly different if introduction of nitrogen-fixing genes in man can dispense with the habit of eating daily!

Despite several possibilities and optimistic predictions, the ***success in the genetic engineering in relation to nitrogen-fixation is very limited***, and briefly described below.

GENETIC ENGINEERING OF NITROGENASE GENE

It is absolutely necessary to identify, isolate and characterize the ***ni***trogen-***f***ixing genes, ***nif*** genes to undertake any kind of genetic manipulations.

Genetic complementation is the common technique used for the isolation *nif* genes. The procedure basically involves the identification and characterization of clones from a wild-type library to restore nitrogen fixation in the various mutants of the original organism.

The *nif* genes were first isolated from the clone banks of the diazotroph *Klebsiella pneumonia.* This organism is found in soil, water and human intestine, and its molecular biology is well known. The isolation of *nif* genes by genetic complementation from *K. pneumonia* is depicted in ***Fig. 52.4***, and involves the following steps.

1. The wild-type DNA of *K. pneumonia* (Nif^+) was cut with restriction endonucleases.

   A clone bank was constructed with a vector and maintained in *E.coli.*

2. *K. pneumonia* cells are exposed to a mutagenic agent. This may result in the mutation of *nif* genes to form Nif^- cells.

3. The Nif^- *K. pneumonia* cells are then conjugated with *E.coli* cells, carrying the clone bank on a vector.

4. The transformants of *K. pneumonia* possessing Nif^+ phenotype can be selected by growing the cells on a minimal medium that does not contain fixed nitrogen.

5. The DNA fragment in the plasmid that contains *nif* genes, which complements Nif^- mutation in *K. pneumonia* can be isolated.

The isolation of *nif* genes will be more effective if a series of independently derived Nif^- mutants are employed in genetic complementation experiments. This approach increases the likelihood of different *nif* genes isolation. Further, by using DNA hybridization probes of *nif* genes, DNA clone bank of *K. pneumonia* can be screened. This allows the identification of additional genes that are involved in nitrogen fixation.

Nitrogenase gene cluster

The entire set of nitrogenase genes from *K. pneumonia* has been identified. Some highlights are listed.

- The nitrogenaes (*nif*) genes are located as a single cluster, occupying approximately 24kb of the bacterial genome.
- There are seven distinct operons that encode 20 different proteins.

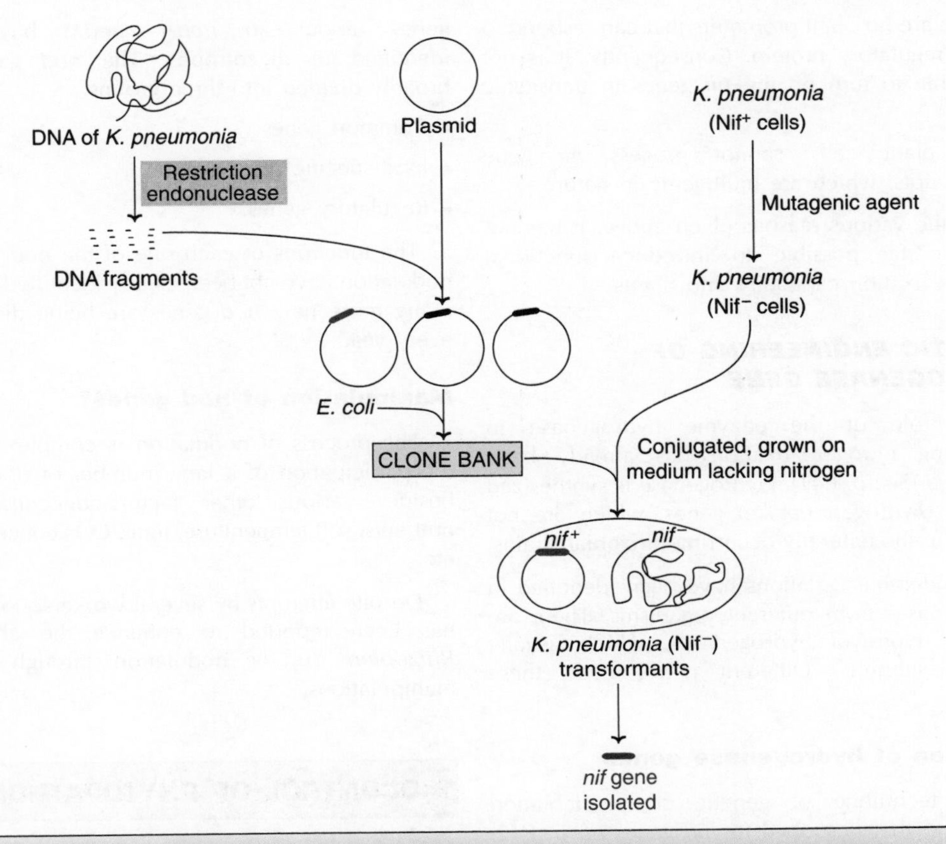

***Fig. 52.4 :** An outline of the method for the isolation of* nif *genes from* K. pneumonia *by genetic complementation.*

- All the *nif* genes transcribe and translate in a well-coordinated fashion.
- The *nif* genes are under the regulatory control of two genes namely *nifA and nifL*.

Although the *nif* genes have been characterized from *K. pneumonia,* for technical reasons, the contribution of this organism for biological nitrogen fixation is almost insignificant. However, the *nif* genes of *K. pneumonia* have been used as hybridization probes to identify *nif* genes from the DNA clone banks of diazotrophic organisms (particularly *Rhizobium* sp). It is now known that almost all the nitrogen-fixing bacteria possess similar type of *nif* gene clusters.

Manipulation of *nif* genes

Some workers have been successful in introducing extra copies of nitrogenase regulatory genes namely *nifA* and *nifL* into diazotrophs. For instance, insertion of more *nifA* genes into *Rhizobium meliloti* resulted in an increased biomass production in alfalfa plants. This is due to the fact that nitrogen fixation in these plants is much increased. But the major limitation of this approach is that the genetically engineered bacteria have a diminished growth rate. As a result, these newly developed bacteria loss their efficiency as plant-growth promoting agents.

Despite continuous efforts by several groups of workers, no significant success has been reported in the transfer of *nif* genes into plants. The major limitations are listed.

- Transfer of 24 kb *nif* gene cluster has not been effective since the normal cellular concentration of oxygen would inactivate nitrogenase enzyme. Any reduction in O_2 results in cell death.
- Transfer of one or two genes of *nif* gene cluster is useless.

- There are no plant promoters that can respond to *nifA* regulatory protein. Consequently, it is not possible to turn on the *nif* genes in transgenic plants.
- The plant cells cannot process *nif* gene transcripts, which are multigenic in nature.

For the various reasons given above, it has not been so far possible to introduce functional nitrogen fixation capability into plants.

GENETIC ENGINEERING OF HYDROGENASE GENE

The role of the enzyme hydrogenase in promoting nitrogen fixation has already been described (See p. 641). Hydrogenase is synthesized by ***hup*** (***h***ydrogen ***up***take) genes, which are not present in the naturally occurring Rhizobial strains.

Considerable variations have been identified in hydrogenases from different organisms. There are different types of hydrogenases, which usually contain subunits. Different genes code these subunits.

Isolation of hydrogenase genes

The technique of genetic complementation (similar to that described for *nif* genes on p. 642) can be successfully employed for this isolation of hydrogenase (*hup*) genes. In fact, *hup* genes were first isolated from *E.coli* by this approach. Later, *hup* genes from *B.japonicum* have also been isolated.

Manipulation of *hup* genes

The hydrogenase (*hup*) genes have been introduced into *R.leguminosarum.* These ***Hup***$^+$ strains of bacteria, when inoculated into legumes, resulted in higher nitrogen fixation.

GENETIC ENGINEERING OF NODULATION GENES

Establishment of nodules on the roots of leguminous plants is a prerequisite for nitrogen fixation. Certain genes involved in nodulation namely ***nod genes*** have been identified in *Rhizobium melitoti.* The technique of genetic complementation (similar to that described for *nif* genes on p. 642) has been used to isolate *nod* genes from *R. melitoti.* A large number of *nod* genes (about 20 *nodA — nodX*) have been identified in diazotrophs. The *nod* genes are broadly divided into three groups.

- Common genes
- Host-specific genes
- Regulatory genes.

The functions of each one of the *nod* genes in nodulation have not been clearly identified. Further, many more new *nod* genes are being discovered every year.

Manipulation of *nod* genes?

The process of nodulation is complex through the participation of a large number of *nod* genes, besides various other factors-concentration of nutrients, soil temperature, light, CO_2 concentration etc.

Despite attempts by several workers, no success has been reported to enhance the ability of *Rhizobium* sp for nodulation through genetic manipulations.

BIOCONTROL OF PHYTOPATHOGENS

Phytopathogens can drastically reduce the crop yield, which may be in the range of 25–100%. Chemical agents are commonly used to control them. This is associated with ill-health affects on humans, besides environmental pollution.

There are certain bacteria that can lessen or prevent the deleterious effects of plant pathogens-fungi or bacteria. And thus, they promote plant growth by indirect means.

Plant growth-promoting bacteria are capable of producing a wide range of substances that can restrict the damage caused by phytopathogens to plants. The important plant growth-promoting substances are ***siderophores, antibiotics*** and certain ***enzymes.***

SIDEROPHORES

There are some bacteria in the soil that can synthesize a low molecular weight (400–1,000 Daltons) ***iron-binding peptides***, collectively referred to as siderophores. Siderophores have high affinity to bind to iron in the soil and transport it to the microbial cell. This is required since iron is essential, and cannot directly enter the bacteria due to a very low solubility.

The growth-promoting bacteria, through siderophores can take up large quantities of iron from the soil, and make it unavailable for the growth and existence of fungal pathogens. This is possible since the siderophores produced by fungi have a very low affinity when compared to siderophores of bacteria.

There is no harm to the plants since they can grow at a much lower concentration of iron in the soil.

Genetic manipulations for siderophores

It is now clearly established that siderophores can prevent the proliferation of phytopathogens. It is therefore logical to think of siderophore genes for more effective biocontrol of plant pathogens.

Pseudobactin is a siderophore synthesized by plant growth-promoting bacteria *Pseudomonas putida*. By genetic complementation and other techniques of molecular biology, at least five separate gene clusters involved in pseudobactin production have been identified.

Genetic manipulation for improved synthesis of siderophore is not an easy job, since it is a complex process involving a large number of genes. Some success, however, has been reported in cloning the genes for iron siderophore receptors from certain plant growth-promoting bacteria, and introducing them into other bacteria.

ANTIBIOTICS

Certain antibiotics produced by plant growth-promoting bacteria, can prevent the growth and proliferation of plant pathogens. Some of the antibiotics synthesized by pseudomonads are agrocin 84, agrocin 434, herbicolin, phenazine, oomycin, pyrrolinitrin.

Genetic manipulations for antibiotics

It is possible to enhance the growth-promoting activity of the bacteria by inserting genes encoding the synthesis of antibiotics.

In fact, a genetically engineered biocontrol bacterium of *Agrobacterium radiobacter* has been developed, and is being marked commercially since 1989. This transgenic organism produces the antibiotic agrocin 84 that is toxic to crown gall disease-causing *Agrobacterium tumefaciens*. By this biocontrol approach, the crop yield of almond trees and peach trees can be improved by preventing crown gall disease.

ENZYMES

Certain plant growth-promoting bacteria are capable of synthesizing some enzymes that can ***degrade fungal cell walls and lyse them***. These enzymes include ***chitinase, β-1,3-glucanase, protease*** and ***lipase***.

Genetic manipulation for enzymes

The genes responsible for encoding the enzyme namely chitinase and β-glucanase have been isolated and characterized. Chitinase gene has been isolated from *Serralia mercescens* and introduced into *Rhizobium meliloti* and *Trichoderma harzianum.* The genetically engineered organisms displayed an increased antifungal activity. By this biocontrol approach, the phytopathogen *Rhizoctonia solani* has been effectively controlled.

BIOFERTILIZERS

It is estimated that more than 100 million tons of fixed nitrogen are needed for global food production. The use of chemical/synthetic fertilizers is the common practice to increase crop yields. Besides the cost factor, the use of fertilizers is associated with environmental pollution.

Scientists are on a constant look for alternate, cheap and environmental-friendly sources of nitrogen and other nutrients for plants. The term biofertilizers is used to refer to the ***nutrient inputs of biological origin to support plant growth***. This can be achieved by the addition of ***microbial inoculants*** as a source of biofertilizers.

Biofertilizers broadly includes the following categories.

- Symbiotic nitrogen fixers
- Asymbiotic nitrogen fixers
- Phosphate solubilising bacteria
- Organic fertilizers.

The most important microorganisms used as biofertilizers along with the crops are listed in *Table 52.2.*

Some of the important features of these biofertilizers are briefly described.

SYMBIOTIC NITROGEN FIXERS

The ***diazotrophic microorganisms*** are the symbiotic nitrogen fixers that serve as biofertilizers. e.g. *Rhizobium* sp and *Bradyrhizobium* sp. The details on these bacteria with special reference to nitrogen fixation must be referred now. Many attempts are being made (although the success has been limited) to genetically modify the symbiotic bacteria for improving nitrogen fixation.

Green manuring

It is a farming practice wherein the leguminous plants which are benefited by the symbiotic nitrogen fixing bacteria are ploughed into the soil and a non-leguminous crop is grown to take benefits from the already fixed nitrogen. Green manuring has been in practice in India for several centuries. It is a ***natural way of enriching the soil with nitrogen***, and minimizing the use of chemical fertilizers. *Rhizobium* sp can fix about 50-150 kg nitrogen/hectare/annum.

ASYMBIOTIC NITROGEN FIXERS

The asymbiotic nitrogen-fixing bacteria can directly convert the gaseous nitrogen to nitrogen-rich compounds. When these asymbiotic nitrogen fixers die, they enrich the soil with nitrogenous compounds, and thus serve as biofertilizers e.g. *Azobacter* sp, *Azospirillum* sp.

Blue-green algae (cynobacteria)

Blue-green algae multiply in water logging conditions. They can fix nitrogen in the form of organic compounds (proteins, amino acids). The term ***algalization*** is used to the process of cultivation of blue-green algae in the field as a source of biofertilizer.

Blue-green algae, besides fixing nitrogen, accumulate biomass, which improves the physical properties of the soil. This is useful for reclamation of alkaline soils besides providing partial tolerance to pesticides. Cynobacteria are particularly useful for paddy fields. The most common blue-green algae are *Azobacter* sp and *Azospirillum* sp.

TABLE 52.2 A selected list of microorganisms used as biofertilizers along with the crops

Category/microorganism	*Useful for crops*
Symbiotic nitrogen fixers	Legumes (pulses, oilseeds)
Rhizobium leguminosarum, R. meliloti, R. ciceri, Bradyrhizobium japonicum	
Asymbiotic nitrogen fixers	
Azobacter, Azospirillum	Wheat, rice, sugarcane, jower, vegetables
Blue green algae (Anabaena, Nostic, Plectonemia)	Rice
Phosphate solubilizing bacteria	Pulses
Thiobacillus, Bacillus	
Mycorrhiza (Glomus)	Pulses

Azolla

Azolla is an aquatic fern, which contains an endophytic cynobacterium *Anabaena azollae* in the leaf cavities providing a symbiotic relationship. *Azolla* with *Anaebaena* is useful as biofertilizer. But due to certain limitation (listed below), the use of *Azolla* has not become popular.

- Azolla plant requires adequate supply of water.
- It can be easily damaged by pest diseases.
- Azolla cultivation is labour intensive.

PHOSPHATE SOLUBILIZING BACTERIA

Certain bacteria (e.g. *Thiobacillus, Bacillus*) are capable of converting non-available inorganic phosphorus present in the soil to utilizable (organic or inorganic) form of phosphate. These bacteria can also produce siderophores, which chelates with iron, and makes it unavailable to pathogenic bacteria. Thus, besides making phosphate available, the plants are protected from disease - causing microorganisms.

Mycorrhizas

Mycorrhizas are the ***fungus roots*** (e.g. *Glomus* sp) with distinct morphological structure. They are developed as a result of mutual symbiosis between certain root-inhabiting fungi and plant roots. Mycorrhizas are formed in plants, which are limited with nutrient supply. These plants may be herbs, shrubs and trees.

For the development of mycorrhizas, the fungus may be located on the root surface (***ectomycorrhizas***) or inside the root (***endo-mycorrhizas***).

In recent years, an artificially produced inoculum of mycorrhizal fungi is used in crop fields. This practice improves plant growth and yield, besides providing ***resistance against biotic*** (pathogens) and ***abiotic*** (climatic changes) ***stress.*** Mycorrhizas also produce plant growth-promoting substances.

ORGANIC FERTILIZERS

There are several organic wastes, which are useful as fertilizers. These include animal dung, urine, urban garbage, sewage, crop residues and oil cakes. A majority of these wastes remain unutilized as organic fertilizers. There exists a good potential for the development of organic manures from these wastes.

BENEFITS OF BIOFERTILIZERS

- Low cost and easy to produce. Small farmers are immensely benefited.
- Fertility of the soil is increased year after year.
- Free from environmental pollution.
- Besides nutrient supply, some other compounds, which promote plant growth, are also produced e.g. plant growth hormones, antibiotics.
- Biofertilizers increase physico-chemical properties of the soil, soil texture, and water holding capacity.
- Reclaimation of saline or alkaline soil is possible by using biofertilizers.
- Biofertilizers improve the tolerance of plants against toxic heavy metals.
- Plants can better withstand biotic and abiotic stresses and improve in product yield.

LIMITATIONS OF BIOFERTILIZERS

- Biofertilizers cannot meet the total needs of the plants for nutrient supply.
- They cannot produce spectacular results, as is the case with synthetic fertilizers.

Considering the advantages and disadvantages of biofertilizers, a realistic and pragmatic approach is to use combination of biofertilizers and synthetic fertilizers for optimum crop yield.

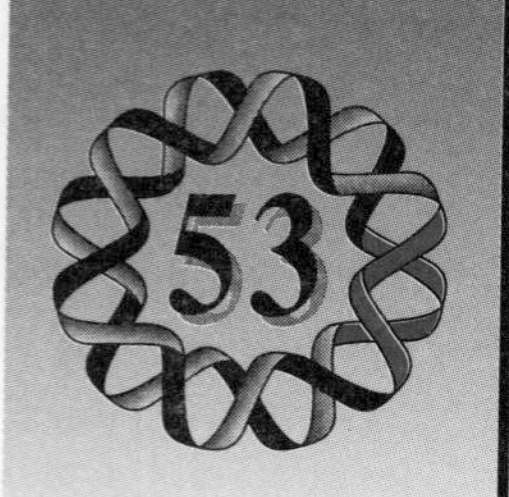

Molecular Marker-Aided Plant Breeding

Plant breeders are always interested to improve the agricultural production. This is possible to produce new/improved plant varieties with the desired characters. An important task of plant breeders is the correct identification, and continued maintenance of the plants with improved characters. There are different types of markers used for this purpose. The basic requirement of a ***marker*** is that it ***must be polymorphic*** i.e. it must exist in different forms. The polymorphism can be detected by three different types of markers

1. Morphological markers
2. Biochemical markers
3. Molecular markers.

Morphological markers

The morphological or phenotype markers represent the quantitative traits that can be visually detected e.g. altered leaf morphology, albinism, dwarfism etc. Morphological markers may be dominant or recessive. These markers are not widely used to detect polymorphism these days due to the following ***limitations***.

- Morphological markers influenced by the environment, and thus may not represent the desired genetic variation.
- Majority of the visible markers may not be required in the plant improvement programmes.

Biochemical markers

The proteins produced by gene expression are also used as markers in plant breeding programmes. The most commonly used are ***isoenzymes***, the different molecular forms of the same enzyme. The isoenzymes can be separated by electrophoresis and identified. However, the polymorphism of isoenzymes is rather poor. Hence, they are not widely used as markers.

MOLECULAR MARKERS

A molecular marker is a ***DNA sequence in the genome which can be located and identified***. As a result of genetic alterations (mutations, insertions, deletions), the base composition at a particular location of the genome may be different in different plants. These differences, collectively called as polymorphisms can be mapped and identified. Plant breeders always prefer to detect the gene as the molecular marker, although this is not always possible. The alternative is to have markers which are closely associated with genes and inherited together.

The molecular markers are highly reliable and ***advantageous*** in plant breeding programmes

- Molecular markers provide a true representations of the genetic make up at the DNA level.

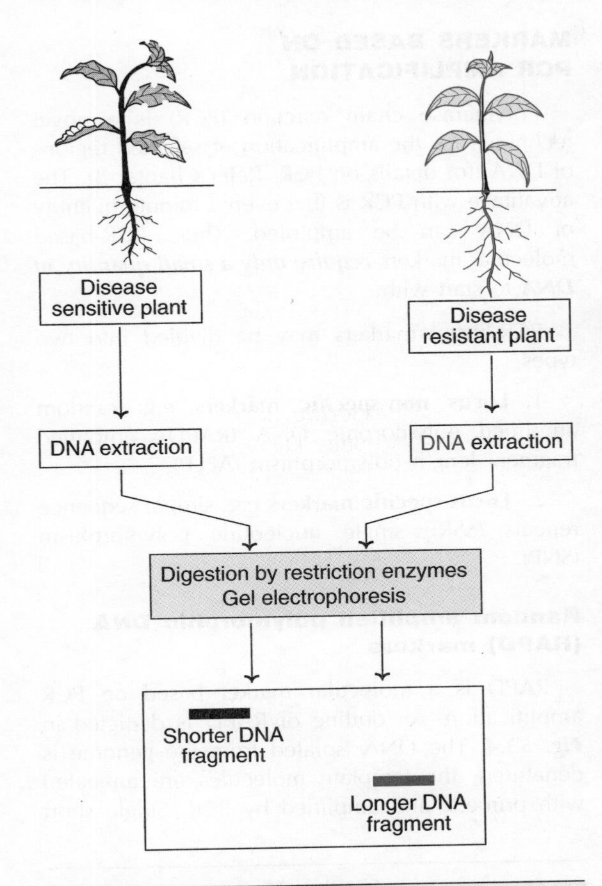

Fig. 53.1 : Basic principle of molecular marker detection (screening of genotypes for the identification of DNA markers).

- They are consistent and not affected by environmental factors.
- Molecular markers can be detected much before development of plants occur.
- A large number of markers can be generated as per the needs.

Basic principle of molecular marker detection

Let us assume that there are two plants of the same species—one with disease sensitivity and the other with disease resistance. If there is DNA marker that can identify these two alleles, then the genome can be extracted, digested by restriction enzymes, and separated by gel electrophoresis. The DNA fragments can be detected by their separation. For instance, the disease resistant plant may have a shorter DNA fragment while the disease — sensitive plant may have a longer DNA fragment (***Fig. 53.1***). Molecular markers are of two types.

1. Based on nucleic acid (DNA) hybridization (non-PCR based approaches).

2. Based on PCR amplification (PCR-based approaches).

MARKERS BASED ON DNA HYBRIDIZATION

The DNA piece can be cloned, and allowed to hybridize with the genomic DNA which can be detected. Marker-based DNA hybridization is widely used. The major ***limitation*** of this approach is that it requires ***large quantities of DNA*** and the use of radioactivity (labeled probes).

Restriction fragment length polymorphism (RFLP)

RFLP was the very first technology employed for the detection of polymorphism, based on the DNA sequence differences. RFLP is mainly ***based on the altered restriction enzyme sites,*** as a result of mutations and recombinations of genomic DNA.

An outline of the RFLP analysis is given in ***Fig. 53.2,*** and schematically depicted in ***Fig. 53.3.***

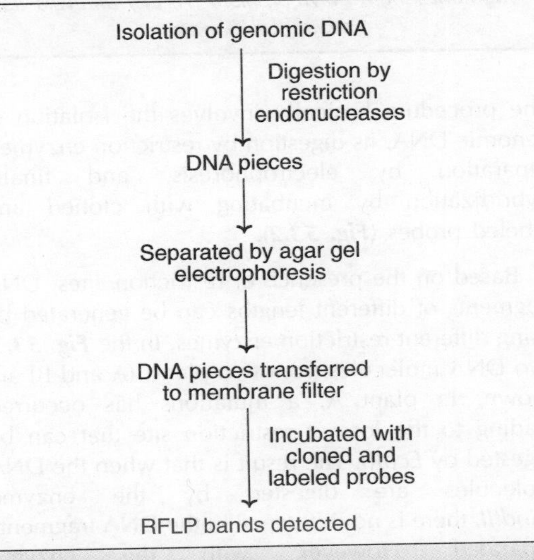

Fig. 53.2 : An outline of restriction fragment length polymorphism (RFLP) analysis as a molecular marker in plant breeding.

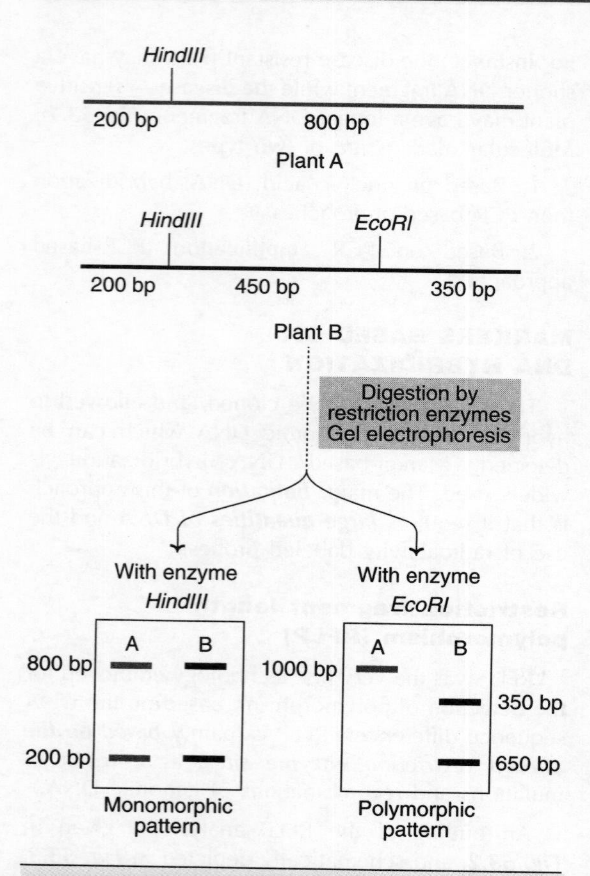

Fig. 53.3 : A schematic representation of restriction fragment length polymorphism (RFLP) analysis as molecular marker.

The procedure basically involves the isolation of genomic DNA, its digestion by restriction enzymes, separation by electrophoresis, and finally hybridization by incubating with cloned and labeled probes (***Fig. 53.2***).

Based on the presence of restriction sites, DNA fragments of different lengths can be generated by using different restriction enzymes. In the ***Fig. 53.3***, two DNA molecules from two plants (A and B) are shown. In plant A, a mutations has occurred leading to the loss of restriction site that can be digested by *EcoRI*. The result is that when the DNA molecules are digested by the enzyme *HindIII*, there is no difference in the DNA fragments separated. However, with the enzyme *EcoRI*, plant A DNA molecules is not digested while plant B DNA molecule is digested. This results in a polymorphic pattern of separation.

MARKERS BASED ON PCR AMPLIFICATION

Polymerase chain reaction (PCR) is a novel technique for the amplification of selected regions of DNA (for details on PCR, Refer Chapter 8). The advantage with PCR is that even a minute quantity of DNA can be amplified. Thus, PCR-based molecular markers ***require only a small quantity of DNA*** to start with.

PCR-based markers may be divided into two types.

1. **Locus non-specific markers** e.g. random amplified polymorphic DNA (RAPD); amplified fragment length polymorphism (AFLP).

2. **Locus specific markers** e.g. simple sequence repeats (SSR); single nucleotide polymorphism (SNP).

Random amplified polymorphic DNA (RAPD) markers

RAPD is a molecular marker based on PCR amplification. An outline of RAPD is depicted in ***Fig. 53.4***. The DNA isolated from the genome is denatured, the template molecules are annealed with primers, and amplified by PCR. Single short

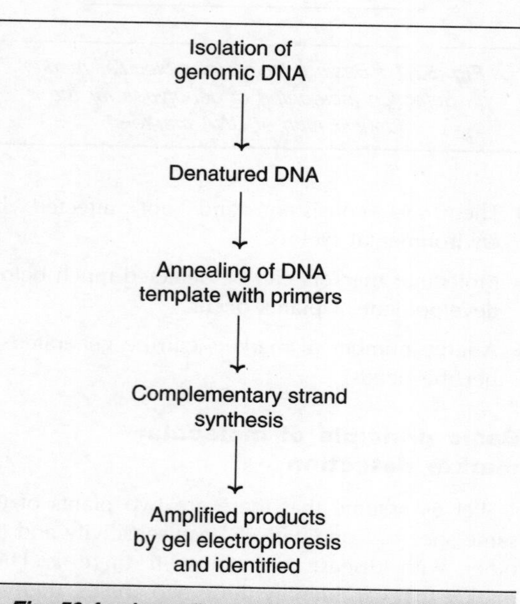

Fig. 53.4 : An outline of random amplified polymorphic DNA (RAPD) analysis as a molecular marker in plant breeding.

oligonucleotide primers (usually a 10-base primer) can be arbitrarily selected and used for the amplification DNA segments of the genome (which may be in distributed throughout the genome). The amplified products are separated on electrophoresis and identified.

Based on the nucleotide alterations in the genome, the polymorphisms of amplified DNA sequences differ which can be identified as bends on gel electrophoresis. Genomic DNA from two different plants often results in different amplification patterns i.e. RAPDs. This is based on the fact that a particular fragment of DNA may be generated from one individual, and not from others. This represents polymorphism and can be used as a molecular marker of a particular species.

Amplified fragment length polymorphism (AFLP)

AFLP is a novel technique involving a ***combination of RFLP and RAPD***. AFLP is based on the principle of generation of DNA fragments using restriction enzymes and oligonucleotide adaptors (or linkers), and their amplification by PCR. Thus, this technique combines the usefulness of restriction digestion and PCR.

The DNA of the genome is extracted. It is subjected to restriction digestion by two enzymes (a rare cutter e.g. *MseI;* a frequent cutter e.g. *EcoRI*). The cut ends on both sides are then ligated to known sequences of oligonucleotides (***Fig. 53.5***).

PCR is now performed for the preselection of a fragment of DNA which has a single specific nucleotide. By this approach of preselective amplification, the pool of fragments can be reduced from the original mixture. In the second round of amplification by PCR, three nucleotide sequences are amplified. This further reduces the pool of DNA fragments to a manageable level (< 100). Autoradiography can be performed for the detection of DNA fragments. Use of radiolabeled primers, and fluorescently labeled fragments quickens AFLP.

AFLP analysis is tedious and requires the involvement of skilled technical personnel. Hence some people are not in favour of this technique. In recent years, commercial kits are made available for AFLP analysis.

AFLP is very sensitive and reproducible. It does not require prior knowledge of sequence

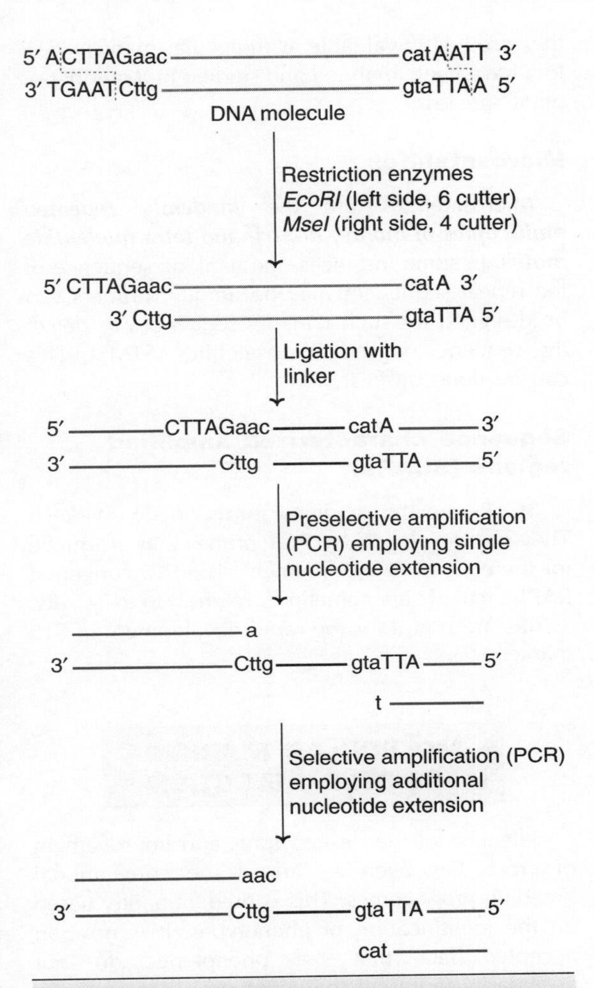

Fig. 53.5 : *A diagrammatic representation of the amplified fragment length polymorphism (AFLP)* ***(Note :*** *The lower case letters represent the sequences found within the amplified region; the coloured lines indicate linkers).*

information. By AFLP, a large number of polymorphic bands can be produced and detected.

Sequence tagged sites (STS)

Sequence tagged sites represent unique ***simple copy segments of genomes***, whose DNA sequences are known, and which can be amplified by using PCR. STS markers are based on the polymorphism of simple nucleotide repeats e.g. $(GA)_n$, $(GT)_n$, $(CAA)_n$ etc. on the genome. STS have been recently developed in plants. When the STS loci contain ***simple sequence length polymorphisms (SSLPs),*** they are highly valuable as molecular markers. STS loci have been analysed and studied in a number of plant species.

Microsatellites

Microsatellites are the ***tandemly repeated multicopies of mono-, di-, tri- and tetra nucleotide motifs***. In some instances, the flanking sequence of the repeat sequences may be unique. Primers can be designed for such flanking sequences to detect the sequence tagged microsatellites (STMS). This can be done by PCR.

Sequence characterized amplified regions (SCARs)

SCARs are the modified forms of STS markers. They are developed by PCR primer that are made for the ends of RAPD fragment. The STS-converted RAPD markers are sometimes referred to as SCARs. SCARs are useful for the rapid development of STS markers.

MOLECULAR MARKER ASSISTED SELECTION

Selection of the desired traits and improvement of crops has been a part of the conventional breeding programmes. This is predominantly based on the identification of phenotypes. It is now an accepted fact that the phenotypes do not necessarily represent the genotypes. Many a times the environment may mark the genotype. Thus, the plant's genetic potential is not truely reflected in the phenotypic expression for various reasons.

The molecular marker assisted selection is based on the identification of DNA markers that link/represent the plant traits. These traits include resistance to pathogens and insects, tolerance to abiotic stresses, and various other qualitative and quantitative traits. The advantage with a molecular marker is that a plant breeder can select a ***suitable marker*** for the desired trait which ***can be detected well in advance***. Accordingly, breeding programmes can be planned.

The following are the ***major requirements*** for the molecular marked selection in plant breeding

- The marker should be closely linked with the desired trait.
- The marker screening methods must be efficient, reproducible and easy to carry out.
- The analysis should be economical.

MOLECULAR BREEDING

With rapid progress in molecular biology and genetic engineering, there is now a possibility of improving the crop plants with respect to yield and quality. The term molecular breeding is frequently used to represent the ***breeding methods that are coupled with genetic engineering techniques***.

Improved agriculture to meet the food demands of the world is a high priority area. For several years, the conventional plant breeding programmes (although time consuming) have certainly helped to improve grain yield and cereal production. The development of dwarf and semi-dwarf varieties of rice and wheat have been responsible for the ***'Green Revolution'***, which has helped to feed millions of poverty-stricken people around the world.

Many development on the agriculture front are expected in the coming years as a result of molecular breeding.

Linkage analysis

Linkage analysis basically deals with studies to ***correlate the link between the molecular marker and a desired trait***. This is an important aspect of molecular breeding programmes. Linkage analysis has to be carried out among the populations of several generations to establish the appropriate linkage.

In the earlier years, linkage analysis was carried out by use of isoenzymes and the associated polymorphisms. Molecular markers are now being used. The techniques employed for this purpose have already been described.

QUANTITATIVE TRAIT LOCI

These are many characteristics controlled by several genes in a complex manner. Some good examples are growth habit, yield, adaptability to environment, and disease resistance. These are referred to as ***quantitative traits***. The ***locations on the chromosomes for these genes*** are regarded as quantitative trait loci (QTL).

The major problem, the plant breeder faces is how to improve the a complex character controlled by many genes. It is not an easy job to manipulate multiple genes in genetic engineering. Therefore, it is a very difficult and time consuming process. For instance, development of Golden Rice (with enriched provitamin A) involving the insertion of just three genes took about seven years.

ARID AND SEMI-ARID PLANT BIOTECHNOLOGY

The terms ***arid zone*** is used to refer to ***harsh environmental conditions with extreme heat and cold***. The fileds have limited water and minerals. It is different task to grow plants and achieve good crop yield in arid zones.

Semi-arid regions are characterized by ***unpredictable weather***, inconsistent rainfall, long dry seasons, and poor nutrients in the soil. Most parts of India and many other developing countries (Africa, Latin America, Southeast Asia) have semi-arid regions.

Crops like sorghum, millet, groundnut and cowpea are mostly grown in semi-arid tropics. Besides unpredictable weather, biotic and abiotic stresses contribute to crop loss in these areas.

The biotechnological approaches for the breeding programmes in the semi-arid regions should cover the following areas.

- Development of crops that are tolerant to drought and salinity.
- Improvements to withstand various biotic and abiotic stresses.
- Micropropagation techniques to spread economically important plants which can withstand harsh environmental conditions.

Some success has been achieved in improving sorghum, milllet and legume crops that are grown in semi-arid regions. Genetic transformation in sorghum was possible by using microprojectile method (For details, Refer Chapter 49).

GREENHOUSE AND GREENHOME TECHNOLOGY

Greenhouse literally means a building made up of glass to grow plants. Green houses are required to ***grow regenerated plants for further propagation, and for growing plants to maturity***. Greenhouses are the intermediary stages involving the transitional step between the plant cultures and plant fields. The purpose of greenhouses is to acclimatize and test the plants before they are released into the natural environment.

The plants are grown in greenhouse to develop adequate root systems and leaves so as to withstand the field environment. The greenhouses are normally equipped with cooling systems to control temperature.

Greenhouses have chambers fitted with artificial lights. It is possible to subject the plants to different lighting profiles. In recent years many improvements have been made in the development of more suitable greenhouses. These include the parameters such as soil, and humidity.

The major limitation of greenhouse technology is an increase in CO_2 production that in turn increases temperature. Some approaches are available to control temperature.

Greenhome technology is a recent development. In this case, ***temperature is controlled by using minimum energy***.

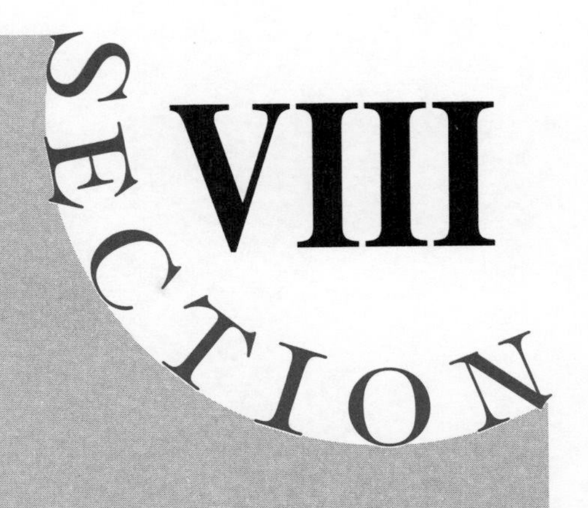

ENVIRONMENTAL BIOTECHNOLOGY

CONTENTS

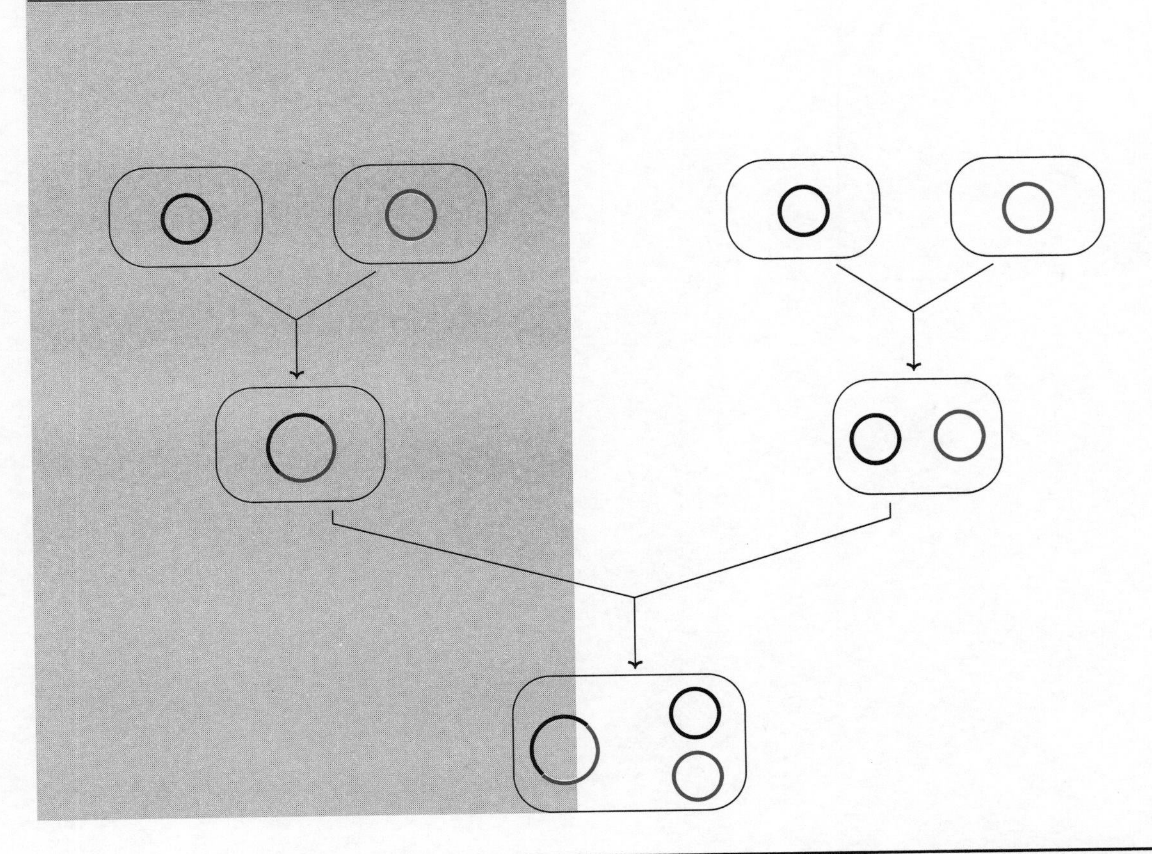

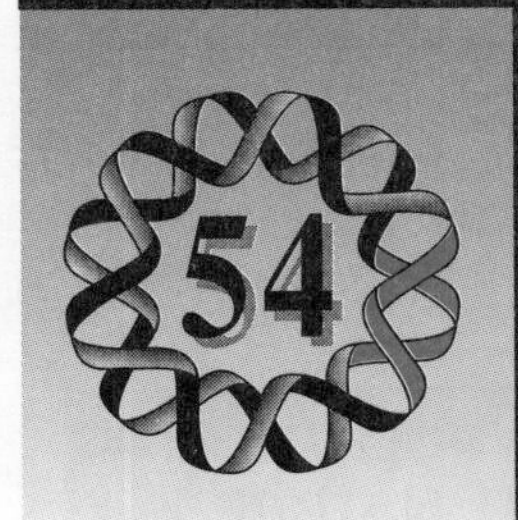

Environmental Pollution — General

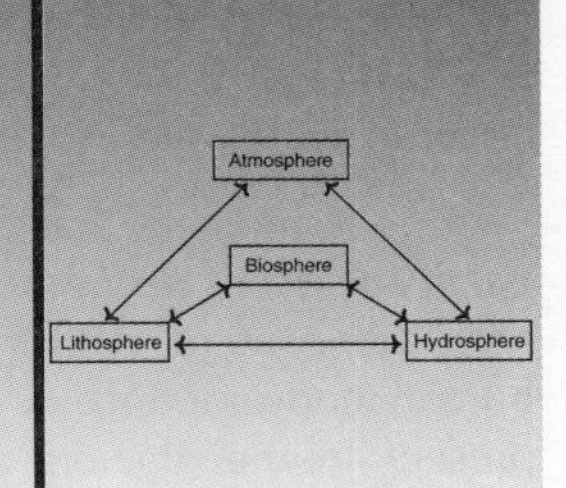

Environment may be considered as our surroundings which includes everything around us, i.e. the ***non-living*** (***abiotic***) and ***living*** (***biotic***) ***environment***. The abiotic environment consists of air, water and soil, while the biotic environment includes all the living organisms (plants, animals, microorganisms) that we regularly come in contact.

ENVIRONMENT — BASIC CONCEPTS

The environment is composed of four basic components.

- Atmosphere
- Hydrosphere
- Lithosphere
- Biosphere.

There is a continuous interaction among the various components of the environment (***Fig. 54.1***). And ultimately, it is the biosphere that gets influenced by the other components.

The four components of the environment are briefly described.

ATMOSPHERE

The atmosphere consists of a blanket of gases, suspended liquids and solids that envelope the earth. The atmosphere is basically derived from the earth itself by various chemical and biochemical

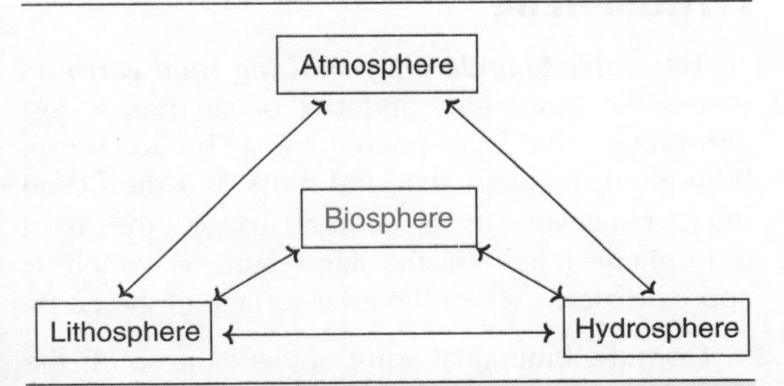

Fig. 54.1 : *Interaction of environmental components.*

reactions. The major components of the atmosphere include the gases nitrogen, oxygen, argon, carbon dioxide, water vapour, and suspended particulates (dust, soot). The composition of the atmosphere depends on time and space, and is highly variable. A liter of air weights around 1.3 g.

The atmosphere is vertically divided into four layes — ***troposphere***, ***stratosphere***, ***mesosphere***, and ***thermosphere***. This division is mainly based on the increase in the temperature.

HYDROSPHERE

The hydrosphere primarily consists of the ***water on the earth's surface***. Thus, the hydrosphere includes oceans, seas, rivers, streams, lakes, reservoirs and polar ice caps. Water is the most abundant substance on the earth's surface, which may be present as ice, liquid and vapour. Approximately, 71% of the earth's surface is covered with water, mainly in the form of oceans.

It is estimated that ***about 97% of the total earth's water is in the oceans and inland seas*** with high salt content. And this water is not useful for human consumption. Around 2% of the water is present in the glaciers and ice caps. The actual water available for human consumption is around 1% of the total earth's water. This includes the ground water, water from lakes and rivers and soil moisture.

Humans uses water in the homes, industries, agriculture and recreation. There is a continuous decrease in the consumable global water. Therefore, there is a need for precious use of water, and its conservation.

LITHOSPHERE

The ***outer boundary layer of the solid earth*** on which the continents and the ocean basins rest constitutes the lithosphere. In a broad sense, lithosphere includes the land mass and the ocean floor. However, in a general usage, the term lithosphere refers to the land surface which is approximately $\frac{3}{10}$th of the total surface of the earth.

From the biological point of view, the soil is the most important part of the lithosphere because it contains the organic matter and supports growth of plants and microorganisms. Lithosphere is involved in the production of food for humans and animals, besides the decomposition of organic wastes.

BIOSPHERE

The biosphere comprises of all the ***zones on earth in which life is present***. Biosphere is spread over the lower part of the atmosphere, the top of the lithosphere and the entire hydrosphere. In other words, the broad spectrum of ***bioresources of the earth***, supporting life constitutes the biosphere. It is estimated that the biosphere contains more than 3.5 lakh species of plants (including algae, fungi, mosses and higher plants) and more than 110 lakh species of animals (unicellular, multicellular and higher animals). The biosphere provides the essential requisites (water, light, heat, air, food, space etc.) for the existence of life.

The biosphere is very vast, and for the sake of understanding, it is divided into smaller units namely ***ecosystems***. An ecosystem may be considered as the smallest unit of biosphere that possesses the requisite characteristics to sustain life e.g., ponds, seas, deserts, cities.

ENVIRONMENTAL POLLUTION — SOURCES AND NATURE

Man lives in two worlds—a ***natural world*** of the native environment and a ***built-world*** created by himself. The built-world, an outcome of the advances made in the science and technology, is associated with environmental pollution. Environmental pollution is a global phenomenon, and therefore a matter of concern for everyone.

Pollution broadly refers to the presence of undesirable substances in the environment which are harmful to man and other organisms. The presence of unwanted substances in the environment may occur due to human activity discharging byproducts, a wide spectrum of waste products and several harmful secondary products (**Note :** It must be remembered that the natural world of environment is not totally free from impurities or undesirable substances. However, such impurities are usually not harmful).

SOURCES OF POLLUTION

As already stated, environmental pollution is mostly due to direct or indirect human activities, arising out of the built-world created by him. There are six ***major sources of environmental pollution***.

1. Industrial sources
2. Agricultural sources
3. Biogenic sources
4. Anthropogenic sources
5. Unnatural sources
6. Extra-terrestrial sources.

The relative importance of each one of these sources depends on the site-specific situation. For instance in cities, anthropogenic sources are the major contributors while in rural areas, agricultural sources significantly add to pollution.

Types of pollution

The environmental pollution may be categorized into six major groups.

1. Air/atmosphere pollution
2. Water pollution
3. Land/soil pollution
4. Noise pollution
5. Thermal pollution
6. Radioactive pollution.

The details of air pollution and water pollution are described elsewhere (Chapters 55 and 56).

NATURE OF POLLUTANTS

The pollutants that occur in the environment may be chemical, biological and physical in their nature.

Chemical pollutants : Gaseous pollutants (sulfur dioxide, nitrogen dioxide), toxic metals, pesticides, herbicides, hydrocarbons, toxins, acidic substances, carcinogens.

Biological pollutants : Pathogenic organisms, products of biological origin.

Physical pollutants : Heat (thermal), sound, odours, radiation and radioactive substances.

POLLUTION MONITORING/ MEASUREMENT

Environmental pollution poses a big threat to the healthy existence of humankind. The Governments worldover pay serious attention to continuously monitor and minimize pollution. The public and non-governmental organizations (NGOs) are also actively involved in this venture. Broadly, there are ***four levels of pollution monitoring agences or environmental protection agencies (EPAs)***.

Primary level : This is at the district or block level. The non-governmental organizations and the rural development agencies are involved in pollution monitoring.

Secondary level : Existing at the state level, the monitoring is done by the respective state pollution control boards.

Tertiary level : This is at the national/country level. Each country has its own environmental protection agency to monitor pollution.

Quaternary level : International/inter-Governmental bodies are closely associated with monitoring of pollution which is a global phenomenon. World Health Organization and United Nation Environmental Programme are actively involved.

BIOTECHNOLOGICAL METHODS FOR MEASUREMENT OF POLLUTION

In recent years, environmental pollution detection and monitoring is being done by approaches involving ***biosystems***. For this, purpose, several groups of plants, animals and microorganisms are utilized. The environmental protection agencis (EPAs) consider ***biomonitoring*** of pollution as a useful device to monitor environmental pollution from the point of diagnostic, preventive and remedial measures.

CRITERIA FOR BIOMONITORING OF POLLUTION

The parameters or the criteria chosen for biomonitoring of pollution are very crucial. They should be reliable, reproducible and cost-effective. Three types of criteria are mostly adopted for biomonitoring of pollution-visual rating, genotoxicity rating and metabolic rating.

Visual rating

In the visual rating, the ***growth rate and productivity*** are considered. When microorganisms are used in the test assay, the growth can be measured by turbidometric analysis. In case of higher plants, growth rate of different parts, visual damage to leaves, seed viability and germination frequency are taken into account.

As regards animals (fishes are commonly used), the concept of LD_{50} is used i.e. the dose at which 50% of the test organism is affected.

Sometimes, the presence or absence of a particular species of an organism serves as an indicator for the environmental pollution.

Genotoxicity rating

Genotoxicity tests ***measure the extent of damage caused to an organism by environmental pollution at the cellular and sub-cellular levels.*** The genotoxic lesions may be detected on the cellular organelles (membranes commonly used), genomes, immune systems, biomolecules, etc.

Cytotoxic tests such as measurement of chromosomal damage (including breakage), sister chromatid exchange (SCE) and micronuclei counting are also useful for pollution detection. The cell viability can be measured by detecting *in vitro* lysosomal viability. In recent yeas, DNA probes are in use for the identification of disease-causing organisms in water.

Metabolic rating

The ***biochemical changes*** with environmental pollution can be measured (qualitatively and quantitatively) in selected organisms. In fact, certain metabolic parameters can be used as ***biomarkers to assess the pollution stress***. The biomarkers used in metabolic rating include chlorophyll, proteins, nucleic acids (DNA and RNA) and changes in enzyme activities.

The biotechnological methods adopted for pollution measurement are briefly described in the following order.

1. General bioassays
2. Cell biological assays
3. Molecular biological assays
4. Biosensors.

BIOASSAYS IN ENVIRONMENTAL MONITORING

In the early years, the conventional physical and chemical methods were used for the detection of environmental pollution. Bioassays are preferred these days, since the biological responses that reflect the damages to the living organisms are very crucial for the actual assessment of pollution.

The organisms employed in the bioassays for pollution detection are expected to satisfy the following criteria.

- It should readily take up the pollutant (absorption or adsorption).
- The organism should be sensitive to the pollutant.
- It should possess measurable features to detect pollution.
- The organism should have wide occurrence, and available round the year.
- The bioassay should be simple, reproducible and cost-effective.

The most commonly used plants and animals in the bioassays are briefly described.

Plant test systems in bioassays

Certain algae, bacteria, lichens, mosses and vascular macrophytes are commonly used in bioassays.

Algal bioassays : Among the plant systems, algal bioassays are the most commonly used. Algae are considered to be reliable indicators of pollution due to their high sensitivity and easy availability, besides simple culturing techniques. The criteria adopted for algal bioassays are the growth rate, biomass accumulation and photosynthetic efficiency.

The algae used in the test assays include *Chlorella, Microcystis, Spirulina, Navicula, Scenedesmus, Anabaena, Ulva, Codium, Fucus* and *Laminaria*. In water, organic pollution can be detected by using the blue green algae, *Microcystis*, while metal pollution can be measured by *Navicula*.

Bacterial bioassays : These are commonly used for the detection of fecal pollution in potable water, the most widely employed test being ***coliform test***. ***Ames test*** that detects mutagenic pollutants is carried out by the bacterium *Salmonella*.

Bacterial bioluminescence is a recent technique used for the measurement of gaseous pollutants and other compounds e.g. sulfur dioxide, formaldehyde, ethylacetate. *Photobacterium phosphoreum* is the organism of choice for bacterial bioluminescence.

Lichens in bioassays : Lichens are widely used for the detection of atmospheric gas pollution, particularly in cities. Lichens are very sensitive for the measurement of sulfur dioxide.

Mosses in bioassays : Environmental metal pollution can be detected by using certain forest and aquatic mosses e.g. *Stereophyllum, Sphagnum, Brynus*.

Vascular macrophytes in bioassays : Water hyacinth (*Eichormia crassipes*) and duck weed (*Lemna minor*) are in use to detect aquatic metal pollution. In fact, certain biochemical parameters of macrophytes are used to serve as ***biomarkers*** of pollution e.g., peroxidase activity increases due to metal pollution; inhibition of nitrate reductase activity by mercury. The other commonly used bioassay parameters are the estimation of soluble proteins, nucleic acids, chlorophyll, and assay of enzyme (e.g. catalase, peroxidase) activities.

Pollution-induced peptides in bioassays : Very recently, some workers have identified the presence of small peptides within the plant cells which are pollution-induced. These peptides, referred to as ***phytochelatins***, are formed as a result of metal pollution. They are reasonably reliable ***for the detection of metal pollution***.

Animal test systems in bioassays

Among the animals, certain fishes, protozoa and helminths are employed in bioassays.

Fishes in bioassays : Toxic effects of environmental pollutants on fishes have been in use for quite some time as a measure of bioassays. In fact, the concept of LD_{50} (i.e. the dose of the pollutant at which 50% of the test organisms are affected) has originated from the studies on fishes. The criteria or parameters used for assessment of fish bioassays include changes in the morphology and organs, behavioural pattern and modifications in metabolisms. The alterations in the ***enzyme acetylcholine esterase serves as a reliable marker for pesticide pollution***.

The most commonly used fishes in bioassays are *Catla, Teleost, Labeo* and *Channa*.

Protozoa in bioassays : The ciliated protozoa serve as good bioassay systems for the detection of environmental pollution. The toxic effects of the pollutants can be measured by the ***changes in the behavioural patterns*** of protozoa, recorded on an ***ethogram***.

Helminths in bioassays : Rotifers are a group of helminths that grow on aquatic vegetation. They are used for the detection of organic matter in water (given by BOD). Rotifers, with round the year availability, easy cultivation, slow growth rate and easy recognition are used for biomonitoring of water.

Pollution-induced peptides in bioassays : As already described in case of plant bioassays (above), pollution-induced small peptides are found in animal cells also. They are collectively referred to as ***metallothioneins*** (comparable to phytochelatins in plants). Metallothioneins are useful ***for the detection of metal pollution***.

Biomonitoring of pollution with multiple species

Most often, bioassays using a single organism are not adequate to detect pollution. In such a case, multiple species of organisms are used.

CELL BIOLOGY IN ENVIRONMENTAL MONITORING

Cell biology deals with the study of the structural and functional aspects of cells and the cellular organelles. It is successfully exploited for environmental pollution detection, particularly with reference to mutagens and carcinogens.

The cell biological methods primarily aim to trace the harmful effects of pollutants on different cellular components — membranes, chloroplasts, mitochondria, chromosomes. In addition, the macromolecules namely nucleic acids (particularly DNA) and proteins are also used. Further, cell biological methods help in understanding the mechanisms of toxicity of pollutants.

Some important cell biological methods used in environmental pollution monitoring are described.

Membrane damage in bioassay

The plasma membrane, an envelope surrounding the cell, protects the cell from hostile environment. It is the first cellular component to be directly exposed to pollutants. Many toxic substances that cause damage to cell structure and its functions are known.

For the purpose of bioassay, the physical damages caused by pollutants or their deposition on the membranes can be detected by light, phase contrast and electron microscopy. This approach may not be always practicable. The alterations in the semipermeable properties of the membranes due to pollutants can be detected by leakage of enzymes (e.g., lactate dehydrogenase), efflux of electrolytes or uptake of trypan blue. ***Lysosomes*** are also useful as ***biomarkers for measurement of cell viability***. This can be done by ***neutral red retention test***. The damaged lysosomes cannot retain this dye.

In recent years, animal and plant tissue culture techniques are also used for pollution monitoring. This is made possible by measuring cellular damages observed in cell cycles. A good example is the use of human lymphocyte culture to monitor the persons exposed to toxic pollutants.

Cytogenetic bioassays

The genetic damages of the cells, as reflected by changes in the chromosomes, can be effectively used in biomonitoring of pollution. For this purpose, animals (e.g. insect *Drosophila*) and plants (e.g. *Arabidiopsis*) with shorter life cycles are preferred. Other plants such as pea, maize and soy bean are also used in cytogenetic bioassays.

Chromosomal damage : The pollutants may cause several types of chromosomal damages-fragmentation, bridge formation, disruption in cell division. The ***chromosomal alterations can be effectively used for pollution detection.*** It has been clearly established that the severity of chromosomal damage depends on the chemical nature of the pollutant.

Micronucleus test : Severe damage to chromosomes by pollutants may result in large scale fragmentation of chromosomes, followed by micronuclei formation. The degree of micronuclei development is directly related to the severity of the damage. Micronucleus test (MNT) is used for ***screening of mutagenic compounds***.

Sister-chromatid exchange : The damages caused by pollutants results in misexchange of chromosomal segments (chromatids) during cell division. The sister chromated exchange (SCE) can be detected by using a fluorescent dye technique.

Ames test in bioassays

Ames test can be used for the ***detection of chemical mutagens and their carcinogenecity***. This is very widely used bioassay for screening of various pollutants, drugs, cosmotics, food additives and metals.

Ames test employs the use of a special mutant strain of bacterium namely *Salmonella typhimurium* (His^-). This organism cannot synthesize histidine, hence the same should be supplied in the medium for its growth. Addition of chemical carcinogens causes mutations (reverse mutation) restoring the ability of this bacterium to synthesize histidine (His^+). By detecting the strain of *Salmonella* (His^+) in the colony of agar plates, the chemical mutagens can be identified. The ***Ames assay can detect about 90% of the chemical carcinogens***.

Recently, the yeast cells (*Saccharomyces cerevisae*) are also used for the detection of chemical carcinogens.

MOLECULAR BIOLOGY IN ENVIRONMENTAL MONITORING

The use of ***molecular probes*** and ***immunoassays*** in monitoring of environmental pollution is gaining importance in recent years. Molecular biological bioassays are particularly useful for the detection of bacteria, viruses and other pathogenic organisms that cause diseases.

DNA probes

DNA probes and ***polymerase chain reaction (PCR)*** can be effectively used for water quality monitoring, particularly potable water. However, these techniques are expensive and not practicable at all places. For more details on DNA probes and PCR, Refer Chapters 9 and 8 respectively.

Immunoassays

Immunological techniques are useful for the detection of pollutants (pesticides, herbicides) and identification of pathogens that exhibit immunological properties. Immunoassays are in use for the measurement of several pesticides e.g. aldrin, triazines DDT, glyphosate. Metabolic products of certain bacteria can also be detected by immunoassays. For instance, assay systems have been developed for the detection of toxins of *cholera* and *Salmonella*.

In recent years, use of ***monoclonal antibodies (MAbs)*** in the detection and biomonitoring of environmental pollution is gaining importance. In fact, assay techniques are available for detection of pesticide and herbicide contamination in water.

Bioluminescent bioassays using Lux reporter genes

Certain genes, referred to as Lux reporter genes, on the plasmids produce assayable signals. Whenever these genes are expressed in luminescent bacteria like *Photobacterium* and *Vibrio*. Some bacterial strains have been developed through gene cloning (employing Lux reporter genes) for the detection of pollutants and their degradation. For instance, genetically altered *Pseudomonas* can be used for detecting naphthalene, xylene, toluene and salicylate.

BIOSENSORS IN ENVIRONMENTAL MONITORING

A biosensor is an ***analytical device containing an immobilized biological material*** (enzyme, organelle, cell) which can specifically interact with an analyte (a compound whose concentration is to be determined) and produce physical, chemical or electrical signals that can be measured. Biosensors are highly specific and accurate in their function.

The details on biosensors—principles of working, types, various applications are described elsewhere (Refer Chapter 21). Some of the important biosensors used in environmental pollution monitoring are briefly described.

BOD biosensor

Biological oxygen demand (BOD_5) is a widely used test for the detection of organic pollution. This test requires five days of incubation. A BOD biosensor using the yeast *Trichosporon cutaneum* with oxygen probe takes just 15 minutes for detecting organic pollution.

Gas biosensors

Microbial biosensors for the detection of gases such as sulfur dioxide (SO_2), methane and carbon dioxide have been developed. *Thiobacillus*-based biosensor can detect the pollutant SO_2, while methane (CH_4) can be detected by immobilized *Methalomonas.* For carbon dioxide monitoring, a particular strain of *Pseudomonas* is used.

Immunoassay biosensors

Immunoelectrodes as biosensors are useful for the detection of low concentrations of pollutants. Pesticide specific antibodies can detect the presence of low concentrations of triazines, malathion and carbamates, by employing immunoassays.

Other biosensors

Biosensors employing ***acetylcholine esterase*** (obtained from bovine RBC) can be used for the detection of organophosphorus compounds in water. In fact, portable pesticide monitors are commercially available in some developed countries.

TABLE 54.1 A selected list of pollutants measured by employing biosensors

Pollutant measured	*Biosensor–biological component*
BOD	*Trichosporon cutaneum*
SO_2	*Thiobacillus* sp
CH_4	*Methanomonas flagellae*
CO_2	*Pseudomonas* sp
Nitrate	*Azobacter vinelandi*
NH_3 and NO_2	Mixed nitrifying bacteria
Nerve gas	Acetylcholine esterase
Ethanol	NADH and dehydrogenase
Phenol	Phenol oxidase
Parathion	Antibody to parathion
Herbicide–induced electron transport chain inhibition	*Synechococcus*

Biosensors for the detection of polychlorinated biphenyls (PCBs) and chlorinated hydrocarbons and certain other organic compounds have been developed.

Phenol oxidase enzyme (obtained from potatoes and mushrooms) containing biosensor is used for the detection of phenol.

A graphite electrode with *Cynobacterium* and *Synechococcus* has been developed to measure the degree of electron transport inhibition during photosynthesis due to certain pollutants e.g. herbicides.

A selected list of environmental pollutants measured by employing biosensors is given in ***Table 54.1***.

BIOTECHNOLOGICAL METHODS FOR MANAGEMENT OF POLLUTION

The different approaches for the management of environmental pollution are described in the respective chapters for air pollution, refer Chapter 55, and for water pollution Chapter 56.

The general concepts of the biotechnological approaches for the abatement of pollution with special reference to the following aspects are described in this chapter.

1. Atmospheric CO_2 reduction.
2. Sewage treatment by bacteria and algae.
3. Eutrophication and phosphorus pollution.
4. Management of metal pollution.
5. Immobilized cells in the management of pollution.

ATMOSPHERIC CO_2 REDUCTION

The lower atmosphere contains CO_2 at a concentration of 0.0314% by volume. There is a continuous addition of CO_2, particularly coming from industrial processes. Any increase in the content CO_2 has to be viewed very seriously, since it is the principal gas that causes ***green house effect*** and rises atmospheric temperature. It is suggested that the global temperature will increase by around 2-5°C on doubling the atmospheric concentration of CO_2. The present belief is that during the past 100–150 years, the CO_2 level increased by about 25% with an increase in the atmospheric temperature by about 0.5%. Thus, CO_2 is closely linked with ***global warming***.

For the reasons stated above, the reduction in atmospheric CO_2 concentration assumes significance. There are mainly two approaches for the biotechnological reduction of CO_2 in the atmosphere.

1. Photosynthesis
2. Biological calcification.

PHOTOSYNTHESIS TO REDUCE ATMOSPHERIC CO_2

Utilization of CO_2 for photosynthesis by plants is the most significant process to reduce CO_2 content in the atmosphere. Photosynthesis may be represented by the following equation.

$$6CO_2 + 6H_2O \xrightarrow[\text{Chlorophyll}]{\text{Sunlight}} C_6H_{12}O_6 + 6O_2$$

Higher plant photosynthesis

The fast growing trees are more efficient in utilizing CO_2 for photosynthesis, hence their propagation is advocated. Further, ***micro-propagation*** and ***synthetic seed*** production through plant tissue culture techniques are also important. The major problem is the continuous deforestation that is associated with a possible increase in atmospheric CO_2. The conservation of forests and plantations is the need of the hour.

Certain biotechnological approaches have also been made to improve the CO_2 utilization by enhancing photosynthesis. The enzyme ***ribulose-bisphosphate carboxylase*** (RUBP-case) is closely linked with CO_2 fixation. There are some attempts to genetically manipulate this enzyme so that the photosynthetic efficiency is increased.

Microalgal photosynthesis

Certain microalgae are more efficient than higher plants in utilizing atmospheric CO_2 for photosynthesis e.g. *Chlorella pyrenodiosa, Spirulina maxima*. These organisms are capable of generating more O_2 than the amount of CO_2 consumed.

It is advocated that growing microalgae in the vicinity of industries and power plants where the production CO_2 is very high will help to minimise the polluting effects of CO_2. In addition, these microalgae, appropriately regarded as ***photobioreactors***, accumulate as ***biomass*** which can be utilized for the extraction of protein for use as food or feed.

Genetic manipulations are in progress to develop new strains of microalgae that can tolerate high concentrations of CO_2, and yield larger biomass. Some success has been reported in the mutants of *Anacystis nidulans* and *Oocystis* sp.

BIOLOGICAL CALCIFICATION TO REDUCE ATMOSPHERIC CO_2

Certain organisms present in the deep sea (corals, green and red algae) are capable of storing CO_2 through a process of biological calcification. The overall process of calcification may be represented as follows.

$$H_2O + CO_2 \longrightarrow H_2CO_3$$

$$H_2CO_3 + Ca^{2+} \longrightarrow CaCO_3 + CO_2 + H_2O$$

As the $CaCO_3$ gets precipitated, more and more atmospheric CO_2 can be utilized for its formation.

SEWAGE TREATMENT BY BACTERIA AND ALGAE

The ***waste water*** resulting from various human activities (domestic), agricultural and industrial is technically referred to as sewage. The sewage is mostly composed of organic and inorganic compounds, toxic substances, heavy metals and pathogenic organisms.

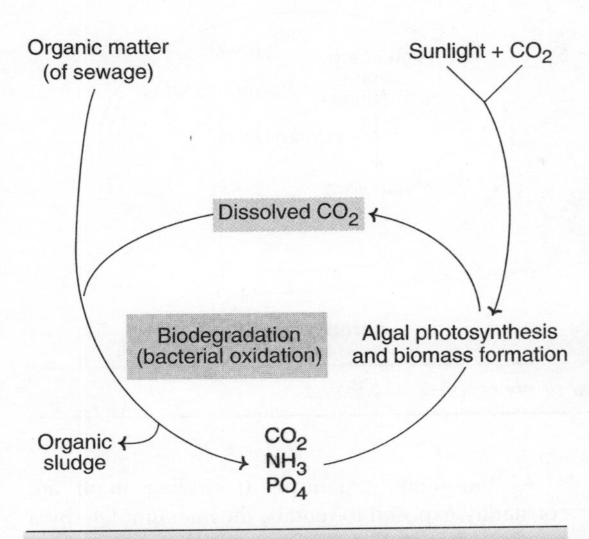

Fig. 54.2 : Sewage treatment by algae.

In the biological treatment of sewage, the organic matter is subjected to ***biodegradation*** or bacterial oxidation. In this way, the organic matter is degraded to smaller molecules (CO_2, NH_3, PO_4 etc.), Biodegradation requires a constant supply of O_2. This can be done by continuous bubbling of atmospheric O_2 through a specially designed equipment. This is an expensive process, besides the involvement of manpower.

A continuous supply of O_2 can be achieved by growing microalgae in the ponds where sewage treatment is being carried out. The algae are very efficient in photosynthesis and they release O_2 in to the ponds. This is the form of dissolved O_2 (***Fig. 54.2***). Thus, ***algal-bacterial symbiosis is responsible for photosynthetic oxygenation and the biodegradation of sewage organic matter***. This is a natural and inexpensive process.

In addition to the supply of CO_2, the algae used in sewage treatment can adsorb certain toxic heavy metals also. This is possible due to the negative charges on the algal cell surface which can take up the positively charged metals. The algal treatment of sewage is useful in several other ways.

- Support fish growth, as the algal cells are good food for fishes, besides supplying dissolved O_2.
- The algal cells, rich in protein, serve as good food and feed.
- Certain metals (that are adsorbed from the sewage) can be recovered.
- The load of pathogenic microorganisms is very much reduced (they either die or settle at the bottom of the pond).

The algal species of different genera ideally suited for sewage treatment are *Chlorella, Euglene, Chlamydomonas, Scenedesmus, Ulothrix* and *Thribonima.*

EUTROPHICATION AND PHOSPHORUS POLLUTION

Sewage, and waste waters from industries and agriculture are rich in organic and inorganic nutrients, containing phosphorus and to a lesser extent nitrogen. These nutrients favour ***excessive growth of algae*** which results in ***oxygen depletion (deoxygenation)*** and this phenomenon is referred to as ***eutrophication***. Eutrophication results in the death of non-resistant organisms (e.g. fishes), and foul smell.

Water blooms : Certain species of algae (particularly blue green algae e.g. *Lynhbia, Microcystis, Oscillatoria, Anabaena*) that can tolerate eutrophication, grow well and form water blooms in waste/sewage water. From the extensive formation of water blooms, one can predict that pond has accumulation of very high quantities of phosphorus. The algae are capable of absorbing phosphorus, and store them as polyphosphates. Phosphorus is a strong promoter of algal growth and water bloom formation. Water blooms are associated with the production of certain toxins (e.g. lipopolysaccharides) that are harmful to fishes and birds. These toxins may also cause certain diseases in humans e.g. diarrhea, gastroenteritis, nausea.

Control of eutrophication : There are broadly two ways of controlling algal growth resulting in eutrophication. In the ***chemical approach***, algicides such are copper sulfate, sodium arsenate and 2, 3-dichloronaphthoquinone are used. But the chemical treatment is associated with increase in sludge volume. In the ***biological approach, cyanophages*** (i.e. the viruses that can kill algal cells) can be used to contain eutrophication.

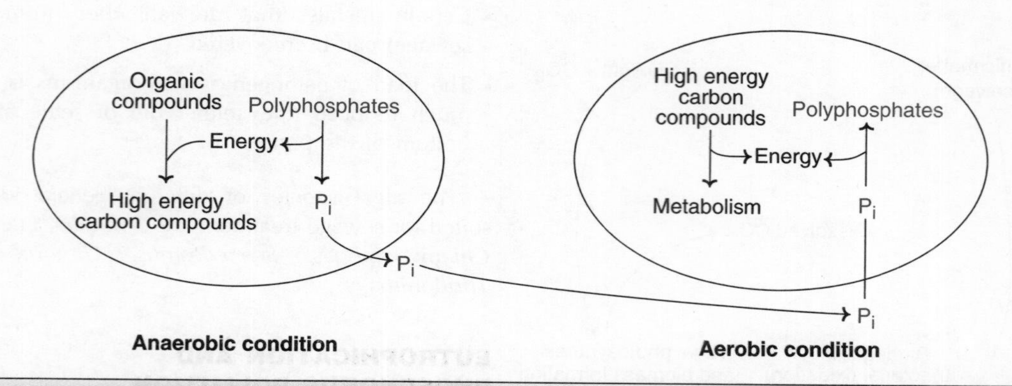

Fig. 54.3 : Biological removal of phosphorus by bacteria.

BIOLOGICAL REMOVAL OF PHOSPHORUS

As stated above, phosphorus significantly contributes to algal growth in waste water. Removal of phosphorus therefore can protect from eutrophication. It is possible to precipitate phosphorus with salts of calcium, magnesium and aluminium. This however, is not practicable on large scale. In addition, ***chemical methods*** add to the sludge volume. Hence, biological methods are preferred.

Biological removal of phosphorus by bacteria is carried out through aerobic and anaerobic processes, as depicted in ***Fig. 54.3***. Under anaerobic conditions, certain organic compounds (e.g. acetate) obtain their energy from polyphosphates to store as carbon reserves. In this process, free inorganic phosphorus is released. In the subsequent aerobic process, the organic carbon reserve compounds are oxidized to generate energy. A small portion of this energy is utilized for the conversion of phosphates to polyphosphates. The net effect is that phosphorus accumulates in the bacterial cell in the form of polyphosphates.

MANAGEMENT OF METAL POLLUTION

Environmental pollution with heavy metals (e.g., lead, cadmium, mercury) causes several toxic manifestations in living organisms, including cancer. Bioaccumulation, biomagnification and biomethylation are some of the characteristic features of metal pollution.

As the living organisms (including man) are constantly exposed to metals, they accumulate by a process referred to as ***bioaccumulation***. Continuous exposure and accumulation of a given metal in the organisms results in its increased concentration, a phenomenon referred to as ***biomagnification***. Biomagnification usually occurs ***through food chain*** and man is the ultimate victim.

Biomethylation is the process of transfer of methyl groups from organic compounds to metals. This is carried out by microorganisms in the soil and water. Although it is true that some metals get detoxified by methylation (e.g. arsenic), some of them may even become more toxic (mercury).

BIOSCAVENGERS OF METALS

Certain aquatic plants namely ***phytoplanktons*** (plants that freely float on water surface) or ***benthics*** (plants attached to some substratum at the bottom of aquatic reservoirs) and microorganisms can take up the metals from the bathing media (waste water, ponds) and act as ***natural bioscavengers***. Besides combating the pollution effects of metals, this process is also useful for the recovery of industrially important metals from the bioscavengers.

In the recent years, environmental protection agencies (EPAs) worldover are advocating the use of aquatic plants and microorganisms as low cost bioabsorbants for the removal of toxic metals from the environmental pollution.

Some of the plants and microorganisms useful for the management of metal pollution are briefly described.

Plants in metal pollution management

Water hyacinth : This is the most common weed found in tropical waters and its control is a major problem. This plant can absorb and accumulate cadmium, mercury, lead and even silver to a significant extent.

Water lettuce : This is a floating aquatic weed, and is also a good metal bioscavenger. It can take up large quantities of lead, cadmium, mercury and arsenic.

Cat-tails : These plants possess long erect leaves and grow in marshy areas. Cat-tail leaves have been shown to be useful for the absorption of nickel, copper, besides calcium and magnesium salts. Water spinach that accumulates lead and chromium is eaten in some areas by poor people. The toxic metals are certainly toxic to humans.

Ferns : The fern namely *Azolla filicoides* accumulates cadmium, copper and uranium. *Salvinia* sp can absorb several metals including lead, nickel and chromium.

Microorganisms in metal pollution management

Algae : Several metals from the fresh water can be absorbed by ***algal blooms***. For instance, *Chlorella vulgaris* can take up copper, mercury and uranium. The marine microalgae (e.g., *Ulva, Laminaria*) are also useful for the abatement of metal pollutants.

Fungi : Certain fungal species are good absorbers of heavy metals (Pb, Hg). e.g. *Rhizopus, Aspergillus, Penicillum, Neurospora.*

Bacteria : A few bacterial species can accumulate metals on their cell walls. For instance, *E. coli* can take up mercury while *Bacillus circulans* can accumulate copper.

Attempts are being made to improve the strains of bacteria (through genetic manipulations) for more efficient uptake and accumulation of toxic metals. Further, such species will also be useful for the recovery of metals from the bacterial biomass.

MECHANISMS OF METAL SCAVENGING

The aquatic plants and microorganisms may take up the metal pollutants through absorption and/or adsorption. The mechanism of accumulation of metals by the bioscavengers is very complex and may involve one or more of the following processes.

Binding of metals to cell walls

Bioaccumulation of metals on the cell walls is commonly observed in lower plants-algae, fungi and bacteria. Even some higher plants can concentrate metals on the cell walls. There is some evidence to show that metals are held to certain organic biopolymers on the cell walls, till the binding sites get saturated.

Accumulation of metals in cellular compartments

Plants are capable of transporting metals to intracellular and intercellular free spaces, and the cellular organelles (lysosomes, vacuoles). Certain metals occur as immobilized metal containing crystals. For instance, heavy metal complexes of calcium oxalate crystals have been detected in algae.

Synthesis of metal binding proteins

Several algae and certain fungal species are known to synthesize metal binding proteins or peptides. ***Phytochelatin*** is an ubiquitious protein present in all the plants. It is a metal chelating protein and is regared as a common buffering molecule for the homeostasis of metals. Phytochelatin is rich in cysteine and can form salt metal complexes through sulfhydryl (SH) groups. It is comparable in its functions to ***metallothionein*** found in animals.

Certain metals are known to induce the synthesis of phytochelatin. Some workers, in recent years, have suggested ***phytochelatin*** can be used as a ***biomarker*** for metal pollution detection.

IMMOBILIZED CELLS IN THE MANAGEMENT OF POLLUTION

The use of immobilized cells, paticularly microbial whole cells, for the abatement of environmental pollution is a recent development. The general aspects of cell immobilization, techniques involved, and their applications are described elsewhere (Chapter 21).

The immobilized cells are useful for the waste water treatment, and for the recovery of metals

TABLE 54.2 A selected list of pollutants and the corresponding immobilized microorganisms used for their abatement

Pollutant	*Immobilized microorganism*
Phenol	*Pseudomonas putida*
	Cryptococcus elinovii
Triethyl lead	*Arthrobacter* sp
4-Chlorophenol	*E. coli*
	Enterobacter sp
	Alcaligenes sp
Ammonia	*Thiosphaera* sp
Copper	*Rhizopus arrhizus*

from industrial effluents. A selected list of the pollutants and the immobilized microorganisms used for their abatement is given in ***Table 54.2***. For instance, phenol and triethyl lead can be removed respectively by immobilized *Pseudomonas putida* and *Arthrobacter* sp.

For more efficient management of a group of environmental pollutants simultaneously, immobilized systems with more than one type of microorganisms are used. In the recent past, ***genetically engineered microorganisms*** (***GEMs***) are being developed for the treatment of polluted water and soils. Some details on this aspect are described in Chapter 59.

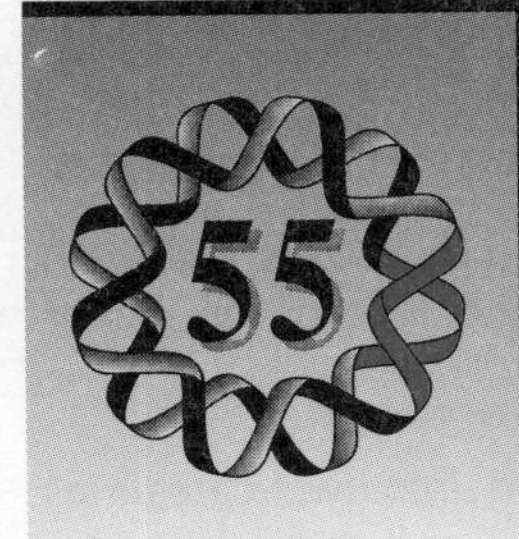

Air Pollution and Control

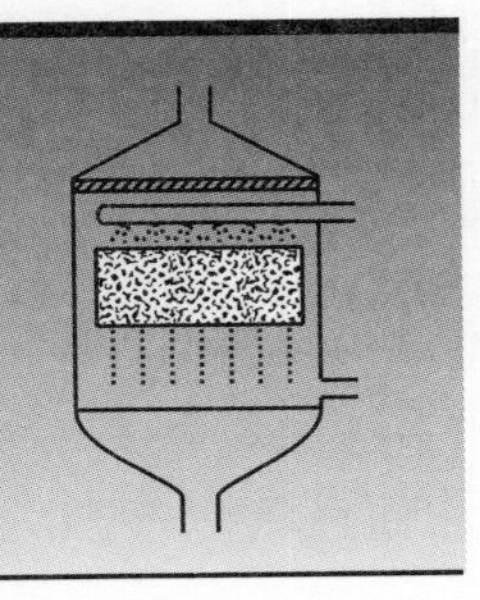

The earth's atmosphere contains various gases, water vapor and suspended particles. The ***dry air*** of the atmosphere is composed of four major gases ***nitrogen***, ***oxygen***, ***argon*** and ***carbon dioxide***, that account for more than 99.5% (***Table 55.1***). The other gases found in traces in the air include helium, methane, krypton, hydrogen, carbon monoxide, nitrous oxide (N_2O), nitrogen dioxide (NO_2), ammonia, ozone, sulfur dioxide and hydrogen sulfide. The lower part of the atmosphere (up to about 12 km) also contains water vapor at a concentration, ranging from 0.01 to 5.0%. This water is mostly contributed by evaporation from the hydrosphere.

The air is getting contaminated by pollution due the natural and unnatural activities of man. '***Air pollution*** is basically the ***presence of foreign substances in the air*** at a concentration that will ***adversely affect the health and property*** of the individual.

As per the World Health Organization (WHO) criteria, air pollution refers to 'the substances put into the air by the activity of mankind into concentration sufficient to cause harmful effects to his health, vegetables, property or to interfere with the enjoyment of his property.'

According to Indian Standards Institution 'air pollution is the presence in ambient atmosphere of substances generally resulting from the activity of man, in sufficient concentration, present for sufficient time and under circumstances which interfere significantly with the comfort, health or welfare of a person or with the full use or enjoyment of his property.'

TABLE 55.1 Composition of the dry air in the lower atmosphere

Gas	*Composition (% by volume)*
Nitrogen	78.08
Oxygen	20.95
Argon	0.93
Carbon dioxide	0.03
Trace gases (He, CH_4, Kr, H_2, CO, N_2O, NO_2, NH_3, O_3, SO_2, H_2S)	> 0.02

The term ***pollutant*** refers to a substance which increases in quantity in the air and adversely affects the environment e.g. carbon monoxide, sulfur dioxide, lead. On the other hand, a ***contaminant*** is a substance which is ***not present in nature***, but released due to human activity e.g. methyl isocyanate. DDT, malathion. However, this distinction is not very rigid, and most authors use the term pollutant to represent both (pollutant as well as contaminant).

SOURCES OF AIR POLLUTANTS

The sources that contribute to air pollution may be broadly categorized into two types.

TABLE 55.2 Major industrial sources of air pollution

Industry	*Major air pollutants*
Thermal power plants	NO_2, N_2O, SO_2, particulates
Steel industries	Smoke, particulates, CO, fluoride
Petroleum refineries	SO_2, smoke, particulates
Metal smelters	SO_2, NO_2, N_2O, smoke, particulates
Fertilizer plants	SO_2, NO_2, N_2O, NH_3, fluoride
Acid plants	SO_2, NO_2, N_2O
Cement plants	SO_2, smoke, particulates
Soap and detergent plants	Particulates, odour
Paper mills	SO_2, particulates, odour

1. **Natural sources :** These include volcanic eruptions, sand storms, decomposition of organic matter, forest fire, pollen grains and cormic dust. The problem of pollution due to natural sources in general, is considered to be minimal.

2. **Anthropogenic (man-made) sources :** Air pollution due to human-induced activities is very high. The sources of pollution include industries, burning of fossil fuels, emissions from vehicles, agricultural activities and warfares.

The sources of air pollution may also considered as ***stationary*** (industries, open combustion) or ***mobile*** (motor vehicles, trains, aircraft) in nature.

Industrial pollutants

The major problem of air pollution is due to industrial activities. Among the several industries, nine types of industries are considered to be the major air pollutant generating industries (***Table 55.2***). Among these, thermal power plants, steel industries, petroleum refineries and metal smelters are the most dangerous polluting industries.

CLASSIFICATION OF AIR POLLUTANTS

Air pollutants are classified based on their origin, chemical composition and the state of the matter.

Classification based on origin

Air pollutants are divided into two categories, based on their origin-primary and secondary.

Primary air pollutants : These pollutants are ***directly emitted into the atmosphere*** and present there as such (i.e. in the form they are originally emitted). Primary air pollutants contribute to as much as ***90% global air pollution***. Particulates, carbon monoxide, (CO), oxides of sulfur (SO_x), oxides of nitrogen (NO_x), hydrocarbons (HCs), radioactive compounds, pollen and bacteria are the major primary air pollutants.

Secondary air pollutants : These are ***produced*** in the air ***as a result of interaction among the primary pollutants***, or by a reaction that occurs between a primary pollutant and a normal constituent of the atmosphere. Good examples of secondary air pollutants are ozone (O_3), peroxyacetyl nitrate (PAN), formaldehyde and smog.

Classification based on chemical composition

According to chemical composition, air pollutants are categorized as organic and inorganic.

Organic air pollutants : These pollutants are mainly composed of carbon and hydrogen. In addition, oxygen, nitrogen, sulfur and phosphorus may also be present e.g. hydrocarbons, organic sulfur compounds, aldehydes, ketones, carboxylic acids.

Inorganic air pollutants : These are purely inorganic in nature e.g. carbon dioxide, carbon monoxide, oxides of sulfur, oxides of nitrogen, ozone.

Classification based on the state of matter

Air pollutants may be divided into two types, based on the state in which they exist-particulate and gaseous.

Particulate air pollutants : The solids and liquids dispersed in the atmosphere constitute the particulate air pollutants. ***Solid particulates*** e.g. smoke, dust, fly ash. ***Liquid particulates*** e.g. mist, fog, spray.

Gaseous air pollutants : These are the organic and inorganic gases that are present in the air as pollutants. ***Organic gases*** e.g. methane, butane, aldehydes. ***Inorganic gases*** e.g. CO_2, SO_2, NO_2, NH_3, H_2S.

EFFECTS OF AIR POLLUTION

Majority of the air pollutants are present normally in the atmosphere, although at low concentrations. Such pollutants are unlikely to cause any significant harmful effects. When the concentrations of the air pollutants go beyond the acceptable limits (variable for each pollutant) they are dangerous and cause several harmful effects. The WHO has set guidelines and fixed ***threshold limit values*** (***TLV***) for each air pollutant. The general effects of air pollutants on humans, plants, animals, materials and global climate are briefly described.

Effects of air pollutants on humans

On an average, man breathes around 22,000 times and inhales about 16 kg of air each day. Primarily, the air we breath is life sustaining. However, pollutants present in the air ***often cause harmful effects***. The nature of the pollutant, its concentration and duration of exposure are among the factors that affect the health of humans. In general, ***infants, elderly people and those with respiratory diseases are more susceptible to air pollution***. Further, adverse health effects of air pollutants are maximum during winter compared to other seasons.

Some of the important air pollutants and their effects on human health are given in ***Table 55.3***. ***Sulfur dioxide is the most dangerous pollutant gas to man***. It is produced in many industries and causes respiratory disorders. Oxides of nitrogen and carbon monoxide reduce O_2 supply to the tissues. Lead pollution is associated with tissue damage and abnormal behavioural pattern. Suspended particulate matter (SPM) mainly causes chronic pulmonary diseases. Prolonged exposure to radioactive isotopes results in anemia, besides a heavy risk of cancer and genetic defects.

Effects of air pollutants on plants

At low concentration, the air pollutants may not cause any visible damage to the plants. However, even at this level, the pollutants may be stored and introduced into the food chain. This in turn, may affect animals as well as humans.

TABLE 55.3 Health effects of some of the air pollutants

Pollutant	*Effects*
Sulfur dioxide (SO_2)	Nose and throat irritation, respiratory illness. Prolonged exposure may lead to chronic bronchitis.
Nitrogen dioxide (NO_2) and nitric oxide (NO)	Irritation of eyes, nose and throat. NO combines with O_2 and reduces supply of O_2 to tissues.
Carbon monoxide (CO)	Binds to hemoglobin and drastically reduces O_2 supply to tissues. May result in cardiovascular and pulmonary diseases.
Heavy metals (Pb)	Damage to liver, kidney and brain; causes anemia, neurobehavioural changes, abnormalities in fertility and pregnancy.
Aliphatic hydrocarbons and polycyclic organic compounds	Cancer
Suspended particulate matter (SPM)	Chronic pulmonary diseases–bronchitis, asthma.
Radioactive isotopes (I^{131}, P^{32}, Co^{60})	Anemia, cancer and genetic defects.

The entry of the gas air pollutants (SO_2, NO_2) predominantly occurs through the stomata, openings on the leaves. Stomata are located at the bottom of the leaves through which CO_2 enters for photosynthesis. In the same way as CO_2 enters the leaves, the gaseous pollutants also enter and cause various effects.

The solid particles are adsorbed on the surfaces of leaves. This may result in clogging of the stomata and a reduced intake of CO_2. Further, the suspended particles deposited on the leaves, may adversely affect the leaf functions (reduced exposure to sun light, decrease in chlorophyll content, interruption of gaseous exchange).

The effects of common air pollutants on leaves are given in ***Table 55.4***. The sensitivity of plants to pollutants depends on many factors such as climatic conditions (light, temperature, humidity),

TABLE 55.4 Effects of air pollutants on plants

Pollutant	*Effects*
Sulfur dioxide	Bleaching of leaves and necrosis (killing of leaves)
Nitrogen dioxide	Bleaching and suppressed growth
Ozone	Bleaching and necrosis
Fluorides	Marginal necrosis
Ammonia	Leaves become dull green
Ethylene and propylene	Leaf curling and leaf dropping
Peroxyacetylnitrate (PAN)	Suppressed growth and silvering of lower leaf surfaces
Particulates (with toxic metals)	Bleaching and necrosis

soil and water, and the individual plant's response to a particular pollutant. The major ***air pollutants affecting plants are SO_2, NO_2, O_3, fluorides, ammonia and ethylene***, besides the ***particulates***. They may damage the plants to varying degrees as outlined in ***Table 55.4***.

The sensitivity of certain selected plants to air pollutants can be used for biomonitoring of air pollution (details given later).

Effects of air pollutants on animals

The effect of air pollution on animals is mostly indirect, as it occurs after they eat polluted plants or foliage. Fluorine, lead and arsenic are three main air pollutants that cause harmful effects to livestock.

Fluorine : Fluorine causes loss of weight, muscular weakness, diarrhea, wearing of teeth, and even death. Fluorosis mainly affects the ruminants, particularly dairy cows.

Lead : Lead poisoning is commonly observed in animals grazing near lead mines. It is associated with loss of appetite, difficulty in breathing, diarrhea and paralysis.

Arsenic : Arsenic toxicity in animals is associated with increased salivation, thirst, irregular pulses, abnormal body temperature and paralysis. Chronic poisoning may result in anemia, diarrhea, paralysis and even death.

Effects of air pollutants on materials

Air pollutants cause immense damage to various materials — stone, metal, paint work, fibre materials, glass, ceramic, textiles, rubber, architecture etc. The adverse effects of air pollution on materials and properties are associated with ***severe economic losses throughout the world***.

Effects of air pollutants on global climatic changes

Air pollution is associated with significant changes in global climate and the related processes e.g., ozone depletion, green house effects, acid rain (Refer Chapter 60).

BIOMONITORING OF AIR POLLUTION

Plants are used to ***monitor*** (biomonitoring) air pollution and such plants are referred to as ***indicator plants***. This is based on the principle of sensitivity and response of the plants to air pollutants. A list of the plants used for biomonitoring and the corresponding air pollutants is given in ***Table 55.5***. Among these, lichens and mosses are most commonly used to check the quality of air. The pattern of occurrence of patches on lichens serves as an index for biomonitoring of air pollution.

Bioluminescence in air pollution monitoring

Bioluminescence is the phenomenon of emission of visible light by an organism. It occurs as an enzymatically catalysed light emitting

TABLE 55.5 Air pollutants and the plants for their biomonitoring

Air pollutant	*Plant(s)*
Sulfur dioxide	Lichens, moss, white pine
Ozone	Tobacco, garden bean
Peroxyacetylnitrate (PAN)	Lettuce, bean
Ethylene	Orchids, marigold, cucumber
Fluoride	Apricot, peach
Heavy metals	Moss, lichens

reaction in living cells. Bioluminescence is an indicator for the analysis of atmospheric gases such as SO_2, formaldehyde and ethyl acetate. The microorganism, *Photobacterium phosphoreum* can be used as a special photodetector. The changes in the emission of light due to a pollutant can be detected by a sensor, amplified and recorded.

AIR POLLUTION CONTROL

The air pollution load particularly from industries, can be reduced by several measures-replacement of burning fuel by electricity or solar energy, improvement in fuel burning process, dispersion and dilution of pollutants, and reduction at source by using control equipment. These measures, however, are useful only to a limited extent.

In the nature itself, there are certain devices, commonly referred to as ***atmospheric self-cleansing processes*** for the removal of air pollutants. These natural processes are very slow and limited, and cannot cope up with the present increased demands of pollution control. However, the artificially devised pollution control measures are based on the same principles of atmosphere self-cleansing processes. These principles include ***dispersion, gravitational settling, flocculation, absorption*** and ***rain out***.

There are ***two categories*** of ***air control devices***—devices to control ***particulate pollutants***, and to control ***gaseous pollutants***.

CONTROL DEVICES FOR PARTICULATE POLLUTANTS

In general, greater emphesis is given to control particulate pollutants, may be because they are visible. It may however, be noted that in terms of volume of air pollution, gaseous pollutant contribution is much higher.

The important devices/equipment used to control particulate pollutants are listed.

- Gravity settling chambers
- Cyclone collectors
- Dynamic precipitators
- Spray towers
- Electrostatic precipitators
- Fabric filters.

Gravity settling chambers

Settling chambers are the oldest and very simple type of equipment used for collection of solid particles (***Fig. 55.1A***). As the air is passed through the chambers at a low velocity, the ***dust particles*** (size 40–100 μm diameter) ***settle by gravity*** and the clean air comes out. Although this technique is simple, inexpensive with low cost of maintenance, it is not possible to settle smaller size dust particles.

Cyclone collectors

Cyclone collectors also operate on the ***principle of gravity settlement***. The equipment mainly consist of a vertically placed cylinder with an inverted cone attached to its base (***Fig. 55.1B***). As the air enters the cylinder, it takes a helical path downwards. Due to rapid spiralling movement of the air, the particles are thrown towards the walls by centrifugal force. These dust particles settle down in the hopper at the bottom, while the dust free air passes through a pipe and comes out.

The cyclone collectors are simple, low cost and easy for maintenance. They are ideal for separation of dust particles with sizes 15–50 μm. Cyclone collectors cannot settle particles less than 10 μm size.

Dynamic precipitators

Dynamic precipitators work on the ***principle of centrifugal force, generated by rotating blades*** (***Fig. 55.1C***). The dust particles of the air are concentrated on the rotating blades from where they are collected in a concentrated stream. By employing this equipment, dust particles of 5–20 μm size can be separated. However, dynamic precipitators are not suitable for sticky or fibrous dust particles, as they stick to the blades.

Spray towers

In spray towers, the ***dust particles*** (10 μm in size) are made to ***settle down by spraying water*** (***Fig. 55.1D***). This technique is particularly useful for separating a heavy load of particles.

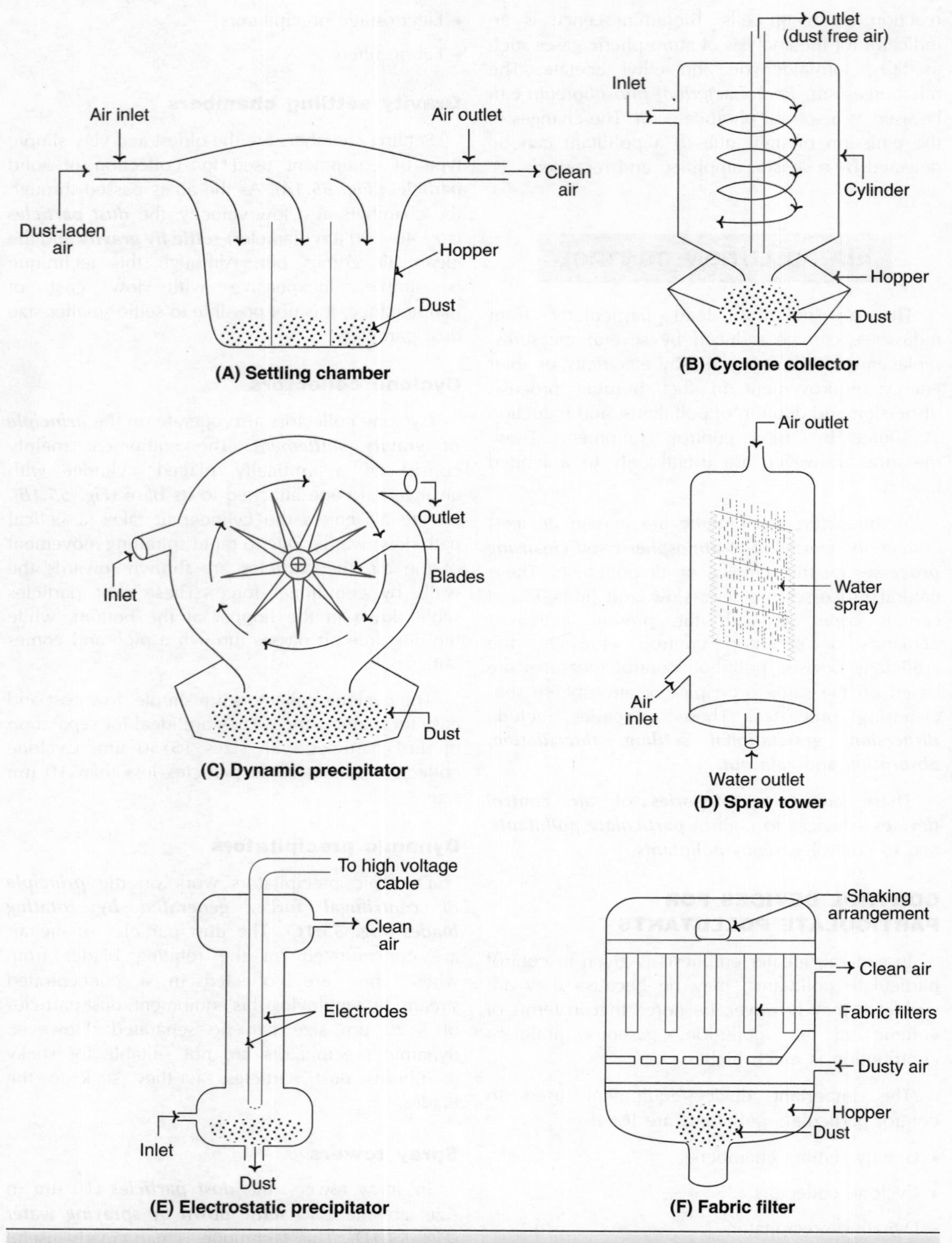

Fig. 55.1 : Control devices for particulate pollutants.

Electrostatic precipitators

Electrostatic precipitators (***ESPs***) are very efficient and versatile. They work on the ***basis of electrostatic attraction***. An ESP consists of a thick cylinder fitted with an inlet at bottom and an outlet at the top (***Fig. 55.1E***). An electrode (more than one electrode are commonly used) fitted at the centre of the cylinder is connected to a high voltage cable. As the dust laden air passes through ESP, larger sized particles settle down due to gravity. The smaller charged particles are attached to the oppositively charged electrodes which gradually fall down to the bottom. The dust free air comes out.

Electrostatic precipitators are said to be ***dry precipitators*** if the dust particles can be removed by scrapping. In case of ***wet electrostatic precipitators***, the particles are removed by using water or any other fluid. Wet precipitators are more efficient, however, dry precipitators are preferably used for practical reasons.

Fabric filters

Fabric filters (***Fig. 55.1F***) are the most efficient and can separate particles with sizes less than 0.5 μm in diameter. As the air or gas is passed over fabric like mats of wool, celluloss etc., ***the dust is trapped while the gas passes out***. Collection of dust on the fabric filter results in the formation of a dust layer (commonly referred to as filter cake). This in turn serves as a more efficient dust collector and helps to capture even fine dust particles. The fabric filters have to be frequently cleaned. Several models of fabric filters have been developed for commercial applications.

CONTROL DEVICES FOR GASEOUS POLLUTANTS

The principle gas pollutants are SO_2, NO_2, N_2O, CO, hydrocarbons, and organic and inorganic acid gases. The control devices used for gaseous pollutants are based on the ***principles of adsorption, absorption, condensation and combustion***. The important aspects of selected devices for controlling gaseous pollutants are briefly described.

Adsorption

When a stream of gas is passed through a porous solid material (absorbent), it can attract and hold the gas (adsorbate) molecules.

TABLE 55.6 A selected list of adsorbents and their major applications

Adsorbent	*Major application(s)*
Silicate or zeolates (as molecular sieves)	Control of SO_2, NO_2 and mercury
Activated alumina	Drying air, gases and liquids
Activated carbon	Removing odours, purification of gases
Silica gel	Drying and purifying gases
Bauxite	Drying of gases and liquids, treatment of petroleum fractions
Fuller's earth	Refining of oils and fats

If the adsorption is purely a physical phenomenon (held by van der Waal's forces), it is referred to as ***physical adsorption***. This process is rapid and easily ***reversible***. In ***chemical adsorption*** (***chemisorption***), the pollutant gas molecules form chemical bonds with the adsorbent. Chemisorption is very slow, usually requires the supply of energy and is irreversible. Pressure and temperature significantly influence chemical adsorption.

In the ***Table 55.6***, a selected list of the commonly used adsorbents along with their major applications is given. The equipment used for adsorption, referred to as ***adsorbers***, may be fixed, moving or fluidized beds.

Multiple fixed bed adsorber : In this, adsorbent is arranged in the form of beds or layers as depicted in ***Fig. 55.2A***. As the adsorption occurs, the adsorbent gets saturated with the adsorbate. For reuse, the gas collected on the adsorbent must be removed. If this is not possible, the adsorbent must be replaced.

Absorption

The pollutant gas (absorbate), when brought in contact with a solvent or liquid (absorbent), gets adsorbed. The process of absorption may occur due to physical or chemical phenomena.

Absorption process is used to control the pollutants SO_2, NO_2, H_2S and hydrocarbons. Ammonia is used as an absorbent for controlling SO_2.

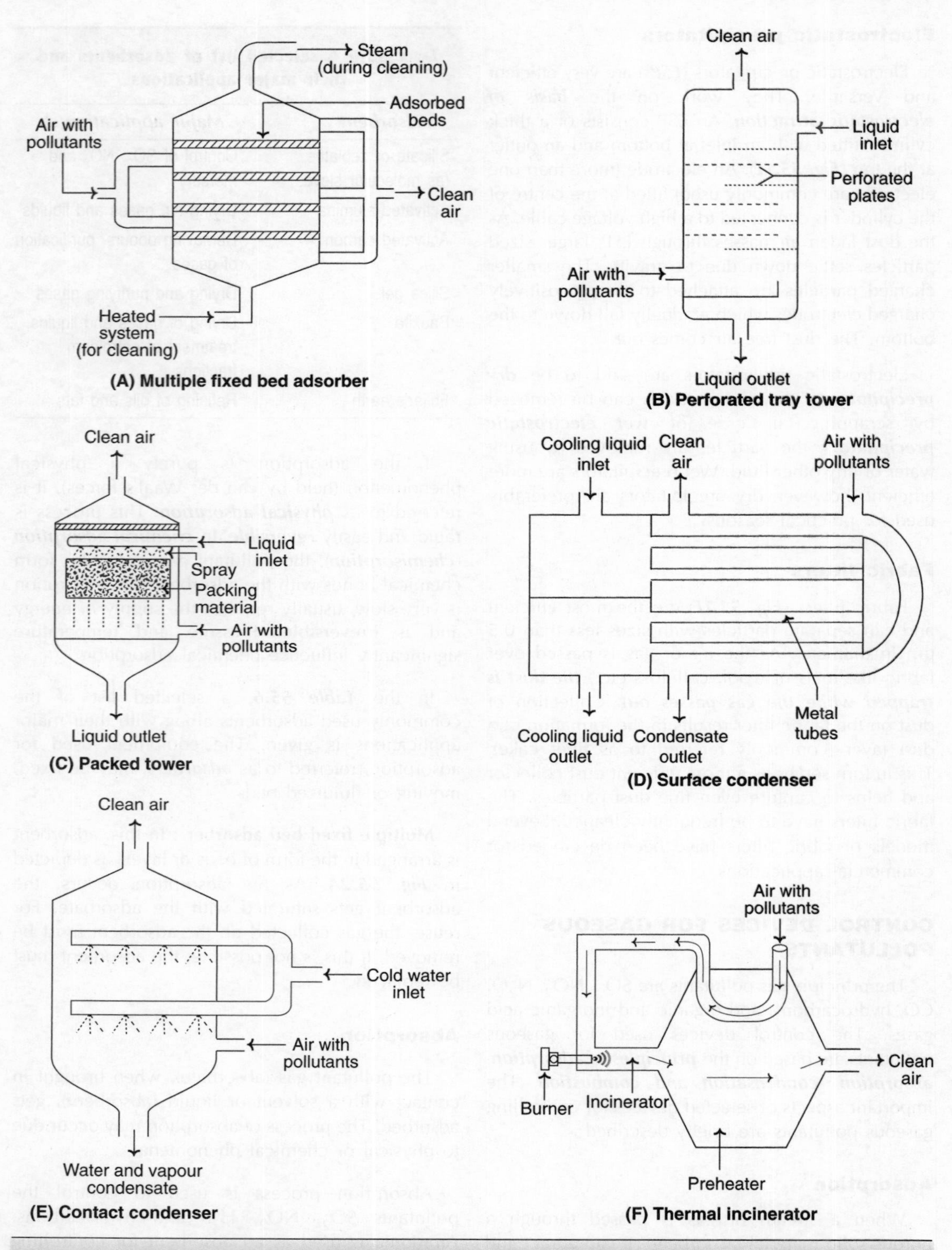

Fig. 55.2 : Control devices for gaseous pollutants.

Different types of ***absorbers*** are used for control of gaseous pollutants. These include spray towers, plate or tray towers and packed towers. The gas absorption units are so designed that there occurs an intimate contact between the gas and the liquid. This will ensure optimal absorption of gas into the liquid.

Spray towers (Refer ***Fig. 55.1D***) : They can efficiently remove gaseous pollutants, besides the particulates. These devices are particularly useful for the removal of pollutant gases with high concentrations of particulates.

Plate or tray towers : These absorbers are designed with horizontal trays or plates so as to provide large liquid-gas interfacial surface (***Fig. 55.2B***). In the perforated tray tower, the absorbent enters the column from the top, spills and flows in a zig zag fashion. The polluted air enters the column from an inlet at the side of the bottom. As the air passes through the openings of the trays, it gets in close contact with liquid due to repeated exposure. This enables the removal of gaseous as well as particulate pollutants. The clean gas emerges at the top.

Packed towers : In this case, the liquid (absorbent) is sprayed over a packing material (e.g. all rings, Berl saddles) with large surface to volume ratio (***Fig. 55.2C***). The air with gaseous pollutants enters from the side of the bottom of the tower and the clean air comes out from the top.

Condensation

When the temperature of a gaseous compound is reduced, its condensation occurs. There are two devices commonly used to control gaseous pollutants, based on the principle of condensation.

Surface condenser : In this device, the cooling medium is passed through metal tubes over which the gas with pollutants is passed (***Fig. 55.2D***). The vapour condenses on the surface of the tubes. This gets collected as a film of liquid which can be drained off.

Contact condenser : In contact condenser, the cooling medium and the gaseous pollutants are made to have a direct contact with each other (***Fig. 55.2E***). As the vapors get cooled, they condense and are easily removed along with the water, and the clean gas comes out from the top of the condenser.

Combustion

It is a fact that combustion or incineration is a major source of air pollution. And surprisingly, the same combustion processes effectively serve to control air pollutants. This is carried out by converting certain pollutants (e.g., hydrocarbons, carbon monoxide) to carbon dioxide and water. For efficient oxidation during combustion, supply of oxygen, optimal temperature and time are necessary. There are different types of combustion processes depending on the pollutant to be oxidized. The most important ones are ***direct-flame combustion, thermal combustion*** and ***catalytic combustion***.

Direct-flame combustion : In this device, the waste gases are directly burnt with or without the addition of auxillary fuels. Direct-flame combustions are most often used in petrochemical plants and refineries.

Thermal combustion : This process usually becomes necessary when the gaseous pollutant concentration is too low, and it is difficult to carry out direct-flame combustion. Thermal combustion is carried out by a ***thermal incinerator*** or ***after burner*** (***Fig. 55.2F***). An heat exchanger preheats the air/gas with gaseous pollutants. This preheated gas is passed over to the incineration equipped with a burner. The temperature of the incinerator may be in the range 500–1000°C, and this actually depends on the nature of the pollutant to be oxidized. Combustion with thermal incinerators has to be carefully carried out so that the oxidation process is efficient and complete. Incomplete combustion may produce more pollutants e.g. carbon monoxide.

Catalytic combustion : This is required when the ***gaseous pollutants are too low in concentration***. By employing a catalyst, the combustion can be made faster and complete, and the catalyst can be used again and again.

Catalytic combustion is used for the removal of NO_2 (in the tail gas) from the nitric acid plants. Here platinum catalyst is used. Carbon monoxide can be removed by using copper (Cu^{2+}) catalyst.

The major limitation of catalytic combution is the high cost of the catalyst and maintenance of the catalytic combustion.

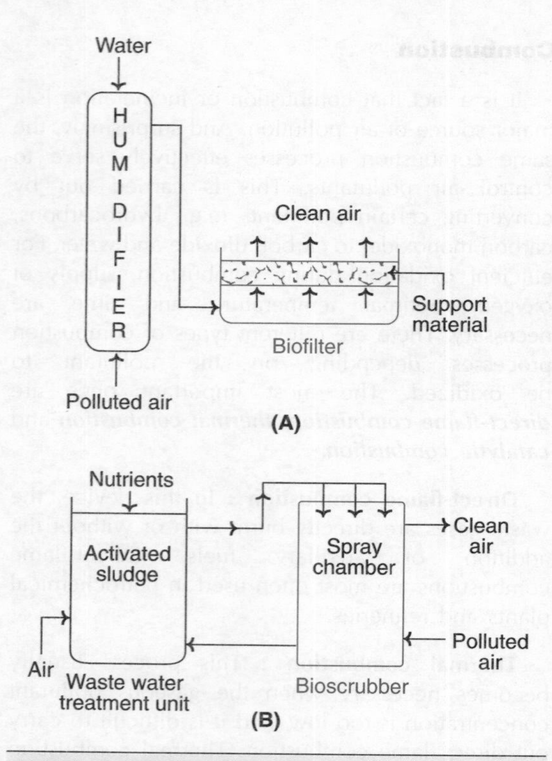

Fig. 55.3 : Treatment processes for the removal of volatile organic compounds (A) Biofilter (B) Bioscrubber.

CONTROL DEVICES FOR VOLATILE ORGANIC COMPOUNDS (VOCs)

There are several volatile organic compounds, arising from industrial and domestic activities, that cause air pollution. Good examples of VOCs are alcohols, ketones, organic acids, phenols and organic solvents. The conventional methods (e.g. combustion, adsorption) of treatment VOCs require large quantities of energy, besides creating secondary pollution.

Biodegradation by microorganisms is a preferred method for controlling air pollution of VOCs. The efficiency of biodegradation depends on the individual compounds and based on this, VOCs are broadly categorized as follows :

- ***Rapidly degraded VOCs***— alcohols, ketones, aldehydes, organic acids.
- ***Slowly degraded VOCs***— hydrocarbons, phenols, organic solvents (chloroethene).
- ***Very slowly degraded VOCs***— polyaromatic hydrocarbons, polyhalogenated hydrocarbons.

There are mainly two types of reactor designs for the biodegradation of VOCs — biofilters and bioscrubbers (***Fig. 55.3***).

Biofilters

A biofilter is composed of a porous medium (of compost, wood chips) that supports the microorganisms forming a film. The polluted air is first passed through a humidifier and then through the biofilter. A great majority of VOCs in the air (approximately 90%) get biodegraded, and clean air comes out of the biofilter (***Fig. 55.3A***).

Advantages of biofilters : They are simple and cost-effective. Certain poorly ***soluble pollutants*** (hydrocarbons) can ***be easily removed*** by this approach. Biofilters can be successfully used for the biodegradation of several xenobiotics e.g. chloromethane.

Disadvantages of biofilters : It is rather difficult to control process conditions (pH, temperature). When compost is used as support material, it generates unpleasant odours. Biofilters require large areas.

Bioscrubbers

Bioscrubber is an improvement over biofilter (***Fig. 55.3B***). When the polluted air is passed through a liquid stream in a spray chamber, the pollutant (VOC) gets transferred to the liquid. The sprayed liquid contains a suspension of microorganisms which cycles between the spray chamber and waste water treatment unit (activated sludge unit). The microbial biodegradation of VOC occurs in the waste water treatment unit. The clean air comes out, after recycle, from the spray chamber. Besides a continuous nutrient supply, it is essential to maintain the pH in the activated sludge unit.

Biotrickle filters

Biotrickle filter is a recent development for more efficient biodegradation of VOCs. It ***works on the principles of adsorption, followed by biodegradation***. The pollutant gases are adsorbed on a solid surface (e.g. activated carbon) and then subjected to biodegradation by a stream of medium containing the desired microorganisms. As of now, biotrickle filters are at an experimental stage, and soon they may be available for use.

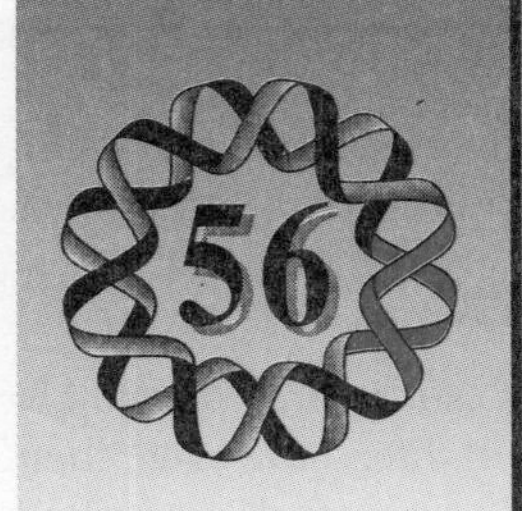

Water Pollution and Sewage

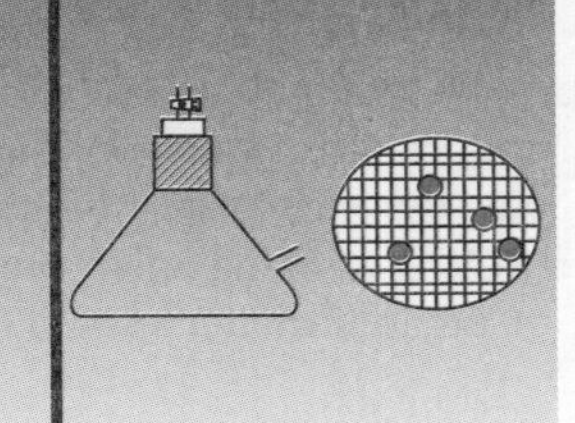

Water is absolutely ***essential for the existence of life*** (animal or plant). It provides a wonderful chemical medium in which all biological and biochemical processes occur. Water dissolves various nutrients, distributes them to cells and removes waste products.

About 60% of the human body is composed of water. One can survive without food for some weeks, but cannot survive without water for more than a few days. Besides drinking, man requires water for bathing, washing, livestock raising, industrial, agricultural and various other purposes.

Water-a scarce natural resource

Water, covering more than 70% of the earth's surface, exists in all three states-liquid, solid and gas. Most of the water on earth is salt water, and is unsuitable for drinking and other needs of man. It is estimated that ***only around 0.007% of the earth's water is available for direct human consumption***. Thus, ***consumable water is a scarce natural resource.***

Water is required for development and progress of people, and therefore a nation. In fact historically, the places of availability of water were the major determinants for the settlement of people. This is because besides regular use, water is essential to raise the crops. It is an accepted fact that a community with good water supply has good growth, progress and prosperity.

For the reasons stated above, it is well recognized worldover that there is an ***urgent need for water conservation and management***. The Governmental policies also support this concept.

DISSOLVED OXYGEN

Oxygen is soluble in water, and this dissolved oxygen (DO) is ***essential to support fish and other aquatic life in water***. The solubility of atmospheric oxygen in fresh water is around 7–15 mg/dl, depending on the temperature and pressure. Increase in temperature and salts in water decreases O_2 solubility.

Oxygen gets dissolved in water by one or more of the following ways.

- Direct entry from the atmosphere.
- By aquatic plant (algae) photosynthesis.
- Introduction by artificial means (aerators).

Importance of dissolved oxygen

A minimum level of dissolved oxygen at a concentration around 4 mg/dl is considered to be necessary to support healthy aquatic life. If good aerobic conditions are not maintained, anaerobic microorganisms take over and cause harmful effects. And this is what happens in polluted waters, particularly from the industrial and municipal wastes.

Determination of dissolved oxygen is very important in water pollution. This is mostly carried out by measuring ***biochemical oxygen demand*** (***BOD***), utilizing microorganisms for the oxidation of organic matter (See p. 683).

WATER POLLUTION

Several kinds of natural, and man made activities (domestic, industrial, agricultural etc.) contribute to water pollution. Water pollution is characterized by certain ***observable disturbances in the normal properties and functions of fresh water***. These include offensive odours, decrease in aquatic life (e.g. fishes), bad taste and unchecked growth of aquatic weeds.

Ground water pollution

The ground water is generally considered to be safe and is useful for drinking, agricultural and industrial purposes. In fact, ***ground water is less prone to pollution***. However, in recent years, it is recognized that contamination with fluoride, arsenic and nitrate in the ground water poses a serious threat to human health.

Surface water pollution

The rivers, lakes and reservoirs are highly susceptible for pollution due to natural and man-made activites (industrial, domestic, agricultural etc.). The routes for the entry of pollutants include sewage outfalls, industrial outfalls, and outfalls from nuclear stations. Surface water pollution is a major threat for the survival of life itself. It is therefore necessary that regular monitoring of various routes of water contamination is done and effective protective measures are taken to minimise the pollution.

NATURE OF WATER POLLUTANTS

There are a large number of water pollutants which may be in dissolved, suspended or colloidal state. The pollutants may be broadly categorized as follows.

- Organic pollutants
- Inorganic pollutants
- Microbiological pollutants
- Radioactive pollutants.

The salient features of these pollutants and the sources of their contribution are briefly described.

ORGANIC POLLUTANTS

Organic compounds as such are absolutely essential for the existence of life. However, their entry into water causes pollution resulting in bad odour and unpleasant taste. In addition, some of the organic compounds may be toxic or even carcinogenic to humans.

Sources of organic pollutants

There are several natural sources of organic pollutants. These include the decay of leaves, plants, and dead animals, besides the release of organic materials from aquatic plants and microorganisms.

Several synthetic organic pollutants (e.g. pesticides, herbicides, ethylbenzene) and synthetic volatile organic chemicals (e.g. carbon tetrachloride, tetrachloroethylene) pollute water. Certain organic pollutants such as dioxin and polychlorinated biphenyls (PCBs) are very toxic, besides being carcinogenic to humans.

INORGANIC POLLUTANTS

In the natural fresh water (source may be ground or surface), there occurs varying concentrations of inorganic chemicals. Most of them, in general, are within the acceptable limits.

Sources of inorganic pollutants

The industrial and agricultural outflows pollute water with inorganic compounds e.g. metal complexes, inorganic salts, mineral acids, trace elements. Among these, water pollution due to toxic metals assumes significance e.g. lead, mercury, cadmium, nickel, arsenic and aluminium.

MICROBIOLOGICAL POLLUTANTS

A wide range of microorganisms (viruses, bacteria, protozoa, algae, helminths) contribute to water pollution. A majority of these organisms are harmless to humans. However, there are certain organisms that cause diseases, referred to as ***water borne diseases***. Such organisms causing some form of sickness in humans are referred to as ***pathogens*** or ***pathogenic organisms***. A selected list of pathogenic organisms and the corresponding diseases is given in ***Table 56.1***.

TABLE 56.1 Common pathogenic organisms found in water (domestic waste water) and the respective diseases

Organism	*Disease*	*Major disease symptom*
Bacteria		
Escherichia coli (*enteropathogenic*)	Gastroenteritis	Diarrhea
Salmonella typhi	Typhoid	High fever, diarrhea
Salmonella paratyphi	Paratyphoid	Fever
Salmonella sp	Salmonellosis	Food poisoning
Vibrio cholerae	Cholera	Diarrhea, dehydration
Shigella sp	Shigellosis	Bacillary dysentery
Legionella pneumophila	Legionellosis	Acute respiratory illness
Viruses		
Adenovirus	Respiratory diseases	Breathing difficulty
Enteroviruses	Gastroenteritis	Diarrhea
Reovirus	Gastroenteritis	Diarrhea
Rotavirus	Gastroenteritis	Diarrhea
Hepatitis A	Infectious hepatitis	Jaundice
Protozoa		
Entamoeba histolytica	Amoebic dysentery	Prolonged diarrhea
Giardia lamblia	Giardiasis	Mild diarrhea, nausea
Balantidium coli	Balantidiasis	Dysentery
Helminths		
Ascaris lumbricoides	Ascariasis	Roundworm infestation
Schistosoma sp	Schistosomiasis	Hematuria, diarrhea
Fasciola hepatica	Fascioliasis	Jaundice
Taenia saginata	Taeniasis	Intestinal infection
Algae		
Microcystis aeruginosa	Gastroenteritis	Diarrhea
Aphanizomenon flosaquae	Gastroenteritis	Diarrhea
Shizothrix calciola	Gastroenteritis	Diarrhea

Sources of pathogens

The pathogens are mainly present in the waste water and for most of them ***human feces are the prime source of pollution***. The human waste can pollute the water from sewage outfalls or from a flow of waste from ground (mostly from failed septic system).

The best way to control water contamination with pathogenic organisms is to prevent the human wastes (particularly feces) from entering potable water.

RADIOACTIVE POLLUTANTS

Water may get polluted with radioactive materials arising from nuclear plants, radioisotopes used in medical, industrial and research purposes, besides the processing of ores to produce radioisotpes. The radioactive pollutants are carcinogenic e.g. uranium, radium, thorium.

TABLE 56.2 Typical composition of domestic waste water or sewage (untreated)

Constituent(s)	*Concentration (mg/l)**		
	Weak	*Medium*	*Strong*
Total solids (TS)	350	700	1,250
Dissolved solids (DS)	250	500	900
Suspended solids (SS)	100	200	350
Total nitrogen	20	45	90
Organic N	10	15	40
Inorganic N (as free NH_3)	10	30	50
Total phosphorus	4	8	16
Organic	1	3	6
Inorganic	3	5	9
Chlorides	25	50	100
Alkalinity (as $CaCO_3$)	50	100	200
Grease	50	50	100 150
Volatile organic compounds (μg / l)	<100	100–400	>400
Biochemical oxygen demand (BOD)	100	200	400
Chemical oxygen demand (COD)	250	500	1000
Total coliform (no/dl)	10^6–10^7	10^7–10^8	10^8–10^9

* *The units for volatile organic compounds and total coliform are given along with them.*

WASTE WATER OR SEWAGE

Sewage is the ***liquid waste*** or waste arising mainly ***from domestic*** (residential, institutional, commercial) and ***industrial sources***.

COMPOSITION OF SEWAGE

The actual composition of sewage depends on the source from which it comes. In general, about 97–99% of sewage is composed of water while the rest (1-3%) is solids. The most important organic, inorganic compounds, and living organisms found in waste water are listed below.

Organic—carbohydrates, fats, proteins, amino acids and urea, besides the products of their degradation.

Inorganic—sand, mud, mineral ash, mineral salts, lead, arsenic, mercury and cyanides.

Living organisms — bacteria, viruses, algae, fungi and protozoa. Some details on pathogenic organisms and the corresponding diseases are given in ***Table 56.1***.

TYPES OF SEWAGE

The waste water (sewage) is broadly categorized as ***weak***, ***medium*** and ***strong***, based on the composition (***Table 56.2***). It must however, be noted that the composition of sewage is highly variable which mostly depends on the local conditions. The sewage mainly consists of solids, organic and inorganic compounds of nitrogen and phosphorus, chlorides, grease and volatile organic compounds. In ***Table 56.2***, the data on biochemical oxygen demand (BOD), chemical oxygen demand (COD) and total coliform for the three types of sewage are also given.

MEASUREMENT OF WATER POLLUTION

The measurement of water pollution in sewage waste water with special reference to organic matter and pathogenic organisms is described.

MEASUREMENT OF ORGANIC MATTER OF SEWAGE

The organic matter present in the sewage is regarded as ***biologically active***, if it can be ***oxidized by the bacteria***. On the other hand, the organic matter resistant ***to bacterial degradation*** is considered as ***biologically inactive***. For the purpose of sewage treatment, the biologically active organic matter is important.

The commonly used laboratory methods for the measurement of organic matter in sewage are given below.

- Biochemical oxygen demand (BOD)
- Chemical oxygen demand (COD)
- Total organic carbon (TOC)
- Theoretical oxygen demand (ThOD).

Biochemical oxygen demand (BOD)

Biochemical oxygen demand is the most widely used parameter to ***measure the organic pollution*** in sewage as well as surface water. BOD basically involves ***the measurement of dissolved oxygen (DO) utilized by the microorganisms for the biochemical oxidation of organic matter***. The demand for oxygen and the process of oxidation depends on the type and quantity of organic matter, temperature and type of the organism used.

In general, biochemical oxygen demand is measured for an ***incubation period of five days*** (hence appropriately referred to as ***BOD_5***) at a temperature of 20°C. If the organic content of the sewage is high, it needs to be diluted for the measurement of BOD. Further, for waste water with less population of microorganisms, seeding with bacterial culture is necessary.

BOD indicates the amount of organic matter present in the sewage. Thus, the more is organic content, the higher is the BOD (Refer ***Table 56.2*** for BOD values of different types of sewages). If the available oxygen (dissolved O_2) is less than the BOD, the organic matter decomposes anaerobically, putrifies and produces foul smell. Thus, ***BOD is a measure of nuisance potential of sewage***.

Limitations of BOD

1. BOD measures only biodegradable organic matter.

2. A high concentration of bacterial load is required.

3. For measuring BOD of toxic waste water, pretreatment is necessary.

4. Requires long period of incubation i.e. 5 days.

Despite these drawbacks, BOD is very widely used worldover for practical and economic reasons.

Chemical oxygen demand (COD)

Chemical oxygen demand refers to the ***oxygen equivalents of organic matter that can be oxidized by using strong chemical oxidizing agents***. Usually, potassium dichromate in the presence of a catalyst, in acidic medium is employed for this purpose. The overall reaction is given below.

$$\text{Organic matter} + Cr_2O_7^{2-} + H^+ \longrightarrow Cr^{3+} + CO_2 + H_2O$$

When compared with BOD, COD oxidizes more organic compounds, hence COD values are higher than BOD values. Chemical oxygen demand can be determined in just three hours, in contrast to BOD requiring five days. Some workers determine COD and calculate BOD. This is possible since there exists a reasonably good correlation between COD and BOD.

Total organic carbon (TOC)

Measurement of total organic carbon is required when the concentration of organic matter is very low. TOC can be determined by oxidizing organic carbon, in the presence of a catalyst to CO_2, which can be measured.

Theoretical oxygen demand (ThOD)

The organic matter of sewage is mainly composed of carbohydrates, proteins, fats and products of their decomposition. If the chemical formulae of the organic matter (i.e. individual compounds) are known, the theoretical oxygen demand can be calculated.

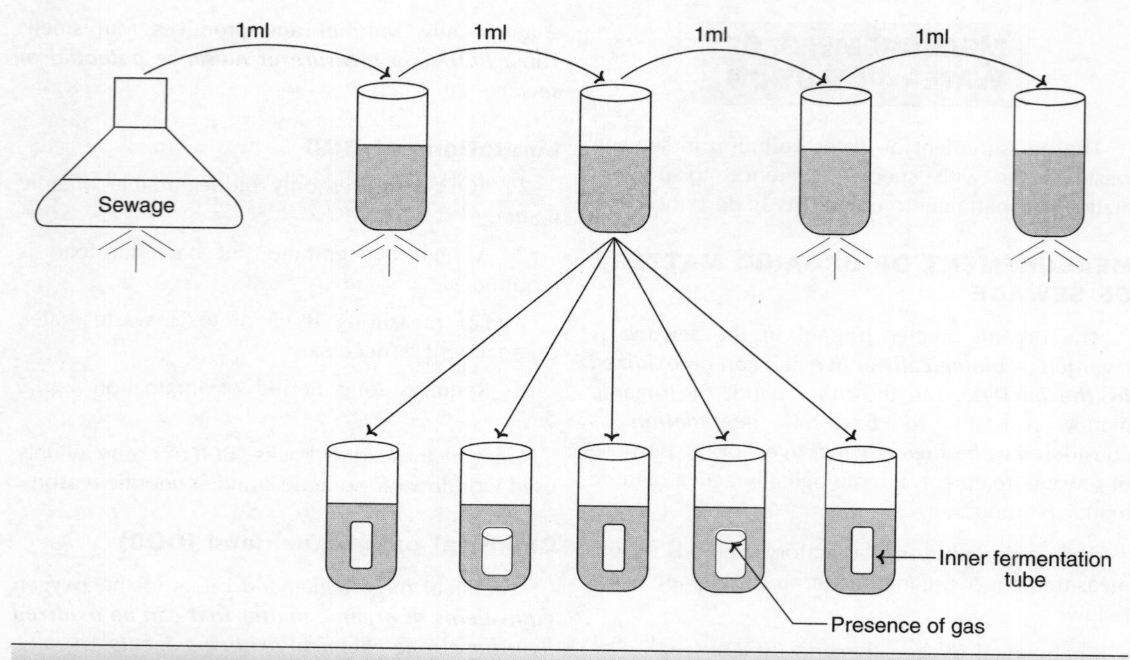

Fig. 56.1 : Multiple-tube fermentation technique for the detection of coliform bacteria.

DETECTION OF PATHOGENIC ORGANISMS OF SEWAGE

Human beings infected with disease-causing microorganisms (i.e. pathogens) are the carriers and they can discharge pathogenic organisms in waste water. Several species of bacteria, viruses, protozoa and helminths are responsible for diseases in humans. A selected list of the pathogenic organisms and the major diseases is given in (***Table 56.1***). Among the diseases (water-borne diseases) originating from sewage, typhoid, paratyphoid, cholera, gastroenteritis, diarrhea, and dysentery are important. All these diseases are highly infectious and are responsible for the death of thousands of people in countries (particularly developing ones) with poor sanitation.

Indicator or index organisms of sewage

It is tedious and time consuming to isolate and identify pathogenic organisms in water waste. Some other non-pathogenic bacteria of sewage polluted water are employed for this purpose e.g. *E. coli, Streptococus faecalis, Clostridium perfingens, Klebisella* sp. These organisms are collectively referred to as ***indicator*** or ***index organisms***.

Among the indicator organisms, the rod-shaped bacteria, commonly known as ***coliform organisms*** (*E. coli, Aerobacter* sp) are the most commonly used. The intestinal tract of man is very rich in coliform bacteria. It is estimated that each person discharges about 100–400 billions of coliform organisms per day. Therefore, the detection of coliform organisms is a clear indication of fecal contamination and thus the presence of pathogenic organisms. On the other hand, the absence of these organisms indicates that the water is free from disease-causing organisms. Detection of coliform organisms is based on the fact that a ***great majority of water-borne diseases have fecal origin***.

LABORATORY METHODS FOR DETECTION OF COLIFORM ORGANISMS

There are three methods commonly employed for the detection of coliform organisms in water samples-multiple tube-fermentation technique, membrane filter technique and colilert technique.

Multiple-tube fermentation (MTF) technique

This is basically a test that involves acid fermentation. Lactose broth fermentation is tested at around 35°C for 1-2 days in a series of tubes,

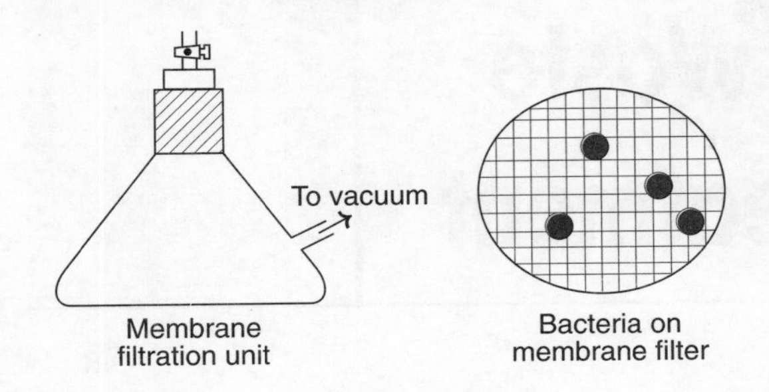

Fig. 56.2 : Membrane filtration technique for the detection of coliform bacteria.

involving sequential tests-presumptive test, confirmed test and completed test.

Presumptive test : The waste water sample is serially diluted. One ml of the sample of each dilution is then transferred to each of the five fermentation tubes. These tubes contain lactose culture medium and inverted gas collection tubes (***Fig. 56.1***). At the end of 24 hour incubation period, if there occurs ***gas collection in the inverted tube, the test is positive indicating the presence of coliform organisms.***

Confirmed test : If no gas formation occurs in the presumptive test, the incubation is continued for another 24 hours. If gas formation is detected now, the test confirms the presence of coliform bacteria. And if no gas is produced even in the confirmed test, it can be assumed that the samples are free from coliform.

Completed test : In this, a sample from positive coliform test is grown on eosin methylene blue (EMD) agar. The incubation is carried out at 35°C for 24 hours. The presence of ***E. coli*** can be ***detected*** by the ***occurrence*** of ***greenish metallic sheen*** on the plates.

Membrane filtration technique (MFT)

The presence of coliform organisms in water can be detected by using cellulose acetate ester with a pore size of 0.3 to 0.5 μm. For this purpose, the membrane is first sterilized for 20 minutes at 80°C. The filtration is carried out in aseptic conditions under vacuum.

As the filtration occurs, the ***bacteria are held on the membrane surface*** (***Fig. 56.2***). The trapped bacteria are dried and stained with a dye such as erythrosine, and detected.

Advantages and disadvantages : The membrane filtration technique is rapid and can be carried out outside the laboratory (fields) also. This is in contrast to multiple tube fermentation technique. The major limitation MFT is that it cannot be used for turbid and/or heavily polluted water. This is because the membrane pores get clogged.

Colilert technique

Although commonly used, both the tests described above (MFT and MF) sometimes give false-positive and false-negative results. Colilert technique is a recent and novel technique designed to specifically detect *E. coli* and other coliform bacteria. This is based on the principle that when ***certain substrates are digested by microorganisms, chromogens*** (coloured substances) ***are produced***. Thus, when O-nitrophenyl β-D-galactopyranoside (ONPG) is used, it is converted to a yellow compound by coliform bacteria. With the substrate 4-methylumbelliferyl β-D-glucuronide, *E. coli* produces a fluorescent compound.

TECHNIQUES TO DISTINGUISH FECAL FROM NON-FECAL BACTERIA

A positive laboratory test for coliform bacteria need not necessarily be due to pathogenic organisms, originating from intestines. For instance, *Enterobacter* (*Aerobacter*) *aerogenes,* found in decaying plant materials can ferment lactose and give a positive coliform test. Thus, the presence of *E. aerogenes* in water does not indicate contamination with coliform bacteria.

A series of laboratory tests are available to differentiate fecal from non-fecal organisms. These techniques are collectively referred to as ***IMViC test***, with the following connotations.

I stands for ***indole test***

M represents ***methy red test***

V is for ***Voges-Proskauer test***

C stands for ***citrate test***

(**Note :** ***i*** is used only for phonetic purpose).

These four tests are used to distinguish *E. coli* from *Enterobacter aerogenes. E. coli* gives positive indole and methyl red tests, and indicates that the source of pollution is of fecal origin. On the other hand, *Enterobacter aerogenes* gives positive Voges-Proskauer and citrate tests which shows that the water pollution is due to non-fecal origin.

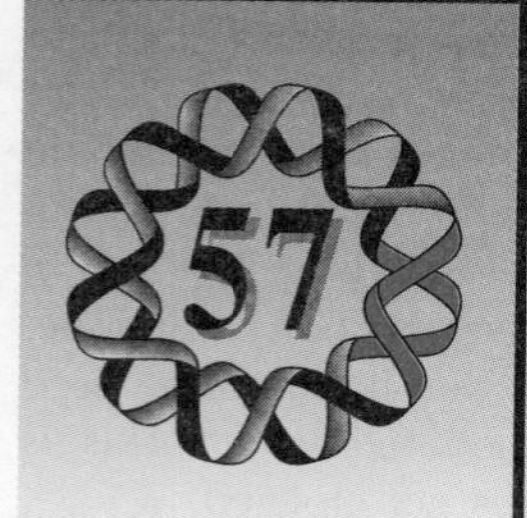

Sewage/Waste Water treatment

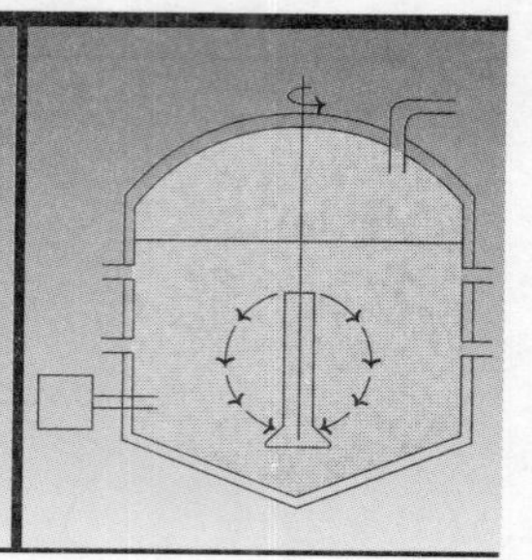

The water pollutants, composition of sewage/ waste water, and the measurement of pollution in sewage are described in the previous chapter. Discharge of ***sewage or waste water*** to the environment is a matter of concern, as it poses ***serious threat to public health.***

In the rural communities, recycling of wastes (human, animal, vegetable) has been practised for centuries. Such recycling processes provide fertilizers and fuel. However, these waste and the crude recycling processes are very dangerous, as they are the major sources of disease-causing pathogens. And in many developing countries, crude, and unscientific recycling of wastes is still in use ***exposing the people to health hazards***. In some countries, the wastes (of rural or urban origin) are carefully treated and disposed off. Waste water/ sewage treatment was started in 19th century (150 years ago), and certainly it is the most important factor for the well being of present day man, besides increasing the life expectancy.

The process designed for the treatment of sewage should have the following objectives.

- Removal of floatable and suspended particles.
- Treatment of biodegradable organic materials.
- Elimination of disease-causing (pathogenic) organisms.

CLASSIFICATION OF TREATMENT PROCESSES

The sewage treatment methods may be classified in two different ways based on the principle of operation or the stages of treatment process.

Based on the principle of operation

Physical unit operations : These methods involve the applications of physical forces for sewage treatment. The physical processes involved include screening, mixing, sedimentation, flocculation and filtration.

Chemical unit operations : These processes operate on the principles of chemical reactions that may involve precipitation, disinfection, adsorption etc.

Biological unit operations : The removal of pollutants, particularly the biodegradable organic materials, can be carried out through biological processes.

Based on the treatment process

The sewage treatment processes are more conveniently classified based on the stages of treatment as ***preliminary, primary, secondary*** and ***tertiary*** treatments.

Preliminary treatment : This process basically involves the removal of floating materials (leaves, rags, papers, animals etc.) settleable inorganic solids (sand, grit etc.), and grease, fats and oils.

Primary treatment : This process, usually carried out by sedimentation, involves the removal of suspended organic solids from the sewage.

Secondary or biological treatment : The removal of fine suspended and dissolved organic material present in the sewage constitutes secondary treatment. This process can be carried out by ***aerobic*** or ***anaerobic biological units***.

Tertiary or advanced treatment : This is the final treatment process of sewage, and is carried out mostly in the developed countries. In general, sewage is disposed off after the secondary treatment. When needed, the tertiary treatment is carried out by disinfection (i.e. chlorination).

Some details on the various treatment processes are briefly described, in the following pages

PRELIMINARY TREATMENT

As already stated, preliminary treatment involves the removal of floating materials (leaves, papers, rags) and settleable inorganic solids (sand, grit), besides oily substances (fats, oils, greases). The three major types of equipment-screeners, grit chambers, and skimming tanks, employed in preliminary screening are briefly described.

Screeners

A screener is a device with openings (usually uniform in size) to remove the floating materials and suspended particles. The process of screening can be carried out by passing sewage through different types of screeners (with different pore sizes). The screeners are classified as ***coarse***, ***medium*** or ***fine***, depending on the size of the openings. The coarse screen has larger openings (75–150 mm). The openings for medium and fine screens respectively are 20–50 mm and less than 20 mm.

Different types of screens-fixed bar screen (coarse or medium) disc type fine screen, drum type fine screen are in use. A diagrammatic representation of a ***fixed bar screen*** is shown in ***Fig. 57.1A***.

A ***shredder*** **or** ***comminutor*** is a special screen that can cut and retain the floating and suspended materials (***Fig. 57.1B***).

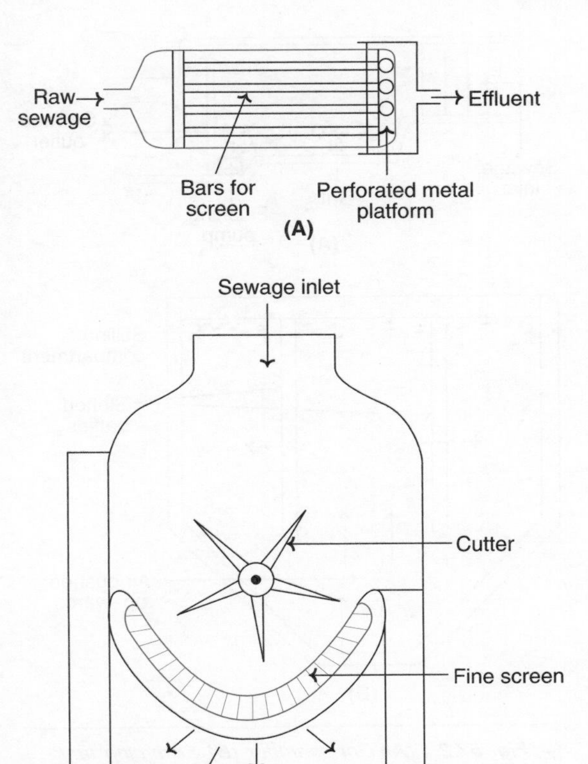

Fig. 57.1 : Diagrammatic representation of screeners (A) Fixed bar screen (coarse or medium) (B) Shredder.

Grit chambers

The heavy ***inorganic materials*** (specific gravity 2.4-2.7) like sand, ash and others ***can be removed*** by using grit chambers. This technique is based on the process of sedimentation due to gravitational forces. Grit chambers may be kept either before or after the screens (described above). A diagrammatic representation of a typical grit chamber is depicted in ***Fig. 57.2A***.

Skimming tanks

Several ***greasy and oily materials*** (fats, oils, waxes, soaps etc.) from the domestic or industrial outlets find their entry into the sewage. They ***can be removed by*** using a skimming tank which is fitted with baffle walls that divide the tank (***Fig. 57.2B***). The skimming tank is divided into

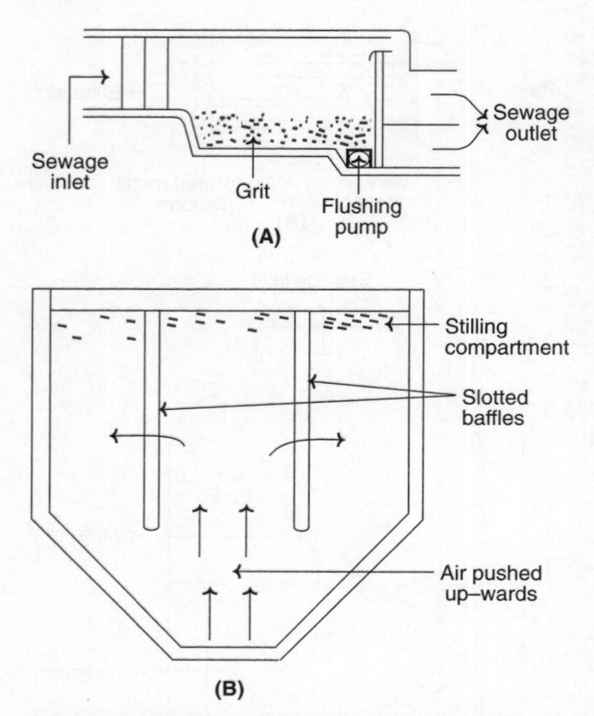

Fig. 57.2 : (A) Grit chamber (B) Skimming tank (cross section).

three compartments that are interconnected. As the compressed air is pushed from the floor of the tank, the raising air bubbles coagulate and solidify the oily and greasy materials present in the sewage. This material is pushed to the side compartment referred to as stilling compartment from where it can be removed manually or mechanically.

PRIMARY TREATMENT

Primary treatment is aimed at the removal of fine suspended organic solids that cannot be removed in the preliminary treatment. Primary treatment basically involves the process of ***sedimentation*** or ***settling***. In the normal process of sewage treatment, sedimentation is usually carried out twice-once before the secondary treatment, referred to as ***primary sedimentation***, and then after the secondary treatment is complete, a process known as ***secondary sedimentation***. It is sometimes necessary to use chemical coagulants to facilitate or aid sedimentation, and this process is referred to as ***chemical precipitation*** or ***coagulation-aided sedimentation***.

Principle of sedimentation

The solid particle of the sewage tend to settle down due to gravity. However, most of the solid particles of organic compounds remain in a suspended state in a flowing sewage. If the flow of the sewage is stopped and if it is stored in a tank referred to as ***sedimentation tank***, the solid particles can settle down at the bottom.

The process of sedimentation is influenced by several factors. These include the size, shape and specific gravity of particles, besides viscosity and flow velocity of sewage.

Types of settling

There ar four major types of settling—discrete settling, flocculant settling, hindered or zone settling and compression. This categorization is mainly based on the tendency of the particles to interact and form solids.

Discrete settling : The particles which do not change their size, shape and weight are referred to as discrete particles or ***granular particles***. The use of grit in sewage may be considered as an example of discrete settling.

Flocculant settling : The flocculant particles can change their size, shape and weight, and thus lose their identity. These particles actually coalesce during settling. Settling of bioflocs, and chemical flocs in secondary sedimentation tanks are good examples of flocculant settling.

Hindered or zone settling : The particles as such, tend to remain in a fixed position with respect to each other. When flocculated, the whole mass of particles settle as a unit or a zone. In the hindered settling the concentration of particles increases from top to the bottom and this results in the thickening of the sludge. Zone settling is employed in conjuction with biological treatment facilities.

Compression : Settlement of particles in the lower layers can occur by compression of the weight of the particles on the upper layers. This process facilitates sludge thickening at the bottom.

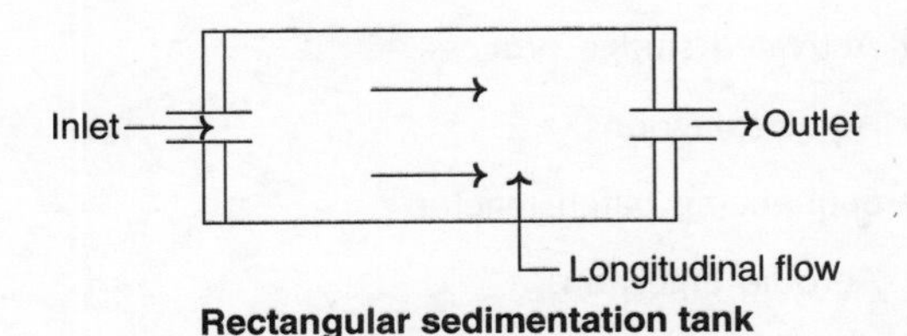

Rectangular sedimentation tank

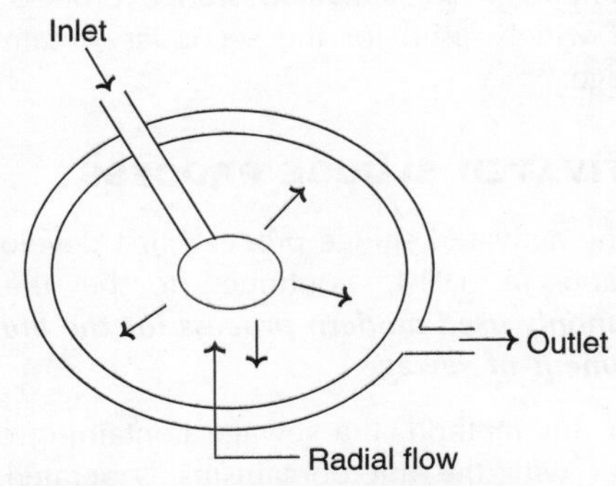

Center–fed circular sedimentation tank

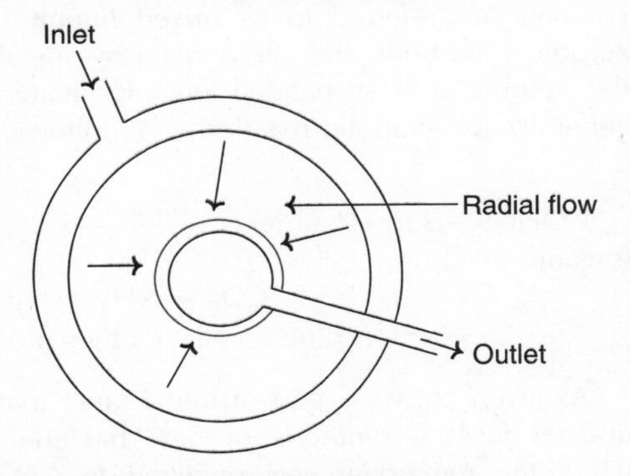

Peripheral–fed sedimentation tank

Fig. 57.3 : Selected examples of sedimentation tanks.

Types of sedimentation tanks (clarifiers)

There are different ways of classifying sedimentation tanks.

Based on the shape — rectangular, circular and square.

Based on the flow of sewage — longitudinal, vertical, radial and spiral.

Based on the purpose and position — primary, secondary, coagulation-cum-sedimentation tanks, grit chambers, septic and Imhoff tanks.

Based on the operation — batch type and continuous flow type.

For the sake of illustration, some sedimentation tanks are depicted in ***Fig. 57.3***.

Chemical-aided sedimentation

It is not always possible to remove the colloidal wastes in sewage by plain sedimentation. However, addition of certain chemicals aids sedimentation, a process referred to as ***chemical precipitation*** or chemical-aided sedimentation. By this technique, about 60–80% of the suspended particles can be removed. Chemical precipitation ***involves three stages—coagulation, flocculation*** and ***sedimentation.***

Coagulation is mainly a chemical process wherein the charged particles are destabilized (by the addition of chemical agents). On the other hand, flocculation involves the physical phenomena of aggregating the destabilized particles to finally form settleable solids (i.e. sedimentation).

The chemicals used in chemical-aided sedimentation are of two types-coagulants and coagulant aids.

Coagulants : These are the chemicalls (normally positively charged) which form insoluble and gelatinous precipitates with colloidal particles (negatively charged ones present in sewage). The most commonly used coagulants in sewage treatment are ***alum*** (aluminium sulfate) ***iron salts*** (ferric sulfate, ferrous sulfate, ferric chloride), ***lime and soda ash*** (sodium carbonate), sodium silicate and sodium aluminate.

Coagulant-aids : These chemicals aid or facilitate the process of coagulation. This is brought out by enchancing the action of coagulants and reducing the amount of sludge formed. The common coagulant aids are ***activated silica, weighting agents*** (e.g. powdered lime stone or silica) and ***polyelectrolytes.***

SECONDARY OR BIOLOGICAL TREATMENT

Biological treatment of sewage is required for the removal of dissolved and fine colloidal organic matter. This process involves the use of microorganisms (bacteria, algae, fungi, protozoa, rotifers, nematodes) that decompose the unstable organic matter to stable inorganic forms.

TABLE 57.1 A list of major biological (secondary) treatment processes used for sewage treatment

Category	*Common process(s)*
Aerobic processes	
Suspended-growth systems	Activated sludge process Plug-flow process Sequencing batch reactor Contact stabilization Oxidation ditch Deep shaft Suspended-growth nitrification Aerobic lagoons Aerobic digestion
Attached-growth systems	Trickling filters Roughing filters Rotating biological contactors (RBC) Packed-bed reactors
Suspended-attached growth combined systems	Activated biofilters (e.g. trickling filter solids-contact process)
Anaerobic processes	
Suspended-growth systems	Anaerobic digestion (single-stage/two-stage) Anaerobic contact process
Attached-growth systems	Anaerobic filter process Expanded-bed process
Pond processes	
	Aerobic ponds Anaerobic ponds Facultative ponds

The biological treatment processes of sewage are broadly classified as ***aerobic***, ***anaerobic*** and ***pond processes***. Depending on the nature of the use of the microorganisms, the biological processes are categorized as ***suspended growth systems*** and ***attached growth systems***. A list of the major secondary (biological) treatment processes is given in ***Table 57.1***, and the most important ones are briefly described.

AEROBIC SUSPENDED-GROWTH TREATMENT PROCESSES

The most important suspended-growth biological treatment systems used for the removal of organic matter are listed.

- Activated sludge process
- Aerated lagoons
- Sequencing batch reactor
- Aerobic digestion.

Among these, activated sludge process is the most widely used for the secondary treatment of sewage.

ACTIVATED SLUDGE PROCESS

The activated sludge process, first developed in England in 1914, continues to be the ***most commonly used modern process for the biological treatment of sewage***.

In this method, the sewage containing organic matter with the microorganisms is aerated (by a mechanical aerator) in an aeration tank. The reactor contents are referred to as ***mixed liquor***. Under aerobic conditions, the microorganisms metabolise the soluble and suspended organic matter. The generalized metabolic reaction is as follows.

$$\underset{\text{(organic matter)}}{COHNS} + O_2 + \text{Nutrients} \xrightarrow{\text{Bacteria}} \underset{\text{(new cells + other products)}}{CO_2 + NH_3 + H_2O}$$

As given above, a part of the organic matter is utilized for the synthesis of new bacterial cells while the remaining gets oxidized to CO_2 and H_2O. The newly formed ***microorganisms are agglomerated to form flocs, technically referred to as sludge***. The separated sludge which is not in contact with organic matter becomes activated. It is separated from the settling tank, and returned to the aeration tank, and recycled. The ***activated sludge recycled*** in aeration tank serves as a ***seed*** or ***inoculum***. The excess and waste sludge can be removed.

For efficient operation of activated sludge process, it is necessary to maintain a constant supply of O_2 which can be done by mechanical aeration or through the use of rotating paddles. Growth of protozoa in a sludge is an indication of its healthy condition.

The disposal of a waste sludge is a problem. It may be used as a fertilizer in crop lands or as landfills, after drying.

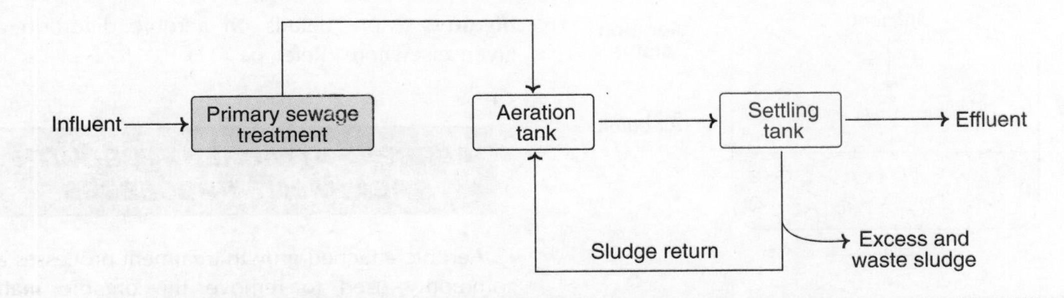

Fig. 57.4 : Flow diagram of activated–sludge process.

Factors affecting performance : There are several factors that influence the efficiency of activated sludge process, the most important being the type of the reactor, aeration, food microorganism (F/M) ratio, nutrients, sludge recirculation rate, besides pH and temperature.

Advantages : The activated sludge process is a very compact, low-cost and an efficient biological treatment system for sewage treatment. It is worked out that under ideal conditions, up to 95% of BOD_5, 98% of bacteria (particularly coliform) and 95% of suspended solids can removed by activated sludge process. The excess and waste sludge has a higher fertilizer value compared to other treatment processes.

Disadvantages : There is production of large volumes of sludge which sometimes becomes difficult to handle. Power consumption is relatively high for operation. Supervision by skilled personnel is necessary.

Conventional activated sludge process

In the normal treatment of sewage, the activated sludge is preceeded by primary sedimentation tank. The conventional activated sludge system consists of a separation tank, settling or sedimentation tank and sludge removal line (***Fig. 57.4***). The sewage after the primary treatment is introduced at the head of the tank. It is desirable to supply O_2 uniformly throughout the tank.

Modified activated sludge processes

For increasing the performance of the activated sludge system, several modifications have been done in the recent years. Most of them are directed to bring out efficient aeration. Aeration can be done by ***step aeration***, ***tapered aeration***, ***high rate aeration by complete mixing and extended aeration***.

AERATED LAGOONS

Aerated lagoons, also called as ***aerated ponds***, are the faculative stabilization ponds wherein surface aerators are installed to overcome the bad adours (due to overload of organic materials). The microbiological treatment of aerated ponds is comparable to the activated sludge process. The major difference is the large surface area in aerated ponds and this is more susceptible for temperature effects.

It is possible to carry out continuous nitrification in aerated lagoons. This however, depends on the design and operating conditions of the pond (particularly the temperature).

SEQUENCING BATCH REACTOR

Sequencing batch reactor (SBR) is a modification of activated sludge treatment system. The processes namely aeration and sedimentation are carried out in both the systems. The major difference is that while in the conventional activated sludge system, aeration and sedimentation occur simultaneously in separate tanks, these two processes are carried out sequentially in the same tank in SBR. Thus, the sequencing batch reactor may be regarded as ***fill-and-draw activated sludge process***.

The operating sequence of a typical SBR is depicted in ***Fig. 57.5***. The process is carried out in a sequence of five steps — ***filling, aeration*** (reacting) ***sedimentation*** (settling), ***decanting*** and ***idle***. Several modifications and improvements have been made in the SBR for more efficient operation.

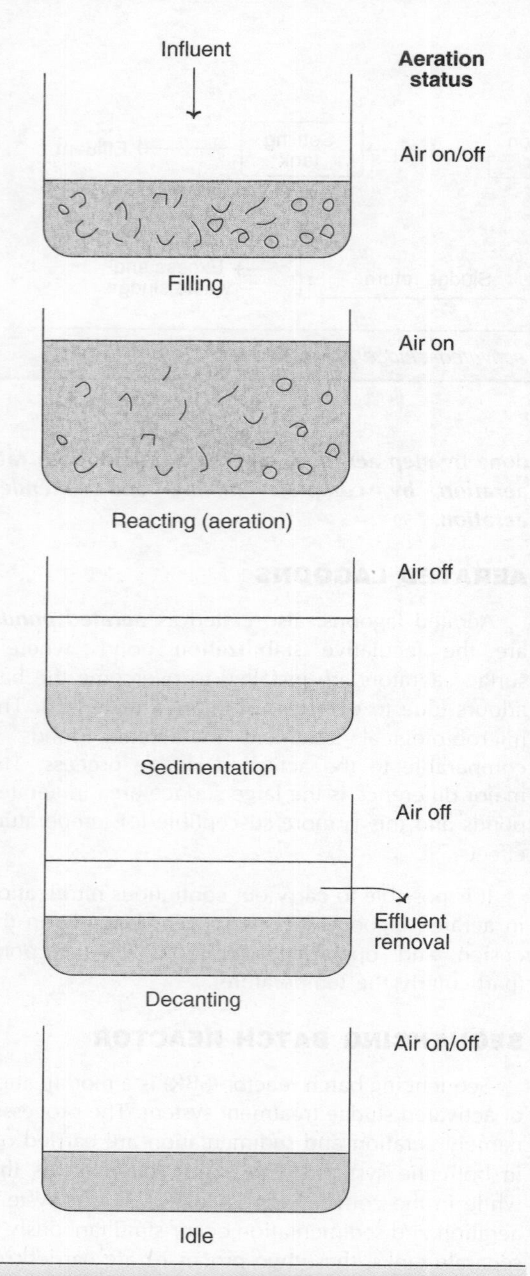

Fig. 57.5 : Operating sequence of a typical sequencing batch reactor (SBR).

AEROBIC DIGESTION

The organic sludges produced from various treatment processes (activated sludge treatment, trickling filter-sludge) are subjected to aerobic digestion in special reactors referred to as ***aerobic digesters***. More details on aerobic digestion are given elsewhere (Refer p. 711).

AEROBIC ATTACHED — GROWTH TREATMENT PROCESSES

Aerobic attached-growth treatment processes are commonly used to remove the organic matter found in the sewage. These processes are also useful for the ***nitrification*** (conversion of ammonia to nitrate). The commonly used attached-growth processes are listed.

- Trickling filters
- Roughing filters
- Rotating biological contractors
- Packed bed reactors.

Among these, trickling filter is most widely used.

TRICKLING FILTERS

Trickling filters, also known as ***percolating*** or ***sprinkling filters***, are commonly used for the biological treatment of domestic sewage and industrial waste water. In a strict sense, trickling filters are not filters, but they are ***oxidation units***.

A diagrammatic representation of trickling filter is depicted in ***Fig. 57.6***. It has a bed of coarse, hard and porous material over which sewage is sprayed. In about two weeks time, the biomass attached to the media surface grows and forms a layer, referred to as ***biological film*** or ***microbial slime***. This film has a thickness of 0.1 to 2.0 mm and is rich in microorganisms. As the liquid (sewage) trickles through the biofilm, the organic matter gets oxidized to CO_2 and NO_2 by the microbial metabolism. This oxidation is carried out by the aerobic organisms (particularly bacteria) that are present on the upper portion of the biological film.

The biological film is rich in the bacteria-*Pseudomonas, Flavobacterium, Alcaligenes,* and algae-*Chlorella, Utothrix,* and *Stigeoclonium,* besides some fungi and yeasts. Biofilms with a thickness in the range of 70–100 μm are efficient for the treatment process.

As the biofilm ages, its thickness increases and it automatically settles to the bottom of the tank.

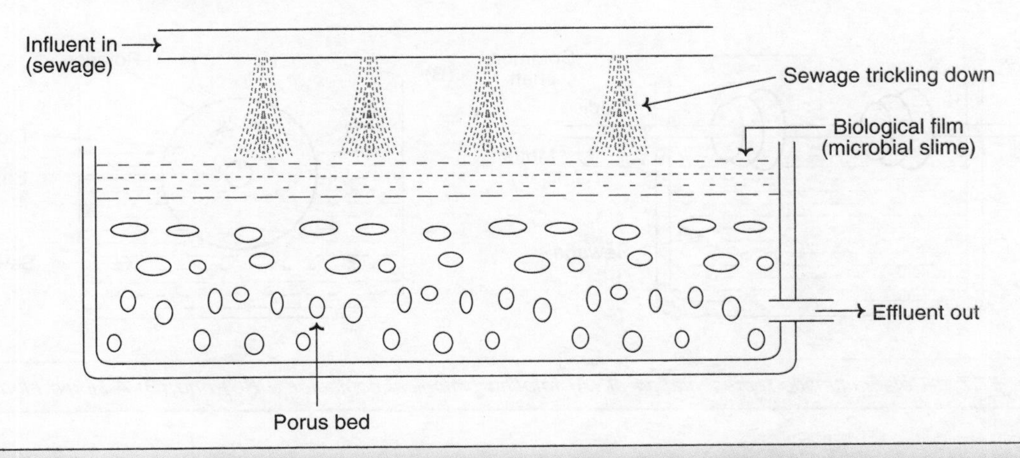

Fig. 57.6 : A diagrammatic representation of trickling filter.

The ***waste waters obtained in milk processing, paper mills*** and ***pharmaceutical industries are treated by trickling filters***.

Types of trickling filters

The trickling filters are classified as ***low rate*** (the conventional one), ***high rate*** and ***super rate***. This categorization is mainly based on the hydraulic and organic loading rates of the sewage. The low rate filters are suitable for the treatment of domestic sewage, while high rate filters and super rate filters are useful for industrial sewage.

Factors affecting performance of trickling filters

The type of the media and its depth, organic and hydraulic loading, filter staging, recirculation rate and flow distribution are the important factors that influence the performance of the trickling filters.

Advantages : Trickling filters are simple, occupy less space and the operating costs are low. They operate efficiently in hot climate and thus are ***suitable for most developing countries*** (like India).

Disadvantages : Removal of BOD is moderate (around 70%), and disposal of excess sludge is necessary. Primary sedimentation is required, since trickling filters cannot handle raw sewage.

ROUGHING FILTERS

Roughing filters are a special type of trickling filters that are designed to operate at high hydraulic loading rates. These filters are mostly used to reduce the organic matter in downstream processing, besides nitrification applications. Due to high hydraulic loading, there is a continuous sloughing of the biological film. In such a case, the unsettled filter effluent can be recycled, and this increases the efficiency of the treatment process. The retention time on the biofilm being less, organic materials that are not readily degradable remain unaffected.

ROTATING BIOLOGICAL CONTACTORS (RBC)

Rotating biological contactor (RBC) is a recent device for the biological treatment of sewage. It operates on the ***principle of aerobic attached-growth system operated on the moving media***. RBC are suitable for the treatment of domestic and industrial sewage in small and medium towns.

A rotating biological contactor is composed of a series of closely spaced and light weight circular discs (***Fig. 57.7***). They are made up of inert materials such s polystyrene or polyvinyl chloride (PVC) or polyethylene. These discs are mounted on a horizontal shaft in a tank through which waste water flows. The shaft is rotated slowly (less than 10 revolutions per minute) by a low speed motor. The discs of the shaft, referred to as ***biodiscs***, are partially (40–60%) submerged in sewage. As the biodiscs are rotated, the biomass attached to them is alternately submerged in sewage. This enables the discs to pick up a thin layer of sewage, and then to ***oxidize the absorbed substrates***. The unoxidized substrates fall back into the sewage.

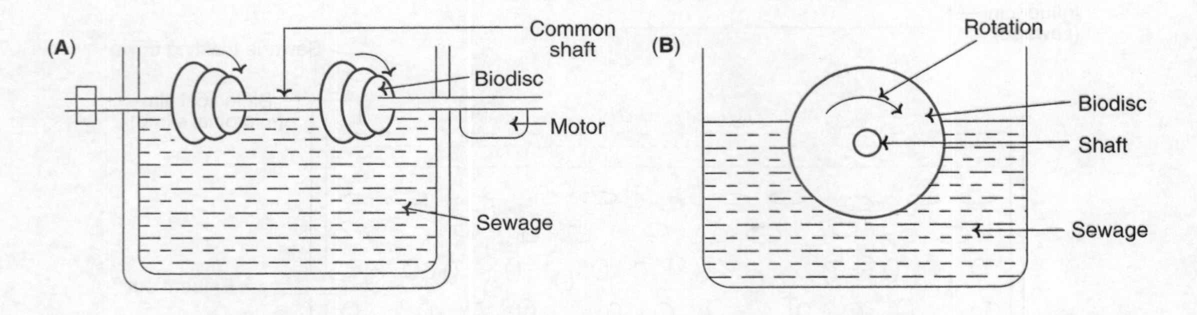

*Fig. 57.7 : A diagrammatic representation of (**A**) rotating biological contactor (RBC) and (**B**) A single biodisc.*

And this process in repeated again and again by the rotating biodiscs.

Rotating biological contractor is basically a ***film flow bioreactor***. The ***microbial biofilm*** is built upon the partly submerged support medium containing biodiscs.

The RBC is very efficient for the removal of organic matter in the sewage (about 90% of BOD). As and when there is an excess growth of biomass, it has to be removed. This process can be carried in a similar fashion, as it is done for the trickling filter (described already).

RBC are commonly used for the ***treatment of municipal waste water***. In addition, they are widely used for the biological processing of ***industrial wastes***, coming from several industries such as ***vegetables***, ***pulp***, ***meat*** and ***textiles***.

Factors affecting performance of RBC : The treatment process in RBC is influenced by rotation speed of shaft, waste water retention time, temperature, disc submergence, organic loading, media density, and number of stages.

Advantages : RBC is compact and requires moderate energy input. It has ***high BOD removal efficiency***.

Disadvantages : Disposal of sludge formed is a major problem with RBC. The treatment process is frequently associated with odour formation. RBC operation requires skilled personnel.

PACKED-BED REACTORS

Packed-bed reactors or ***fluidized bed reactors*** are used for the removal of BOD and nitrification. A reactor is packed with a medium to which the microorganisms get attached and form biofilms. The sewage along with air (or pure oxygen) is introduced from the bottom of the reactor (***Fig. 57.8***). The main advantage with packed bed reactors is that they have high surface area of biofilms for unit of reactor.

ANAEROBIC SUSPENDED — GROWTH TREATMENT PROCESSES

Anaerobic processes basically involve the decomposition of organic and inorgnic matter in the absence of oxygen. Anaerobic processing systems are important for the treatment of sludges,

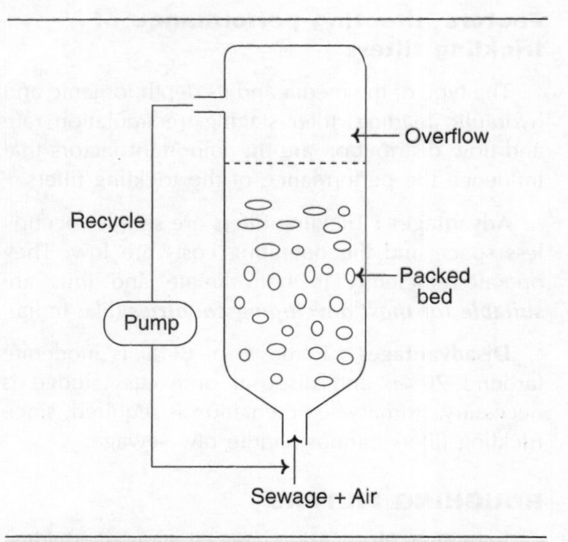

Fig. 57.8 : A diagrammatic representation of a packed-bed reactor.

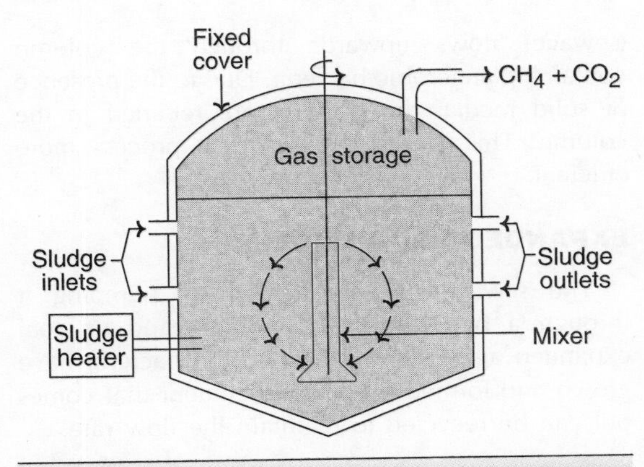

Fig. 57.9 : High-rate complete mix, single-stage anaerobic digester.

and high strength organic sewage. Several reactor systems for anaerobic suspended-growth treatment process have been developed. Among these, the ***complete-mix anaerobic digestion process*** is most widely used for the treatment of sewage.

ANAEROBIC DIGESTION

Anaerobic digestion is mostly useful for the stabilization of concentrated sludges that are produced on the treatment of industrial sewage. A diagrammatic representation of a typical high-rate, complete mix, single stage digester is depicted in ***Fig. 57.9***.

The process of anaerobic digestion is carried out in an air tight reactor. Sludge is introduced continuously or intermittently. In the high-rate digestion system, the contents of the digester are heated and mixed completely. And it takes about 15 days for the process to be complete.

Biodegradation of organic matter of sludge (or sewage)

The biological degradation of organic matter of sludge occurs in three stages (***Fig. 57.10***) — hydrolysis, acidogenesis and methanogenesis.

Hydrolysis : In the enzyme-catalysed reactions, high molecular weight compounds (proteins, polysaccharides, lipids and nucleic acids) are degraded to low molecular weight compounds (amino acids, monosaccharides, fatty acids, purines and pyrimidines). The latter serve as substrates for energy supply and microbial growth.

Acidogenesis : The low molecular weight compounds (referred above) are converted to acidic products (propionate, butyrate, lactate).

Methanogenesis : This is the third and final stage and involves the production of methane and carbon dioxide, from the intermediates formed in

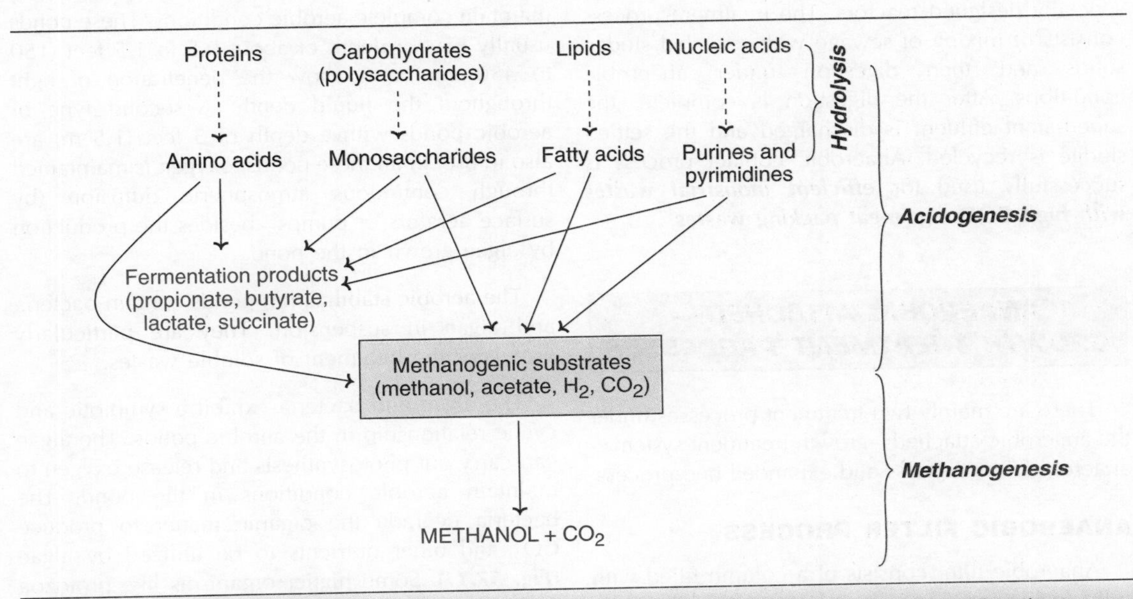

Fig. 57.10 : A diagrammatic view of the degradation of organic materials in anaerobic digestion.

acidogenesis. Methane gas is highly insoluble and its departure from the digester represents the stabilization of sewage or sludge.

Microorganisms to degrade organic matter of sludge (or sewage)

A consortium of anearobic microorganisms work together for degradation of sludge (or sewage) organic matter. They may be categorized into two types.

1. **Acid-forming bacteria :** These are also known as ***acidogens*** or ***non-methanogenic bacteria***. They bring out the hydrolysis of macromolecules (e.g. carbohydrate) to simple substrates (e.g. monosaccharides), and the latter to acids e.g. *Clostridium* sp, *Corynebacterium* sp, *Lactobacillus* sp, *Actinomyces* sp, *Staphylococcus* sp, *Peptococcus anaerobus*, *Escherichia coli*.

2. **Methanogenic bacteria :** These bacteria, also referred to as ***methanogens*** or ***methane formers*** are responsible for the conversion of acetic acid and hydrogen to methane and carbon dioxide. The most important methanogens belong to the genera *Methanobacterium*, *Methanobacillus*, *Methanococcus* and *Methanosarcina*.

ANAEROBIC CONTACT PROCESS

Anaerobic contact process is carried out in a specially designed reactors. The treatment process consists of mixing of sewage with recycled sludge solids and then digestion under anaerobic conditions. After the digestion is complete, the supernatant effluent is discharged and the settled sludge is recycled. Anaerobic contact process is successfully used for ***efficient industrial wastes with high BOD*** e.g. ***meat packing wastes***.

ANAEROBIC ATTACHED— GROWTH TREATMENT PROCESSES

There are mainly two treatment processes under the anaerobic attached—growth treatment system— anaerobic filter process and expanded bed process.

ANAEROBIC FILTER PROCESS

Anaerobic filter consists of a column filled with solid media for the treatment of organic matter in sewage. In this process system, waste water (sewage) flows upwards through the column containing anaerobic bacteria. Due to the presence of solid media, the bacteria are retained in the column. This makes the treatment process more efficient.

EXPANDED-BED PROCESS

The sewage can be treated by pumping it through a bed of inert materials (sand or coal expanded aggregates) on which the bacteria have grown and formed a film. The effluent that comes out can be recycled to maintain the flow rate.

POND TREATMENT PROCESSES

Pond treatment processes for the treatment of sewage (containing biodegradable wastes) are carried out by specially designed and constructed ponds. These ponds, referred to as ***stabilization ponds***, are large, shallow earthen basins. The treatment process is a natural one involving the combined use of bacteria and algae. The stabilization ponds are classified as ***aerobic***, ***anaerobic*** and ***facultative ponds***.

AEROBIC PONDS

The aerobic ponds, as the name indicates, maintain complete aerobic conditions. These ponds usually have a depth of about 0.5 to 1.5 feet (150 to 450 mm) and allow the penetration of light throughout the liquid depth. A second type of aerobic ponds with a depth of 5 feet (1.5 m) are also in use. In all these ponds, oxygen is maintained through continuous atmospheric diffusion (by surface aerators or pumps), besides the production by algae grown in the pond.

The aerobic stabilization ponds contain bacteria and algae in suspension. They are particularly useful for the treatment of soluble wastes.

The algae and bacteria exhibit a symbiotic and cyclic relationship in the aerobic ponds. The algae can carry out photosynthesis and release oxygen to maintain aerobic conditions in the pond. The bacteria degrade the organic matter to produce CO_2 and other nutrients to be utilized by algae (***Fig. 57.11***). Some higher organisms like protozoa and rotifers present in the pond are responsible for the polishing of the effluent.

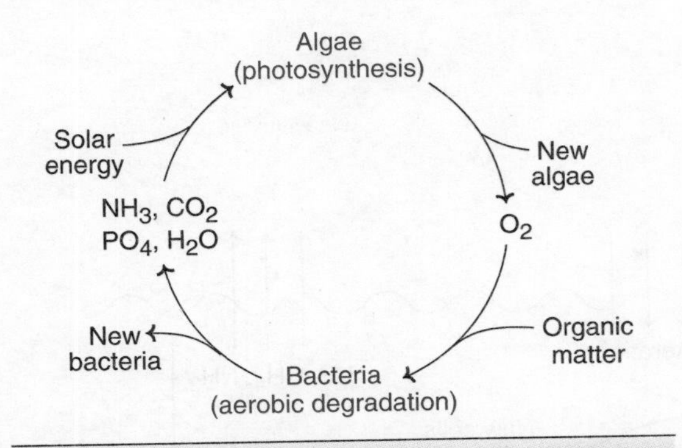

Fig. 57.11 : The symbiotic relationship between algae and bacteria in an aerobic pond.

Factors affecting aerobic ponds

The species of the algae and bacteria present in the pond significantly influence the efficiency of the aerobic ponds. The other factors such as the quality and quantity of organic material, degree of pond mixing, nutrients, sunlight, pH and temperature are also important for the successful operation of these ponds.

ANAEROBIC PONDS

Anaerobic ponds are useful for the ***treatment of high-strength organic matter and solid*** containing sewage/waste water. These ponds are completely devoid of dissolved O_2. They are very deep (up to 30 feet i.e. about 9 m), so that heat conservation is possible, besides requiring minimum land area (for pond construction).

When the sewage is added to the pond, precipitation and anaerobic conversion of organic waste to CO_2, methane and other gases, organic acids etc. occurs. Under suitable conditions, 75% of the BOD can be removed in anaerobic ponds. The clarified effluent is usually discharged for further treatment.

FACULTATIVE PONDS

In facultative ponds, the treatment of sewage is carried out by a combination of both aerobic and anaerobic processes. Three types of microorganisms ***aerobic***, ***anaerobic*** and ***facultative*** (both aerobic and anaerobic) are employed in facultative ponds.

The term ***oxidation pond*** or ***stabilization pond*** is frequently used for facultative ponds.

A diagrammatic view of a facultative pond is depicted in ***Fig. 57.12***. It consists of three zones.

1. **The surface aerobic zone :** It has the aerobic bacteria and algae, existing in a symbiotic relation (as explained on p. 696).

2. **The bottom anaerobic zone :** It contains anaerobic bacteria and solids that undergo decomposition.

3. **Intermediate facultative zone :** This zone is partly aerobic and partly anaerobic and contains both types (aerobic and anaerobic) of bacteria.

Processes that occur in facultative ponds

The sewage organic matter is stabilized by both aerobic and anaerobic processes. The algae present in the aerobic zone carry out photosynthesis and release O_2. This oxygen is utilized by the aerobic and facultative bacteria to oxidize soluble and colloidal organic matter. The organic solids present in the anaerobic zone (bottom sludge) are degraded to dissolved organic compounds (organic acids) and gases such as CO_2, CH_4 and H_2S. The organic acids can be oxidized by the aerobic bacteria while the gases produced (CO_2, CH_4, H_2S, NH_3) may be vented to the atmosphere. In fact, most of CO_2 is utilized by the algae for photosynthesis, while H_2S combines with O_2 to form sulfuric acid.

$$H_2S + 2O_2 \longrightarrow H_2SO_4$$

In the absence of adequate O_2 in the upper layers of the pond, gases with unpleasant and foul odours (H_2S) are vented to the atmosphere. These foul smells often cause nuisance to the surroundings.

It is generally possible to maintain good O_2 supply by the algae and facultative bacteria. Sometimes, surface aerators are used to enhance the efficiency of facultative ponds (particularly when the sewage contains high organic content).

Advantages : For the facultative ponds, the initial and operating costs are low. There is no need for skilled personnel.

Disadvantages : Unpleasant odours and mosquite breeding are frequently seen in facultative ponds. The requirement of land area for construction of these ponds is more.

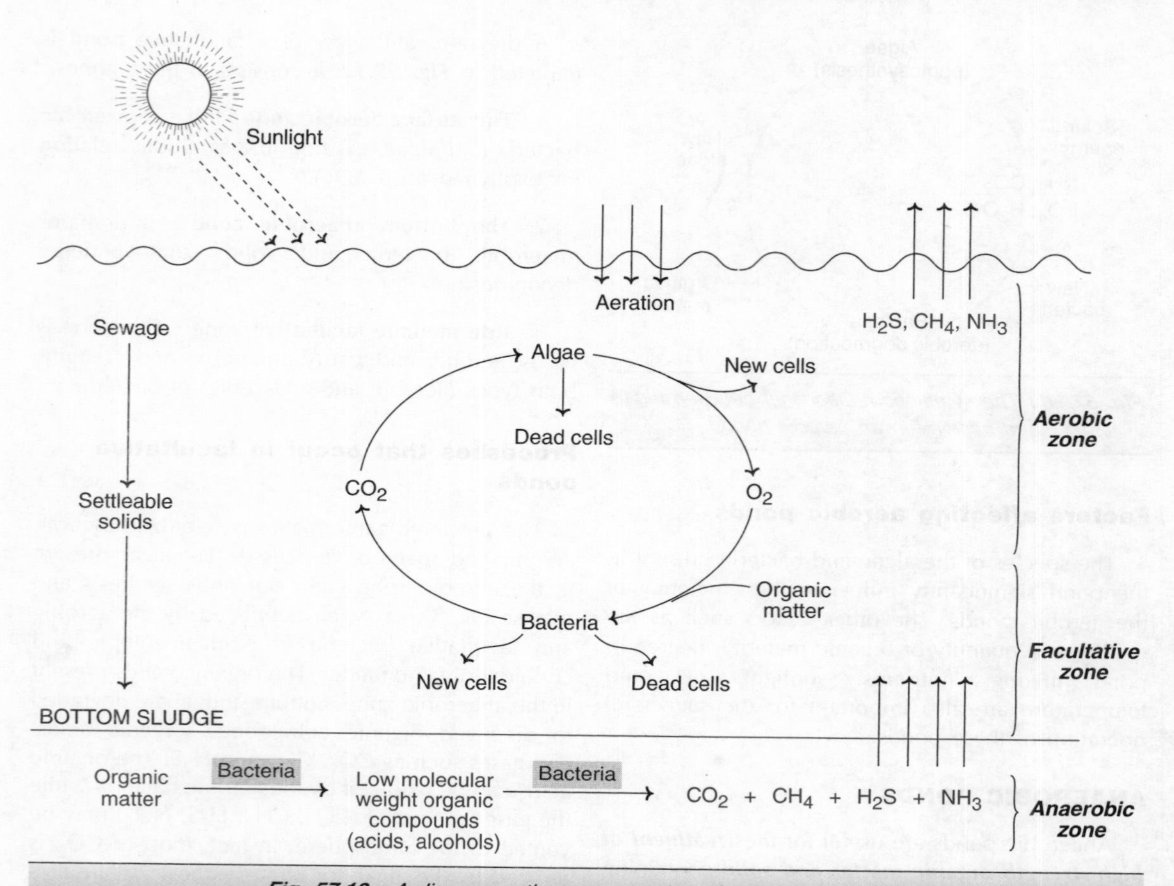

Fig. 57.12 : A diagrammatic representation of a facultative pond.

TERTIARY TREATMENT

Tertiary treatment or ***advanced treatment*** is sometimes needed ***for the removal of suspended and dissolved substances***, after the conventional primary and secondary treatments. In general, the effluent of the sewage obtained after secondary treatment can be conveniently disposed without causing any nuisance. However, tertiary treatment is needed under the following circumstances.

- When the quality of the effluent to be discharged does not meet the standard requirements (particularly in the developed countries).
- When there is a necessary to reuse the sewage/ waste water (***reclamation of water*** is quite expensive, but is required in certain situations of water shortage).
- For the removal of nitrogen and phosphorus compounds.

Tertiary treatment process broadly involves the removal of suspended and dissolved solids, nitrogen, phosphorus and pathogenic organisms. In the conventional heirarchy of sewage treatment, the unit operations are carried out in the order of preliminary, primary, secondary and finally tertiary treatment. However, sometimes advanced (tertiary) treatment process may be directly carried out bypassing the other unit operations. This mainly depends on the composition of waste water and the requirements.

There are four major processes under the tertiary treatment.

1. Solids removal
2. Biological nitrogen removal
3. Biological phosphorus removal
4. Disinfection.

Some authors use the term ***biological nutrient removal for the removal of nitrogen and phosphorus***.

SOLIDS REMOVAL

The techniques for the removal of suspended and dissolved solids in waste water treatment are comparable with those employed for the processing of potable (drinking) water.

Removal of suspended solids

The effluents obtained from secondary treatment may contain suspended solids in the size 0.1 to 100 μm. The concentration of these solids is variable, and is usually 20–40 mg/l. The removal of suspended solids is carried out by ***granular medium (sand) filtration*** and ***microscreening***. Sometimes, diatomaceous earth filters and coagulation-cum sedimentation techniques are also used.

Removal of dissolved solids

The dissolved solids can be removed mainly by two techniques—***adsorption*** and ***ion-exchange***.

Adsorption by activated carbon : Activated carbon is highly porous and provides large surface area for the adsorption of dissolved solids in the advanced treatment. The compounds that can be removed by adsorption include ***organic materials*** (herbicides, pesticides, tannins, lignins, colour and odour producing substances), ***inorganic materials*** (toxic trace metals) and several other pollutants.

Granular activated carbon contactors

Granular activated carbon contactors (***GAC***) are the most widely used for the advanced treatment of sewage. The GAC consists of a tank (usually cylindrical) which is loaded with granular activated carbon (***Fig. 57.13***). The waste water/sewage (influent) is passed from top through the activated carbon bed and the effluent comes out from the bottom. The solids attached to the carbon bed hamper further adsorption process. These particles can be removed by backwashing.

The activated carbon requires periodical regeneration. This can be done by heating in a furnance at about 800°C in the absence of O_2. At this temperature, the adsorbed organic compounds are converted to gases and released. The ***carbon granulates are reactivated for reuse***.

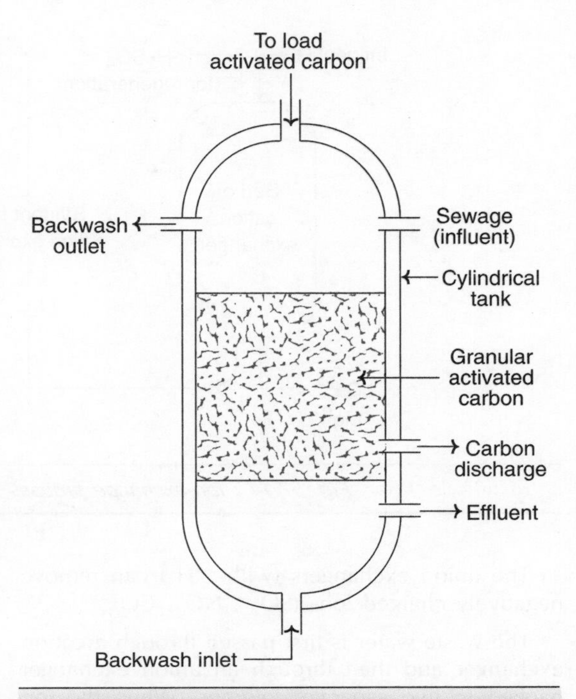

Fig. 57.13 : A diagrammative representation of granular activated carbon contactor (GAC).

Powdered activated carbon (PAC), instead of granulated carbon, is sometimes used for absorption process. PAC is added to an aeration tank (of secondary treatment) which can adsorb several organic compounds.

Ion-exchange for dissolved solids removal

As the name indicates, ion-exchange involves the displacement of one ion by another. The exchange occurs between the ions of insoluble exchange material (ion-exchange materials) and the ions of different species in solution (i.e. waste water for advanced treatment).

The ion-exchange process is carried out by employing two types of ion-exchange materials—cation exchangers and anion exchangers (***Fig. 57.14***). The synthetic resins with strong acidic (H^+) and basic (OH^-) functional groups serve as ion exchangers. The cation exchangers (with H^+ or Na^+) can replace the positively charged ions (Ca^{2+}, Mg^{2+}) in water by hydrogen ions. This is what is done for removing the hardness of water.

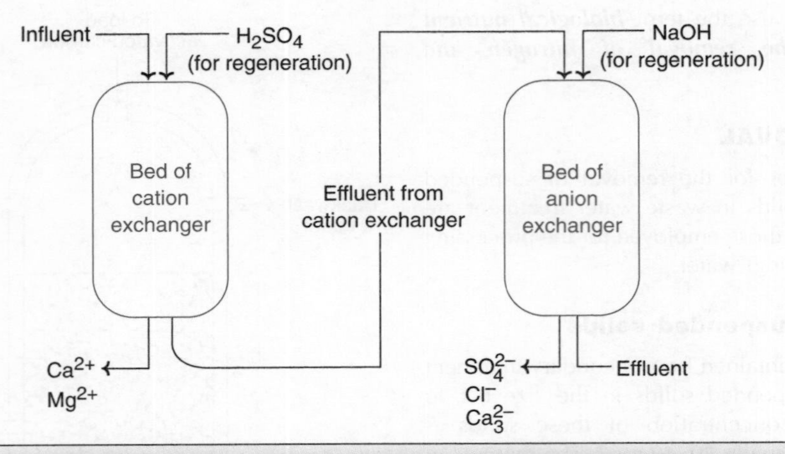

Fig. 57.14 : Ion-exchange process for the removal of dissolved solids.

The anion exchangers (with OH^-) can remove negatively charged ions (SO_4^{2-}, NO_3, CO_3^{2-}).

The waste water is first passed through a cation exchanger and then through an anion exchanger packed in two separate columns. When the ion exchange capacity of the resin is exhausted, it has to be regenerated for further use. For cation-exchange resins, regeneration can be done with strong acids (H_2SO_4, HCl), while for anion exchange resins, alkali (NaOH) is used.

For an effective removal of dissolved solids by ion exchange, the waste water should not contain high concentration of suspended solids as they block the ion exchange beds.

BIOLOGICAL NITROGEN REMOVAL

Decomposition products of proteins and the urea present in sewage are the major constituents of biological nitrogen. Although, nitrogen is a nutrient, its excess concentration causes eutrophication, and thus its removal is required. Biological nitrogen removal (***BNR***) is carried out by the methods based on the following principles (***Fig. 57.15***).

1. Assimilation of nitrogen
2. Nitrification and denitrification.

Assimilation of nitrogen

Since nitrogen is a nutrient, the microorganisms in the sewage can assimilate ammonia nitrogen, and grow. As some of these cells die, a portion of this ammonia nitrogen will be returned to the sewage.

Nitrification and denitrification

Nitrification : Ammonia nitrogen first gets oxidized to nitrite (NO_2^-) by the bacteria *Nitrosomonas* sp. This is followed by further oxidation nitrite (NO_2^-) to nitrate (NO_3^-) by *Nitrobacter* sp.

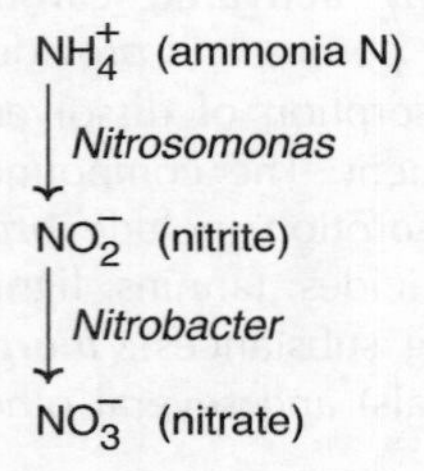

The bacteria involved in nitrification are auxotrophs. The nitrification process is accomplished by aerobic suspended growth and aerobic attached-growth systems. In the general practice, nitrification is carried out along with the BOD removal in the secondary treatment with suitable modifications. Trickling filters, rotating biological contactors and packed towers can be used for nitrification process.

Denitrification : The ***removal of nitrogen*** in the form of nitrate by converting to nitrogen gas is referred to as denitrification. This process ***occurs under anaerobic conditions*** and is brought out by certain genera of bacteria-*Aerobacter, Bacillus, Brevibacterium, Lactobacillus, Micrococcus, Pseudomonas* and *Spirillum.* These bacteria are heterotrophs and require no oxygen, but the

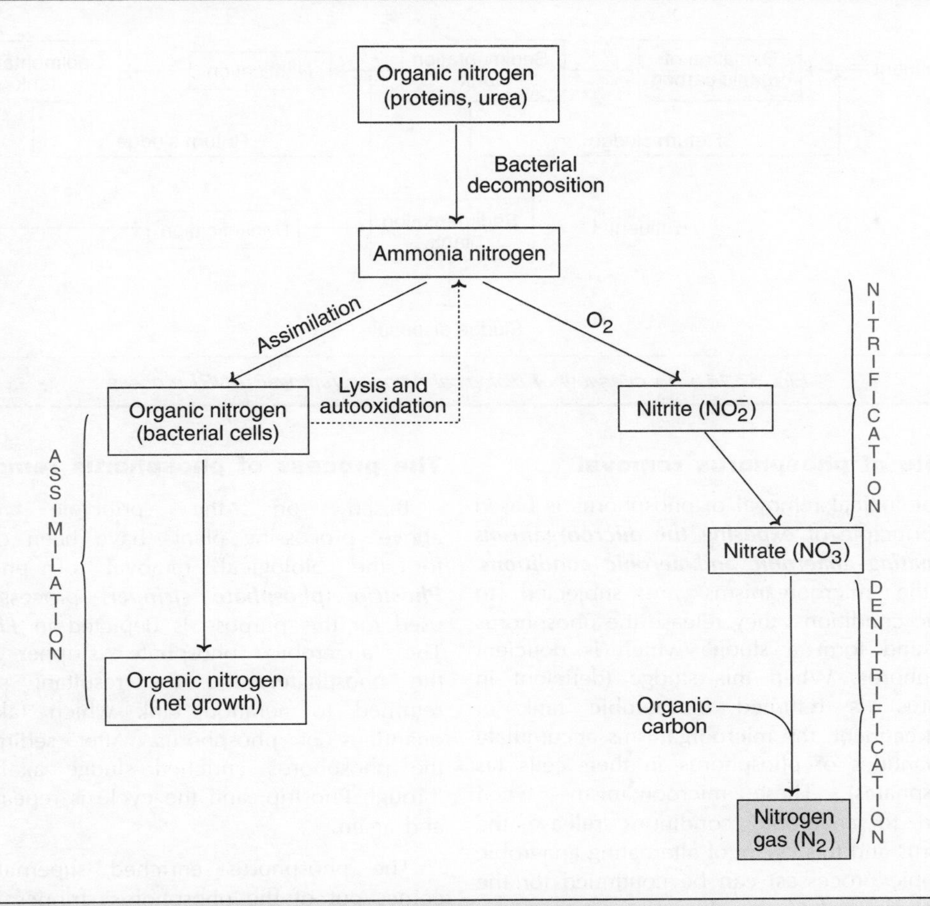

Fig. 57.15 : Biological nitrogen removal.

presence of organic carbon is essential. The presence of even minute quantities of O_2 suppresses denitrification. The heterotrophic bacteria can reduce nitrate in the following stages, to finally nitrogen gas.

NO_3^- (nitrate)
↓
NO_2^- (nitrite)
↓
NO (nitric oxide)
↓
N_2O (nitrous oxide)
↓
N_2 (nitrogen gas)

The process denitrification can be carried out by suspended growth and attached growth systems. The plug flow type of activated sludge system is commonly used.

The flow diagram for the ***removal of biological nitrogen*** is depicted in ***Fig. 57.16***. The process ***primarily consists of the removal of organic carbon (aerobic), followed by nitrification (aerobic) and denitrification (anaerobic).***

BIOLOGICAL PHOSPHORUS REMOVAL

Phosphorus in the sewage is mostly present in the form of orthophosphate (PO_4^{3-}), polyphosphate (P_2O_7) and organic bound phosphorus. In fact, phosphorus is an essential nutrient for microorganisms. Thus, during the normal secondary treatment process, 10–30% of the sewage phosphorus is utilized by the microorganisms for growth and energy purposes.

Phosphorus removal from waste water is required to control eutrophication and to maintain water quality.

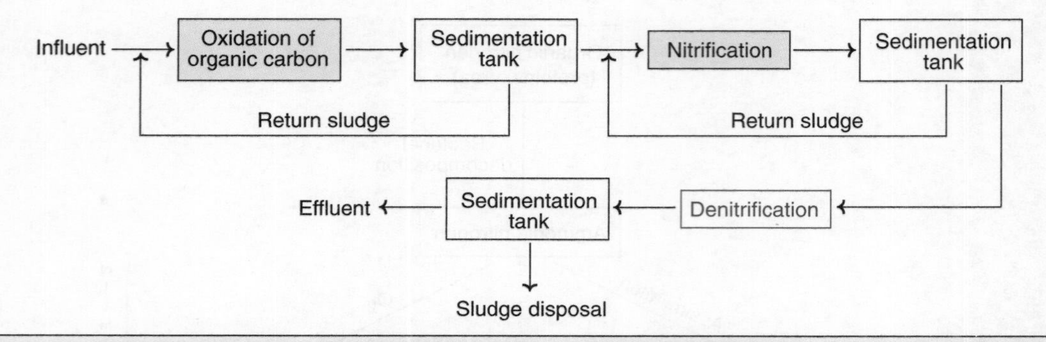

Fig. 57.16 : An overview of biological nitrogen removal (BNR) process.

Principle of phosphorus removal

The biological removal of phosphorus is based on the principle of ***exposing the microorganisms to alternating anaerobic and aerobic conditions***. When the microorganisms are subjected to anaerobic conditions, they release the phosphorus content and form a sludge which is deficient in phosphorus. When this sludge (deficient in phosphorus) is returned to aerobic tank of sewage treatment, the microorganisms accumulate large quantities of phosphorus in their cells (as polyphosphates). These microorganisms when subjected to anaerobic conditions release the phosphorus and this cycle (of alternating anaerobic and aerobic processes) can be continued for the biological removal of phosphorus.

Acinetobacter sp are mainly responsible for the biological removal of phosphorus.

The process of phosphorus removal

Based on the principle described above, processing plants have been developed for the biological removal of phosphorus. ***Phostrip*** (***phosphate stripper***) process system, used for this purpose is depicted in ***Fig. 57.17***. The anaerobic phosphate stripper removes the phosphate, and the resultant sludge is returned to aeration tank which takes large quantities of phosphorus. After sedimentation, the phosphorus enriched sludge again passes through Phostrip, and the cycle is repeated again and again.

The phosphorus enriched supernatant that comes out of the phosphorus stripper is treated with lime to precipitate the phosphorus. The resultant liquid supernatant can be returned to the aeration tank for further treatment.

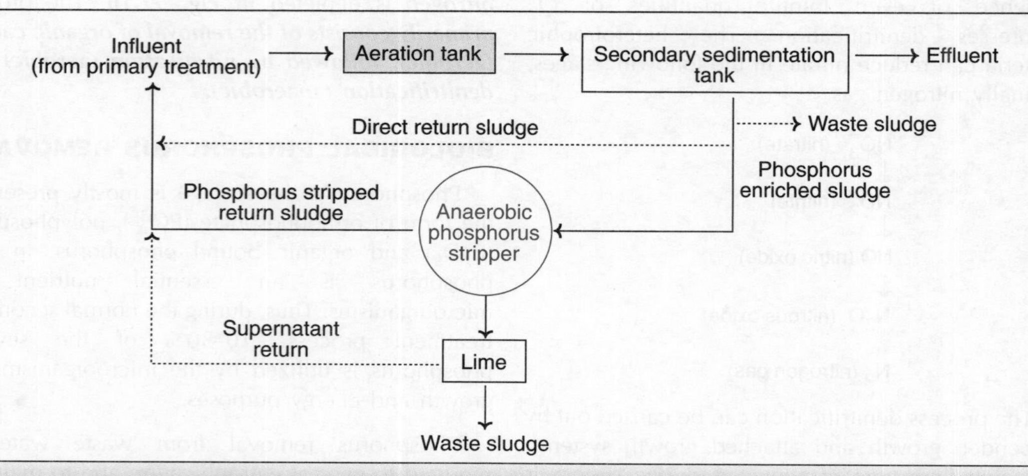

Fig. 57.17 : Biological phosphorus removal by Phostrip (phosphate stripper) process.

DISINFECTION

Disinfection broadly refers to the ***selective destruction*** or ***inactivation of disease-causing*** (pathogenic) ***organisms***. In the process of disinfection, all the organisms are not destroyed. This is in contrast to sterilization which involves the destruction of all the organisms.

There are several water borne diseases (typhoid, cholera, dysentery) caused by bacteria, viruses and other pathogens (Refer ***Table 56.1***). The very purpose of disinfection is to control these diseases.

Agents for disinfection

Disinfection is accomplished by using chemical and physical agents, besides mechanical and radiation means.

Chemical agents : Chlorine and its compounds are most commonly used. The other chemicals— bromine, iodine, ozone, alcohols, phenols, heavy metals, hydrogen peroxide, alkalies and acids are sometimes employed. After ***chlorine*** (regarded as ***most universal disinfectant***), bromine and iodine are in use. In recent years, ozone as a disinfectant is gaining importance, since it is very effective.

Physical agents : Heat and light can be effectively used as disinfectants. Sunlight (particularly ultra-violet rays) is in fact a good disinfectant.

Mechanical means : The pathogenic organisms can also be removed by mechanical means, during the course of waste water treatment. The processes involving screens (coarse and fine), grit chambers and sedimentation can partly remove the disease-causing organisms.

Radiation means : The gamma rays emitted from radioisotopes can serve as effective disinfectants.

Characteristics of an ideal disinfectant

An ideal disinfectant should possess the following characteristics.

- Toxic to pathogens at low concentration
- Soluble and stable in water
- Non-toxic to man and higher organisms
- Cheap and easily available.

Disinfection with chlorine

Chlorine is a very widely used disinfectant, as it satisfies the criteria (listed above) of an ideal disinfectant. The most commonly used chlorine compounds are — chlorine gas (Cl_2), calcium hypochloride [$Ca(COCl_2)$], sodium hypochlorite ($NaOCl$) and chlorine dioxide (ClO_2).

The disinfection efficiency of chlorine depends on the number of microorganisms in the water being treated, pH and temperature.

SEWAGE/WASTE WATER TREATMENT — A SUMMARY

The various treatment processes of sewage i.e. preliminary, primary, secondary and tertiary (with details of operations processing units in each category), have been described in this chapter. The treatment of sludge is dealt with in the next chapter. They were, however, discussed as independent operations.

A conventional sewage treatment plant has the requisite operating units arranged one after another for treatment and final disposal of sewage. The flow chart of a conventional sewage treatment plant is depicted in ***Fig. 57.18***.

WASTE WATER TREATMENT OF SOME INDUSTRIES

The characteristics of waste water are highly variable depending on the industrial source, which in turn depends on the industrial activity. Thus, treatment of waste water differs, and this is largely dependent on the industry. The treatment schemes of waste waters of dairy, distillery, tannery, sugar and antibiotic industries are briefly described.

WASTE WATER TREATMENT FOR DAIRIES

Dairy waste water is polluted at various stages by the activities of dairy operation. This has to be appropriately treated before being discharged. This is essential to avoid water pollution. A schematic represntation of dairy waste water treatment is depicted in ***Fig. 57.19***, and briefly described below.

The processing of dairy waste water is carried out ***by a two-stage pond system***. The treatment is first done in an anaerobic pond, and then in an

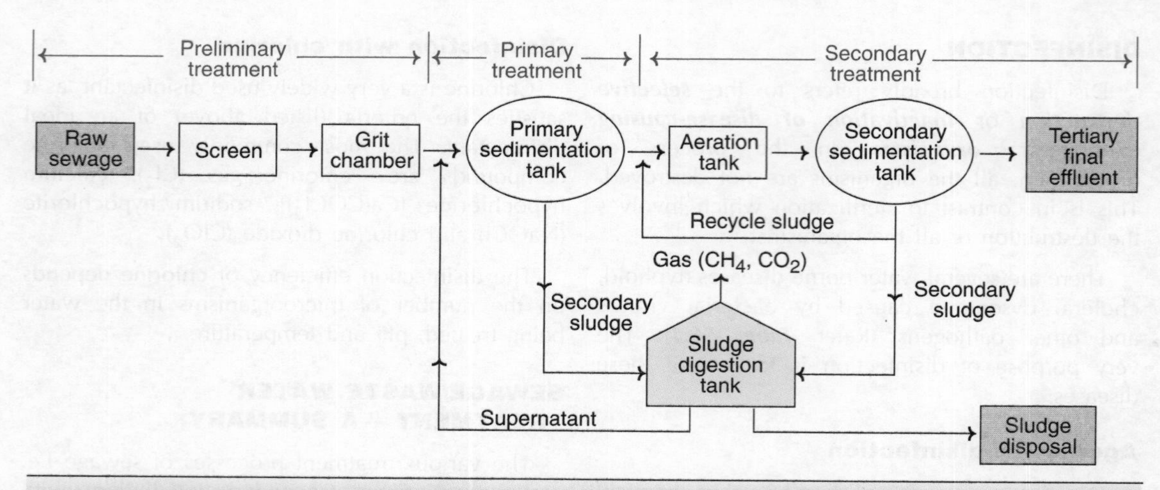

Fig. 57.18 : A diagrammatic representation of a flow chart of conventional sewage treatment plant.

aerobic pond. The treated water coming out of the anaerobic pond is rich in nutrients, hence is useful for irrigation purposes. At the end of the two-stage treatment, about 95% of the BOD material is removed from the waste water.

WASTE WATER TREATMENT FOR DISTILLERY

The waste water from distilleries mostly consists of dissolved O_2 and organic wastes (predominantly fermented starches and organic nitrogen). The treatment is carried out by a ***two-stage bacterial oxidation in anaerobic reactors***. The complex organic wastes are first degraded to organic molecules (acids, aldehydes, alcohols, ketones etc.). These molecules are further oxidized to smaller organic (CH_4) and inorganic (CO_2, NH_3, H_2S, H_2O) compounds (***Fig. 57.20***).

The products formed in the first stage of bacterial oxidation will promote the growth and multiplication of new bacterial cells. This is advantageous for more efficient bacterial oxidation.

WASTE WATER TREATMENT FOR TANNERY

Tanneries are industries involved in the processing of animal skins. For the transformation of skins to leathers, a large number of chemicals, dyes, tanning agents etc., are used. Tannery waste water poses a serious environmental threat since many of the ingradients have low biodegradability. The treatment process is carried out in two phases (***Fig. 57.21***).

Phase I : This phase involves ***biological acidification*** and production of sulfides from sulfates present in the waste water. The sulfide recovered in the form of sodium hydrogen sulfide is reused in tanneries.

Phase II : This is carried out in an anaerobic sludge blanket reactor. In this phase, the ***organic***

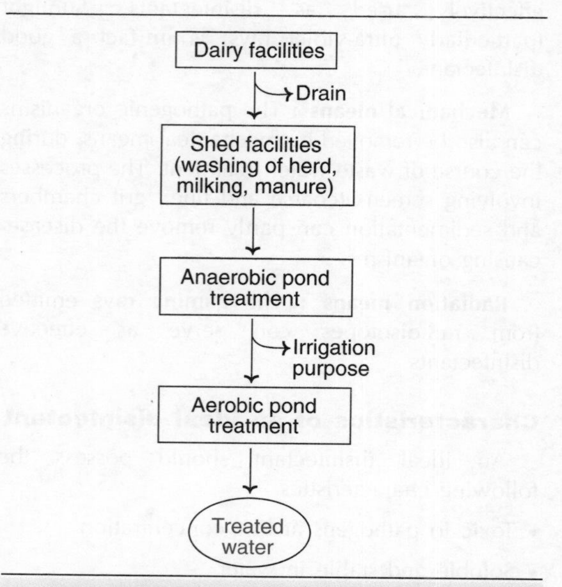

Fig. 57.19 : A diagrammatic representation of dairy waste water treatment.

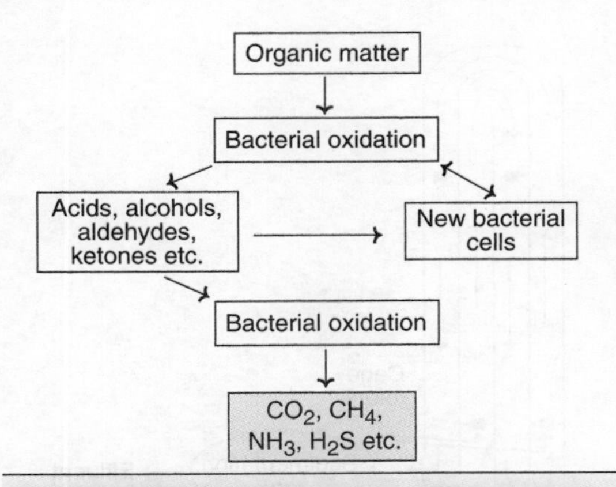

Fig. 57.20 : A diagrammatic representation of distillery organic waste water treatment.

acids are converted into gases. The left over sulfide from phase I is converted into solution, and processed to produce sulfur which will be useful in chemical industries.

With the two phase systems for waste water treatment of tanneries, it is possible to remove 20% of chemical oxygen demand (COD) and 90% of the sulfur compounds. Sometimes, additional aerobic bioreactors are used to remove more COD.

WASTE WATER TREATMENT FOR SUGAR INDUSTRY

The waste water from sugar industries contains high COD materials which are biodegradable. The treatment process is comparable to that described for waste water treatment of distillery (***Fig. 57.20***).

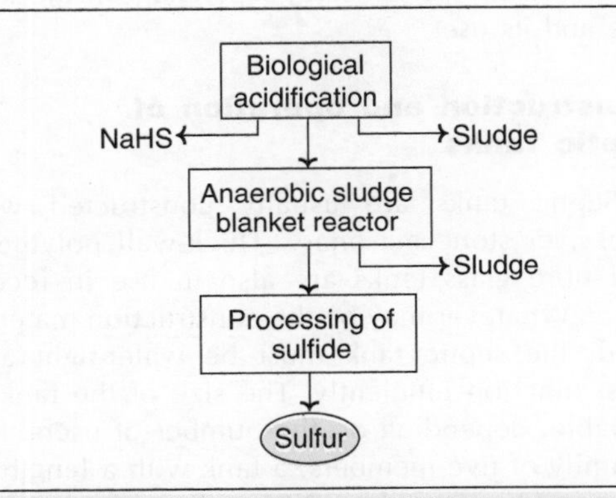

Fig. 57.21 : A diagrammatic representation of tannery waste water treatment.

TREATMENT OF ANTIBIOTICS IN WASTE WATER

There is a widespread use of antibiotics in human healthcare, animal husbandry and agriculture. In addition, the drug and antibiotic industries also directly contribute to pollution. Antibiotic pollution has become a major environmental threat. This is mostly due to the development of antibiotic resistance by the pathogenic bacteria. The conventional waste water treatment processes are ineffective in removing the antibiotics.

Special tertiary treatment processes are required to remove the antibiotic pollutants. The treatment involves the degradation of target molecules by oxidation, exposure to ultraviolet light etc. Some pharmaceutical industries have introduced a new technique namely ***membrane filtration*** to remove even trace amounts of antibiotics from the waste water.

WATER RECYCLING

There is shortage of water throughout the world. Therefore, there is a need for recycling of waste water (i.e. the use of reclaimed waste water) wherever, possible.

Approximately two thirds of world's water is utilized for irrigation purposes. In the developing countries at some places, the raw domestic sewage (completely untreated) is directly used for irrigation of crop land. Such practices expose the people to risk of infections by pathogenic bacteria, viruses and prions. It is therefore desirable to develop low-cost ***technologies to produce irrigation water from waste waters.***

Large quantities of water is also utilized in industries. For instance, to make one ton of steel, about 300 tones of water is needed. Consumption of water is also high for many other industries such as food, paper and textiles. At some places, and for some industries, processes for recycling of water have been developed. The technology for the recycling of water is variable, and this mainly depends on the industry.

Recycling of waste water is useful for agriculture, horticulture and watering of lawns and golf courses, besides supplying to lakes (fishing and boating purposes). However, the use of recycled water for drinking purposes should be avoided.

SMALL SEWAGE/WASTE WATER TREATMENT SYSTEMS

The large scale sewage/waste water of treatment processes have been described. They are not suitable for the treatment of small sewage or waste water, particularly coming from small communities.

The on-site systems of sewage treatment for individual residences (or communities) with special reference to oxidation ditch, septic tanks and Imhoff tanks are briefly described.

OXIDATION DITCH

Oxidation ditch method, first developed in Netherlands, is a suitable method for the treatment of sewage in small communities. This is basically an ***aeration type of activated sludge process*** (See p. 690) with a mechanical system of aeration. However, there is no primary sedimentation of sewage, consequently the problem of handling and treatment of primary sludge is eliminated.

Oxidation ditch consists of aeration units, namely ditch channels (2 or more) constructed side by side (***Fig. 57.22***). The sizes of the ditch channels are variable-length 150–1000 m, width 1-5 m and depth 1-5 m. They are constructed with brick or stone masonary. A special type of rotors (cage rotors) are fitted into each ditch channel for continuously agitating and circulating the sludge, besides supplying O_2. The sludge is allowed to settle down in a separate sedimentation tank. The activated sludge is returned to ditch channels.

Instead of using a separate sedimentation tank, the sewage may be allowed to settle down in the ditch channels by stopping the rotors (usually during night). The supernatant from the ditch channels can be taken out. The excess sludge collected (in the sedimentation tank or at the bottom of ditch channels) can be stabilized.

SEPTIC TANKS

Septic tanks are recommended for individual houses and for small communities and institutions with a contributing population around 300.

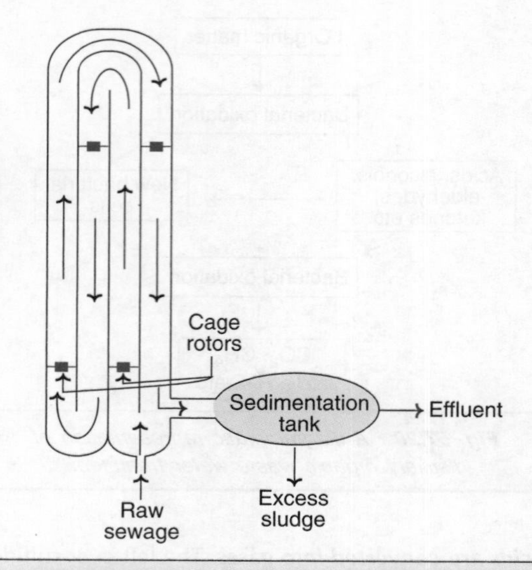

Fig. 57.22 : A diagrammatic representation of oxidation ditch.

Septic tanks work on the principle of ***anaerobic digestion***. This occurs as the solids of the sewage settle at the bottom of the tank. Under anaerobic conditions, the biodegradable organic matter is converted to gases (CH_4, CO_2, H_2S etc.) and liquid compounds. This results in a drastic reduction in the volume of sludge. A thick crust of scum formed on the surface of septic tank maintains anaerobic conditions. The effluent coming out of the septic tank contains some organic solids and pathogens. Therefore, disposal of the effluent from septic tank has to be dealt with very carefully. The septic tanks are desludged and cleaned at regular intervals, usually once in 2-5 years (depending on the tank size and its use).

Construction and operation of septic tanks

Septic tanks are usually constructed with bricks, or stone masonary. Thick-wall polythene and fibre glass tanks are also in use in recent years. Whatever may be the construction material used, the septic tank must be water-tight and must function efficiently. The size of the tank is variable, depending on the number of users. For a family of five members, a tank with a length of 1.5 m and a breadth of 0.75 m is recommended. For such a tank, the cleaning interval is 2-3 years.

A conventional septic tank has two compartments, the first compartment being twice the size of the second one (***Fig. 57.23***). For effective sedimentation of solids, the tank should be designed to prevent the short-circuiting at the top and the bottom of the tank. Further, the location of inlet and outlet should be such that the contents of the septic tank are not disturbed while the sewage enters or effluent leaves. Septic tank should be provided with a ventilation pipe, the top of which should be covered with a mosquito proof wire mesh.

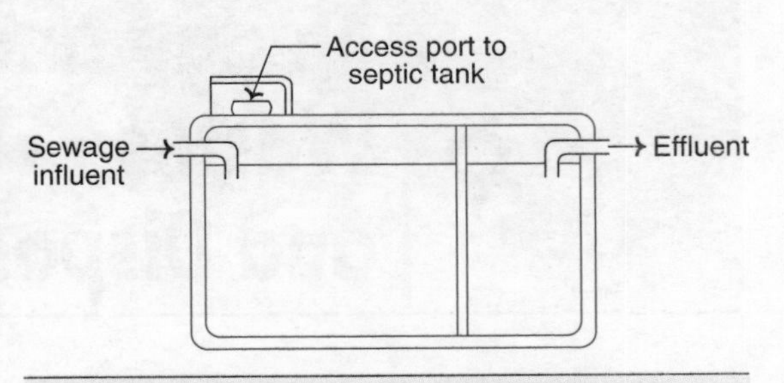

Fig. 57.23 : Schematic representation of a conventional two-compartment septic tank.

As the sewage enters the septic tank, the solids settle to the bottom while grease and other light materials float on the surface, and form a scum. The ***bottom-settled organic material undergoes facultative and anaerobic decomposition to form more stable compounds and gases*** (CH_4, CO_2, H_2S). In this way, there is a continuous reduction of solids of sewage entering the septic tank. However, sludge accumulates at the bottom of the tank. Desludging of septic tank has to be carried out periodically (once in 2-5 years).

IMHOFF TANKS

Imhoff tank is an ***improved septic tank.*** It basically consists of a two storey tank in which the sedimentation (settling) occurs in the upper tank while the digestion of the settled solids takes place in the lower compartment (***Fig. 57.24***).

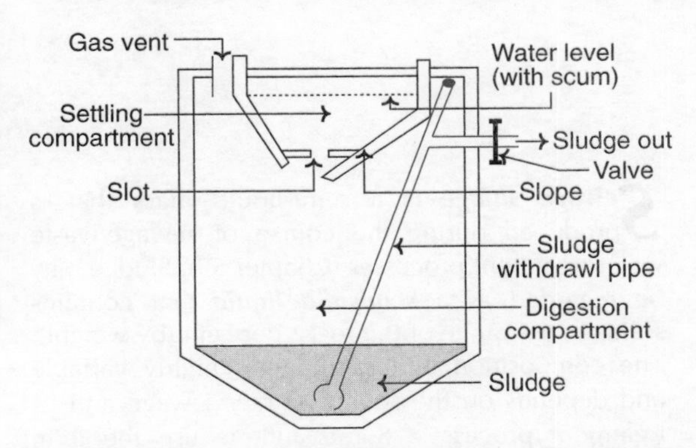

Fig. 57.24 : A diagrammatic view of imhoff tank.

As the sewage enters the sedimentation tank, the solids settle down to the bottom and the sewage flows into the digestion tank through slopes and slot of the sedimentation tank. Gas produced in the digestion process escapes through gas vent. The sedimentation tank is designed in such a way that the gases and the gas-buoyed sludge particles raising from the sludge layer do not enter into it. The sludge collection at the bottom can be withdrawn periodically.

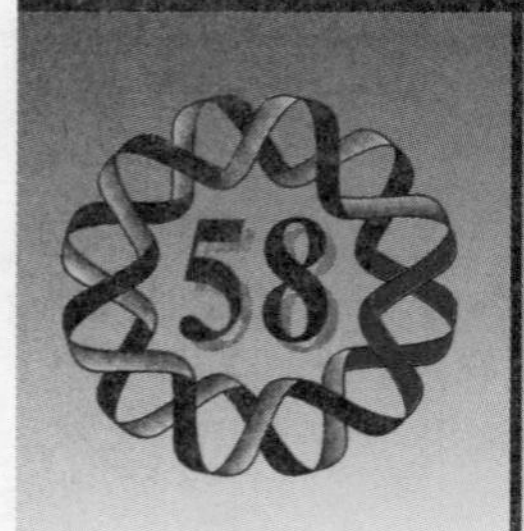

Sludge and Solid Wastes — Treatment and Disposal

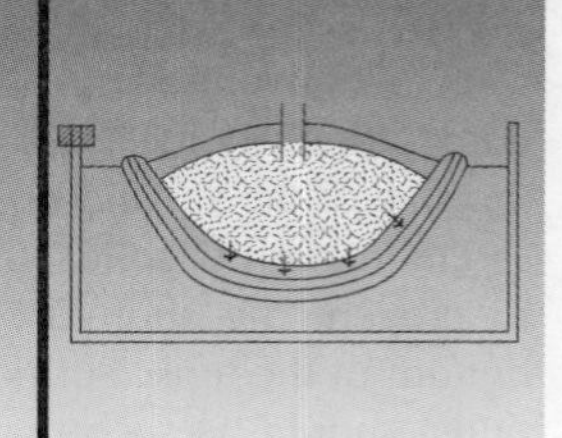

Sewage sludge is a semi-liquid mass that is produced during the course of sewage/waste water treatment processes (Chapter 57). Sludge may be regarded as a ***semisolid liquid*** that contains solids in the range of 0.5 to 12 per cent (by weight). The composition of the sludge is highly variable and depends on the source of raw sewage and its treatment processes. Some authors use the term ***organic slurries*** for sewage sludge.

SOURCES AND CHARACTERISTICS OF SLUDGE

The following unit operations are the ***major sources*** of sludge.

- Screening
- Grit removal
- Primary sedimentation
- Secondary sedimentation
- Sludge-processing units.

The details on the above processes have already been described. The ***important sludges*** and their ***characteristics*** are given in ***Table 58.1***. The characters of sludge are variable and depend on the origin of the sludge, and the aging after it is produced.

Chemical composition of sludge

The chemical composition of sludge is variable. The major constituents of sludge are proteins and other nitrogen containing compounds, grease and fats, cellulose, hydrocarbons, phosphorus, iron, silica, organic acids, heavy metals, pathogens and pesticides.

The various ***methods of sludge treatment and disposal*** are given ***in Table 58.2***. The important aspects of selected processes are briefly described.

PRELIMINARY OPERATIONS

The preliminary operations are carried out to provide a constant and homogeneous sludge for further processing.

Sludge grinding

Grinding of sludge is carried out to cut a large mass of sludge into small pieces. For this purpose, hardended steel cutters and overload sensors are used.

Sludge degritting

Sometimes, removal of grit (degritting) is necessary for the effective treatment of sludge. Degritting can be carried out by applying centrifugal force to the flowing sludge. Cyclone degritters are usually employed for this purpose to separate grit particles from the organic sludge.

Sludge blending

Sludge produced in ***primary*** (settleable solids), ***secondary*** (settleable solids and biological solids) and ***tertiary*** (biological solids and chemical solids) treatments is mixed (blended) to produce a uniform mixture.

TABLE 58.1 Major sludges and their characteristics

Sludge	*Characteristics*
Screenings	Contains organic and inorganic materials that can be easily removed.
Grit	Rich in heavier inorganic solids and a good quantity of organic matter (fats, grease).
Primary sludge	Obtained from the primary settling tanks, grey in colour and offensive in odour.
Activated sludge	Brownish to dark in colour with flocculant appearance, usually has earthy odour and can be digested easily.
Trickling-filter sludge	Brownish in colour with inoffensive odour (fresh sludge), easily digestible.
Scum	Floatable materials skimmed from the surfaces of primary and secondary settling tanks. Scum contains oils, fats, food wastes, plastic materials, cotton etc.
Aerobically digested sludge	Brownish to black in colour with flocculant appearance. No offensive odour.
Anaerobically digested sludge	Dark brown to black in colour, contains large quantities of gas. On drying the sludge, the gases escape.
Septage	Sludge of septic tanks, black in colour. Usually well digested due to long storage. Offensive odour due to hydrogen sulfide.

Sludge storage

Storage of sludge becomes necessary when the processing units are not in operations (night shifts, weekends). Short-term storage of sludge is accomplished in settling tanks while for long-term storage, specially designed tanks have to be used.

SLUDGE THICKENING (CONCENTRATION)

The solid content of the sludge is variable and may range from 0.5 to 12%. It is necessary to concentrate the sludge (particularly with low solid content) by removing some amount of liquid. Physical methods are employed for sludge thickening.

Gravity thickening

Gravity thickening is the most commonly used method for the thickening of primary sludge. It can be carried out in the conventional sedimentation tank (circular tank is preferred). As the sludge gets concentrated by gravity, the supernatant can be returned to the treatment plant (i.e. primary settling tank).

TABLE 58.2 Sludge treatment and disposal methods

Type of process	*Treatment methods*
Preliminary operations	Grinding, degritting, blending, storage
Thickening	Gravity thickening Flotation thickening Centrifugal thickening Rotary drum thickening
Stabilization	Lime stabilization Heat treatment Anaerobic digestion Aerobic digestion Composting
Conditioning	Chemical method Heat treatment method
Disinfection	Pasteurization
Dewatering	Vacuum filter Centrifuge Sludge drying beds
Heat drying	Flash dryer Slow dryer Rotary dryer
Thermal reduction	Multiple-hearth incinerator Fluidized bed incinerator
Ultimate disposal	Land application Distribution and marketing Landfill Lagooning

Flotation thickening

Flotation thickening is the technique of choice for the treatment of sludges from suspended-growth biological treatment processes. There are three types of flotation thickening processes — ***dissolved air flotation***, ***dispersed-air flotation***, and ***vacuum flotation***. Among these, dissolved-air flotation is widely used. In this technique, air is passed through the sludge that is held at high pressure. The air raises to the top of the sludge in the form of bubbles along with attached particles to form a sludge blanket. This can be skimmed off at regular intervals. The efficiency of flotation thickening depends on the air to solids ratio.

Centrifugal thickening

Centrifugal thickening is based on the principle of settlement of sludge particles under the influence of centrifugal forces. Two types of centrifuges — ***solid bowl centrifuge*** and ***basket centrifuge*** are used for this purpose. Although concentration of sludge by centrifugal thickening is efficient, it involves high cost of maintenance and power consumption.

Rotary drum thickening

Thickening of the sludge can be carried out by use of rotary drums. As the sludge is passed over the rotating screen drums, the solids separate from the water and the thickened sludge rolls out at the drum ends.

SLUDGE STABILIZATION

Sludge requires stabilization to achieve the following objectives.

- To reduce the load of disease-causing organisms (pathogens).
- To inhibit the potential for putrefaction.
- To eliminate offensive odours.

Sludge stabilization can be carried out by appropriate biological and chemical means. The ***techniques used for sludge stabilization are — lime stabilization, heat treatment, anaerobic digestion, aerobic digestion and composting***. They are briefly described.

Lime stabilization

When lime, in the form of hydrated lime [$Ca(OH)_2$] or quick lime (CaO) is added to the sludge, the pH raises to 12 or higher. At high pH, the microorganisms cannot grow. Consequently, the sludge will not putrify, create unpleasant odours and does not pose health hazards.

In the ***lime pretreatment***, addition of lime is done prior to dewatering, while in ***lime post-treatment***, it is done after dewatering.

Heat treatment

Heat treatment involves heating of sludge for a short period (250°C for about 30 minutes) under pressure. By this process, sludge is dewatered and sterilized. Heat treatment helps in stabilization and conditioning (discussed later) of the sludge. However, due to high cost, it is less frequently used.

Anaerobic sludge digestion

Anaerobic digestion of sewage is one of the oldest forms of biological treatment processes. The same operating unit is equally useful for the stabilization of sludge. There are different ways of carrying out anaerobic sludge digestion — standard rate digestion, single-stage high rate digestion and two-stage digestion.

Standard rate digestion : This is a single-stage digestion process (Refer ***Fig. 57.9***). The sludge is added and heated by external heat exchangers. As the sludge gets digested, the gas released comes out to the surfaces. Along with the gas, certain sludge particles (fats, oils, grease) also raise to the top to form a scum which can be removed.

Single-stage high rate digestion : This is characterized by high rate of sludge loading, and its digestion under anaerobic conditions. The sludge is continuously mixed by gas, heated and recirculated for optimal digestion.

Two-stage digestion : There are two digestion tanks used in this process of high-rate digestion. The first tank is used for digestion proper (with mixing and heating facilities) while the second digester is employed for storage and concentration.

Thermophilic anaerobic digestion : Sometimes, sludge digestion can be carried out at relatively ***higher temperature*** (45–60°C) by ***thermophilic bacteria***. In fact, the digestion process is faster with increased bacterial destruction and improved dewatering at higher temperature. But the major limitation is the requirement of high energy for continuous heating. For this reason, thermophilic anaerobic digestion process is not widely used.

Aerobic sludge digestion

Aerobic digestion of sludges from various sources (primary, secondary and tertiary treatments) is becoming popular in recent years for the following reasons.

- The digestion of volatile solids is as effective as in anaerobic digestion.
- Fertilizer value of the sludge is much higher.
- Lower capital and operational costs.

However, the major limitation in aerobic digestion is the continuous supply of O_2 which is a costly affair.

The process, aerobic digestion of sludge is comparable to activated sludge process (Refer p. 690).

Principle of aerobic digestion : When the nutrient (substrates) supply to the microorganisms is depleted, they start oxidizing their own cellular (protoplasmic) materials for energy supply and maintenance. About 70–80% of the cellular organic matter can be oxidized aerobically to produce carbon dioxide, nitrate (NO_3^-) and water. Approximately 20–30% of the cellular organic matter cannot be oxidized, as it is not biodegradable.

A diagrammatic representation of an ***aerobic digester*** is depicted in ***Fig. 58.1***. The process can be carried out by batch or continuous flow system of operation. With regard to the aeration process, aerobic digestion is of two types—conventional aerobic digestion and high purity oxygen aerobic digestion.

Conventional aerobic digestion : Atmospheric air is used in the conventional digester for the process of aerobic digestion.

High-purity oxygen aerobic digestion : In this case, a pure grade of oxygen instead of air is used. The digestion process is usually carried out in closed tanks.

Thermophilic aerobic digestion : This is refinement of the above two techniques, and can effectively digest up to 20% of the biodegradable organics. The procers is carried out by thermophilic bacteria at a temperature around 45°C. There are certain advantages of thermophilic aerobic digestion. These include killing of more pathogenic organisms and digestion of more solids, with minimal unpleasent odours in stabilized sludge.

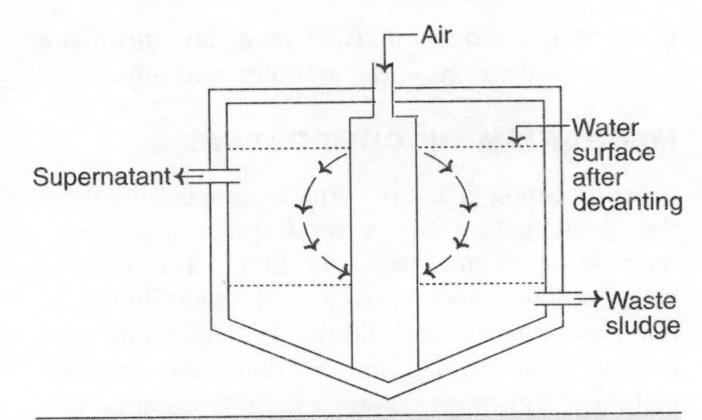

Fig. 58.1 : Diagrammatic representation of an aerobic digester.

COMPOSTING

Composting basically involves ***the process of biological degradation of solid organic waste material to stable end products***. Although composting can be carried out under aerobic and anaerobic conditions, aerobic composting is more frequently used. Thus, composting may be considered as an ***aerobic microbiological process*** for converting solid organic wastes into stable sanitary, nuisance free, humus like material that can be safely disposed into the environment.

Composting is a cost-effective and ***environment friendly process for stabilization and ultimate disposal of sludge***. The product of composting is useful for soil improvement and the production of mushrooms. Thus, composting is ultimately helpful for reuse and recycling of organic waste materials from domestic, agriculture and industry.

Organisms involved in composting

A wide variety of organisms (both unicellular and multicellular) are involved in the process composting. The bacteria make up 80–90% of the microorganisms found in the compost. These bacteria possess a broad range of enzymes to degrade a wide range of organic compounds.

The other organisms actively involved in composting are ***actinomycetes*** (a filamentous type of bacteria), ***fungi*** (molds, yeasts), and ***protozoa***, besides earthworms, insects, mites and ants.

MECHANISM OF COMPOSTING

Composting is a very complex process involving the participation of several microorganisms—bacteria, actinomycetes and fungi. The bacteria bring out the decomposition of macromolecules namely proteins and lipids, besides generating energy (heat). Fungi and actinomycetes degrade cellulose and other complex organic compounds.

Composting may be divided into three stages with reference to changes in temperature—mesophilic, thermophilic and cooling.

Mesophilic stage : The fungi and acid-producing bacteria are active in this stage, and the temperature increases from ambient to about 40°C.

Thermophilic stage : As the composting proceeds, the temperature raises from 40°C to 70°C. Thermophilic bacteria, thermophilic fungi and actinomycetes are active in this stage. Thermophilic stage is associated with high rate and maximum degradation of organic materials.

Cooling stage : The microbial degradative activity slows down and the thermophilic organisms are replaced by mesophilic bacteria and fungi. Cooling stage is associated with formation of water, pH stabilization and completion of humeic acid formation.

METHODS OF COMPOSTING

The operation of composting involves the following steps.

- Mixing of dewatered sludge with a bulking agent (saw dust, rice hulls, straw or recycle compost). The bulking agent improves the porosity of the mixture for good aeration.
- Creating aerobic conditions (aeration) by mechanical or other means. This is needed for the supply of oxygen, to control temperature, and for the removal of water (moisture).
- Removal of the bulking agent, if possible.
- Storage and disposal of the compost.

There are three major methods of composting—***aerated static pile, windrow, and in-vessel systems***. As per a recent survey, the approximate distribution of different composting methods is given.

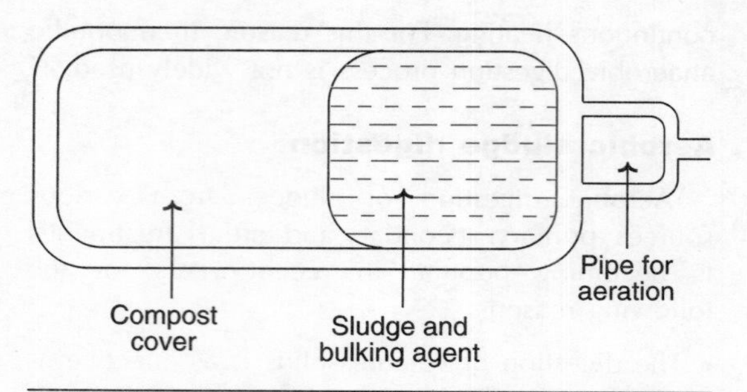

***Fig. 58.2** : A diagrammatic representation of aerated static pole of composting.*

Aerated static pile	–	55%
Windrow	–	30%
In-vessel	–	15%

Aerated static pile system

The ***dewatered sludge*** is mixed with a bulking agent (wood chips) and ***placed over a grid of aeration*** or ***exhaust piping***. Air is supplied through blowers for efficient aeration. A layer of compost is kept over the top of the aerated static pile for insulation and good aeration (***Fig. 58.2***). It takes about 3-4 weeks for composting, and another 4-5 weeks for curing. The cured compost is screened to reduce the quantity, besides the recovery of the bulking agent.

Windrow system

Windrows are a type of static piles with periodical turning and mixing of sludge during the composting period (3-4 weeks). The mixing is usually carried out at weekly intervals and is associated with release of unpleasant and offensive odours. The windrows may be open or covered and the aeration is carried out by mechanical means.

In-vessel system

In the in-vessel composting system, the process is ***carried out in a closed vessel*** or container. This is an advanced method and is designed to control the environmental conditions (temperature, air flow and O_2 supply), besides minimizing the release of offensive odours. The advantages of in-vessel system include higher efficiency of composting, with lower labour costs, and smaller area for the plant.

There are two major systems of in-vessel composting — plug flow and dynamic.

Plug-flow in-vessel composting reactors : There are two types of plug-flow in-vessel reactors— ***cylindrical tower*** and ***tunnel*** (***Fig. 58.3A*** and ***58.3B***). In both the cases, the relationship between the particles in the composting mass is maintained the same throughout the process. As the sewage is fed, the composting occurs on the principle of first in and first out.

Dynamic in-vessel composting reactors : These are also known as ***agitated bed in-vessel composting reactors***. In these units, the composting material is mechanically mixed during the period of processing. ***Dynamic circular reactors*** and ***dynamic rectangular reactors*** (***Fig. 58.3C and 58.3D***) are in common use. In circular reactors, the ***augurs*** rotate around the centre of the reaction vessel and mix the composting material. As regards the rectangular reactors, ***extraction conveyor*** is responsible for mixing the compost, and for the discharge of the compost to the outlet conveyor.

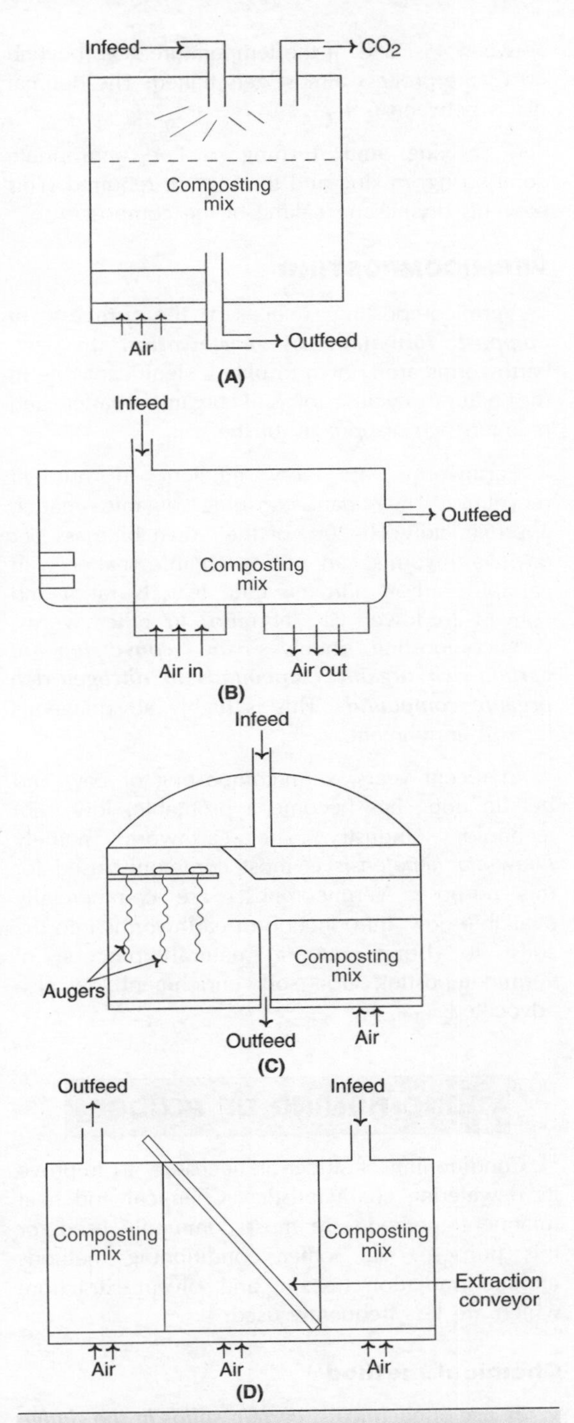

Fig. 58.3 : *Diagrammatic representation of composting reactors (A) Plug-flow cylindrical tower (B) Plug-flow tunnel (C) Dynamic circular reactor (D) Dynamic rectangular reactor.*

Factors affecting aerobic composting

There are several factors that influence the sludge-composting process. The important ones are briefly discussed.

1. **Type of sludge :** Both untreated and digested sludges can be composted. However, untreated sludge requires more oxygen, and emits unpleasant odours.

2. **Carbon nitrogen ratio :** For efficient composting, the carbon nitrogen ratio should be in the range of 25 : 1 to 35 : 1. It is desirable to periodically check and maintain this ratio.

3. **Bulking agents :** Cheap and readily available bulking agents (saw dust, wood chips) are used. Their particle size and moisture content influence composting.

4. **Moisture content :** A moisture content of sludge less than 60% is ideal for composting.

5. **Aeration :** It is desirable that the oxygen supply is constantly maintained, and it properly reaches the composting material.

6. **Temperature and pH :** Best results of composting are seen when the temperature is

between 45–55°C. If the temperature goes beyond 60°C, the process almost gets halted. The optimal pH is between 6-9.

7. **Mixing and turning :** For appropriate composting, mixing and turning are required. This prevents drying and caking of the compost.

VERMICOMPOSTING

Vermicomposting refers to the ***process of compost formation by earthworms***. In fact, earthworms are known to play a significant role in the natural cycling of soil organic matter and maintenance of porosity of the soil.

Earthworms are very efficient in nutrient recycling. They can consume organic matter, approximately 10–20% of their own biomass per day. Earthworms can utilize organic matter with variable carbon nitrogen ratio (C : N ratio) and convert to lower C : N ratio. In other words, vermicomposting involves the ***conversion of carbon-rich organic compounds to nitrogen-rich organic compounds***. This is highly advantageous for soil enrichment.

In recent years, vermicomposting of cow and buffalo dung has become a profitable, low (bio) technology industry. The earthworm namely *Drawidia nepalensis* is most commonly used for this purpose. Vermicomposts are commercially available now. Introduction of earthworms into the soils to bring out a natural process of vermicomposting (for soil enrichment) is also advocated.

CONDITIONING OF SLUDGE

Conditioning of sludge is necessary to improve its dewatering characteristics. Chemical and heat treatment methods are most commonly used for this purpose. The other conditioning methods include irradiation, freezing and solvent extraction, which are less frequently used.

Chemical method

By use of chemicals, ***certain solids in the sludge can be coagulated*** with a release of absorbed water. Chemical conditioning can reduce the moisture content of the sludge by about 15–30% (i.e. from about 95% to about 65%). The most commonly used chemicals are alum, lime, ferric chloride and organic polymers.

Heat treatment method

Heat treatment ***can stabilize and condition the sludge***. This process is carried out for a short period under pressure. Heat treatment results in the coagulation of solids, besides reducing the water affinity of sludge solids.

DISINFECTION OF SLUDGE

In recent years, disinfection of sludge is becoming significant due to its reuse or its application on the land. This is because the ***pathogenic organisms of the sludge*** should be ***destroyed*** to protect the health of the inhabitants who are exposed to it. There are a large number of disinfection methods to choose.

- Pasteurization
- Heat drying
- Irradiation
- High pH treatment
- Addition of chlorine
- Long-term storage of digested sludge
- Complete composting.

DEWATERING

Dewatering basically involves the process of ***reducing the moisture content of sludge***. Dewatering can be carried out by vacuum filters, centrifuges and sludge drying beds.

Vacuum filtration

Dewatering by vacuum filtration is rather old, but has been discontinued in recent years due to high operating and maintenance costs, besides the complexicity of the process. In fact, improved and more efficient alternative methods have been developed during the past ten years.

Centrifugation

Centrifugation is commonly used for the dewatering of sludges obtained from industries. By the process of centrifugation, it is possible to remove liquids from solids. Different types of centrifuges (solid bowel centrifuge, basket centrifuge) are commercially available for sludge dewatering.

Sludge drying beds

Drying beds are widely used in developed countries (USA, Britain) to dewater the digested sludge. This method produces high solid containing dried product which can be easily disposed off (in a landfill or as soil conditioner). Sludge drying beds are cost-effective.

HEAT DRYING

When the sludge is subjected to mechanical heat drying, the water content can be substantially reduced. The ultimate purpose of heat drying is to prepare a sludge, free from moisture that can be incinerated efficiently. Mechanical heat drying can be carried out by flash dryers, spray dryers, rotary dryers and multiple hearth dryers.

THERMAL REDUCTION OF SLUDGE

Thermal reduction basically involves the total or partial conversion of organic solids to oxidized end products such as carbon dioxide and water. This may be carried out by incineration or by wet-air oxidation. Thermal reduction of sludge is associated with destruction of pathogenic organisms, detoxification of toxic compounds and reducing the volume of disposable sludge.

The major processes employed for thermal reduction of sludge are multiple-hearth incineration, fluidized-bed incineration and wet-air oxidation.

ULTIMATE DISPOSAL OF SLUDGE

While considering the final disposal of sludge, its beneficial uses are first taken into account. Sludge is useful for the supply of nutrients to the soil, besides possessing the properties of soil conditioning. Thus, attempts are made to dispose the sludge in a beneficial manner. If this is not possible, alternates are considered.

Land applications of sludge (as a fertilizer)

The ***spreading of sludge on*** or ***just below the soil surface*** is considered as land applications of sludge. Sludge may be used in the agricultural lands, forest lands, and dedicated land disposal sites. The pathogens and toxic organic compounds present in the sludge can be respectively destroyed by sunlight and soil microorganisms. Sludge applied to land is thus useful as a soil conditioner to improve the characteristics of land-nutrient transport facilitation and increased water retention. Thus, ***sludge can replace the expensive fertilizers***.

The quantity of organic materials and the pathogens must be reduced before the sludge is applied on the land. A high content of organic matter will result in offensive odours while the pathogens spread diseases. There are in fact regulatory requirements to control pathogens of sludge by various means.

Distribution and marketing

Distribution and marketing of sludge for beneficial purposes is gaining importance in recent years. It is estimated that about 10–20% of the total sludge produced is utilized in this fashion. The marketed sludge is used as substitution for topsoil and peat on parks, lawns, golf courses and in ornamental and vegetable gardens.

There are regulatory requirements to reduce the pathogenic organisms for distribution and marketing of sludge.

LANDFILLING

Landfilling is a method for the ***final disposal of sludge*** that is not useful any more. The ***sanitary landfill method*** is most suitable for the disposal of solid domestic wastes. This involves a low-cost ***anaerobic technology***. In this method, the sludge or solid wastes are deposited in low-lying and low value sites. The deposition is done almost daily and the deposits are covered with a layer of soil (***Fig. 58.4***). With the coverage of the new waste deposits, nuisance conditions such as bad odours and flies are minimized.

It is desirable that the sludge is dewatered so that its transportation becomes easy. Further, the generation of ***leachate*** (***liquid that percolates out due to leaching***) is minimal from a dewatered sludge.

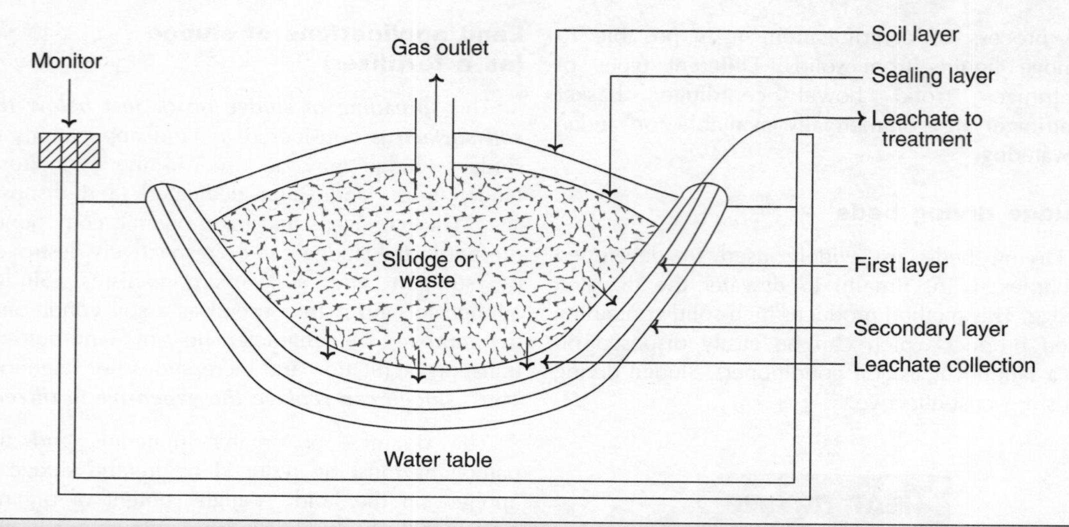

Fig. 58.4 : A diagrammatic representation of a landfill.

At lease two impermeable layers are built below the landfill to prevent the leakage of leachate to the surrounding lands. The accumulated leachate can be taken out and treated by appropriate methods.

The complete filling of landfills may take several months or even years, depending on the size of the site and the quantity of waste being deposited. Landfills can be used for the ***generation of methane gas*** for commercial use. However, methane production usually commences several months after the landfill is completely filled.

In some countries, there are strict regulations to use landfills for sewage disposal. These include the air- and water tight sites to protect the environment.

LAGOONING

A lagoon is a ***shallow lake*** (or earth basin) ***usually located near a river or a sea***. Lagooning (disposal of sludge into lagoons) is a convenient method of sludge disposal if the treatment plant is located at a remote place. In lagooning, the sludge is stabilized by anaerobic and aerobic decomposition which is accompanied by release of objectionable odours. For this reason, lagoons should be located away from dwelling areas and high ways to avoid nuisance conditions.

The stabilized solids of the sludge settle to the bottom of lagoon and accumulate. The sludges can be stored indefinitely in lagoons or may be removed periodically.

SEPTAGE AND SEPTAGE DISPOSAL

Septage is a ***combination of sludge, scum and liquid coming out from a septic tank*** (Refer Chapter 57). It must be disposed under controlled conditions to avoid environmental pollution.

The most commonly used methods of septage disposal are listed below.

- ***Land application*** (surface or subsurface).
- ***Co-treatment with waste water*** (biological or chemical treatment processes).
- ***Co-disposal with solid wastes*** (composting and landfilling).
- ***Independent processing facilities*** (composting, biological treatment, chemical oxidation, lime stabilization).

For more details on these treatment processes, the reader must refer the preceeding pages.

TREATMENT AND DISPOSAL OF SOLID WASTES

Solid wastes are mostly being treated by incineration and landfilling, although these methods have certain limitations.

Incineration : This requires costly equipment and high power consumption. Incinerators do not allow recovery of any useful materials. Further, it is frequently associated with environmental pollution.

Landfilling : The various aspects of landfilling have been described (Refer p. 715). The major limitation of landfills is the problem of leachates and gas emissions which pollute the environment. Further, they are not efficient producers of ***biogas***. It is not possible to recycle the reusable products (paper, plastic, construction materials etc.) in landfilling.

SEPARATION AND COMPOSTING PLANTS

The industrial and municipal solid wastes can be effectively treated by separation, followed by composting. In fact, huge plants are constructed to serve the dual purposes.

Separation

It is possible to recover several useful materials from the solid wastes by employing physical processes.

- Plastic materials for reuse.
- Sand and gravel for construction purposes.
- Paper and cardboard for use in paper industry.
- Iron and aluminium for metallurgy.

After the separation of the important reusable materials, the left out in the solid wastes is mainly the ***biodegradable organic matter.***

Composting

A good account on the principles and processes of composting have already been described (See p. 711). The solid wastes are mostly composted by anaerobic process and to a lesser extent by aerobic means.

Dry anaerobic composting (DRANCO) process

In recent years, some companies have developed specific anaerobic digesters for composting solid wastes. The designing of digester is mainly based on the solid content of the waste, the temperature (from 35°C to 55°C) and the number of stages (1 or 2).

Dry anaerobic composting process is a commercially designed anaerobic digester. It is employed for composting of high solid (200–400 g/l) wastes at thermophilic temperature (around 55°C) by using a single stage reactor. The main advantage of DRANCO process is the ***high rate of composting under controlled conditions***. This is evident from the fact that the composting of solids can be completed in about two weeks time. This is in contrast to a landfill which takes several years, sometimes even decades (10–30 years)!

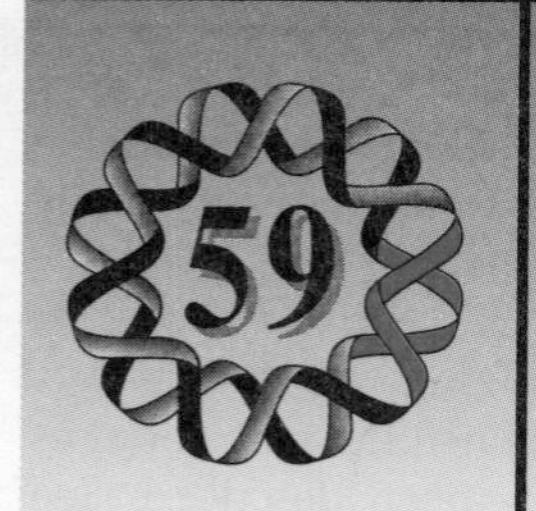

Biodegradation and Bioremediation

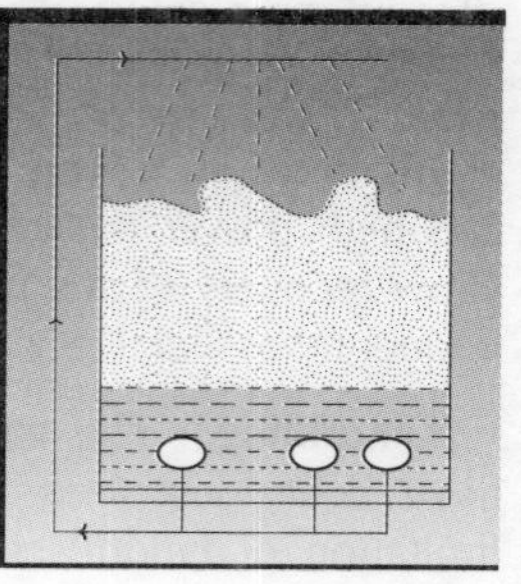

Biodegradation or biological degradation is the ***phenomenon of biological transformation of organic compounds*** by ***living organisms, particularly the microorganisms***. Biodegradation basically involves the conversion of complex organic molecules to simpler (and mostly non-toxic) ones. The term ***biotransformation*** is used for ***incomplete biodegradation*** of organic compounds involving one or a few reactions. Biotransformation is employed for the synthesis of commercially important products by microorganisms. For details on biotransformation, refer Chapter 22.

Bioremediation refers to the ***process of using microorganisms to remove the environmental pollutants*** i.e. the toxic wastes found in soil, water, air etc. The ***microbes serve as scavengers*** in bioremediation. The removal of organic wastes by microbes for ***environmental clean-up*** is the essence of bioremediation. The other names used (by some authors) for bioremediation are ***biotreatment***, ***bioreclamation*** and ***biorestoration***.

It is rather difficult to show any distinction between biodegradation and bioremediation, hence they are considered together in this chapter. Further, in biotechnology, most of the reactions of biodegradation/bioremediation involve xenobiotics. Thus, this chapter may be appropriately considered as microbial degradation of xenobiotics. For the bioremediation of metal pollutants, the reader must Refer Chapter 32).

Xenobiotics

Xenobiotics (xenos-foregin) broadly refer to the unnatural, foreign and synthetic chemicals such as pesticides, herbicides, refrigerants, solvents and other organic compounds. Microbial degradation of xenobiotics assumes significance, since it provides an effective and economic means of disposing of toxic chemicals, particularly the environmental pollutants.

PSEUDOMONAS — THE PREDOMINANT MICROORGANISM FOR BIOREMEDIATION

Members of the genus *Pseudomonas* (a soil microorganism) are the most predominant microorganisms that degrade xenobiotics. Different strains of *Pseudomonas,* that are capable of detoxifying more than 100 organic compounds, have been identified. The examples of organic compounds are several hydrocarbons, phenols, organophosphates, polychlorinated biphenyls (PCBs) and polycylic aromatics and naphthalene.

About 40–50 microbial strains of micro-organisms, capable of degrading xenobiotics have been isolated. Besides *Pseudomonas,* other good examples are *Mycobacterium, Alcaligenes,* and *Nocardia.* A selected list of microorganisms and the xenobiotics degraded is given in ***Table 59.1***.

Consortia of microorganisms for biodegradation : A particular strain of microorganism may degrade one or more compounds. Sometimes, for the

TABLE 59.1 A selected list of microorganisms and the pollutants (xenobiotics) that are degraded by bioremediation

Microorganism	*Pollutant chemicals*
Pseudomonas sp	Aliphatic and aromatic hydrocarbons— alkylaminoxides, alkylammonium benzene, naphthalene, anthracene xylene, toluene, polychlorinated biphenyls (PCBs), malathion, parathion, organophosphates.
Mycobacterium sp	Benzene, branched hydrocarbons, cycloparaffins
Alcaligenes sp	Polychlorinated biphenyls, alkyl benzene, halogenated hydrocarbons.
Nocardia sp	Naphthalene, alkylbenzenes, phenoxyacetate.
Arthrobacter sp	Benzene, polycyclic aromatics, phenoxyacetate, pentachlorophenol.
Corynebacterium sp	Halogenated hydrocarbons, phenoxyacetate.
Bacillus sp	Long chain alkanes, phenylurea.
Candida sp	Polychlorinated biphenyls
Aspergillus sp	Phenols
Xanthomonas sp	Polycyclic hydrocarbons
Streptomyces sp	Halogenated hydrocarbons, phenoxyacetate.
Fusarium sp	Propanil
Cunninghamella sp	Polycyclic aromatics, polychlorinated biphenyls.

degradation of a single compound, the synergetic action of a few microorganisms (i.e. a consortium or cocktail of microbes) may be more efficient. For instance, the insecticide parathion is more efficiently degraded by the combined action of *Pseudomonas aeruginosa* and *Psudomonas stulzeri*.

Co-metabolism in biodegradation : In general, the metabolism (breakdown) of xenobiotics is not associated with any advantage to the microorganism. That is the pollutant chemical cannot serve as a source of carbon or energy for the organism. The term co-metabolism is often used to indicate the ***non-beneficial*** (***to the microorganism***) ***biochemical pathways concerned with the biodegradation of xenobiotics***. However, co-metabolism depends on the presence of a suitable substrate for the microorganism. Such compounds are referred to ***co-substrates***.

Factors affecting biodegradation

Several factors influence biodegradation. These include the chemical nature of the xenobiotic, the capability of the individual microorganism, nutrient and O_2 supply, temperature, pH and redox potential. Among these, ***the chemical nature of the substrate that has to be degraded is very important***. Some of the relevant features are given hereunder.

- In general, aliphatic compounds are more easily degraded than aromatic ones.
- Presence of cyclic ring structures and length chains or branches decrease the efficiency of biodegradation.
- Water soluble compounds are more easily degraded.
- Molecular orientation of aromatic compounds influences biodegradation i.e. ortho > para > meta.
- The presence of halogens (in aromatic compounds) inhibits biodegradation.

Besides the factors listed above, there are two recent developments to enhance the biodegradation by microorganisms.

Biostimulation : This is a process by which the microbial activity can be enhanced by ***increased supply of nutrients*** or by addition of certain ***stimulating agents*** (electron acceptors, surfactants).

Bioaugmentation : It is possible to increase biodegradation ***through manipulation of genes***. More details on this genetic manipulation i.e. genetically engineered microorganisms (GEMs), are described later. Bioaugmentation can also be achieved by employing a consortium of micro-organisms.

Enzyme systems for biodegradation

Several enzyme systems (with independent enzymes that work together) are in existence in the microorganisms for the degradation of xenobiotics.

TABLE 59.2 A selected list of xenobiotics and the plasmids containing genes (in *Plasmodium*) for biodegradation

Xenobiotic	*Name of plasmid in* Pseudomonas
Naphthalene	NAH
Xylene	XYL
Xylene and toluene	TOL, pWWO, XYL-K
Salicylate	SAL
Camphor	CAM
3-Chlorobenzene	pAC25

The genes coding for the enzymes of biodegradative pathways may be present in the chromosomal DNA or more frequently on the plasmids. In certain microorganisms, the genes of both chromosome and plasmid contribute for the enzymes of biodegradation.

As already described, the microorganism *Pseudomonas* occupies a special place in biodegradation. A selected list of xenobiotics and the plasmids containing the genes for their degradation is given in ***Table 59.2***.

RECALCITRANT XENOBIOTICS

There are certain compounds that ***do not easily undergo biodegradation*** and therefore ***persist in the environment for a long period*** (sometimes in years). They are labeled as recalcitrant. There may be several reasons for the resistance of xenobiotics to microbial degradation.

- They may chemically and biologically inert (highly stable).
- Lack of enzyme system in the microorganisms for biodegradation.
- They cannot enter the microorganisms being large molecules or lack of transport systems.
- The compounds may be highly toxic or result in the formation highly toxic products that kill microorganisms.

There are a large number of racalcitrant xenobiotic compounds e.g. chloroform, freons, insecticides (DDT, lindane), herbicides (dalapon) and synthetic polymers (plastics e.g. polystyrene, polyethylene, polyvinyl chlorine).

It takes about 4-5 years for the degradation of DDT (75–100%) in the soil. A group of microorganisms (*Aspergillus flavus, Mucor aternans, Fusarium oxysporum* and *Trichoderma viride*) are associated with the slow biodegradation of DDT.

Biomagnification : The phenomenon of ***progressive increase in the concentration of a xenobiotic*** compound, as the substance is passed ***through the food chain*** is referred to as biomagnification or ***bioaccumulation***. For instance, the insecticide DDT is absorbed repeatedly by plants and microorganism. When they are eaten by fish and birds, this pesticide being recalcitrant, accumulates, and enters the food chain. Thus, DDT may find its entry into various animals, including man. DDT affects the nervous systems, and it has been banned in some countries.

TYPES OF BIOREMEDIATION

The most important aspect of environmental biotechnology is the effective management of hazardous and toxic pollutants (xenobiotics) by bioremediation. The environmental clean-up process through bioremediation can be achieved in two ways—*in situ* and *ex situ* bioremediation.

In situ bioremediation

In situ bioremediation involves a direct approach for the microbial degradation of xenobiotics at the sites of pollution (soil, ground water). Addition of adequate quantities of nutrients at the sites promotes microbial growth. When these microorganisms are exposed to xenobiotics (pollutants), they develop metabolic ability to degrade them. The growth of the microorganisms and their ability to bring out biodegradation are dependent on the supply of essential nutrients (nitrogen, phosphorus etc.). *In situ* bioremediation has been successfully applied for clean-up of oil spillages, beaches etc. There are two types of *in situ* bioremediation-intrinsic and engineered.

Intrinsic bioremediation : The inherent metabolic ability of the microorganisms to degrade certain pollutants is the intrinsic bioremediation. In fact, the microorganisms can be tested in the laboratory for their natural capability of biodegradation and appropriately utilized.

Engineered *in situ* bioremediation : The inherent ability of the microorganisms for bioremediation is generally slow and limited. However, by using suitable physico-chemical means (good nutrient and O_2 supply, addition of electron acceptors, optimal temperature), the bioremediation process can be engineered for more efficient degradation of pollutants.

Advantages of *in situ* bioremediation

1. Cost-effective, with minimal exposure to public or site personnel.
2. Sites of bioremediation remain minimally disrupted.

Disadvantages of *in situ* bioremediation

1. Very time consuming process.
2. Sites are directly exposed to environmental factors (temperature, O_2 supply etc.).
3. Microbial degrading ability varies seasonally.

Ex situ bioremediation

The waste or toxic materials can be collected from the polluted sites and the bioremediation with the requisite microorganisms (frequently a consortium of organisms) can be carried out at designed places. This process is certainly an improvement over *in situ* bioremediation, and has been successfully used at some places.

Advantages of *ex situ* bioremediation

1. Better controlled and more efficient process.
2. Process can be improved by enrichment with desired microorganisms.
3. Time required in short.

Disadvantages of *ex situ* bioremediation

1. Very costly process.
2. Sites of pollution are highly disturbed.
3. There may be disposal problem after the process is complete.

METABOLIC EFFECTS OF MICROORGANISMS ON XENOBIOTICS

Although it is the intention of the biotechnologist to degrade the xenobiotics by microorganisms to the advantage of environment and ecosystem, it is not always possible. This is evident from the different types of metabolic effects as shown below.

Detoxification : This process involves the microbial conversion of toxic compound to a non-toxic one. Biodegradation involving detoxification is highly advantageous to the environment and population.

Activation : Certain xenobiotics which are not toxic or less toxic may be converted to toxic or more toxic products. This is dangerous.

Degradation : The complex compounds are degraded to simpler products which are generally harmless.

Conjugation : The process of conjugation may involve the conversion of xenobiotics to more complex compounds. This is however, not very common.

TYPES OF REACTIONS IN BIOREMEDIATION

Microbial degradation of organic compounds primarily involves aerobic, anaerobic and sequential degradation.

Aerobic bioremediation

Aerobic biodegradation involves the utilization of O_2 for the oxidation of organic compounds. These compounds may serve as substrates for the supply of carbon and energy to the microorganisms. Two types of enzymes namely monooxygenases and dioxygenases are involved in aerobic biodegradation. Monooxygenases can act on both aliphatic and aromatic compounds while dioxygenases oxidize aliphatic compounds.

Anaerobic bioremediation

Anaerobic biodegradation does not require O_2 supply. The growth of anaerobic microorganisms (mostly found in solids and sediments), and consequently the degradation processes are slow. However, anaerobic biodegradation is cost-effective, since the need for continuous O_2 supply is not there. Some of the important anaerobic reactions and examples of organic compounds degraded are listed below.

Hydrogenation and dehydrogenation — benzoate, phenol, catechol.

Dehalogenation — Polychlorinated biphenyls (PCBs), chlorinated ethylenes. The term ***dechlorination*** is frequently used for dehalogenation of chlorinated compounds.

Carboxylation and decarboxylation — toluene, cresol and benzoate.

Sequential bioremediation

In the degradation of several xenobiotics, both aerobic and anaerobic processes are involved. This is often an effective way of reducing the toxicity of a pollutant. For instance, tetrachloromethane and tetrachloroethane undergo sequential degradation.

BIODEGRADATION OF HYDROCARBONS

Hydrocarbon are mainly the pollutants from oil refineries and oil spills. These pollutants can be degraded by a consortium or cocktail of microorganisms e.g. *Pseudomonas, Corynebacterium, Arthrobacter, Mycobacterium* and *Nocardia.*

Biodegradation of aliphatic hydrocarbons

The uptake of aliphatic hydrocarbons is a slow process due to their low solubility in aqueous medium. Both aerobic and anaerobic processes are operative for the degradation of aliphatic hydrocarbons. For instance, unsaturated hydrocarbons are degraded in both anaerobic and aerobic environments, while saturated ones are degraded by aerobic process.

Some aliphatic hydrocarbons which are reclacitrant to aerobic process are effectively degraded in anaerobic environment e.g. chlorinated aliphatic compounds (carbon tetrachloride, methyl chloride, vinyl chloride).

Biodegradation of aromatic hydrocarbons

Microbial degradation of aromatic hydrocarbons occurs through aerobic and anaerobic processes. The most important microorganism that participates in these processes is *Pseudomonas.*

The biodegradation of aromatic compounds basically involves the following sequence of reactions.

1. Removal of the side chains.
2. Opening of the benzene ring.

Most of the non-halogenated aromatic compounds undergo a series of reactions to produce ***catechol*** or ***protocatechuate.*** The bioremediation of toluene, L-mandelate, benzoate, benzene, phenol, anthracene, naphthalene, phenanthrene and salicylate to produce catechol is shown in ***Fig. 59.1***. Likewise, ***Fig. 59.2***, depicts the bioremediation of quinate, p-hydroxymandelate, p-hydroxybenzoyl formate, p-toluate, benzoate and vanillate to produce protocatechuate. Catechol and protocatechuate can undergo oxidative cleavage pathways. In ***ortho-cleavage pathway***, catechol and protocatechuate form acetyl CoA (***Fig. 59.3***), while in ***metacleavage pathway*** (***Fig. 59.4***), they are converted to pyruvate and acetaldehyde. The degraded products of catechol and protocatechuate are readily metabolised by almost all the organisms.

BIODEGRADATION OF PESTICIDES AND HERBICIDES

Pesticides and herbicides are regularly used to contain various plant diseases and improve the crop yield. In fact, they are a part of the modern agriculture, and have significantly contributed to ***green revolution***. The common herbicides and pesticides are propanil (anilide), propham (carbamate), atrazine (triazine), picloram (pyridine), dichlorodiphenyl trichloroethane (DDT) monochloroacetate (MCA), monochloropropionate (MCPA) and glyphosate (organophosphate).

Most of the pesticides and herbicides are toxic and are recalcitrant (resistant to biodegradation). Some of them are ***surfactants*** (active on the surface) and retained on the surface of leaves.

Biodegradation of halogenated aromatic compounds

Most commonly used herbicides and pesticides are aromatic halogenated (predominantly chlorinated) compounds. The biodegradative pathways of halogenated compounds are comparable with that described for the degradation of non-halogenated aromatic compounds (***Figs. 59.1, 59.2, 59.3*** and ***59.4***). The rate of degradation of halogenated compounds is inversely related to the number of halogen atoms that are originally present on the target molecule i.e. compounds with higher number of halogens are less readily degraded.

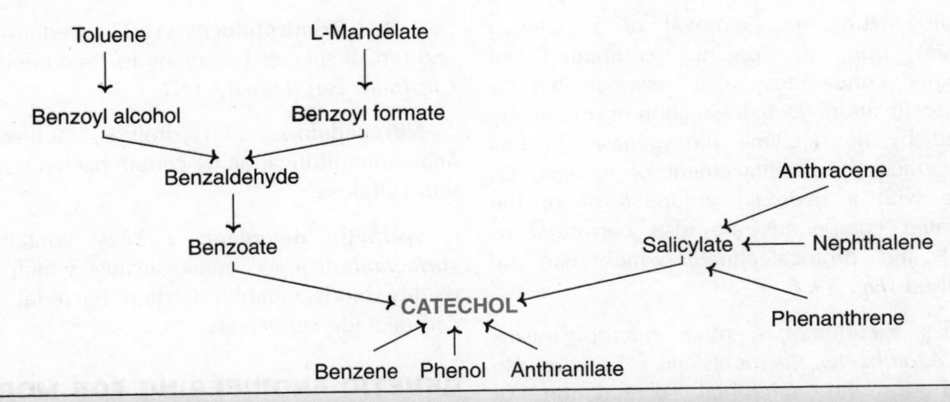

Fig. 59.1 : Bioremediation of certain aromatic compounds by bacteria to produce catechol.

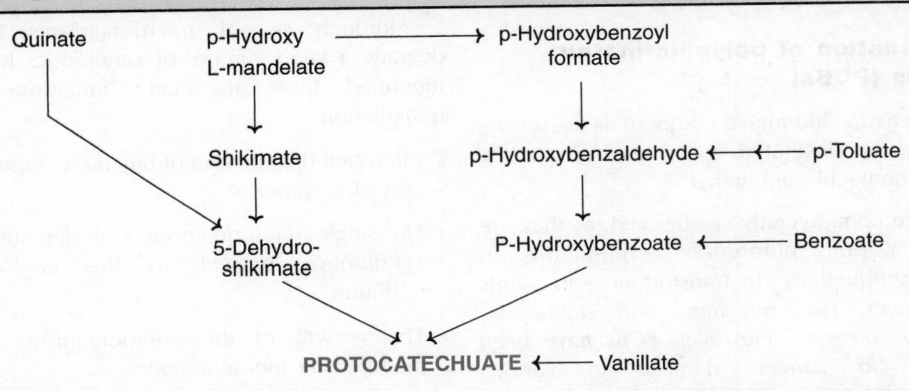

Fig. 59.2 : Bioremediation of certain organic compounds by bacteria to produce protocatechuate.

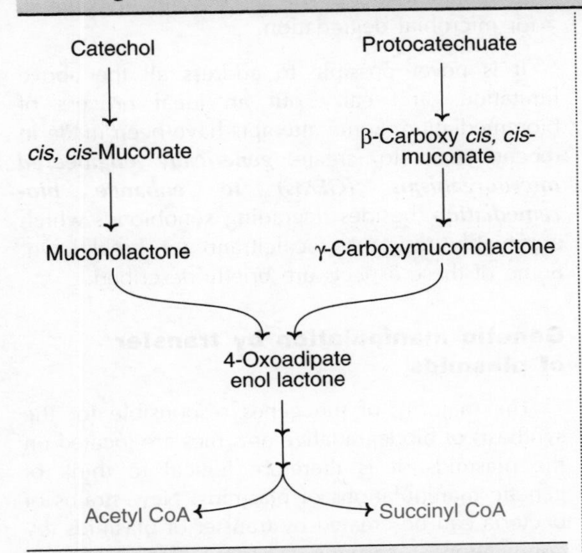

Fig. 59.3 : Conversion of catechol and protocatechuate to acetyl CoA and succinate by ***ortho–cleavage pathway****.*

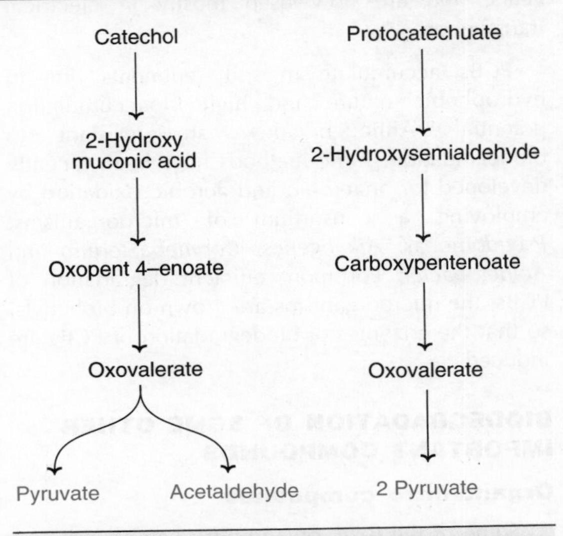

Fig. 59.4 : Conversion of catechol and protocatechuate to pyruvate and acetaldehyde by ***meta–cleavage pathway****.*

Dehalogenation (i.e. removal of a halogen substituent from an organic compound) of halogenated compounds is an essential step for their detoxification. Dehalogenation is frequently catalysed by the enzyme dioxygenase. In this reaction, there is a replacement of halogen on benzene with a hydroxyl group. Most of the halogenated compounds are also converted to catechol and protocatechuate which can be metabolised (***Fig. 59.4***).

Besides *Pseudomonas,* other microorganisms such as *Azotobacter, Bacilluefs* and *E. coli* are also involved in the microbial degradation of halogenated aromatic compounds.

Biodegradation of polychlorinated biphenyls (PCBs)

The aromatic chlorinated compounds possessing biphenyl ring (substituted with chlorine) are the PCBs e.g. pentachlorobiphenyl.

PCBs are commercially synthesized, as they are useful for various purposes — as pesticides, in electrical conductivity (in transformers), in paints and adhesives. They are inert, very stable and resistant to corrosion. However, ***PCBs have been implicated in cancer***, damage to various organs and impaired reproductive function. Their commercial use has been restricted in recent years, and are now used mostly in electrical transformers.

PCBs accumulate in soil sediments due to hydrophobic nature and high bioaccumulation potential. Although they are resistant to biodegradation, some methods have been recently developed for anaerobic and aerobic oxidation by employing a consortium of microorganisms. *Pseudomonas, Alkaligenes, Corynebacterium* and *Acinetobacter.* For more efficient degradation of PCBs, the microorganisms are grown on biphenyls, so that the enzymes of biodegradation of PCBs are induced.

BIODEGRADATION OF SOME OTHER IMPORTANT COMPOUNDS

Organo-nitro compounds

Some of the toxic organo-nitro compounds can be degraded by microorganisms for their detoxification.

2, 4, 6-Trinitrotoluene (TNT) : Certain bacteria and fungal species belonging to *Pseudomonas* and *Clostrium* can detoxify TNT.

Nitrocellulose : Hydrolysis, followed by anaerobic nitrification by certain bacteria, degrades nitrocellulose.

Synthetic detergents : They contain some ***surfactants*** (surface active agents) which are not readily biodegradable. Certain bacterial plasmid can degrade surfactants.

GENETIC ENGINEERING FOR MORE EFFICIENT BIOREMEDIATION

Although several microorganisms that can degrade a large number of xenobiotics have been identified, there are many limitations in bio-remediation.

- Microbial degradation of organic compounds is a very slow process.
- No single microorganism can degrade all the xenobiotics present in the environmental pollution.
- The growth of the microorganisms may be inhibited by the xenobiotics.
- Certain xenobiotics get adsorbed on to the particulate matter of soil and become unavailable for microbial degradation.

It is never possible to address all the above limitations and carry out an ideal process of bioremediation. Some attempts have been made in recent years to create ***genetically engineered microorganisms (GEMs) to enhance bio-remediation,*** besides degrading xenobiotics which are highly resistant (recalcitrant) for breakdown. Some of these aspects are briefly described.

Genetic manipulation by transfer of plasmids

The majority of the genes responsible for the synthesis of biodegradative enzymes are located on the plasmids. It is therefore logical to think of genetic manipulations of plasmids. New strains of bacteria can be created by transfer of plasmids (by conjugation) carrying genes for different degradative pathways. If the two plasmids contain homologous regions of DNA, recombination occurs

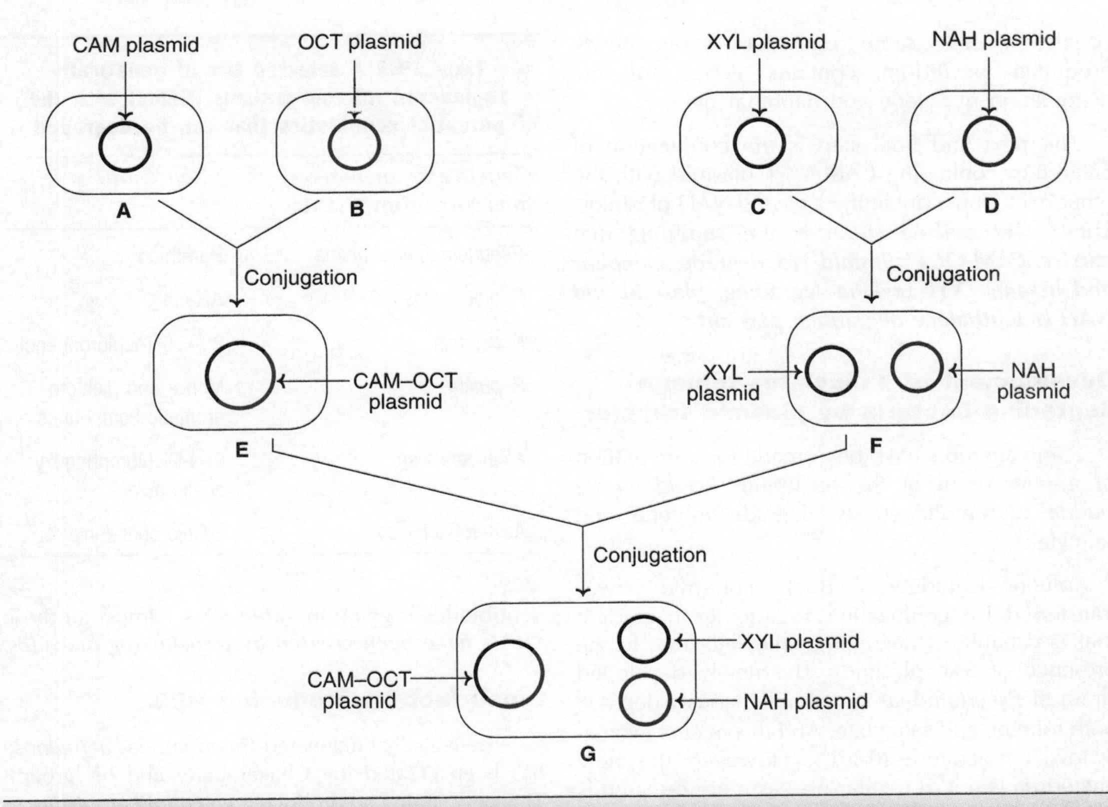

Fig. 59.5 : Creation of the superbug by transfer of plasmids (A, B, C, D, E, F and G are the different strains of bacteria containing the plasmids shown. Strain G is the superbug.)

between them, resulting in the formation of a larger fused plasmid (with the combined functions of both plasmids). In case of plasmids which do not possess homologous regions of DNA, they can coexist in the bacterium (to which plasmid transfer was done).

The first successful development of a new strain of bacterium (*Psuedomonas*) by manipulations of plasmid transfer was done by Chakrabarty and his co-workers in 1970s. They used different plasmids and constructed a ***new bacterium*** called as ***superbug***, that can degrade a number of hydrocarbons of petroleum simultaneously. United States granted patent to this superbug in 1981 (as per the directive of American Supreme Court). Thus, ***superbug*** became ***the first genetically engineered microorganism to be patented***. Superbug has played a significant role in the development of biotechnology industry, although it has not been used for large scale degradation of oil spills.

Creation of superbug by transfer of plasmids

Superbug is a bacterial strain of *Pseudomonas* that can degrade camphor, octane, xylene and naphthalene. Its creation is depicted in ***Fig. 59.5***.

The bacterium containing CAM (camphor-degrading) plasmid was conjugated with another bacterium with OCT (octane-degrading) plasmid. These plasmids are not compatible and therefore, cannot coexist in the same bacterium. However, due to the presence of homologous regions of DNA, recombination occurs between these two plasmids resulting in a single CAM-OCT plasmid. This new bacterium possesses the degradative genes for both camphor and octane.

Another bacterium with XYL (xylene-degrading) plasmid is conjugated with NAH (naphthalene-degrading) plasmid containing bacterium. XYL and NAH plasmids are compatible and therefore can coexist in the same bacterium. This newly produced bacterium contains genes for the degradation of xylene and naphthalene.

The next and final step is the conjugation of bacterium containing CAM-OCT plasmid with the other bacterium containing XYL and NAH plasmids. The newly created strain is the ***superbug*** that ***carries CAM-OCT plasmid (to degrade camphor and octane), XYL (xylene-degrading) plasmid and NAH (naphthalene-degrading) plasmid***.

Development of salicylate—toluene degrading bacteria by plasmid transfer

Some attempts have been made for the creation of a new strain of the bacterium *Pseudomonas putida* to simultaneously degrade toluene and salicylate.

Toluene-degrading (TOL) plasmid was transferred by conjugation to another bacterium that is capable of degrading salicylate (due to the presence of SAL plasmid). The newly developed strain of *Pseudomonas* can simultaneously degrade both toluene and salicylate. And this occurs even at a low temperature (0-5°C). However, the new bacterium is not in regular use, as more research is being conducted on its merits and demerits.

Genetic manipulation by gene alteration

Work is in progress to manipulate the genes for more efficient biodegradation. The plasmid pWWO of *Pseudomonas* codes for 12 different enzymes responsible for the meta-cleavage pathway (for the conversion of catechol and protocatechuate to pyruvate and acetaldehyde, See ***Fig. 59.4***) for degradation of certain aromatic compounds. Some success has been reported to alter the genes of plasmid pWWO for more efficient degradation of toluene and xylene.

GENETICALLY ENGINEERED MICROORGANISMS (GEMs) IN BIOREMEDIATION

Superbug (described already) is the first genetically engineered microorganism. Several workers worldover have been working for the creation of GEMs, specifically designed for the detoxification of xenobiotics. A selected list of GEMs with a potential for the degradation of xenobiotics is given in ***Table 59.3***. Almost all these ***GEMs have been created by transferring plasmids***.

TABLE 59.3 A selected list of genetically engineered microorganisms (GEMs) with the potential xenobiotics that can be degraded

Genetically engineered microorganism (GEMs)	*Xenobiotic*
Pseudomonas diminuta	Parathion
P. oleovorans	Alkane
P. cepacia	2, 4, 5-Trichlorophenol
P. putida	Mono- and dichloro-aromatic compounds
Alcaligenes sp	2, 4-Dichlorophenoxy acetic acid
Acinetobacter sp	4-Chlorobenzene

Biosurfactant producing GEM

A genetically engineered *Pseudomonas aeruginosa* has been created (by Chakarabarty and his group). This new strain can produce a ***glycolipid emulsifier*** (a biosurfactant) which can reduce the surface tension of an oil water interface. The reduced interfacial tension promotes biodegradation of oils.

GEM for degradation of vanillate and SDS

A new strain of *Pseudomonas* sp (strain ATCC 1915) has been developed for the degradation of vanillate (waste product from paper industry) and sodium dodecyl sulfate (SDS, a compound used in detergents).

GEMs and environmental safety

The genetically engineered microorganisms (GEMs) have now become handy tools of biotechnologists. The risks and health hazards associated with the use of GEMs are highly controversial and debatable issues. The fear of the biotechnologists, and even the general public is that the new organism (GEM), once it enters the environment, may disturb the ecological balance and cause harm to the habitat. Some of the GEMs may turn virulant and become ***genetic bombs***, causing great harm to humankind.

Because of the risks involved in the use of GEMs, so far no GEM has been allowed to enter the environmental fields. Thus, the use of GEMs has been confined to the laboratories, and fully controlled processes of biodegradation (usually employing bioreactors). Further, several precautionary measures are taken while creating GEMs, so that the risks associated with their use are minimal.

Some researchers are of the opinion that GEMs will create biotechnological wonders for the environmental management of xenobiotics, in the next few decades. This may be possible only if the associated risks of each GEM is thoroughly evaluated, and fully assured of its biosafety.

BIOREMEDIATION OF CONTAMINATED SOILS AND WASTE LANDS

Due to industrialization and extensive use of insecticides, herbicides and pesticides, the solids and waste lands worldover are getting polluted. The most common pollutants are hydrocarbons, chlorinated solvents, polychlorobiphenyls and metals.

Bioremediation of soils and waste lands by the use of microorganisms is gaining importance in the recent years. In fact, some success has been reported for the detoxification of certain pollutants (e.g. hydrocarbons) in the soil by microorganisms.

Bioremediation of soils can be done by involving two principles-biostimulation and bioaugmentation.

Biostimulation in soil bioremediation

Biostimulation basically involves the ***stimulation of microorganisms already present in the soil***, by various means. This can be done by many ways.

- Addition of nutrients such as nitrogen and phosphorus.
- Supplementation with co-substrates e.g. methane added to degrade trichloroethylene.
- Addition of surfactants to disperse the hydrophobic compounds in water.

Addition of nutrient and co-substrates promote microbial growth while surfactants expose the hydrophobic molecules. In all these situations, the result is that there occurs biostimulation by effective bioremediation of polluted soil or waste land.

Bioaugmentation in soil bioremediation

Addition of specific microorganisms to the polluted soil constitutes bioaugmentation. The pollutants are very complex molecules and the native soil microorganisms alone may not be capable of degrading them effectively. The examples of such pollutants include polychlorobiphenyls (PCBs), trinitrotoluene (TNT), polyaromatic hydrocarbons (PAHs) and certain pesticides.

Based on the research findings at the laboratory level (with regard to biodegradation), it is now possible to add a ***combination of microorganisms*** referred to as ***consortium or cocktail*** of microorganisms, to achieve bioaugmentation.

With the development of genetically engineered microorganisms (GEMs), they can be also used to bioaugment soils for very efficient bioremediation. But the direct use of GEMs in the soils is associated with several risks and health hazards.

TECHNIQUES OF SOIL BIOREMEDIATION

The most commonly used methods for the bioremediation are soils are *in situ* bioremediation, land farming and slurry phase bioreactors.

In situ bioremediation of soils

In situ bioremediation broadly involves the biological clean-up of soils without excavation. This technique is used for the bioremediation of sub-surfaces of soils, buildings and road ways that are polluted. Sometimes, water (oxygenated) is cycled through the sub-surfaces for increasing the efficiency of microbial degradation. There are two types of *in situ* soil bioremediation techniques-bioventing and phytoremediation.

Bioventing : This is very efficient and cost-effective technique for the bioremediation of petroleum contaminated soils. Bioventing involves ***aerobic biodegradation of pollutants by circulating air through sub-surfaces of soil.*** Although, it takes some years, bioventing can be used for the degradation of soluble paraffins and polyaromatic hydrocarbons. The major limitation of this technique is air circulation which is not always practicable.

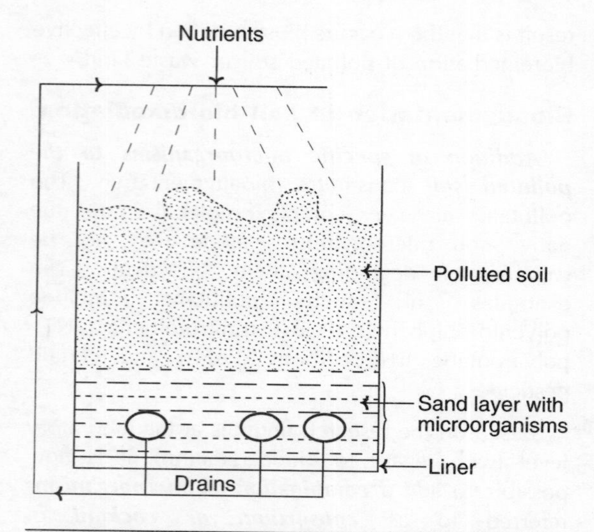

Fig. 59.6 : A diagrammatic representation of landfarming system.

Phytoremediation : Bioremediation by ***use of plants*** constitutes phytoremediation. Specific plants are cultivated at the sites of polluted soil. These plants are capable of stimulating the biodegradation of pollutants in the soil adjacent to roots (rhizosphere). although phytoremediation is a cheap and environmental friendly clean-up process for the biodegradation of soil pollutants, it takes several years.

Landfarming in soil bioremediation

Landfarming is a technique for the bioremediation of hydrocarbon contaminated soils. A diagrammatic representation of land farming system (also referred to as ***solid phase soil reactor***) is depicted in ***Fig. 59.6***.

The soil is excavated, mixed with microorganisms and nutrients and spread out on a liner, just below the polluted soil. The soil has to be regularly ploughed for good mixing and aeration. If the soil is mixed with compost and/or temperature is increased the efficiency of biodegradation increases. Addition of co-substrates, and anaerobic pretreatment of polluted soils also increases the degradation process.

Landfarming has been successfully used for the bioremediation of soils polluted with chloroethane ***b***enzene, ***t***oluene and ***x***ylene. The last three compounds are often referred to as ***BTX aromatics***.

Slurry-phase bioreactors in soil bioremediation

Slurry-phase bioreactors are improved land farming systems. In these cases, the ***excavated polluted soil is subjected to bioremediation under optimally controlled conditions*** in specifically designed bioreactors. Due to a close contact between the xenobiotics and the microorganisms, and the optimal conditions (nutrient supply, temperature, aeration etc.), the degradation is very rapid and efficient. Slurry-phase bioreactors, however, are not suitable for widespread use due to high cost.

BIOREMEDIATION OF GROUND WATER

Environmental pollution also results in the contamination of ground water at several places. The commonly found pollutants are the petroleum hydrocarbons (aliphatic, aromatic, cyclic and substituted molecules). Bioremediation of ground water can be carried out by two methods pump- and -treat technique and biofencing technique.

Pump- and -treat technique for bioremediation of ground water

Bioremediation of underground water by pump- and -treat technology is mostly based on physico-chemical principles to remove the pollutants. The treatment units are set up above the ground. Strip columns and activated carbon filters can remove most of the ground water pollutants. Treated water is recycled through injection well several times so that the pollutants are effectively removed.

For removal of certain organic pollutants, biological reactors (bioreactors) have to be installed (***Fig. 59.7A***). For instance, for the biodegradation of tetrachloroethane, a bioreactor with granular methogenic sludge is found to be effective. In recent years, bioreactors with both aerobic and anaerobic bacteria have been developed for better bioremediation of highly polluted ground waters.

It is however, not possible to achieve good clean up of ground water by pump- and -treat technology, for various reasons (sub-surface heterogenecities, strongly adsorbed compounds, low permeability of pollutants etc.).

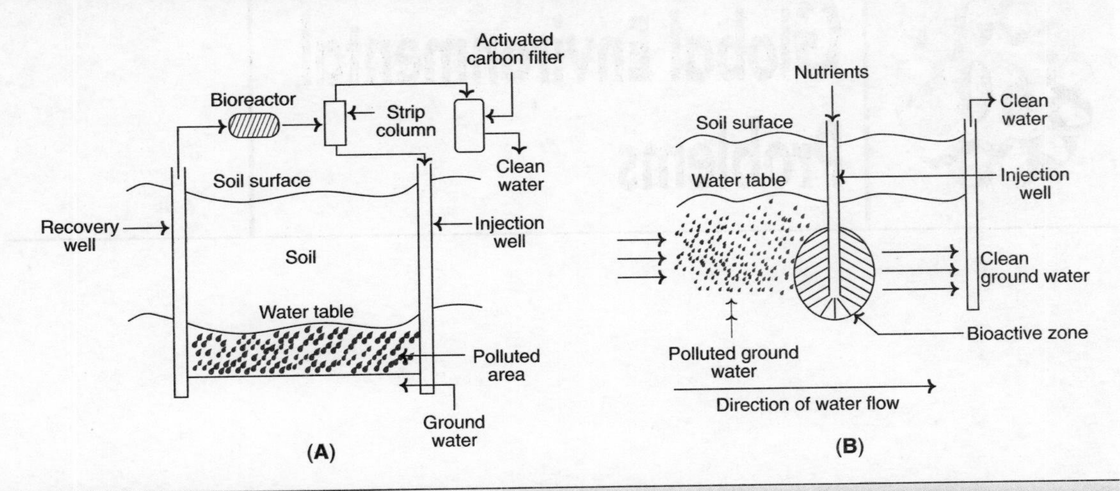

*Fig. 59.7 : Bioremediation of ground water **(A)** Pump- and -treat technique **(B)** Biofencing technique.*

Biofencing technique for bioremediation of ground water

Biofencing is an improved technique for the bioremediation of ground water. It consists of installation of a bioactive zone at the down-gradient edge of a contaminated ground water area. Nutrients are injected through a well to the bioactive zone (***Fig. 59.7B***). As the ground water passes through the bioactive zone (by the impact of natural direction of flow), the pollutants are biodegraded, and clean ground water comes out.

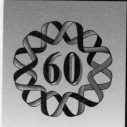

Global Environmental Problems

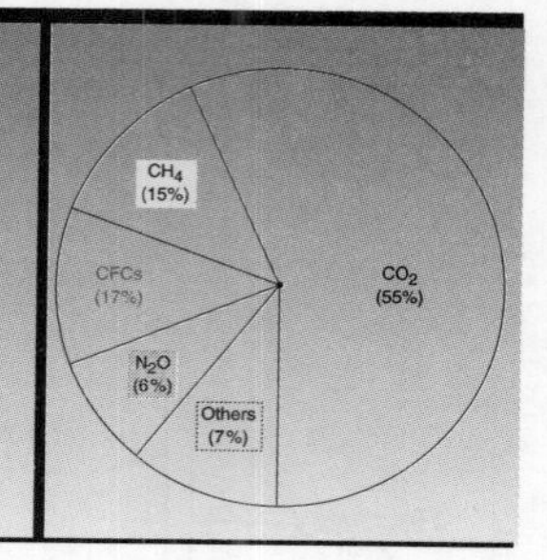

Some of the environmental issues attract world-wide attention, as they are the global problems. These include ***green house effect and global warming***, ***depletion of ozone*** and ***acid rain.*** The global environmental problems along with the environmental sustainability are briefly described in the following pages.

GREEN HOUSE EFFECT AND GLOBAL WARMING

The earth receives solar energy from the sun in the form of short wave radiations (mostly visible light). This solar energy is absorbed by the earth's surface and emitted into the space as long-wave (infra red) radiations. If the incoming radiations from the sun and the outgoing radiations from the earth are equal, then a good balance between the absorbed and emitted energy by the earth is maintained. But this does not happen.

The incoming short-wave radiations (from the sun) can easily pass through the atmosphere while the outgoing long-wave radiations (from the earth) are partially absorbed by certain gases in the atmosphere. ***Green house effect refers to the phenomenon of retention of earth's heat by the atmosphere***. The ***consequence of green house effect is global warming***.

GREEN HOUSE GASES

The ***gases that cause green house effect*** are collectively referred to as green house gases (***Fig. 60.1***). The most important green house gases are ***carbon dioxide*** (55%), ***methane*** (15%), ***chlorofluorocarbons*** (17%), ***nitrous oxide*** (6%) and several other gases like carbon monoxide, nitrous oxide, ozone, sulfur dioxide, fluorine, bromine and iodine (7%). The presence of water vapour in the atmosphere in association with green house gases significantly contributes to global warming.

Sources of green house gases

The important sources of major green house gases are given in the ***Table 60.1***. Fossil-fuel combustion, decompostion of organic wastes, deforestation and industries largely contribute to green house gases. Chlorofluoro-carbons (CFCs) are synthetic chemicals widely used in the preparation of refrigerants, solvents and aerosol propellants. ***CFCs are dangerous environmental pollutants*** that significantly contribute to green house effect. The global warming potential of CFCs is around 7,000 in comparison to CO_2 taken as 1, methane 11 and nitrous oxide 260.

The relative contribution of total green house gases from the major contributing sources is given in the next page.

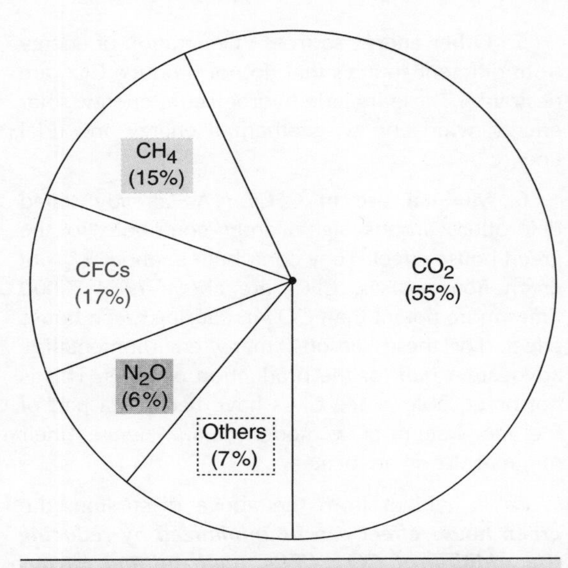

Fig. 60.1 : Approximate contribution of green house gases in global warming (CFCs-Chlorofluorocarbons)

Fossil-fuel combustion and anaerobic decomposition of organics	–	57%
Chlorofluorocarbons	–	17%
Agriculture	–	15%
Deforestation	–	8%
Others	–	3%

Effects of green house gases and global warming

The natural occurrence of green house effect is essential for the existence of life on earth. For instance, it is only due to the presence of CO_2 and water vapour, the mean temperature of the earth's surface is around 17°C. In their total absence, the temperature would have been around –17°C, where life cannot exist!

The main problem is the ever increasing concentrations of the green house gases in the atmosphere that are resulting in irreversible and highly dangerous climatic changes. The effects of global warming contributed by green house gases are listed below.

1. **Increase in temperature :** There occurs a general warming up of the atmosphere due to green house gases. It is estimated that the temperature increases by about 0.3°C per decade.

2. **Changes in sea level :** Due to a rise in temperature, there occurs thermal expansion of oceans and melting of glaciers, ice sheets and ice caps. The net result is an increase in sea level. It is estimated that during the last 100 years, the average sea level has risen by about 20 cm. As per the present prediction, the sea level is expected to rise by 20–30 cm in the next 2-3 decades. Rise in sea levels may be disastrous to some low-lying areas e.g. Netherlands, Maldives.

3. **Water imbalance :** The warmer world would have less water available on the earth and this may lead to water crisis.

4. **Crop yield :** Due to a rise in temperature, the agricultural production may be reduced. There may also occur dislocation of crop lands. Some researchers however, predict that the crop yield may be higher in some areas due to increased availability of CO_2.

5. **Ecosystem :** Some disturbances in the ecosystem and the existence of living organisms may not be ruled out.

TABLE 60.1 Important sources of major green house gases

Green house gas	*Sources*
Carbon dioxide (CO_2)	Fossil-fuel burning Deforestation Respiration Emissions from industries
Methane (CH_4)	Anaerobic decomposition of organic wastes Gas, oil and coal production Burning of biomass Wetland cultivation
Chlorofluorocarbons (CFCs)	Refrigerants Solvents Aerosol propellants Foam packagings
Nitrous oxide (N_2O)	Fertilizers Natural soils Fossil-fuel combustion
Ozone (O_3)	Photochemical reactions in troposphere
Carbon monoxide (CO)	Fossil-fuel combustion Biomass burning

6. **Human health :** The changing climatic conditions, due to global warming, may adversely affect human health. For instance, the risk of spreading major tropical diseases (malaria, filariasis, schistosomiasis, dengue fever, yellow fever) would be higher.

MEASURES TO CONTROL GREEN HOUSE EFFECT

The major contribution of green house gases comes from the developed countries. Thus, with a world's population of about 15%, these countries contribute to as much as 65% of green house gases. This is mostly because of industrialization and changing life styles of people. It is therefore, natural to expect that the developed countries significantly contribute (finances and resources) for the containment of global warming.

There is a worldwide concern on the alarming impact of global warming due to green house effect. Several steps are being taken at the international and national levels for the protection of environment with particular reference to green house effect.

Some of the important approaches for the management of green house effect with special reference to biotechnology are briefly described.

1. **Renewable forms of energy :** The various forms of energy generation (fossil-fuel burning, fuel wood combustion) are intimately linked to the production of green house gases. Switching over to renewable froms of energy (the best being solar source) is highly desirable.

2. **Reforestation :** Deforestation is major concern. Growing of plants wherever possible and reforestation are the need of the hour. Plants will take up atmospheric CO_2 and generate O_2, and thus significantly help to reduce the green house effect.

3. **Development of energy-efficient industries :** Attention should be directed for the technological advancement of industries with low energy consumption. And wherever possible, renewable sources of energy should be used.

4. **Nuclear power industries :** Cost-effective installation of nuclear power stations is advocated. This will certainly help to solve energy crisis, besides minimizing the green house effect. But care should be taken for a safe disposal of nuclear wastes.

5. **Other energy sources :** Generation of energy from different sources that do not produce CO_2 are desirable. These include hydroelectric energy, solar energy, wind energy, geothermal energy and tidal energy.

6. **Minimal use of CFCs :** As already stated chloroflurocarbons significantly contribute to the green house effect. They contribute to about 17% of green house gases. CFCs are about 4,000–7,000 times more potent than CO_2 in causing green house effect. For these reasons, many environmentalists advocate a halt for the production of CFCs. This is not practicable, since CFCs have become a part of the life system of a modern man. Hence, their minimal use is advocated.

As is evident from the above discussion, the ***green house effect can be minimized by reducing the addition of CO_2, CFCs, methane and nitrous oxide to the environment.***

THE PROBLEM OF OZONE

Ozone (O_3) is a blue coloured gas with a pungent smell. It forms a thick layer in the stratosphere of the atmosphere (16 to 40 km). The concentration of ozone is in the range of 2-8 ppm (parts per million by volume) depending on the distance.

Generation of ozone

Ozone is produced naturally when oxygen is dissociated by solar ultraviolet radiations (80–240 nm).

$$O_2 \xrightarrow[\text{(80–240 nm)}]{\text{UV radiation}} O + O$$

$$O + O_2 + M \longrightarrow O_3 + M$$

(M represents a third body molecule like N_2 or O_2).

Beneficial affects of ozone

Ozone is capable of absorbing ultraviolet radiations from the sun (200–300 nm) so that they do not reach the earth and cause health hazards (described later). In this process, ozone dissociation occurs as follows.

$$O_3 \xrightarrow[\text{(200–300 nm)}]{\text{UV radiation}} O_2 + O$$

Thus, ozone is constantly being generated and destroyed in the stratosphere.

DEPLETION OF OZONE

There are a number of pollutant gases in the stratosphere-nitric oxide (NO), nitrous oxide (N_2O), chlorine (Cl) and chlorofluorocarbons (CFCs like chlorofluoromethane or freon) that can react with ozone to produce oxygen. The net result is that the ozone gets depleted in the stratosphere of the atmosphere.

There are three major mechanisms for the destruction of ozone-nitrogen system, hydrogen system and chlorine system.

Nitrogen system

About 60% of the ozone destruction occurs by nirogen system. Nitrous oxide (N_2O), produced by the microbial action in soils and oceans enters the atmosphere and reaches the stratosphere. Here, in the presence of light, N_2O reacts with nascent oxygen (O) to form nitric oxide (NO). The latter is a powerful destroyer of ozone.

$$N_2O + O \xrightarrow{\text{UV radiation}} 2NO$$

$$N_2O \xrightarrow{\text{UV radiation}} NO + O$$

$$NO + O_3 \longrightarrow NO_2 + O_2$$

Hydrogen system

Approximately 10% of the ozone is destroyed by hydrogen system. The hydroxyl (OH) group that reacts with ozone is mostly derived from water, and to a lesser extent from methane.

The reactions involving H_2O are shown below.

$$H_2O + O \xrightarrow{\text{UV radiation}} 2OH$$

$$OH + O_3 \longrightarrow H_2O + O_2$$

Chlorine system

Chlorofluorocarbons (CFCs) and natural chlorine can also destroy ozone to a significant extent. CFCs on dissociation form Cl which acts on ozone, as shown below.

$$CFCl_2, CF_2Cl_2 \xrightarrow{\text{UV radiation}} Cl_2 + Cl$$

$$Cl + O_3 \longrightarrow ClO + O_2$$

Other systems

Besides the major systems described above, there are several other compounds that can destroy ozone. A group of chemicals namely halons, widely used in fire extinguishers, are important in this regard. The major halons are bromochlorofluro-carbons and bromofluorocarbons.

OZONE HOLE

It was in 1987, the first evidence for the depletion of ozone over the entire Antarctic content came to light. This is regarded as ozone hole, and the depletion of O_3 was observed between 12 to 24 km altitude. Later evidence indicated that the occurrence of ozone hole over Antarctic continent is an annual phenomenon, during August and September. The factors for the causation of ozone hole are not clearly known.

The present belief that the chlorine and chlorine radicals are mainly responsible for ozone hole. It is feared that more ozone holes may develop which is highly dangerous.

EFFECTS OF OZONE DEPLETION

Ozone acts as a filter of ultraviolet radiations from the sun with a result that the hazardous UV rays do not reach the earth. The ***biologically active UV radiations (UV-B)*** are in the range of 2.9×10^{-7} nm to 3.2×10^{-7} nm. They are highly senstive for ozone depletion.

UV-B radiations cause several harmful effects to the living (humans, animals, plants) and non-living (materials) systems on earth. Some of them are briefly described.

Effects on human health

1. The incidence of skin cancer (melanoma) is very high in the population exposed to UV-B radiations. Melanoma is associated with overexposure to sunlight-mostly found in people who spend more time outdoors. It is estimated that with every 1% decrease in ozone layer, there would be an increase of about 3% in the skin cancers of people.

2. UV-B radiations may damage DNA and cause mutations that may result in various types of cancers.

3. Exposure to UV-B radiation is also associated with several other health complications-damage to eyes, decreased immune response, increased incidence of several infections.

Effects on terrestrial plants

1. Exposure to UV-B radiations in some plants may result in reduced growth and smaller leaves, with a reduced efficiency of photosynthesis.

2. The quality and quantity of foods are adversely affected.

3. Retardation in the growth of forests.

Effects on aquatic ecosystems

1. The aquatic life is very vulnerable to UV-B radiations, particularly up to a depth of 20 m in clear waters and a depth of 5m in unclear waters.

2. Harmful effects have been observed in fishes, crabs, shrimp and zooplanktons.

3. There occurs a reduction in the photosynthetic efficiency of phytoplankton.

MEASURES TO CONTROL OZONE DEPLETION

The only effective way of controlling ozone depletion is the complete elimination of the factors responsible for it. As already described oxides of nitrogen, chlorofluorocarbons and halons largely contribute to ozone destruction. These are the environmental pollutants and reduction in their production/utilization will largely help to control ozone depletion.

ACID RAIN

The normal rain water is slightly acidic with a pH in the range of 6-7. This acidity is contributed by the naturally occurring CO_2 which gets dissolved in the rain water to form carbonic acid.

$$CO_2 + H_2O \longrightarrow H_2CO_3$$

The lowest pH of the normal rain is around 5.6.

When the ***pH of the rain water is less than 5.5, it is considered as acid rain***. This acidity is predominantly contributed by two acids namely ***sulfuric acid*** and ***nitric acid***, and to a lesser extent by hydrochloric acid and organic acids.

DEVELOPMENT OF ACID RAIN

As the industrialization worldover increases, there is an increase in the environmental pollution by oxides of sulfur and nitrogen. These gaseous pollutants are light and they can be carried away (from the site of production) to hundreds and thousands of kilometers by the winds. Thus, the export of the acid forming pollutants may occur from one region to another region, and from one country to another country. For this reason, acid rain is a global problem.

The following reactions summarise the formation of acid rain from the oxides of sulfur (SO_x) and oxides of nitrogen (NO_x).

$$SO_x + O_2 + H_2O \longrightarrow \underset{\text{(Sulfurous acid)}}{H_2SO_3} + \underset{\text{(Sulfuric acid)}}{H_2SO_4}$$

$$NO_x + O_2 + H_2O \longrightarrow \underset{\text{(Nitrous acid)}}{HNO_2} + \underset{\text{(Nitric acid)}}{HNO_3}$$

In the development of acid rain, there occurs diffusion of SO_2, and diffusion of HNO_3 gas into the cloud particles/droplets.

EFFECTS OF ACID RAIN

Acid rain disturbs the environment. The actual effects of acid rain depends on the degree of the acidity and the nature of the environment-aquatic, terrestrial, human population and materials. Some of the important aspects are described.

Effects on aquatic environment

The aquatic system is very sensitive to acid rain. With periodical falls of acid rains, the lakes become more and more acidic.

1. The fishes and other aquatic organisms including microorganisms are very sensitive to pH. At a pH below 4, most of them die.

2. The surving fishes contain high concentrations of toxic metals such as mercury, aluminium, lead and zinc (these metals find their entry into lakes by leaching of surrounding rocks by acid rain).

Effects on terrestrial environment

1. Acid rain damages forests and all forms of vegetation.

2. Soil acidification, due to acid rain, may lead to necrosis of leaves.

3. Plants also accumulate several toxic metals e.g. aluminium, cadmium, mercury, lead.

Effects on human health

1. Sulfuric acid of acid rain is very dangerous, as it causes breathing problems.

2. The toxic metals (Cd, Zn, Hg, Cu, Al) liberated from rocks and soils by acid rain may ultimately reach the human body through plants and animals through food chain or drinking water. The toxic effects of these metals on humans are well known.

Effects on materials

The acid rain causes deterioration of buildings, marble rocks, limestones etc. Thus, acid rains have become a big threat to preservation of monuments and cultural heritages throughout the world.

MEASURES TO CONTROL ACID RAIN

The most effective measure to control acid rain is to drastically reduce the production of acid-forming gases i.e. the ***industrial emission of oxides of sulfur and nitrogen should be minimized***.

Some measures have been taken to reduce the SO_2 emission into atmosphere-desulfurification of the fuels used in industries, recovery of SO_2 as H_2SO_4.

More concrete measures need to be taken globally for effective control of acid rain.

ENVIRONMENTAL SUSTAINABILITY AND BIOTECHNOLOGY

The various aspects of environment and their impact on earth with special reference to human beings have been described (Chapter 54). Some of the important global environmental problem are described in this chapter.

Despite the occurrence of a complex and sometimes dangerous alterations in the environment, the life processes should go on, normally as far as possible. Environmental sustainability broadly deals with ***the sustenance*** (***support and maintenance***) ***of the environment to continue life on earth in a normal way***.

Biotechnology significantly contributes to environmental sustainability. There are three different approaches in this regard.

1. **Pollution protection :** Environment can be protected from pollution by using renewable raw materials, recycling the processes, appropriate methods for degradation of wastes.

2. **Pollution clean-up :** This can be done by employing biotechnological methods for clean up of oil spills, detoxification of contaminated soils, and purification of water supplies.

3. **Pollution control :** Once pollution has occurred, biotechnological methods can be used for control. For instance, heavy metals can be recovered from polluted water.

It is a fact that the various activities of humans are exceeding the sustainable capacity of the earth. Increased industrialization and urbanisation are adversely affecting the environment (with heavy pollution).

The biotechnologists are expected to improve the existing biological, chemical and various other industrial processes to make them environmental friendly. They should develop integrated systems which are efficient, controllable and clean. It is the duty of the environmental biotechnologists to achieve a maximum global environmental safety.

Eco-Tech : This is a new environmental technology concept. International Organisation for Biotechnology and Bioengineering in 1994, defined Eco-Tech as follows :

"Embedding technology into ecosphere and human culture by using the whole range of biodiversity in a holistic and low-invasive way in order to achieve benefits for humankind obeying ecological principles".

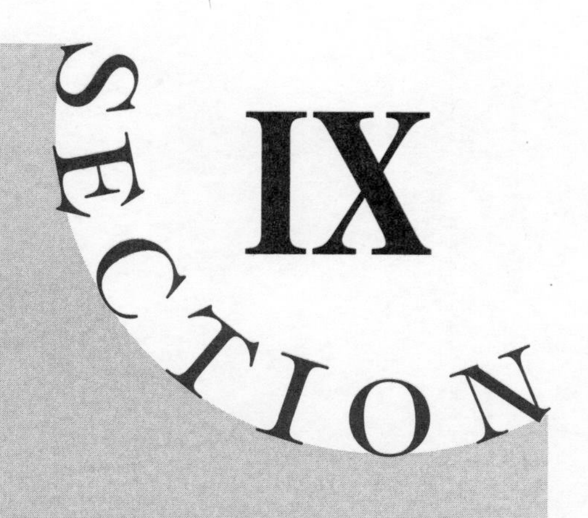

BIOTECHNOLOGY AND SOCIETY

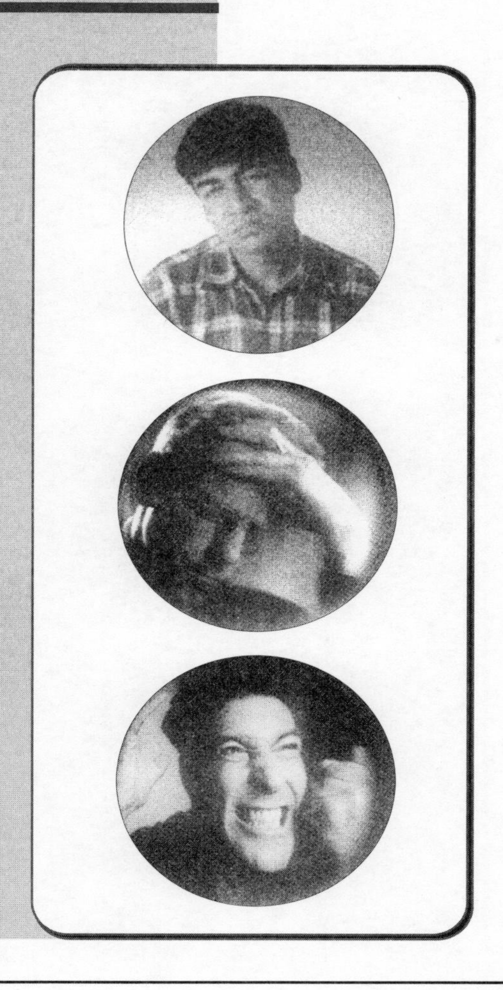

CONTENTS

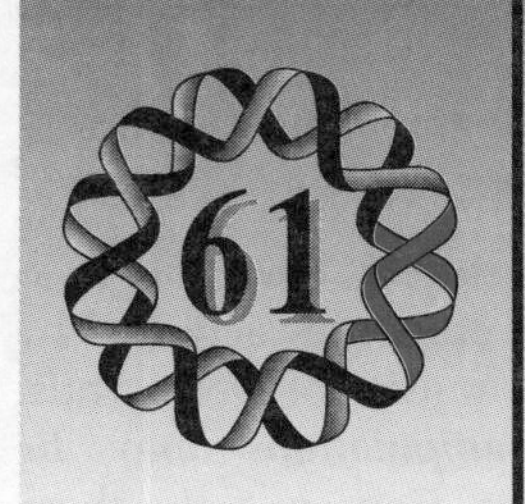

Biotechnology — Society, Risks, Ethics, Patenting

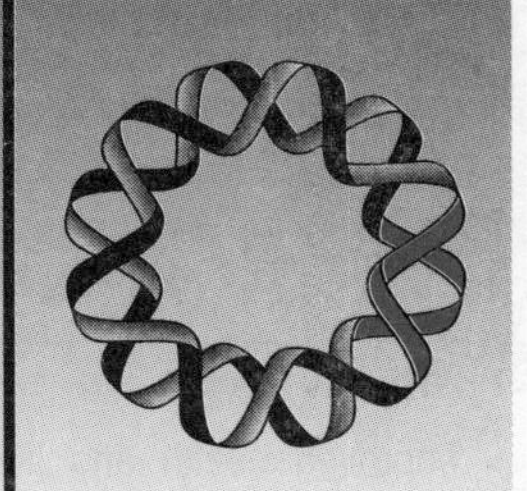

Advances in biotechnology, and their applications are most frequently associated with controversies. Based on their perception to biotechnology, the people may be grouped into three broad categories.

1. ***Strong opponents*** who oppose the new technology, as it will give rise to problems, issues and concerns humans have never faced before. They consider biotechnology as an unnatural manipulative technology.

2. ***Strong proponents*** who consider that the biotechnology will provide untold benefits to society. They argue that for centuries the society has safely used the products and processes of biotechnology.

3. A ***neutral group*** of people who have a balanced approach to biotechnology. This group believes that research on biotechnology (with regulatory systems), and extending its fruits to the society should be pursued with a cautious approach. The risks and benefits of the developments of biotechnology may not be much different from that of any other branch of science.

BENEFITS OF BIOTECHNOLOGY

The fruits of biotechnology are beneficial to the fields of healthcare, agriculture, food production, manufacture of industrial enzymes and appropriate environmental management.

It is a fact that modern technology in various forms is woven tightly into the fabric of our lives. Our day-to-day life is inseparable from technology. Imagine life about 1-2 centuries ago where there was no electricity, no running water, sewage in the streets, unpredictable food supply and an expected life span of less than 40 years. Undoubtedly, technology has largely contributed to the present day world we live in. Many pepople consider biotechnology as a technology that will improve the quality of life in every country, besides maintaining living standards at a reasonably higher level.

The probable positive and negative effects of biotechnology, with special reference to developing countries are given in ***Table 61.1***.

ELSI OF BIOTECHNOLOGY

Why so much uproar and negativity to biotechnology? This is mainly because the major part of the modern biotechnology deals with genetic manipulations. These unnatural genetic manipulations, as many people fear, may lead to unknown consequences.

ELSI is the short form to represent the ***ethical, legal and social implications of biotechnology***. ELSI broadly covers the relationship between biotechnology and society with particular reference to ethical and legal aspects.

TABLE 61.2 The probable positive and negative effects of biotechnology (particularly in the developing countries)

Positive effects

- Improved health and life span (through more effective pharmaceuticals, vaccines etc.).
- Increased crop production and more food.
- Decreased dependence on import of food, fertilizers and chemicals.
- Enhanced biomass production for energy.
- Use of plants and animals as bioreactors.
- Improved food storage facilities.
- Increased production and health of livestock.

Negative effects

- More dependence on developed countries and private companies for technology and resources.
- Increase in unemployment as the labour requirement is less.
- Reduction in natural biodiversity and natural ecosystems.
- More legal and financial complications.
- Increased growing of cash crops at the cost of food crops.
- Production of more and more herbicide resistant plants.

Risks and ethics of biotechnology

The modern biotechnology deals with genetic manipulations of viruses, bacteria, plants, animals, fish and birds. Introduction of foreign genes into various organisms raises concerns about the safety, ethics and unforeseen consequences. Some of the popular phrases used in the media while referring to experiments on recombinant DNA technology are listed.

- Manipulation of life
- Playing with God
- Man-made evolution

The major apprehension of genetic engineering is that through recombinant DNA experiments unique microorganisms or viruses (either inadvertently or sometimes deliberately for the purpose of war) may be developed that would cause epidemics and environmental catastrophes. Due to these fears, the regulatory guidelines for research dealing with DNA manipulation were very stringent in the earlier years.

So far, risk assessment studies have failed to demonstrate any hazardous properties acquired by host cells/organisms due to transfer of DNA. Thus, ***the fears of genetic manipulations may be unfounded*** to a large extent. Consequently, there has been some relaxation in the regulatory guidelines for recombinant DNA research (For more details, Refer Chapter 6).

It is now widely accepted that biotechnology is certainly beneficial to humans. But it should not cause problems of safety to people and environment, and create unacceptable social, moral and ethical issues. The public fears of biotechnology, besides some of the risks, social and ethical issues can be better understood with special reference to the following.

1. Therapeutic products for use in healthcare.
2. Genetic modifications of foods and food ingradients and their consumption.
3. Release of genetically engineered organisms into the environment.
4. Applications of human genetic research.

RECOMBINANT THERAPEUTIC PRODUCTS FOR HUMAN HEALTHCARE

It is fortunate that there is ***no serious criticism*** about the use recombinant products for medical applications. This is mostly because the therapeutic products and strategies are designed to cure diseases, alleviate sufferings and improve the quality of life. Further, the products are used under the medical supervision. In general, the recombinant products designed for human healthcare are more readily acceptable by the public. Good examples are the use of insulin, interferons, tissue plasminogen activator and various vaccines (for more details, Refer Chapters 15 and 16).

GENETIC MODIFICATIONS AND FOOD CONSUMPTION

The overall objectives of genetic modifications with reference to foods are listed

- To increase the quality and quantity of existing foods.

- To produce new products.
- To improve the financial returns.

Each country has its own regulations for introducing foods into the market. For instance, in USA, the Food and Drug Administration (FDA) regulates the introduction of foods, drugs, pharmaceuticals, and medical devices into the marketplace.

As regards the foods and food ingradients developed by genetic engineering, the FDA believes that no new regulations are needed. The existing regulations for the assessment foods for safety by toxicity, allergenicity and impurity testing are adequate. If the chemical composition of the existing food is altered by genetic modification, it should be specified, and the new product should be accordingly labeled.

To highlight the public perception of genetically modified foods, some selected examples of food ingradients and their acceptance, or certain controversies related to their use, are briefly described.

Chymosin

Chymosin is milk clotting proteolytic enzyme that hydrolyses the milk protein casein to produce curd, which in turn is processed into ***cheese***. Traditionally, chymosin is derived from the stomach of calves in the form of rennet.

By genetic engineering techniques, the chymosin gene was cloned and expressed in *E. coli*. This resulted in a large scale and cost-effective production of chymosin. The chemical composition, structure and biological activity of recombinant chymosin were identical to the chymosin of rennet. FDA gave license to chymosin for its commercial use, and it is now widely used in cheese making.

Tryptophan

In 1989–90, an unusually high incidence of the disease ***eosinophilia-myalgia syndrome (EMS)*** was reported in USA. EMS is a rare disease with muscular pain and respiratory complications, and may be fatal. Investigations revealed that the victims of EMS were consuming large quantities of food supplement tryptophan (obtained from one company). This tryptophan was produced by genetically engineered microorganisms. Chemical analysis of the commercial preparations revealed the presence of certain metabolic derivative of tryptophan. The most important among them was 1-1′ ethylene — bis (tryptophan) which was responsible for EMS (based on the results of animal experiments). It was concluded that the pharmaceutical company did not take adequate care for purification of tryptophan. Consequently, recombinant tryptophan (even without the impurities!) was banned for human consumption in USA.

Bovine somatotropin story

Bovine somatotropin (BST, also known as bovine growth hormone), when injected to dairy cattle, increases the milk production significantly. By recombinant DNA technology, the gene for BST was cloned and expressed in *E. coli*. The recombinant BST (rBST) so produced, when injected to cows was found to increase milk production by 20–25%.

The effect of rBST was considered from two aspects — on the animals and consumers.

1. **Effect of rBST on animals :** Administration of rBST can produce localized swelling at the site of injection. There may be some other adverse effects like increased susceptibility to infection, decreased reproductive capability. The proponents of rBST argue that these problem could occur even in normal animals.

2. **Effect on human health :** The natural BST or even rBST increases the body levels of ***insulin-like growth factor-I*** (IGF-I) which in turn enhances milk production. There is evidence that IGF-I stimulates growth of cancer cells. This causes concern among the consumers of milk produced by using rBST. The counter argument is that rBST injection, after about 100 days of lactation begins, is not associated with increased levels of IGF-I. The opponents of rBST strongly feel that since milk is consumed by most people, any inherent risk, however small is unacceptable.

Recombinant BST was licensed in USA, for use in dairly cattle in 1994. Some countries in fact have banned the use of rBST. There are some people (particularly among the scientists) who believe that the hue and cry raised against rBST is more due to economic and political reasons. It is feared that by rBST use, the dairy industry may be controlled by large industrial groups and the small dairy farms may become unprofitable.

The rBST story is an interesting illustration of the problems surrounding the use of genetic engineering.

RECOMBINANT FOODS AND RELIGIOUS BELIEFS

Some of the ethical concerns of the use of recombinant foods are related to religious beliefs, besides food habits. For instance

- Transfer of pig genes into sheep may offend the sentiments of Jews and Muslims.
- Introduction of animal genes into food plants may invite opposition by strict vegetarians.
- Transfer of human genes to food animals may be unacceptable to some people.
- Feeding of human gene — containing organisms to animals sounds in bad taste (at present, the genetically modified yeast that produce recombinant proteins after their use, are fed to animals).

The religious groups, in general, are selective about the foods to be eaten. However, they are not so rigid when it comes to the use of medically-derived products. For instance — Jews and Muslims may accept pig-derived insulin for use in diabetic patients. This is due to the fact that ***all religious faiths consider human life is the most valuable, and its preservation the first priority***. Further, the general belief is that the human body is violated only by oral consumption and not by injection or surgical interventions.

Eating genes everyday!

Everyday, we eat plants and animals and various products derived from them, besides a large number of bacteria. In other words, we regularly consume genetic material, the DNA, organized into genes in various organisms! So far no one has attempted to categorize genes as vegetarian and non-vegetarian, as we do for foods!!

ARE GM FOODS SAFE?

The production of transgenic plants and animals by genetic engineering techniques has now become routine. These organisms will enter the food chain in the form of ***genetically modified foods*** (GM foods). Some social and environmental groups are against the consumption of GM foods. These people insist that the GM foods should be specifically labeled.

As regards the safety of GM foods, opinions range from one extreme that they are absolutely safe, and improve human nutrition to the other that they should not be consumed at all. Most of the people have opinions somewhere between these two extremes.

RELEASE OF GENETICALLY ENGINEERED ORGANISMS

The release of genetically engineered organisms (***GEOs***), also called as ***genetically manipulated organisms (GMOs)*** into the environment has been a controversial issue; and continues to be so. It is feared that the release of GEOs into the environment could have far-reaching consequences. This is due to the fact that the living GEOs proliferate, persist, disperse, and sometimes may transfer their DNA into other organisms. It is further feared that there exists a possibility of GEOs displacing the existing organisms, besides creating new species. This may lead to severe environmental damage.

For the reasons stated above, the regulatory authories are very careful in permiting the field trails of GEOs. Further, the release of GEOs into the environment has to be carefully monitored and recorded.

Ice-minus *Pseudomonas syringae*

A genetically modified strain of ***Pseudomonas syringae*** was the first GEO that was given permission for field trails (in 1987). This organism is a genetically engineered ice-minus strain, when sprayed onto the leaves could prevent frost damage to the plants (Refer Chapter 50).

Field trails with other GEOs

A number of open-field trails have been conducted with several GEOs during the past two decades or so. The studies concluded that the genetically modified micororganisms do not persist in environment for long, do not transfer the genes into other organism and do not exhibit any abnormal biological functions. Thus, the ***initial apprehensions on the use of GEOs appear to be unfounded***.

Release of transgenic plants and animals

The transgenic plants developed for higher quality and quantity of foods, in general, are more liberally permitted to go to fields. It is generally believed that the transgenic plants do not significantly differ from the natural cultivars (traditional plants) obtained by plant breeding experiments.

The ***transgenic Bt-plants*** such as cotton, corn, soybean and potato were ***approved for cultivation in USA***. However, some countries did not allow Bt-plants in their fields e.g. Bt-rice was not allowed in Philippines, Bt-cotton in France.

The transgenic animals have not posed as big a problem as the transgenic plants. This is due to the fact that animals can be much easily identified and contained (since copulation is animals can be done as derised, unlike in plants where pollination is difficult to control). A majority of transgenic animals are used for medical purposes, hence they are generally appreciated. But the major problem for transgenic animals comes from animal activists.

Many people, and also some Governments, are suspicious of the use of GEOs due to various reasons-risks, societal beliefs and economic concerns.

Biological warfare

The most serious hazard associated with genetic engineering is the construction of harmful biological agents (viruses, microorganisms) either deliberately or otherwise. However, so far there have been no records of any new infectious agents created by recombinant DNA technology.

Most of the countries of the world are signatories to the Biological Weapons Conventions of 1972. As a signatory, a nation pledges 'never to produce microbial or other biological agents, or toxins, whatever may be their method of production, for use in wars'. Many people are, however concerned about the possible use of gene manipulations for military purposes.

APPLICATIONS OF HUMAN GENETIC rDNA RESEARCH

The ultimate goal of advances in biotechnology is for the benefit of mankind (either direct or indirect). Biotechnology largely contributes to human genetic research involving the following areas

- Genetic testing and screening for diseases
- Genetic portfolios
- Human gene therapy.

Genetic testing and screening

Techniques are now available for prenatal testing to specifically detect whether a fetus carries genetic defects. This will help the parents to be better prepared for the future baby.

The negative aspect of prenatal testing is that the couple may opt for abortion even for a minor genetic defect or sometimes for gender bias.

Genetic portfolios

The elucidation of the entire human genome sequence and identification of genes has now become a reality. It may soon be possible to have individual genetic portfolios that will diagnose future health complications e.g. risk for cancer, heart disease. The ***genetic portfolios*** (based on the genes) ***will fortell the individuals' future*** which is now being predicted through stars (astrology).

Genetic portfolios of individual may pose certain problems with regard to marriages, insurances. Who would like to be a spouse of someone who will soon be a victim of cancer or heart attack? Which insurance company would insure a person with a very high risk of diseases? Many ethical committes are of the opinion that insurance companies should not require, or should not be allowed to have access to individuals' genetic portfolios.

Human gene therapy

Theoretically, correction of genetic defects is possible by gene therapy. The present status of human gene therapy has been described (Chapter 13). From the ethical perspective, gene therapy involving introduction of genes into a patient is comparable to the practice of transplation of organs (e.g., heart, liver, lungs). Therefore, there is not much controversy over gene therapy, as long as it is intended to be used to alleviate serious medical disorders. However, the gene therapy must be under a close supervision to satisfy medical, legal, ethical and safety implications, besides addressing the public concerns.

Germ line gene therapy : This is not being carried out at present due to technical, ethical and social reasons. Manipulation of germ cells will lead to serious problems and complications.

At one international meeting on biotechnology the following was the final message given to biotechnology companies on the applications of genetic engineering to humans.

'*Provide the information and listen to the public*'.

HUMAN EMBRYONIC STEM CELL RESEARCH

The human embryonic stem cell (ESC) lines were established in November 1998. These cells are capable of giving rise to any human cell type. ESC lines open the possibilities of treating diseases with cell therapy. Disorders that involve the loss of normal cells such as diabetes mellitus, Parkinson's disease, Alzheimer's disease could perhaps be corrected with cell therapy. This may however, take more time.

There are many ethical and legal issues involved in ESC research, besides several objections raised by the public. In fact, the U.S. Federal Government has banned the use of federal funds for human embryo research for over 20 years. At present, most of research on ESC is being supported by private companies.

CLONING HUMANS ?

After the cloning of the sheep Dolly (in February, 1997), some groups of researchers naturally became interested to eplore the possibilities of cloning humans. The very thought of human cloning has become a highly charged and controversial issue.

A such, considering the biomedical ethics, most of the countries have banned research related to human cloning. It cannot be predicted at present whether some day human cloning may become invitable!

Scientists who were awarded Britain's first licence for human cloning have recently (2005) created an early stage of human cloned embryo by using nuclear transfer. The researchers, as such, are not interested to make babies by cloning. Instead, they wish to create test-tube embryos to supply stem cells that can give rise to every tissue in the body. By this approach, it might be one day possible to repair tissue damages and cure many diseases e.g. Parkinson's disease, diabetes mellitus.

PATENTING BIOTECHNOLOGY INVENTIONS

Biotechnology involves the production of a large number of commercial products of economic importance. Broadly, biotechnology inventions can be categorized into two forms — products and processes.

BIOTECHNOLOGY PRODUCTS

1. **Living entities :** The various forms of life-existing and life-supporting systems derived from living organisms are regarded as living entities. These include microorganism, animals and plants, cell lines, organelles, plasmids and genes.

2. **Naturally occurring products :** The primary and secondary metabolites produced by living systems e.g. alcohol, antibiotics.

BIOTECHNOLOGY PROCESSES

Biotechnology involves development of several processes — isolation, purification, cultivation, bioconversion etc. Novel, innovative, simple and cost-effective processes are developed for the isolation and creation of the above products. Some examples are listed

- Production of monoclonal antibodies
- Bioconversion of sugar to alcohol
- Microbial production of antibiotics.

WHAT IS A PATENT?

A patent is a government (or patent office) — issued document that allows the holder (patentee) the exclusive right to manufacture, use, or sell an invention for a defined period, usually 20 years. The patent may be regarded as a ***legal document safeguarding the previleges and rights of an invention/inventor***.

The very purpose of patenting in biotechnology is to ensure the just financial returns for those who have invested heavily — the finances, intellectual abilities, besides the hard work.

INTELLECTUAL PROPERTY RIGHTS

Patent is the most important form of ***intellectual property rights*** (***IPRs***) in biotechnology. The other IPRs are trade secrets, copyrights, and trade marks.

Trade secrets : The private information pertaining to specific formulations and technical procedures that a company wishes to protect from others are regarded as trade secrets. The best known trade secret is the formula for coca-cola. Only five persons in the world are said to know the formula which has been kept in a bank in Atlanta, Georgia. The trade secret of coca-cola has remained a secret for more than 100 years!

Copyrights : The protection of authorships of published work comes under copyrights of IPRs.

Trade marks : The specific symbols or words to identify a particular product or process of a company constitute trade marks.

THE PROCESS OF PATENTING

As regards patenting of biotechnology inventions, the ***products or processes*** (described on p. 744) are ***patentable***. For patenting, the following criteria must be satisfied.

- The invention must be novel
- It must be useful
- The patent application must provide the full description of the invention.

In contrast to various other technology inventions, biotechnology inventions most often relate to living materials. For this reason, the patenting of biotechnology inventions is often associated with difficulties. Patenting, in general, is a commercial decision, assisted by legal advice.

The patent application must be prepared by an expert with the assistance of a patent lawyer. It must contain the detailed information about the invention — background, description explaining the nature of the invention with figures and illustrations, its utility etc. The patent office, after a thorough scrutiny of the application, may reject or grant the patent. If rejected, the applicant may appeal to the Patent Appeals Board. If again rejected, the decision may be challenged legally. Many a times, the process of patenting becomes a frustrating experience. Thomas Edison, probably the only individual in the world with more than 1000 patents to his credit, once said about patenting 'an invitation to a lawsuit'.

Patenting in different countries

Patenting laws are very complex and vary between different countries. It is interesting to note that a patent application rejected in one country may be given patent in other country. The best example is the production of recombinant human tissue plasminogen activator (tPA) in *E. coli*. Genentech company was awarded patent for tPA production in USA, while it was first rejected in UK. After appeals and legal battles, patent was finally granted in UK also.

Patenting microorganisms

A genetically engineered strain of the bacterium *Pseudomonas* called ***superbug*** was ***the first micro-organism to be patented***. Superbug is capable of breaking down the multiple impuries of crude oil. It took almost 10 years of procedural delays, and legal battles to get the superbug patented. Now, many microrganisms are patented.

Patenting multicellular organisms

A genetically manipulated mouse namely the ***oncomouse*** was the first and probably, to date the only ***animal to be patented*** in both USA and UK. This transgenic mouse carries a gene that makes it susceptible to tumor formation.

Patenting genes?

The human genome projects (HGPs) have elucidated almost the entire sequence of human genome, besides identifying the genes. Patenting of DNA sequences and genes has become a controversial and debatable issue. Some researchers and institutions in fact have approached the patent offices for grant of patents. So far, patents have not been granted for genes. The most important reason being that the genes are natural, universal and inherent biological functional units of all individuals.

Patenting, and cell/tissue donor's rights

While dealing with human tissues/cells, the involvement of the donor of source material becomes very important. John Moore was a victim of hairy-cell leukemia, a rare form of cancer. His spleen was removed, and Mo cell lines developed. These cell lines were patented by the researchers and their associated organizations. Moore, however was not involved in the patenting.

Moore filed a suit in the court on the ground that he should also be a party to the profits derived by using his tissue. The court allowed his claim to share the profits.

PLANT BREEDERS' RIGHTS

Agriculture for the first time was included (in 1994) in the ***trade-related intellectual property rights (TRIPS)***. TRIPS is a major concern for developing countries.

The plant varieties in many countries (not in India) are protected through plant breeders' rights (PBR) or ***plant variety rights (PVR)***. PVR provides legal protection to the original breeder or owner of the plant variety. It is believed that PBR will ***encourage innovative research and plant breeding programmes***, in view of the expected financial returns.

Plant breeders' rights are comparable to the patent rights. Under TRIPS agreement, plant breeder possesses the exclusive rights over the plant developed. It prevents the third parties from using the plant without the owner's consent.

Although PBR will increase competition and development of good plant varieties, the owner's motto would be profit making. Therefore, PBR will prohibit the free exchange of plant materials, besides threatening the farmer's rights. It is feared that PBR will benefit rich farmers and developed countries only.

PATENTING AND BIOTECHNOLOGY RESEARCH

In the earlier years, research used to be mostly for academic interest and worthwhile scientific contributions. And researchers were purely academic-oriented with not much interest in financial gains from what they do. Further, unlike now, the research used to be supported mostly by Governments/Universities.

There used to be no secrecy in research. Academic recognition and outstanding research publications (open to all) were adequate to satisfy the researchers. Watson and Crick who discovered DNA structure never had a thought of patenting!

The situation has now changed. A good proportion of research is either being conducted or financially supported by private companies/ universities. It is quite natural for these companies to expect returns for their investments. There is a lot of change in the attitude of researchers also. For many scientists, ***financial gains have become more important than academic recognition***. Consequently, some people carry out research secretly and opt for patenting of their discoveries rather than publishing.

We have to accept the fact that the progress of research is usually much faster in private companies compared to many government organizations. This may be due to the higher financial returns and efficient administration.

Probably, the biotechnological research might not have progressed to the same extent as it is today without the dreams of getting the patents by scientists and research funding organizations.

BIOTECHNOLOGY AND THE DEVELOPING COUNTRIES

A major proportion of research related to biotechnology is carried out by the developed countries. The fruits of biotechnology are probably, more useful and relevant to developing countries, as illustrated with the following applications

- Increased levels of nutrition with improved nutrient composition in the foods (through transgenic plants).
- Prevention of child deaths by appropriate immunization (using recombinant vaccines).
- Supply of clean drinking water, and improved sewage disposal (by appropriate biotechnological treatments).

Despite the known benefits, some of the developing countries are reluctant to open doors for the advances made in biotechnology. This may be more due to political considerations rather the economic reasons.

The applications of biotechnology, particularly to human healthcare, may someday be regarded as a barometer to evaluate the progress of a nation.

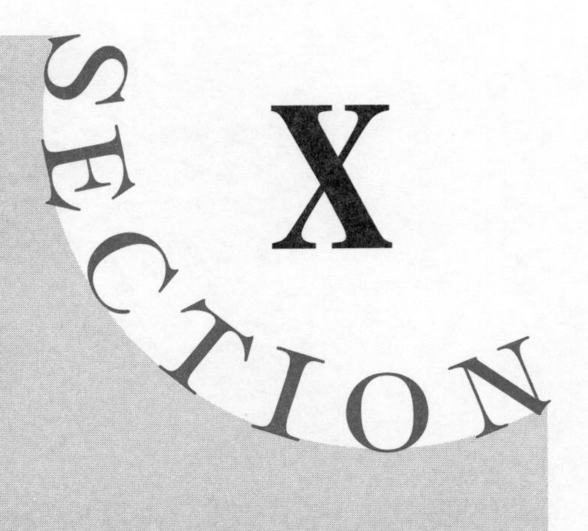

BASICS TO LEARN BIOTECHNOLOGY

CONTENTS

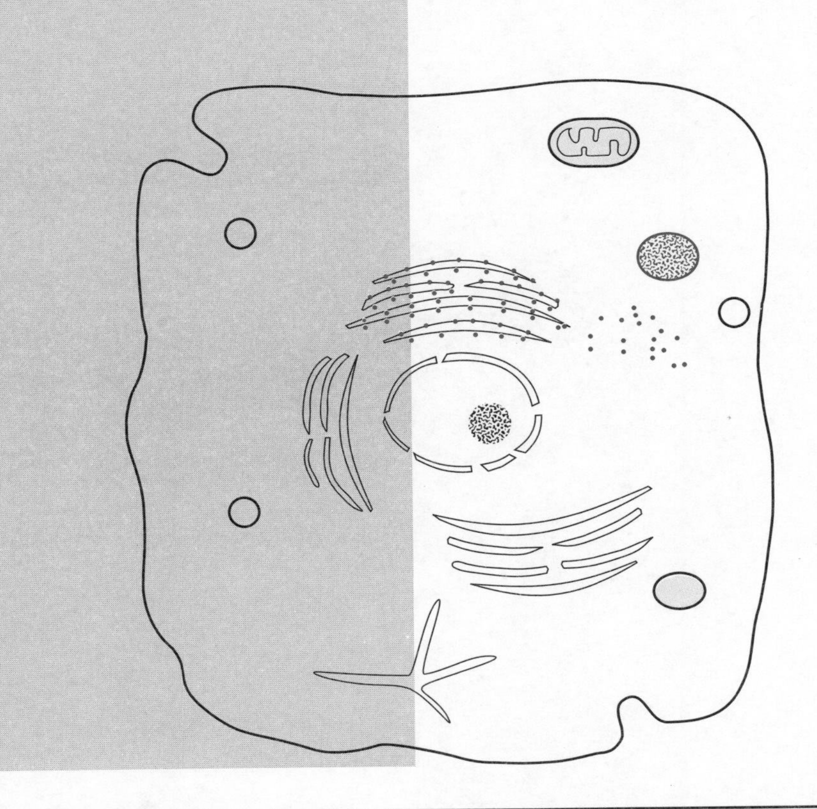

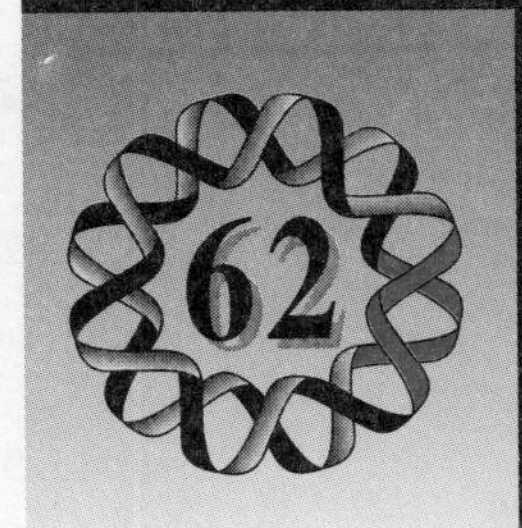

Cell — The Basic Unit of Life

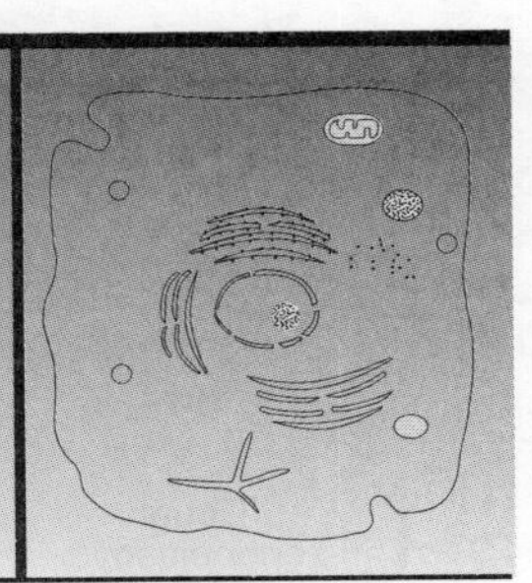

The cell is the structural and functional unit of life. It may be also regarded as the ***basic unit of biological activity.***

The concept of cell originated from the contributions of Schleiden and Schwann (1838). However, it was only after 1940, the complexities of cell structure were exposed.

PROKARYOTIC AND EUKARYOTIC CELLS

The cells of the living kingdom may be divided into two categories

1. **Prokaryotes** (*Greek* : pro-before; karyon – nucleus) lack a well defined nucleus and possess relatively simple structure. These include the various bacteria.

2. **Eukaryotes** (*Greek* : eu-true; karyon-nucleus) possess a well defined nucleus and are more complex in their structure and function. The higher organisms (animals and plants) are composed of eukaryotic cells.

A comparison of the characteristics between prokaryotes and eukaryotes is listed in ***Table 62.1***.

TABLE 62.1 Comparison between prokaryotic and eukaryotic cells

Character	*Prokaryotic cell*	*Eukaryotic cell*
Size	Small (generally 1-10 μm)	Large (generally 10-100 μm)
Cell membrane	Cell is enveloped by a rigid cell wall	Cell is enveloped by a flexible plasma membrane
Sub-cellular organelles	Absent	Distinct organelles are found (e.g. mitochondria, nucleus, lysosomes)
Nucleus	Not well defined; DNA is found as nucleoid, histones are absent	Nucleus is well defined, surrounded by a membrane; DNA is associated with histones
Energy metabolism	Mitochondria absent, enzymes of energy metabolism bound to membrane	Enzymes of energy metabolism are located in mitochondria
Cell division	Usually fission and no mitosis	Mitosis
Cytoplasm	Organelles and cytoskeleton absent	Contains organelles and cytoskeleton (a network of tubules and filaments)

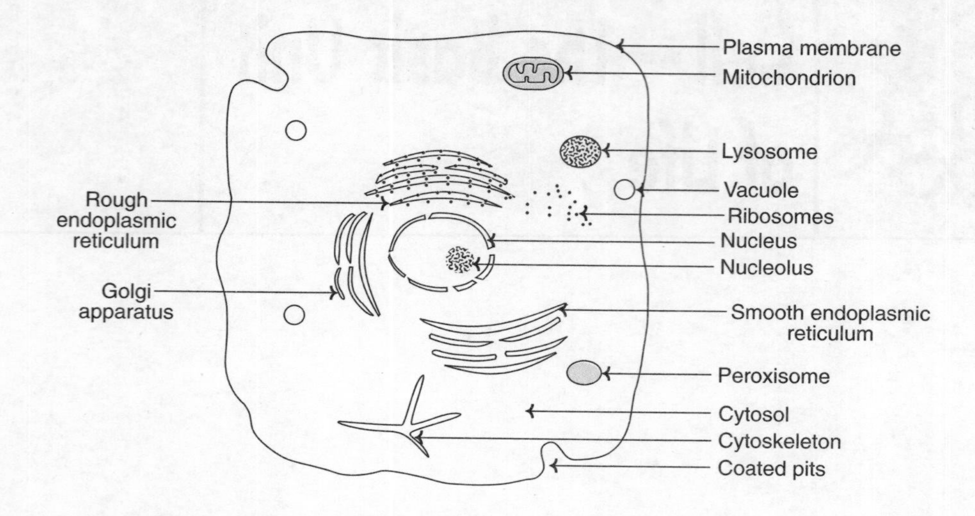

Fig. 62.1 : A diagrammatic representation of a rat liver cell.

EUKARYOTIC CELL

The salient features of an animal cell and a plant cell are briefly described

ANIMAL CELL

The human body is composed of about 10^{14} cells. An eukaryotic cell is generally 10 to 100 μm in diameter. A diagrammatic representation of a typical rat liver cell is depicted in ***Fig. 62.1***.

The cell consists of well defined subcellular organelles, enveloped by a plasma membrane. By differential centrifugation of tissue homogenate, it is possible to isolate each cellular organelle in a relatively pure form (Refer Chapter 64). The subcellular organelles are briefly described in the following pages.

Nucleus

Nucleus is the largest cellular organelle, surrounded by a double membrane nuclear envelope. The outer membrane is continuous with the membranes of endoplasmic reticulum. At certain intervals, the two nuclear membranes have nuclear pores with a diameter of about 90 nm. These pores permit the free passage of the products synthesized in the nucleus into the surrounding cytoplasm.

Nucleus contains ***DNA***, the repository of genetic information. Eukaryotic DNA is associated with basic protein (histones) in the ratio of 1 : 1, to form ***nucleosomes***. An assembly of nucleosomes constitutes ***chromatin*** fibres of chromosomes (*Greek*: chroma-colour; soma-body). Thus, a single human chromosome is composed of about a million nucleosomes. The number of chromosomes is a characteristic feature of the species. Humans have 46 chromosomes, compactly packed in the nucleus.

The nucleus of the eukaryotic cell contains a dense body known as ***nucleolus***. It is rich in RNA, particularly the ribosomal RNA which enters the cytosol through nuclear pores.

The ground material of the nucleus is often referred to as ***nucleoplasm***. It is rich in enzymes such as DNA polymerases and RNA polymerases. To the surprise of biochemists, the enzymes of glycolysis, citric acid cycle and hexose monophosphate shunt have also been detected in the nucleoplasm.

Mitochondria

The mitochondria (*Greek*: mitos-thread; chondros-granule) are the centres for the cellular respiration and energy metabolism. They are regarded as the ***power houses of the cell*** with variable size and shape. Mitochondria are rod-like or filamentous bodies, usually with dimensions of

1.0 × 3 μm. About 2,000 mitochondria, occupying about $^1/_5$th of the total cell volume, are present in a typical cell.

The mitochondria are composed of a double membrane system. The outer membrane is smooth and completely envelops the organelle. The inner membrane is folded to form ***cristae*** (*Latin*-crests) which occupy a larger surface area. The internal chamber of mitochondria is referred to as ***matrix***.

The components of electron transport chain and oxidative phosphorylation (flavoprotein, cytochromes b, c_1, c, a and a_3 and coupling factors) are buried in the inner mitochondrial membrane. The matrix contains several enzymes concerned with the energy metabolism of carbohydrates, lipids and amino acids (e.g., citric acid cycle, β-oxidation). The matrix enzymes also participate in the synthesis of heme and urea. Mitochondria are the principal producers of ATP in the aerobic cells. ATP, the energy currency, generated in mitochondria is exported to all parts of the cell to provide energy for the cellular work.

The mitochondrial matrix contains a circular double-stranded DNA (mtDNA), RNA and ribosomes. Thus, the mitochondria are equipped with an independent protein synthesizing machinery. It is estimated that about 10% of the mitochondrial proteins are produced in the mitochondria.

The ***structure and functions of mitochondria closely resemble prokaryotic cells***. It is hypothesized that mitochondria have evolved from aerobic bacteria. Further, it is believed that during evolution, the aerobic bacteria developed a symbiotic relationship with primordial anaerobic eukaryotic cells that ultimately led to the arrival of aerobic eukaryotes.

Endoplasmic reticulum

The network of membrane enclosed spaces that extends throughout the cytoplasm constitutes endoplasmic reticulum (ER). Some of these thread-like structures extend from the nuclear pores to the plasma membrane.

A large portion of the ER is studded with ribosomes to give a granular appearance which is referred to as ***rough endoplasmic reticulum***. Ribosomes are the factories of protein biosynthesis. During the process of cell fractionation, rough ER is disrupted to form small vesicles known as ***microsomes***. It may be noted that microsomes as such do not occur in the cell.

The smooth endoplasmic reticulum does not contain ribosomes. It is involved in the synthesis of lipids (triacylglycerols, phospholipids, sterols) and metabolism of drugs, besides supplying Ca^{2+} for the cellular functions.

Golgi apparatus

Eukaryotic cells contain a unique cluster of membrane vesicles known as ***dictyosomes*** which, in turn, constitute Golgi apparatus (or Golgi complex). The newly synthesized proteins are handed over to the Golgi apparatus which catalyse the addition of carbohydrates, lipids or sulfate moieties to the proteins. These chemical modifications are necessary for the transport of proteins across the plasma membrane.

Certain proteins and enzymes are enclosed in membrane vesicles of Golgi apparatus and secreted from the cell after the appropriate signals. The digestive enzymes of pancreas are produced in this fashion.

Golgi apparatus are also involved in the membrane synthesis, particularly for the formation of intracellular organelles (e.g. peroxisomes, lysosomes).

Lysosomes

Lysosomes are spherical vesicles enveloped by a single membrane. Lysosomes are regarded as the digestive tract of the cell, since they are actively involved in digestion of cellular substances—namely proteins, lipids, carbohydrates and nucleic acids. Lysosomal enzymes are categorized as ***hydrolases***. These include the following enzymes (with substrate in brackets)

- α-Glucosidase (glycogen)
- Cathepsins (proteins)
- Lipases (lipids)
- Ribonucleases (RNA)

The pH of the lysosomal matrix is more acidic (pH < 5) than the cytosol (pH~7) and this facilitates the degradation of different compounds. The lysosomal enzymes are responsible for maintaining the cellular compounds in a dynamic state, by their

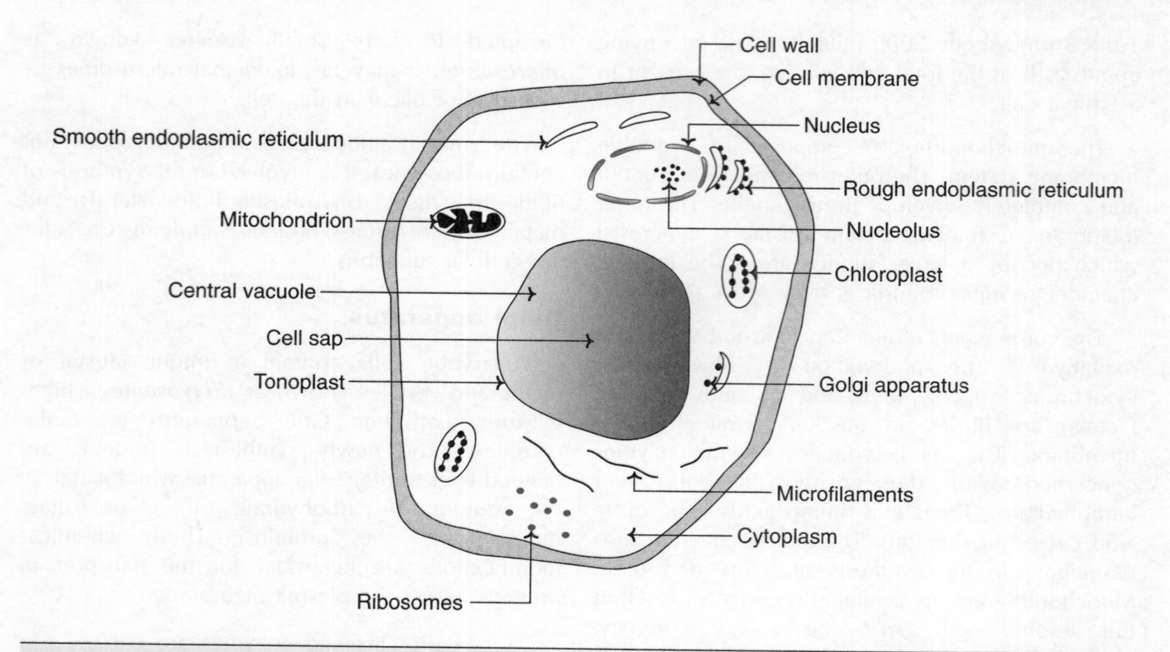

Fig. 62.2 : A diagrammatic representation of a plant cell.

degradation and recycling. The degraded products leave the lysosomes, usually by diffusion, for reutilization by the cell. Sometimes, however, certain residual products, rich in lipids and proteins, collectively known as ***lipofuscin*** accumulate in the cell. Lipofuscin is the age pigment or wear and tear pigment which has been implicated in ageing process.

The digestive enzymes of cellular compounds are confined to the lysosomes in the best interest of the cell. Escape of these enzymes into cytosol will destroy the functional macromolecules of the cell and result in many complications. The occurrence of several diseases (e.g. arthritis, muscle diseases, allergic disorders) has been partly attributed to the release of lysosomal enzymes.

Peroxisomes

Peroxisomes, also known as microbodies, are single membrane cellular organelles. They are spherical or oval in shape and contain the enzyme ***catalase***. Catalase protects the cell from the toxic effects of H_2O_2 by converting it to H_2O and O_2. Peroxisomes are also involved in the oxidation of long chain fatty acids ($>C_{18}$) and synthesis of plasmalogens and glycolipids. Plants contain ***glyoxysomes***, a specialized type of peroxisomes, which are involved in the glyoxylate pathway.

Cytosol and cytoskeleton

The cellular matrix is collectively referred to as cytosol. Cytosol is basically a compartment containing several enzymes, metabolites and salts in an aqueous gel like medium. More recent studies however, indicate that the cytoplasm actually contains a complex network of protein filaments, spread throughout, that constitutes cytoskeleton. The cytoplasmic filaments are of three types- microtubules, actin filaments and intermediate filaments. The filaments which are polymers of proteins are responsible for the structure, shape and organization of the cell.

PLANT CELL

A diagrammatic representation of a typical plant cell is depicted in ***Fig. 62.2***. The cell wall, chloroplasts and vacuoles are the most important and distinguishing components of plant cells when compared to animal cells.

In the ***Table 62.2***, a comparison between plant and animal cells is given. The salient features of plant cell organelles are briefly described.

Table 62.2 A comparison between plant and animal cells

Character	*Plant cell*	*Animal cell*
Size	Generally larger	Smaller than plant cells
Cell wall	Surrounded by rigid cell wall of cellulose	Absent
Vacuole	Mature plant cells possess a large vacuole	Absent
Plastids	Chloroplasts found in green plants	Absent
Cell division	Division of cytoplasm during cell division occurs by the formation of a cell plate	Division occurs by constriction

Cell wall

The plant cell wall is usually rigid, non-living and permeable component, surrounding the plasma membrane. Cell walls are of two types — primary and secondary.

The ***primary cell wall*** is the one that is formed during the course of cell division. It is mainly composed of cellulose, and is flexible in nature. The ***secondary cell wall*** is rigid and more complex in nature. Chemically, it is made up of more cellulose, and high content of lignin. Lignin is the major component of wood. The secondary cell wall is inextensible and determines the final shape and size of the plant cell.

Besides cellulose and lignin, hemicelluloses, pectins, and extensins (oligosaccharides) are also present in the cell wall.

Chloroplasts

The chloroplasts are found only in the plant cells, and are the sites of photosynthesis. The general term ***plastids*** is often used to collectively represent chloroplasts (green plastids containing chlorophylls), ***chromoplasts*** (yellow to reddish colour plastids containing carotenoids) and ***leucoplasts*** (colourless plastids).

Chloroplasts have a double membrane system. Internally, chloroplasts contain a system of flattened membranous discs called ***thylakoids***. Piles of thylakoids are located in the central region called ***stroma***. Chlorophyll, the sunlight-capturing green pigment is present in the thylakoids.

Vacuoles

Plant cells have membrane-bound, liquid filled vesicles called vacuoles, which may occupy as much as 90% of the cells total volume. The vacuoles may contain wide range of dissolved molecules such as salts, sugars, pigments and toxic wastes. The pigments of vacuoles contribute to the colours of flowers and leaves. The physical support of plant tissues comes from the high internal pressure of water maintained within the vacuoles.

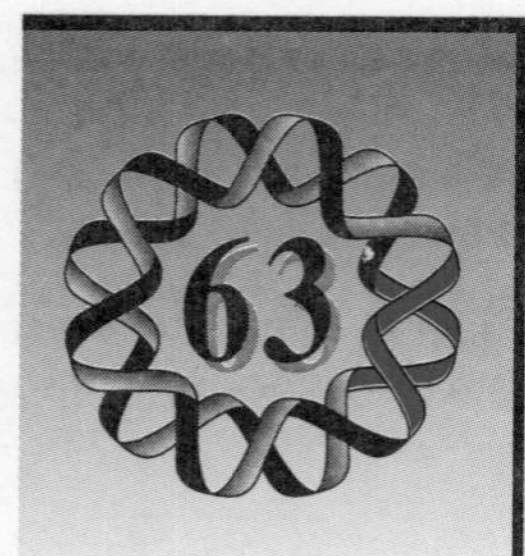

Microorganisms

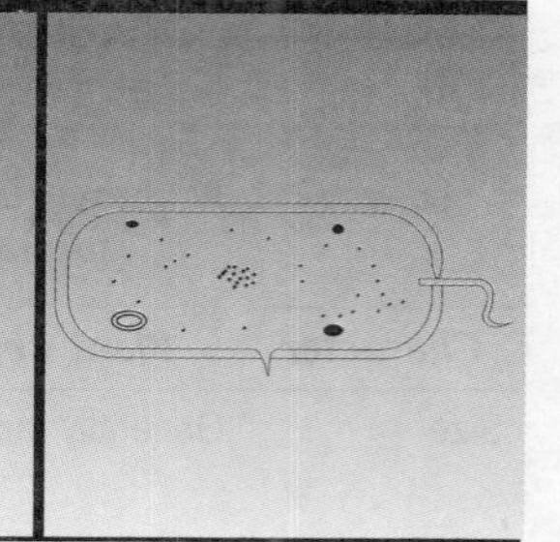

Microbiology (Greek, mikros—small; bios–life) is the ***science of small*** or ***microscopic organisms***. The most important microorganisms relevant to biotechnology include bacteria, fungi, and viruses. Microorganisms are very widely distributed, and are found almost everywhere in nature. In general, the conditions for their growth and multiplication (food, temperature, moisture etc.) are similar to that of humans. Hence, they are most abundantly present at places where people live.

A very brief description of the microorganisms, relevent to biotechnology is given in this chapter.

BACTERIA

Bacteriology, the study of bacteria, forms a major part of microbiology. The population of bacteria exceeds all other organisms. For instance, one kg of a soil may contain more bacteria than the entire human population! Bacteria are very important in biotechnology for the following reasons

- Diseases they cause
- Domestic uses
- Industrial applications
- Agricultural processes.

CHARACTERISTICS OF BACTERIA

Bacteria are ***prokaryotic unicellular organisms***. They lack organized nucleus, but possess a rigid cell wall comparable to that found in plants. The average size of a bacterium is around 2 μm. The bacteria may be spherical, rod-like, spirally coiled or filament like. Certain bacteria may occur in more than one form. A typical structure of a rod-shaped bacterium is depicted in ***Fig. 63.1***.

Gram-positive and Gram-negative bacteria

Based on the response to Gram's stain, the bacteria are grouped as Gram +ve or Gram –ve. By Gram's stain, several distinguishing features of bacteria can be identified. For instance, Gram +ve bacteria possess single-layered cell wall while Gram –ve bacteria have a double-layered one.

Aerobic, anaerobic and facultative bacteria

On the basis of respiration (i.e. response to O_2), the bacteria are grouped into three categories

1. **Aerobic bacteria :** These bacteria require O_2 for their growth e.g. *Pseudomonas* sp, *Mycobacterium* sp.

2. **Anaerobic bacteria :** These bacteria do not require O_2 to obtain energy, and to grow. In fact, the presence of O_2 is toxic to them e.g. *Peptococcus* sp.

3. **Facultative bacteria :** The bacteria that can grow in both aerobic and anaerobic conditions are regarded as facultative bacteria. e.g. *Shigella* sp, *Salmonella* sp.

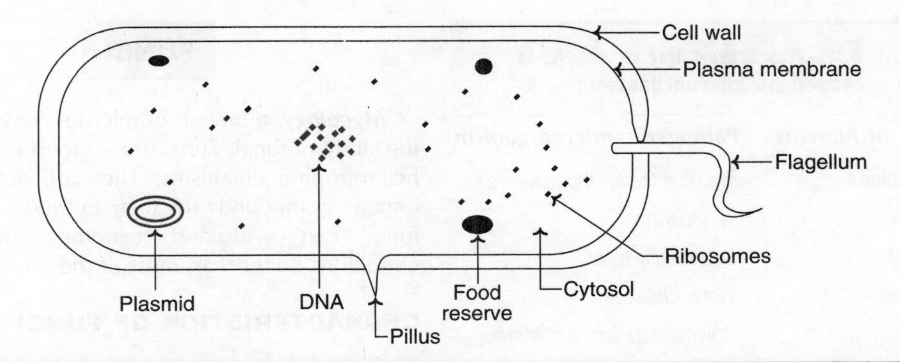

Fig. 63.1 : A typical structure of a rod-shaped bacterium.

Nutritional aspects of bacteria

Based on their nutrition, the bacteria are categorized as autotrophic or heterotrophic.

1. **Autotrophic bacteria :** These bacteria are capable of synthesizing their own food from inorganic substances. They are compable to higher plants in this aspect. Autotrophic bacteria utilize different hydrogen compounds (not H_2O as in the case of higher plants). These include hydrogen, ammonia, hydrogen sulfide and methane e.g. *Hydrogenomonas* sp, *Nitrosomonas* sp, *Methanomonas* sp.

2. **Heterotrophic bacteria :** These bacteria cannot synthesize their own food, and are therefore dependent on the outside source. Heterotrophs are of two types—sporophytes and parasites.

Sporophytes obtain their food from sources of animal or plant origin. These include organic remains like corpses, animal excreta, meats, fruits and various other products of plant and animal origin. Sporophytes secrete digestive enzymes that break the complex organic molecules into simpler and easily absorbable forms. These heterotrophic bacteria are ***useful for the disposal of sewage***, cleansing of leather, and manufacture of certain compounds (alcohols, organic acids). Sporophytes can also spoil foods, and damage soils (by denitrification).

Parasites are the bacteria that obtain their food from living organisms, namely the hosts. They may be either harmless (non-pathogenic) or harmful (pathogenic) to the hosts. *E. coli* is a good example of non-pathogenic bacteria which has a symbiotic relationship in the human intestine. The pathogenic bacteria may cause serious diseases either by destroying the host's cells or releasing toxins e.g. *Clostridium tetani.*

IMPORTANCE OF BACTERIA

Bacteria play a very important and crucial role in the continuous sustenance of life on earth. They are both friends and enemies of humans. Bacteria are important due to the diseases they cause, industrial and agricultural applications.

Diseases caused by bacteria

The bacteria pose a serious threat to humans, animals and plants due to various diseases they cause. A selected list of the important diseases and the corresponding organisms is given in ***Table 63.1***.

Industrial uses of bacteria

An important aspect of biotechnology is the industrial use of bacteria for the production of several compounds. Traditionally, bacteria are in use for the preparation of curd, vinegar, pickles, curing tea and tobacco leaves. In recent years, large-scale production of amino acids, organic solvents, vitamins and antibiotics is being carried out by employing bacteria.

Bacteria play a significant role in the decay and disposal of dead plants and animals. Appropriate sewage disposal requires bacteria. Bacteria are also needed for the disposal of animal dung and human excreta.

Agricultural applications of bacteria

Nitrogen fixation by converting free nitrogen into nitrogenous compounds is very important in agriculture. This is exclusively carried out by

TABLE 63.1 A selected list of diseases caused by microorganisms

Diseases of humans	*Pathogenic microorganism*
Tuberculosis	*Mycobacterium tuberculosis*
Leprosy	*M. leparae*
Typhoid	*Salmonella typhi*
Cholera	*Vibrio cholerae*
Diptheria	*Corynebacterium diphtheriae*
Syphillis	*Treponema pallidum*
Tetanus	*Clostridium tetani*
Bacterial dysentery	*Shigella dysenteriae*
Gonorrhoea	*Neisseria gonorrhoeae*
Diseases of animals	
Anthrax	*Bacillus anthracis*
Pneumonia	*Diplococcus pneumoniae*
Black leg of cattle	*Clostridium chauvei*
Diseases of plants	
Crown galls	*Agrobacterium tumefaciens*
Pear blight	*Pseudomonas amylovorus*
Ring rot of potato	*Corynebacterium sependonicum*
Citrus canker	*Xanthomonas citri*
Black rot of cabbage	*X. campestris*

symbiotic nitrogen-fixing bacteria. In addition, ***nitrifying bacteria*** (convert ammonia to nitrates) and ***ammonifying bacteria*** (convert amino acids to ammonia) also contribute to agricultural practices.

CONTROL OF PATHOGENIC BACTERIA

As already stated above, bacteria cause several diseases. There are different approaches to control pathogenic bacteria

- Use of antibiotics
- Treatment with antiseptics and disinfectants.
- Sterilization and autoclaving
- Radiation treatment
- Biological control.

In addition to the above, vaccines have been developed against certain pathogens to control diseases in humans and animals.

FUNGI

Mycology, a branch of microbiology, deals with the study of fungi. Fungi are a group of eukaryotic, heterotrophic organisms. They are dependent on organic compounds for their nutrition. In general, fungi can withstand extreme environmental conditions better than most of the microorganisms.

CHARACTERISTICS OF FUNGI

Fungi cells are usually larger than the bacteria. The sizes may range 1-5 μm in width and 5–35 μm in length. Fungal cells may be elongated or spherical.

The fungi are heterotrophic, since they cannot synthesize their own food from the inorganic compounds.

IMPORTANCE OF FUNGI

As is the case with bacteria, fungi are both friends and enemies of humans.

Beneficial aspects of fungi

The ***yeasts are useful*** for the following

- Alcohol fermentation e.g. *Saccharomyces cerevisiae*
- Production of vitamins e.g. *Ashbya gossypii.*
- Citric acid fermentation e.g. *Candida* sp.
- Baker's yeast e.g. *S. cerevisiae.*

The ***application of molds*** are listed

- Production of enzymes e.g. *Aspergillus* sp.
- Citric acid fermentation e.g. *Aspergillus niger.*
- Penicillin production e.g. *Penicillium notatum.*
- Steroid transformation e.g. *Rhizopus* sp.
- Gluconic acid production e.g. *Aspergillus niger.*

Harmful aspects of fungi

- Spoilage of foods e.g. moldy bread, rot of fruits and vegetables.
- Deterioration of textiles made up of cotton.
- Damage to paper.
- Diseases caused by fungi e.g. ring worm of the scalp in children caused by *Microsporum audouinii.*

CONTROL OF FUNGI

The fungal growth can be controlled by using phenol and its derivatives e.g. cresol, ethylphenol, propylphenol, butylphenol. Chlorine and chlorine compounds are also useful in this regard.

Vegetative cells of yeasts and other fungi can be destroyed by moist heat at 50–60°C for about 5–10 minutes. Spores, however require higher temperature 20–80°C.

VIRUSES

A virus may be regarded as a small microorganism with a nucleoprotein entity which lives and multiplies in the living cells of other organisms. Thus, viruses as are unable to live in a cell-free environment, and become active and multiply as they enter living cells.

CHARACTERISTICS OF VIRUSES

Viruses are the smallest living entities. They do not possess the usual cellular structures. Viruses are composed of either DNA or RNA, and not both of them together. ***Retroviruses*** is the name given to viruses containing RNA as the genetic material.

Viruses do not possess independent metabolisms, and further they also lack respiratory machinery.

BIOLOGICAL STATUS OF VIRUSES

Organismal theory : Viruses are considered as primitive living microorganisms as they possess genetic material, biosynthetic machinery and certain enzymes, besides being infective.

TABLE 63.2 A selected list of common viral diseases

Diseases of humans	***Virus***
Common cold	*Rhinoviruses*
Small pox	*Pox virus*
Rabies	*Rabies virus*
Infectious hepatitis	*Hepatitis virus*
Measles	*Measles virus*
Poliomyelitis	*Polio virus*
Influenza	*Influenza virus*
Encaphalitis	*Encephalitis virus*
Mumps	*Mumps virus*
Diseases of plants	
Tobacco mosaic	*Tobacco mosaic virus*
Potato leaf roll	*Potato leaf roll virus*
Tomato leaf curl	*Tomato leaf curl virus*

Molecular theory : Some people consider viruses are non-living chemical molecules rather than living beings. They argue that viruses do not possess any cellular structures, cannot respire and cannot live independently.

IMPORTANCE OF VIRUSES

Viruses are associated with several diseases in humans and plants (***Table 63.2***). Besides the common diseases such as common cold, and rabies, viruses cause diseases such as AIDS. i.e. human immunodeficiency virus (HIV) is responsible for AIDS, the dreaded and incurable disease.

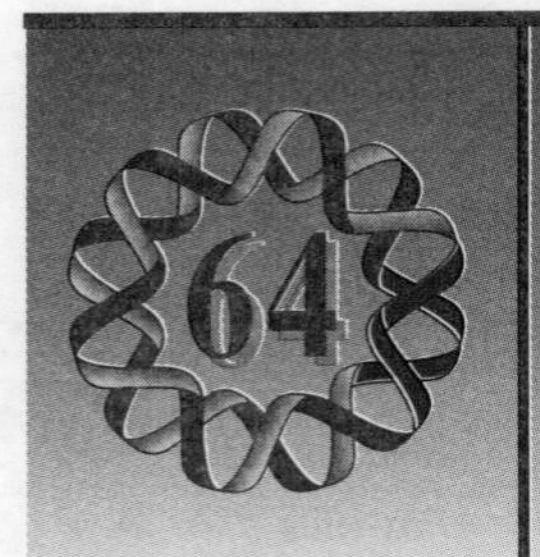

Bioorganic and Biophysical Chemistry, and Biochemistry Tools

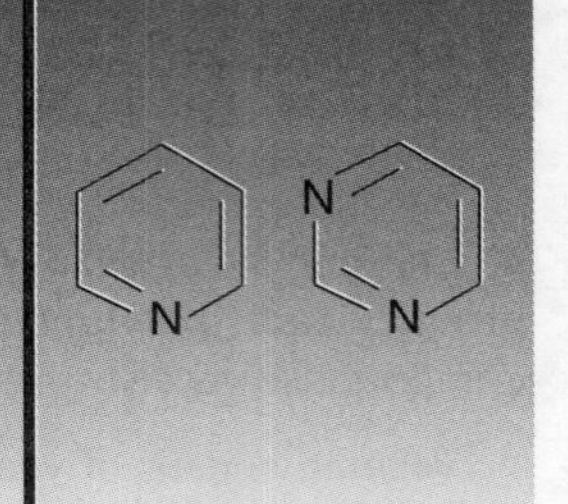

The fundamental principles of bioorganic and biophysical chemistry, besides the common tools employed in biochemistry are briefly described in this chapter.

INTRODUCTION TO BIOORGANIC CHEMISTRY

As life comes from previous life, it was believed for a long that the carbon compounds of organisms (hence the name organic) arose from life only. This is referred to as ***vital force theory***. Friedrich Wohler (1825) first discovered that urea (NH_2—CO—NH_2), the organic compound, could be prepared by heating ammonium cyanate (NH_4NCO), in the laboratory. Thereafter, thousands and thoushands of organic compounds have been synthesized outside the living system.

Organic chemistry broadly deals with the chemistry of carbon compounds, regardless of their origin. Biochemistry, however, is concerned with the ***carbon chemistry of life only***. The general principles of organic chemistry provide strong foundations for understanding biochemistry. However, biochemistry exclusively deals with the reactions that occur in the living system in aqueous medium.

MOST COMMON ORGANIC COMPOUNDS FOUND IN LIVING SYSTEM

The organic compounds, namely carbohydrates, lipids, proteins, nucleic acids and vitamins are the most common organic compounds of life.

COMMON FUNCTIONAL GROUPS IN BIOCHEMISTRY

Most of the physical and chemical properties of organic compounds are determined by their functional groups. Biomolecules possess certain functional groups which are their reactive centres. The common functional groups of importance in biomolecules are presented in ***Table 64.1***.

COMMON RING STRUCTURES IN BIOCHEMISTRY

There are many homocyclic and heterocyclic rings, commonly encountered in biomolecules. A selected list of them is given in ***Fig. 64.1***.

Homocyclic rings

Phenyl ring derived from benzene is found in several biomolecules (phenylalanine, tyrosine, catecholamines). Phenanthrene and cyclopentane form the backbone of steroids (cholesterol, aldosterone). Coenzyme Q is an example of benzoquinone while vitamin K is a naphthoquinone.

Heterocyclic rings

Furan is the ring structure found in pentoses. Pyrrole is the basic unit of porphyrins found in many biomolecules (heme) while pyrolidine is the ring present in the amino acid, proline. Thiophen ring is a part of the vitamin biotin. The amino acid histidine contains imidazole.

TABLE 64.1 Common functional groups of importance in biomolecules

Functional group: Name	Functional group: Group	General structural formula	Type of compound	Examples of biomolecule(s)
Hydroxyl	—OH	R—OH	Alcohol	Glycerol, ethanol
Aldehyde	$-\overset{O}{\overset{\Vert}{C}}-H$	$R-\overset{O}{\overset{\Vert}{C}}-H$	Aldehyde	Glyceraldehyde, glucose
Keto	$-\overset{O}{\overset{\Vert}{C}}-$	$R_1-\overset{O}{\overset{\Vert}{C}}-R_2$	Ketone	Fructose, sedoheptulose
Carboxyl	$-\overset{O}{\overset{\Vert}{C}}-OH$	$R-\overset{O}{\overset{\Vert}{C}}-OH$	Carboxylic acid	Acetic acid, palmitic acid
Amino	$-NH_2$	$R-NH_2$	Amino acid	Alanine, serine
Imino	$-\overset{H}{\overset{\vert}{N}}-$	$R-\overset{H}{\overset{\vert}{N}}-$	Imino acid	Proline, hydroxyproline
Sulfhydryl	—SH	R—SH	Thiol	Cysteine, coenzyme A
Ether	—O—	R_1-O-R_2	Ether	Thromboxane A_2
Ester	$-\overset{O}{\overset{\Vert}{C}}-O-R_1$	$R_2-\overset{O}{\overset{\Vert}{C}}-O-R_1$	Ester	Cholesterol ester
Amido	$-\overset{O}{\overset{\Vert}{C}}-N(R_1)(R_2)$	$R_3-\overset{O}{\overset{\Vert}{C}}-N(R_1)(R_2)$	Amide	N-Acetylglucosamine

Pyran structure is found in hexoses. Pyridine nucleus is a part of the vitamins-niacin and pyridoxine. Pyrimidines (cytosine, thymine) and purines (adenine, guanine) are the constituents of nucleotides and nucleic acids. Indole ring is found in the amino acid tryptophan. Purine and indole are examples of fused heterocyclic rings.

ISOMERISM

The compounds possessing identical molecular formulae but different structures are referred to as ***isomers.*** The phenomenon of existence of isomers is called isomerism (*Greek* : isos—equal; meros—parts). Isomers differ from each other in physical and chemical properties. ***Isomerism is partly responsible for the existence of a large number of organic molecules.***

Consider the molecular formula—C_2H_6O. There are two important isomers of this—ethyl alcohol (C_2H_5OH) and diethyl ether (CH_3OCH_3) as shown below :

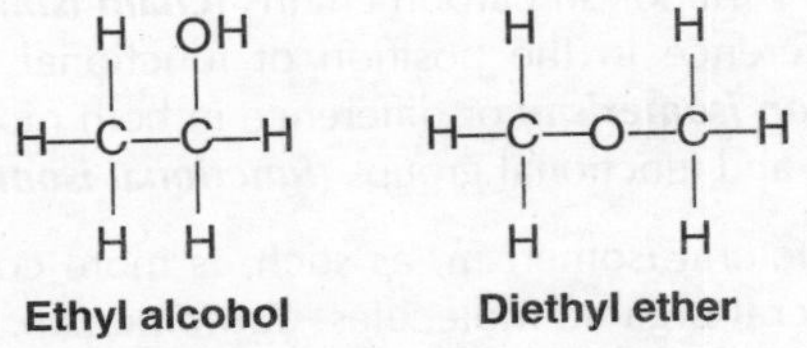

```
   H  OH           H       H
   |  |            |       |
H—C—C—H        H—C—O—C—H
   |  |            |       |
   H  H            H       H
```

Ethyl alcohol **Diethyl ether**

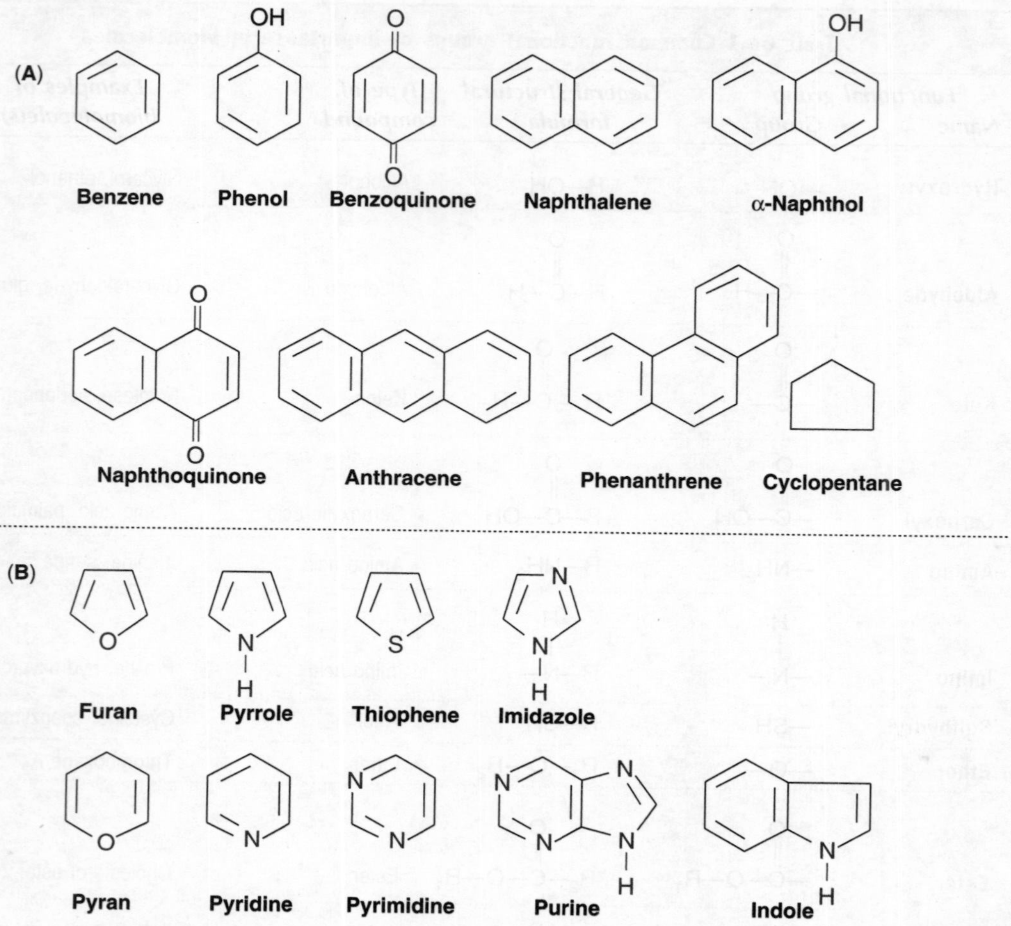

(A)

Benzene Phenol Benzoquinone Naphthalene α-Naphthol

Naphthoquinone Anthracene Phenanthrene Cyclopentane

(B)

Furan Pyrrole Thiophene Imidazole

Pyran Pyridine Pyrimidine Purine Indole

*Fig. 64.1 : Common ring structures found in biomolecules **(A)** Homocyclic rings **(B)** Heterocyclic rings.*

Isomerism is broadly divided into two categories — structural isomerism and stereo-isomerism.

Structural isomerism

The difference in the arrangement of the atoms in the molecule (i.e. molecular framework) is responsible for structural isomerism. This may be due to variation in carbon chains ***(chain isomerism)*** or difference in the position of functional groups ***(position isomerism)*** or difference in both molecular chains and functional groups ***(functional isomerism)***.

Structural isomerism, as such, is more common in general organic molecules. ***Tautomerism,*** a type of structural isomerism, occurs due to the migration of an atom or group from one position to the other e.g. purines and pyrimidines.

Stereoisomerism

Stereoisomerism (*Greek* : stereos—space occupying) is, perhaps, more relevant and important to biomolecules. The differential space arrangement of atoms or groups in molecules gives rise to stereoisomerism. Thus, stereoisomers have the same structural formula but differ in their spacial arrangement.

Stereoisomerism is of two types—***geometric isomerism*** and ***optical isomerism.***

Geometrical isomerism : This is also called *cis-trans* isomerism and is exhibited by certain molecules possessing double bonds. Geometrical isomerism is due to restriction of freedom of rotation of groups around a carbon-carbon double bond (C = C). Maleic acid and fumaric acid are classical examples of *cis-trans* isomerism.

```
H—C—COOH        H—C—COOH
  ||              ||
H—C—COOH     HOOC—C—H
```

Maleic acid *(cis)* **Fumaric acid** *(trans)*

When similar groups lie on the same side, it is called *cis* isomer (*Latin* : cis—on the same side). On the other hand, when similar groups lie on the opposite sides, it is referred to as *trans* isomer (*Latin* : trans—across). As is observed from the above structure, maleic acid is a *cis* form while fumaric acid is a *trans* form.

Geometric isomerism is also observed in sterols and porphyrins. *cis-trans* isomers differ in physical and chemical properties.

Optical isomerism : Optical isomers or enantiomers occur due to the presence of an ***asymmetric carbon*** (a chiral carbon). Optical isomers differ from each other in their optical activity to rotate the plane of polarized light.

What is an asymmetric carbon?

An object is said to be symmetrical if it can be divided into equal halves e.g. a ball. Objects which cannot be divided into equal halves are asymmetric, e.g. hand. An asymmetric object cannot coincide with its mirror image. For instance, left hand is the mirror image of right hand and these two can never be superimposed. In contrast, a symmetrical object like a ball superimposes its image.

A carbon is said to be ***chiral*** (*Greek* : hand) or asymmetric when it is attached to four different groups. Their mirror images do not superimpose with each other.

```
    B     :     B
    |     :     |
  A—C—D   :   D—C—A
    |     :     |
    E     :     E
        Mirror
```

The number of possible optical isomers of a molecule depends upon the specific number of chiral carbon (n). It is given by 2^n.

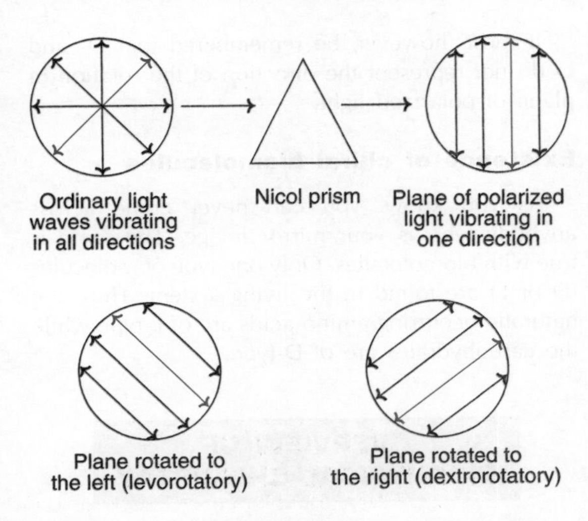

Fig. 64.2 : Diagrammatic illustration of optical activity.

What is optical activity?

The ordinary light propagates in all directions. However, on passing ordinary light through a Nicol prism, the plane of polarized light vibrates in one direction only (***Fig. 64.2***).

Certain organic compounds (optical isomers) which are said to exhibit optical activity rotate the plane of polarized light either to the left or to the right.

The term ***levorotatory*** (indicated by 1 or (–) sign) is used for the substances which rotate the plane of polarized light to the left. On the other hand, the term ***dextrorotatory*** (indicated by d or (+) sign) is used for substances rotating the plane of polarized light to right (***Fig. 64.2***).

The term ***racemic*** mixture represents equal concentration of d and l forms which cannot rotate the plane of polarized light.

Configuration of chiral molecules

While representing the configuration of chiral molecules, the configuration of ***glyceraldehyde*** is taken as a ***reference standard.***

```
    CHO            CHO
    |              |
  H—C—OH       HO—C—H
    |              |
   CH2OH          CH2OH
```

D-Glyceraldehyde **L-Glyceraldehyde**

It must, however, be remembered that D- and L- do not represent the direction of the rotation of plane of polarized light.

Existence of chiral biomolecules

As you know, you can never come across anybody who is your mirror image. The same is true with biomolecules. Only one type of molecules (D or L) are found in the living system. Thus, the naturally occurring amino acids are of L-type while the carbohydrates are of D-type.

OVERVIEW OF BIOPHYSICAL CHEMISTRY

The general laws and principles of chemistry and physics are applicable to biochemistry as well. It is, therefore, worthwhile to have a brief understanding of some of the basic chemical and physical principles that have direct relevance to life.

It must, however, be remembered that all these aspects are quite unrelated to each other.

ACIDS AND BASES

According to Lowry and Bronsted, an acid is defined as a substance that gives off protons while a base is a substance that accepts protons. Thus, ***an acid is a proton (H^+) donor and a base is a proton acceptor.***

Alkalies : The metallic hydroxides such as NaOH and KOH are commonly referred to as alkalies. These compounds do not directly satisfy the criteria of bases. However, they dissociate to form metallic ion and OH^- ion. The latter, being a base, accepts H^+ ions.

Ampholytes : The substances which can function both as acids and bases are referred to as ampholytes. Water is the best example for ampholytes.

Hydrogen ion concentration (pH)

The acidic or basic nature of a solution is measured by H^+ ion concentration. The strength of H^+ ions in the biological fluids is exceedingly low. For this reason, the conventional units such as moles/l or g/l are not commonly used to express H^+ ion concentration.

Sorenson (1909) introduced the term pH to express H^+ ion concentration. ***pH is defined as the negative logarithm of H^+ ion concentration.***

$$pH = -\log [H^+]$$

BUFFERS

The pH of a given solution can be easily altered by the addition of acids or bases. ***Buffers are defined as the solutions which resist change in pH by the addition of small amounts of acids or bases.*** A buffer usually consists of a weak acid and its salt (e.g. acetic acid and sodium acetate) or a weak base and its salt (e.g. ammonium hydroxide and ammonium chloride). Several buffers can be prepared in the laboratory. Nature has provided many buffers in the living system.

Mechanism of buffer action

Let us consider the buffer pair of acetic acid and sodium acetate. Acetic acid, being a weak acid, feebly ionizes. On the other hand, sodium acetate ionizes to a large extent.

$$CH_3COOH \rightleftharpoons CH_3COO^- + H^+$$
$$CH_3COONa \rightleftharpoons CH_3COO^- + Na^+$$

When an acid (say HCl) is added, the acetate ions of the buffer bind with H^+ ions (of HCl) to form acetic acid which is weakly ionizing. Therefore, the pH change due to acid is resisted by the buffer.

$$H^+ + CH_3COO^- \longrightarrow CH_3COOH$$

When a base (say NaOH) is added the H^+ ions of the buffer (acetic acid) combine with OH^- ions to form water, which is weakly dissociated. Thus, the pH change due to base addition is also prevented by the buffer.

$$OH^- + H^+ \longrightarrow H_2O$$

Buffering capacity : The efficiency of a buffer in maintaining a constant pH on the addition of acid or base is referred to as buffering capacity. It mostly depends on the concentration of the buffer components.

SOLUTIONS

Solutions may be regarded as mixtures of substances. In general, a solution is composed of two parts — ***solute*** and ***solvent.*** The substance that is dissolved is solute and the medium that dissolves the solute is referred to as solvent. The particle size of a solute in solution is < 1 nm.

The relative concentrations of substances in a solution can be measured by several ways.

Per cent concentration : This represents parts per 100. The most frequently used is weight per volume (w/v) e.g. 9% saline (9 g/100 ml solution).

Parts per million (ppm) : This refers to the number of parts of a substance in one million parts of the solution. Thus 10 ppm chlorine means 10 µg of chlorine in 1 g of water.

Molarity (M) : It is defined as the number of moles of solute per liter solution. NaCl has a molecular weight of 58.5. To get one molar (1 M) or one mole solution of NaCl, one gram molecular weight (58.5 g) of it should be dissolved in the solvent (H_2O) to make to a final total volume of 1 liter. For smaller concentrations, millimole and micromole are used.

Molality : It represents the number of moles of solute per 1,000 g of solvent. One molal solution can be prepared by dissolving 1 mole of solute in 1,000 g of solvent.

Normality : Molarity is based on molecular weight while normality is based on equivalent weight. One gram equivalent weight of an element or compound represents its capacity to combine or replace 1 mole of hydrogen.

COLLOIDAL STATE

Thomas Graham (1861), regarded as the 'father of colloidal chemistry', divided substances into two classes—***crystalloids*** and ***colloids.***

Crystalloids are the substances which in solution can freely pass (diffuse) through parchment membrane e.g. sugar, urea, NaCl. Colloids (*Greek* : glue-like), on other hand, are the substances that are retained by parchment membrane e.g. gum, gelatin, albumin. The above classification of Graham is no longer tenable, since any substance can be converted into a colloid by suitable means. For instance, sodium chloride in benzene forms a colloid.

Colloidal state : As such, there are no group of substances as colloids, rather, substances can exist in the form of ***colloidal state*** or ***colloidal system.*** Colloidal state is characterized by the particle size of 1 to 100 nm. When the particle size is <1 nm, it is in true solution. For the particle sizes >100 nm, the matter exists as a visible precipitate. Thus, the colloidal state is an intermediate between true solution and precipitate.

Phases of colloids : Colloidal state is heterogeneous with two phases.

1. **Dispersed phase** (internal phase) which constitutes the colloidal particles.

2. **Dispersion medium** (external phase) which refers to the medium in which the colloidal particles are suspended.

Classification of colloids

Based on the affinity of dispersion medium with dispersed phase, colloids are classified as ***lyophobic*** and ***lyophilic*** colloids.

1. **Lyophobic** (*Greek* : solvent-hating) **:** These colloids do not have any attraction towards dispersion medium. When water is used as dispersion medium, the colloids are referred to as ***hydrophobic.***

2. **Lyophilic** (*Greek* : solvent-loving) **:** These colloids have distinct affinity towards dispersion medium. The term ***hydrophilic*** is used for the colloids when water is the dispersion medium.

Biological importance of colloids

1. **Biological fluids as colloids :** These include blood, milk and cerebrospinal fluid.

2. **Biological compounds as colloidal particles :** The complex molecules of life, the high molecular weight proteins, complex lipids and polysaccharides exist in colloidal state.

3. **Fat digestion and absorption :** The formation of emulsions, facilitated by the emulsifying agents bile salts, promotes fat digestion and absorption in the intestinal tract.

4. **Formation of urine :** The filtration of urine is based on the principle of dialysis.

DIFFUSION

The molecules in liquids or gases are in continuous motion. ***Diffusion may be regarded as the movement of solute molecules from a higher concentration to a lower concentration.*** Diffusion is more rapid in gases than in liquids. The smaller particles diffuse faster than the larger ones. The greater the temperature, the higher is the rate of diffusion.

Applications of diffusion

1. Exchange of O_2 and CO_2 in lungs and in tissues occurs through diffusion.

2. Certain nutrients are absorbed by diffusion in the gastrointestinal tract e.g. pentoses, minerals, water soluble vitamins.

3. Passage of the waste products namely ammonia, in the renal tubules occurs due to diffusion.

OSMOSIS

Osmosis (*Greek* : push) refers to the ***movement of solvent*** (most frequently water) ***through a semipermeable membrane.***

The flow of solvent occurs from a solution of low concentration to a solution of high concentration, when both are separated by a semipermeable membrane.

Osmotic pressure

Osmotic pressure may be defined as the excess pressure that must be applied to a solution to prevent the passage of solvent into the solution, when both are separated by a semipermeable membrane.

The solutions that exert the same osmotic pressure are said to be ***isoosmotic.*** The term ***isotonic*** is used when a cell is in direct contact with an isoosmotic solution (0.9% NaCl) which does not change the cell volume and, thus, the cell tone is maintained. A solution with relatively greater osmotic pressure is referred to as ***hypertonic.*** On the other hand, a solution with relatively lower pressure is ***hypotonic.***

Units of osmotic pressure : Osmotic pressure of biological fluids is frequently expressed as ***milliosmoles.*** The osmotic pressure of plasma (of human blood) is 280-300 milliosmoles/l.

Applications of osmosis

1. **Fluid balance and blood volume :** The fluid balance of the different compartments of the body is maintained due to osmosis.

2. **Red blood cells and fragility :** When the RBC are kept in ***hypotonic solution*** (say 0.4% NaCl), the cells bulge due to entry of water which often causes rupture of plasma membrane of RBC ***(hemolysis).***

3. **Transfusion :** Isotonic solutions of NaCl (0.9%) or glucose (5%) or a suitable combination of these two are commonly used in transfusion in hospitals for the treatment of dehydration, burns etc.

4. **Action of purgatives :** The mechanism of action of purgatives is mainly due to osmotic phenomenon. For instance, epson ($MgSO_4$ $7H_2O$) or Glauber's (Na_2SO_4 $10H_2O$) salts withdraw water from the body, besides preventing the intestinal water absorption.

5. **Edema due to hypoalbuminemia :** Disorders such as kwashiorkor and glomerulonephritis are associated with lowered plasma albumin concentration and edema. Edema is caused by reduced oncotic pressure of plasma, leading to the accumulation of excess fluid in tissue spaces.

VISCOSITY

Liquid or fluid has a tendency to flow which is referred to as fluidity. The term viscosity may be defined as the ***internal resistance offered by a liquid or a gas to flow***. The property of viscosity is due to frictional forces between the layers while their movement occurs.

Viscosity of colloidal solutions, particularly lyophilic colloids, is generally higher than true solutions.

Units of viscosity : The unit of viscosity is ***poise,*** after the scientist Poiseuille, who first systematically studied the flow of liquids. A poise represents dynes/cm^2.

Applications of viscosity

1. **Viscosity of blood :** Blood is about 4 times more viscous than water. The viscosity of blood is mainly attributed to suspended blood cells and colloidal plasma proteins.

2. **Viscosity change in muscle :** Excitation of the muscle is associated with increase in the viscosity of the muscle fibres. This delays the change in the tension of the contracting muscle.

SURFACE TENSION

A molecule in the interior of a liquid is attracted by other molecules in all directions. In contrast, a molecule on the surface is attracted only downwards and sideways and not upwards. Due to this, the surface layer behaves like a stretched film. ***Surface tension is the force with which the molecules on the surface are held together.*** It is expressed as dynes/cm. Surface tension decreases with increase in temperature.

Applications of surface tension

1. **Digestion and absorption of fat :** Bile salts reduce the surface tension. They act as detergents and cause emulsification of fat, thereby allowing the formation of minute particles for effective digestion and absorption.

2. **Surfactants and lung function :** The low surface tension of the alveoli keeps them apart and allows an efficient exchange of gases in lungs. In fact, certain surfactants, predominantly dipalmitoyl phosphatidyl choline (dipalmitoyl lecithin), are responsible for maintaining low surface tension in the alveoli. Surfactant deficiency causes respiratory distress syndrome in the infants.

ADSORPTION

Adsorption is a surface phenomenon. It is the process of accumulation of a substance (adsorbate) on the surface of another substance (adsorbent). Adsorption differs from absorption, as the latter involves the diffusion into the interior of the material.

Applications of adsorption

1. **Formation of enzyme-substrate complex :** For the catalysis to occur in biological system, formation of enzyme-substrate complex is a prerequisite. This happens by adsorption of substrate on the enzyme.

2. **Action of drugs and poisons :** On adsorption at the cell surface, drugs and poisons exert their action.

3. **Adsorption in analytical biochemistry :** The principle of adsorption is widely employed in the chromatography technique for the separation and purification of compounds (enzymes, immunoglobulins).

ISOTOPES

Isotopes are defined as the elements with same atomic number but different atomic weights. They possess the same number of protons but differ in the neutrons in their nuclei. Therefore, isotopes (*Greek* : iso—equal; tope—place) occupy the same place in the periodic table. The chemical properties of different isotopes of a particular element are identical.

Isotopes are of two types—***stable*** and ***unstable.*** The latter are more commonly referred to as radioactive isotopes and they are of particular interest to biochemists.

Stable isotopes

They are naturally occurring and do not emit radiations (non-radioactive) e.g. deuterium (heavy hydrogen) ^{2}H; ^{13}C; ^{15}N; ^{18}O. Stable isotopes can be identified and quantitated by mass spectrometry or nuclear magnetic resonance (NMR). They are less frequently used in biochemical investigations.

Radioactive isotopes

The atomic nucleus of radioactive isotopes is unstable and, therefore, undergoes decay. The radioactive decay gives rise to one of the following 3 ionizing radiations.

1. **α-Rays** — an α particle possessing 2 protons i.e. helium nuclei.

2. **β-Rays** — due to the emission of electrons.

3. **γ-Rays** — due to emission of high energy photons.

The β and γ emitting radioisotopes are employed in biochemical research.

Applications of radioisotopes in biochemistry

Radioactive isotopes have become indispensable tools of biochemistry. They can be conveniently used as tracers in biochemical research since the chemical properties of different isotopes of a particular element are identical. Therefore, the living cells cannot distinguish the radioactive isotope from a normal atom. A few important application of radioisotopes are listed

1. By the use of isotope tracers, the metabolic origin of complex molecules such as heme, cholesterol, purines and phospholipids can be determined.

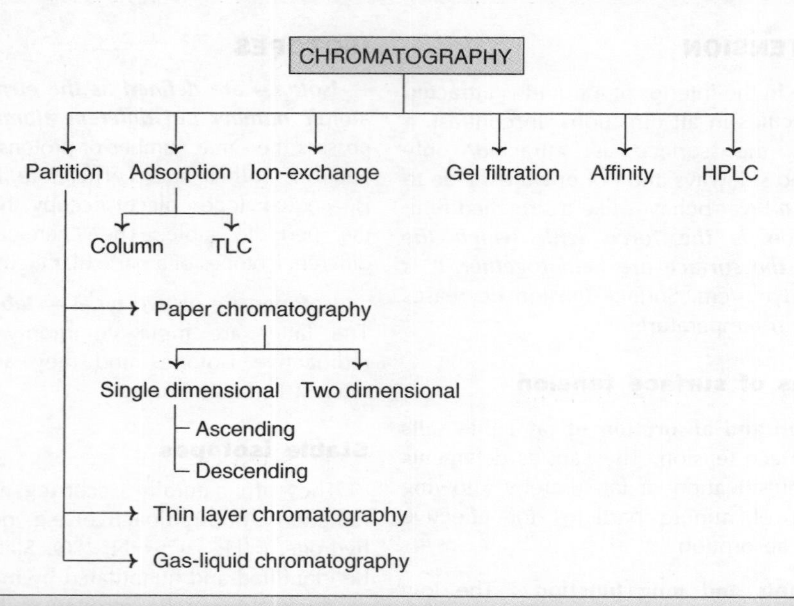

Fig. 64.3 : Important types of chromatography
(HPLC—High performance liquid chromatography; TLC—Thin layer chromatography)

2. The precursor-product relationship in several metabolic pathways has been investigated by radioisotopes. e.g. Krebs cycle, β-oxidation of fatty acids, urea cycle, fatty acid synthesis.

3. Radioisotopes are conveniently used in the study of metabolic pools (e.g. amino acid pool) and metabolic turnovers (e.g. protein turnover).

4. Certain endocrine and immunological studies also depend on the use of radioisotopes e.g. radioimmunoassay.

5. Radioisotopes are employed in elucidating drug metabolism.

TOOLS OF BIOCHEMISTRY

The foundations for the present (and the future, of course!) knowledge of biochemistry are based on the laboratory tools employed for biochemical experimentation. The basic principles of some of the commonly employed tools are described here.

CHROMATOGRAPHY

Chromatography is one of the most useful and popular tools of biochemistry. It is an analytical technique dealing with the ***separation of closely related compounds from a mixture***. These include proteins, peptides, amino acids, lipids, carbohydrates, vitamins and drugs.

Principles and classification

Chromatography (*Greek* : chroma — colour; graphein — to write), usually consists of a ***mobile phase*** and a ***stationary phase.*** The mobile phase refers to the mixture of substances (to be separated), dissoved in a liquid or a gas. The stationary phase is a porous solid matrix through which the sample contained in the mobile phase percolates. The interaction between the mobile and stationary phases results in the separation of the compounds from the mixture. These interactions include the physicochemical principles such as ***adsorption, partition, ion-exchange, molecular sieving*** and ***affinity.***

The interaction between stationary phase and mobile phase is often employed in the classification chromatography e.g. partition, adsorption, ion-exchange. Further, the classification of chromatography is also based either on the nature of the stationary phase (paper, thin layer, column), or on the nature of both mobile and stationary phases (gas-liquid chromatography). A summary of the different methods (classes) of chromatography is given in ***Fig. 64.3***.

1. **Partition chromatography :** The molecules of a mixture get partitioned between the stationary phase and mobile phase depending on their relative affinity to each one of the phases.

2. **Adsorption column chromatography :** The adsorbents such as silica gel, alumina, charcoal powder and calcium hydroxyapatite are packed into a column in a glass tube. This serves as the stationary phase. The sample mixture in a solvent is loaded on this column. The individual components get differentially adsorbed on to the adsorbent. The elution is carried out by a buffer system (mobile phase). The individual compounds come out of the column at different rates which may be separately collected and identified. For instance, amino acids can be identified by ninhydrin colorimetric method. An automated column chromatography apparatus — ***fraction collector*** — is frequently used nowadays.

3. **High performance liquid chromatography (HPLC) :** In general, the chromatographic techniques are slow and time consuming. The separation can be greatly improved by applying high pressure in the range of 5,000-10,000 psi (pounds per square inch), hence this technique is also referred (less frequently) to as high pressure liquid chromatography.

More information on chromatography with special reference to ***gel-filtration chromatography, ion-exchange chromatography, affinity chromatography and hydrophobic interaction chromatography*** is given under downstream processing (Chapter 20).

ELECTROPHORESIS

The ***movement of charged particles*** (ions) ***in an electric field*** resulting in their migration towards the oppositely charged electrode is known as electrophoresis. Molecules with a net positive charge (cations) move towards the negative cathode while those with net negative charge (anions) migrate towards positive anode. Electrophoresis is a widely used analytical technique for the separation of biological molecules such as plasma proteins, lipoproteins and immunoglobulins.

Different types of electrophoresis

1. **Zone electrophoresis :** An inert supporting material such as paper or gel are used.

2. **Isoelectric focussing :** This technique is primarily based on the ***immobilization of the molecules at isoelectric pH*** during electrophoresis. Stable pH gradients are set up (usually in a gel) covering the pH range to include the isoelectric points of the components in a mixture. Isoelectric focussing can be conveniently used for the purification of proteins.

3. **Immunoelectrophoresis :** This technique involves combination of the principles of electrophoresis and immunological reactions. Immunoelectrophoresis is useful for the analysis of complex mixtures of antigens and antibodies.

PHOTOMETRY—COLORIMETER AND SPECTROPHOTOMETER

Photometry broadly deals with the study of the phenomenon of light absorption by molecules in solution. The specificity of a compound to absorb light at a particular wavelength (monochromatic light) is exploited in the laboratory for quantitative measurements. From the biochemist's perspective, photometry forms an important laboratory tool for accurate estimation of a wide variety of compounds in biological samples. Colorimeter and spectrophotometer are the laboratory instruments used for this purpose. They work on the principles discussed below.

When a light at a particular wavelength is passed through a solution (incident light), some amount of it is absorbed and, therefore, the light that comes out (transmitted light) is diminished. The nature of light absorption in a solution is governed by ***Beer-Lambert law.***

Beer's law states that the amount of transmitted light decreases exponentially with an increase in the concentration of absorbing material (i.e. the amount of light absorbed depends on the concentration of the absorbing molecules). And according to Lambert's law, the transmitted light decreases exponentially with increase in the thickness of the absorbing molecules (i.e. the amount of light absorbed is dependent on the thickness of the medium).

The ratio of transmitted light (I) to that of incident light (I_O) is referred to as transmittance (T).

$$T = \frac{I}{I_O}$$

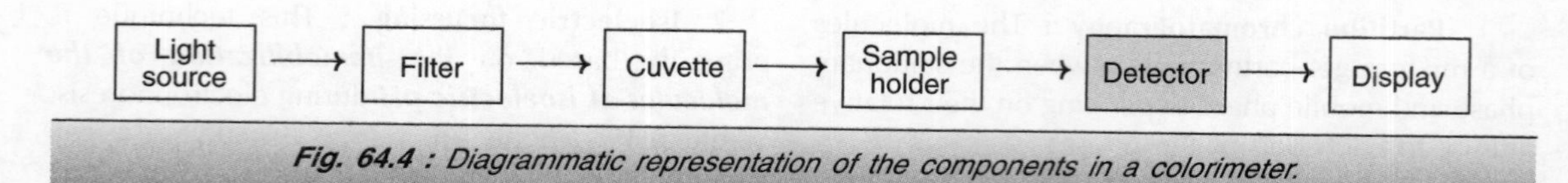

Fig. 64.4 : Diagrammatic representation of the components in a colorimeter.

Absorbance (A) or optical density (OD) is very commonly used in laboratories. The relation between absorbance and transmittance is expressed by the following equation.

$$A = 2 - \log_{10}T$$
$$= 2 - \log\% \, T$$

Colorimeter

Colorimeter (or photoelectric colorimeter) is the instrument used for the measurement of coloured substances. This instrument is operative in the visible range (400-800 nm) of the electromagnetic spectrum of light. The working of colorimeter is based on the principle of Beer-Lambert law.

The colorimeter, in general consists of light source, filter sample holder and detector with display (meter or digital). A filament lamp usually serves as a light source. The filters allow the passage of a small range of wave length as incident light. The sample holder is a special glass cuvette with a fixed thickness. The photoelectric selenium cells are the most common detectors used in colorimeter. The diagrammatic representation of a colorimeter is depicted in ***Fig. 64.4***.

Spectrophotometer

The spectrophotometer primarily differs from colorimeter by covering the ultraviolet region (200-400 nm) of the electromagnetic spectrum. Further, the spectrophotometer is more sophisticated with several additional devices that ultimately increase the sensitivity of its operation severalfold when compared to a colorimeter. A precisely selected wavelength (say 234 nm or 610 nm) in both ultra violet and visible range can be used for measurements. In place of glass cuvettes (in colorimeter), quartz cells are used in a spectrophotometer.

The spectrophotometer has similar basic components as described for a colorimeter (***Fig. 64.4***) and its operation is also based on the Beer-Lambert law.

ULTRACENTRIFUGATION

Ultracentrifugation is an indispensable tool for the isolation of subcellular organelles, proteins and nucleic acids. In addition, this technique is also employed for the determination of molecular weights of macromolecules.

The rate at which the sedimentation occurs in ultracentrifugation primarily depends on the size and shape of the particles or macromolecules (i.e. on the molecular weight). It is expressed in terms of ***sedimentation coefficient***(s).

The sedimentation coefficient has the units of seconds. It was usually expressed in units of 10^{-13} s (since several biological macromolecules occur in this range), which is designated as one ***Svedberg unit.*** For instance, the sedimentation coefficient of hemoglobin is 4×10^{-13} s or 4S; ribonuclease is 2×10^{-13} s or 2S. Conventionally, the subcellular organelles are often referred to by their S value e.g. 70S ribosome.

Isolation of subcellular organelles by centrifugation

The cells are subjected to disruption by sonication or osmotic shock or by use of homogenizer. This is usually carried out in an isotonic (0.25 M) sucrose. The advantage with sucrose medium is that it does not cause the organelles to swell. The subcellular particles can be separated by differential centrifugation. The most commonly employed laboratory method separates subcellular organelles into 3 major fractions—nuclear, mitochondrial and microsomal (***Fig. 64.5***).

When the homogenate is centrifuged at 700 g for about 10 min, the nuclear fraction (includes plasma membrane) gets sedimented. On centrifuging the supernatant (I) at 15,000 g for about 5 min mitochondrial fraction (that includes lysosomes, peroxisomes) is pelleted. Further centrifugation of the supernatant (II) at 100,000 g for about 60 min separates microsomal fraction (that includes ribosomes and endoplasmic reticulum). The supernatant (III) then obtained corresponds to the cytosol.

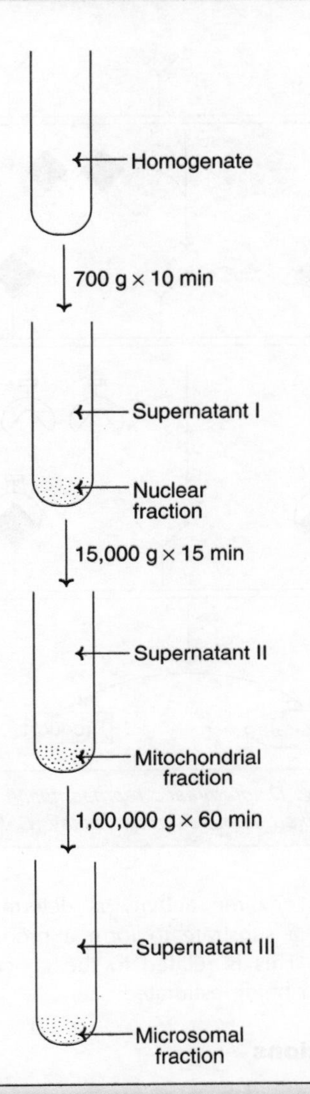

Fig. 64.5 : Separation of subcellular fractions by differential centrifugation.

The purity (or contamination) of the subcellular fractionation can be checked by the use of ***marker enzymes.*** DNA polymerase is the marker enzyme for nucleus, while glutamate dehydrogenase and glucose 6-phosphatase are the markers for mitochondria and ribosomes, respectively. Hexokinase is the marker enzyme for cytosol.

RADIOIMMUNOASSAY

Radioimmunoassay (RIA) was developed in 1959 by Solomon, Benson and Rosalyn Yalow for the estimation of insulin in human serum. This technique has revolutionized the estimation of several compounds in biological fluids that are found in exceedingly low concentrations (nanogram or picogram). RIA is a highly sensitive and specific analytical tool.

Principle

Radioimmunoassay combines the principles of ***radioactivity*** of isotopes and ***immunological*** reactions of antigen and antibody, hence the name.

The principle of RIA is primarily based on the competition between the labeled and unlabeled antigens to bind with antibody to form antigen-antibody complexes (either labelled or unlabeled). The unlabeled antigen is the substance (say insulin) to be determined. The antibody to it is produced by injecting the antigen to a goat or a rabbit. The specific antibody (Ab) is then subjected to react with unlabeled antigen in the presence of excess amounts of isotopically labeled (^{131}I) antigen (Ag^+) with known radioactivity. There occurs a competition between the antigens (Ag^+ and Ag) to bind the antibody. Certainly, the labeled Ag^+ will have an upper hand due to its excess presence.

$$Ag^+ + Ab \longrightarrow Ag^+Ab$$

$$Ag \rightarrow Ag^+ \quad \downarrow \quad Ag\text{-}Ab$$

As the concentration of unlabeled antigen (Ag) increases the amount of labelled antigen-antibody complex (Ag^+-Ab) decreases. Thus, the concentration of Ag^+-Ab is inversely related to the concentration of unlabeled Ag i.e. the substance to be determined. This relation is almost linear. A standard curve can be drawn by using different concentrations of unlabeled antigen and the same quantities of antibody and labeled antigen.

The labeled antigen-antibody (Ag^+-Ab) complex is separated by precipitation. The radioactivity of ^{131}I present is Ag^+-Ab is determined.

Applications

RIA is no more limited to estimating of hormones and proteins that exhibit antigenic properties. By the use of ***haptens*** (small molecules such as dinitrophenol, which, by themselves, are not antigenic), several substances can be made antigenic to elicit specific antibody responses. In this way, a wide variety of compounds have been brought under the net of RIA estimation. These include peptides, steroid hormones, vitamins, drugs, antibiotics, nucleic acids, structural proteins and hormone receptor proteins.

Radioimmunoassay has tremendous application in the diagnosis of hormonal disorders, cancers and therapeutic monitoring of drugs, besides being useful in biomedical research.

ENZYME-LINKED IMMUNOSORBANT ASSAY

Enzyme-linked immunosorbant assay (ELISA) is a non-isotopic immunoassay. An enzyme is used as a label in ELISA in place of radioactive isotope employed in RIA. ELISA is as sensitive as or even more sensitive than RIA. In addition, there is no risk of radiation hazards (as is the case with RIA) in ELISA.

Principle

ELISA is based on the immunochemical principles of antigen-antibody reaction. The stages of ELISA, depicted in ***Fig. 64.6***, are summarized.

1. The antibody against the protein to be determined is fixed on an inert solid such as polystyrene.

2. The biological sample containing the protein to be estimated is applied on the antibody coated surface.

3. The protein antibody complex is then reacted with a second protein specific antibody to which an enzyme is covalently linked. These enzymes must be easily assayable and produce preferably coloured products. Peroxidase, amylase and alkaline phosphatase are commonly used.

4. After washing the unbound antibody linked enzyme, the enzyme bound to the second antibody complex is assayed.

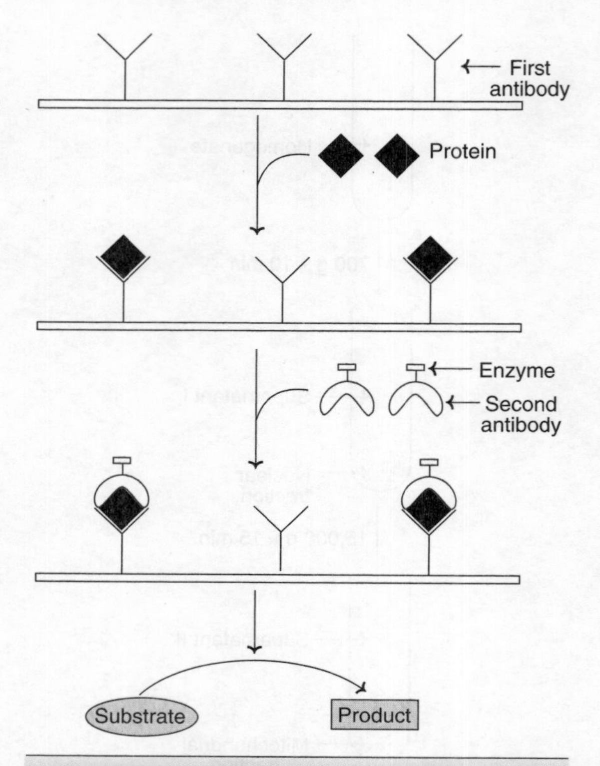

***Fig. 64.6 :** Diagrammatic representation of enzyme-linked immunosorbant assay (ELISA).*

5. The enzyme activity is determined by its action on a substrate to form a product (usually coloured). This is related to the concentration of the protein being estimated.

Applications

ELISA is widely used for the determination of small quantities of proteins (hormones, antigens, antibodies) and other biological substances. The most commonly used pregnancy test for the detection of human chorionic gonadotropin (hCG) in urine is based on ELISA. By this test, pregnancy can be detected within few days after conception. ELISA is also useful for the diagnosis of AIDS.

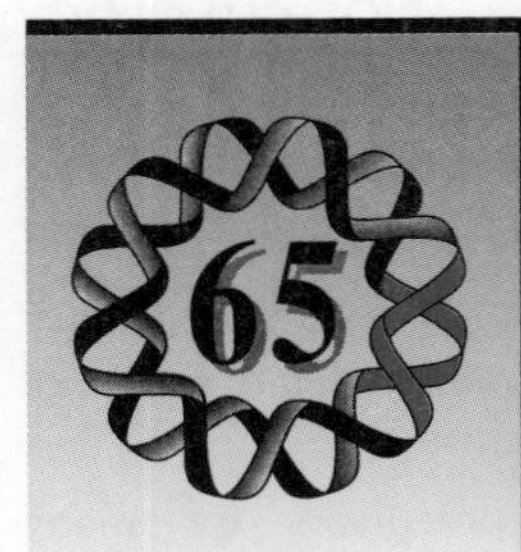

Biomolecules

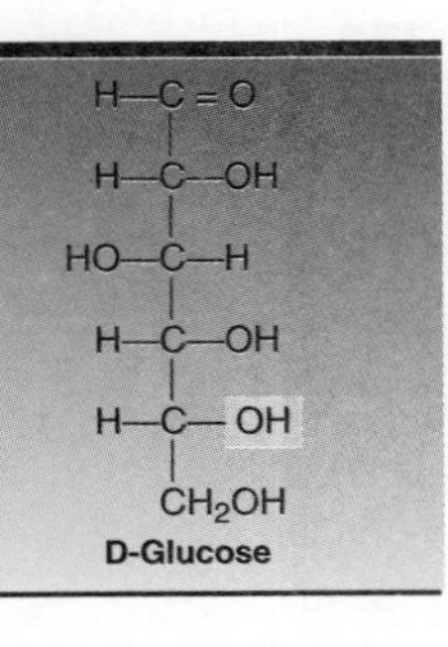

The living matter is composed of mainly six elements — ***carbon***, ***hydrogen***, ***oxygen***, ***nitrogen***, ***phosphorus*** and ***sulfur***. These elements together constitute about 90% of the dry weight of the human body. Several other functionally important elements are also found in the cells. These include Ca, K, Na, Cl, Mg, Fe, Cu, Co, I, Zn, F, Mo and Se.

Carbon—a unique element of life

Carbon is the most predominant and versatile element of life. It possesses a unique property to form infinite number of compounds. This is attributed to the ability of carbon to form stable covalent bonds and C—C chains of unlimited length. It is estimated that about 90% of compounds found in living system invariably contain carbon.

CHEMICAL MOLECULES OF LIFE

Life is composed of lifeless chemical molecules. A single cell of the bacterium, *Escherichia coli* contains about 6,000 different organic compounds. It is believed that man may contain about 100,000 different types of molecules although only a few of them have been characterized.

Complex biomolecules

The organic compounds such as amino acids, nucleotides and monosaccharides serve as the ***monomeric units*** or building blocks of complex biomolecules — proteins, nucleic acids (DNA and RNA) and polysaccharides, respectively. The important biomolecules (macromolecules) with their respective building blocks and major functions are given in ***Table 65.1***. As regards lipids, it may be

TABLE 65.1 The major complex biomolecules of cells

Biomolecule	*Building block (repeating unit)*	*Major functions*
Protein	Amino acids	Fundamental basis of structure and function of cell (static and dynamic functions).
Deoxyribonucleic acid (DNA)	Deoxyribonucleotides	Repository of hereditary information.
Ribonucleic acid (RNA)	Ribonucleotides	Essentially required for protein biosynthesis.
Polysaccharide (glycogen)	Monosaccharides (glucose)	Storage form of energy to meet short term demands.
Lipids	Fatty acids, glycerol	Storage form of energy to meet long term demands; structural components of membranes.

Table 65.2 Chemical composition of a normal man (weight 65 kg)

Constituent	*Percent (%)*	*Weight (kg)*
Water	61.6	40
Protein	17.0	11
Lipid	13.8	9
Carbohydrate	1.5	1
Minerals	6.1	4

noted that they are not biopolymers in a strict sense, but majority of them contain fatty acids.

Structural heirarchy of an organism

The macromolecules (proteins, lipids, nucleic acids and polysaccharides) form supramolecular assemblies (e.g. membranes) which in turn organize into organelles, cells, tissues, organs and finally the whole organism.

Chemical composition of man

The chemical composition of a normal man, weighing 65 kg, is given in ***Table 65.2***. Water is the solvent of life and contributes to more than 60% of the weight. This is followed by protein (mostly in muscle) and lipid (mostly in adipose tissue). The carbohydrate content is rather low which is in the form of glycogen.

The basic information on the various biomolecules is essential for a better understanding of the concepts of biotechnology. An overview of the chemistry of carbohydrates, lipids and proteins (amino acids) is described in this Chapter. The ***biomolecules namely nucleic acids (DNA and RNA) which are directly relevant to biotechnology are described in Chapter 11.***

CARBOHYDRATES

Carbohydrates are the most abundant organic molecules in nature. They are primarily composed of the elements ***carbon, hydrogen and oxygen***. The name carbohydrate literally means 'hydrates of carbon.'

Carbohydrates may be defined as polyhydroxy-aldehydes or ketones or compounds which produce them on hydrolysis. The term 'sugar' is applied to carbohydrates soluble in water and sweet to taste.

Functions of carbohydrates

Carbohydrates participate in a wide range of functions

1. They are the most abundant dietary source of energy (4 Cal/g) for all organisms.

2. Carbohydrates are precursors for many organic compounds (fats, amino acids).

3. Carbohydrates (as glycoproteins and glycolipids) participate in the structure of cell membrane and cellular functions such as cell growth, adhesion and fertilization.

4. Carbohydrates also serve as the storage form of energy (glycogen) to meet the immediate energy demands of the body.

CLASSIFICATION OF CARBOHYDRATES

Carbohydrates are often referred to as saccharides (*Greek* : sakcharon-sugar). They are broadly classified into 3 groups—***monosaccharides, oligosaccharides*** and ***polysaccharides***. This categorization is based on the number of sugar units. Mono- and oligosaccharides are sweet to taste, crystalline in character and soluble in water, hence they are commonly known as ***sugars***.

Monosaccharides

Monosaccharides (*Greek* : mono-one) are the simplest group of carbohydrates and are often referred to as simple sugars. They have the general formula $C_n(H_2O)_n$, and they cannot be further hydrolysed.

Based on the number of carbon atoms, the monosaccharides are regarded as trioses (3C), tetroses (4C), pentoses (5C), hexoses (6C) and heptoses (7C). These terms along with functional groups are used while naming monosaccharides. For instance, ***glucose is a aldohexose while fructose is a ketohexose.***

Oligosaccharides

Oligosaccharides (*Greek* : oligo-few) contain 2-10 monosaccharide molecules which are liberated on hydrolysis. Based on the number of monosaccharide units present, the oligosaccharides are further subdivided to ***disaccharides, trisaccharides*** etc.

Polysaccharides

Polysaccharides (*Greek* : poly-many) are polymers of monosaccharide units with high molecular weight (up to a million). They are usually tasteless (non-sugars) and form colloids with water. Polysaccharides are of two types—***homopolysaccharides*** and ***heteropolysaccharides***.

MONOSACCHARIDES

Stereoisomerism is an important character of monosaccharides. Stereoisomers are the compounds that have the same structural formulae but differ in their spatial configuration.

A carbon is said to be asymmetric when it is attached to four different atoms or groups. The number of asymmetric carbon atoms (n) determines the possible isomers of a given compound which is equal to 2^n. Glucose contains 4 asymmetric carbons and thus has 16 isomers.

Glyceraldehyde—the reference carbohydrate

Glyceraldehyde (triose) is the simplest monosaccharide with one asymmetric carbon atom. It exists as two stereoisomers, and has been chosen as the reference carbohydrate to represent the structure of all other carbohydrates.

D- and L-isomers

The D- and L-isomers are mirror images of each other. The spacial orientation of —H and —OH groups on the carbon atom (C_5 for glucose) that is adjacent to the terminal primary alcohol carbon determines whether the sugar is D- or L-isomer. If the —OH group is on the right side, the sugar is of D-series, and if on the left side, it belongs to L-series. The structures of D- and L-glucose based on the reference monosaccharide, D- and L-glyceraldehyde (glycerose) are depicted in ***Fig. 65.1***.

It may be noted that the naturally occurring monosaccharides in the mammalian tissues are mostly of D-configuration. The enzyme machinery of cells is specific to metabolise D-series of monosaccharides.

Optical activity of sugars

Optical activity is a characteristic feature of compounds with asymmetric carbon atom. When a beam of polarized light is passed through a solution

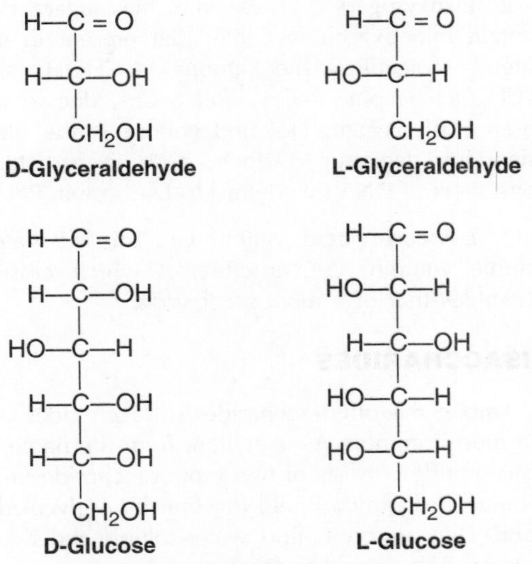

H—C = O
H—C—OH
CH_2OH
D-Glyceraldehyde

H—C = O
HO—C—H
CH_2OH
L-Glyceraldehyde

H—C = O
H—C—OH
HO—C—H
H—C—OH
H—C—OH
CH_2OH
D-Glucose

H—C = O
HO—C—H
H—C—OH
HO—C—H
HO—C—H
CH_2OH
L-Glucose

Fig. 65.1 : D- and L-forms of glucose compared with D- and L-glyceraldehydes (the reference carbohydrate).

of an optical isomer, it will be rotated either to the right or left. The term ***dextrorotatory*** (+) ***and levorotatory*** (–) are used to compounds that respectively rotate the plane of polarized light to the right or to the left.

GLYCOSIDES

Glycosides are formed when the hemiacetal or hemiketal hydroxyl group (of anomeric carbon) of a carbohydrate reacts with a hydroxyl group of another carbohydrate or a non-carbohydrate (e.g. methyl alcohol, phenol, glycerol). The bond so formed is known as ***glycosidic bond*** and the non-carbohydrate moiety (when present) is referred to as ***aglycone***.

DERIVATIVES OF MONOSACCHARIDES

There are several derivatives of monosaccharides, some of which are physiologically important

1. **Amino sugars :** When one or more hydroxyl groups of the monosaccharides are replaced by amino groups, the products formed are amino sugars e.g. D-glucosamine, D-galactosamine. They are present as constituents of heteropolysaccharides.

2. **Deoxysugars :** These are the sugars that contain one oxygen less than that present in the parent molecule. The groups —CHOH and —CH_2OH become —CH_2 and —CH_3 due to the absence of oxygen. D-2-Deoxyribose is the most important deoxysugar since it is a structural constituent of DNA (in contrast to D-ribose in RNA).

3. **L-Ascorbic acid** (vitamin C) **:** This is a water-soluble vitamin, the structure of which closely resembles that of a monosaccharide.

DISACCHARIDES

Among the oligosaccharides, disaccharides are the most common. As is evident from the name, a disaccharide consists of two monosaccharide units (similar or dissimilar) held together by a ***glycosidic bond***. They are crystalline, water-soluble and sweet to taste. The disaccharides are of two types

1. **Reducing** disaccharides with free aldehyde or keto group e.g. maltose, lactose.

2. **Non-reducing** disaccharides with no free aldehyde or keto group e.g. sucrose, trehalose.

POLYSACCHARIDES

Polysaccharides (or simply glycans) consist of repeat units of monosaccharides or their derivatives, held together by glycosidic bonds. They are primarily concerned with two important functions-structural, and storage of energy.

Polysaccharides are of two types

1. **Homopolysaccharides** which on hydrolysis yield only a single type of monosaccharide. They are named based on the nature of the monosaccharide unit. Thus, ***glucans*** are polymers of glucose whereas ***fructosans*** are polymers of fructose.

2. **Heteropolysaccharides** on hydrolysis yield a mixture of a few monosaccharides or their derivatives.

HOMOPOLYSACCHARIDES

Starch

Starch is the carbohydrate reserve of plants which is the most important dietary source for higher animals, including man. High content of starch is found in cereals, roots, tubers, vegetables etc. Starch is a homopolymer composed of D-glucose units held by α-glycosidic bonds. It is known as ***glucosan or glucan***.

Starch consists of two polysaccharide components-water soluble ***amylose*** (15-20%) and a water insoluble ***amylopectin*** (80-85%). Chemically, amylose is a long unbranched chain with 200–1,000 D-glucose units held by α (1 → 4) glycosidic linkages. Amylopectin, on the other hand, is a branched chain with α (1 → 6) glycosidic bonds at the branching points and α (1 → 4) linkages everywhere else. Amylopectin molecule containing a few thousand glucose units looks like a branched tree (20–30 glucose units per branch).

Glycogen

Glycogen is the carbohydrate reserve in animals, hence often referred to as ***animal starch***. It is present in high concentration in liver, followed by muscle, brain etc. Glycogen is also found in plants that do not possess chlorophyll (e.g. yeast, fungi).

The structure of glycogen is similar to that of amylopectin with more number of branches. Glucose is the repeating unit in glycogen joined together by α (1 → 4) glycosidic bonds, and α (1 → 6) glycosidic bonds at branching points.

Cellulose

Cellulose occurs exclusively in plants and it is the most abundant organic substance in plant kingdom. It is a predominant constituent of plant cell wall. Cellulose is totally absent in animal body.

Cellulose is composed of β-D-glucose units linked by ***β (1 → 4) glycosidic bonds***. Cellulose cannot be digested by mammals—including man—due to lack of the enzyme that cleaves β-glycosidic bonds (α amylase breaks α bonds only). Certain ruminants and herbivorous animals contain microorganisms in the gut which produce enzymes that can cleave β-glycosidic bonds. Hydrolysis of cellulose yields a disaccharide ***cellobiose,*** followed by ***β-D-glucose***.

Cellulose, though not digested, has great importance in human nutrition. It is a major constituent of ***fiber***, the ***non-digestable carbohydrate***. The functions of dietary fiber include decreasing the absorption of glucose and cholesterol from the intestine, besides increasing the bulk of feces.

HETEROPOLYSACCHARIDES

When the polysaccharides are composed of different types of sugars or their derivatives, they are referred to as heteropolysaccharides or ***heteroglycans***.

Mucopolysaccharides

These are heteroglycans made up of repeating units of sugar derivatives, namely amino sugars and uronic acids. Mucopolysaccharides are more commonly known as ***glycosaminoglycans (GAG)***. Acetylated amino groups, besides sulfate and carboxyl groups are generally present in GAG structure.

Some of the mucopolysaccharides are found in combination with proteins to form ***mucoproteins*** or ***mucoids*** or ***proteoglycans***. Mucoproteins may contain up to 95% carbohydrate and 5% protein.

Mucopolysaccharides are essential components of tissue structure. The extracellular spaces of tissue (particularly connective tissue-cartilage, skin, blood vessels, tendons) consist of collagen and elastin fibers embedded in a matrix or ground substance. The ground substance is predominantly composed of GAG.

The important mucopolysaccharides include hyaluronic acid, chondroitin 4-sulfate, heparin, dermatan sulfate and keratan sulfate.

LIPIDS

Lipids (*Greek* : lipos-fat) are of great importance to the body as the chief concentrated storage form of energy, besides their role in cellular structure and various other biochemical functions. As such, lipids are a heterogeneous group of compounds.

Lipids may be regarded as organic substances relatively insoluble in water, soluble in organic solvents (alcohol, ether etc.), actually or potentially related to fatty acids and utilized by the living cells.

Unlike the polysaccharides, proteins and nucleic acids, lipids are not polymers. They are mostly small molecules.

CLASSIFICATION OF LIPIDS

Lipids are broadly classified (modified from Bloor) into simple, complex, derived and miscellaneous lipids, which are further subdivided.

1. **Simple lipids :** Esters of fatty acids with alcohols. These are mainly of two types

   (a) **Fats and oils** (triacylglycerols) **:** These are esters of fatty acids with glycerol. The difference between fat and oil is only physical. Thus, oil is a liquid while fat is a solid at room temperature.

   (b) **Waxes :** Esters of fatty acids (usually long chain) with alcohols other than glycerol. Cetyl alcohol is most commonly found in waxes.

2. **Complex (or compound) lipids :** Esters of fatty acids with alcohols containing additional groups such as phosphate, nitrogenous base, carbohydrate, protein etc. They are further divided :

   (a) **Phospholipids :** Lipids containing phosphoric acid and frequently a nitrogenous base. This is in addition to alcohol and fatty acids.

   (b) **Glycolipids :** These lipids contain a fatty acid, carbohydrate and nitrogenous base. The alcohol is sphingosine, hence they are also called as glycosphingolipids. Glycerol and phosphate are absent e.g., cerebrosides, gangliosides.

   (c) **Lipoproteins :** Macromolecular complexes of lipids with proteins.

   (d) **Other complex lipids :** Sulfolipids, aminolipids and lipopolysaccharides are among the other complex lipids.

3. **Derived lipids :** These are the derivatives obtained on the hydrolysis of group I and group 2 lipids which possess the characteristics of lipids. These include glycerol and other alcohols, fatty acids, mono- and diacylglycerols, lipid soluble vitamins, steroid hormones, hydrocarbons and ketone bodies.

4. **Miscellaneous lipids :** These include a large number of compounds possessing the characteristics of lipids e.g., carotenoids, squalene, hydrocarbons such as pentacosane (in bees wax), terpenes etc.

5. **Neutral lipids :** The lipids which are uncharged are referred to as neutral lipids. These are mono-, di-, and triacylglycerols, cholesterol and cholesteryl esters.

Functions of lipids

Lipids perform several important functions

1. They are the concentrated fuel reserve of the body (triacylglycerols).

2. Lipids are the constituents of membrane structure and regulate the membrane permeability (phospholipids and cholesterol).

3. They serve as a source of fat soluble vitamins (A, D, E and K).

4. Lipids are important as cellular metabolic regulators (steroid hormones and prostaglandins).

FATTY ACIDS

Fatty acids are carboxylic acids with hydrocarbon side chain. They are the simplest form of lipids.

Even and odd carbon fatty acids

Most of the fatty acids that occur in natural lipids are of even carbons (usually 14C–20C). This is due to the fact that biosynthesis of fatty acids mainly occurs with the sequential addition of 2 carbon units. Palmitic acid (16C) and stearic acid (18C) are the most common. Among the odd chain fatty acids, propionic acid (3C) and valeric acid (5C) are well known.

Saturated and unsaturated fatty acids

Saturated fatty acids do not contain double bonds, while unsaturated fatty acids contain one or more double bonds. Both saturated and unsaturated fatty acids almost equally occur in the natural lipids. Fatty acids with one double bond are known as monounsaturated and those with 2 or more double bonds are collectively known as ***polyunsaturated fatty acids (PUFA)***.

Shorthand representation of fatty acids

Instead of writing the full structures, biochemists employ shorthand notations (by numbers) to represent fatty acids. The general rule is that the total number of carbon atoms is written first, followed by the number of double bonds and finally the (first carbon) position of double bonds, starting from the carboxyl end. Thus, saturated fatty acid, palmitic acid is written as 16 : 0, oleic acid as 18 : 1; 9, arachidonic acid as 20 : 4; 5, 8, 11, 14.

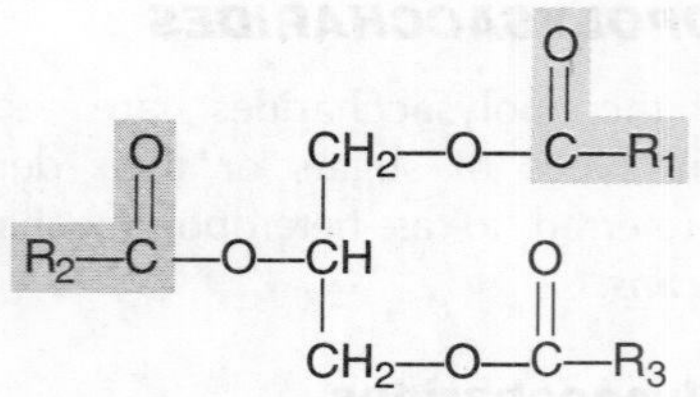

$$\begin{array}{l} CH_2-O-\overset{O}{\overset{\|}{C}}-R_1 \\ R_2-\overset{O}{\overset{\|}{C}}-O-CH \\ CH_2-O-\overset{O}{\overset{\|}{C}}-R_3 \end{array}$$

Triacylglycerol

Fig. 65.2 : General structure of triacylglycerol.

Essential fatty acids

The fatty acids that cannot be synthesized by the body and, therefore, should be supplied in the diet are known as essential fatty acids (EFA). Chemically, they are polyunsaturated fatty acids, namely ***linoleic acid*** (18 : 2; 9, 12) and ***linolenic acid*** (18 : 3; 9, 12, 15). ***Arachidonic acid*** (20 : 4; 5, 8, 11, 14) becomes essential, if its precursor linoleic acid is not provided in the diet in sufficient amounts.

TRIACYLGLYCEROLS

Triacylglycerols (formerly triglycerides) are the esters of glycerol with fatty acids. The fats and oils that are widely distributed in both plants and animals are chemically triacylglycerols. They are insoluble in water and non-polar in character and commonly known as neutral fats.

Fats as stored fuel : Triacylglycerols are the most abundant group of lipids that primarily function as fuel reserves of animals. The fat reserve of normal humans (men 20%, women 25% by weight) is sufficient to meet the body caloric requirements for 2-3 months.

Structures of acylglycerols : Monoacylglycerols, diacylglycerols and triacylglycerols, respectively consisting of one, two and three molecules of fatty acids esterified to a molecule of glycerol, are known. Among these, triacylglycerols are the most important biochemically.

Triacylglycerols of plants have higher content of unsaturated fatty acids compared to that of animals.

PHOSPHOLIPIDS

These are complex or compound lipids containing phosphoric acid, in addition to fatty

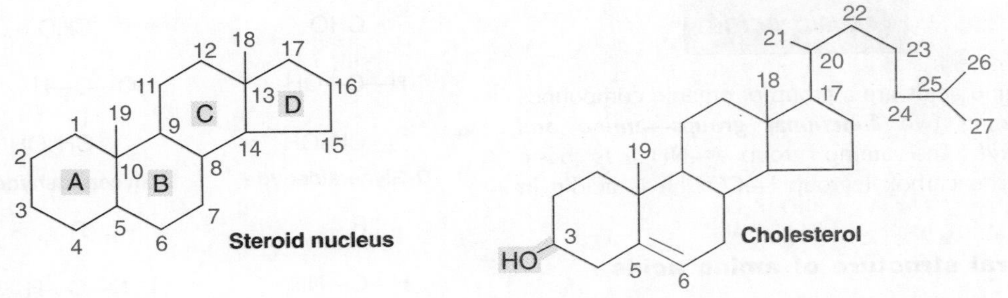

Steroid nucleus

Cholesterol

Fig. 65.3 : Structures of steroids (A, B, C-Perhydrophenanthrene; D-Cyclopentane).

acids, nitrogenous base and alcohol. There are two classes of phospholipids

1. Glycerophospholipids (or phosphoglycerides) that contain glycerol as the alcohol. e.g. lecithins, cephalins, phosphatidylinositol, phosphatidylserine, plasmalogens.

2. Sphingophospholipids (or sphingomyelins) that contain sphingosine as the alcohol. e.g. ceramide.

LIPOPROTEINS

Lipoproteins are molecular complexes of lipids with proteins. They are the transport vehicles for lipids in the circulation. There are five types of lipoproteins, namely ***chylomicrons, very low density lipoproteins (VLDL), low density lipoproteins (LDL), high density lipoproteins (HDL) and free fatty acid-albumin complexes.***

STEROIDS

Steroids are the compounds containing a cyclic steroid nucleus (or ring) namely cyclopentanoperhydrophenanthrene (CPPP). It consists of a phenanthrene nucleus (rings A, B and C) to which a cyclopentane ring (D) is attached.

There are several steroids in the biological system. These include ***cholesterol, bile acids, vitamin D, sex hormones*** and ***adrenocortical hormones***. If the steroid contains one or more hydroxyl groups it is commonly known as ***sterol*** (means solid alcohol). The structures of steroid nucleus and cholesterol are depicted in ***Fig. 65.3***.

PROTEINS AND AMINO ACIDS

Proteins are the most abundant organic molecules of the living system. They occur in every part of the cell and constitute about 50% of cellular dry weight. Proteins form the fundamental basis of structure and function of life.

Functions of proteins

Proteins perform a great variety of specialized and essential functions in the living cells. These functions may be broadly grouped as ***static*** (*structural*) and ***dynamic***.

Structural functions : Certain proteins perform 'brick and mortar' roles and are primarily responsible for structure and strength of body. These include ***collagen*** and ***elastin*** found in bone matrix, vascular system and other organs and ***α-keratin*** present in epidermal tissues.

Dynamic functions : The dynamic functions of proteins are more diversified in nature. These include proteins acting as ***enzymes, hormones, blood clotting factors, immunoglobulins***, membrane receptors, storage proteins, besides their function in genetic control, muscle contraction, respiration etc. Proteins performing dynamic functions are appropriately regarded as '***the working horses***' of cell.

Proteins are polymers of amino acids

Proteins on complete hydrolysis (with concentrated HCl for several hours) yield L-α-amino acids. This is a common property of all the proteins. Therefore, proteins are the polymers of ***L-α-amino acids.***

AMINO ACIDS

Amino acids are a group of organic compounds containing two ***functional groups—amino and carboxyl***. The amino group (—NH_2) is basic while the carboxyl group (—COOH) is acidic in nature.

General structure of amino acids

The amino acids are termed as α-amino acids, if both the carboxyl and amino groups are attached to the same carbon atom, as depicted below

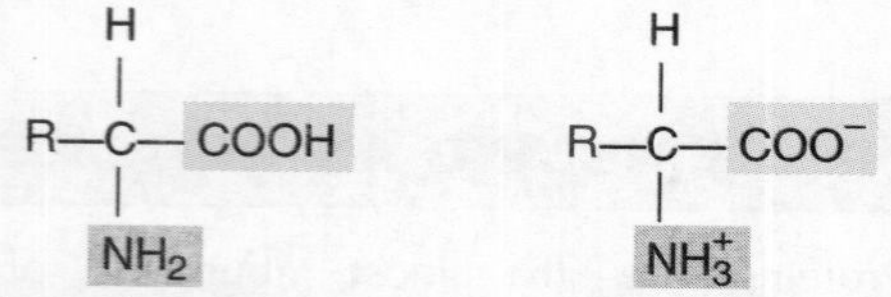

$$R{-}\overset{H}{\underset{NH_2}{C}}{-}COOH \qquad R{-}\overset{H}{\underset{NH_3^+}{C}}{-}COO^-$$

General structure **Exists as ion**

The α-carbon atom binds to a side chain represented by R which is different for each of the 20 amino acids found in proteins. The amino acids mostly exist in the ionized form in the biological system (shown above).

Optical isomers of amino acids

If a carbon atom is attached to four different groups, it is asymmetric and therefore exhibits optical isomerism. The amino acids (except glycine) possess four distinct groups (R, H, COO^-, NH_3^+) held by α-carbon. Thus all the amino acids (except glycine where R = H) have optical isomers.

The structures of L- and D-amino acids are written based on the configuration of L- and D-glyceraldehyde as shown in ***Fig. 65.4***. The proteins are composed of L-α-amino acids

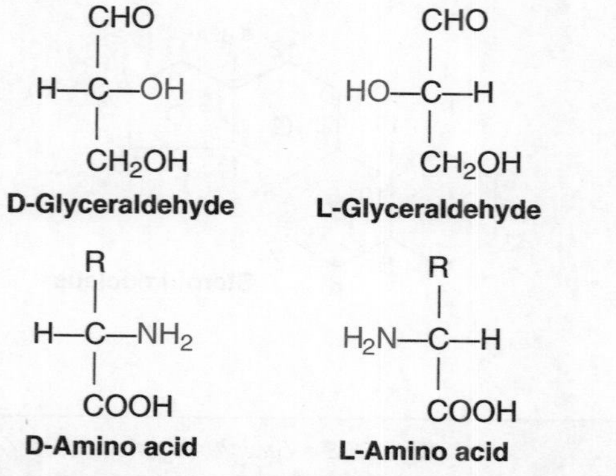

CHO / H—C—OH / CH_2OH — **D-Glyceraldehyde**

CHO / HO—C—H / CH_2OH — **L-Glyceraldehyde**

R / H—C—NH_2 / COOH — **D-Amino acid**

R / H_2N—C—H / COOH — **L-Amino acid**

Fig. 65.4 : *D- and L-forms of amino acid based on the structure of glyceraldehyde.*

Classification of amino acids

There are different ways of classifying the amino acids based on the structure and chemical nature, nutritional requirement, metabolic fate etc.

A. Amino acid classification based on the structure : A comprehensive classification of amino acids is based on their structure and chemical nature. Each amino acid is assigned a 3 letter or 1 letter symbol. These symbols are commonly used to represent the amino acids. The 20 amino acids found in proteins are divided into seven distinct groups.

In ***Table 65.3***, the different groups of amino acids, their symbols and structures are given.

B. Nutritional classification of amino acids : The twenty amino acids (Table 65.3) are required for the synthesis of variety of proteins, besides other biological functions. However, all these 20 amino acids need not be taken in the diet. Based on the nutritional requirements, amino acids are grouped into two classes—essential and non-essential.

1. **Essential or indispensable amino acids :** The amino acids which cannot be synthesized by the human body and, therefore, need to be supplied through the diet are called essential amino acids. They are required for proper growth and maintenance of the individual. The ten amino acids listed below are essential for humans (and also rats) :

   Arginine, **V**aline, **H**istidine, **I**soleucine, **L**eucine, **L**ysine, **M**ethionine, **P**henylalanine, **T**hreonine, **T**ryptophan.

   [The code ***A.V. HILL, MP., T. T.*** (first letter of each amino acid) may be memorized to recall essential amino acids. Other useful codes are H. VITTAL, LMP and MATTVILPhLy.]

2. **Non-essential or dispensable amino acids :** The body can synthesize about 10 amino acids to meet the biological needs, hence they need not be consumed in the diet. These are — glycine, alanine, serine, cysteine, aspartate, asparagine, glutamate, glutamine, tyrosine and proline.

TABLE 65.3 Structural classification of L-α-amino acids found in proteins

Name	*Symbol*		*Structure*	*Special group present*
	3 letters	*1 letter*		
I. Amino acids with aliphatic side chains				
1. Glycine	Gly	G	$H{-}CH(NH_3^+){-}COO^-$	
2. Alanine	Ala	A	$CH_3{-}CH(NH_3^+){-}COO^-$	
3. Valine	Val	V	$(H_3C)_2CH{-}CH(NH_3^+){-}COO^-$	Branched chain
4. Leucine	Leu	L	$(H_3C)_2CH{-}CH_2{-}CH(NH_3^+){-}COO^-$	Branched chain
5. Isoleucine	Ile	I	$CH_3{-}CH_2{-}CH(CH_3){-}CH(NH_3^+){-}COO^-$	Branched chain
II. Amino acids containing hydroxyl (—OH) groups				
6. Serine	Ser	S	$CH_2(OH){-}CH(NH_3^+){-}COO^-$	Hydroxyl
7. Threonine	Thr	T	$H_3C{-}CH(OH){-}CH(NH_3^+){-}COO^-$	Hydroxyl
Tyrosine	Tyr	Y	See under aromatic	Hydroxyl

Table 65.3 contd. next page

Name	Symbol 3 letters	Symbol 1 letter	Structure	Special group present
III. Sulfur containing amino acids				
8. Cysteine	Cys	C	$CH_2-CH-COO^-$ SH NH_3^+	Sulfhydryl
Cystine	—	—	$CH_2-CH-COO^-$ S NH_3^+ S $CH_2-CH-COO^-$ NH_3^+	Disulfide
9. Methionine	Met	M	$CH_2-CH_2-CH-COO^-$ $S-CH_3$ NH_3^+	Thioether
IV. Acidic amino acids and their amides				
10. Aspartic acid	Asp	D	β α $^-OOC-CH_2-CH-COO^-$ NH_3^+	β-Carboxyl
11. Asparagine	Asn	N	$H_2N-C(=O)-CH_2-CH-COO^-$ NH_3^+	Amide
12. Glutamic acid	Glu	E	γ β α $^-OOC-CH_2-CH_2-CH-COO^-$ NH_3^+	γ-Carboxyl
13. Glutamine	Gln	Q	$H_2N-C(=O)-CH_2-CH_2-CH-COO^-$ NH_3^+	Amide
V. Basic amino acids				
14. Lysine	Lys	K	ε δ γ β α $CH_2-CH_2-CH_2-CH_2-CH-COO^-$ NH_3^+ NH_3^+	ε-Amino
15. Arginine	Arg	R	$NH-CH_2-CH_2-CH_2-CH-COO^-$ $C=NH_2^+$ NH_3^+ NH_2	Guanidino
16. Histidine	His	H	(imidazole ring: HN, N)$-CH_2-CH-COO^-$ NH_3^+	Imidazole

Table 65.3 contd. next page

Name	Symbol 3 letters	Symbol 1 letter	Structure	Special group present
VI. Aromatic amino acids				
17. Phenylalanine	Phe	F	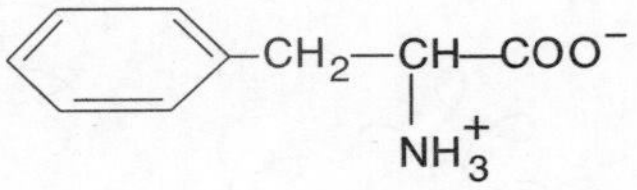 C_6H_5–CH_2–CH(NH_3^+)–COO^-	Benzene or phenyl
18. Tyrosine	Tyr	Y	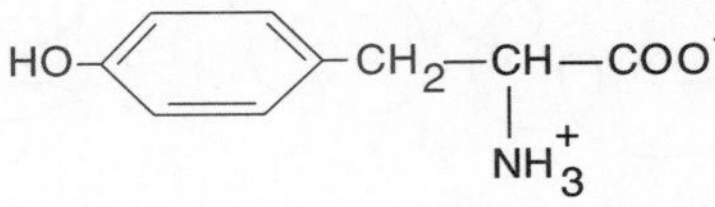 HO–C_6H_4–CH_2–CH(NH_3^+)–COO^-	Phenol
19. Tryptophan	Trp	W	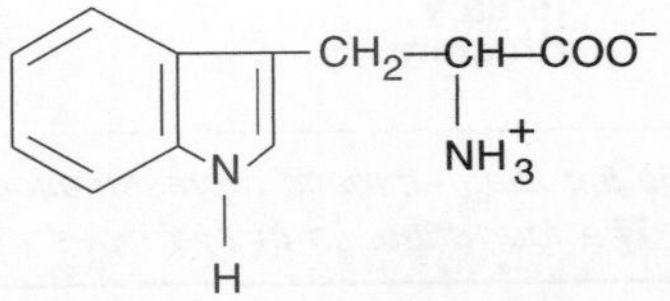 Indole(N–H)–CH_2–CH(NH_3^+)–COO^-	Indole
VII. Imino acid				
20. Proline	Pro	P	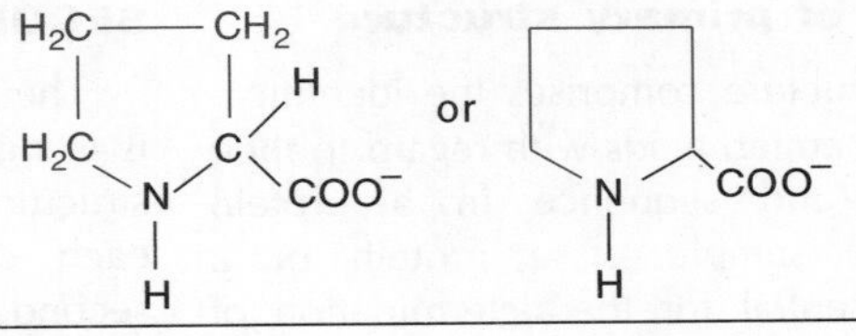 H_2C–CH_2, H_2C–C(H)–COO^-, N–H (ring) or pyrrolidine ring N(H)–COO^-	Pyrrolidine

(***Note*** : *R group is shown in colour*)

STRUCTURE OF PROTEINS

Proteins are the polymers of L-α-amino acids. The structure of proteins is rather complex which can be divided into 4 levels of organization (***Fig. 65.5***) :

1. **Primary structure :** The linear sequence of amino acids forming the backbone of proteins (polypeptides).

2. **Secondary structure :** The spacial arrangement of protein by twisting of the polypeptide chain.

3. **Tertiary structure :** The three dimensional structure of a functional protein.

4. **Quaternary structure :** Some of the proteins are composed of two or more polypeptide chains referred to as subunits. The spacial arrangement of these subunits is known as quaternary structure.

PRIMARY STRUCTURE OF PROTEIN

Each protein has a unique sequence of amino acids which is determined by the genes contained in DNA. The primary structure of a protein is largely responsible for its function.

Peptide bond

The amino acids are held together in a protein by covalent peptide bonds or linkages. These bonds are rather strong and serve as the cementing material between the individual amino acids.

Formation of a peptide bond : When the amino group of an amino acid combines with the carboxyl group of another amino acid, a peptide bond is formed (***Fig. 65.6***). Note that a dipeptide will have two amino acids and one peptide (not two) bond. Peptides containing more than 10 amino acids (decapeptide) are referred to as polypeptides.

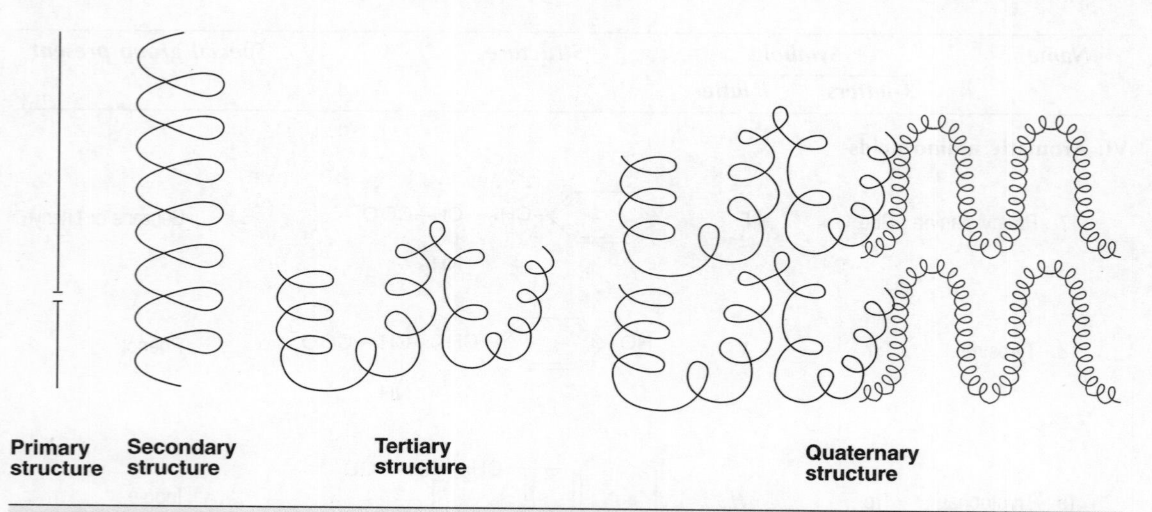

*Fig. 65.5 : Diagrammatic representation of protein structure (**Note** : The four subunits of two types in quaternary structure).*

Determination of primary structure

The primary structure comprises the identification of constituent amino acids with regard to their quality, quantity and sequence in a protein structure. A pure sample of a protein or a polypeptide is essential for the determination of primary structure which involves 3 stages.

1. Determination of amino acid composition.
2. Degradation of protein or polypeptide into smaller fragments.
3. Determination of the amino acid sequence.

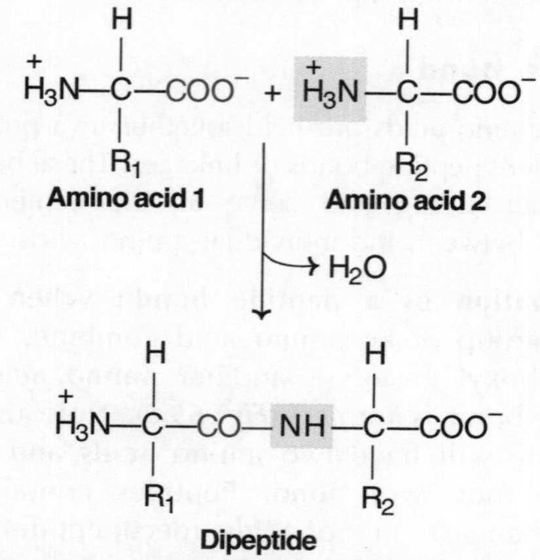

$$H_3\overset{+}{N}-\underset{R_1}{\overset{H}{C}}-COO^- + H_3\overset{+}{N}-\underset{R_2}{\overset{H}{C}}-COO^-$$

Amino acid 1 Amino acid 2

$$\downarrow \rightarrow H_2O$$

$$H_3\overset{+}{N}-\underset{R_1}{\overset{H}{C}}-CO-NH-\underset{R_2}{\overset{H}{C}}-COO^-$$

Dipeptide

Fig. 65.6 : Formation of a peptide bond.

SECONDARY STRUCTURE OF PROTEIN

The conformation of polypeptide chain by twisting or folding is referred to as secondary structure. The amino acids are located close to each other in their sequence. Two types of secondary structures, ***α-helix*** and ***β-sheet***, are mainly identified.

α-Helix

α-Helix is the ***most common spiral structure of protein***. It has a rigid arrangement of polypeptide chain. α-Helical structure was proposed by Pauling and Corey (1951) which is regarded as one of the milestones in the biochemistry research. The salient features of a right-handed α-helix which is a stable and more commonly found structure, in the living system (***Fig.** 65.7*) are given below

1. The α-helix is a tightly packed coiled structure with amino acid side chains extending outward from the central axis.

2. The α-helix is ***stabilized by hydrogen bonding***. It is formed between H atom attached to peptide N, and O atom attached to peptide C.

3. All the peptide bonds except the first and last in a polypeptide chain participate in hydrogen bonding.

4. Each turn of α-helix contains 3.6 amino acids and travels a distance of 0.54 nm. The spacing of each amino acid is 0.15 nm.

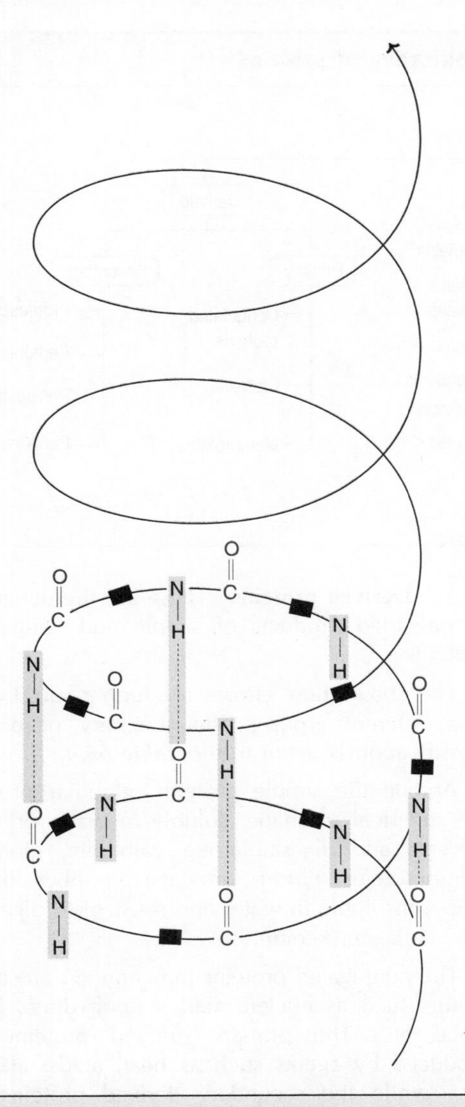

Fig. 65.7 : Diagrammatic representation of secondary structure of protein — a right handed α-helix

(■-Indicate $-\overset{\displaystyle H}{\overset{|}{C}}-R$ groups of amino acids; dotted coloured shades are hydrogen bonds; Note that only a few hydrogen bonds shown for clarity).

5. α-Helix is a stable conformation formed spontaneously with the lowest energy.

β-Pleated sheet

This is the second type of structure (hence β after α) proposed by Pauling and Corey. β-Pleated sheets (or simply β-sheets) are composed of two or more segments of fully extended peptide chains. In the β-sheets, the hydrogen bonds are formed between the neighbouring segments of polypeptide chain(s).

TERTIARY STRUCTURE OF PROTEIN

The ***three-dimensional arrangement of protein*** structure is referred to as tertiary structure. It is a compact structure with hydrophobic side chains held interior while the hydrophilic groups are on the surface of the protein molecule. This type of arrangement ensures stability of the molecule.

Bonds of tertiary structure : Besides the hydrogen bonds, disulfide bonds (—S—S), ionic interactions (electrostatic bonds) and hydrophobic interactions also contribute to the tertiary structure of proteins.

Domains : The term domain is used to represent the basic units of protein structure (tertiary) and functions. A polypeptide with 200 amino acids normally consists of two or more domains.

QUATERNARY STRUCTURE OF PROTEIN

A great majority of the proteins are composed of single polypeptide chains. Some of the proteins, however, consist of two or more polypeptides which may be identical or unrelated. Such proteins are termed as ***oligomers*** and possess quaternary structure. The individual polypeptide chains are known as ***monomers, protomers*** or ***subunits***. A ***dimer*** consits of ***two*** polypeptides while a tetramer has four.

Bonds in quaternary structure : The monomeric subunits are held together by non-convalent bonds namely hydrogen bonds, hydrophobic interactions and ionic bonds.

CLASSIFICATION OF PROTEINS

Proteins are classified in several ways. Three major types of classifying proteins based on their function, chemical nature and solubility properties and nutritional importance are discussed here.

Functional classification of proteins

Based on the function they perform, proteins are classified into different groups (with examples)

TABLE 65.4 Summary of classification of proteins

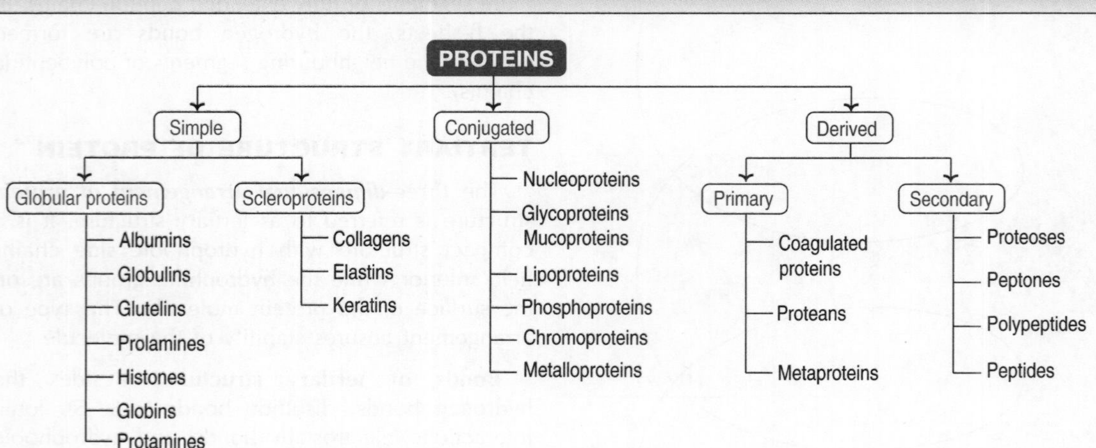

1. **Structural proteins :** Keratin of hair and nails, collagen of bone.

2. **Enzymes or catalytic proteins :** Hexokinase, pepsin.

3. **Transport proteins :** Hemoglobin, serum albumin.

4. **Hormonal proteins :** Insulin, growth hormone.

5. **Contractile proteins :** Actin, myosin.

6. **Storage proteins :** Ovalbumin, glutelin.

7. **Genetic proteins :** Nucleoproteins.

8. **Defense proteins :** Snake venoms, Immunoglobulins.

9. **Receptor proteins** for hormones, viruses.

Protein classification based on chemical nature and solubility

This is a more comprehensive and popular classification of proteins. It is based on the amino acid composition, structure, shape and solubility properties. Proteins are broadly classified into 3 major groups (***Table 65.4***).

1. **Simple proteins :** They are composed of only amino acid residues.

2. **Conjugated proteins :** Besides the amino acids, these proteins contain a non-protein moiety known as prosthetic group or conjugating group.

3. **Derived proteins :** These are the denatured or degraded products of simple and conjugated proteins.

The above three classes are further sub-divided into different groups. The summary of protein classification is given in the ***Table 65.4***.

Among the simple proteins, globular proteins are spherical in shape, soluble in water or other solvents and digestable e.g., albumin, globulin. Scleroproteins (fibrous proteins) are fiber like in shape, insoluble in water and resistant to digestion e.g., collagen, keratin.

The conjugated proteins may contain prosthetic groups such as nucleic acid, carbohydrate, lipid, metal etc. The primary derived proteins are produced by agents such as heat, acids, alkalies etc., while the secondary derived proteins are hydrolytic products of proteins.

ISOPRENOIDS AND PIGMENTS

Isoprenoids and pigments are organic compounds mostly distributed in plant kingdom. They perform a wide variety of functions.

ISOPRENOIDS

Isoprenoids are also called as ***terpenoids or (terpenes)*** as they are found in turpentine oil in high concentrations. The naturally occurring isoprenoids are composed of a ***five carbon isoprene***

TABLE 65.5 Classification of terpenes with selected examples

Class	Basic structure		Example
	Isoprene units	Structure	
Hemiterpenes	1	C_5H_8	Isoprene
Monoterpenes	2	$C_{10}H_{16}$	Limonene
Sesquiterpenes	3	$C_{15}H_{24}$	Abscisic acid
Diterpenes	4	$C_{20}H_{32}$	Gibberellin
Triterpenes	6	$C_{30}H_{48}$	Stigmasterol
Tetraterpenes	8	$C_{40}H_{64}$	Carotenes
Polyterpenes	n	$(C_5H_8)_n$	Rubber

unit. A majority of the isoprenoids are formed by joining of isoprene units head to tail as depicted below

```
    C            C
    |            |
C—C—C—C——C—C—C—C
 Head   Tail   Head   Tail
```

Classification of terpenes

The classification of terpenes is mainly based on the number of isoprene (C_5H_8) units present. The major classes of terpenes with selected examples are given in ***Table 65.5***.

PIGMENTS

Pigments are cloured organic compounds found in the living organisms, mostly in plants, and to a minor extent in animals. Chemically, pigments are high molecular weight molecules, mostly composed of unsaturated hydrocarbons. Some of the pigments also contain cyclic structures. The major groups of pigments are briefly described.

Tetrapyrroles

The most abundant coloured compound in the world is chlorophyll, the photosynthetic pigment. There are different types of chlorophylls (c, d, e, a) with slight variation in colours — green, greenish blue, greenish yellow.

Structurally, chlorophylls are composed of tetrapyrroles (pyrrole rings) with their nitrogen linked to magnesium.

Tetrapyrroles are also found in heme in certain proteins. These include hemoglobin, cytochromes, catalase and peroxidase.

Tetraterpenes (carotenoids)

The colour of carotenoids is variable, generally yellow, orange or red. A large number of carotenoids (about–600) have been identified in plant kingdom e.g. β-carotene, xanthophylls, lycopene.

Anthocyanins

Anthocyanins are a group of flavonoids which represent the natural phenolic products. Anthocyanins are coloured compounds, mostly found in flowers and fruits. They contain a common ring structure called ***anthocyanidin***.

Quinoid pigments

Being present in trace amounts, quinoid pigments do not significantly contribute to visible colours. They however, perform some other functions e.g. involvement in electron transport chain, antioxidant functions etc. The most common quinoid pigments are benzoquinones, naphthoquinones, anthraquinones, tannins and lignins.

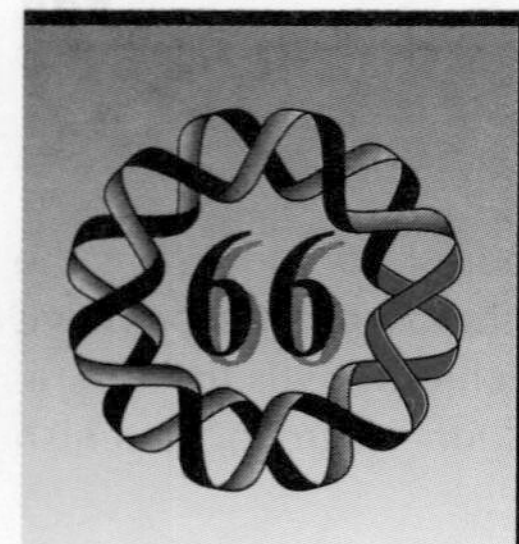

Enzymology

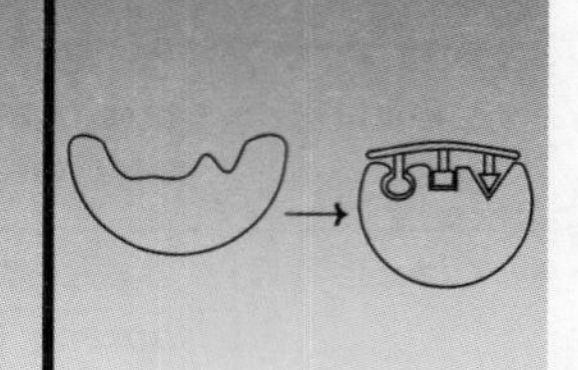

Enzymes are biocatalysts — the catalysts of life. A ***catalyst*** is defined as a ***substance that increases the velocity*** or rate of a chemical reaction without itself undergoing any change in the overall process.

Enzymes may be defined as biocatalysts synthesized by living cells. They are protein in nature, colloidal and thermolabile in character, and specific in their action.

In recent years, certain non-protein enzymes (chemically RNA) have also been identified.

NOMENCLATURE AND CLASSIFICATION

In the early days, the enzymes were given names by their discoverers in an arbitrary manner. For example, the names pepsin, trypsin and chymotrypsin convey no information about the function of the enzyme or the nature of the substrate on which they act.

Enzymes are sometimes considered under two broad categories : (a) **Intracellular enzymes**—They are functional within cells where they are synthesized. (b) **Extracellular enzymes**—These enzymes are active outside the cell; all the digestive enzymes belong to this group.

The International Union of Biochemistry (IUB) appointed an Enzyme Commission in 1961. This committee made a thorough study of the existing enzymes and devised some basic principles for the classification and nomenclature of enzymes. Since 1964, the ***IUB system of enzyme classification*** has been in force. Enzymes are divided into ***six major classes*** (in that order). Each class on its own represents the general type of reaction brought about by the enzymes of that class.

1. **Oxidoreductases :** Enzymes involved in oxidation-reduction reactions.

2. **Transferases :** Enzymes that catalyse the transfer of functional groups.

3. **Hydrolases :** Enzymes that bring about hydrolysis of various compounds.

4. **Lyases :** Enzymes specialised in the addition or removal of water, ammonia, CO_2 etc.

5. **Isomerases :** Enzymes involved in all the isomerization reactions.

6. **Ligases :** Enzymes catalysing the synthetic reactions (*Greek* : ligate—to bind) where two molecules are joined together and ATP is used.

[The word ***OTHLIL*** (first letter in each class) may be memorised to remember the six classes of enzymes in the correct order].

Each class in turn is subdivided into many sub-classes which are further divided. A four digit ***Enzyme Commission (E. C.) number*** is assigned to each enzyme representing the class (first digit), sub-class (second digit), sub-sub class (third digit) and the individual enzyme (fourth digit).

In the ***Table 66.1***, selected examples for the six classes of enzymes are given.

CHEMICAL NATURE OF ENZYMES

All the enzymes are invariably proteins. In recent years, however, a few RNA molecules have been shown to function as enzymes. Each enzyme has its own tertiary structure and specific conformation which is very essential for its catalytic activity. The functional unit of the enzyme is known as ***holoenzyme*** which is often made up of ***apoenzyme*** (the protein part) and a ***coenzyme*** (non-protein organic part).

$$\underset{\text{(active enzyme)}}{\text{Holoenzyme}} \longrightarrow \underset{\text{(protein part)}}{\text{Apoenzyme}} + \underset{\text{(non-protein part)}}{\text{Coenzyme}}$$

FACTORS AFFECTING ENZYME ACTIVITY

The contact between the enzyme and substrate is the most essential pre-requisite for enzyme activity. The important factors that influence the velocity of the enzyme reaction are discussed hereunder

1. Concentration of enzyme

As the concentration of the enzyme is increased, the velocity of the reaction proportionately increases (***Fig. 66.1***). In fact, this property of enzyme is made use in determining the activities of serum enzymes for diagnosis of diseases.

2. Concentration of substrate

Increase in the substrate concentration gradually ***increases the velocity of enzyme reaction*** within the limited range of substrate levels. A rectangular hyperbola is obtained when velocity is plotted against the substrate concentration (***Fig. 66.2***). Three distinct phases of the reaction are observed in the graph.

Enzyme kinetics and K_m value : The enzyme (E) and substrate (S) combine with each other to form

Table 66.1 Classification of enzymes

*Enzyme class with examples**	*Reaction catalysed*
1. **Oxidoreductases**	
Alcohol dehydrogenase (alcohol : NAD^+ oxidoreductase E. C. 1.1.1.1.), cytochrome oxidase, L- and D-amino acid oxidases	Oxidation ⟶ Reduction $AH_2 + B \longrightarrow A + BH_2$
2. **Transferases**	
Hexokinase (ATP : D-hexose 6-phosphotransferase, E. C. 2.7.1.1.), transaminases, transmethylases, phosphorylase	Group transfer $A - X + B \longrightarrow A + B - X$
3. **Hydrolases**	
Lipase (triacylglycerol acyl hydrolase E. C. 3.1.1.3), choline esterase, acid and alkaline phosphatases, pepsin, urease	Hydrolysis $A - B + H_2O \longrightarrow AH + BOH$
4. **Lyases**	
Aldolase (ketose 1-phosphate aldehyde lyase, E. C. 4.1.2.7), fumarase, histidase	Addition ⟶ Elimination $A - B + X - Y \longrightarrow AX - BY$
5. **Isomerases**	
Triose phosphate isomerase (D-glyceraldehyde 3-phosphate ketoisomerase, E.C. 5.3.1.1), retinol isomerase, phosphohexose isomerase	Interconversion of isomers $A \longrightarrow A'$
6. **Ligases**	
Glutamine synthetase (L-glutamate ammonia ligase, E. C. 6.3.1.2), acetyl CoA carboxylase, succinate thiokinase	Condensation (usually dependent on ATP) $A + B \xrightarrow[\text{ATP} \quad \text{ADP + Pi}]{} A - B$

* *For one enzyme in each class, systematic name along with E.C. number is given in the brackets.*

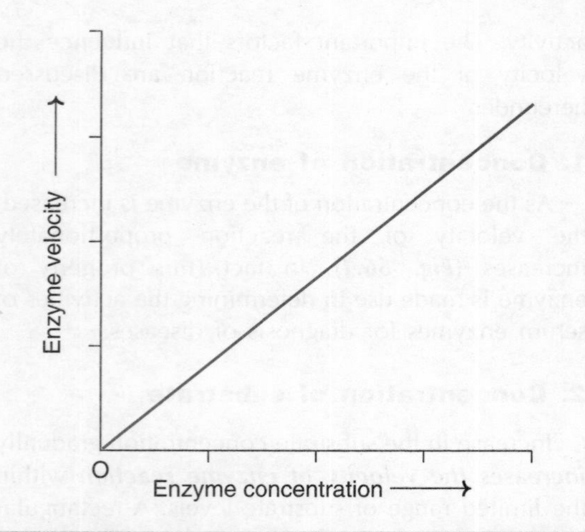

Fig. 66.1 : Effect of enzyme concentration on enzyme velocity.

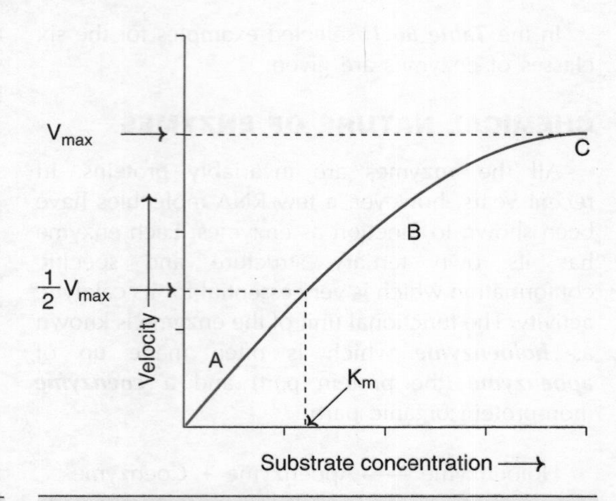

Fig. 66.2 : Effect of substrate concentration on enzyme velocity (A–linear; B–curve; C–almost unchanged).

an unstable enzyme-substrate complex (ES) for the formation of product (P).

$$E + S \underset{k_2}{\overset{k_1}{\rightleftharpoons}} ES \xrightarrow{k_3} E + P$$

Here k_1, k_2 and k_3 represent the velocity constants for the respective reactions, as indicated by arrows.

K_m, the Michaelis-Menten constant (or Brig's and Haldane's constant), is given by the formula

$$K_m = \frac{k_2 + k_3}{k_1}$$

The following equation is obtained after suitable algebraic manipulation.

$$v = \frac{V_{max}\,[S]}{K_m + [S]} \qquad \text{equation (1)}$$

where v = Measured velocity,

V_{max} = Maximum velocity,

S = Substrate concentration,

K_m = Michaelis-Menten constant.

K_m or the ***Michaelis-Menten constant*** is defined as the ***substrate concentration*** (expressed in moles/lit) ***to produce half-maximum velocity*** in an enzyme catalysed reaction. It indicates that half of the enzyme molecules (i.e. 50%) are bound with the substrate molecules when the substrate concentration equals the K_m value.

K_m value is a constant and a characteristic feature of a given enzyme. It is a representative for measuring the strength of ES complex. A ***low K_m value indicates a strong affinity between enzyme and substrate***, whereas a high K_m value reflects a weak affinity between them. For majority of enzymes, the K_m values are in the range of 10^{-5} to 10^{-2} moles.

Lineweaver-Burk double reciprocal plot : For the determination of K_m value, the substrate saturation curve (***Fig. 66.2***) is not very accurate since V_{max} is approached asymptotically. By taking the reciprocals of the equation (1), a straight line graphic representation is obtained.

The Lineweaver-Burk plot is shown in ***Fig. 66.3***. It is much easier to calculate the K_m

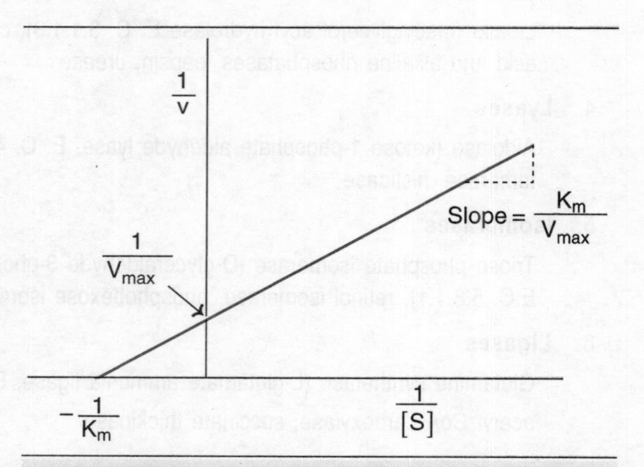

Fig. 66.3 : Lineweaver-Burk double reciprocal plot.

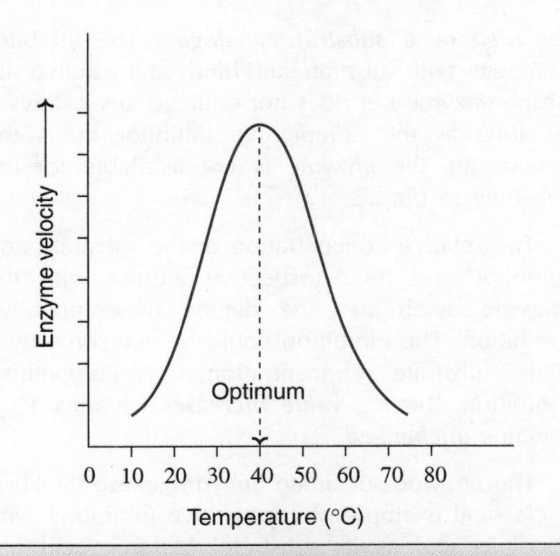

Fig. 66.4 : Effect of temperature on enzyme velocity.

from the intercept on x-axis which is $-(1/K_m)$. Further, the double reciprocal plot is useful in understanding the effect of various inhibitions (discussed later).

3. Effect of temperature

Velocity of an enzyme reaction increases with increase in temperature up to a maximum and then declines. A bell-shaped curve is usually observed (***Fig. 66.4***).

The optimum temperature for most of the enzymes is between 40°C–45°C. However, a few enzymes (e.g. venom phosphokinases, muscle adenylate kinase) are active even at 100°C.

In general, when the enzymes are exposed to a temperature above 50°C, ***denaturation*** leading to derangement in the native (tertiary) structure of the protein and active site are seen. Majority of the enzymes become inactive at higher temperature (above 70°C).

4. Effect of pH

Increase in the hydrogen ion concentration (pH) considerably influences the enzyme activity and a bell-shaped curve is normally obtained (***Fig. 66.5***). Each enzyme has an optimum pH at which the velocity is maximum.

Most of the enzymes of higher organisms show optimum activity around neutral pH (6-8). There are, however, many exceptions like pepsin (1-2), acid phosphatase (4-5) and alkaline phosphatase (10-11) for optimum pH.

5. Effect of product concentration

The accumulation of reaction products generally decreases the enzyme velocity. For certain enzymes, the products combine with the active site of enzyme and form a loose complex and, thus, inhibit the enzyme activity. In the living system, this type of inhibition is generally prevented by a quick removal of products formed.

6. Effect of activators

Some of the enzymes require certain inorganic ***metallic cations*** like Mg^{2+}, Mn^{2+}, Zn^{2+}, Ca^{2+}, Co^{2+}, Cu^{2+}, Na^{+}, K^{+} etc. for their optimum activity. Rarely, anions are also needed for enzyme activity e.g. chloride ion (Cl^{-}) for amylase.

ACTIVE SITE

Enzymes are big in size compared to substrates which are relatively smaller. Evidently, a small portion of the huge enzyme molecule is directly involved in the substrate binding and catalysis.

The active site (or active centre) of an enzyme is defined as the small region at which the substrate(s) binds and participates in the catalysis.

Salient features of active site

1. The existence of active site is due to the tertiary structure of protein resulting in three-dimensional native conformation.

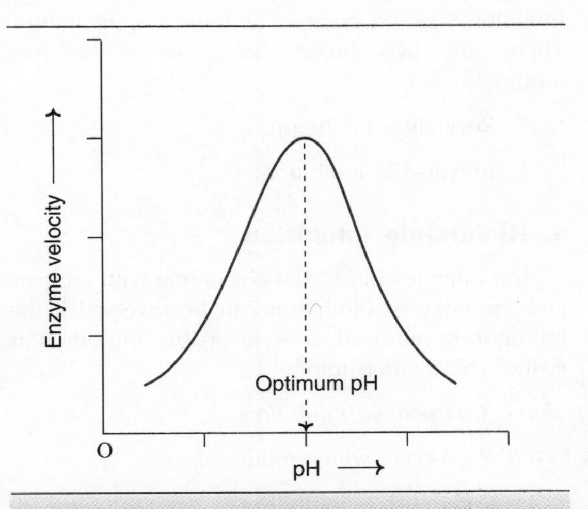

Fig. 66.5 : Effect of pH on enzyme velocity.

2. The active site is made up of amino acids (known as catalytic residues) which are far from each other in the linear sequence of amino acids (primary structure of protein). For instance, the enzyme lysozyme has 129 amino acids. The active site is formed by the contribution of amino acid residues numbered 35, 52, 62, 63 and 101.

3. The active site is not rigid in structure and shape. It is rather ***flexible*** to promote the specific substrate binding.

4. Generally, the active site possesses a ***substrate binding site*** and a ***catalytic site.*** The latter is for the catalysis of the specific reaction.

5. Of the 20 amino acids that could be present in enzyme structure, only some of them are repeatedly found at the active sites of various enzymes. These amino acids are serine, aspartate, histidine, cysteine, lysine, arginine, glutamate, tyrosine etc. Among these amino acids, ***serine*** is the most frequently found.

6. The substrate[S] binds the enzyme (E) at the active site to form enzyme-substrate complex (ES). The product (P) is released after the catalysis and the enzyme is available for reuse.

$$E + S \rightleftharpoons ES \longrightarrow E + P$$

ENZYME INHIBITION

Enzyme inhibitor is defined as a substance which binds with the enzyme and brings about a decrease in catalytic activity of that enzyme. The inhibitor may be organic or inorganic in nature. There are two broad categories of enzyme inhibition

1. Reversible inhibition.
2. Irreversible inhibition.

1. Reversible inhibition

The inhibitor binds non-covalently with enzyme and the enzyme inhibition can be reversed if the inhibitor is removed. The reversible inhibition is further sub-divided into

I. Competitive inhibition

II. Non-competitive inhibition

I. **Competitive inhibition :** The inhibitor (I) which closely resembles the real substrate (S) is regarded as a ***substrate analogue***. The inhibitor competes with substrate and binds at the active site of the enzyme but does not undergo any catalysis. As long as the competitive inhibitor holds the active site, the enzyme is not available for the substrate to bind.

The relative concentration of the substrate and inhibitor and their respective affinity with the enzyme determines the degree of competitive inhibition. The inhibition could be overcome by a high substrate concentration. In competitive inhibition, the ***K_m value increases*** whereas V_{max} remains ***unchanged.***

The enzyme succinate dehydrogenase (SDH) is a classical example of competitive inhibition with succinic acid as its substrate. Malonic acid has structural similarity with succinic acid and compete with the substrate for binding at the active site of SDH.

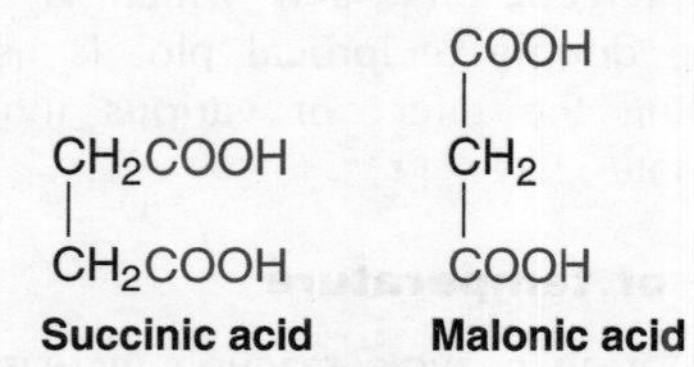

Some more examples of the enzymes with substrates and competitive inhibitors of biological significance are given in ***Table 66.2***.

Antimetabolites : These are the chemical compounds that block the metabolic reactions by their inhibitory action on enzymes. Antimetabolites are usually structural analogues of substrates and thus are competitive inhibitors (***Table 66.2***). They are in use for the treatment of cancer, gout etc. The term ***antivitamins*** is used for the antimetabolites which block the biochemical actions of vitamins causing deficiencies. e.g., sulphanilamide, dicumarol.

II. **Non-competitive inhibition :** The inhibitor binds at a site other than the active site on the enzyme surface. This binding impairs the enzyme function. The inhibitor has no structural resemblance with the substrate. However, there usually exists a strong affinity for the inhibitor to bind at the second site. In fact, the inhibitor does not interfere with the enzyme-substrate binding. But the catalysis is prevented, possibly due to a distortion in the enzyme conformation.

TABLE 66.2 Selected examples of enzymes with their respective substrates and competitive inhibitors

Enzyme	*Substrate*	*Inhibitor*	*Significance of inhibitor*
Xanthine oxidase	Hypoxanthine Xanthine	Allopurinol	Used in the control of gout to reduce excess production of uric acid from hypoxanthine.
Monoamine oxidase	Catecholamines (epinephrine, norepinephrine)	Ephidrene, amphetamine	Useful for elevating catecholamine levels.
Dihydrofolate reductase	Dihydrofolic acid	Aminopterin, amethopterin, methotrexate	Employed in the treatment of leukemia and other cancers.
Acetylcholine esterase	Acetylcholine	Succinyl choline	Used in surgery for muscle relaxation, in anaesthetised patients.
	Para aminobenzoic acid (PABA)	Sulphanilamide	Prevents bacterial synthesis of folic acid.
	Vitamin K	Dicumarol	Acts as an anticoagulant.
	Pyridoxine (vitamin B_6)	Isonicotinic acid hydrazide (INH)	INH is an antituberculosis drug, its prolonged use leads to B_6 deficiency.

The inhibitor generally binds with the enzyme as well as the ES complex.

For non-competitive inhibition, the ***K_m* value is unchanged** while ***V_{max}* is lowered**.

Heavy metal ions (Ag^+, Pb^{2+}, Hg^{2+} etc.) can non-competitively inhibit the enzymes by binding with cysteinyl sulfhydryl groups.

2. Irreversible inhibition

The inhibitors bind covalently with the enzymes and inactivate them, which is irreversible. These inhibitors are usually toxic substances which may be present naturally or man-made.

Iodoacetate is an irreversible inhibitor of the enzymes like papain and glyceraldehyde 3-phosphate dehydrogenase. Iodoacetate combines with sulfhydryl (–SH) groups at the active site of these enzymes and makes them inactive.

Diisopropyl fluorophosphate (DFP) is a ***nerve gas*** developed by the Germans during Second World War. DFP irreversibly binds with enzymes containing serine at the active site, e.g. ***serine proteases, acetylcholine esterase***.

Suicide inhibition : In this type of irreversible inhibition, the original inhibitor is converted to a more potent form by the same enzyme that ought to be inhibited e.g., allopurinol, an inhibitor of xanthine oxidase, gets converted to alloxanthine, a more effective inhibitor of the enzyme.

ENZYME SPECIFICITY

Enzymes are highly specific in their action when compared with the chemical catalysts. The occurrence of thousands of enzymes in the biological system might be due to the specific nature of enzymes. Three types of enzyme specificity are well-recognised

1. Stereospecificity, 2. Reaction specificity,
3. Substrate specificity,

Specificity is a characteristic property of the active site.

1. Stereospecificity or optical specificity

Stereoisomers are the compounds which have the same molecular formula, but differ in their structural configuration.

The ***enzymes act only on one isomer*** and, therefore, exhibit stereoisomerism.

e.g. L-amino acid oxidase and D-amino acid oxidase act on L- and D-amino acids respectively.

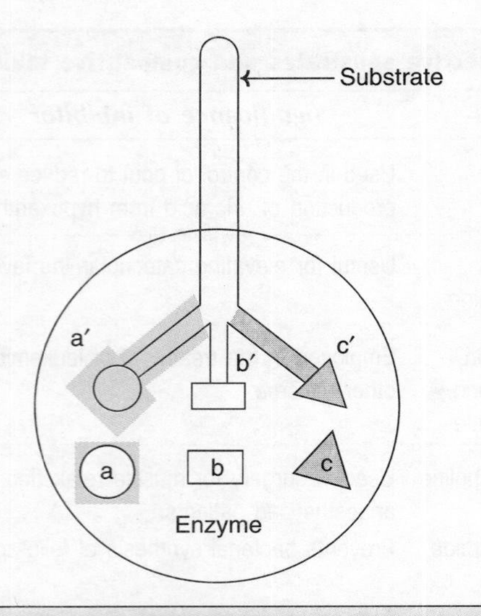

Fig. 66.6 : Diagrammatic representation of stereo-specificity (a′,b′,c′)—three point attachment of substrate to the enzyme (a, b, c).

Hexokinase acts on D-hexoses;
Glucokinase on D-glucose;
Amylase acts on α-glycosidic linkages;
Cellulase cleaves β-glycosidic bonds.

Stereospecificity is explained by considering three distinct regions of substrate molecule specifically binding with three complementary regions on the surface of the enzyme (***Fig. 66.6***). The class of enzymes belonging to ***isomerases do not exhibit stereospecificity***, since they are specialized in the interconversion of isomers.

2. Reaction specificity

The same substrate can undergo different types of reactions, each catalysed by a separate enzyme and this is referred to as reaction specificity. An amino acid can undergo transamination, oxidative deamination, decarboxylation, racemization etc. The enzymes however, are different for each of these reactions.

3. Substrate specificity

The substrate specificity varies from enzyme to enzyme. It may be either absolute, relative or broad.

(a) **Absolute substrate specificity :** Certain enzymes act only on one substrate e.g. glucokinase acts on glucose to give glucose 6-phosphate, urease cleaves urea to ammonia and carbon dioxide.

(b) **Relative substrate specificity :** Some enzymes act on structurally related substances. This, in turn, may be dependent on the specific group or a bond present. The action of trypsin and chymotrypsin is a good example for group specificity. Trypsin hydrolyses peptide linkage involving arginine or lysine. Chymotrypsin cleaves peptide bonds attached to aromatic amino acids (phenylalanine, tyrosine and tryptophan). Examples of bond specificity-glucosidases acting on glycosidic bonds of carbohydrates, lipases cleaving ester bonds of lipids etc.

(c) **Broad specificity :** Some enzymes act on closely related substrates which is commonly known as broad substrate specificity, e.g. hexokinase acts on glucose, fructose, mannose and glucosamine and not on galactose.

COENZYMES

Many enzymes require certain non-protein small additional factors, collectively referred to as cofactors for catalysis. The cofactors may be organic or inorganic in nature.

The non-protein, organic, low molecular weight and dialysable substance associated with enzyme function is known as coenzyme.

The functional enzyme is referred to as ***holoenzyme*** which is made up of a protein part ***(apoenzyme)*** and a non-protein part ***(coenzyme)***. The term ***activator*** represents the inorganic cofactor (like Ca^{2+}, Mg^{2+}, Mn^{2+} etc.) necessary to enhance enzyme activity.

Coenzymes are second substrates : Coenzymes are often regarded as the second substrates or ***cosubstrates***, since they have affinity with the enzyme comparable with that of the substrates. Coenzymes undergo alterations during the enzymatic reactions, which are later regenerated. This is in contrast to the substrate which is converted to the product.

Coenzymes participate in various reactions involving transfer of atoms or groups like hydrogen, aldehyde, keto, amino, acyl, methyl, carbon

TABLE 66.3 Coenzymes of B-complex vitamins

Coenzyme (abbreviation)	*Derived from vitamin*	*Atom or group transferred*	*Dependent enzyme (example)*
Thiamine pyrophosphate (TPP)	Thiamine	Aldehyde or keto	Transketolase
Flavin mononucleotide (FMN)	Riboflavin	Hydrogen and electron	L-Amino acid oxidase
Flavin adenine dinucleotide (FAD)	Riboflavin	"	D-Amino acid oxidase
Nicotinamide adenine dinucleotide(NAD^+)	Niacin	"	Lactate dehydrogenase
Nicotinamide adenine dinucleotide phosphate ($NADP^+$)	"	"	Glucose 6-phosphate dehydrogenase
Lipoic acid	Lipoic acid	"	Pyruvate dehydrogenase complex
Pyridoxal phosphate (PLP)	Pyridoxine	Amino or keto	Alanine transaminase
Coenzyme A (CoA)	Pantothenic acid	Acyl	Thiokinase
Tetrahydrofolate (FH_4)	Folic acid	One carbon	Formyl transferase (formyl, methenyl etc.)
Biotin coenzyme	Biotin	CO_2	Pyruvate carboxylase
Methylcobalamin; Deoxyadenosyl cobalamin	Cobalamin	Methyl/isomerisation	Methylmalonyl CoA mutase

dioxide etc. Coenzymes play a decisive role in enzyme function.

Coenzymes from B-complex vitamins : Most of the coenzymes are the derivatives of water soluble B-complex vitamins. In fact, the biochemical functions of B-complex vitamins are exerted through their respective coenzymes. The chapter on vitamins gives the details of structure and function of the coenzymes. In ***Table. 66.3***, a summary of the vitamin related coenzymes with their functions is given.

Non-vitamin coenzymes : Not all coenzymes are vitamin derivatives. There are some other organic substances, which have no relation with vitamins but function as coenzymes. They may be considered as non-vitamin coenzymes e.g. ATP, CDP, UDP etc.

Nucleotide coenzymes : Some of the coenzymes possess nitrogenous base, sugar and phosphate. Such coenzymes are, therefore, regarded as nucleotides e.g. NAD^+, $NADP^+$, FMN, FAD, coenzyme A, UDPG etc.

Coenzymes do not decide enzyme specificity : A particular coenzyme may participate in catalytic reactions along with different enzymes. For instance, NAD^+ acts as a coenzyme for lactate dehydrogenase and alcohol dehydrogenase. In both the enzymatic reactions, NAD^+ is involved in hydrogen transfer. The ***specificity of the enzyme is mostly dependent on the apoenzyme and not on the coenzyme.***

MECHANISM OF ENZYME ACTION

Catalysis is the prime function of enzymes. The nature of catalysis taking place in the biological system is similar to that of non-biological catalysis. For any chemical reaction to occur, the reactants have to be in an activated state or a transition state.

Enzymes lower activation energy : The energy required by the reactants to undergo the reaction is known as ***activation energy.*** The reactants when heated attain the activation energy. The catalyst (or the enzyme in the biological system) reduces the activation energy and this causes the reaction to proceed at a lower temperature. Enzymes do not alter the equilibrium constants, they only enhance the velocity of the reaction.

The role of a catalyst or an enzyme is comparable with a tunnel made in a mountain to reduce the barrier as illustrated in ***Fig. 66.7***. The enzyme lowers energy barrier of reactants, thereby making the reaction go faster. The enzymes reduce the activation energy of the reactants in such a way that all the biological systems occur at body temperature (below 40°C).

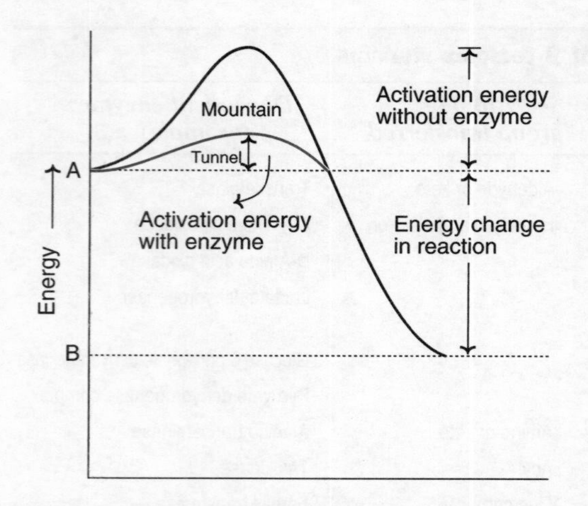

Fig. 66.7 : Effect of enzyme on activation energy of a reaction (A is the substrate and B is the product. Enzyme decreases activation energy).

Enzyme-substrate complex formation

The prime requisite for enzyme catalysis is that the substrate (S) must combine with the enzyme (E) at the active site to form enzyme-substrate complex (ES) which ultimately results in the product formation (P).

$$E + S \rightleftharpoons ES \longrightarrow E + P$$

A few theories have been put forth to explain mechanism of enzyme-substrate complex formation (***Fig. 66.8***).

Lock and key model or Fischer's template theory

According to this model, the structure or conformation of the enzyme is rigid. The substrate fits to the binding site (now active site) just as a key fits into the proper lock or a hand into the proper glove. Thus the active site of an enzyme is a rigid and pre-shaped template where only a specific substrate can bind. This model does not give any scope for the flexible nature of enzymes, hence the model totally fails to explain many facts of enzymatic reactions, the most important being the effect of allosteric modulators.

Induced fit theory or Koshland's model

Koshland, in 1958, proposed a more acceptable and realistic model for enzyme-substrate complex formation. As per this model, the active site is not rigid and pre-shaped. The essential features of the substrate binding site are present at the nascent active site. The interaction of the substrate with the enzyme induces a fit or a conformation change in the enzyme, resulting in the formation of a strong substrate binding site. Further, due to induced fit, the appropriate amino acids of the enzyme are repositioned to form the active site and bring about the catalysis (***Fig. 66.8***).

Induced fit model has sufficient experimental evidence from the X-ray diffraction studies. Koshland's model also explains the action of allosteric modulators and competitive inhibition on enzymes.

Substrate strain theory

In this model, the substrate is strained due to the induced conformation change in the enzyme. It is also possible that when a substrate binds to the preformed active site, the enzyme induces a strain to the substrate. The strained substrate leads to the formation of product. The concept of substrate strain explains the role of enzyme in increasing the rate of reaction.

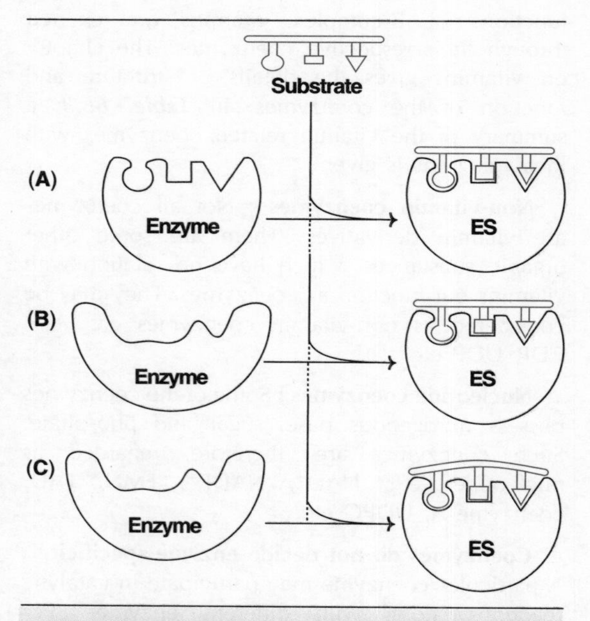

*Fig. 66.8 : Mechanism of enzyme–substrate (ES) complex formation **(A)** Lock and key model; **(B)** Induced fit theory **(C)** Substrate strain theory.*

66.4 Important enzymes in the diagnosis of diseases

Serum enzyme (elevated)	*Disease (most important)*
Amylase	Acute pancreatitis
Serum glutamate pyruvate transaminase (SGPT)	Liver diseases (hepatitis)
Serum glutamate oxaloacetate transaminase (SGOT)	Heart attacks (myocardial infarction)
Alkaline phosphatase	Rickets, obstructive jaundice
Acid phosphatase	Cancer of prostate gland
Lactate dehydrogenase (LDH)	Heart attacks, liver diseases
Creatine phosphokinase (CPK)	Myocardial infarction (early marker)
Aldolase	Muscular dystrophy
5′-Nucleotidase	Hepatitis
γ-Glutamyl transpeptidase (GGT)	Alcoholism

In fact, a combination of the induced fit model with the substrate strain is considered to be operative in the enzymatic action.

Mechanism of enzyme catalysis

The formation of an enzyme-substrate complex (ES) is very crucial for the catalysis to occur. It is estimated that an enzyme catalysed reaction proceeds 10^6 to 10^{12} times faster than a non-catalysed reaction. It is worthwhile to briefly understand the ways and means through which the catalytic process takes place leading to the product formation. The enhancement in the rate of the reaction is mainly due to four processes :

1. *Acid-base catalysis;*
2. *Substrate strain;*
3. *Covalent catalysis;*
4. *Entropy effects.*

DIAGNOSTIC IMPORTANCE OF ENZYMES

Estimation of enzyme activities in biological fluids (particularly plasma/serum) is of great clinical importance. Enzymes in the circulation are divided into two groups.

1. **Plasma specific or plasma functional enzymes :** Certain enzymes are normally present in the plasma and they have specific functions to perform. Generally, these enzyme activities are higher in plasma than in the tissues. They are mostly synthesized in the liver and enter the circulation e.g. lipoprotein lipase, plasmin, thrombin, choline esterase, ceruloplasmin etc.

Impairment in liver function or genetic disorders often leads to a fall in the activities of plasma functional enzymes e.g. deficiency of ceruloplasmin in Wilson's disease.

2. **Non-plasma specific or plasma non-functional enzymes :** These enzymes are either totally absent or present at a low concentration in plasma compared to their levels found in the tissues. The digestive enzymes of the gastrointestinal tract (e.g. amylase, pepsin, trypsin, lipase etc.) present in the plasma are known as ***secretory enzymes.*** All the other plasma enzymes associated with metabolism of the cell are collectively referred to as ***constitutive enzymes*** (e.g. lactate dehydrogenase, transaminases, acid and alkaline phosphatases, creatine phosphokinase).

Estimation of the activities of non-plasma specific enzymes is very important for the diagnosis and prognosis of several diseases.

A summary of the important enzymes useful for the diagnosis of specific diseases is given in ***Table 66.4***.

ISOENZYMES

The ***multiple forms of an enzyme*** catalysing the same reaction are ***isoenzymes*** or ***isozymes.*** They, however, differ in their physical and chemical properties which include the structure, electrophoretic and immunological properties, K_m and V_{max} values, pH optimum, relative susceptibility to inhibitors and degree of denaturation. e.g. lactate dehydrogenase (5 isoenzymes), creatine kinase (3 isoenzymes).

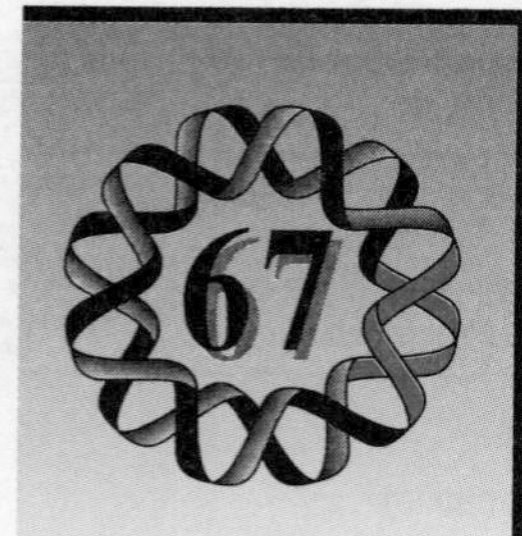

Metabolisms

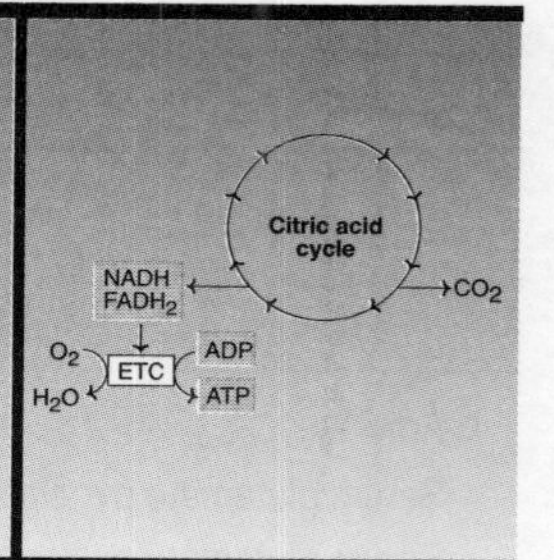

Hundreds of reactions simultaneously take place in a living cell, in a well-organized and integrated manner. The entire spectrum of ***chemical reactions, occurring in the living system,*** are collectively referred to as ***metabolism.***

A ***metabolic pathway*** (or metabolic map) constitutes a series of enzymatic reactions to produce specific products. The term ***metabolite*** is applied to a substrate or an intermediate or a product in the metabolic reactions.

Some salient features of metabolisms with special reference to higher organisms, particularly humans are given in this chapter.

INTRODUCTION TO METABOLISM

Metabolism is broadly divided into two categories (***Fig. 67.1***).

1. **Catabolism :** The degradative processes concerned with the breakdown of complex molecules to simpler ones, with a concomitant release of energy.

2. **Anabolism :** The biosynthetic reactions involving the formation of complex molecules from simple precursors.

A clear demarcation between catabolism and anabolism is rather difficult, since there are ***several intermediates common to both the processes.***

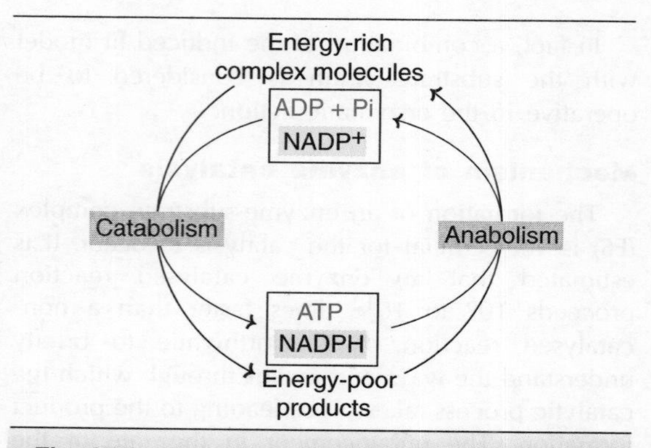

Fig. 67.1 : An outline of catabolism and anabolism.

Catabolism

The very purpose of catabolism is to trap the energy of the biomolecules in the form of ATP and to generate the substances (precursors) required for the synthesis of complex molecules. Catabolism occurs in three stages (***Fig. 67.2***).

1. **Conversion of complex molecules into their building blocks :** Polysaccharides are broken down to monosaccharides, lipids to free fatty acids and glycerol, and proteins to amino acids.

2. **Formation of simple intermediates :** The building blocks produced in stage (1) are degraded to simple intermediates such as pyruvate and acetyl CoA. These intermediates are not readily identifiable as carbohydrates, lipids or proteins. A small quantity of energy (as ATP) is captured in stage 2.

3. **Final oxidation of acetyl CoA :** Acetyl CoA is completely oxidized to CO_2, liberating NADH

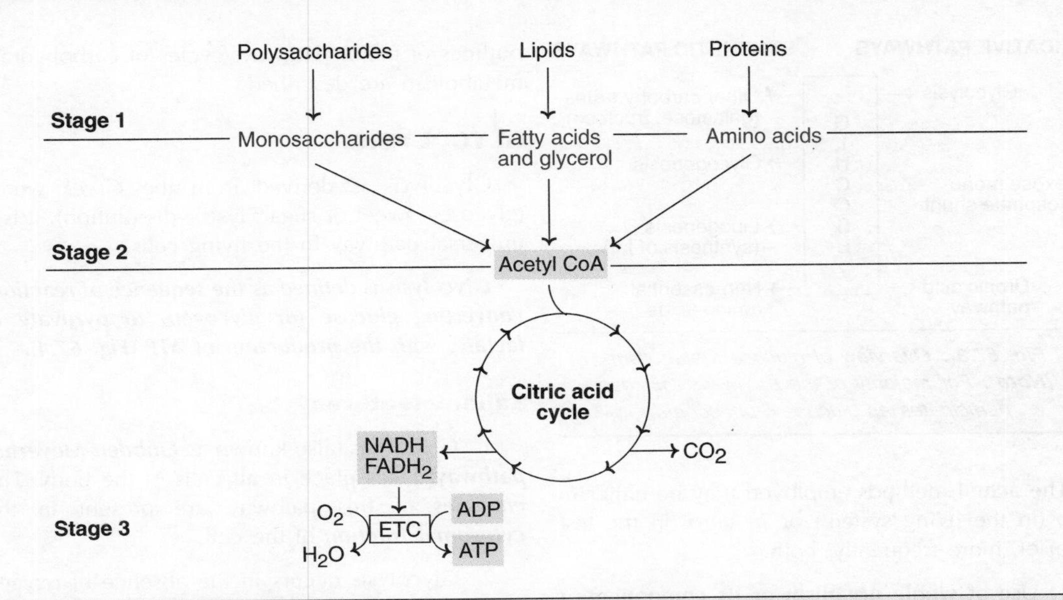

Fig. 67.2 : The three stages of catabolism (ETC-Electron transport chain).

and $FADH_2$ that finally get oxidized to release large quantity of energy (as ATP). ***Krebs cycle*** (or citric acid cycle) is the common metabolic pathway involved in the final oxidation of all energy-rich molecules. This pathway accepts the carbon compounds (pyruvate, succinate etc.) derived from carbohydrates, lipids or proteins.

Anabolism

For the synthesis of a large variety of complex molecules, the starting materials are relatively few. These include pyruvate, acetyl CoA and the intermediates of citric acid cycle. Besides the availability of precursors, the anabolic reactions are dependent on the ***supply of energy*** (as ATP or GTP) and reducing equivalents (as NADPH + H^+).

The anabolic and catabolic pathways are not reversible and operate independently. As such, the metabolic pathways occur in specific cellular locations (mitochondria, microsomes etc.) and are controlled by different regulatory signals.

The terms—intermediary metabolism and energy metabolism—are also in use. ***Intermediary metabolism*** refers to the entire range of catabolic and anabolic reactions, not involving nucleic acids. ***Energy metabolism*** deals with the metabolic pathways concerned with the storage and liberation of energy.

Types of metabolic reactions

The biochemical reactions are mainly of four types

1. Oxidation-reduction.
2. Group transfer.
3. Rearrangement and isomerization.
4. Make and break of carbon-carbon bonds.

These reactions are catalysed by specific enzymes—more than 2,000 known so far.

Methods employed to study metabolism

The metabolic reactions do not occur in isolation. They are interdependent and integrated into specific series that constitute ***metabolic pathways.*** It is, therefore, not an easy task to study metabolisms. Fortunately, the ***basic metabolic pathways in most organisms are essentially identical.***

Several methods are employed to elucidate biochemical reactions and the metabolic pathways. These experimental approaches may be broadly divided into 3 categories :

1. Use of whole organisms or its components.
2. Utility of metabolic probes.
3. Application of isotopes.

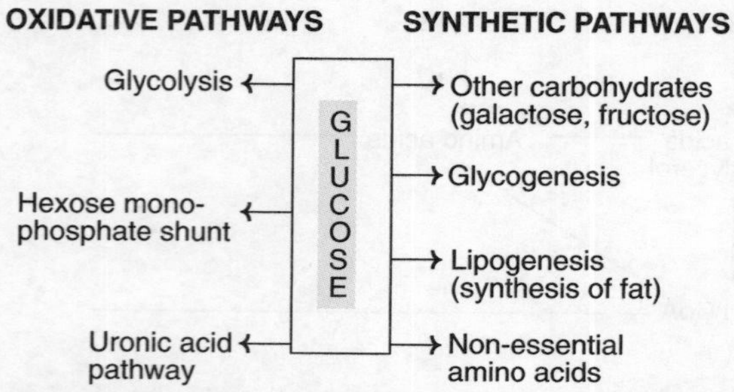

Fig. 67.3 : Overview of glucose metabolism. (Note : For majority of the pathways, glucose participates as glucose 6-phosphate).

The actual methods employed may be either *in vivo* (in the living system) or *in vitro* (in the test tube) or, more frequently, both.

1. **Use of whole organism or its components :**

(a) **Whole organisms :** Glucose tolerance test (GTT).

(b) **Isolated organs, tissue slices, whole cells,** subcellular organelles etc., to elucidate biochemical reactions and metabolic pathways.

2. **Utility of metabolic probes :** Two types of metabolic probes are commonly used to trace out biochemical pathways. These are metabolic ***inhibitors*** and ***mutations.***

3. **Application of isotopes.**

METABOLISM OF CARBOHYDRATES

Carbohydrates are the major source of energy for the living cells. The monosaccharide ***glucose is the central molecule in carbohydrate metabolism*** since all the major pathways of carbohydrate metabolism are connected with it (***Fig. 67.3***). Glucose is utilized as a source of energy, it is synthesized from non-carbohydrate precursors and stored as glycogen to release glucose as and when the need arises. The other monosaccharides important in carbohydrate metabolism are fructose, galactose and mannose.

The ***fasting blood glucose*** level in normal humans is ***60-100 mg/dl*** (4.5-5.5 mmol/l) and it is very efficiently maintained at this level. The outlines of major pathways/cycles of carbohydrate metabolism are described.

GLYCOLYSIS

Glycolysis is derived from the *Greek* words (glycose—sweet or sugar; lysis—dissolution). It is a universal pathway in the living cells.

Glycolysis is defined as the sequence of reactions converting glucose (or glycogen) to pyruvate or lactate, with the production of ATP (***Fig. 67.4***).

Salient features

1. Glycolysis (also known as ***Embden-Meyerhof pathway***) takes place in all cells of the body. The ***enzymes*** of this pathway are present in the ***cytosomal fraction*** of the cell.

2. Glycolysis occurs in the absence of oxygen (anaerobic) or in the presence of oxygen (aerobic). Lactate is the end product under anaerobic condition. In the aerobic condition, pyruvate is formed, which is then oxidized to CO_2 and H_2O.

3. Glycolysis is a major pathway for ATP synthesis in tissues lacking mitochondria, e.g. erythrocytes, cornea, lens etc.

4. Glycolysis is very ***essential for brain*** which is dependent on glucose for energy. The glucose in brain has to undergo glycolysis before it is oxidized to CO_2 and H_2O.

5. Glycolysis (anaerobic) may be summarized by the net reaction

$$\text{Glucose} + 2\text{ADP} + 2\text{Pi} \longrightarrow 2\text{ Lactate} + 2\text{ATP}$$

6. Reversal of glycolysis along with the alternate arrangements made at the irreversible steps will result in the synthesis of glucose (gluconeogenesis).

CONVERSION OF PYRUVATE TO ACETYL COA

Pyruvate is converted to acetyl CoA by ***oxidative decarboxylation***. This is an irreversible reaction, catalysed by a multienzyme complex, known as ***pyruvate dehydrogenase complex*** (PDH), which is found only in the mitochondria. High concentrations of PDH are found in cardiac muscle and kidney. The enzyme PDH requires five cofactors (coenzymes), namely — TPP, lipoamide, FAD, coenzyme A and NAD^+ (lipoamide contains

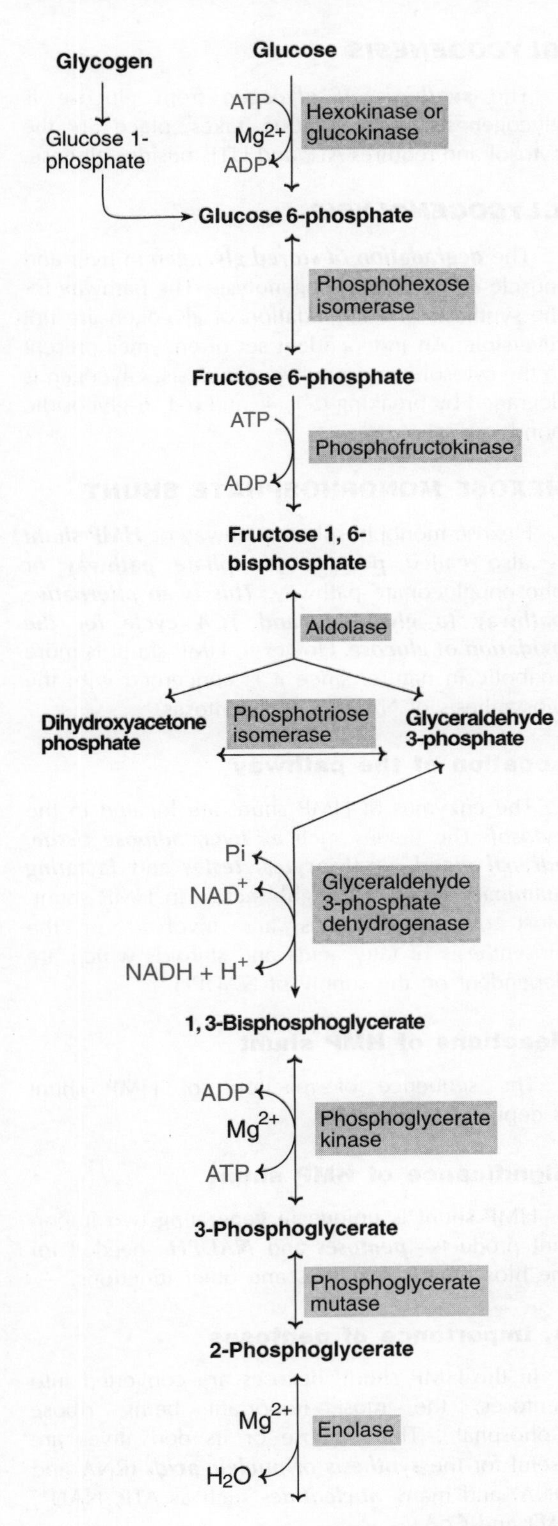

Fig. 67.4 contd. next column

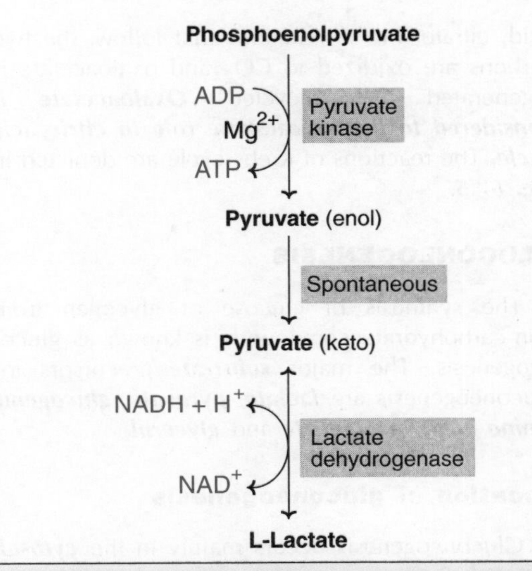

Fig. 67.4 : The reactions in the pathway of glycolysis (The three steps catalysed by hexokinase, phosphofructokinase and pyruvate kinase are irreversible).

lipoic acid linked to ε-amino group of lysine). The overall reaction of PDH is

$$\text{Pyruvate} + NAD^+ + \text{CoA} \xrightarrow{\text{PDH}} \text{Acetyl CoA} + CO_2 + NADH + H^+$$

CITRIC ACID CYCLE

The citric acid cycle (Krebs cycle or tricarboxylic acid—TCA cycle) is the most important metabolic pathway for the energy supply to the body. About 65-70% of the ATP is synthesized in Krebs cycle. ***Citric acid cycle essentially involves the oxidation of acetyl CoA to CO_2 and H_2O.***

The citric acid cycle is the final common oxidative pathway for carbohydrates, fats and amino acids. This cycle not only supplies energy but also provides many intermediates required for the synthesis of amino acids, glucose, heme etc. Krebs cycle is the most important central pathway connecting almost all the individual metabolic pathways (either directly or indirectly).

The enzymes of TCA cycle are located in ***mitochondrial matrix***, in close proximity to the electron transport chain.

Krebs cycle basically involves the combination of a two carbon acetyl CoA with a four carbon oxaloacetate to produce a six carbon tricarboxylic acid, citrate. In the reactions that follow, the two carbons are oxidized to CO_2 and oxaloacetate is regenerated and recycled. ***Oxaloacetate is considered to play a catalytic role in citric acid cycle.*** The reactions of Krebs cycle are depicted in ***Fig. 67.5***.

GLUCONEOGENESIS

The synthesis of glucose or glycogen from non-carbohydrate compounds is known as gluconeogenesis. The major ***substrates***/precursors for gluconeogenesis are ***lactate***, ***pyruvate***, ***glucogenic amino acids***, ***propionate*** and ***glycerol.***

Location of gluconeogenesis

Gluconeogenesis occurs mainly in the ***cytosol***, although some precursors are produced in the mitochondria. Gluconeogenesis mostly takes place in liver and, to some extent, in kidney matrix (about one-tenth of liver capacity).

Reactions of gluconeogenesis

Gluconeogenesis closely resembles the reversed pathway of glycolysis, although it is not the complete reversal of glycolysis. Essentially, 3 (out of 10) reactions of glycolysis are irreversible. The seven reactions are common for both glycolysis and gluconeogenesis. The ***three irreversible steps*** of glycolysis are catalysed by the enzymes, namely ***hexokinase***, ***phosphofructokinase*** and ***pyruvate kinase***.

GLYCOGEN METABOLISM

Glycogen is the storage form of glucose in animals, as is starch in plants. It is stored mostly in liver (6-8%) and muscle (1-2%). Due to more muscle mass, the quantity of glycogen in muscle (250 g) is about three times higher than that in the liver (75 g).

Functions of glycogen

The prime function of liver glycogen is to maintain the blood glucose levels, particularly between meals. Liver glycogen stores increase in a well-fed state which are depleted during fasting. Muscle glycogen serves as a fuel reserve for the supply of ATP during muscle contraction.

GLYCOGENESIS

The ***synthesis of glycogen*** from glucose is glycogenesis. Glycogenesis takes place in the cytosol and requires ATP and UTP, besides glucose.

GLYCOGENOLYSIS

The ***degradation of stored glycogen*** in liver and muscle constitutes glycogenolysis. The pathway for the synthesis and degradation of glycogen are not reversible. An independent set of enzymes present in the cytosol carry out glycogenolysis. Glycogen is degraded by breaking α-1, 4- and α-1, 6-glycosidic bonds.

HEXOSE MONOPHOSPHATE SHUNT

Hexose monophosphate pathway or ***HMP shunt*** is also called ***pentose phosphate pathway*** or phosphogluconate pathway. ***This is an alternative pathway to glycolysis and TCA cycle for the oxidation of glucose.*** However, HMP shunt is more anabolic in nature, since it is concerned with the biosynthesis of NADPH and pentoses.

Location of the pathway

The enzymes of HMP shunt are located in the ***cytosol***. The tissues such as ***liver, adipose tissue, adrenal gland, erythrocytes, testes*** and ***lactating mammary gland***, are highly active in HMP shunt. Most of these tissues are involved in the biosynthesis of fatty acids and steroids which are dependent on the supply of NADPH.

Reactions of HMP shunt

The sequence of reactions of HMP shunt is depicted in ***Fig. 67.6***.

Significance of HMP shunt

HMP shunt is unique in generating two important products—***pentoses*** and ***NADPH***—needed for the biosynthetic reactions and other functions.

A. Importance of pentoses

In the HMP shunt, hexoses are converted into pentoses, the most important being ribose 5-phosphate. This pentose or its derivatives are useful for the ***synthesis of nucleic acids*** (RNA and DNA) and many ***nucleotides*** such as ATP, NAD^+, FAD and CoA.

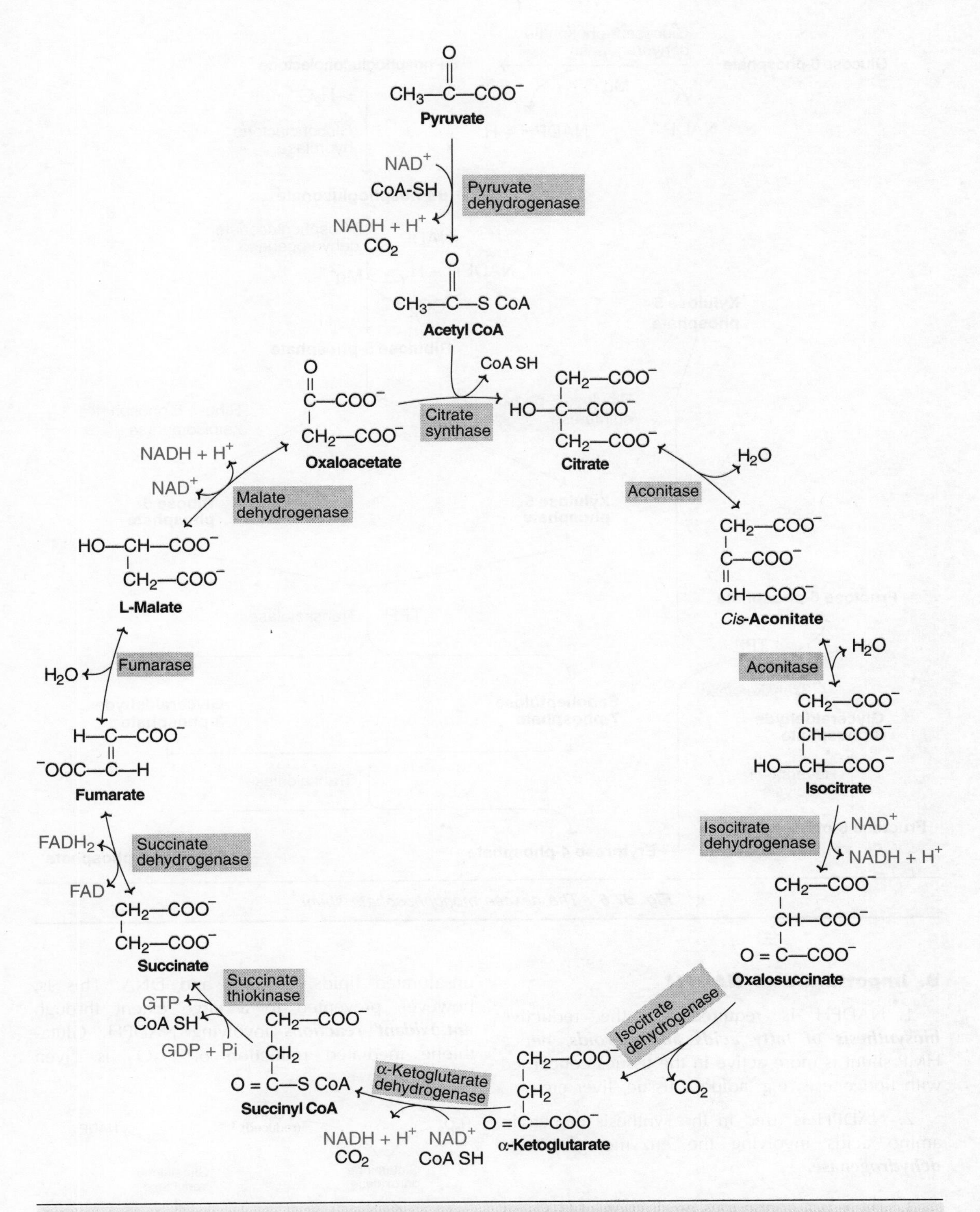

Fig. 67.5 : The citric acid (Krebs) cycle.

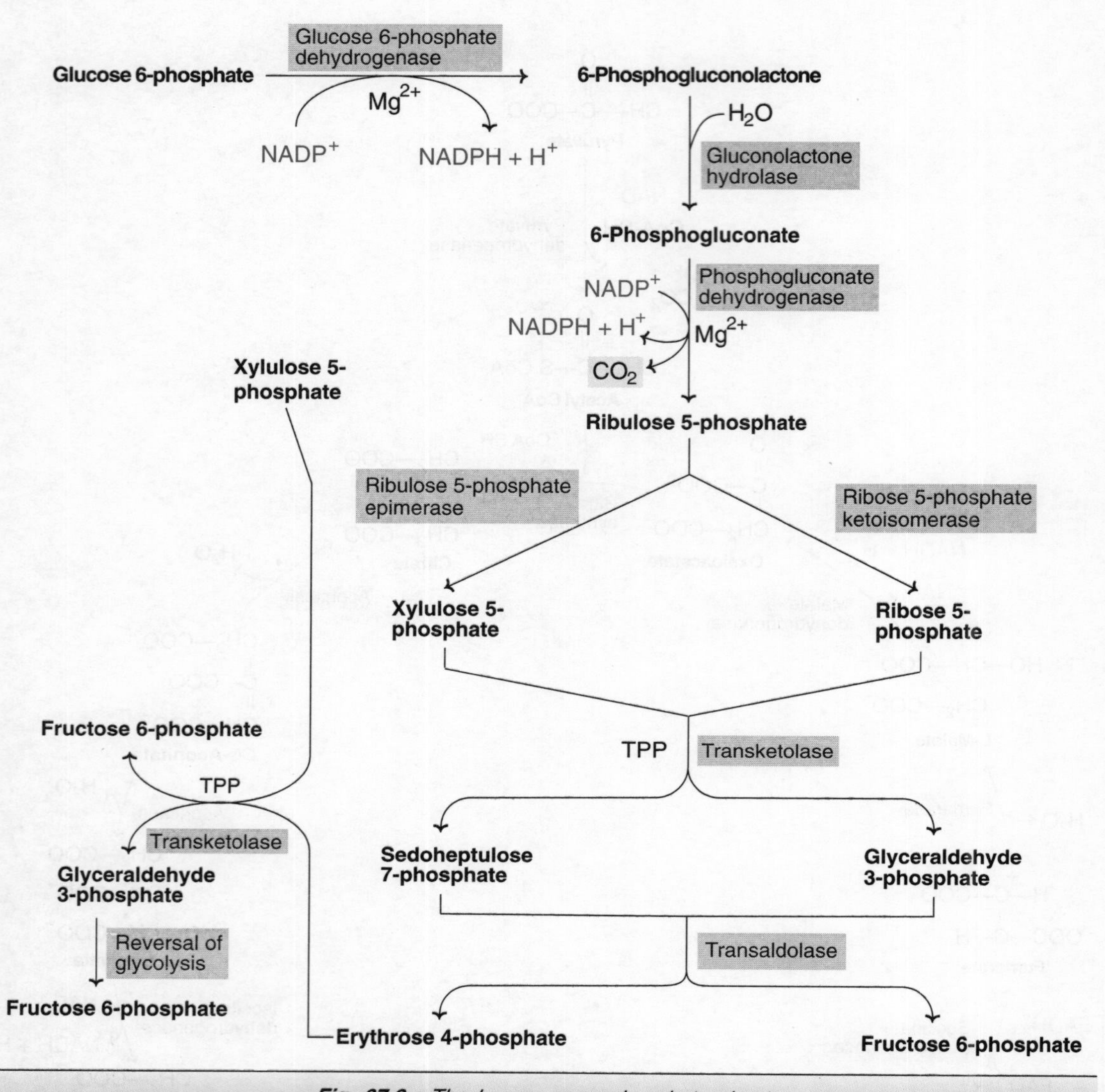

Fig. 67.6 : The hexose monophosphate shunt.

B. Importance of NADPH

1. NADPH is required for the reductive ***biosynthesis of fatty acids and steroids***, hence HMP shunt is more active in the tissues concerned with lipogenesis, e.g. adipose tissue, liver etc.

2. NADPH is used in the synthesis of certain amino acids involving the enzyme ***glutamate dehydrogenase.***

3. There is a continuous production of H_2O_2 in the living cells which can chemically damage unsaturated lipids, proteins and DNA. This is, however, prevented to a large extent through ***antioxidant reactions*** involving NADPH. Glutathione mediated reduction of H_2O_2 is given hereunder

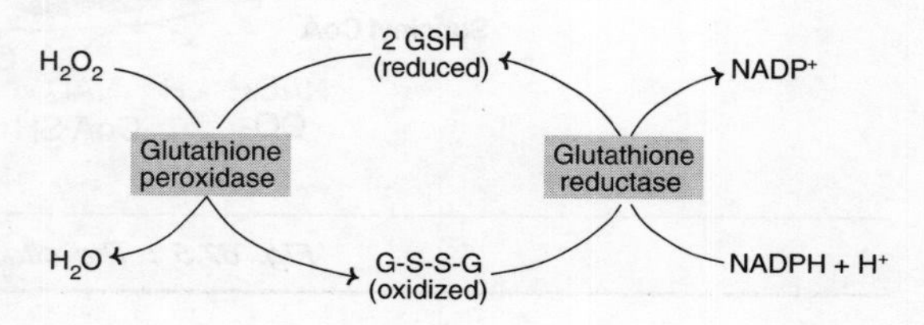

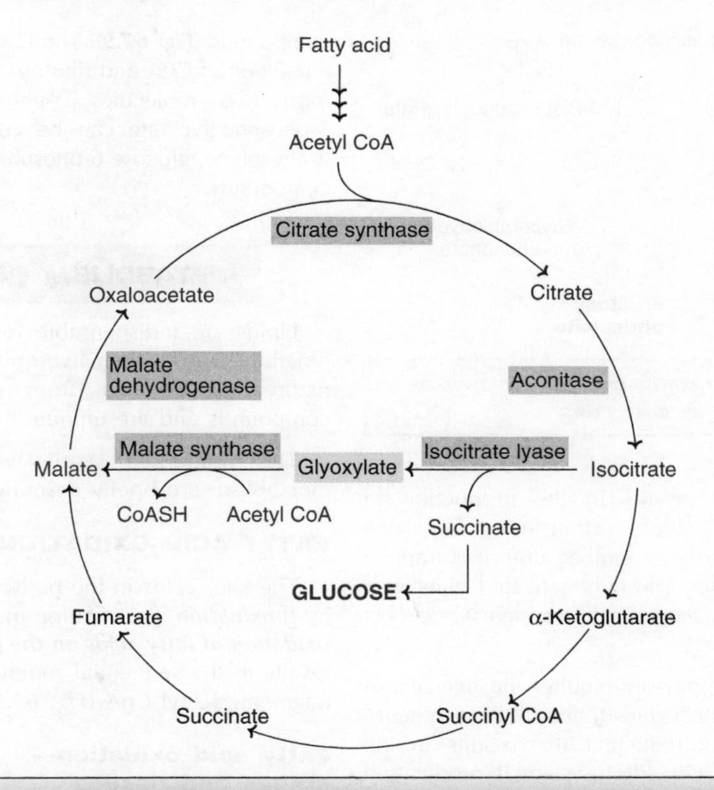

Fig. 67.7 : The glyoxylate cycle (represented in green colour).

Glutathione (reduced, GSH) detoxifies H_2O_2, peroxidase catalyses this reaction. NADPH is responsible for the regeneration of reduced glutathione from the oxidized one.

GLYOXYLATE CYCLE

The animals, including man, cannot carry out the net synthesis of carbohydrate from fat. However, the ***plants*** and many ***microorganisms*** are equipped with the metabolic machinery—namely the glyoxylate cycle—to convert fat into carbohydrates. This pathway is very significant in the germinating seeds where the stored triacylglycerol (fat) is converted to sugars to meet the energy needs.

The glyoxylate cycle is regarded as an anabolic variant of citric acid cycle and is depicted in ***Fig. 67.7***.

PHOTOSYNTHESIS

The ***synthesis of carbohydrates in green plants*** by assimilation of carbon dioxide is referred to as photosynthesis. It is now recognized that photosynthesis primarily involves the process of energy transduction in which ***light energy is converted into chemical energy*** (in the form of oxidizable carbon compounds).

It is an established fact that all the energy consumed by the biological systems arises from the solar energy, that is trapped in the photosynthesis. The basic equation of photosynthesis is given below.

$$CO_2 + H_2O \xrightarrow[\text{chlorophyll}]{\text{light}} (CH_2O)$$

In the above equation, (CH_2O) represents carbohydrate. Photosynthesis in the green plants occurs in the chloroplasts, a specialized organelles. The mechanism of photosynthesis is complex, involving many stages, and participation of various macromolecules and micromolecules.

The role of photosystems

The initial step in the photosynthesis is the absorption of light by chlorophyll molecules in the

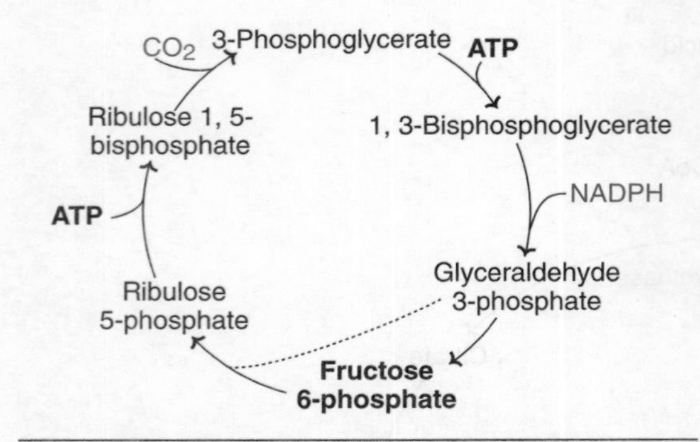

Fig. 67.8 : An outline of the Calvin cycle of photosynthesis.

chloroplasts. This results in the production of excitation energy which is transferred from one chlorophyll molecule to another, until it is trapped by a reaction center. The light-activated transfer of an electron to an acceptor (photosystems) occurs at the reaction center.

Photosynthesis primarily requires the interactions of two distinct photosystems (I and II). Photosystem I generates a strong reductant that results in the formation of NADPH. Photosystem II produces a strong oxidant that forms O_2 from H_2O. Further, the generation of ATP occurs as electrons flow from photosystem II to photosystem I (***Fig. 67.8***). Thus, light is responsible for the flow of electrons from H_2O to NADPH with a concomitant generation of ATP.

The Calvin cycle

The ***dark phase of photosynthesis*** is referred to as Calvin cycle. In this cycle, the ATP and NADPH produced in the light reaction (described above) are utilized to convert CO_2 to hexoses and other organic compounds (***Fig. 67.9***). The Calvin cycle starts with a reaction of CO_2 and ribulose 1, 5-bisphosphate to form two molecules 3-phosphoglycerate. This 3-phosphoglycerate can be converted to fructose 6-phosphate, glucose 6-phosphate and other carbon compounds.

METABOLISM OF LIPIDS

Lipids are indispensable for cell structure and function. Due to their hydrophobic and non-polar nature, lipids differ from rest of the body compounds and are unique in their action.

The important pathways/cycles of lipid metabolism are briefly described.

FATTY ACID OXIDATION

The fatty acids in the body are mostly oxidized by ***β-oxidation***. β-Oxidation may be defined as the ***oxidation of fatty acids on the β-carbon atom***. This results in the sequential removal of a two carbon fragment, acetyl CoA (***Fig. 67.10***).

Fatty acid oxidation—stages and tissues

The β-oxidation of fatty acids involves three stages

I. Activation of fatty acids occurring in the cytosol;

II. Transport of fatty acids into mitochondria;

III. β-Oxidation proper in the mitochondrial matrix.

Fatty acids are oxidized by most of the tissues in the body. However, ***brain, erythrocytes and adrenal medulla cannot utilize fatty acids for energy requirement.***

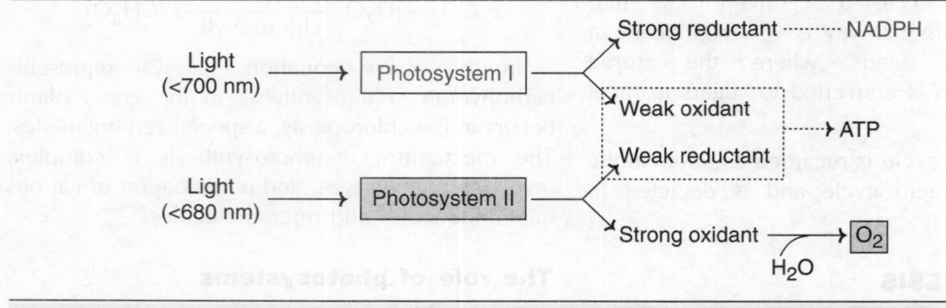

Fig. 67.9 : Interaction between two photosystems in photosynthesis.

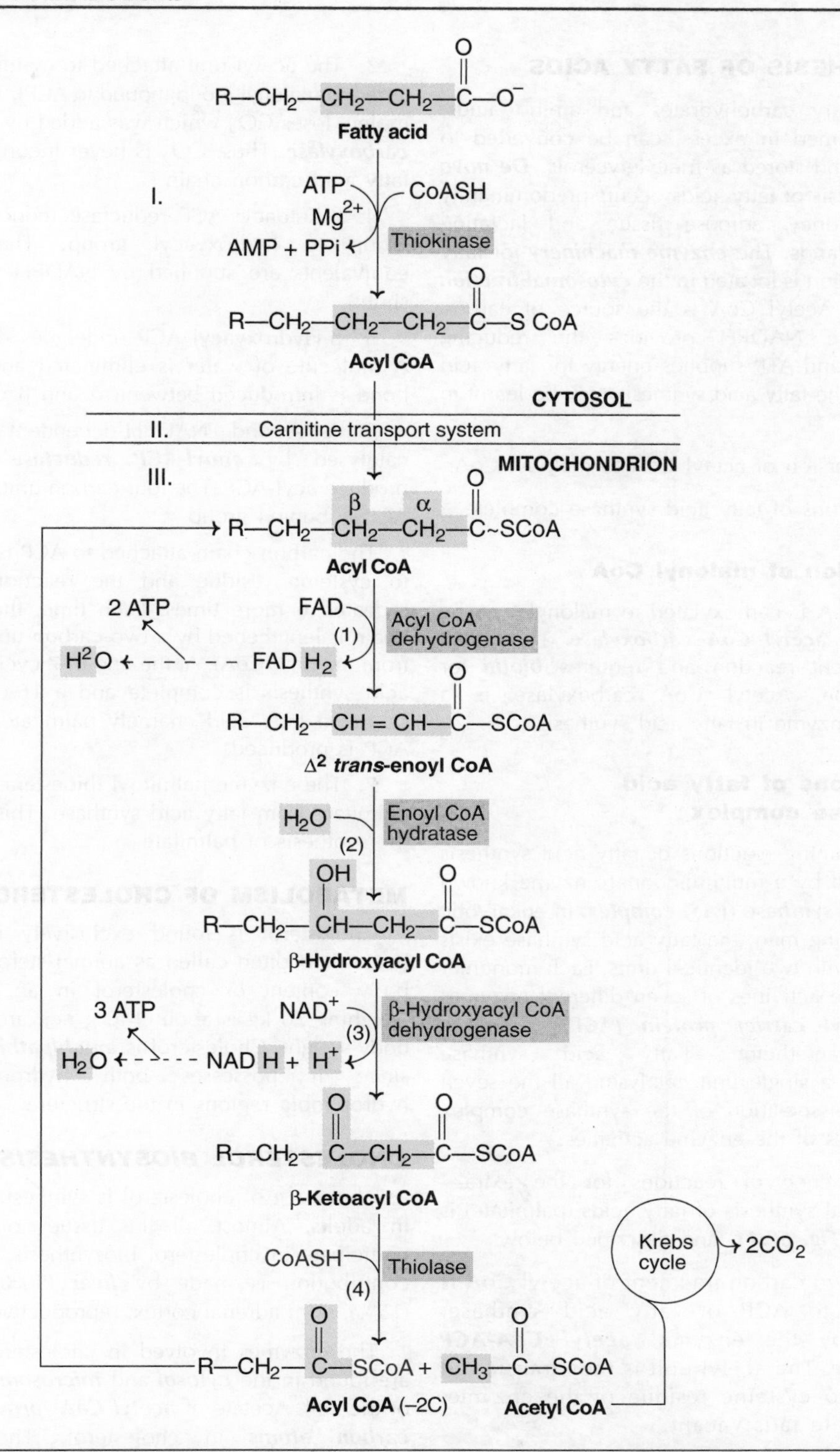

***Fig. 67.10 :** β-Oxidation of fatty acids : Palmitoyl CoA (16 carbon) undergoes seven cycles to yield 8 acetyl CoA [I-Activation; II-Transport; III-β Oxidation proper—(1) Oxidation, (2) Hydration, (3) Oxidation and (4) Cleavage]*

BIOSYNTHESIS OF FATTY ACIDS

The dietary carbohydrates and amino acids, when consumed in excess, can be converted to fatty acids and stored as triacylglycerols. ***De novo*** (new) synthesis of fatty acids occurs predominantly in liver, kidney, adipose tissue and lactating mammary glands. The ***enzyme machinery*** for fatty acid production is located in the ***cytosomal fraction*** of the cell. Acetyl CoA is the source of carbon atoms while NADPH provides the reducing equivalents and ATP supplies energy for fatty acid formation. The fatty acid synthesis may be learnt in 2 stages

I. Conversion of acetyl CoA to malonyl CoA.

II. Reactions of fatty acid synthase complex.

I. Formation of malonyl CoA

Acetyl CoA is carboxylated to malonyl CoA by the enzyme ***acetyl CoA carboxylase.*** This is an ATP-dependent reaction and requires ***biotin*** for CO_2 fixation. Acetyl CoA carboxylase is a regulatory enzyme in fatty acid synthesis.

II. Reactions of fatty acid synthase complex

The remaining reactions of fatty acid synthesis are catalysed by a multifunctional enzyme known as ***fatty acid synthase (FAS) complex.*** In eukaryotic cells, including man, the fatty acid synthase exists as a dimer with two identical units. Each monomer possesses the activities of seven different enzymes and an ***acyl carrier protein (ACP)*** bound to 4′-phosphopantetheine. Fatty acid synthase functions as a single unit catalysing all the seven reactions. Dissociation of the synthase complex results in loss of the enzyme activities.

The sequence of reactions for the extra—mitochondrial synthesis of fatty acids (palmitate) is depicted in ***Fig. 67.11***, and described below

1. The two carbon fragment of acetyl CoA is transferred to ACP of fatty acid synthase, catalysed by the enzyme, ***acetyl CoA-ACP transacylase***. The acetyl unit is then transferred from ACP to cysteine residue of the enzyme. Thus ACP site falls vacant.

2. The enzyme ***malonyl CoA-ACP transacylase*** transfers malonate from malonyl CoA to bind to ACP.

3. The acetyl unit attached to cysteine is transferred to malonyl group (bound to ACP). The malonyl moiety loses CO_2 which was added by ***acetyl CoA carboxylase.*** Thus, CO_2 is never incorporated into fatty acid carbon chain.

4. β-Ketoacyl ACP reductase reduces ketoacyl group to hydroxyacyl group. The reducing equivalents are supplied by NADPH (from HMP shunt).

5. β-Hydroxyacyl ACP undergoes dehydration. A molecule of water is eliminated and a double bond is introduced between α and β carbons.

6. A second NADPH-dependent reduction, catalysed by ***enoyl-ACP reductase*** occurs to produce acyl-ACP. The four-carbon unit attached to ACP is butyryl group.

The carbon chain attached to ACP is transferred to cysteine residue and the reactions 2-6 are repeated 6 more times. Each time, the fatty acid chain is lengthened by a two-carbon unit (obtained from malonyl CoA). At the end of 7 cycles, the fatty acid synthesis is complete and a 16-carbon fully saturated fatty acid—namely palmitate—bound to ACP is produced.

7. The enzyme palmitoyl thioesterase separates palmitate from fatty acid synthase. This completes the synthesis of palmitate.

METABOLISM OF CHOLESTEROL

Cholesterol is found exclusively in animals, hence it is often called as animal sterol. The total body content of cholesterol in an adult man weighing 70 kg is about 140 g i.e., around 2 g/kg body weight. Cholesterol is ***amphipathic*** in nature, since it possesses both hydrophilic and hydrophobic regions in the structure.

CHOLESTEROL BIOSYNTHESIS

About 1 g of cholesterol is synthesized per day in adults. Almost all the tissues of the body participate in cholesterol biosynthesis. The largest contribution is made by ***liver*** (50%), ***intestine*** (15%), skin, adrenal cortex, reproductive tissue etc.

The enzymes involved in cholesterol synthesis are found in the ***cytosol*** and ***microsomal fractions*** of the cell. Acetate of ***acetyl CoA provides*** all the ***carbon atoms*** in cholesterol. The reducing equivalents are supplied by ***NADPH*** while ***ATP*** provides energy. The key intermediates of cholesterol formation are depicted in ***Fig. 67.12***.

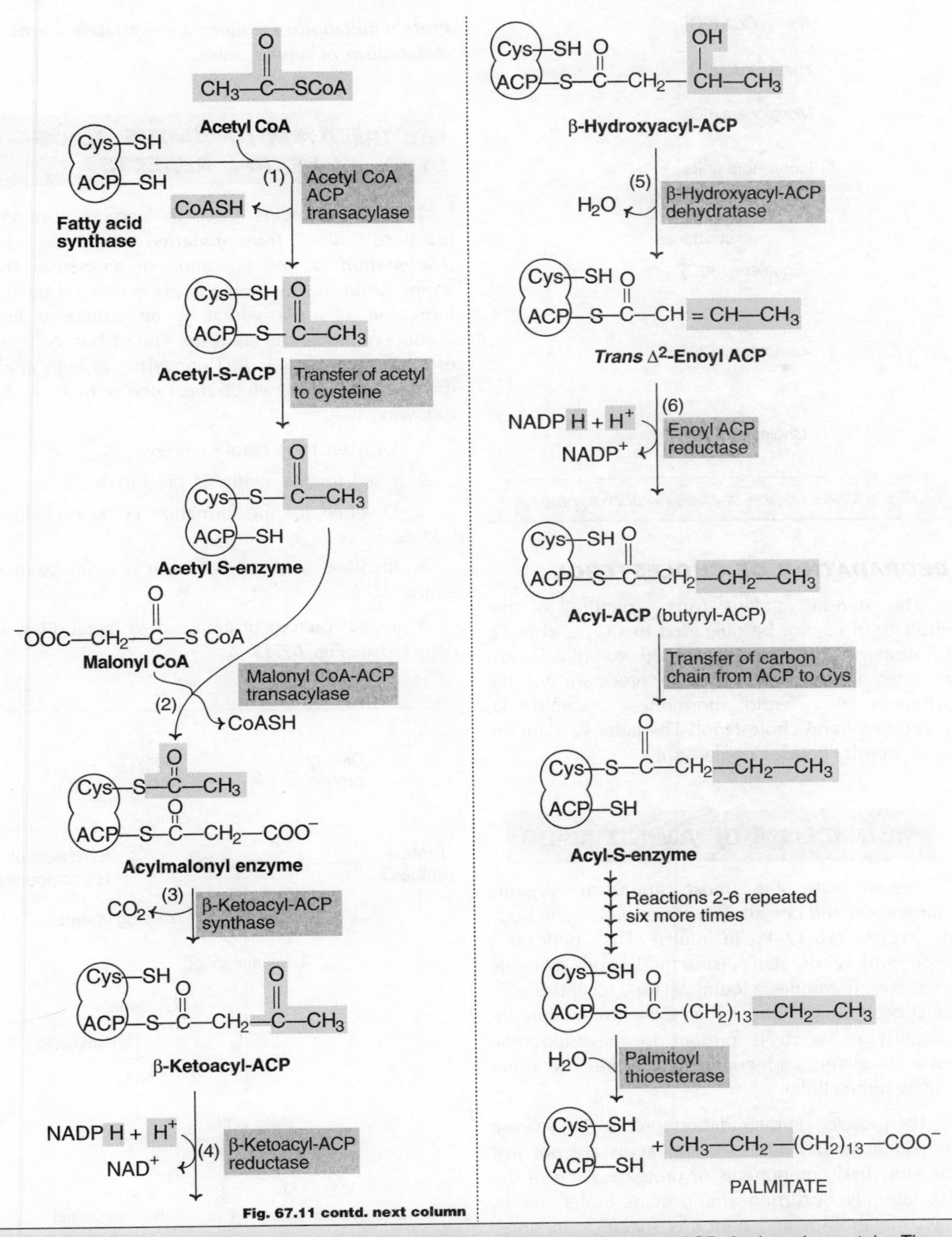

Fig. 67.11 : Biosynthesis of long chain fatty acid–palmitate. (Cys–Cysteine; ACP–Acyl carrier protein; The pathway repeats 7 times to produce palmitate; the first two carbons at the methyl end are directly from acetyl CoA, the rest of the carbons come from malonyl CoA).

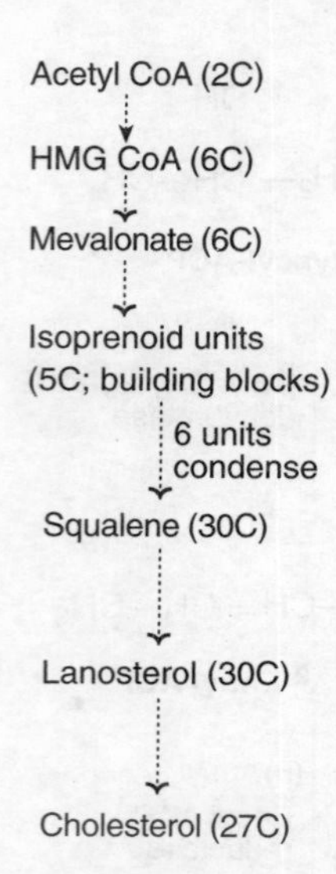

Fig. 67.12 : Outline of cholesterol biosynthesis.

DEGRADATION OF CHOLESTEROL

The steroid nucleus (ring structure) of the cholesterol cannot be degraded to CO_2 and H_2O. Cholesterol (50%) is converted to bile acids, excreted in feces, serves as a precursor for the synthesis of steroid hormones, vitamin D, coprostanol and cholestanol. The latter two are the fecal sterols, besides cholesterol.

METABOLISM OF AMINO ACIDS

Proteins are the ***most abundant organic compounds*** and constitute a major part of the body dry weight (10-12 kg in adults). They perform a wide variety of static (structural) and dynamic (enzymes, hormones, clotting factors, receptors etc.) functions. About half of the body protein (predominantly collagen) is present in the supportive tissue (skeleton and connective) while the other half is intracellular.

The proteins on degradation (proteolysis) release individual amino acids. Amino acids are not just the structural components of proteins. Each of the 20 naturally occurring amino acids undergoes its own metabolism and performs specific functions. Some of the amino acids also serve as precursors for the synthesis of many biologically important compounds (e.g. melanin, serotonin, creatine etc.), ***Protein metabolism is more appropriately learnt as metabolism of amino acids.***

METABOLISM OF AMINO ACIDS— GENERAL ASPECTS

The amino acids undergo certain common reactions like ***transamination*** followed by ***deamination*** for the liberation of ***ammonia***. The amino group of the amino acids is utilized for the formation of ***urea*** which is an excretory end product of protein metabolism. The carbon skeleton of the amino acids is first converted to keto acids (by transamination) which meet one or more of the following fates.

1. Utilized to generate energy.
2. Used for the synthesis of glucose.
3. Diverted for the formation of fat or ketone bodies.
4. Involved in the production of non-essential amino acids.

A general picture of amino acid metabolism is depicted in ***Fig. 67.13***.

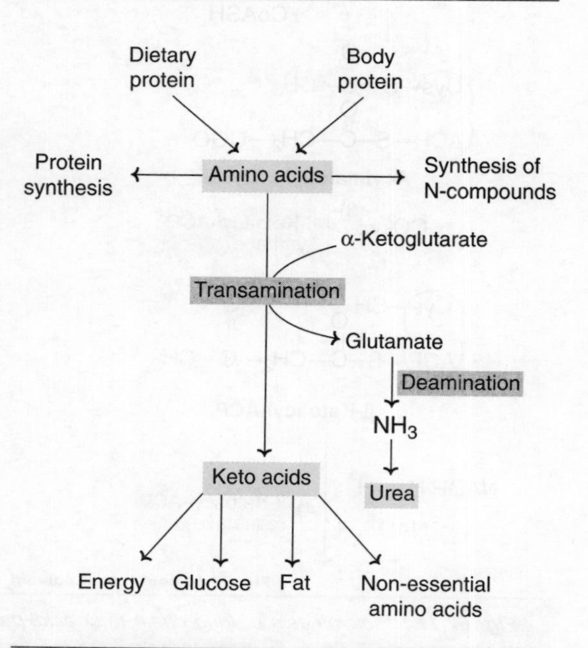

Fig. 67.13 : An overview of amino acid metabolism.

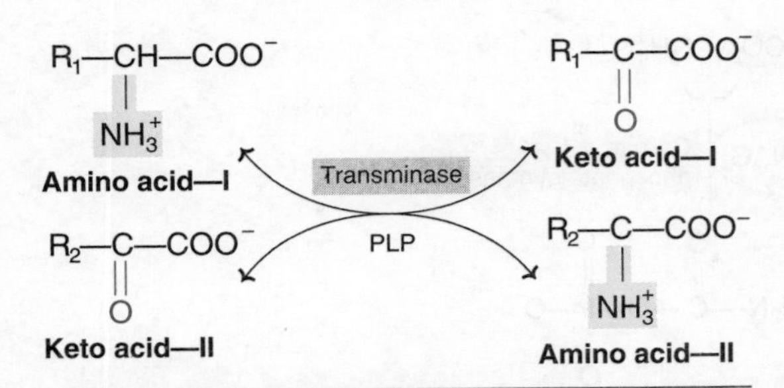

Fig. 67.14 : Transamination reaction.

TRANSAMINATION

The transfer of an amino (–NH_2) group from an amino acid to a keto acid is known as transamination (***Fig. 67.14***). This process involves the interconversion of a pair of amino acids and a pair of keto acids, catalysed by a group of enzymes called ***transaminases*** (recently, ***aminotransferases***).

The salient features of transamination are :

1. All transaminases require ***pyridoxal phosphate*** (PLP), a coenzyme derived from vitamin B_6.

2. There is no free NH_3 liberated, only the transfer of amino group occurs.

3. Transamination is ***reversible***.

4. It involves both catabolism (degradation) and anabolism (synthesis) of amino acids. Transamination is ultimately responsible for the synthesis of non-essential amino acids.

5. Transamination diverts the excess amino acids towards ***energy generation***.

6. The amino acids undergo transamination to finally concentrate nitrogen in glutamate. ***Glutamate*** is the only amino acid that undergoes oxidative deamination to a significant extent to liberate free NH_3 for urea synthesis.

7. All amino acids except lysine, threonine, proline and hydroxyproline participate in transamination.

DEAMINATION

The removal of amino group from the amino acids as NH_3 is deamination. It results in the liberation of ammonia for urea synthesis. Deamination may be either oxidative or non-oxidative.

UREA CYCLE

Urea is the end product of protein metabolism (amino acid metabolism). The nitrogen of amino acids converted to ammonia (as described above) is toxic to the body. It is converted to urea and detoxified. As such, urea accounts for 80-90% of the nitrogen containing substances excreted in urine.

Urea is ***synthesized in liver*** and transported to kidneys for excretion in urine. Urea cycle is the ***first metabolic cycle*** that was elucidated by Hans Krebs and Kurt Henseleit (1932), hence it is known as ***Krebs-Henseleit cycle***. The individual reactions, however, were described in more detail later on by Ratner and Cohen.

Urea has ***two amino (—NH_2) groups***, one derived ***from NH_3*** and the other ***from aspartate.*** Carbon atom is supplied by CO_2. Urea synthesis is a five-step cyclic process, with five distinct enzymes. The first ***two enzymes*** are present in ***mitochondria*** while the ***rest*** are localized in ***cytosol***. The reactions of urea cycle are depicted in ***Fig. 67.15***.

METABOLISM OF INDIVIDUAL AMINO ACIDS

The metabolisms of certain individual amino acids are very briefly given in the form of overviews.

GLYCINE

Glycine (Gly, G) is a non-essential, optically inactive and ***glycogenic*** (precursor for glucose) amino acid. It is indispensable for chicks. The outline of glycine metabolism is depicted in ***Fig. 67.16***. Glycine is actively involved in the synthesis of many specialized products (heme, purines, creatine etc.) in the body, besides its incorporation into proteins, synthesis of serine and glucose and participation in one-carbon metabolism.

PHENYLALANINE AND TYROSINE

Phenylalanine (Phe, F) and tyrosine (Tyr, Y) are structurally related aromatic amino acids. Phenylalanine is an essential amino acid while tyrosine is non-essential. Besides its incorporation into proteins, the only function of phenylalanine is its conversion to tyrosine. For this reason, ingestion of tyrosine can reduce the dietary requirement of phenylalanine. This phenomenon is referred to as ***'sparing action' of tyrosine on phenylalanine.***

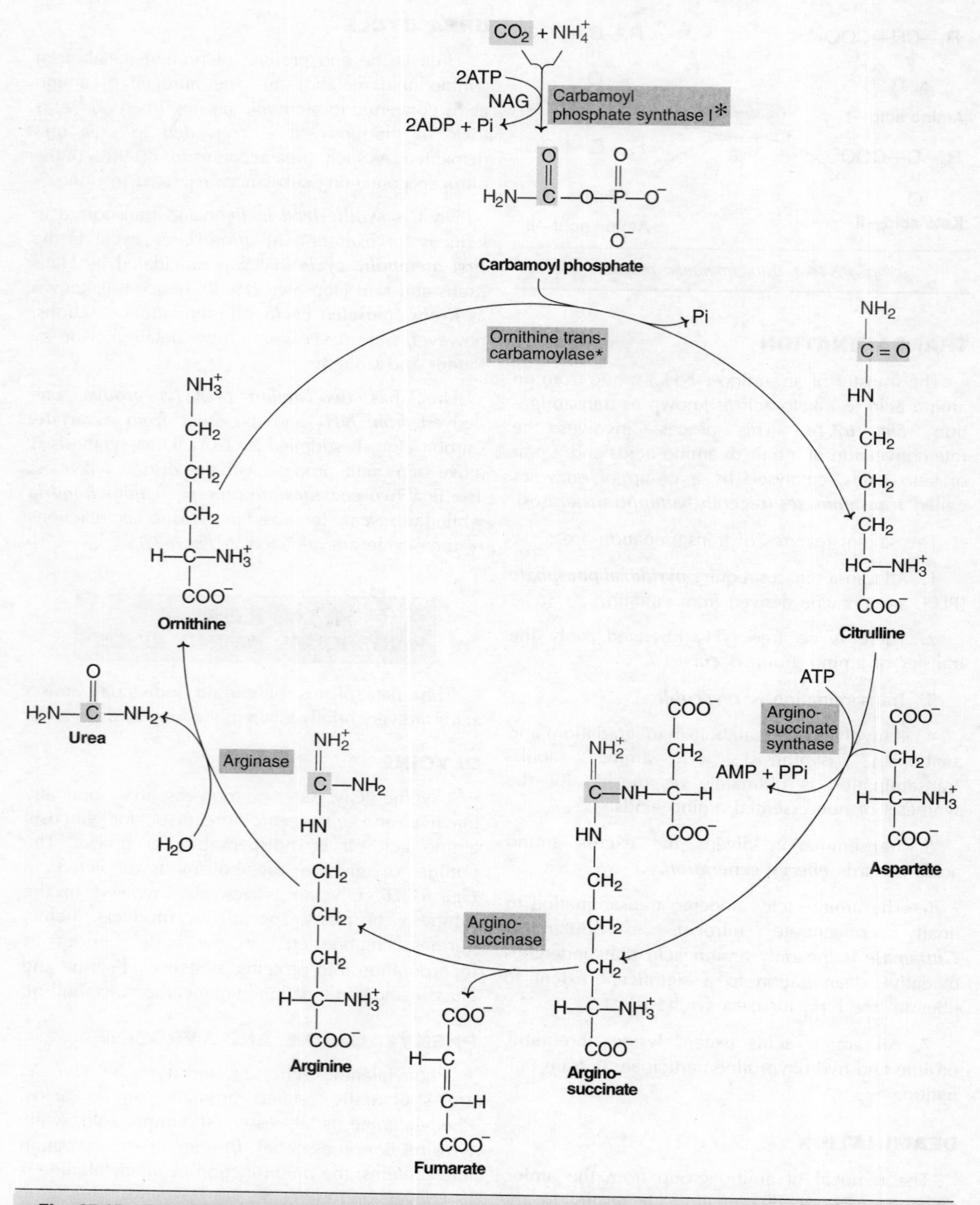

*Fig. 67.15 : Reactions of urea cycle (NAG–N-acetylglutamate; (in the formation of urea, one amino group is derived from free ammonium ion while the other is from aspartate; carbon is obtained from CO_2; * mitochondrial enzymes, the rest of the enzymes are cytosomal).*

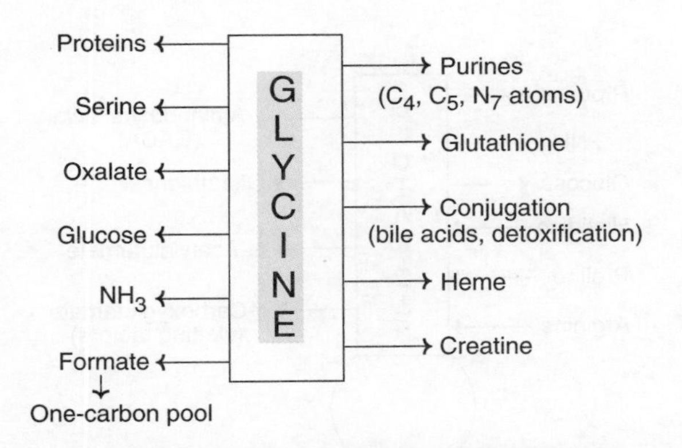

Fig. 67.16 : Overview of glycine metabolism.

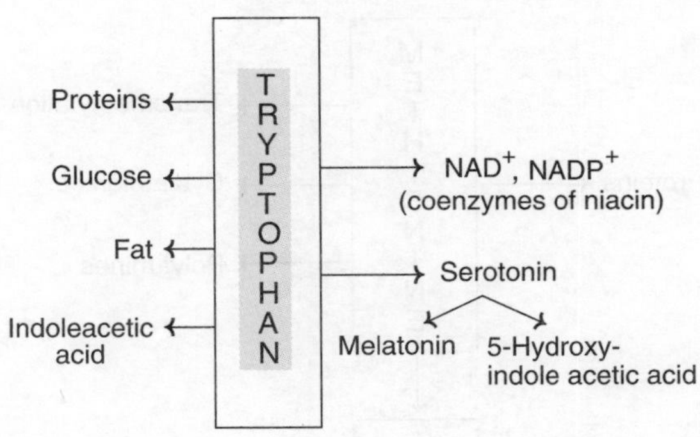

Fig. 67.18 : Overview of tryptophan metabolism.

The predominant metabolism of phenylalanine occurs through tyrosine. Tyrosine is incorporated into proteins and is involved in the synthesis of a variety of biologically important compounds—***epinephrine, norepinephrine, dopamine*** (catecholamines), ***thyroid hormones***—and the pigment ***melanin*** (***Fig. 67.17***). During the course of degradation, phenylalanine and tyrosine are converted to metabolites which can serve as precursors for the synthesis of glucose and fat. Hence, these amino acids are both ***glucogenic*** and ***ketogenic***.

TRYPTOPHAN

Tryptophan (Trp, W) was the first to be identified as an essential amino acid. It contains an indole ring and chemically it is α-amino β-indole propionic acid. Tryptophan is both ***glucogenic*** and ***ketogenic*** in nature. It is a precusor for the synthesis of important compounds, namely ***NAD^+*** and ***$NADP^+$*** (coenzymes of niacin), ***serotonin*** and ***melatonin*** (***Fig. 67.18***).

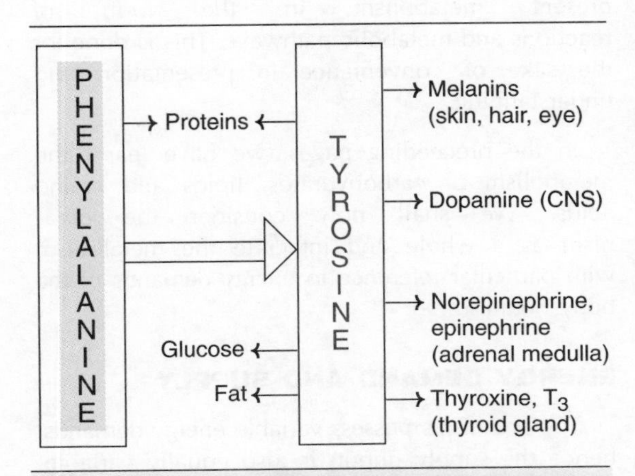

Fig. 67.17 : Overview of phenylalanine and tyrosine metabolism (CNS—Central nervous system; T_3—Triiodothyronine).

SULFUR AMINO ACIDS

The sulfur-containing amino acids are methionine, cysteine and cystine. Among these, only ***methionine*** is ***essential***. It serves as a precursor for the synthesis of cysteine and cystine which are, therefore, non-essential. An overview of the metabolism of the sulfur amino acids is depicted in ***Fig. 67.19***.

GLUTAMATE AND GLUTAMINE

Glutamate and glutamine are non-essential glycogenic amino acids. Both of them play a predominant role in the amino acid metabolism and are directly involved in the final transfer of amino group for urea synthesis. In ***Fig. 67.20***, an outline of glutamate and glutamine metabolism is given.

FATE OF CARBON SKELETON OF AMINO ACIDS

After the removal of amino groups, the carbon skeleton of amino acids is converted to intermediates of TCA cycle or their precursors. The carbon skeleton finally has one or more of the following fates :

1. Oxidation via TCA cycle to produce energy (about 10-15% of body needs).

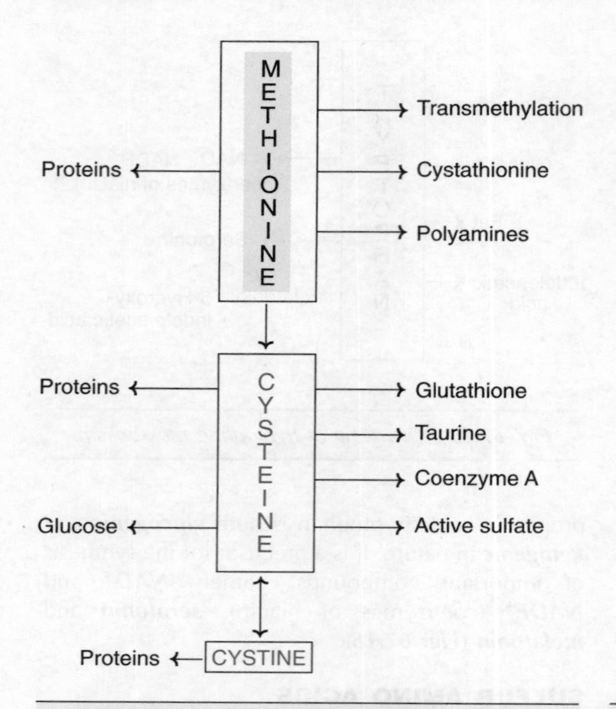

Fig. 67.19 : Overview of the metabolism of sulfur amino acids.

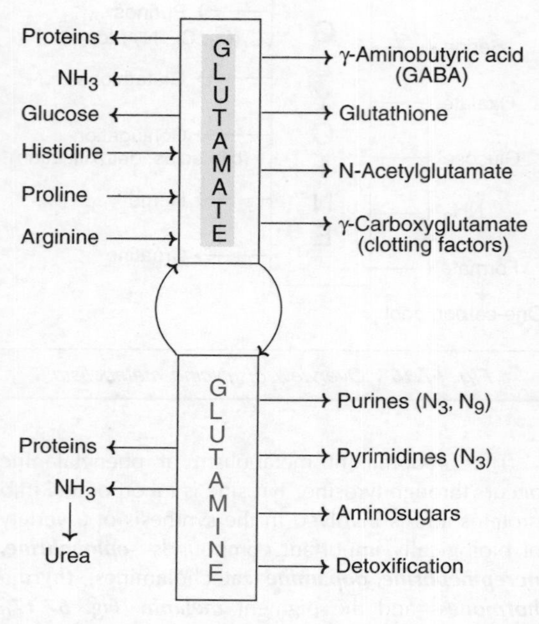

Fig. 67.20 : Overview of glutamate and glutamine metabolism.

2. Synthesis of glucose.

3. Formation of lipids—fatty acids and ketone bodies.

4. Synthesis of non-essential amino acids.

The carbon skeletons of the 20 standard amino acids (or the amino acids of proteins) are degraded to one of the following seven products—***pyruvate***, ***α-ketoglutarate***, ***succinyl CoA***, ***fumarate***, ***oxaloacetate***, ***acetyl CoA*** and ***acetoacetate***. Some authors use the term amphibolic (*Greek*: amphiboles—uncertain) intermediates to these compounds due to their multiple metabolic functions.

The amino acids are classified into three groups, based on the nature of the metabolic end products of carbon skeleton (***Table 67.1***).

Inborn errors of amino acid metabolism—a summary

Several inherited disorders are associated with amino acid metabolism. In ***Table 67.2***, a summary of major diseases and the enzyme defects is given.

INTEGRATION OF METABOLISM

Metabolism is a continuous process, with thousands of reactions, simultaneously occurring in the living cell. However, biochemists prefer to present metabolism in the form of reactions and metabolic pathways. This is done for the sake of convenience in presentation and understanding.

In the preceeding pages, we have learnt the metabolism of carbohydrates, lipids and amino acids. We shall now consider the organism as a whole and integrate the metabolism with particular reference to energy demands of the body organism.

ENERGY DEMAND AND SUPPLY

The organisms possess variable energy demands, hence the supply (input) is also equally variable. The consumed metabolic fuel may be burnt (oxidized to CO_2 and H_2O) or stored to meet the energy requirements as per the body needs. ***ATP***

TABLE 67.1 Classification of amino acids based on the fate of carbon skeleton

Glycogenic (glucogenic)	*Glycogenic and Ketogenic*	*Ketogenic*
Alanine	Phenylalanine*	Leucine*
Arginine*	Isoleucine*	Lysine*
Aspartate	Tyrosine	
Cysteine	Tryptophan*	
Glutamine		
Glutamate		
Glycine		
Histidine*		
Hydroxyproline		
Methionine*		
Proline		
Serine		
Threonine*		
Valine*		

**Essential amino acids; (Helpful tips to recall—ketogenic amino acids start with letter 'L'; PITT for glyco-and ketogenic amino acids; rest of the 20 amino acids are only glycogenic).*

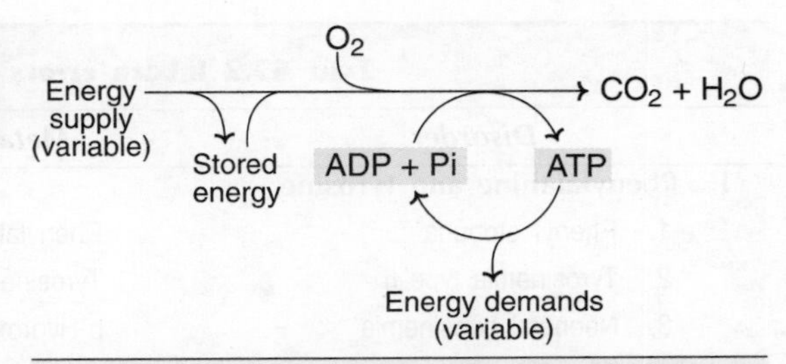

***Fig. 67.21** : A summary of body's energy supply and demands. (**Note** : ATP serves as the energy currency).*

serves as the ***energy currency of the cell*** in this process (***Fig. 67.21***).

The humans possess enormous capacity for food consumption. It is estimated that one can consume as much as 100 times his/her basal requirements! Obesity, a disorder of overnutrition mostly prevalent in affluent societies, is primarily a consequence of overconsumption.

INTEGRATION OF MAJOR METABOLIC PATHWAYS OF ENERGY METABOLISM

An overview of the interrelationship between the important metabolic pathways, concerned with fuel metabolism depicted in ***Fig. 67.22***, is briefly

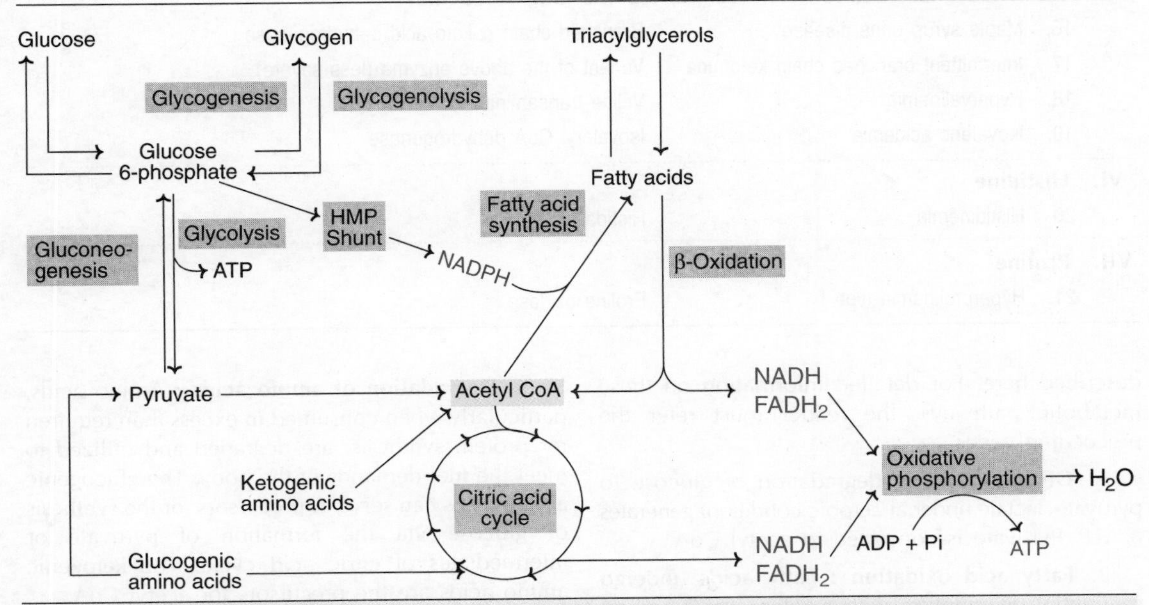

***Fig. 67.22** : An overview of integration of metabolic pathways of energy metabolism (HMP shunt—Hexose monophosphate shunt).*

TABLE 67.2 Inborn errors of amino acid metabolism

Disorder	Metabolic defect (enzyme/other)
I. Phenylalanine and tyrosine	
1. Phenylketonuria	Phenylalanine hydroxylase
2. Tyrosinemia type II	Tyrosine transaminase
3. Neonatal tyrosinemia	p-Hydroxy phenylpyruvate dioxygenase
4. Alkaptonuria	Homogentisate oxidase
5. Tyrosinosis (tyrosinemia type I)	Maleyl acetoacetate isomerase or fumaryl acetoacetate hydrolase
6. Albinism	Tyrosinase
II. Sulfur amino acids (methionine, cysteine and cystine)	
7. Cystinuria	Defect in renal reabsorption
8. Cystinosis	Impairment in cystine utilization (defect in lysosomal function)
9. Homocystinuria type I	Cystathionine synthetase
10. Homocystinuria type II	N^5, N^{10}-Methylene THF reductase
11. Homocystinuria type III	N^5-Methyl THF-homocysteine methyltransferase
12. Cystathionuria	Cystathioninase
III. Glycine	
13. Glycinuria	Defect in renal reabsorption
14. Primary hyperoxaluria	Glycine transaminase
IV. Tryptophan	
15. Hartnup's disease	Defective intestinal absorption
V. Branched chain amino acids (valine, leucine and isoleucine)	
16. Maple syrup urine disease	Branched chain α-keto acid dehydrogenase
17. Intermittent branched chain ketonuria	Variant of the above enzyme (less severe)
18. Hypervalinemia	Valine transaminase
19. Isovaleric acidemia	Isovaleryl CoA dehydrogenase
VI. Histidine	
20. Histidinemia	Histidase
VII. Proline	
21. Hyperprolinemia type I	Proline oxidase

described here. For detailed information on these metabolic pathways, the reader must refer the preceeding pages.

1. **Glycolysis :** The degradation of glucose to pyruvate (lactate under anaerobic condition) generates 8 ATP. Pyruvate is converted to acetyl CoA.

2. **Fatty acid oxidation :** Fatty acids undergo sequential degradation with a release of 2-carbon fragment, namely acetyl CoA. The energy is trapped in the form of NADH and $FADH_2$.

3. **Degradation of amino acids :** Amino acids, particularly when consumed in excess than required for protein synthesis, are degraded and utilized to meet the fuel demands of the body. The glucogenic amino acids can serve as precursors for the synthesis of glucose via the formation of pyruvate or intermediates of citric acid cycle. The ketogenic amino acids are the precursors for acetyl CoA.

4. **Citric acid cycle :** Acetyl CoA is the key and common metabolite, produced from different fuel

sources (carbohydrates, lipids, amino acids). ***Acetyl CoA*** enters citric acid cycle and gets oxidized to CO_2. Thus, citric acid cycle is the final common metabolic pathway for the oxidation of all foodstuffs. Most of the energy is trapped in the form of NADH and $FADH_2$.

5. **Oxidative phosphorylation :** The NADH and $FADH_2$, produced in different metabolic pathways, are finally oxidized in the electron transport chain (ETC). The ETC is coupled with oxidative phosphorylation ***to generate ATP.***

6. **Hexose monophosphate shunt :** This pathway is primarily concerned with the liberation of NADPH and ribose sugar. NADPH is utilized for the biosynthesis of several compounds, including fatty acids. Ribose is an essential component of nucleotides and nucleic acids (note—DNA contains deoxyribose).

7. **Gluconeogenesis :** The synthesis of glucose from non-carbohydrate sources constitutes gluconeogenesis. Several compounds (e.g. pyruvate, glycerol, amino acids) can serve as precursors for gluconeogenesis.

8. **Glycogen metabolism :** Glycogen is the storage form of glucose, mostly found in liver and muscle. It is degraded (glycogenolysis) and synthesized (glycogenesis) by independent pathways. Glycogen effectively serves as a ***fuel reserve*** to meet body needs, ***for a brief period*** (between meals).

REGULATION OF METABOLIC PATHWAYS

The metabolic pathways, in general, are controlled by four different mechanisms

1. *The availability of substrates*
2. *Covalent modification of enzymes*
3. *Allosteric regulation*
4. *Regulation of enzyme synthesis.*

The details of these regulatory processes are discussed under the individual metabolic pathways, in the preceeding pages.

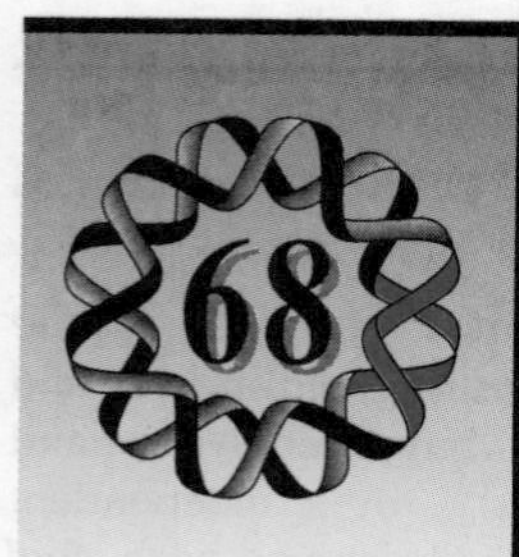

Immunology

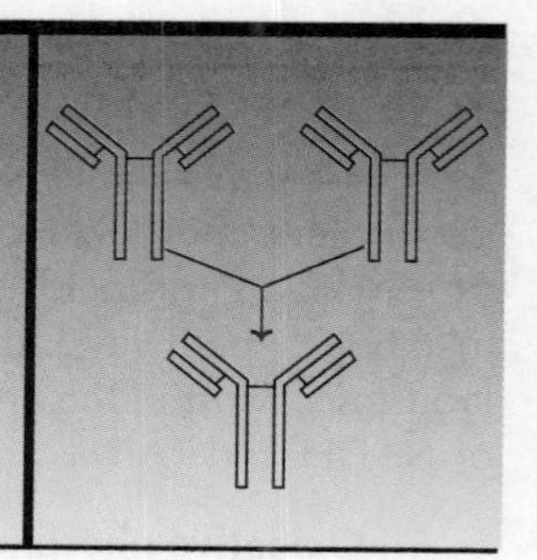

Immunology deals with the study of immunity and immune systems of vertebrates. Immunity (immunis literally means exempt/free from burden) broadly involves the ***resistance shown***, and ***protection offered by the host organism against the infectious diseases***. The immune system consists of a complex network of cells and molecules, and their interactions. It is specifically designed to eliminate infectious organisms from the body. This is possible since the organism is capable of distinguishing the self from non-self, and eliminate non-self.

Immunity is broadly divided into two types — innate (non-specific) immunity and adaptive or acquired (specific) immunity.

INNATE IMMUNITY

Innate immunity is non-specific, and represents the inherent capability of the organism to offer resistance against diseases. It consists of defensive barriers.

First line of defense

The ***skin*** is the largest organ in the human body, constituting about 15% of the adult body weight. The skin provides mechanical barrier to prevent the entry of microorganisms and viruses. The acidic (pH 3-5) environment on the skin surface inhibits the growth of certain microorganisms. Further, the sweat contains an enzyme lysozyme that can destroy bacterial cell wall.

Second line of defense

Despite the physical barriers, the microorganisms do enter the body. The body defends itself and ***eliminates the invading organisms by non-specific mechanisms*** such as sneezing and secretions of the mucus. In addition, the body also tries to kill the pathogens by phagocytosis (involving macrophages and complement system). The inflammatory response and fever response of the body also form a part of innate immunity.

THE IMMUNE SYSTEM

The immune system represents the third and most potent defense mechanism of the body. Acquired (adaptive or specific) immunity is capable of specifically recognizing and eliminating the invading microorganisms and foreign molecules (antigens). In contrast to innate immunity, the acquired immunity displays four distinct characteristics

- Antigen specificity
- Recognition diversity
- Immunological memory
- Discrimination between self and non-self.

The ***body*** possess tremendous capability to specifically ***identify various antigens*** (antigen is a foreign substance, usually a protein or a carbohydrate that elicits immune response). Exposure to an antigen leads to the development of immunological memory. As a result, a second encounter of the body to the same antigen results in a heightened state of immune response. The immune system recognizes and responds to foreign antigens as it is capable of distinguishing self and non-self. Autoimmune diseases are caused due to a failure to discriminate self and non-self antigens.

ORGANIZATION OF IMMUNE SYSTEM

The immune system consists of several organs distributed throughout the body (***Fig. 68.1***). These lymphoid organs are categorized as primary and secondary.

Primary lymphoid organs

These organs provide appropriate micro-environment for the development and maturation of antigen-sensitive lymphocytes (a type of white blood cells). The ***thymus*** (situated above the heart) and bone marrow are the central or primary lymphoid organs. T-lymphocyte maturation occurs in the thymus while B-lymphocyte maturation takes place in the bone marrow.

Secondary lymphoid organs

These are the sites for the initiation of immune response. e.g. spleen, tonsils, lymph nodes, appendix, Peyers patches in the gut. Secondary lymphoid organs provide the microenvironment for interaction between antigens and mature lymphocytes.

CELLS OF THE IMMUNE SYSTEM

Two types of lymphocytes namely B-cells and T-cells are critical for the immune system. In addition, several accessory cells and effector cells also participate.

B-lymphocytes

The site of development and maturation of B-cells occurs in ***b***ursa fabricus in birds, and ***b***one marrow in mammals. During the course of immune response. B-cells mature into plasma cells and secrete antibodies (immunoglobulins).

The B-cells possess the capability to specifically recognize each antigen and produce antibodies against it. B-lymphocytes are inimately associated with ***humoral immunity***.

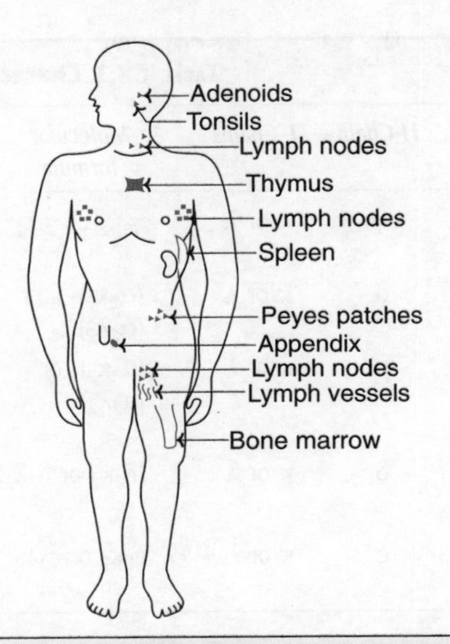

Fig. 68.1 : *A diagrammatic representation of human lymphatic system.*

T-lymphocytes

The maturation of T-cells occurs in the ***t***hymus, hence the name. The T-cells can identify viruses and microorganisms from the antigens displayed on their surfaces. There are at least four different types of T-cells.

- ***Inducer T-cells*** that mediate the development of T-cells in the thymus.
- ***Cytotoxic T-cells*** (T_C), capable of recognizing and killing the infected or abnormal cells.
- ***Helper T-cells*** (T_H) that initiate immune responses.
- ***Suppressor T-cells*** mediate the suppression of immune response.

T-lymphocytes are responsible for the ***cell-mediated immunity***.

IMMUNOGLOBULINS

The humoral immunity is mediated by a special group of proteins called immunoglobulins or ***antibodies***, produced by B-lymphocytes.

STRUCTURE OF IMMUNOGLOBULINS

All the immunoglobulin (Ig) molecules basically consist of two identical ***heavy (H) chains*** (mol. wt. 53,000 to 75,000 each) and two identical ***light (L) chains*** (mol. wt. 23,000 each) held together by disulfide linkages and non-covalent interactions

TABLE 68.1 Characteristics of human immunoglobulins

Type	H-Chain	L-Chains	Molecular formula	Molecular weight	Percentage carbohydrate	Serum conc. mg/dl	Major function(s)
IgG	γ	κ or λ	$\gamma_2\kappa_2$ or $\gamma_2\lambda_2$	~150,000	3	800–1,500	Mostly responsible for humoral immunity
IgA	α	κ or λ	$(\alpha_2\kappa_2)_{1-3}$ or $(\alpha_2\lambda_2)_{1-3}$	$\sim(160{,}000)_{1-3}$	8	150–400	Protects the body surfaces
IgM	μ	κ or λ	$(\mu_2\kappa_2)_5$ or $(\mu_2\lambda_2)_5$	~900,000	12	50–200	Humoral immunity, serves as first line of defense
IgD	δ	κ or λ	$(\delta_2\kappa_2$ or $\delta_2\lambda_2)$	~180,000	13	1–10	B-cell receptor ?
IgE	ε	κ or λ	$\varepsilon_2\kappa_2$ or $\varepsilon_2\lambda_2$	~190,000	12	0.02–0.05	Humoral sensitivity and histamine release.

(***Fig. 68.2***). Thus, immunoglobulin is a Y-shaped tetramer (H_2L_2). Each heavy chain contains approximately 450 amino acids while each light chain has 212 amino acids. The heavy chains of Ig are linked to carbohydrates, hence immunoglobulins are ***glycoproteins***.

Constant and variable regions : Each chain (L or H) of Ig has two regions (domains), namely the constant and the variable. The amino terminal half of the light chain is the variable region (V_L) while the carboxy terminal half is the constant region (C_L). As regards heavy chain, approximately one-quarter of the amino terminal region is variable (V_H) while the remaining three-quarters is constant (C_{H1}, C_{H2}, C_{H3}). The amino acid sequence (with its tertiary structure) of variable regions of light and heavy chains is responsible for the specific binding of immunoglobulin (antibody) with antigen.

CLASSES OF IMMUNOGLOBULINS

Humans have five classes of immunoglobulins — namely ***IgG, IgA, IgM, IgD and IgE*** — containing the heavy chains γ, α, μ, δ and ε, respectively. The type of heavy chain ultimately determines the class and the function of a given Ig.

Two types of light chains — namely kappa (κ) and lambda (λ) — are found in immunoglobulins. They differ in their structure in C_L regions. An immunoglobulin (of any class) contains two κ or two λ light chains and never a mixture. The occurrence of κ chains is more common in human immunoglobulins than λ chains.

The characteristics of the 5 classes of human immunoglobulins are given in ***Table 68.1***.

Immunoglobulin G (IgG)

IgG is the most abundant (75–80%) class of immunoglobulins. IgG is composed of a single Y-shaped unit (monomer). It can traverse blood vessels readily. IgG is the only immunoglobulin that can cross the placenta and transfer the mother's immunity to the developing fetus. IgG triggers ***foreign cell destruction*** mediated by complement system.

Immunoglobulin A (IgA)

IgA occurs as a single (monomer) or double unit (dimer) held together by J chain. It is mostly found in the body secretions such as saliva, tears, sweat, milk and the walls of intestine. IgA is the most predominant antibody in the colostrum, the initial secretion from the mother's breast after a baby is born. The IgA molecules bind with bacterial antigens present on the body (outer epithelial) surfaces and remove them. In this way, IgA ***prevents the foreign substances*** from entering the body cells.

Immunoglobulin M (IgM)

IgM is the largest immunoglobulin composed of 5 Y-shaped units (IgG type) held together by a J polypeptide chain. Thus IgM is a pentamer. Due to its large size, IgM cannot traverse blood vessels, hence it is restricted to the blood stream. IgM is the first antibody to be produced in response to an

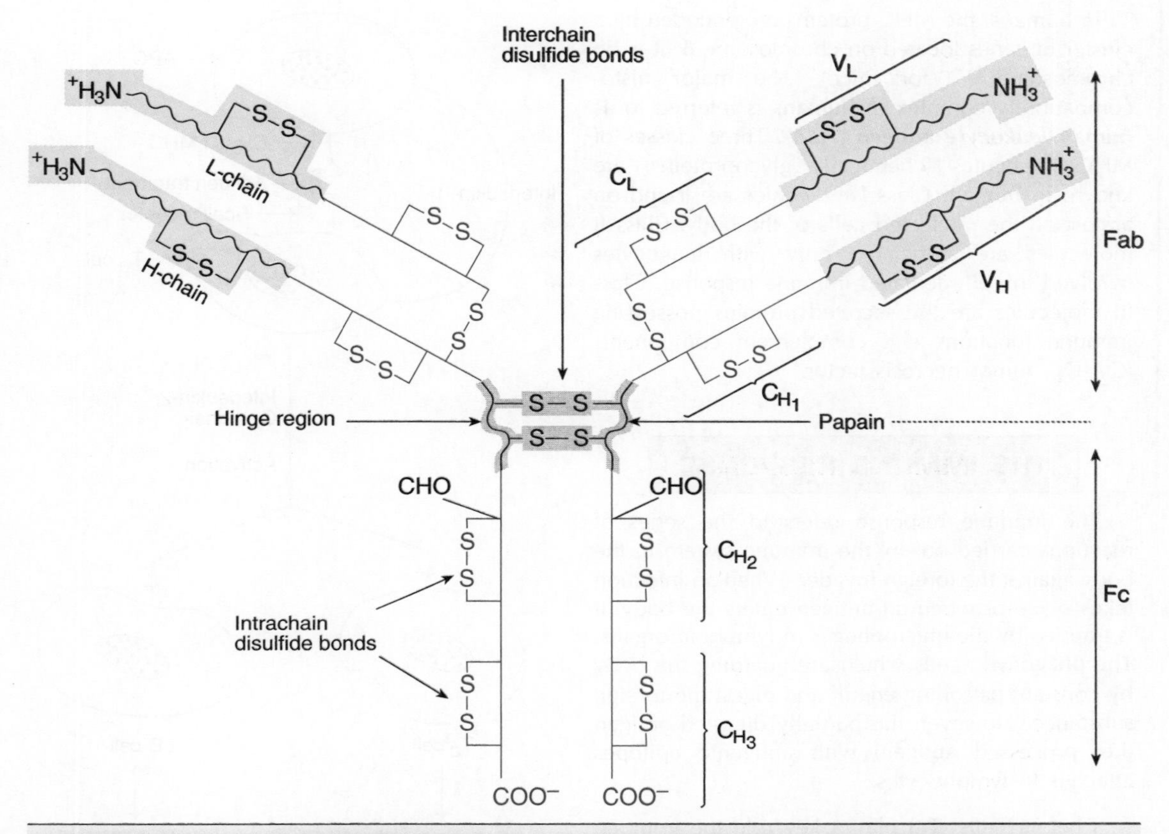

***Fig. 68.2 :** Diagrammatic representation of human IgG molecule (V—Variable region, C—Constant region; CHO—Carbohydrate; Each heavy chain is composed of four units—V_H, C_{H_1}, C_{H_2}, C_{H_3} while light chain consists of two units—V_L, C_L).*

antigen and is the most ***effective against invading microorganisms***.

Immunoglobulin D (IgD)

IgD is composed of a single Y-shaped unit and is present in a low concentration in the circulation. IgD molecules are present on the surface of B cells. Their function, however, is not known for certain. Some workers believe that IgD may function as ***B-cell receptor***.

Immunoglobulin E (IgE)

IgE is a single Y-shaped monomer. It is normally present in minute concentration in blood. IgE levels are elevated in individuals with ***allergies*** as it is associated with the body's allergic responses. The IgE molecules tightly bind with mast cells which release histamine and cause allergy.

SYNTHESIS OF IMMUNOGLOBULINS

There are millions of different antigens. It was a big puzzle for a long time how an individual can produce so many antibodies to protect against antigens. It is now recognized that a gene rearrangement involving a combination of several genes is responsible for generating an extremely large number of antibodies. (For more details Refer Chapter 5).

MAJOR HISTOCOMPATIBILITY COMPLEX

The major histocompatibility complex (*MHC*) represents a special group of ***proteins, present on the cell surfaces of T-lymphocytes***. MHC is involved in the recognition of antigens on T-cells. It may be noted here that the B-cell receptors (antibodies) can recognize antigens and on their own, while T-cells can do so through the mediation of MHC.

In humans, the MHC proteins are encoded by a cluster of genes located on chromosome 6 (it is on chromosome 17 for mice). The major histo-compatibility complex in humans is referred to as ***human leukocyte antigen (HLA)***. Three classes of MHC molecules (chemically glycoproteins) are known in human. Class I molecules are found on almost all the nucleated cells of the body. Class II molecules are associated only with leukocytes involved in cell-mediated immune response. Class III molecules are the secreted proteins possessing immune functions e.g. complement components (C_2, C_4), tumor necrosis factor.

THE IMMUNE RESPONSE

The immune response refers to the series of reactions carried out by the immune system in the body against the foreign invader. When an infection takes place or when an antigen enters the body, it is trapped by the macrophages in lymphoid organs. The phagocytic cells which are guarding the body by constant patrolling engulf and digest the foreign substance. However, the partially digested antigen (i.e. processed antigen) with antigenic epitopes attaches to lymphocytes.

T-helper cells (T_H) play a key role the immune response (***Fig. 68.3***). This is brought out through the participation of antigen presenting cell (APC), usually a macrophage. Receptors of T_H cell bind to class II MHC-antigen complex displayed on the surface of APC. APC secretes interleukin-I, which activates the T_H cell. This activated T_H cell actively grows and divides to produce clones of T_H cells. All the T_H cells possess receptors that are specific for the MHC-antigen complex. This facilitates triggering of immune response in an exponential manner. The T_H cells secrete interleukin-2 which promotes the prolifiration of cytotoxic T cells (T_C cells) to attack the infected cells through cell-mediated immunity. Further, interleukin-2 also activates B-cells to produce immunoglobulins which perform humoral immunity.

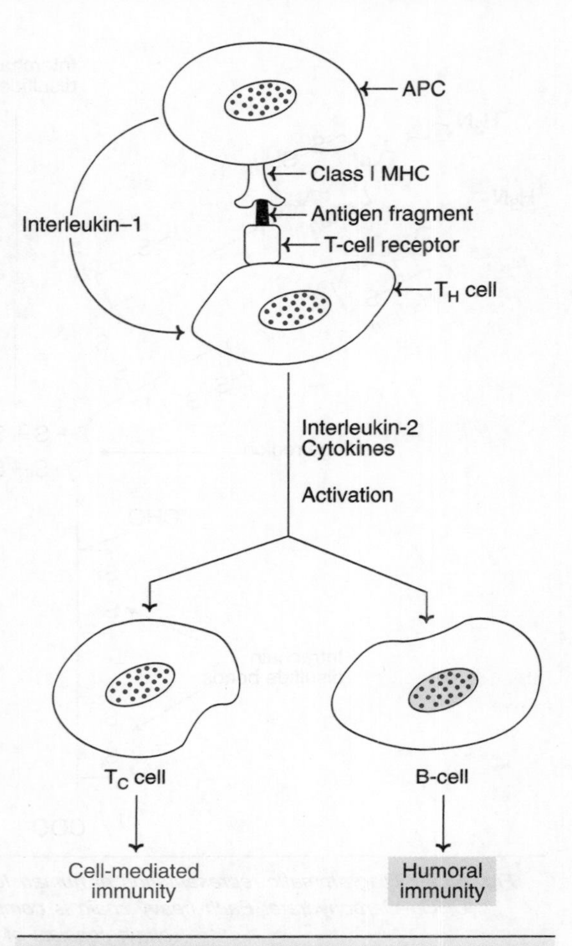

Fig. 68.3 : *A diagrammatic representation of the central role of helper T cells (T_H cells) in immune response (APC—Antigen presenting cell; T_C cell—Cytotoxic T-cell).*

CYTOKINES

Cytokines are a group of ***proteins*** that ***bring*** about ***communication between different cell types*** involved in immunity. They are low molecular weight glycoproteins and are produced by lymphoid and non-lymphoid cells during the course of immune response. Cytokines may be regarded as soluble messenger molecules of immune system. They can act as short messengers between the cells or long range messengers by circulating in the blood and affecting cells at far off sites. The latter function is comparable to that of hormones.

The term ***interleukin (IL)*** is frequently used to represent cytokines. There are more than a dozen interleukins (IL-I......IL_{12}), produced by different cells with wide range of functions. The main function (directly or indirectly) of cytokines is to ***amplify immune responses*** and inflammatory responses.

Therapeutic uses of cytokines

It is now possible to produce cytokines *in vitro*. Some of the cytokines have potential applications in the practice of medicine. For instance, IL-2 is used in cancer immunotherapy, and in the treatment of immunodeficiency diseases. IL-2 induces the proliferation and differentiation of T-and B-cells, besides increasing the cytotoxic capacity of natural killer cells.

A group of cytokines namely interferons can combat viral infection by inhibiting their replication.

IMMUNITY IN HEALTH AND DISEASE

The prime function of imune system is to protect the host against the invading pathogens. The body tries its best to overcome various strategies of infectious agents (bacteria, viruses), and provides immunity.

Some of the important immunological aspects in human health and disease are briefly described.

AUTOIMMUNE DISEASES

In general, the immune system is self-tolerant i.e. not responsive to cells or proteins of self. Sometimes, for various reasons, the ***immune system fails to discriminate between self and non-self***. As a consequence, the cells or tissues of the body are attacked. This phenomenon is referred to as ***autoimmunity*** and the diseases are regarded as autoimmune diseases. The antibodies produced to self molecules are regarded as ***autoantibodies***. Some examples of autoimmune diseases are listed.

- Insulin-dependent diabetes (pancreatic β-cell autoreactive T-cells and antibodies).
- Rheumatoid arthritis (antibodies against proteins present in joints).
- Myasthenia gravis (acetylcholine receptor autoantibodies).
- Autoimmune hemolytic anemia (erythrocyte autoantibodies).

Mechanism of autoimmunity : It is widely accepted that autoimmunity generally occurs as a consequence of body's response against bacterial, viral or any foreign antigen. Some of the epitopes of foreign antigens are similar (homologous) to epitopes present on certain host proteins. This results in cross reaction of antigens and antibodies which may lead to autoimmune diseases.

ORGAN TRANSPLANTATION

The phenomenon of transfer of cells, tissues or organs from one site to another (in the same organism, ***autograft*** or from another organism ***allograft***) is regarded as organ transplantation. In case of humans, majority of organ transplantations are allografts (between two individuals). The term ***xenograft*** is used if tissues/ organs are transferred from one species to another e.g. from pig to man (For more details on xenotransplantation Refer Chapter 41).

Organ transplantation is associated with immunological complications, and tissue rejection. This is because the host body responds to the transplanted tissue in a similar way as if it were an invading foreign organism. Major histocompatibility complex (MHC) is primarily involved in allograft rejection. This is due to the fact that MHC proteins are unique to each individual, and the immune system responds promptly to foreign MHCs.

Organ transplantation between closely related family members is preferred, since their MHCs are also likely to be closely related. And major immunological complications can be averted.

CANCERS

Growth of tumors is often associated with the formation novel antigens. These ***tumor antigens*** (also referred to as oncofetal antigens e.g. α-fetoprotein) are recognized as non-self by the immune systems. However, tumors have developed several mechanisms to evade immune responses.

AIDS

Acquired immunodeficiency syndrome (AIDS), caused by human immunodeficiency virus, is characterized by immunosuppression, secondary neoplasma and neurological manifestations. AIDS primarily affects the cell-mediated immune system which protects the body from intracellular parasites such as viruses, and bacteria. Most of the immunodeficiency symptoms of AIDS are associated with a reduction in CD_4 (cluster determinant antigen 4) cells.

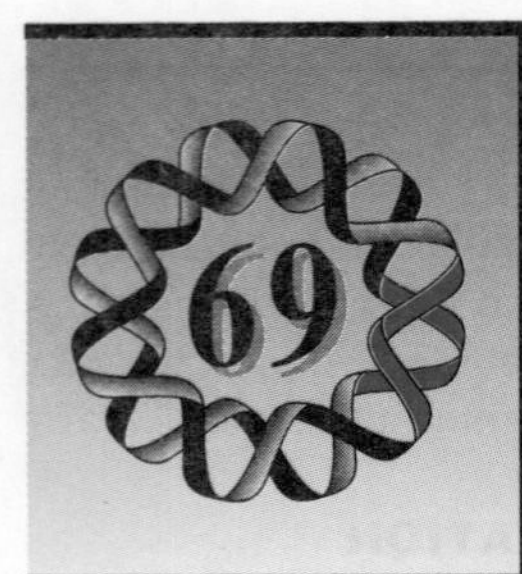

Genetics

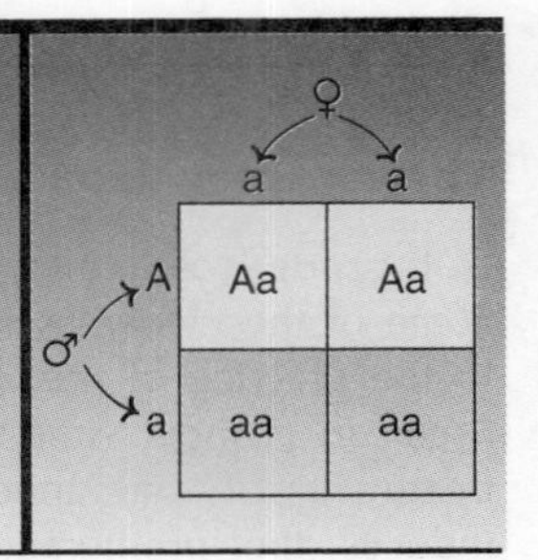

Genetics is the ***study of heredity***. It is appropriately regarded as the science that explains the similarities and differences among the related organisms.

The blood theory of inheritance in humans

For many centuries, it was customary to explain inheritance in humans through blood theory. People used to believe that the children received blood from their parents, and it was the union of blood that led to the blending of characteristics. That is how the terms 'blood relations', 'blood will tell', and 'blood is thicker than water' came into existence. They are still used, despite the fact that blood is no more involved in inheritance. With the advances in genetics, the more appropriate terms should be as follows

- ***Gene relations*** in place of blood relations.
- ***Genes will tell*** instead of blood will tell.

BRIEF HISTORY AND DEVELOPMENT OF GENETICS

Genetics is relatively young, not even 150 years. The blood theory of inheritance was questioned in 1850s, based on the fact that the semen contained no blood. Thus, blood was not being transferred to the offspring. Then the big question was what was the hereditary substance.

Mendel's experiments : It was in 1866, an Austrian monk named Gregor Johann Mendel, for the first time reported the fundamental laws of inheritance. He conducted several experiments on the breeding patterns of pea plants. Mendel put forth the ***theory of transmissible factors*** which states that inheritance is controlled by ***certain factors*** passed from parents to offsprings. His results were published in 1866 in an obscure journal Proceedings of the Society of Natural Sciences.

For about 35 years, the observations made by Mendel went unnoticed, and were almost forgotten. Two European botanists (Correns and Hugo de Vries) in 1900, independently and simultaneously rediscovered the theories of Mendel. The year 1900 is important as it marks the beginning the modern era of genetics.

The origin of the word gene : In the early years of twentieth century, it was believed that the Mendel's inheritance factors are very closely related to chromosomes (literally coloured bodies) of the cells. It was in 1920s, the term ***gene*** (derived from a Greek word *gennan* meaning to produce) was introduced by Willard Johannsen. Thus, ***gene replaced the earlier terms inheritance factor or inheritance unit***.

Chemical basis of heredity : There was a controversy for quite sometime on the chemical basis of inheritance. There were two groups—the protein supporters and DNA supporters. It was in 1944, Avery and his associates presented convincing evidence that the chemical basis of heredity lies in DNA, and not in protein. Thus, ***DNA*** was finally identified as ***the genetic material***. Its structure was elucidated in 1952 by Watson and Crick.

Importance of genes in inheritance—studies on twins

Monozygotic or identical twins contain the same genetic material — DNA or genes. Studies conducted on identical twins make starting revelations with regard to inheritance. One such study is described here.

Oskar Stohr and Jack Yufe were identical twins separated at birth. Oskar was taken to Germany where he was brought up by his grandmother as a Christian. Jack was raised by his father in Israel as a Jew. The two brothers were reunited at the age of 47. Despite the different environmental influences, their behavioural patterns and personalities were remarkably similar

- Both men had moustaches, wore two pocket shirts, and wire-rimmed glasses.
- Both loved spicy foods and tended to fall asleep in front of television.
- Both flushed the toilet before using.
- Both read maganizes from back to front.
- Both stored rubber bands on their wrists.
- Both liked to sneeze in a room of strangers.

Besides Oskar and Jack, many other studies conducted on identical twins point out the importance of genes on the inherited characters related to personality and mannerisms.

BASIC PRINCIPLES OF HEREDITY IN HUMANS

The understanding of how genetic characteristics are passed on from one generation to the next is based on the principles developed by Mendel.

As we know now, the human genome is organized into a diploid (2n) set of 46 chromosomes. They exist as ***22 pairs of autosomes*** and ***one pair of sex chromosomes (XX/XY)***. During the course of meiosis, the chromosome number becomes haploid (n). Thus, haploid male and female gametes — sperm and oocyte respectively, are formed. On fertilization of the oocyte by the sperm, the diploid status is restored. This becomes possible as the zygote receives one member of each chromosome pair from the father, and the other from the mother. As regards the sex chromosomes, the males have X and Y, while the females have XX. The sex of the child is determined by the father.

Monogenic and polygenic traits

The genetic traits or characters are controlled by single genes or multiple genes. The changes in genes are associated with genetic diseases.

Monogenic disorders : These are the single gene disease traits due to alterations in the corresponding gene e.g. Sickle-cell anemia, phenylketonuria. Inheritance of monogenic disorders usually follows the Mendelian pattern of inheritance.

Polygenic disorders : The genetic traits conferred by more than on gene (i.e multiple genes), and the disorders associated with them are very important e.g. height, weight, skin colours, academic performance, blood pressure, aggressiveness, length of life.

PATTERNS OF INHERITANCE

The heredity is transmitted from parent to offspring as individual characters controlled by genes. The genes are linearly distributed on chromosomes at fixed positions called ***loci***.

A gene may have different forms referred to as ***alleles***. Usually one allele is transferred from the father, and the other from the mother. The allele is regarded as ***dominant*** if the trait is exhibited due to its presence. On the other hand, the allele is said to be ***recessive*** if its effect is masked by a dominant allele. The individuals are said to be ***homozygous*** if both the alleles are the same. When the alleles are different they are said to be ***heterozygous***.

The pattern of inheritance of monogenic traits may occur in the following ways (***Fig. 69.1***).

1. Autosomal dominant
2. Autosomal recessive
3. Sex-linked.

1. **Autosomal dominant inheritance :** A normal allele may be designated as ***a*** while an autosomal dominant disease allele as ***A*** (***Fig. 69.1A***). The male with Aa genotype is an affected one while the female with aa is normal. Half of the genes from the affected male will carry the disease allele. On mating, the male and female gametes are mixed in different combinations. The result is that ***half of the children*** will be heterozygous (Aa) and ***have the disease***. Example of autosomal dominant inherited diseases are familial hypercholesterolemia, β-thalassemia, breast cancer genes.

(A) Autosomal dominant

PARENTS

Male (♂)
Genotype - Aa
Phenotype - Affected male

Female (♀)
Genotype - aa
Phenotype - Normal female

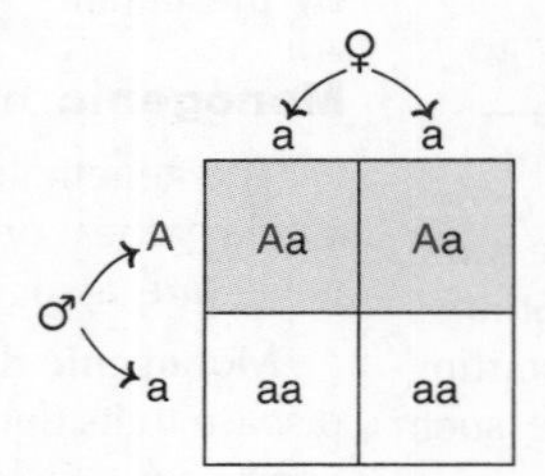

CHILDREN
Genotype ratio - 1 : 1 Aa to aa
Phenotype - 50% affected
- 50% normal

(B) Autosomal recessive

PARENTS

Male (♂)
Genotype - Bb
Phenotype - Carrier male

Female (♀)
Genotype - Bb
Phenotype - Carrier female

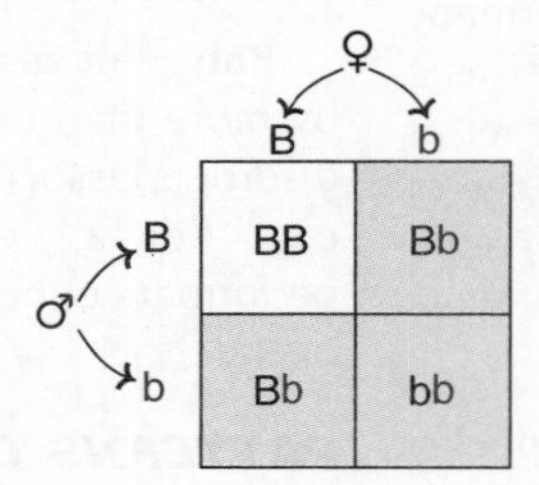

CHILDREN
Genotype ratio - 1 : 2 : 1 BB/Bb/bb
Phenotype - 25% affected
- 25% normal
- 50% carriers

(C) X-chromosome (sex chromosome)–linked inheritance

PARENTS

Male (♂)
Genotype - XY
Phenotype - Normal male

Female (♀)
Genotype - X^cX
Phenotype - Carrier female

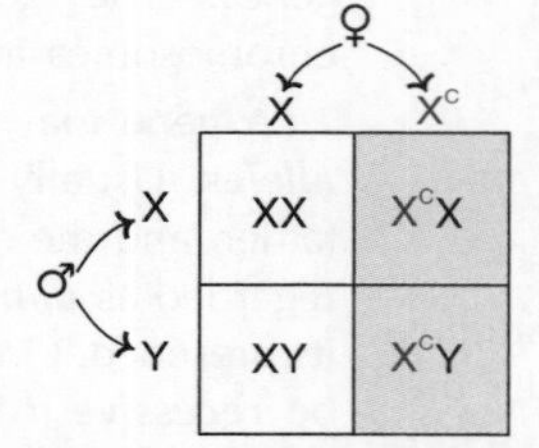

CHILDREN
Genotype ratio - 1 : 1 : 1 : 1 XX/XY/X^cX/X^cY
Phenotype - 50% of males affected

*Fig. 69.1 : Patterns of inheritance-autosomal dominant, autosomal recessive and X-linked (**Note** : Genotype refers to the description of genetic composition, while phenotype represents the observable character displayed by an organism).*

2. **Autosomal recessive inheritance :** In this case, the normal allele is designated as ***B*** while the disease-causing one is ***a*** (***Fig. 69.1B***). The gametes of carrier male and carrier female (both with genotype Bb) get mixed. For these heterozygous carrier parents, there is one fourth chance of having an affected child. Cystic fibrosis, sickle-cell anemia and phenylketonuria are some good examples of autosomal recessive disorders.

3. **Sex (X)-linked inheritance :** In the ***Fig. 69.1C***, sex-linked pattern of inheritance is depicted. A normal male (XY) and a carrier female (X^CY) will produce children wherein, half of the male children are affected while no female children is affected. This is due to the fact that the male children possess only one X chromosome, and there is no dominant allele to mark its effects (as is the case with females). Colour blindness and hemophilia are good examples of X-linked diseases.

A selected list of genetic disorders (monogenic traits) due to autosomal and sex-linked inheritance in humans is given in ***Table 69.1***.

GENETIC DISEASES IN HUMANS

The pattern of inheritance and monogenic traits along with some of the associated disorders are described above (***Table 69.1***). Besides ***gene mutations, chromosomal abnormalities*** (aberrations) also result in genetic diseases.

TABLE 69.1 Selected examples of genetic disorders (monogenic traits) in humans

Inherited pattern/disease	*Estimated incidence*	*Salient features*
Autosomal dominant		
Familial hypercholesterolemia	1 : 500	High risk for heart diseases
Huntington disease	1 : 5000	Nervous disorders, dementia
Familial retinoblastoma	1 : 12000	Tumors of retina
Breast cancer genes (*BRAC 1 and 2*)	1 : 800	High risk for breast and ovarian cancers
β-Thalassemia	1 : 2500 (in people of Mediterranean descent)	A blood disorder; the blood appears to be blue instead of red
Autosomal recessive		
Sickle-cell anemia	1 : 100 (in Africans)	Severe life threatening anemia; confers resistance to malaria
Cystic fibrosis	1 : 2500 (in Caucasians)	Defective ion transport; severe lung infections and early death (before they reach 30 years)
Phenylketonuria	1 : 2000	Mental retardation due to brain damage
α_1-Antitrypsin deficiency	1 : 5000	Damage to lungs and liver
Tay-Sachs disease	1 : 3000 (in Ashkenazi Jews)	Nervous disorder; blindness and paralysis
Severe combined immunodeficiency disease (SCID)	Rare (only 100 cases reported worldwide)	Highly defective immune system; early death
Sex-linked		
Colour blindness	1 : 50 males	Unable to distinguish colours
Hemophilia (A/B)	1 : 10,000 males	Defective blood clotting
Duchenne muscular dystrophy	1 : 7000 males	Muscle wastage
Mitochondrial		
Leber hereditary optic neuropathy	Not known	Damage to optic nerves, may lead to blindness

Aneuploidy : The presence of ***abnormal number of chromosomes*** within the cells is referred to as aneuploidy. The most common aneuploid condition is ***trisomy*** in which three copies of a particular chromosome are present in a cell instead of the normal two e.g. trisomy-21 causing ***Down's syndrome***; trisomy-18 that results in ***Edward's syndrome***. These are the examples of autosomal aneuploidy.

In case of sex-linked aneuploidy, the sex chromosomes occur as three copies. e.g. phenotypically male causing Klinefelter's syndrome has XXY; trisomy-X is phenotically a female with XXX.

Selected examples of chromosomal disorders along the with the syndromes and their characteristic features are given in ***Table 69.2***.

EUGENICS

Eugenics is a ***science of improving human race based on genetics***. Improving the traits of plants and animals through breeding programmes has been in practice for centuries.

Eugenics is a highly controversial subject due to social, ethical, and political reasons. The proponents of eugenics argue that people with

Table 69.2 Selected examples of chromosomal disorders in humans

Condition	*Chromosome*	*Syndrome*	*Salient features*
Normal			
Females	2n (46, XX)	—	—
Males	2n (46, XY)	—	—
Autosomal aneuploidy	**2n + specific chromosome**		
Trisomy-21	47, XY, +21	Down's syndrome	IQ<50; Congenital heart disease, low life expectancy
Trisomy-18	47, XY, +21	Edward's syndrome	Malformation of heart, kidney and other organs
Trisomy-13	47, XY, +13	Patau's syndrome	Small head, polydactyly, congenital heart diseases
Sex-linked aneuploidy			
Phenotypically male	47, XXY	Klinefelter's syndrome	Small testes, infertility
	47, XYY	Jacob's syndrome	Usually asymptomatic, often tall
Phenotically female	47, XXX	Triplo-X (trisomy-X)	Usually asymptomatic, about 20% mentaly handicapped
	47, XO (missing Y)	Turner's syndrome	Short stature.

desirable and good traits (good blood) should reproduce while those with undersirable characters (bad blood) should not. The advocates of eugenics, however, do not force any policy, but they try to convince the people to perform their duty voluntarily. The object of eugenics is to limit the production of people who are unfit to live in the society.

Eugenics in Nazi Germany

Germany developed its own eugenic programme during 1930s. A law on eugenic sterilization was passed in 1933. In a span of three years, compulsory sterilization was done on about 250,000 people, who allegedly suffered from hereditary disabilities, feeble mindedness, epilepsy, schizophrenia, blindness, physical deformaties, and drug or alcohol addition.

The German Government committed many atrocities in the name of racial purity. Other countries, however do not support this kind of eugenics.

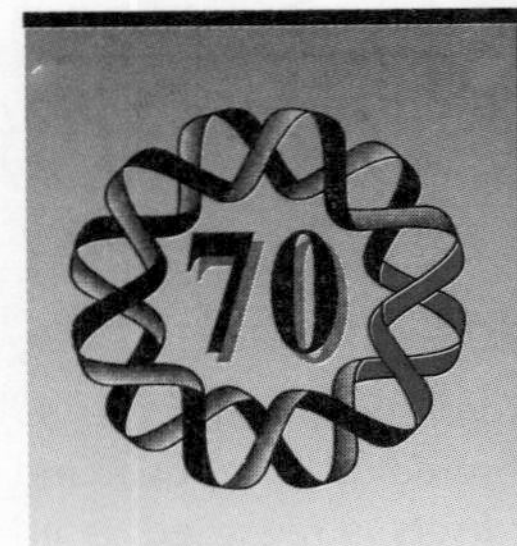

Bioinformatics

Bioinformatics is ***the combination** (**or marriage**!) **of biology and information technology***. Basically, bioinformatics is a recently developed science using information to understand biological phenomenon. It broadly involves the computational tools and methods used to manage, analyse and manipulate volumes and volumes of biological data.

Bioinformatics may also be regarded as a part of the ***computational biology***. The latter is concerned with the application of quantitative analytical techniques in modeling and solving problems in the biological systems. Bioinformatics is an interdisciplinary approach requiring advanced knowledge of computer science, mathematics and statistical methods for the understanding of biological phenomena at the molecular level.

History and relevance of bioinformatics

The term bioinformatics was first introduced in 1990s. Originally, it dealt with the management and analysis of the data pertaining to ***DNA, RNA and protein sequences***. As the biological data is being produced at an unprecedented rate, its management and interpretation invariably requires bioinformatics. Thus, bioinformatics now includes many other types of biological data. Some of the most important ones are listed below

- Gene expression profiles
- Protein structure
- Protein interactions
- Microarrays (DNA chips)
- Functional analysis of biomolecules
- Drug designing.

Bioinformatics is largely (not exclusively) a computer-based discipline. Computers are in fact very essential to handle large volumes of biological data, their storage and retrieval.

We have to accept the fact that there is no computer on earth (however advanced) which can store information, and perform the functions like a living cell. Thus a highly complex information technology lies right within the cells of an organism. This primarily includes the organism's genes and their dictates for the organisms biological processes and behaviour.

BROAD COVERAGE OF BIOINFORMATICS

Bioinformatics covers many specialized and advanced areas of biology.

Functional genomics : Identification of genes and their respective functions.

Structural genomics : Predictions related to functions of proteins.

Comparative genomics : For understanding the genomes of different species of organisms.

DNA microarrays : These are designed to measure the levels of gene expression in different tissues, various stages of development and in different diseases.

Medical informatics : This involves the management of biomedical data with special referece to biomolecules, *in vitro* assays and clinical trials.

COMPONENTS OF BIOINFORMATICS

Bioinformatics comprises three components

1. **Creation of databases** : This involves the organizing, storage and management the biological data sets. The databases are accessible to researchers to know the existing information and submit new entries. e.g. protein sequence data bank for molecular structure. Databases will be of no use until analysed.

2. **Development of algorithms and statistics** : This involves the development of tools and resources to determine the relationship among the members of large data sets e.g. comparison of protein sequence data with the already existing protein sequences.

3. **Analysis of data and interpretation** : The appropriate use of components 1 and 2 (given above) to analyse the data and interpret the results in a biologically meaningful manner. This includes DNA, RNA and protein sequences, protein structure, gene expression profiles and biochemical pathways.

BIOINFORMATICS AND THE INTERNET

The internet is an ***inter***national computer ***net***work. A computer network involves a group of computers that can communicate (usually over a telephone system) and exchange data between users.

It is the ***internet protocol*** (IP) that determines how the packets of information are addressed and routed over the network. To access the internet, a computer must have the correct hardware (modem/ network card), appropriate software and permission for access to network. For this purpose, one has to subscribe to an ***internet service provider*** (ISP).

World wide web (www) : www involves the exchange of information over the internet using a programme called ***browser***. The most widely used browsers are Internet explorer and Netscape navigator.

www works on the basis of ***Uniform resource locator*** (URL) which is a document with a unique address. URLs takes the format ***http.//*** (***h***yper***t***ext ***t***ransfer ***p***rotocol) that can identify the protocol for communication over www.

BIOLOGICAL DATABASES

The collection of the ***biological data*** on a computer which can be manipulated to appear in ***varying arrangements and subsets*** is regarded as a database. The biological information can be stored in different databases. Each database has its own website with unique navigation tools.

The biological databases are, in general, publicly accessible. Selected examples of biological databases are briefly described (***Table 70.1***).

Nucleotide sequence databases

The nucleotide sequence data submitted by the scientists and genome sequencing groups is at the databases namely GenBank, EMBL (European Molecular Biology Laboratory) and DDBJ (DNA Data Bank of Japan). There is a good coordination between these three databases as they are synchronized on daily basis.

Besides the primary nucleotide databases (referred above), there are some other databases also to provide information on genes, genomes and ongoing research projects.

Protein sequence databases

Protein sequence databases are usually prepared from the existing literature and/or in consultation with the experts. In fact, these databases represent the translated DNA databases.

Molecular structure of databases

The three dimensional (3-D) structures of macromolecules are determined by X-ray crystallography and nuclear magnetic resonance (NMR). PDB and SCOP are the primary databases of 3-D structures of biological molecules.

Other databases

KEGG database is an important one that provides information on the current knowledge of molecular biology and cell biology with special reference to information on metabolic pathways, interacting molecules and genes.

TABLE 70.1 Selected examples of biological databases in bioinformatics

Database	*Salient features*
Primary nucleotide sequence databases	
GenBank (www.ncbi.nih.gov/GeneBank/)	Provides nucleotide sequence databases maintained by the National Center for Biotechnology Information (NCBI), USA.
EMBL (www.ebi.ac.uk/embl/)	European Molecular Biology Laboratory (EMBL) maintains nucleotide sequence databases under the aegis of European Bioinformatics Institue (EBI), UK.
Other nucleotide sequence databases	
UniGene (www.ncbi.nih.gov/UniGene/)	The nucleotide sequences of GenBank in the form of clusters, representing genes are available.
Genome Biology (www.ncbi.nlm.nih.gov/Genomes/)	The information about the completed genomes is available.
EBI Genomes (www.ebi.uk./genomes/)	Provides data and statistics for the completed genomes, besides the information on the ongoing projects.
Protein sequence database	
SWISS-PROT (www.expasy.ch/sport)	Provides the description of the structure of a protein, its domains structure, post-translational modifications, variants etc. It has high level of integration with other databases and minimal level of redundancy.
PIR (pir.georgetown.edu)	Protein information resource (PIR) is a database provided by the National Biomedical Research Foundation (NBRF) in USA.
Protein sequence motif databases	
PROSITE (www.expasy.ch/prosite/)	Provides information on protein families and domains. It also has patterns and profiles for sequences and biological functions.
Pfam (www.cgr.ki.se/Pfam/)	A database of protein families defined in the form of domains. It has multiple alignment of a set of sequences.
Macromolecular databases	
PDB (www.rcsb.org/pdb)	This is the primary database for 3-dimensional (3-D) structures of biological macromolecules (determined by X-ray and NMR studies).
SCOP (www.mrc.lmb.cam.ac.uk/scop/)	Provides information on the structural classification of proteins (SCOP). The proteins are classified on the basis of 3-D structures.
Other databases	
KEGG (www.genome.ad.jp/kegg/)	The Kyoto Encyclopedia of Genes and Genomes (KEGG) is a database with latest computerised information on biomolecules and cell biology. KEGG provides details on information pathways, interacting molecules and the connecting links with genes.

APPLICATIONS OF BIOINFORMATICS

The advent of bioinformatics has revolutionized the advancements in biological science. And biotechnology is largely benefited by bioinformatics. The best example is the sequencing of human genome in a record time which would not have been possible without bioinformatics. A selected list of applications of bioinformatics is given below.

- Sequence mapping of biomolecules (DNA, RNA, proteins).
- Identification of nucleotide sequences of functional genes.
- Finding of sites that can be cut by restriction enzymes.
- Designing of primer sequence for polymerase chain reaction.
- Prediction of functional gene products.
- To trace the evolutionary trees of genes.
- For the prediction of 3-dimensional structure of proteins.
- Molecular modelling of biomolecules.
- Designing of drugs for medical treatment.
- Handling of vast biological data which otherwise is not possible.
- Development of models for the functioning various cells, tissues and organs.

The above list of applications however, may be treated as incomplete, since at present there is no field in biological sciences that does not involve bioinformatics.

APPENDICES

CONTENTS

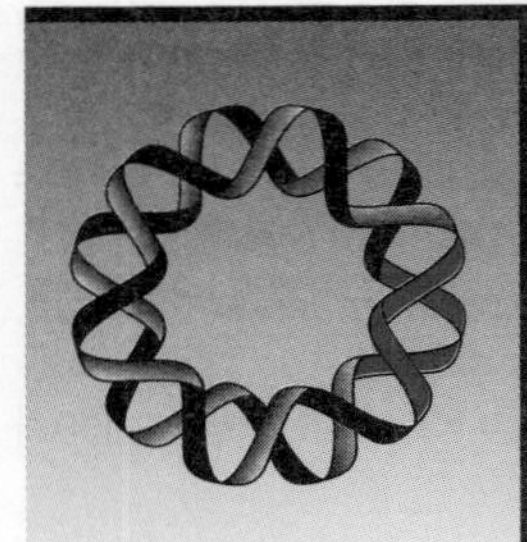

Glossary

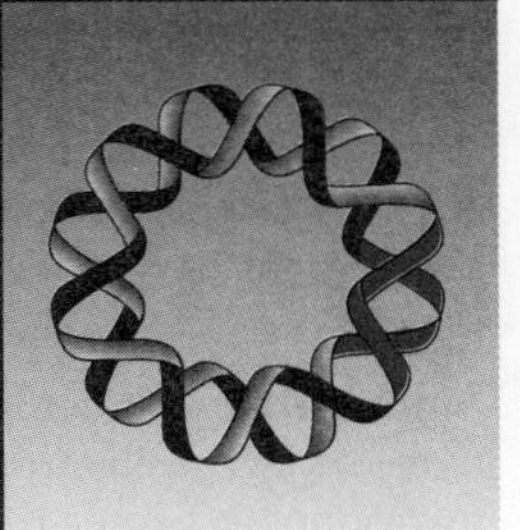

A

Abzymes The catalytic antibodies or ***anti**b**ody** en**zymes***.

Abiotic stress The stress caused to plants due to herbicides, water deficiency, ozone, intense light etc.

Abscisic acid An important plant growth regulator for the induction of embryogenesis.

Acid rain When the pH of the rain water is less than 5.5, it is considered as acid rain.

Active site The site on the enzyme at which the substrate binds.

Adaptor A synthetic, double-stranded oligonucleotide used to attach sticky ends to a blunt ended molecule.

Aerated lagoons (aerated ponds) Facultative stabilization ponds with surface aerators to overcome bad odours (due to overload of organic materials).

Aerated ponds See aerated lagoons.

Aerobe A microorganism dependent on O_2 for its growth.

Affinity chromatography A type of chromatography in which the matrix contains chemical groups that can selectively bind (ligands) to the molecules being purified.

Affinity tag The tagged amino acid sequence which forms a part of the recombinant protein and acts as an identification tag.

Agarose gel electrophoresis Electrophoresis carried out on agarose gel to separate DNA fragments.

Agrobacterium tumefaciens A rod shaped bacterium that causes crown gall disease by inserting its DNA into plant cells.

AIDS ***A**cquired **i**mmuno**d**eficiency **s**yndrome*, a disease caused by a retrovirus resulting in diminished immune response, and increased susceptibility to various infections and cancers.

Aleurone The outmost layer of the endosperm in a seed.

Algalization The process of cultivation of blue-green algae (cynobacteria) in the fields as a source of biofertilizer.

Allele Alternative forms (one or more) of a gene occupying a given locus on the chromosome.

Allogeneic cells The cells taken from a person other than the patient for use in culture, tissue engineering etc.

Allosteric regulation An enzyme regulating process in which binding of a small effector molecule at one site (allosteric site) affects of the activity at other site (active site) of an enzyme.

Ames test A test used for the detection of chemical mutagens and their carcinogenecity.

Amino acid The building blocks or monomeric units of proteins.

Aminoglycosides Oligosaccharide (carbohydrate) antibiotics.

Amplified fragment length polymorphism (AFLP) A sensitive method for the detection of polymorphism in the genome. It is based on the principle of RFLP and RAPD.

Amphipathic Structures or molecules possessing two surfaces, hydrophilic (water loving) and hydrophobic (water hating).

Anaerobe A microorganism that can grow in the absence of O_2.

Androgenesis Development of plants from male gametophytes.

Aneuploidy An abnormal condition of chromosomes, differing from the usual diploid constitution. This may be due to a loss or gain of chromosomes.

Annealing The pairing of complementary single strands of DNA to form a double helix.

Antibiotic A biological molecule that is produced by one organism which can kill/inhibit the growth of another organism.

Antibody A protein (immunoglobulin) synthesized by B-lymphocytes that recognizes antigen.

Anticodon A set of three nucleotides in tRNA molecule that are complementary to a set of three nucleotides (codon) in mRNA.

Antigen A substance that elicits immune response and induces the production of antibodies.

Antioxidants A group of substances that can prevent oxidation e.g. vitamin E.

Antisense therapy The *in vivo* treatment of a genetic disease by blocking translation (protein synthesis) with a DNA or RNA sequence that is complementary to specific mRNA.

Apoptosis Programmed cell death.

Aptamers A special type of oligonucleotides that can specifically bind to target proteins and not to nucleic acids.

Aspartame A low-calorie artificial sweetener used in soft-drink industry. Chemically, it is aspartyl-phenylalanine methyl ester.

Assisted reproductive technology (ART) The manipulations of reproduction in animals and humans.

Attenuation A regulatory process used by some bacteria to control the expression of certain amino acid operons.

Autoimmunity An abnormal immune response against his/her body's own components.

Autologous cells Cells taken from an individual, cultured/stored, and (sometimes) genetically manipulated, and infused back into the original donor.

Autoradiography The process of detection of radioactively labeled molecules by exposure of an X-ray sensitive film.

Autosomes Chromosomes that are not involved in sex determination.

Autotroph An organism that is capable of synthesizing its own food e.g. plants through photosynthesis.

Auxins A group of plant growth regulators which are involved in cell elongation, root initiation etc. e.g. indole acetic acid.

Auxotroph A mutant microorganism that can grow when a nutrient is supplied (this nutrient is not needed by the wild type).

B

Bacillus thuringiensis A rod shaped bacterium whose toxic crystals act as an insecticide against certain species of arthropods.

Bacterial artificial chromosome (BAC) : A vector system based on the F-factor plasmid of *E. coli.* BAC is used for cloning large (100–300 kb) DNA segments.

Bacteriophage A virus that infects a bacterium. Also called ***phage.***

Baker's yeast The living cells of aerobically grown yeast, *Saccharomyces cerevisiae,* used in bread making.

Base pair (bp) The hydrogen bonded structure formed between two complementary nucleotides (i.e. partnership of A with T or of C with G) in DNA structure.

Base ratio The ratio of A to T, or C to G in a double-stranded DNA.

Batch culture (batch fermentation) A cell or microbial culture that is grown for a limited time. It follows a sigmoid pattern of growth.

Bergmann's plating technique The most widely used method for culture of isolated single plant cells.

Binary vector system A two plasmid vector system for transferring T-DNA into plant cells. The virulence genes are on one plasmid while the engineered T-DNA region is on the other plasmid.

Bioaccumulation (biomagnification) Increasing the concentration of chemical agents by way of increasing the quantities in the organisms of a food chain.

Biodegradation Biological transformation of organic compounds by living organisms, particularly the microorganisms.

Biofertilizers The nutrient inputs of biological origin that support plant growth.

Bioaugmentation The addition of microorganisms to waste sites so that the hazardous wastes are rendered harmless.

Biofiltration The process of removing complex wastes (from domestic or industrial sources) by using microorganisms.

Biogas A mixture of gases mainly composed of methane, CO_2, nitrogen and hydrogen sulfide. It is used for cooking purposes, generation of electricity etc.

Biohazards The accidents or risks associated with biological materials.

Bioinformatics A science of using information technology to understand biological phenomena. It may be regarded as a marriage between biology and information technology.

Bioleaching The use of bacteria to recover valuable metals from ores.

Biolistics The process of introducing DNA into plant and animal cells, and organelles by bombardment of DNA-coated pellets under pressure at high speed. This is also called as ***microprojectile bombardment***.

Biochemical oxygen demand (BOD) The oxygen required to meet the metabolic needs of aerobic organisms in water containing organic compounds.

Biological databases The collection of biological data on a computer in different arrangements and subsets.

Biomass The organic mass that can be used as a source of energy. Biomass also refers to the cell mass produced by a population of living organisms.

Biometry Application of statistical methods to study biological problems.

Biopesticides The toxic compounds produced by living organisms that can specifically kill a particular pest species.

Bioplastics The biodegradable plastics, chemically composed of polyhydroxy alkanoates (PHAs).

Biopol A biodegradable plastic composed of polyhydroxybutyric acid and valeric acid.

Bioprocess technology A more recent usage to replace fermentation technology that involves large-scale cultivation of microorganisms for industrial purposes.

Bioprosthesis materials The natural materials modified to become biologically inert e.g. collagen-based connective tissue forming porcine heart valves.

Bioreactor A growth chamber or a vessel (fermenter) for cells or microorganisms. The cells or cell extracts carry out biological reactions in a bioreactor.

Bioremediation The biological process involving living organisms to remove unwanted substances (contaminants or pollutants) from soil or water.

Biosensor An analytical device containing an immobilized biological material (enzyme, antibody, organelle or whole cell) which reacts with an analyte to produce signals that can be measured.

Biosorption The process of microbial cell surface adsorption of metals.

Biosphere All the zones on the earth in which life is present.

Biostimulation Addition of specific nutrients to enhance the growth of naturally occurring microorganisms that convert toxic compounds to non-toxic compounds.

Biotechnology The applications of biological principles, organisms and products to practical purposes.

Biotic stress The stress caused to plants by insects, pathogens (viruses, fungi, bacteria), wounds etc.

Biotransformation The use of biological systems for the conversion of biomolecules.

Blastoderm A stage in embryogenesis in which a layer of nuclei or cells around the embryo surround the internal mass of yolk.

Blotting The transfer of macromolecules by capillary action from a gel to a membrane.

B-lymphocytes Also called ***B-cells***, mature in bone marrow, and are the precursors for the antibody producing cells (plasma cells).

BOD See biochemical oxygen demand.

Brewer's yeast A strain of yeast usually belonging to *Saccharomyces cerevisiae* that is used for the production of beer.

Broth Any fluid medium supporting the growth of microorganisms.

Bt plants The plant carrying the toxin producing gene from *Bacillus thuringiensis,* and capable of protecting themselves from insect attack.

Bystander effect The phenomenon of the death of unmodified cells by a cytotoxic metabolite that is produced by genetically modified cells.

C

CAAT box A promoter sequence of DNA for eukaryotic transcription units.

Callus A mass of undifferentiated plant tissues formed from plant cells or tissue cuttings when grown in culture.

Cancer Uncontrolled growth of cells of a tissue or an organ in higher organisms.

Cap The chemical modification at the 5′ end of eukaryotic mRNA molecules.

Capsases A group of protease enzymes that are associated with apoptosis (programmed cell death).

Capsid The external protein coat of a virus particle.

Casettee mutagenesis Replacement of a wild type DNA by a synthetic double-stranded oligonucleotide (a small DNA fragment).

Catabolite repression The phenomenon of the decreased expression of bacterial operons by extracellular glucose.

cDNA (complementary DNA) A double-stranded DNA synthesized *in vitro* from an mRNA by using reverse transcriptase and DNA polymerase.

cDNA library A collection of cDNA clones, generated *in vitro* from mRNA sequences of a single cell (or tissue) population.

Cell cloning The production of a population of cells derived from a single cell.

Cell culture The culture of dispersed (or disaggregated) cells obtained from the original tissue, or from a cell line.

Cell cycle The series of events that occur in a cell between one division and the next.

Cell immortalization The acquisition of an infinite life span by a cell.

Cell lines Animal or plant cells that can be cultivated under laboratory conditions.

Cell-mediated immune response The activation of the T-lymphocytes of the immune system in response to a foreign antigen.

Cell synchronization Manipulation of cells at different stages of cell cycle in a culture so that the cells will be at the same phase.

Cell transformation A change in the phenotype of a cell due to a new genetic material.

Cell viability The capability of cellular existence, survival and development.

Cellular senescence See senescence.

Central dogma The statement regarding the unidirectional transfer of information from DNA to RNA to protein.

Chaperone A protein required for the proper assembly or folding of other proteins or polypeptides *in vivo.*

Chaperonin A multisubunit protein which forms a structural conformation to facilitate the folding of other proteins *in vivo.*

Chemical oxygen demand (COD) Oxygen equivalents of organic matter that can be oxidized by using strong chemical oxidizing agents.

Chemiluminescence The phenomenon of emission of light from a chemical reaction.

Chimeric antibodies Antibodies in which the individual polypeptide chains are composed of segments from two different species (usually man and mouse).

Chimera A recombinant DNA molecule that contains sequences from different organisms.

Chloroplast The photosynthetic organelle of a plant cell.

Chromatin The complex of DNA and protein in a cell.

Chromatography An analytical technique dealing with the separation of closely related compounds from a mixture.

Chromosome A physically distinct unit of the genome, carrying many genes.

Chromosome jumping A technique used for the identification of two segments of DNA in a chromosome separated by thousands of base pairs.

Chromosome walking It is a technique used to identify the overlapping sequences of DNA in a chromosome in order to identify a particular locus of interest.

Cistron The smallest functional unit (sequence) of DNA) that encodes a polypeptide chain.

Clean gene technology The process of developing transgenic plants without the presence of selectable marker genes or by use of more acceptable genes.

Clonal propagation See micropropagation.

Clone A population of cells or, organisms, or molecules that are identical to the parent cell (organism) or precursor molecule.

Cloning vector (vehicle) A plasmid or a phage that carries an inserted foreign DNA to be introduced into a host cell.

Codon A triplet nucleotide sequence of mRNA coding for an amino acid in a polypeptide.

Coenzyme See cofactor.

Cofactor A low-molecular weight non-protein compound required for an enzymatic reaction.

Cofermentation Fermentation carried out by simultaneously growing two microorganisms in a bioreactor.

Cointegrate vector The modified Ti plasmid in combination with an intermediate cloning vector.

Colchicine An alkaloid used to block mitosis by arresting spindle formation.

Colony hybridization A technique that employs nucleic acid probe to identify a bacterial colony with a vector carrying specific gene(s).

Complement system A group of serum proteins that help in the formation of membrane attack complex to destroy invading pathogens.

Composting The process of biological degradation of solid organic wastes to stable end products.

Concatemer A DNA molecule composed of a number of individual pieces (or sequences) joined together via cohesive ends.

Congenital The term used to describe genetic abnormalities present at birth.

Conjugation The transfer of DNA from one bacterium to another through cell-to-cell contact.

Constitutive genes Also called as house-keeping genes. They are expressed as a function of interaction between RNA polymerase and the promoter without any additional regulation.

Contaminant A substance not present in nature but released due to human activities e.g. methyl-isocyanate.

Contig map A chromosome map in which various DNA segments have been joined together to form a continuous DNA molecule.

Continuous fermentation Fermentation carried out by continuous addition of fresh medium that balances with the removal of cell suspension (from the bioreactor).

Copy number The number of plasmids in a bacterial cell. It also refers to the number of copies of a gene in a genome of an organism.

Cosmids A high capacity cloning vector consisting of the λ cos site inserted into a plasmid.

Crossing-over The reciprocal exchange of genetic material between chromosomes during meiosis.

Crown gall disease A plant disease caused by Ti plasmid of *Agrobacterium tumefaciens*.

Cryopreservation Storage and preservation at very low temperatures (–196°C).

Cryoprotectant A chemical agent or a compound that can prevent damage to cells while they are frozen or defrosted.

Cultivar A term used to refer to the plants found only under cultivation.

Culture A population of microorganisms or cells (from plants/animals) that are grown under controlled conditions.

Culture medium The nutrients prepared in the form of a fluid (broth) or solid for the growth of cells/tissues in the laboratory.

Cybrid (cytoplasmic hybrid) A viable cell formed by the fusion of a cytoplast with a whole cell.

Cybridization The process of formation of cybrids.

Cyclins The proteins that accumulate during the cell cycle and regulate the biochemical events in a cell cycle specific manner.

Cynophages The viruses that can kill algal cells.

Cystic fibrosis A disease affecting lungs and other tissues due to defects in ion transport. It is caused by the deficiency of *CFTR* gene.

Cytoplasmic hybrid See cybrid.

Cytoplasmic inheritance Inheritance as a property of genes located in the cytosol (in mitochondria or chloroplasts).

Cytoplasmic transfer The transfer of cytoplasm from a donor (with active mitochondria) into the oocytes.

Cytoprotoplasts The sub-protoplasts containing the original cytoplasmic material (in part or full) but lack nucleus.

Cytoskeleton The network of fibres in the cytoplasm of a eukaryotic cell.

Cytotoxicity The toxic effects on cells that result in metabolic alterations including the death of cells.

Cytotoxic T-cells (T_C) The lymphocytes that mediate the lysis of target cells.

D

Dedifferentiation The process of differentiated cells getting reverted to non-differentiated cells.

Degeneracy This term is used in relation to genetic code representing the fact that there may be more than one codon for most amino acids.

Denaturation The process of unfolding of a protein, or separation of the two complementary strands of DNA.

Diabetes mellitus A disease characterized by increased blood glucose concentration (hyperglycemia).

Diazotrophs The microorganisms involved in diazotrophy.

Diazotrophy The process of fixation of atmospheric nitrogen by microorganisms.

Differentiation The development of cells or tissues or organs.

Diploid A cell or an organism that has a set of all pairs (i.e. two sets) of chromosomes.

Diploidization The process of doubling chromosomes of a cell.

DNA chip A DNA microarray that consists of oligonucleotide sequences immobilized on a chip. It is used for the analysis of gene structure and function.

DNA fingerprinting A technique for the identification of individuals based on the small differences in DNA sequences.

DNA hybridization The pairing of two DNA molecules used to detect the specific sequence in the sample DNA.

DNA marker A DNA sequence that exists in two or more readily identifiable forms (polymorphic forms) which can be used to mark a map position on a genome map.

DNA microarray See DNA chip.

DNA probe (gene probe) A segment of DNA that is tagged with a label (i.e. isotope) so as to detect a complementary base sequence in the DNA sample after a hybridization reaction.

DNA profiling The term used to describe different methods for the analysis of DNA to establish the identity of an individual.

DNA repair The biochemical processes that correct mutations occurring due to replication errors or as a consequence of mutagenic agents.

DNA sequencers The machines that are used for the determination of specific sequences of nucleotides in a given DNA molecule.

DNA vaccine A gene or DNA sequence, encoding an antigenic protein, incorporated into the cells of a target animal.

Dolly The first mammal (sheep) cloned by Wilmut and Campbell in 1997.

Domain A segment of a polypeptide or protein that has specific conformation and function.

Dot-blot A technique in which small dots (or spots) of nucleic acid are immobilized on a nitrocellulose or nylon membrane for hybridization.

Double helix The double-stranded DNA structure in the native form in a cell.

Doubling time The time required to double the number of cells in a tissue culture.

Downstream Towards the 3′-end of polynucleotide or DNA sequence.

Downstream processing The methods/procedures used to isolate and purify the products (e.g. proteins) of fermentation processes.

Dry anaerobic composting (DRANCO) An anaerobic digesting process for the composting of solid wastes.

E

Edible vaccines The vaccines produced in plants which can enter the body on eating them.

Electrophoresis An analytical technique that separates charged molecules in an electrical field.

Electroporation The technique of introducing DNA into cells by inducing transient pores by electric pulse.

Elicitors The compounds of biological origin that stimulate the production of secondary metabolites.

ELISA See enzyme-linked immunosorbent assay.

ELSI The ***e***thical, ***l***egal, and ***s***ocial ***i***mplications that arise as a result of developments in genetic engineering or biotechnology.

Embryo An organism in the early stages of development. In humans, the first two months in the uterus.

Embryogenesis The process by which an embryo develops from a fertilized egg cell, or asexually from a group of cells.

Embryonic stem cells (ES cells) The cells of an early embryo that can give rise to all differentiated cells, including germ cells.

Embryo rescue The culture of immature embryos to rescue them from unripe or hybrid seeds which fail to germinate.

Embryo transfer The process of implantation of embryos from a donor animal, or developed by *in vitro* fertilization into the uterus of a recipient animal.

Endomitosis The process of doubling chromosomes without division of the nucleus. This results in polyploidy.

Endosperm The nutritive tissue that develops in the embryo sac of most angiosperm plants.

Energy-rich crops The plants which are very efficient in converting CO_2 into biomass.

Enhancer A regulatory sequence of DNA that enhances the rate of transcription of a gene or genes that are located at distant places.

Enzyme A biocatalyst synthesized by living cells.

Enzyme-linked immunosorbent assay (ELISA) A technique for the detection of small quantities of proteins by utilizing antibodies linked to enzymes, which in turn catalyse the formation of coloured products.

Enzyme technology Involves the production, isolation, purification and use of enzymes.

Epitopes The specific antigen determinants located on the antigens.

Eutrophication Excess growth of algae (in sewage/ waste waters) which leads to oxygen depletion.

Exon A region of the eukaryotic gene that is expressed as mRNA which is translated into a protein.

Exosome A multiprotein complex that is involved in the degradation of mRNA in eukaryotes.

Explant A piece of tissue isolated from the intact plant that is used to initiate culture or development of plant.

Exponential phase This refers to a phase in culture in which cells divide at a maximum rate.

Expressed sequence tag (EST) A cDNA that is sequenced in order to gain rapid access to the genes in a genome.

Extein The functional component of a discontinuous protein.

Ex vivo Outside the body. This term is commonly used to describe the manipulations of genes outside the body for gene therapy i.e. *ex vivo* gene therapy.

Eugenics The science of improving human stock by selective breeding. It involves giving better chances for more suitable people in the society to reproduce than the less suitable people.

Eukaryotes The organisms with a well defined and membrane bound nucleus.

F

F_1 Also called first filial generation, refers to the first generation of offsprings from a cross.

F_2 The second generation of offsprings from a cross with at least one F_1 parent. F_2 is also called second filial generation.

Familial traits The traits shared by members of a family. These include the hereditary as well as the environmentally influenced traits e.g. social and behavioural traits.

Fed-batch fermentation The process of fermentation by growing cells or microorganisms during which nutrients are added periodically (to the bioreactor).

Fermentation The growth of cells or microorganisms in bioreactors (fermenters) to synthesize special products. Fermentation in biochemistry refers to the degradation of carbon compounds by cells or organisms under anaerobic (lack of oxygen) conditions.

Fermenter A containment system for the cultivation of prokaryotic cells.

Fertilization The fusion of male gamete (sperm) with female gamete (egg) to produce a zygote.

Flavr Savr Transgenic tomato developed by using antisense technology. (Note : It was not a commercial success).

Flow cytometry A method used to sort out cells, organelles or biological materials by passing through apertures of defined sizes.

Fluidized bed reactors See packed bed reactors.

Fluorescent *in situ* hybridization (FISH) The method of employing fluorescent labels for locating markers on chromosomes by detecting the hybridization positions.

F-plasmid It is a *f*ertility plasmid that directs the conjugal transfer of DNA between bacteria.

Frameshift mutation A mutation that occurs as a result of insertion or deletion of a group of nucleotides that are not multiples of three. This results in the alteration of the frame in which the codons are translated into proteins.

Fusion protein A protein that is formed by fusion of two polypeptides, normally coded by separate genes.

Fusogen An agent that induces fusion of protoplasts in somatic hybridization.

G

Gamete The haploid male (sperm) or female (egg) cells that fuse to produce a diploid zygote during sexual reproduction.

Gamete intrafallopian transfer (GIFT) The transfer of both sperm and oocyte into the fallopian tube so as to allow the fertilization to occur naturally *in vivo*.

Gametoclonal variations The variations observed in the regenerated plants from gametic cells (e.g. anther culture).

Gametophyte The haploid stage of the life cycle of plants.

GEMs See genetically engineered microorganisms.

Gene A segment of DNA that encodes a functional protein. It is the basic unit of inheritance located on a chromosome.

Gene amplification Increase in the expression of a gene several fold.

Gene bank A library of genes or clones of an entire genome of a species.

Gene cloning It basically involves the insertion of a gene (a fragment of DNA) or recombinant DNA into a cloning vector, and propagation of the DNA molecule in a host organism.

Gene knockout The process of destroying a specific gene by blocking its function.

Gene map The linear array of genes of a chromosome.

Gene probe See DNA probe.

Generation time See doubling time.

Gene silencing The instability of gene expression in transgenic plants.

Gene therapy Treatment of diseases by use of genes or DNA sequences.

Genetically engineered microorganisms (GEMs) The microorganisms with genetic modifications are collectively referred to as GEMs.

Genetically modified (GM) foods The entry of transgenic plants and animals into the food chain represents GM foods.

Genetically modified organisms (GMOs) A term used to represent an organisms that are genetically engineered. It usually describes the transgenic plants and transgenic animals.

Genetic code The total set of 64 codons that code for 20 amino acids, and three termination codons.

Genetic disease A disease caused by defective gene(s) that can be transmitted from one generation to the next.

Genetic engineering Broadly involves all the *in vitro* genetic manipulations.

Genetic portfolios The identification of all the genes in individuals represents genetic portfolios.

Genetic immunization The immune response of the body stimulated by DNA vaccines.

Genetics A branch of biology involving the study of genes.

Genome The total content of DNA represented by the genes contained in a cell.

Genomic library A collection of clones representing the entire genome of an organism.

Genomics The study of the structure and function of genomes.

Genotype The genetic constitution of an organism. (opposite of phenotype).

Germ cell A reproductive cell which on maturation can be fertilized to produce the organism.

Germ line Reproductive cells that produce gametes which in turn give rise to sperms and eggs.

Germplasm The hereditary material transmitted to the offspring through germ cells.

Gibberellins A group of plant hormones that induce cell elongation and cell division.

Global warming The retention of earth's heat by atmosphere (greenhouse effect) results in global warming.

Glufosinate See phosphinothricin

Glycinin A lysine-rich protein of soybean.

Glyphosate An herbicide used to destroy unwanted plants.

GMOs See ***g***enetically ***m***odified ***o***rganisms.

Golden rice The genetically engineered rice with provitamin A (β-carotene) enrichment.

GRAS This is a short form for ***g***enerally ***r***egarded ***a***s ***s***afe, and is in use in some countries to represent the safety (no history of causing illness to humans) of foods, drugs and other materials. GRAS is also used to represent the host organisms employed in genetic engineering experiments.

Gratuitous inducer A substance that can induce transcription of gene(s), but is not a substrate for the induced enzyme(s).

Greenhouse effect The phenomenon of retention of earth's heat by the atmosphere.

Greenhouse technology The growing of plants in greenhouses before the plant cultures are transfered to fields.

Green revolution The improvement in crop varieties and their management for increase in world's food supply.

Gynogenesis Ovary or ovule culture that results in the production of haploids (gynogenic haploids).

H

Hairy root diseases A plant disease caused by the infection of *Agrobacterium rhizogens.*

Haploid Containing one set of chromosomes (opposite to diploid).

HeLa cells A pure cell line of human cancer cells used for the cultivation of viruses.

Helix-loop-helix motif A domain commonly found in DNA-binding proteins.

Helix-turn-helix motif The structural motif for the attachment of a protein to DNA molecule.

Herbicides The weedkillers that destroy the unwanted and useless plants.

Heritable traits The characteristics that are under the control of genes, and transmitted from one generation to another.

Heterochromatin The relatively more condensed part of chromatin which is believed to contain DNA that is not being transcribed.

Heteroduplex A DNA molecule formed by base pairing between two strands that do not have complete complementary sequences.

Heterogeneous nuclear RNA (hnRNA) The unprocessed nuclear RNA produced in transcription. This is also regarded as ***primary transcript***.

Heterokaryon A cell in which two or more nuclei of different genetic make-up are present.

Heterologous Refers to gene sequences that are not identical, but show variable degrees of similarity.

Heterozygous Having two different alleles for a given trait in a diploid organism (cell/nucleus).

High fructose corn syrup (HFCS) A good substitute for sugar in the preparation of soft drinks, processed foods and baking. HFCS contains equal amounts of glucose and fructose.

Hirudin A natural anticoagulant protein produced by salivary glands of leeches.

Histotypic cultures The growth and propagation of cells in three-dimensional matrix to high cell density.

Hogness box (TATA box) A DNA sequence found in eukaryotic promoters. This has a sequence TATAAAT, and is comparable to Pribnow box found in eukaryotes.

Homologous chromosomes Members of the paired chromosomes in diploid organisms that are identical in DNA sequences (genes) and in their visible structure.

Homozygous Possessing two identical alleles for a given trait in a diploid organism (cell/nucleus).

Host A cell or an organism used to propagate recombinant DNA molecules.

Host cells The living cells in which the carrier of recombinant DNA (or vector) can be propagated.

Holliday structure An intermediate structure formed during recombination between two DNA molecules (or chromosomes).

Homokaryon A cell with two or more identical nuclei as a result of fusion.

Humulin ***Hum***an ins***ulin*** used for the treatment of diabetic patients. It was developed by Eli LiPly company and was approved for human use in 1982.

Human Genome Project (HGP) An international megaproject for the identification of human genome sequences, the genes and their functions.

Humoral immune response The production of antibodies by B-cells of the immune system in response to antigens.

Human mouse The transgenic mouse with human immune system.

Hybrid DNA See heteroduplex DNA.

Hybridization At the molecular level, it refers to joining together of artificially separated nucleic acid strands via hydrogen bonding between complementary bases. It also refers to the production of hybrids or hybrid offsprings from genetically dissimilar parents.

Hybridoma A clone of hybrid cells produced by fusion of a myeloma cell with an antibody producing cell. Each hybridoma produces only one type of monoclonal antibody.

Hydrosphere The water on the earths surface which includes oceans, seas, rivers, polar ice caps etc.

Hypervariable region A region of the genome that possesses variable number of repeated sequences which are useful for the diagnosis of individuals (through DNA fingerprinting).

I

Ice-minus bacteria The bacteria that do not synthesize ice nucleation proteins.

ICI protein The single cell protein produced by the company Imperial Chemical Industries (ICI) from methanol and ammonia.

Imhoff tanks An improved septic tank with two compartments—one for the sedimentation and the other for the digestion.

Immobilized cells The cells that are entrapped in the matrices (of alginate, agarose, polyacrylamide) and used in bioreactors.

Immobilized enzyme An enzyme that is physically localized in a defined region so that it can be reused in a continuous process.

Immune system The network of cells, tissues and organs that defends the body against foreign invaders.

Immunoglobulins The special group of proteins, commonly referred to as antibodies, produced by B-lymphocytes, and involved in humoral immunity.

Indigo A blue pigment extensively used to dye cotton and wool.

Inducer A small molecule that triggers gene transcription by binding to a regulatory protein.

Inducible genes The genes that can be stimulated by inducers.

Innate immunity The inherent capability of an organism to offer resistance against diseases.

Insulin A hormone synthesized by β-cells of the pancreas. It facilitates the uptake and metabolism of glucose.

Insertion sequence (IS) A small transposable element found in bacteria. It carries genes needed for its own transposition.

Intein The part of a polypeptide removed by splicing process after translation.

Interferons A group of glycoproteins that resist viral infections and regulate immune responses.

Intergeneric A cross between two genera.

Interleukins A group of lymphokines important for the function of immune system.

Interspecific A cross between two different species of a genus.

Intron A segment of the DNA that is transcribed, but removed from within the transcript. Thus introns represent the non-coding regions within a discontinuous gene. (Intron is also the trade name for ***in***terfe***ron***-α).

In vitro Literally means 'in glass', refers to biological activities/reactions carried out in the test tube rather than the living cell or organism.

***In vitro* fertilization (IVF)** The fertilization of eggs of a female in the laboratory conditions, and transferring the fertilized eggs (zygotes) into the uterus a few days later.

***In vitro* mutagenesis** The techniques used to produce a specified mutation at a predetermined in a DNA.

In vivo Literally means '*in life*', refers to the natural situation within a cell or organism.

***In vivo* gene therapy** The direct delivery of gene(s) to a tissue or an organ to alleviate genetic disorders.

Isotopes The elements with the same atomic number but different atomic weights.

J

Junk DNA The ***intergenic content of DNA*** is also referred to as junk DNA.

K

Karyotyping The method of photographing the complete set of chromosomes for a particular cell type and organizing them into pairs based on size and shape.

Kilobase (kb) A unit consisting of one thousand nitrogenous bases in a DNA or RNA molecule.

Klenow fragment A fragment of DNA polymerase I that lacks 5′-exonuclease activity.

Knockout mouse A genetically altered mouse lacking the genes for an entire organ or organ system.

Kozak consensus The nucleotide sequence surrounding the initiation codon of eukaryotic mRNA.

L

Lac operon See lactose operon.

Lactose operon (lac operon) The cluster of genes responsible for the coding of enzymes involved in utilization of lactose by *E. coli*.

Lagging strand The DNA strand of a double helix that is copied in a discontinuous fashion during replication.

Landfarming A technique for the bioremediation of hydrocarbon contaminated soils.

Landfilling A method for the final disposal of sludge.

Leading strand The DNA strand of a double helix that is copied in a continuous fashion during replication.

Leghemoglobin A protein present in the nodules of leguminous plants, that is comparable to hemoglobin in animals.

Leucine zipper motif A domain commonly found in DNA-binding proteins.

Linkers The short known sequences of DNAs (or oligonucleotides) that are joined to the ends of DNA molecules during the process of gene cloning.

Lipoplexes The lipid-DNA complexes, also referred to as ***liposomes***.

Lithosphere The outer boundary layer of the solid earth on which the continents and the ocean basins rest.

Locus The site on the chromosome where a specific gene is located.

Long terminal repeats (LTRs) Similar sequences of genetic information that are located at the ends of the genomes of retroviruses.

Lymphoma Cancer of the lymph tissue.

Lytic cycle The replication cycle of bacteria that ultimately results in the lysis of host cells.

M

Macrolides Antibiotics with large lactone rings.

Major histocompatibility complex (MHC) The special group of proteins present on the cell surfaces of T-lymphocytes. MHC is involved in the recognition of antigens on T-cells.

Magnetic resonance imaging (MRI) A medical technology designed to observe the internal organs and structures without invasive procedures.

Marker genes The set of genes used for selecting the transformed plant materials (cells/tissues).

Megabase (Mb) Indicates 10^6 bp of DNA.

Meiosis Nuclear division of germ cells to produce egg cells or sperms containing haploid (half) number of chromosomes.

Melting temperature (T_m) The midpoint of temperature range at which DNA gets denatured.

Meristem A localized region of actively dividing cells in plants i.e. tips of stems and roots.

Mesophile A microorganism that can grow at an optimum temperature around 37°C, and is capable of surviving within the temperature range of 20-50°C.

Messenger RNA (mRNA) A single-stranded RNA that is capable of synthesizing one or more polypeptide chains.

Metabolic load It represents the changes in metabolic and cellular functions of the host cell due to the presence of cloned DNA.

Metabolism The entire range of chemical reactions occurring in a living cell or an organism.

Metabolite A low molecular biological compound essential for cell's or body's metabolism.

Metabolomics The use of genome sequence analysis for determining the capability of a cell/tissue/organisms to synthesize metabolites.

Metallothioneins A group of small peptides produced in animals due to metal pollution.

Michaelis-Menten constant The substrate concentration (moles/liter) to produce half-maximal velocity in an enzyme-catalysed reaction.

Microchromosome See human artificial chromosome.

Microinjection The delivery of DNA or other compounds into eukaryotic cells using a fine microscopic needle.

Microprojectile bombardment See biolistics.

Micropropagation The propagation of a plant in a controlled and artificial environment under aseptic conditions, using a defined growth medium.

Microsatellites A type of sequence length polymorphism that has tandem copies of di-tri-or tetranucleotide repeat units. Microsatellites are also called as short tandem repeats.

Miniprotoplasts The sub-protoplasts containing nucleus, and are capable of regeneration into plants.

Mismatch The absence of base pairing between one or more nucleotides of two hybridized nucleic acid strands.

Mitosis Nuclear division in somatic cells. The parent and the daughter cells contain the same number of chromosomes.

Molasses A byproduct of sugar industry, used as a cheap source of carbohydrates in fermentation industries.

Molecular breeding The plant breeding methods that are coupled with genetic engineering techniques.

Molecula marker A DNA sequence in the genome which can be located and identified.

Monellin A protein found in the fruits of an African plant *Discorephyllum cumminsii* which is about 100,000 times sweeter than sucrose.

Monoclonal antibody (MAb) A specific and single type of antibody that is produced by hybridoma cells. MAb is directed against a specific antigenic determinant (epitope).

Monocotyledons (monocots) A class of plants that possess one seed leaf.

Monoploid (monohaploid) A cell or an organism (usually a plant) with the lowest number of chromosomes, denoted by x e.g. barley n = x – 7.

Morphogenesis The growth and development of an undifferentiated structure to a differentiated form.

MRI See magnetic resonance imaging.

Motif The part of a protein that mediates the binding of regulatory proteins (transcription factors) to DNA.

Multicellular tumor spheroids (MCTS) *In vitro* cellular three-dimensional proliferating models for the study of tumor cells.

Multiple alleles The alternative forms of a gene that has more than two alleles.

Multiple myeloma A cancer of B-lymphocytes.

Multiple ovulation See superovulation.

Mushrooms The fungi belonging to the class basidomycetes. Some of them are edible e.g. *Agaricus bisporus* (button mushroom).

Mutagenesis The changes in the nucleotides of DNA of an organism by physical or chemical treatments.

Mutagens The agents that increase the rate of mutation by inducing changes in DNA.

Mutation The changes in the base sequences of DNA that are heritable.

Muteins The second generation recombinant therapeutic proteins are collectively referred to as muteins.

Myasthenia gravis An autoimmune disease causing neuromuscular disorders. The disease occurs due to the production of antibodies against acetyl choline receptors.

Myeloma A tumor cell line derived from a lymphocyte which usually produces a single type of immunoglobulin.

Mycelium A mass of interwoven thread-like filaments of a fungus or bacteria.

N

Natural selection The preservation of favourable alleles while rejecting the injurious ones in a natural way.

Nick The position in a double-stranded DNA where one of the polynucleotides is broken due to lack of phosphodiester bond.

Nitrogen fixation The process of conversion of atmospheric nitrogen to ammonia. Biological nitrogen fixation occurs in prokaryotes and is catalysed by the enzyme nitrogenase.

Nodulation The formation of nodules on the roots of plants by symbiotic bacteria.

Nodule A tumor like growth on the roots of legumes (beans, peanuts) that contains symbiotic nitrogen fixing bacteria.

Northern blotting The transfer of RNA from an electrophoresis gel to a membrane to perform Northern hybridization.

Northern hybridization The technique used for the detection of specific RNA molecule through Northern blotting.

Nucleoid A term used to represent the DNA-containing region of a prokaryotic cell.

O

Okazaki fragment A short segment of DNA synthesized during replication on the lagging strand of double helix.

Old biotechnology See traditional biotechnology.

Oleosin partition technology The purification of foreign proteins through their production in oil bodies.

Oleosins The oil body proteins that are hydrophobic in nature, and are associated with plant seeds.

Oligonucleotide A small piece of synthetic single-stranded DNA molecule.

Oligonucleotide-directed mutagenesis A technique to alter one or more specific nucleotides in a gene (DNA sequence) so that a protein with specific amino acid change is produced.

Oncogene A gene that promotes cell proliferation to result in uncontrolled growth.

Oncomouse The animal model of mouse for cancer. It was granted U.S. patent in 1988, the first animal to be patented.

Oocyte It is a stage in the development of female gamete or ovum (egg). The words oocyte and ovum are used interchangeably.

Operon A cluster of bacterial genes under the control of a sigle regulatory sequence.

Opine An amino acid derivative formed in some plants by the condensation of an amino acid with a sugar or a keto acid.

Organ culture The *in vitro* culture of an organ so as to achieve the development and/or preservation of the original organ.

Organogenesis The process of morphogenesis that finally results in the formation of organs e.g. shoots, roots.

Osmolyte A compound that is involved in the regulation of osmotic pressure within a cell.

Osmoticum The agent or a compound that increases the osmotic pressure of a liquid.

Ovum The fully mature female gamete or egg cell.

Ozone hole Depletion of ozone layer in the atmosphere may result in ozone hole that may cause harmful effects to living organisms.

P

Packed bed reactors (fluidized bed reactors) Devices used for the removal of BOD, and nitrification.

Packed cell volume (PCV) It is a test for the determination of viability of cells. PCV is expressed as percentage of volume of cells after sedimentation in a low speed centrifuge.

Parthenogenesis Production of an embryo from a female gamete without the participation of male gamete.

Patent A government—issued document that provides the holder the exclusive rights to manufacture, use or sell an invention for a defined period (usually 20 years).

Pathogenesis—related (PR) proteins The low-molecular weight proteins produced by plants to protect themselves against invading pathogens (fungi, bacteria).

Pedigree A chart form depicting the genetic relationships between the members of a human family.

Phage A virus infecting bacterium.

Phage display A technique involving the identification of proteins that interact with one another.

Phagemid A cloning vector created by a mixture of plasmid and phage DNA.

Pharm animal A genetically engineered animal to produce pharmaceutical products.

Phenotype The appearance or other characteristics of an organism that result from an interaction of its genetic constitution with the environment.

Phosphinothricin (glufosinate) A broad spectrum herbicide.

Photosynthesis The synthesis of carbohydrates in green plants by assimilation of carbon dioxide.

Phytoalexins The secondary metabolites produced in plants in response to infection.

Phytochelatins A group of small peptides produced in plants as a result of metal pollution.

Phytohormone The general name used for all the hormones produced by plants.

Phytoplanktons The aquatic plants that freely float on water surface.

Plantibodies The antibodies produced in plants.

Plantlet Small rooted shoot or germinated embryo.

Plasmid An autonomous, circular, self-replicating extrachromosomal DNA, found in bacteria and some other cells.

Plating efficiency The percentage of cells plated which produce cell colonies.

Point mutation A mutation caused by an alteration of a single nucleotide in a DNA molecule.

Pollutant A substance which increases in quantity in the air and adversely affects the environment e.g. CO, lead.

Poly(A) tail A series of A-nucleotides attached to the 3′-end of eukaryotic mRNA.

Polyclonal antibodies Different antibodies which can react with the same antigen.

Polyhydroxyalkanoates (PHA) Intracellular carbon and energy storage compounds. They are biodegradable polymers.

Polymerase chain reaction (PCR) A technique of amplifying DNA *in vitro*.

Polymorphism The allelic variations in the genomes that result in different phenotypes.

Position effect The phenomenon of different levels of gene expression that is observed after insertion of a new gene at different positions in the eukaryotic genome.

Post-transcriptional modifications The changes that occur in the primary transcript (RNAs) after they are synthesized.

Post-translational modifications The changes that take place after the protein is synthesized.

Pribnow box A DNA sequence found in the prokaryotes that is required for transcription initiation.

Primary cells The eukaryotic cells taken directly from an animal for culture purpose.

Primary culture The culture produced by the freshly isolated cells or tissues taken from an organism.

Primary transcript The initial or primary product of transcription of a gene(s). Mature mRNA is produced after processing.

Primer A short sequence of oligonucleotides that hybridizes with template strand and provides initiation for the nucleic acid synthesis.

Primer extension Synthesis of a copy of a nucleic acid from a primer.

Primer walking A technique for sequencing long (>1 kb) pieces of DNA.

Primordium The earliest detectable stage of an organ in plants.

Prion A proteinaceous infectious agent which behaves like an inheritable trait (although no DNA/RNA is present).

Probe A labeled molecule used in hybridization technique.

Prokaryote An organism whose cells lack a membrane bound or distinct nucleus.

Protein engineering Generation of proteins with subtly modified structures conferring improved properties e.g. higher catalytic function, thermostability.

Protein targeting The process of transport of proteins from one compartment to other within a cell. Also called as ***protein sorting***.

Proteome The total population of proteins produced by a cell.

Proteomics The study of proteome.

Protoplast A cell from which the cell wall is completely removed.

Psuedogene An inactivated and non-functional copy of a gene.

Pyrosequencing A DNA sequencing method involving the detection of nucleotide addition from the release of pyrophosphate which emits chemiluminescence.

Q

Quantitative PCR A polymerase chain reaction that is used to estimate the number of DNA molecules in a sample.

R

RAC Recombinant DNA Advisory Committee, a supervisory group that oversees the recombinant DNA experiments.

RACE See rapid amplification of cDNA ends.

Radioimmunoassay (RIA) An analytical techniques based on the principles of radioactivity of isotopes and immunological reactions of antigen and antibody. RIA is a sensitive technique for the estimation of several biological compounds.

Random amplified polymorphic DNA (RAPD) A PCR-based method of DNA profiling. It basically involves the amplification of DNA sequences using random primers, and use of genetic fingerprints to identify individual organisms (mostly plants).

RAPD See random amplified polymorphic DNA.

Rapid amplification of cDNA ends (RACE) A technique that employs reverse transcription and PCR for the rapid amplification of cDNA ends.

Recalcitrant xenobiotics The xenobiotics that do not easily undergo biodegradation, and therefore persist in the environment for a long period.

Recombinant vaccines The new generation of vaccines produced by employing recombinant DNA technology.

Recombination Exchange of genetic information between two different DNA molecules.

Regeneration Development and formation of new organs.

Renaturation The reassociation of two nucleic acid strands after denaturation.

Replication The synthesis of DNA from a parent DNA molecule.

Reading frame A series of triplet codons in a DNA sequence.

Recombinant DNA (rDNA) A DNA molecule created in the laboratory by ligating different pieces of DNA which are not normally joined together.

Recombinant DNA (rDNA) technology The techniques involved in the construction, and use of recombinant DNA molecules.

Recombinant protein A protein that is produced by the expression of a cloned gene of a recombinant cell.

Reporter gene A gene whose phenotype can be assayed which in turn can be used to determine the function of regulatory DNA sequence.

Repression Inhibition of transcription by blocking the binding of RNA polymerase to transcription initiation site.

Restriction endonuclease An enzyme that specifically cuts DNA molecule at specific nucleotide sequences.

Restriction fragment length polymorphism (RFLP) A restriction fragment with variable lengths due to the presence of polymorphic restriction sites at one or both ends.

Restriction mapping The process of determining the restriction sites in a DNA molecule by analysing the sizes of the restriction fragments.

Retrovirus A virus with RNA as genetic material.

Reverse transcription The process of synthesis of DNA from RNA.

RFLP See restriction fragment length polymorphism.

Rheology The ability of a solution to modify its flow characteristics.

Ribosome-inactivating proteins (RIPs) The antifungal/antimicrobial proteins secreted by plants that inhibit protein biosynthesis.

Ribosomes The centres (or factories) for protein biosynthesis.

Ribozyme An RNA molecule that has catalytic activity.

RNA vaccines RNA molecules which can synthesize antigenic proteins and offer immunity.

Rotating biological contactor (RBC) A device for the biological treatment of sewage.

S

Salvage pathway The direct conversion of purines and pyrimidines into the corresponding nucleotides.

Satellite DNA Repetitive DNA that forms a satellite band in a density gradient.

Scale-up The expansion of laboratory experiments to full-sized industrial processes.

SCP See single-cell protein.

Secondary metabolite A metabolite that is not required for the growth and maintenance of cellular functions.

Senescence The biological aging of cells, characterized by loss of functions and degradation of biological molecules.

Septic tanks Anaerobic digesters of solids of the sewage settled at the bottom of tanks.

Sewage The liquid waste arising mainly from domestic and industrial sources.

Sex chromosomes The non-autosomal X and Y chromosomes in humans that determine the set of individuals. Males are XY, females XX.

Short tandem repeats See microsatellites.

Shot gun approach A technique for sequencing of genome in which the molecules to be sequenced are randomly broken down into fragments, which are then individually squenced.

Shoot tip The terminal portion of a shoot comprising the meristem dome and adjoining leaf and stem tissues.

Shuttle vectors The plasmid vectors that are designed to replicate in two different hosts e.g. *E. coli* and *Streptomyces* sp.

Siderophore A low molecular weight compound that can tightly bind to iron. They are produced by certain soil microorganisms and plants to obtain iron from the surroundings.

Signal peptide A short sequence of amino acids at the N-terminal end of some proteins that facilitates the protein to cross membrane.

Single-cell protein (SCP) The cellular mass or protein extracts of microorganisms grown in large quantities. SCP is used as human or animal protein supplement, or food substitute.

Single copy sequence A sequence of nucleotides that occur only once in a genome.

Single-locus probe Probe used in DNA finger-printing that identifies a single sequence (locus) in the genome.

Single nucleotide polymorphisms (SNPs) The positions on the genome where some individuals have one nucleotide (e.g. G) while others have a different nucleotide (e.g. C).

Site-directed mutagenesis The techniques used to produce a specified mutation at a predetermined position in a DNA molecule.

Sludge The semi-solid mass produced during the course of sewage/waste water treatment processes.

SNPs See single nucleotide polymorphisms.

Solid substrate (state) fermentation Fermentation process wherein the growth of the microorganisms is carried out on solid substrates.

Somaclonal variations The genetic variations found in the cultured plant cells when compared to a pure breeding strain.

Somaclones The plants derived from somaclonal variations.

Somatic cell Any body cell as opposed to germ cell. Somatic cell is non-reproductive, and divides by mitosis.

Somatic cell gene therapy The delivery of gene(s) to somatic cells to correct genetic defects.

Somatic embryogenesis Formation of embryos from asexual cells.

Southern hybridization A technique used for the detection of specific DNA sequences (restriction fragments).

Sparger A device that introduces air into a bioreactor in the form of a fine stream.

Splicing A term used to describe the removal of introns and joining of exons in RNA. Thus, introns are spliced out while exons are spliced together.

Stem cell A progenitor cell that is capable of dividing continuously throughout the life of an organism.

Stirred tank fermenter A fermentation vessel in which the cells or microorganisms are mixed by mechanically driven impellers.

Stop codons The three triplets (UAA, UAG, UGA) which terminate protein biosynthesis (translation).

Stuffer DNA The non-essential DNA of a vector that can be replaced by a foreign DNA.

Subculture The transfer of cells from one culture vessel to another culture vessel.

Sub-protoplasts The fragments derived from protoplasts that do not contain all the contents of the plant cells.

Subunit vaccine An immunogenic protein produced from a cloned gene or purified from a disease-causing organism.

Suicide gene A gene that produces a protein which is capable of destroying the cell by direct or indirect means.

Superbug The first genetically engineered organism (bacterial strain of *Pseudomonas*) that was patented. It carries different hydrocarbon-degrading genes on plasmids.

Superovulation The process of inducing more ovarian follicles to ripen and produce more eggs.

Symbiotic The ecological relationship in which two different species or organisms live together for mutual benefit.

Synchronization A term used to represent the cells when they are at the same stage of cell division.

T

Tandem repeat A repeat consisting of an array of DNA sequence that is repeated continuously in the same direction.

T-cells See T-lymphocytes.

T-DNA The part of the Ti plasmid that is transferred to the plant DNA.

Telomere The natural end DNA sequence in a chromosome.

Template The polynucleotide strand (of nucleic acid) that determines the sequence of nucleotides in a newly synthesized nucleic acid. Template is used by polymerases (DNA or RNA) for new strand synthesis.

Termination codons See stop codons.

Thaumatin A protein extracted from berries which is about 3000 times sweeter than sucrose.

Ti plasmid The large-sized *t*umor *i*nducing plasmid found in *Agrobacterium tumefaciens*. It directs crown gall formation in certain plant species.

Tissue culture A process where individual cells, or tissues of plants or animals are grown artificially.

Tissue engineering The application of the principles of engineering to cell culture for the construction of functional anatomical units.

T-lymphocytes (T-cells) The lymphocytes that are dependent on the thymus for their differentiation, and are involved in cell-mediated immune responses.

Totipotent A term used to describe a cell that is not committed to a single developmental pathway, and thus it is capable of forming all types of differentiated cells.

Traditional (old) biotechnology The age old practices for the preparation of foods and beverages, based on the natural capabilities of microorganisms.

Transcript A gene product in the form of RNA.

Transcription The synthesis of RNA from DNA (or gene).

Transcriptome The entire content of RNA molecules in a cell.

Transcriptomics The study of transcriptome.

Transduction Transfer of bacterial genes from one cell to another by packaging in a phage particle.

Transfection The insertion of a purified phage DNA molecule into a bacterial cell.

Transfer RNA (tRNA) The RNA involved in the transfer of amino acids to ribosomes during protein biosynthesis. tRNA, also called as ***soluble RNA*** contains 71-80 nucleotides.

Transformation The acquisition of new genes by a cell through the uptake of naked DNA.

Transgene The target gene responsible for the development of transgenic organisms.

Transgenic An organism that carries a foreign DNA (transgene).

Translation The biosynthesis of a polypeptide, the sequence being determined by codons of mRNA.

Transposon A genetic element that is capable of moving from one position to another in a DNA molecule. It is also called as transposable element.

Trickling filters Oxidation units used for the biological treatment of sewage in small communities.

Triplex A type of DNA structure with three polynucleotides.

Trisomy The occurrence of three copies of a homologous chromosome in a nucleus.

Trypsinization Disaggregation of tissues by the enzyme trypsin.

Tumor An enlargement or swelling of tissue due to pathological overgrowth.

Turbidostat An open continuous culture system into which fresh medium flows in response to an increase in the turbidity of culture.

Upstream Refers to the 5′-end of a polynucleotide.

Vaccine A preparation introduced into the body to stimulate immunity against a pathogen.

Variable number tandem repeats (VNTRs) Repetitive DNA composed of a number of copies of a short sequence. VNTRs are involved in the generation of polymorphic loci which are useful in DNA fingerprinting.

Vector See cloning vector.

Vegetative cell A non-reproductive cell that divides by mitosis.

Vegetative propagation The asexual propagation of plants from the detached parts of plants.

Veggie (vegetable) vaccines See edible vaccines.

Vermicomposting The process of compost formation by earthworms.

Vinegar An aqueous solution containing about 4% acetic acid, and is widely used as a flavouring agent.

Virus An infectious agent that cannot replicate without a host cell.

Vitrification An undesirable condition in *in vitro* tissues, characterized by brittleness and glassy appearance.

VNTRs See variable number tandem repeats.

Western blotting The transfer of protein from a gel to a membrane.

Wild type The term used in genetics to describe a commonly observed phenotype (in the normal/ native state) of an organism.

Wobble hypothesis The process in which a single tRNA can decode more than one codon (of mRNA).

X

Xenobiotics The unnatural, foreign and synthetic chemicals such as pesticides, herbicides and various organic compounds.

Xenogeneic cells The cells taken from different species (e.g. pig source for humans) for use in experiments such as tissue engineering.

Xenotransplantation The replacement of failed human organs by the functional animal organs.

X-ray crystallography A technique used to determine the three-dimensional structure of large molecules.

Y

Yeast artificial chromosome (YAC) A cloning vector constructed from the components of a yeast chromosome.

Yeast two-hybrid system A technique to detect the proteins that interact with each other.

Z

Z-DNA A type of DNA conformation in which two polynucleotides are wound in the form of a left-handed helix.

Zinc finger motif A common structural motif that attaches a protein to a DNA molecule.

Zoo blotting A blotting technique used to determine the genes of related organisms by hybridization.

Zygote The fertilized egg formed by the fusion of two gametes during meiosis.

Zygote intrafallopian transfer (ZIFT) The transfer of the fertilized eggs (zygotes) within 24 hours into the fallopian tube by using laparoscopy.

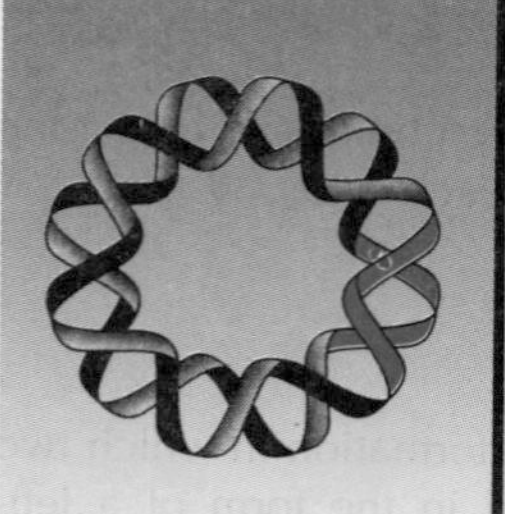

Abbreviations

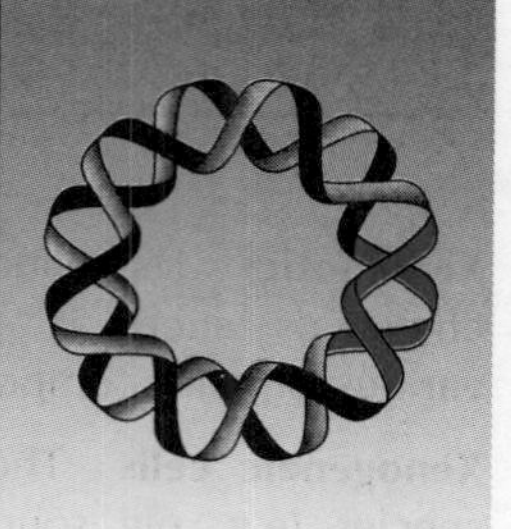

ACC 1-Aminocyclopropane-1 carboxylic acid.

AcMNPV Autographa californica multiple nuclear polyhedrosis virus.

ACP Acyl carrier protein

ADEPT Antibody-directed enzyme prodrug therapy.

ADA Adenosine deaminase.

AFLP Amplified fragment length polymorphism.

AH Assisted hatching.

AIDS Acquired immunodeficiency syndrome.

AK Aspartokinase

ALS Acetolactate synthase.

AP-PCR Arbitrarily primed PCR.

ART Assisted reproductive technology.

ATPS Aqueous two-phase systems.

BAC Bacterial artificial chromosome.

BCG Bacillus Calmette-Guerin.

BNR Biological nitrogen removal.

BOD Biochemical oxygen demand.

bp Base pair.

BPTI Bovine pancreatic trypsin inhibitor.

Bt *Baccillus thuringiensis*

CAMs Cell adhesion molecules.

CaMV Cauliflower mosaic virus

cDNA Complementary DNA.

CDK Cyclin-dependent kinase.

CDRs Complement determining regions.

CF Cystic fibrosis

CFCs Chlorofluorocarbons

CFTR Cystic fibrosis transmembrane regulator.

CHEF Contour-clamped homogeneous electric-field electrophoresis.

CMS Cytoplasmic male sterility

CMV Cucumber mosaic virus

COD Chemical oxygen demand

COH Controlled ovarian hyperstimulation

CPPP Cyclopentenoperhydrophenanthrene

CpTi Cowpea trypsin inhibitor

CSTR Continuous stirred tank reactor

CT Cytoplasmic transfer

CTAB Cetyltrimethyl ammonium

CS Calf serum

DEAE Diethylaminoethyl

DHFR Dihydrofolate reductase

DHPDS Dihydropicolinate synthase

DMD Duchenne's muscular dystrophy

DMEM Dulbecco's modification of Eagle's medium.

DMSO Dimethyl sulfoxide

DNA Deoxyribonucleic acid

DSBs Double-stranded breaks

DVT Deep vein thrombosis

EAAs Essential amino acids

EBV Epstein-Bar virus

E. C. Enzyme commission

EGF Epidermal growth factor

ELISA Enzyme-linked immunosorbant assay

EMEM Eagle's minimal essential medium

EMS Eosinophilia-myalgia syndrome

EPAs Environmental protection agencies

EPSPS 5-Enoyl-pyruvylshikimate 3-phosphate synthase

ES Embryonic stem

ESC Embryonic stem cell

ET Embryo transfer

FACS Fluorescent activated cell sorter

FDA Fluoresein diacetate

FENI Flap endonuclease I

FGF Fibroblast growth factor

FMD Foot and mouth disease

GAG Glycosaminoglycans

Gb Gigabase pair

GBSS Granule-bound starch synthase

GCV Ganciclovir

GDH Glutamate dehydrogenase

GEMs Genetically engineered microorganisms

GEOs Genetically engineered organisms

GFAP Glial fibrillary acidic protein

GH Growth hormone

GIFT Gamete intrafallopian transfer

GLUT Glucose transporter

GM Genetically modified

GMEM Glasgow's modification of Eagle's medium

gp Glycoprotein

HAC Human artificial chromosome

HAT Hypoxanthine aminopterin and thymidine

HBsAg Hepatitis B surface antigen

HDGS Homology-dependent gene silencing

HEAR High erucic acid rape

HFCS High fructose corn syrup

HFS High fructose syrup

hGH Human growth hormone

HGP Human genome project

HGPRT Hypoxanthine-guanine phosphoribosyl transferase.

HIC Hydrophobic interaction chromatography

HIV Human immunodeficiency virus

HLA Histocompatability locus antigen

HMP Hexose monophosphate

HNPCC Hereditary nonpolyposis colon cancer

hnRNA Heterogeneous nuclear RNA

HPLC High performance liquid chromatography

HPV Human papilloma virus

HSV Herpes simplex virus

IC Inhibitory concentration

ICI Imperial Chemical Industries

ICM Inner cell mass

ICP Insecticidal crystalline protein

ICSI Intracytoplasmic sperm injection

Ig Immunoglobulin

IGF Insulin-like growth factor

IHGSC International Human Genome Sequencing Consortium

IL Interleukins

ImviC Indole, methyl red, voges-Proskaver and Citrate tests (i used for phonetic purpose).

IPRs Intellectual property rights

IRES Internal ribosomal entry site

ISFET Ion-selective field effect transistors

IUI Intrauterine insemination

IVC Intravaginal culture

IVF *In vitro* fertilization

IVM *In vitro* maturation

kb Kilobase

kDa Kilodaltons

K_m Michaelis-Menten constant

LDL Low density lipoprotein

LEAR Low-erucic acid rape

LHb Leghemoglobin

LINEs Long interspersed nuclear elements

LOS Low oxygen storage

LPS Low pressure storage

LTR Long terminal repeats

MAb Monoclonal antibody

Mb Megabase pair

MCTS Multicellular tumor spheroids

MEOR Microbial enhanced oil recovery

MFT Membrane filtration technique

MGT Mean generation time

MODY Maturity onset diabetes of the young

MOET Multiple ovulation with embryo transfer

mRNA Messenger RNA
MSG Monosodium glutamate
mtDNA Mitochondrial DNA
MTF Multiple-tube fermentation
NASA National Aeronautics Space Administration
NHGRI National Human Genome Research Institute
NIIDM Non-insulin dependent diabetes mellitus
OHSS Ovarian hyperstimulation syndrome
p Promoter squence
pa Polyadenylation sequence
PAGE Polyacrylamide gel electrophoresis
PBR Plant breeders' rights
PCBs Polychlorinated biphenyls
PCNA Proliferating cell nuclear antigen
PCR Polymerase chain reaction
PCV Packed cell volume
PDGF Platelet-derived growth factor
PDT Population doubling time
PEG Polyethylene glycol
PFGE Pulsed-field gel electrophoresis
PG Prostaglandins; Polygalacturonase
PGD Preimplantation genetic diagnosis
PHA Polyhydroxyalkanoates
PHB Polyhydroxybutyrate
PPi Pyrophosphate
PQQ Pyrroloquinoline quinone
PR Pathogen-related
PTGS Post-transcriptional gene silencing
PUFA Polyunsaturated fatty acids
RAC Recombinant DNA Advisory Committee
RACE Rapid amplification of cDNA ends
RAIT Radioimmunotherapy
RAPD Radom amplified polymorphic DNA
rDNA Recombinant DNA
RFC Replication factor C
RFLP Restriction fragment length polymorphism
RIA Radioimmunoassay
RIPs Ribose-inactivating proteins
RNA Ribonucleic acid
ROSNI Round spermid nucleus injection
RPA Replication protein A
RPMI Roswell Park Memorial Institute
rRNA Ribosomal RNA
RT-PCR Reverse transcription polymerase chain reaction.
SARs Scaffold attachment regions
SCF Silicon carbide fibres
SCF Sister chromatid exchange
SCF Supercritical fluid
SCID Severe combined immunodeficiency
SCS Specialized chromatin structure
SCP Single-cell protein
sIgA Secretory immunoglobin A
SINEs Short interspersed nuclear elements
SIPC Surface immobilized plant cell
SNPs Single nucleotide polymorphisms
SPECT Single photon emission computed tomography
SSB Single-stranded binding
ssDNA Single-stranded DNA
SSF Solid substrate (solid state) fermentation
STRs Short tandem repeats; stirred tank reactors
SUZI Subzonal insertion
T-DNA Transferred DNA
TE Tissue engineering
TELISA Thermometric ELISA
ThOD Theoretical oxygen demand
TGF-β Transforming growth factor β
TGS Transcriptional gene silencing
TILs Tumor infiltrating lymphocytes
TK Thymidine kinase
Tm Melting temperature
TMV Tobacco mosaic virus
TNF Tumor necrosis factor
TOC Total organic carbon
tPA Tissue plasminogen activator
TRIPS Trade-related intellectual property rights
tRNA Transfer RNA
TTC Triphenyl tetrazolium chloride
TUNEL *T*dt-mediated d*U*TP ***n***ick ***e***nd-***l***abeling assay
VEGF Vascular endothelial growth factor
VNTRs Variable number tandem repeats
XP Xeroderma pigmentosum
YAC Yeast artificial chromosome

Index

A

B

C

E

F

G

H

I

N

O

P

Q

R

S

T

W